CURRENT GENITOURINARY CANCER SURGERY

EDITED BY

E. David Crawford, M.D.

Professor of Surgery
Chairman, Division of Urology
Director, Clinical Cancer Center
Associate Director, University of Colorado Cancer Center
University of Colorado Health Sciences Center
Attending Physician
Denver Veterans Administration Medical Center
Rose Medical Center
Denver, Colorado

Sakti Das, M.B.B.S.

Associate Clinical Professor of Urology
University of California School of Medicine
Davis, California
Staff Urologist, Kaiser Permanente Medical Center
Walnut Creek, Calfornia

LEA & FEBIGER PHILADELPHIA • LONDON
1990

Lea & Febiger
200 Chester Field Parkway
Malvern, PA 19355-9725
U.S.A.
(215) 251-2230
800-444-1785

Lea & Febiger (UK) Ltd.
45a Croydon Road
Beckenham, Kent BR3 3RB
U.K.

Chapter and page reprints may be purchased from
Lea & Febiger in quantities of 100 or more.

Library of Congress Cataloging-in-Publication Data
Current genitourinary cancer surgery / [edited by] E. David Crawford,
  Sakti Das.
       p.   cm.
     Includes bibliographical references.
     ISBN 0-8121-1301-2
     1. Genitourinary organs—Cancer—Surgery. I. Crawford, E. David.
II. Das, Sakti.
     [DNLM: 1. Urogenital Neoplasms—surgery. WJ 160 C976]
  RD571.C86   1990
  616.99'46059—dc20
  DNLM/DLC
  for Library of Congress   89-13908
                                                        CIP

PRINTED IN THE UNITED STATES OF AMERICA

Print number: 5   4   3   2   1

To

our most adorable children
Michael, Marc, Ryan
and
Raja

FOREWORD

Since the turn of the century, patients with genitourinary tumors have been primarily managed by urologic surgeons. Recently, remarkable advances have occurred in both the surgical and nonsurgical management of patients having both localized and advanced genitourinary tumors. These advances include a wide array of new therapeutic strategies that combine increased efficacy with decreased morbidity. There have been significant new developments in surgical techniques and in medical and radiation oncology. Newly developed surgical approaches such as nerve-sparing prostatectomy and continent urinary diversion have been major advances that have enabled the treatment of genitourinary cancer patients to be performed with significantly less morbidity. Advances in endoscopic techniques and laser phototherapy have added entirely new therapeutic strategies for the management of patients with urothelial carcinomas.

Major new developments in medical and radiation oncology provide the urologic surgeon the opportunity to implement, in collaboration with specialists from these disciplines, more effective treatments for genitourinary malignancies. It is essential that the urologist be knowledgeable about these new and innovative surgical as well as nonsurgical techniques.

Current Genitourinary Cancer Surgery includes contributions from established authorities in the management of each type of genitourinary cancer, presenting their most up-to-date management techniques for a wide variety of urologic malignancies. The editors have also included contributions on such topics as radioactive isotope implantation for prostate carci-

noma and radiation therapy of bladder, prostate, penile, and renal carcinoma. Authoritative and in-depth analysis of recent advances in chemotherapy, hormonal therapy, and immunotherapy for genitourinary malignancies are also included.

Over the past decade there has been an explosion of knowledge in immunology, molecular aspects of chemotherapy, growth factors, and molecular genetics of genitourinary malignancies. It is imperative that the urologic surgeon continues to be knowledgeable in the surgical as well as nonsurgical options available for the treatment of patients with genitourinary cancer. Urologists should be involved in the development of these new forms of therapy for patients with genitourinary malignancies and actively participate in their administration.

Current Genitourinary Cancer Surgery reflects the collaborative roles of genitourinary surgeons with medical and radiation oncologists in the management of genitourinary cancer patients, as well as in the development of new forms of surgical and nonsurgical therapies. Hopefully, building on the advances presented in this text, even more effective therapies for patients with localized and advanced genitourinary malignancies will be developed in the future.

W. Marston Linehan, M.D.
Head, Urologic Oncology Section
Surgery Branch
National Cancer Institute
Bethesda, MD

P R E F A C E

"Knowledge comes, but wisdom lingers" . . .
Alfred Tennyson

The quantum advances in the understanding of the cellular and biologic behavior of genitourinary malignancies in the last decade have been accompanied by equally dramatic progress in the diagnostic and therapeutic maneuvers. This rapid evolutionary process has provided implications for urologists in all practice settings, as genitourinary cancers account for more than 25% of all cancers in the United States. From the tremendous excitement engendered by the virtually curative potential of a combined modality approach in the management of testicular tumors, to the recent evidences about the responsiveness of advanced prostate cancer to total androgen blockade, the practicing urologist is challenged to keep abreast of a broad spectrum of therapeutic options including chemotherapy, radiation therapy, and hormonal manipulation, while maintaining traditional surgical practice with refinement in surgical techniques.

In the present text, the contents of Genitourinary Cancer Surgery published in 1982 has been expanded to encompass new developments in chemotherapy, radiation therapy, radiologic evaluation, ultrasonography, magnetic resonance, and computerized tomography, as well as addressing areas of continuing and supportive care. The ten sections dealing with surgical therapy of genitourinary cancers elaborate the technical aspects of each surgical procedure through comprehensive il-

lustrations to guide urologists regardless of their level of preparation or training. Each section begins with a comprehensive overview of the neoplasm followed by the description of surgical management, with emphasis on newer modifications of specific procedures. The variety of surgical recommendations encompasses traditional as well as recent techniques, those which generate healthy controversy and scientific curiosity. Modern surgical approaches such as potency-sparing radical prostatectomy and cystoprostatectomy, modifications in retroperitoneal lymph node dissections to preserve ejaculatory function, a full range of continent urinary diversions, endourologic procedures, and laser therapy are discussed from the perspectives of enhancement of traditional surgical procedures. Similarly, alternative approaches to the management of genitourinary tumors are presented by radiation therapists and medical oncologists. The management of genitourinary malignancies is often a multidisciplinary process. Therefore, chemotherapy, immunotherapy, and hormonal therapy are presented from the perspectives of urologic oncologists as well as those of medical oncologists. It behooves all practicing urologists to develop a working knowledge of chemotherapy and biologic response modification because exquisite sensitivity has been demonstrated by genitourinary cancers to a number of conventional and investigative agents.

Perioperative management is extensively discussed with respect to each operative procedure. The sections dealing with pelvic exenteration, vascular and intestinal surgical techniques, nutritional care, psychosexual concerns, and care of the terminally ill constitute special assets to this comprehensive text.

Grateful acknowledgement is extended to the contributing authors for the time and effort they have devoted to sharing their expertise with the readers of this book. We also wish to express our appreciation for the generous support of the Division of Urology of Kaiser Permanente in Walnut Creek, California, as well as the Department of Surgery and the Cancer Center of the University of Colorado Health Sciences Center. Our special thanks to our publishing staff for their constant help, accommodation, and versatility at every step of the production. We are especially grateful to Judith Allen for editorial assistance, Pat Mariani for the preparation of the manuscript, and James Brodale for medical illustrations. Through the collective efforts of these friends and the constant encouragement and good wishes of many others who remain in the background, our dream of producing *Current Genitourinary Cancer Surgery* has materialized.

We thank you all in earnest sincerity.

E. David Crawford, M.D.
Denver, Colorado
Sakti Das, M.B.B.S.
Walnut Creek, California

CONTRIBUTORS

N. SCOTT ADZICK, M.D.

Assistant Professor of Surgery
Division of Pediatric Surgery
University of California School of Medicine
San Francisco, California

ARJAN D. AMAR, M.D.

Associate Clinical Professor of Urology
University of Calfornia School of Medicine
San Francisco, California
Chief of Urology, Kaiser Permanente Medical Center
Walnut Creek, California

RICHARD J. BABAIAN, M.D.

Associate Professor of Urology
M.D. Anderson Cancer Center
Houston, Texas

ROBERT A. BADALAMENT, M.D.

Assistant Professor
Division of Urology
Ohio State University Hospitals
Columbus, Ohio

MALCOLM A. BAGSHAW, M.D.

Professor and Chairman
Department of Radiation Oncology
Stanford University School of Medicine
Stanford, California

EDWARD J. BARTLE, M.D.

Associate Professor of Surgery
Section of Vascular Surgery
University of Colorado Health Sciences Center
Chief of Vascular Surgery
Denver Veterans Administration Medical Center
Denver, Colorado

STEVEN M. BERNSTEIN, M.D.

Division of Urology
Department of Surgery
University of Texas School of Medicine
Houston, Texas

DAVID BLOOM, M.D.

Associate Professor of Surgery
Section of Urology
University of Michigan School of Medicine
Ann Arbor, Michigan

STUART D. BOYD, M.D.

Associate Professor of Urology
Department of Urology
University of Southern California School of Medicine
Los Angeles, California

ELY BRAND, M.D.

Assistant Professor
Division of Gynecologic Oncology
Department of Obstetrics and Gynecology
University of Colorado Health Sciences Center
Denver, Colorado

MICHAEL K. BRAWER, M.D.

Assistant Professor of Urology
Department of Urology
University of Washington School of Medicine
Seattle, Washington

PETER R. CARROLL, M.D.

Assistant Professor of Urology
Department of Urology
University of California School of Medicine
San Francisco, California

GERALD W. CHODAK, M.D.

Associate Professor of Surgery/Urology
Section of Urology
University of Chicago
Chicago, Illinois

E. DAVID CRAWFORD, M.D.

Professor of Surgery
Chairman, Division of Urology
University of Colorado Health Sciences Center
Attending Physician
Denver Veterans Administration Medical Center
Rose Medical Center
Denver, Colorado

KENNETH B. CUMMINGS, M.D.

Professor and Chief
Division of Urology
University of Medicine and Dentistry of New Jersey
Robert Wood Johnson Medical School
New Brunswick, New Jersey

ALFRED A. deLORIMIER, M.D.

Professor of Surgery
Division of Pediatric Surgery
University of California School of Medicine
San Francisco, California

SAKTI DAS, M.B.B.S.

Associate Clinical Professor of Urology
University of California School of Medicine
Davis, California
Staff Urologist, Kaiser Permanente Medical Center
Walnut Creek, California

MARILYN A. DAVIS, R.N., M.S.

Senior Instructor
Division of Urology
University of Colorado Health Sciences Center
Denver, Colorado

JOHN P. DONOHUE, M.D.

Distinguished Professor and Chairman
Department of Urology
Indiana University Hospital
Indianapolis, Indiana

ROBERT E. DONOHUE, M.D.

Associate Professor of Surgery
Division of Urology
University of Colorado Health Sciences Center
Chief of Urology
Denver Veterans Administration Medical Center
Denver, Colorado

F. ANDREW DORR, M.D.

Senior Investigator
Cancer Therapy Evaluation Program
Division of Cancer Treatment
National Cancer Institute
Bethesda, Maryland

JOSEPH R. DRAGO, M.D.

Professor of Surgery
Chief, Division of Urology
Levy Professor of Cancer
Ohio State University Hospitals
Columbus, Ohio

MICHAEL J. DROLLER, M.D.

Professor and Chairman
Department of Urology
The Mount Sinai Medical Center
New York, New York

MARILYN H. DUNCAN, M.D.

Associate Professor
Pediatric Oncology Program
Department of Pediatrics
University of New Mexico School of Medicine
Albuquerque, New Mexico

W. STERLING EDWARDS, M.D.

Emeritus Professor of Surgery
University of New Mexico School of Medicine
Albuquerque, New Mexico

RICHARD M. EHRLICH, M.D.

Professor of Surgery/Urology
Division of Urology
UCLA School of Medicine
Los Angeles, California

MARIO A. EISENBERGER, M.D.

Associate Professor of Medicine/Oncology
University of Maryland Cancer Center
Baltimore, Maryland

DONALD C. FISCHER, M.D.

Professor of Medicine
Department of Medicine
University of Cincinnati College of Medicine
Cincinnati, Ohio

ROBERT C. FLANIGAN, M.D.

Professor and Chairman
Department of Urology
Loyola University Medical Center
Maywood, Illinois

JEFFREY D. FORMAN, M.D.

Assistant Professor
Department of Radiation Oncology
University of Michigan Medical Center
Ann Arbor, Michigan

FUAD S. FREIHA, M.D.

Associate Professor
Chief of Urologic Oncology
Department of Surgery, Division of Urology
Stanford University Medical Center
Stanford, California

GLENN GERBER, M.D.

Department of Urology
University of Chicago
Chicago, Illinois

RUBEN F. GITTES, M.D.

Division of Urology
Scripps Clinic and Research Foundation
LaJolla, California

DONALD R. GOFFINET, M.D.

Professor
Division of Radiation Therapy
Department of Radiation Oncology
Stanford University Medical Center
Stanford, California

EDMOND T. GONZALES, JR., M.D.

Professor of Urology
Scott Department of Urology
Baylor College of Medicine
Director of Pediatric Urology
Texas Children's Hospital
Houston, Texas

JAMES E. GOTTESMAN, M.D.

Associate Clinical Professor of Urology
University of Washington School of Medicine
Seattle, Washington

H. BARTON GROSSMAN, M.D.

Associate Professor of Surgery
Section of Urology
University of Michigan Medical School
Director, Urologic Oncology Program
University of Michigan Cancer Center
Ann Arbor, Michigan

MICHAEL R. HARRISON, M.D.

Professor of Surgery
Division of Pediatric Surgery
University of California School of Medicine
San Francisco, California

MARK B. HAZUKA, M.D.

Assistant Professor of Radiation Oncology
Division of Radiation Oncology
Department of Radiology
University of Colorado Health Sciences Center
Denver, Colorado

RICHARD K. HEPPE, M.D.

Division of Urology
University of Colorado Health Sciences Center
Denver, Colorado

MARTIN A. KOYLE, M.D.

Associate Professor of Surgery/Urology
Division of Urology
University of Colorado Health Sciences Center
Pediatric Urologist
The Children's Hospital
Denver, Colorado

J. PHILIP KUEBLER, M.D., PH.D.

Assistant Professor of Medicine
Department of Medicine/Oncology
University of Oklahoma Health Science Center
Oklahoma City, Oklahoma

DONALD L. LAMM, M.D.

Professor and Chairman
Department of Urology
West Virginia Medical Center
Morgantown, West Virginia

PAUL H. LANGE, M.D.

Professor and Chairman
Department of Urologic Surgery
University of Washington School of Medicine
Seattle, Washington

S. LAWRENCE LIBRACH, M.D.

Associate Professor
Departments of Family and Community Medicine, and
    Behavioral Science
University of Toronto
Toronto, Ontario, Canada

ALLEN S. LICHTER, M.D.

Professor and Chairman
Department of Radiation Oncology
University of Michigan Medical Center
Ann Arbor, Michigan

MICHAEL M. LIEBER, M.D.

Professor of Urology
Mayo Medical School
Rochester, Minnesota

GARY LIESKOVSKY

Associate Professor of Urology
University of Southern California Medical Center
Los Angeles, California

MICHAEL T. MACFARLANE, M.D.

Assistant Professor of Surgery/Urology
Division of Urology
UCLA School of Medicine
Los Angeles, California

FRANK MAYER, M.D.

Department of Surgery
University of Colorado Health Sciences Center
Denver, Colorado

WINSTON K. MEBUST, M.D.

Professor and Chairman
Section of Urology
University of Kansas Medical Center
Kansas City, Kansas

FRED A. METTLER, JR., M.D.

Professor and Chairman
Department of Radiology
University of New Mexico School of Medicine
Albuquerque, New Mexico

WILLIAM R. MORGAN, M.D.

Assistant Professor of Surgery
Section of Urology
Yale University School of Medicine
New Haven, Connecticut

WILLIAM L. NABORS, M.D.

Instructor in Urology
Division of Urology
University of Colorado Health Sciences Center
Denver, Colorado

PERINCHERY NARAYAN, M.D.

Associate Professor of Urology
Department of Urology
University of California School of Medicine
San Francisco, California

CRAIG R. NICHOLS, M.D.

Assistant Professor of Medicine
Department of Medicine
Indiana University School of Medicine
Wishard Memorial Hospital
Indianapolis, Indiana

JORGE C. PARADELO, M.D.

Clinical Assistant Professor of Therapeutic Radiology
University of Missouri
Kansas City School of Medicine
Kansas City, Missouri

PAUL C. PETERS, M.D.

Professor and Chairman
Division of Urology
University of Texas Southwestern Medical School
Dallas, Texas

ROBERT A. READ, M.D., PH.D.

Department of Surgery
University of Colorado Health Sciences Center
Denver, Colorado

JOHN F. REDMAN, M.D.

Professor and Chairman
Department of Urology
University of Arkansas College of Medicine
Little Rock, Arkansas

JEROME P. RICHIE, M.D.

Elliot C. Cutler Professor of Urological Surgery
Harvard Medical School
Chief of Urology
Brigham and Women's Hospital
Boston, Massachusetts

ROBERT ROSENBERG, M.D.

Associate Professor
Department of Radiology
University of New Mexico School of Medicine
Albuquerque, New Mexico

RANDALL G. ROWLAND, M.D., PH.D.

Professor
Department of Urology
University Hospital
Indiana University Medical Center
Indianapolis, Indiana

KENNETH J. RUSSELL, M.D.

Assistant Professor
Department of Radiation Oncology
University of Washington Cancer Center
Seattle, Washington

MICHAEL F. SAROSDY, M.D.

Associate Professor and Chief
Division of Urology
University of Texas Health Science Center
San Antonio, Texas

WILLIAM T. SAUSE, M.D.

Clinical Professor
Radiation Oncology
University of Utah Medical Center
Salt Lake City, Utah

PETER T. SCARDINO, M.D.

Professor and Chairman
Department of Urology
Baylor College of Medicine
Houston, Texas

JOSEPH D. SCHMIDT, M.D.

Professor of Surgery/Urology
Head, Division of Urology
University of California Medical Center
San Diego, California

DONALD G. SKINNER, M.D.

Professor and Chairman
Department of Urology
University of Southern California School of Medicine
Los Angeles, California

ARTHUR D. SMITH, M.D.

Professor and Chairman
Department of Urology
Long Island Jewish Medical Center
New Hyde Park, New York

JOSEPH A. SMITH, JR., M.D.

Professor of Surgery/Urology
Division of Urology
University of Utah Medical Center
Salt Lake City, Utah

RICHARD M. SMITH, M.D.

Clinical Instructor
Department of Medicine
University of Cincinnati College of Medicine
Cincinnati, Ohio

ROBERT B. SMITH, M.D.

Professor of Surgery/Urology
Division of Urology
UCLA Health Science Center
Los Angeles, California

JEFFREY A. SNYDER, M.D.

Assistant Professor of Surgery/Urology
Director of Neurosurgery, Female Urology, and
Reconstructive Surgery
Division of Urology
University of Colorado Health Sciences Center
Denver, Colorado

JACEK T. SOSNOWSKI, M.D.

Department of Urology
West Virginia Medical Center
Morgantown, West Virginia

JOSEPH T. SPAULDING, M.D.

Chairman, Department of Urology
Pacific Presbyterian Medical Center
San Francisco, California

RONALD L. STEPHENS, M.D.

Professor of Medicine
Division of Clinical Oncology
University of Kansas Medical Center
Kansas City, Kansas

GREG VAN STIEGMANN, M.D.

Associate Professor of Surgery
Chief of Endoscopic and Laser Surgery
Department of Surgery
University of Colorado Health Sciences Center
Denver, Colorado

IAN M. THOMPSON, M.D.

Major, Medical Corps
Urology Service
Department of Surgery
Brook Army Medical Center
Fort Sam Houston, Texas

JOHN W. VESTER, M.D.

Professor of Medicine and Clinical Biochemistry
University of Cincinnati College of Medicine
Cincinnati, Ohio

JULIAN WAN, M.D.

Instructor in Urology
Section of Urology
University of Michigan School of Medicine
Ann Arbor, Michigan

MICHAEL WILLIAMSON, M.D.

Associate Professor
Department of Radiology
University of New Mexico School of Medicine
Albuquerque, New Mexico

PHILLIP G. WISE, M.D.

Clinical Instructor
Division of Urology
University of California Medical Center
San Diego, California

CONTENTS

An Anatomic Approach to the Kidneys and Retroperitoneum

"I began to investigate the transversalis fascia. I sought it in books, where its descriptions were vague and unconvincing; in anatomy departments which had no dissection to offer; and in the human body where I failed entirely to find it."

DENIS BROWNE[1]

John F. Redman

A ny surgeon who has pursued the detailed aspects of anatomy has shared Denis Browne's frustrations. Although the transversalis fascia is a vital component in extirpative cancer surgery, many of its aspects have been difficult to define. Anatomy that seemed clear in the dissecting room or in surgical texts can become confused through a developing incision in an actual surgical procedure. This chapter details a careful, thorough anatomic approach to the kidneys and retroperitoneum that can eliminate much of that confusion.

RETROPERITONEAL CONNECTIVE TISSUE

The basis for an understanding of the retroperitoneum is a knowledge of the retroperitoneal connective tissue. There has been much confusion in the literature regarding what lies between the peritoneum, aptly described by Browne as a "membrane hardly thicker than a soap-bubble,"[1] and the lining muscles of the abdominal cavity. This tissue is more complex than just "packing material" between the osteomuscular wall and the peritoneum.

A brief description of its embryologic origins should help in understanding the retroperitoneal connective tissue. Hayes gives a clear description, and his conclusions coincide with

what is seen surgically, in regard to anatomic findings and planes of dissection.[2] The retroperitoneal connective tissue is derived from three separate embryologic origins: (1) a parietal layer, from the young mesenchymal tissue intimately associated with the developing musculature of the abdominal wall, (2) a visceral layer, from loose mesenchymal tissue distributed between the developing intrinsic fascia of the muscles, and (3) the celomic epithelium.

The parietal layer becomes the transversalis fascia, which is the intrinsic investing fascia of the muscular abdominal wall. The celomic epithelium becomes the peritoneum, which is backed by a thin supportive tissue containing nutrient vessels. The intermediate layer derived from loose mesenchyme is intimately related to the supporting backing of the peritoneum. The enlarging kidney, as it grows within this intermediate layer of connective tissue, compresses the tissue to form a limiting fascial-like structure (Gerota's fascia). In like manner, the ureter and spermatic vessels are surrounded by this tissue and thus are held to the serosal surface. This intermediate retroperitoneal connective tissue has been loosely termed the subserosal layer.

The retroperitoneal connective tissue becomes more complex by virtue of what Hayes has termed "fusion fascia." One should recall that the primitive gut, with the structures arising in its mesentery (the pancreas), at one time was covered with peritoneum over most of its circumference as well as its mesentery. With rotation of the gut, the duodenum and pancreas, as well as the ascending and descending colon, come to rest upon the primitive celomic epithelium. The colonic mesentery in part comes to rest against the serosal covering of the duodenum and pancreas. With obliteration of the peritoneum per se, a firm fascia is produced.

Tobin described three "dissectable strata" of the retroperitoneal connective tissue: (1) an inner stratum associated intimately with the peritoneum and with the digestive system with its nerve blood supply, (2) an intermediate stratum embedding the adrenals, urogenital system, and the great vessels, and (3) an outer stratum, which is the intrinsic fascia of the components of the body wall (Fig. 1-1).[3,4] In the region of the kidneys, the intermediate stratum, particularly in obese individuals, may be in the form of two laminae, with local thickenings of the ventral lamina forming the renal (Gerota's) fascia with its contained perirenal fat. The dorsal lamina forms the perirenal fat and the areolar tissue between the ventral (Gerota's) lamina and the tranversalis fascia (Fig. 1-2). In thinner individuals, the intermediate stratum caudal to the region of the kidney will not be laminated.

In keeping with Tobin's belief that "a knowledge of the fascial strata of the abdomen and pelvis is a great asset to the surgeon who operates in these regions," it may be stated that cleavage planes exist theoretically between (1) the transversalis fascia and the intermediate stratum (subserosal layer), (2) between the intermediate stratum and the inner stratum (supporting connective tissue of the peritoneum), (3) between the intermediate stratum and the colon and its mesentery, and (4) between the intermediate stratum and the pancreas and duodenum (Fig. 1-3).[3] Graphic evidence that these planes exist is provided by radiographic studies of extraperitoneal effusions, and by the identification of planes of dissection of retroperitoneal abscesses.[5,6]

SURGICAL APPROACHES TO THE KIDNEY AND RETROPERITONEUM

The incisions used to gain access to the kidneys and retroperitoneum fall basically into four groups: midline abdominal, transverse abdominal, flank, and thoracoabdominal incisions. The placement and execution of the incisions of the body wall are described in the standard urologic surgical texts.[7,8] The following descriptions of the surgical approaches deal primarily with the location and development of retroperitoneal tissue planes.

Midline and Transverse Abdominal Transperitoneal Approaches

This section reviews the salient anatomic points for an incisions that gives wide exposure to the retroperitoneum without disturbing the investments of the kidney, presumably the approach most preferred by the surgeon.

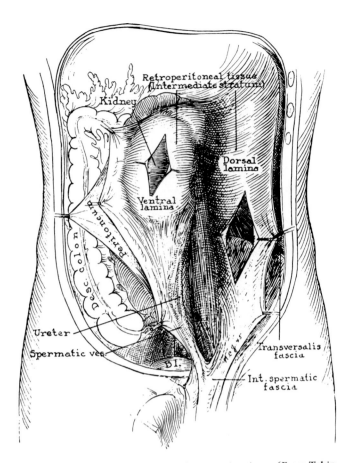

FIG. 1-1. Strata of the retroperitoneal connective tissue. (From Tobin, C. E., Benjamin, J. A., and Wells, J. C.: Continuity of the fasciae lining the abdomen, pelvis and spermatic cord. Surg. Gynecol. Obstet., 83:575, 1946. By permission of Surgery, Gynecology & Obstetrics.)

From within the peritoneal cavity, on exposure of the tissue just lateral to the lateral border of the ascending colon, it may be noted that the peritoneum, along with the thin but adherent underlying tissue containing small vessels, can be moved freely over an underlying layer, which can be seen through the thin peritoneum and its supporting layer. The underlying tissue is the subserosal layer of retroperitoneal connective tissue.

An incision through the peritoneum and its underlying connective tissue along the colonic border opens a tissue plane (fusion fascia) that may be carried medially between the colon per se and the underlying subserosal layer (Gerota's fascia). If the peritoneal incision is carried around the hepatic flexure of the colon and around the cecum, the plane may be developed as it is carried dorsal to the mesentery of the colon. The plane may be further developed by carrying the dissection dorsal to the duodenum (fusion fascia).

Gerota's fascia is contiguous across the midline over the vena cava and aorta, extending over the renal vessels of the left side. If the peritoneal incision is carried cranially from the cecum to the level where the duodenum emerges from its retroperitoneal position, the entirety of the ascending colon and small bowel may be displaced from the abdominal cavity.

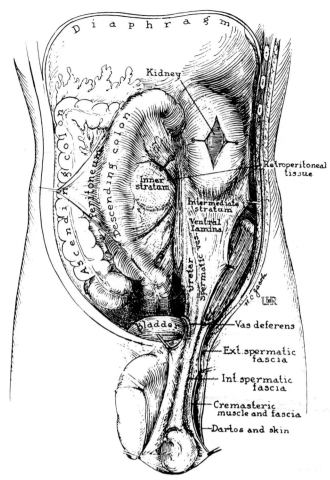

FIG. 1-2. Intermediate stratum of the retroperitoneal tissue in the region of the kidney. (From Tobin, C. E., Benjamin, J. A., and Wells, J. C.: Continuity of the fasciae lining the abdomen, pelvis and spermatic cord. Surg. Gynecol. Obstet., *83*:575, 1946. By permission of Surgery, Gynecology & Obstetrics.)

The right kidney, as well as the right ureter, the gonadal vessels, and the aorta and vena cava, will remain undisturbed, covered with an intact Gerota's fascia. The lymphatics and lymph nodes should also be visible and undisturbed.

On the left side, a similar plane of dissection may be achieved by incision of the peritoneum and its supporting connective tissue on the lateral aspect of the descending colon. The peritoneal incision may be carried around the splenic flexure of the colon. Exposure of the peritoneum that lies between the caudal border of the pancreas and the cranial margin of the transverse colon will be enhanced by division of the omentum to separate the stomach from the transverse colon. With incision of the peritoneum between the transverse colon and the pancreas, the cleavage plane over Gerota's fascia is developed.

The duodenum may be elevated by pursuing the cleavage plane dorsal to that structure. Division of the inferior mesenteric vein as it joins the splenic vein gives even wider exposure. As one moves cranially, the pancreas may be elevated off the subserosal layer to reveal the left kidney and adrenal and

the renal vasculature, which usually can be seen clearly through the thin overlying Gerota's fascia. On the left side, the stomach, pancreas, and spleen may be rolled to the right side of the abdomen by continuation of the peritoneal incision around the lateral aspect of the tail of the pancreas and parietal peritoneal attachment of the greater curvature of the stomach.

Extraperitoneal Transverse Abdominal and Subcostal Flank Exposures

These two incisions are basically the same as those just described. However, instead of being directed through the abdominal and flank musculature directly into the peritoneal cavity, the incisions are deepened through the muscle without incision of the dorsal investing fascia of the transversus abdominis muscle. The aponeurosis of the transversus abdominis may be incised laterally in the direction of its fibers. If the incision is to approach or cross the midline, the posterior rectus sheath may be incised after the rectus itself has been incised.

The further development of the incision along anatomic planes is accomplished more easily if approached in a lateral-to-medial direction. The layer immediately underlying the aponeurosis of the transversus abdominis muscle, the dorsal investing fascia of the transversus abdominis, is the transversalis fascia. A plane may be developed between the subserosal layer and the transversalis fascia if one moves in a lateral-to-medial direction. As the subserosal fascia and underlying peritoneum are reflected, the transversalis fascia can be progressively incised.

From the lateral border of the rectus to the midline, the amount of extraperitoneal connective tissue becomes more scant, and in some individuals the peritoneum becomes frankly adherent to the transversalis fascia. In some, the plane of dissection can be carried between the transversalis fascia and the posterior rectus sheath across the midline. In others, the adherence is so dense that a plane cannot be established.

To gain access to the other side, the surgeon should incise the peritoneum as close to the midline as possible, with closure of the peritoneum once the plane is gained on the contralateral side. Caudally, the peritoneal envelope, surrounded by its retroperitoneal connective tissue, may be swept medially. The correct plane of dissection can be ascertained by examination of the dorsal aspect of the transversus abdominis muscle. If bare muscle fibers are noted, the surgeon may assume that the incision is not deep enough. Identification of fascia over the muscle confirms the correct plane. Laterally, sweeping the retroperitoneal connective tissue from the transversalis fascia becomes more difficult at times because of the adherence of the one structure to the other, particularly laterally at the level of the midaxillary line and at the lateral apposition of the transversus abdominis to the quadratus lumborum.

A similar situation occurs over the psoas muscle. If the surgeon observes bare muscle fibers over the quadratus or psoas muscle, he only has to sharply incise the fibrous tissue he is sweeping medially to again regain the plane between transver-

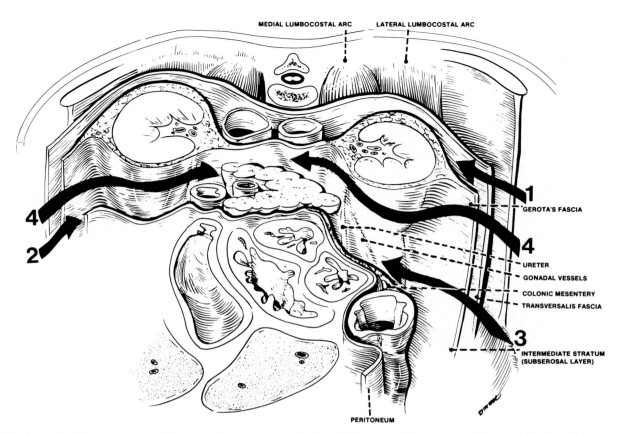

MEDIAL LUMBOCOSTAL ARC   LATERAL LUMBOCOSTAL ARC

GEROTA'S FASCIA

URETER
GONADAL VESSELS
COLONIC MESENTERY
TRANSVERSALIS FASCIA

INTERMEDIATE STRATUM
(SUBSEROSAL LAYER)

PERITONEUM

FIG. 1-3. Anatomic cleavage planes (1) between the transversalis fascia and the intermediate stratum (subserosal layer), (2) between the intermediate stratum and the inner stratum (supporting connective tissue of the peritoneum), (3) between the intermediate stratum and the colon and colonic mesentery, and (4) between the intermediate stratum and the pancreas and duodenum.

salis fascia and the retroperitoneal connective tissue. At first, this may seem risky because of the grossly similar appearance of these glistening surfaces to peritoneum, colon, or dilated ureter. The peritoneal envelope, surrounded by its retroperitoneal connective tissue which encases the ureter and spermatic vessels, can be swept from the posterior abdominal wall, the lateral abdominal wall, and the anterior abdominal wall toward the midline. The only adherence of the peritoneum occurs deep in the pelvis, where it is tethered at the level of the internal ring by the remnants of the patent processus vaginalis peritonei. Cranially, the retroperitoneal connective tissue can be separated from the posterolateral abdominal wall.

At times the retroperitoneal connective tissue adheres to the fibrous tissue arcs over the quadratus lumborum muscle (lateral lumbocostal arc) and over the psoas muscle (medial lumbocostal arc), which represents the point of insertion of the diaphragm over the surface of these muscles. It should be noted that the retroperitoneal connective tissue is scant between the peritoneum and transversalis fascia on the undersurface of the diaphragm. At times, to maintain an extraperitoneal cleavage plane, it is necessary to pursue a plane between the transversalis fascia and the diaphragm.

Generally, in the course of freeing the retroperitoneal connective tissue from the diaphragm, numerous penetrating vessels will be noted. These should be sealed (preferably through electrocautery) to prevent staining of the tissue, which makes the identification of anatomic cleavage planes more difficult.

Remember that, in the case of neoplasms, these vessels may be greatly enlarged.

Following the freeing of the peritoneal envelope with its adherent retroperitoneal connective tissue, a plane of dissection can be started by incising along the lateral border of the colon to obtain the cleavage plane between the colon and its mesentery and the subserosal layer. This plane of dissection can be carried across the midline. To obtain access to the renal vasculature or to the vena cava or aorta, the subserosal layer must be incised over the vessels. The only major vessels that penetrate this subserosal layer from the dorsal to the ventral aspect occur in the midline; these are the inferior mesenteric artery, the superior mesenteric artery, and the celiac axis.

Twelfth-Rib Flank Exposure

Attention to detail is essential for a true subperiosteal resection of the tip of the twelfth rib. To gain a subperiosteal plane of dissection, it is generally easiest to sharply reflect the periosteum from the caudal keel of the rib with a periosteal elevator. Excursions with the periosteal elevator at right angles to the keel penetrate the periosteum in the same manner as if one were to incise the periosteum with a knife. The rib edge is sharp, and to remove the periosteum, one must carefully follow the contours of this edge. Once the inner aspect of the rib has been exposed, it is easy to strip the periosteum from the rib.

It is usually possible to identify a muscular layer immediately under the periosteum. This muscle is the diaphragm. If pleura is present, it will be located between the periosteum and the diaphragm. If the pleura extends beyond the periosteum of the twelfth rib, the incision is best developed from the more medial aspect where transversalis fascia has been incised, and the diaphragm is best exposed from its inner aspect. With incision of the diaphragmatic attachments caudal to the twelfth rib, one can usually strip the pleura from the inner aspect of the periosteum of the twelfth rib using the "snowshoe" principle, peeling the pleura away much as one would peel away a hernia sac from the spermatic cord. An attempt to perform this dissection from the periosteal side generally allows access to the pleural cavity.

Eleventh-Rib Extraperitoneal Flank Exposure

Great lengths of the eleventh rib may be resected and the exposure maintained extrapleurally if attention is given to detail, which is even more important in the case of the eleventh-rib incision than in the twelfth-rib exposure. Almost without exception, the pleura will be seen extending under the periosteum of the eleventh rib. With progression to the medial aspect of the incision, the retroperitoneal connective tissue is swept from the transversalis fascia and the diaphragm can be freed at the level of the lateral lumbocostal arc, i.e., the insertion of the diaphragm over the quadratus lumborum. This incision may be carried caudally and laterally to free the diaphragmatic attachments. The pleura can then be swept from the underside of the periosteum of the eleventh rib with broad-based traction (snowshoe principle).

Thoracoabdominal Transpleural Exposure

Any of the ribs, as high as the seventh, may be chosen for this incision. The incision usually begins at the midaxillary line over the body of the rib and is carried along the axis of the rib. The incision may be carried down to the midline if the exposure is to be transpleural and transperitoneal; if the incision is to be transpleural but extraperitoneal, a paramedian or pararectus incision may be used. The rib is resected subperiosteally. With incision through the periosteum, the pleural cavity is entered.

Prior to incision of the diaphragm of the costochondral junction, if the surgeon wishes to remain extraperitoneal, the caudal portion of the incision should be developed in the manner already described for extraperitoneal exposures. Because of the scant amount of retroperitoneal connective tissue between the peritoneum and its supporting connective tissue and the transversalis fascia overlying the diaphragm, an incision made from the cranial aspect of the diaphragm may well enter directly into the peritoneum if the peritoneum is not freed from the caudal aspect of the diaphragm prior to this maneuver.

The entire peritoneal envelope with its supporting connective tissue may be mobilized from the retroperitoneum as described for the extraperitoneal transverse abdominal and subcostal flank exposures. If the procedure is carried out intraperitoneally on the right side, the liver can be rotated medially for further exposure by careful incision of the right triangular ligament, which represents the reflection of the peritoneum onto the hepatic surface.

Dorsolumbar Flap Incision for Thoracoabdominal Extrapleural Exposure

This incision allows similar exposure to that gained with a transpleural transthoracic exposure. The anatomic key to this incision is the division of the lateral lumbocostal arc of the diaphragm, that is, the attachment of the diaphragm to the quadratus lumborum muscle. The diaphragm can then be retracted upward with the pleural reflection (costophrenic sinus). Nagamatsu states that "if this is performed with care and deliberation, it is entirely possible to avoid pleural injury."[9] Because the ribs are resected at the costal arc, the adherence of the pleura to the periosteum of the ribs is not disturbed; thus, there is less opportunity for injury to the pleura. The remainder of the dissection is carried out as in the previously mentioned extrapleural exposures.

Lumbodorsal Incision

Anatomically, this incision is simple: with the correct placement of the incision, only the lumbodorsal fascia is incised in the direction of the skin incision, along with the latissimus dorsi and the serratus posterior inferior muscle ventrally. The quadratus lumborum is noted in the medial aspect of the incision and is reflected medially, and the iliohypogastric nerve is preserved. With incision of the transversalis fascia, the extraperitoneal connective tissue is visible.

REFERENCES

1. BROWNE, D., and SYDNEY, M. B. Some anatomical points in the operation for undescended testicle. Lancet, 224:460, 1933.
2. HAYES, M. A. Abdominopelvic fasciae. Am. J. Anat., 87:119, 1950.
3. TOBIN, C. E., BENJAMIN, J. A., and WELLS, J. C. Continuity of the fasciae lining the abdomen, pelvis and spermatic cord. Surg. Gynecol. Obstet., 83:575, 1946.
4. TOBIN, C. E. The renal fascia and its relation to the transversalis fascia. Anat. Rec., 89:295, 1944.
5. MEYERS, M. A., WHALEN, J. P., PEELLE, K., and BERNE, A. S. Radiologic features of extraperitoneal effusions. Radiology, 104:249, 1972.
6. STEVENSON, E. O. S., and OZERAN, R. S. Retroperitoneal space abscesses. Surg. Gynecol. Obstet., 128:1202, 1969.
7. GLENN, J. F. Urologic Surgery. 2nd Ed. Hagerstown, Maryland, Harper & Row, 1975.
8. HARRISON, J. H., et al. Campbell's Urology. 4th Ed. Vols. 2, 3. Philadelphia, Saunders, 1979.
9. NAGAMATSU, G. R., LERMAN, P. H., and BERMAN, M. H. The dorsolumbar flap incision in urologic surgery. J. Urol., 67:787, 1952.

SECTION
I

ADRENAL TUMORS

CHAPTER
2

Surgery of the Adrenal Gland

John P. Donohue

Any discussion of surgery of the adrenal gland is best preceded by a review of the diagnosis and pathophysiology of its surgical diseases according to their origin from either cortex or medulla. Then, details of surgical approach may follow in the same logical sequence.

DIAGNOSIS OF SURGICALLY TREATABLE ADRENAL DISORDERS

Adrenal Cortex

Adrenal cortical lesions are classified according to their distinctive hormonal manifestation resulting from the hyperfunction of the specialized cells of the zona glomerulosa, zona fasciculata, and zona reticularis of the adrenal cortex.

ALDOSTERONISM. Primary aldosteronism is characterized by hypertension secondary to inappropriate excessive production of aldosterone by the zona glomerulosa of the adrenal cortex. As a result, it is associated with suppression of plasma renin activity, hypokalemia, and metabolic alkalosis. Although primary aldosteronism here refers to the functional adrenal adenoma, it can also be caused by bilateral micronodular hyperplasia of zona glomerulosa cells. This condition is thought to

occur in about 20% of the patients with chemical aldosteronism.[1]

Diagnosis. Major clinical features are benign hypertension, usually in the absence of severe vascular disease. Urinary aldosterone and potassium excretion are elevated; likewise plasma aldosterone is elevated, but serum potassium is reduced. Although relative hypervolemia exists (secondary to increased sodium resorption at the proximal tubules in exchange for potassium), hypernatremia is only mild and metabolic alkalosis is often not severe. Both normokalemic and nonalkalotic forms have also been recognized. Usually patients are between 30 and 60 years of age. Few children have been reported. The most common symptom is relative muscle weakness, and the most common sign is hypertension.

The key to establishing the diagnosis is finding elevated urinary and plasma aldosterone together with unprovoked hypokalemia. The other major criterion for diagnosis is suppression of renal renin production. The two most reliable tests for primary aldosteronism are: (1) failure to suppress aldosterone output during sodium loading (saline suppression test, i.e., 2 L over 2 to 3 hrs) and (2) failure to stimulate plasma renin activity, even in the presence of sodium deprivation (negative furosemide [Lasix] stimulation test) (Table 2-1). Therefore, the sine qua non of the diagnosis of primary aldo-

TABLE 2-1. *Tests for Diagnosis of Adrenal Surgical Diseases*

TESTS	ALDOSTERONISM	CUSHING'S SYNDROME	VIRILIZATION	PHEOCHROMOCYTOMA	NEUROBLASTOMA	1°/2° CARCINOMA	INCIDENTAL ADENOMA
Plasma renin activity (PRA)	+						−
Lasix stimulation (PRA, Aldo)	−						
Serum electrolytes (K+, CO2)	+						−
Plasma aldosterone (PA)	+						−
Urine aldosterone (UA)	+						−
Differential adrenal venous samples (Diff. Adr. VV)	+	±					−
Isotopic scan (19-iodo cholesterol)	+	+					+
Isotopic scan (M-BIG)				+			
Computed Tomography (CT Scan)	+	+	+	+	+	+	+
Magnetic resonance imaging (MRI)				+			
Plasma cortisol (OHC)		+	+				−
Plasma 17-ketosteroids (17-Ketos)			+				
Serum testosterone (T)			+				
Fractionated ketosteroids (FR. Ketos)			+				
Pregnanetriols (S. Pregnt.)			+				−
Clonidine suppression test				+			−
Catecholamines, (VMA, HVA)				+			−
Serum norepinephrine (NE)				+	+		−
Serum epinephrine (E)				+	+		−
Urine norepinephrine (U/NE)				+	+		−
Urine epinephrine (U/E)				+	+		−
Selective venous IVC/SVC samples				+			
Whole lung tomography (WLTs)					+	+	
Skull, sella x-ray incl. CT scan		+					
Bone scan, incl. skeletal survey					+	+	
Angiography		+	+				
Selective basilar venous samples (ACTH)		+					
Serum ACTH		+					−
Dexamethasone suppression		+					−

steronism is failure to suppress plasma aldosterone after saline loading (2 L in 3 hrs) and failure of plasma renin activity to be stimulated by salt and volume depletion (40 mg furosemide q8h, 10 meq sodium diet for 24 hrs, and 2 hrs of ambulation). These rigid criteria positively identified some 125 patients with primary aldosteronism and surgically removed adrenal adenomas.

Once the diagnosis of aldosteronism is confirmed by a negative saline (aldosterone) suppression test and a negative furosemide (Lasix) (renin) stimulation test, the next step is localization of the disease. The two best localizing techniques in our experience are adrenal venous blood collections for aldosterone (with cortisol levels as a check on the accuracy of the sample) and adrenal venography.[2]

Treatment. Surgical treatment is best reserved for those patients diagnosed as having unilateral disease.[3] The differential adrenal venous sampling and venography can provide diagnostic accuracy in more than 90% of patients. Those with bilateral hyperplasia (excessive aldosterone production from both adrenals in the absence of any adenoma noted on venography) are best treated medically with spironolactone orally, ranging from 100 mg to 400 mg a day.

CUSHING'S SYNDROME. Cushing's syndrome is a general term referring to the clinical presentation of corticosteroid excess. This condition can be produced by administration of glucocorticoid, or may occur naturally from several pathologic dysfunctional states.[3–6] A basophilic pituitary adenoma was originally described by Harvey Cushing as the cause of the syndrome.[7] However, this adenoma is responsible for about 75 to 80% of the syndrome presentations. Other causes include adrenal tumors producing excess cortisol and other benign or malignant tumors producing ACTH.[12–16]

Diagnosis. The clinical presentation is classic. Prominent findings are truncal obesity with peripheral extremity muscle wasting out of keeping with the central obesity. Plethora, hypertension, and increased bruising and striae are also distinctive features. In women, hirsutism and amenorrhea may be present. On physical examination, the classic moon facies and buffalo hump are well known. The moon facies is caused by an increased size of cheek fat pads. Because the changes are often subtle, old photographs are helpful in recognizing them. Hypertension is almost always present. Renin profiles are generally low, because vascular volume is expanded. Major problems with long-term corticosteroid excess are infections and cardiovascular accidents from chronic hypertension.

Laboratory findings vary with the cause of the syndrome. Cushing's syndrome, caused by pituitary adenoma, is associated with elevated plasma ACTH (normal in pg/ml is 95 ± 12). In Cushing's disease, these values are roughly doubled to 164 ± 19. Elevated fasting blood sugar is seen late in the disease, but a diabetic-type glucose tolerance curve is commonly present owing to excess production of glucocorticoid. Adrenal CT scans reveal bilateral symmetric enlargement of the adrenals. Confirmation of pituitary Cushing's syndrome requires demonstration of increased production of corticosteroids by the adrenals and increased production of ACTH from the anterior pituitary. This can be proved by demonstration of increased urinary and plasma cortisol, increased plasma ACTH and corticosteroid suppression with synthetic corticosteroids such as dexamethasone, and administration of blockers of corticosteroid synthesis such as metyrapone.[8] Failure to suppress with low-dose dexamethasone (1 mg), but suppression with high-dose (4 mg) dexamethasone can be taken as evidence for pituitary-dependent Cushing's disease. The ability of metyrapone to inhibit the synthesis of corticosteroid by blocking 11-hydroxylation also makes it a useful diagnostic tool. As 11-hydroxylation is blocked, substance "S" is produced instead of cortisol. Patients with Cushing's disease of pituitary origin have an increased production of substance "S" because of their hyperplastic glands, and they also have an increased ability to produce corticosteroids when stimulated by ACTH. The metyrapone stimulation test is useful in discriminating the pituitary-dependent Cushing's disease where there is a hyperactive response from adrenal tumors with a failure to respond.[9] Patients with ectopic ACTH production also fail to respond to metyrapone stimulation. A single-dose test is carried out by administering 30 mg/kg at midnight and measuring plasma levels of substance "S," cortisol, and ACTH at 8:00 A.M. the following morning.[9]

Cushing's syndrome caused by benign adenomas is best proved by measurement of elevated plasma cortisol with loss of diurnal curve, i.e., persistently elevated plasma values, even in the afternoon and evening. In patients with a primary adrenal disorder, i.e., glucocorticoid excess secondary to tumor, ACTH is suppressed. Furthermore, failure of plasma cortisol to suppress with both the 1- and 4-mg doses of dexamethasone is a characteristic feature of the adrenal tumor. Once these chemical values are confirmed, further diagnostic studies should include arteriography (for many of these tumors can be quite large with massive and variable blood supply), administration of radioactive cholesterol (I 131-C19), ultrasonograms, and CT scans. Usually, differential venous collections and venography are not necessary to localize these tumors. CT scans are helpful in localizing small adrenal adenomas in the 2-cm range. Most secretory adrenal cortical adenomas are associated with hyperaldosteronism. Of 85 cases reviewed, 13 were associated with Cushing's syndrome, 65 with aldosteronism, and 7 with inappropriate virilization.[10] In one series, 149 patients with Cushing's syndrome were analyzed;[11] 121 of these cases were associated with bilateral hyperplasia and presumably extra adrenal pituitary stimulation, 13 were caused by primary adrenal adenoma, and 15 by adrenal carcinoma. Therefore, about one fifth of patients with Cushing's syndrome will have primary adrenal tumors, either adenoma or carcinoma.

Treatment. The treatment of this condition is directed toward the primary dysfunction. Adrenalectomy is indicated in the 20% of cases that are caused by primary adrenal tumors. It is of great importance to identify and localize the source of excess corticosteroid production. Localization techniques that are most practical are the CT scan, radioisotopic study with C-19 I-131 and, in the event of a large tumor, arteriography.

VIRILIZING TUMORS. Adrenal hirsutism and virilization may come from a variety of causes: congenital deficiencies in steroid production (congenital adrenal hyperplasia), adrenal tumors, Cushing's syndrome secondary to increased ACTH production by the pituitary, ovarian tumors, polycystic ovaries, or ill-defined variants thereof. Hirsutism is most commonly idiopathic.[17]

Diagnosis. Virilizing adrenal tumors in the female are characterized by amenorrhea, hirsutism, deep voice, increased muscle mass, enlargement of the clitoris and, sometimes, decrease in breast size. In the male, such tumors may produce precocious puberty, early onset of prostatic enlargement, pubic axillary hair, and beard growth. The testes remain small. In the more adult male, tumors may be recognized only as a space-occupying lesion or by their metastases. These tumors must be differentiated from congenital adrenal hyperplasia, idiopathic hirsutism, Cushing's syndrome, and other ovarian diseases. Generally, adrenal tumors do not produce much testosterone, but ovarian tumors do. Fractionated ketosteroids and measurement of dehydroepiandrosterone elevations are helpful. As noted, testosterone elevations are more likely to be gonadal in origin. In addition, other major androgen precursors, such as delta-5-pregnenolone, progesterone, and 17-hydroxy-progesterone, may be elevated. Most virilizing adrenal tumors are not suppressible by administration of dexamethasone. They also fail to increase secretion in response to ACTH administration. Localization by adrenal radioisotope scanning,[18] CT scans, and sometimes venography, arteriography, and ultrasonography is useful. Usually, if a solitary benign tumor can be located and removed, the prognosis is good. Large tumors are often malignant, however, and prognostic advice to the patient should be guarded.

Adrenal Medulla

PHEOCHROMOCYTOMA. Pheochromocytomas have been found along the distribution of chromaffin tissue, which is laid down during fetal development and has mostly disappeared by late childhood. The largest accumulations of chromaffin tissue are in the adrenal medulla and in the organ of Zuckerkandl at the origin of the inferior mesenteric artery. Most pheochromocytomas are located between the diaphragm and the pelvic floor.[19-22] In the sporadic, nonfamilial pheochromocytoma, about 80% of tumors involve a single adrenal, 10% are extra-adrenal, and 10% are malignant. For this reason, they are sometimes referred to as the "10% tumors."[23] In children, they may be called the 30% tumors.[24] The catecholamines norepinephrine (NE) and epinephrine (E) are synthesized from the precursor amino acid tyrosine. The enzyme phenylethylamine N-methyl transferase (PNMT) converts NE to E; this is almost exclusively a property of the adrenal medulla (85% of adrenal catecholamine is epinephrine). Even though most pheochromocytomas arise in the adrenal medulla, most tumors secrete primarily NE. If, however, it is determined that there is predominant secretion of E, then the tumor is almost invariably located in the adrenal. A purely E-secreting tumor is extremely uncommon and difficult to diagnose because hypertension is minimal; in fact, the presenting symptom in some patients is shock.

The variable complex of symptoms experienced by a patient with a pheochromocytoma probably reflects mostly the proportion of NE to E secreted. Symptoms stem more from secretion of E, while NE determines the level of hypertension. Nearly all patients have troublesome headaches; excessive sweating is almost as common. Other symptoms are palpitations, episodes of uneasiness or anxiety, pallor, flushing, weakness, nausea, tremor, chest pain, shortness of breath, and abdominal cramps. As is well known, any one patient's combination of symptoms occurs in "spells," which may or may not appear related to precipitating events such as smoking, sexual intercourse, pressure on the abdomen, and defecation. Symptoms precipitated by micturition denote a urinary bladder location for the pheochromocytoma. Although the hypertension is famous for its paroxysmal nature, probably more than 50% of patients have sustained hypertension. An orthostatic decrease in blood pressure in an untreated hypertensive patient suggests the diagnosis of pheochromocytoma. (This finding is also suggestive of primary aldosteronism.) In some patients the single clue to the existence of a pheochromocytoma is a hypertensive crisis associated with either pregnancy, the administration of a general anesthetic, surgery, or the use of certain drugs. Drugs like morphine, ACTH, parenteral guanethidine, or parenteral methyl-dopa may release catecholamines from the tumor, whereas propranolol may increase the pressor response to circulating E.

Diagnosis. The diagnosis of pheochromocytoma is made from outpatient biochemical tests. Three kinds of measurements are made in urine: vanillylmandelic acid (VMA), total metanephrines (normetanephrine and metanephrine), and free catecholamines. These tests provide meaningful information, are available to any physician, and are nearly equal in their sensitivity and specificity. If all three are carried out simultaneously, 95% of pheochromocytomas will be detected. The urine must be kept acidic by prior addition of HCL or acetic acid to the collection container.

The quantitation of catecholamines in plasma was formerly carried out by fluorometric methods, procedures that require meticulous technique and large plasma samples and that frequently provided inaccurate results. A major advance in this area was the development of the radioenzymatic assay for measurement of catecholamines. Plasma is incubated with an enzyme that transfers a ^{3}H-containing methyl group from *S*-adenosylmethione (SAM) to the catecholamine. The radiolabeled catecholamine is then isolated and the radioactivity counted. The radioenzymatic assay used at Indiana University School of Medicine (developed by D. P. Henry) utilizes the enzyme PNMT to transfer a ^{3}H-methyl group from SAM to NE to produce ^{3}HE. Employing this assay at this institution, re-

searchers have taken measurements of plasma NE, as well as the urinary excretion of NE, including excretion measured in an easily collected morning urine sample ("sleep NE"), and have clearly delineated patients with pheochromocytoma from other hypertensive patients. NE can be measured in plasma samples from multiple sites of venous drainage to find a tumor whose location has been elusive.[25]

The radioenzymatic assay is making an important impact in investigative studies of the sympathoadrenal system, and it appears that it may in part revise our approach to the diagnosis of pheochromocytoma. Similar assays are under evaluation from important metabolites of catecholamines in plasma, which may further increase our diagnostic accuracy.[26,27]

The clonidine suppression test is another useful aid in the diagnosis of pheochromocytoma.[28] Plasma catecholamines are normally increased through the activation of the sympathetic nervous system. In pheochromocytoma, however, they arise through synthesis by the tumor itself. The excess diffusion into the plasma bypasses normal storage and release mechanisms. Clonidine decreases resting plasma catecholamines by inhibition of centrally mediated adrenergic influences. Because of this central blocking effect, clonidine does not suppress catecholamine release in pheochromocytoma. This fact is useful in diagnosis of patients with essential hypertension whose catecholamine release is thought to be neurogenically mediated but not mediated by tumor. Clonidine should suppress the catecholamine release in essential hypertensives by blocking the central neurogenic release mechanisms. This phenomenon is particularly helpful because clonidine suppression does not occur (i.e., plasma epinephrine and norepinephrine values are not suppressed) in patients with pheochromocytoma. This test is fairly specific (i.e., few false positives). It is an adjunctive test that is useful in patients whose elevated catecholamines need to be distinguished from the subset with essential hypertension.

When the diagnosis of pheochromocytoma is firmly established, the next step is to try to find its location. Occasionally an intravenous pyelogram shows the tumor. In our experience, computerized tomography can delineate most adrenal pheochromocytomas. In the past, the tumor was located by arteriography. (This procedure has been replaced, however, by the safer isotopic scanning with 131-MIBG.)[26,27] Knowing where the tumor resides and the anatomy of its blood supply may allow the surgeon to better plan the approach.

Arteriography is not particularly dangerous when carried out by an experienced radiologist and when patients are pretreated with phenoxybenzamine (Dibenzyline), an alpha adrenergic receptor-blocking drug that has contributed greatly to the management of the pheochromocytoma patient. The dosage of phenoxybenzamine is determined by the antihypertensive response, and treatment should continue for at least one week before adequate receptor blockade is achieved. Total protection against spikes in blood pressure is not attainable. During arteriography and surgery, preparations should be made for the administration of intravenous phenoxybenzamine (and propranolol if problematic tachycardia or arrhythmias occur). Use of propranolol should be limited to situations where alpha blockade has already been established.

Improved techniques of computerized tomography (CT) have greatly simplified the diagnosis (i.e., localization) of pheochromocytoma. Despite these improvements, multiple, asymptomatic, or metastatic pheochromocytomas have remained difficult to locate because prior imaging techniques were nonspecific. The advent of the radiopharmaceutic agent 131-MIBG permits scintigraphic localization based on functional principles. This agent resembles norepinephrine in molecular structure; it is thought to enter adrenergic tissue by the same mechanism as the pressor amine itself. Incorporation in medullary tissue metabolic pathways localizes the isotope effectively for scanning. It has special value in localizing multiple, metastatic, or asymptomatic tumors.

FAMILIAL PHEOCHROMOCYTOMAS. The characteristics of familial pheochromocytomas differ in some ways from those of the more common sporadic type. Fifty percent of familial tumors are bilateral, yet extra-adrenal locations almost never occur. The familial pheochromocytoma is more likely to secrete epinephrine. In some instances, this may be the only biochemical abnormality, which can make the condition difficult to diagnose. These tumors usually occur as part of well-recognized syndromes.

Multiple endocrine adenomatosis type II (MEA-II) or Sipple's syndrome consists of pheochromocytoma, medullary thyroid carcinoma, and primary hyperparathyroidism. Pheochromocytoma is not associated with MEA-I (pituitary, pancreatic, and parathyroid tumors); only hyperparathyroidism is common to MEA-I and -II. A small percentage of patients with von Recklinghausen's neurofibromatosis and von Hippel-Lindau's cerebellar hemangioblastomatosis will have pheochromocytomas.

NEUROBLASTOMA. This tumor, while often adrenal in origin, is the subject of Chapter 41.

PRIMARY ADRENAL CARCINOMA. Primary adrenal cortical carcinoma is relatively uncommon, with a frequency of about 2 per 1,000,000 per year. Although these tumors carry a generally poor prognosis, cure can be achieved with complete surgical resection in those who present early enough without metastases. Five-year cure rates of 25 to 40% are obtained in those patients with the primary tumor thought to be completely resected.

Staging has three levels. Stage I refers to tumor confined to the adrenal gland with no evidence of local or distant spread. Stage II refers to direct extension of tumor into adjacent tissues or spread to the regional lymph nodes. Stage III indicates distant metastases. The most common sites of metastases are liver, lung, peritoneum or pleura, lymph nodes, and renal and venous (i.e., renal venous or vena cava) involvement. Other common points of involvement are bone, pancreas, brain, and direct extension into diaphragm, pancreas, or small intestine.

About half the patients who present with primary adrenal carcinoma have tumors completely resected surgically that are considered low stage. The remainder do less well. The five-year survival rate for stage I is about 50%, for stage II about 15%, and stage III about 5%.

Adrenal carcinoma is associated with several hormonal presentations. These are about evenly distributed. One of the common presentations is Cushing's syndrome with corticosteroid excess. Inappropriate secretion of ketogenic steroids is also well known in carcinomas.

There is no useful chemotherapeutic program for this disease. Although some considered Orthopara-DDD for metastatic disease because of its destructive effect on the adrenal cortex, its clinical usefulness has largely been unproven.

Secondary adrenal carcinomas result from metastatic hematogenous spread, generally from breast or lung. Renal cell carcinoma can directly involve the adrenal, as does a rare case of ureteral or even testicular carcinoma. These are usually postmortem discoveries. Occasionally a clinical decision must be made in a person who has had a single primary tumor treated successfully some years earlier. In such a case, it is appropriate to remove the adrenal if this is the only clinically evident tumor.

INCIDENTAL TUMORS. Nonfunctioning adenomas represent one of the more interesting clinical situations in recent years. Their management is based on evidence of functional activity that is excessive. Critical tests relate to ruling out aldosteronism and Cushing's disease. It is also reasonable to screen for ketogenic steroid excess, although this condition would rarely be present. Table 2-1 indicates the appropriate screening studies, all of which will be negative.

One of the important considerations in the nonfunctioning adenoma is the relationship of size and clinical behavior. In general, adenomas smaller than 2 cm that are nonfunctional can be followed safely with serial ultrasound and CT examinations. If there is evidence of any rapid growth exceeding 3 cm, adrenal resection is indicated. On the other hand, it is known that most will remain stable and, if there is no evidence of growth or functional activity, such patients can be followed safely. It is well known from Conn's early work,[29] and that derived from the Thorndike Laboratories, that about 5% of postmortem examinations will reveal some adrenal corticoadenomatous growth, hence, the rather exaggerated predictions by Conn about the true instance of aldosteronism many years ago.

There is an interesting parallel between the renal corticoadenoma and the adrenal corticoadenoma. Growth kinetics suggest that beyond a certain critical mass tumors must be considered malignant, although they may well have a similar histologic appearance when grossly smaller. A 1-cm renal cortical adenoma may well have the same histology as a well-differentiated renal carcinoma. The same extrapolation holds true for the adrenal. A 1-cm cortical adenoma is invariably benign, yet a 10-cm cortical tumor is invariably malignant. The change from a well-differentiated smaller tumor to a usually poorly differentiated large tumor involves many deregulation factors currently under study. In any case, the nonfunctioning adenoma that is less than 2 cm is generally followed expectantly, and a patient with any tumor over 2½ cm is considered a reasonable candidate for surgery.[30]

SURGICAL APPROACHES AND TECHNIQUES

Surgery for Aldosteronism

In the usual case, the approach is dorsal. With the patient in the prone position, the pyelograms are reviewed and the suitable rib is chosen for subperiosteal excision. Usually this is a twelfth rib, or an eleventh rib in a large patient, particularly on the left. The rib is removed as proximal as possible near its articulation to facilitate exposure (Figs. 2-1, 2-2, 2-3).

A key point in exposure of the adrenal through the dorsal route is the caudal mobilization of the kidney and adrenal without entering Gerota's fascia. With a hand or sponge stick placed medial and caudad in the apex of the wound, the kidney and other contents within Gerota's fascia can be drawn posteriorly and laterally. Such posterolateral retraction of the kidney allows separation of the superior aspect of the adrenal from the diaphragm and hepatic structures on the right, and the pancreas on the left. Very gentle dissection with forceps is satisfactory before Harrington or malleable retractors are placed on the liver or pancreas. Narrow or broad Deaver retractors are sometimes useful medially. Vascular clips and silk ligatures are used for proximal traction on the adrenal. The structures are tied in continuity, passing at right angle below the tissue to be tied and ligated with 2-0 black silk on the proximal or gland side (Fig. 2-4). Vascular clips are used on the body wall or renal side. This technique allows meticulous dissection without blood loss. Every effort must be made not to manipulate the gland itself. Any rough movements can cause swelling within the gland and subsequent difficulty identifying adenomas. Even slight spillage of blood into tissue planes may obscure the edges of the gland. If spillage occurs, copious irrigation may be used to clean off tissue planes.

The common adrenal vein is often the last portion of the dissection, particularly when one is mobilizing the right adrenal. Once the gland has been fully mobilized, the common right adrenal vein is secured between 2-0 silk ligatures. When the vein is more apical, its early division and removal provide better glandular mobilization. Should venous length be a problem, one can doubly clip the venous structures on either side and divide between them. Usually, with gentle elevation, one can achieve enough length for double ligatures (see Fig. 2-4).

If the pleural cavity has been entered, both the parietal and diaphragmatic closures are made with nonabsorbable sutures. Air in the pleural space is evacuated through a small red rubber catheter. During positive pressure lung inflation, the tube is removed. Normally a chest tube is not necessary postoperatively. The only special consideration postoperatively is the need to follow serum potassium determinations twice a day for the first several days. Hyperkalemia secondary to suppression of the contralateral zona glomerulosa is rare. For the same reason, replacement therapy with mineralocorticoids has not been necessary. Over 80% of patients become normotensive within several weeks postoperatively. When a unilateral ade-

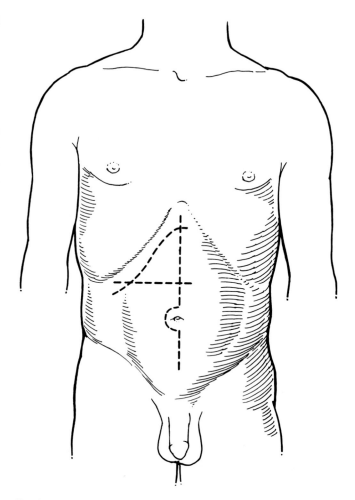

FIG. 2-1. Midline, transverse, or subcostal incisions are suitable for approach to retroperitoneal tumors including adrenal tumors.

noma is clearly localized, a good result can be expected from surgery.[3–6]

Surgery for Cushing's Disease

Once the diagnosis has been established and a primary adrenal cortical tumor has been revealed as the cause of excess cortisol secretion (as opposed to pituitary tumor with excess ACTH production with bilateral adrenal cortical hyperplasia), removal of the tumor-bearing adrenal is the treatment of choice.

It must be emphasized that preoperative preparation requires tissue fixation of corticosteroids. Therefore, cortisone acetate, 50 mg 4 times a day, is recommended for at least one, if not two, days preoperatively. The rate of return of adrenal secretion by the contralateral suppressed adrenal cortex is variable. Therefore, intraoperative corticosteroids are essential, and gradual tapering over a week to a base level of 30 mg of cortisol per day maintenance is a reasonable therapeutic trial. Then gradual tapering to levels as low as 10 to 15 mg a day can be attempted. Weakness, fatigue, hypotension, and hyponatremia are clues that replacement is inadequate.

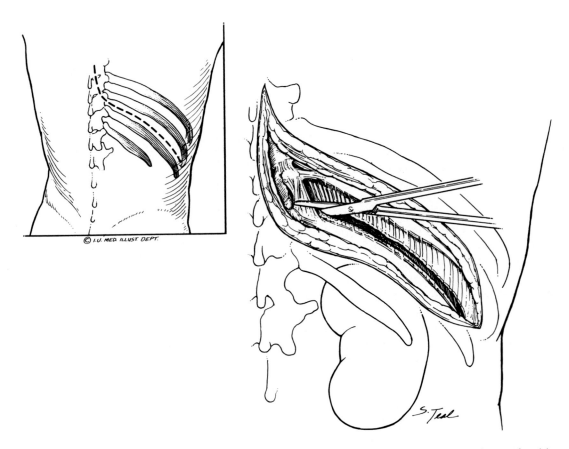

FIG. 2-2. A key component of the dorsal approach is incision of the costovertebral ligament. This incision can be done under vision or blindly by palpation, incising medially on the superior surface of the rib to the level of the vertebra. The key is to stay on the superior and dorsal aspect of the rib and to divide the ligamentous attachments sharply with heavy scissors or a diathermic blade.

TECHNIQUE. The small adrenal adenoma producing Cushing's syndrome can be treated by the dorsal approach as described earlier for primary aldosteronism. However, larger tumors, if localized to one side, are best approached through a transverse upper abdominal or thoracoabdominal incision.[16]

Transabdominal approach. Most surgeons prefer a transverse incision extending across both rectus muscles to the tip of the twelfth rib or resecting the distal twelfth rib. To expose the right adrenal, the liver and gallbladder are retracted cephalad. The distal stomach, duodenum, and hepatic flexure of the colon are retracted medially. Occasionally hepatic and colonic adhesions must be divided. The posterior peritoneum can be reflected medially after incising the mesocolon and separating it from the anterior aspect of Gerota's fascia (Fig. 2-5). Retraction of the duodenum and head of the pancreas medially (Kocher maneuver) is helpful in gaining exposure of the right adrenal (Fig. 2-6). Gentle caudad retraction of the upper pole of the kidney aids in the dissection of the right adrenal gland.

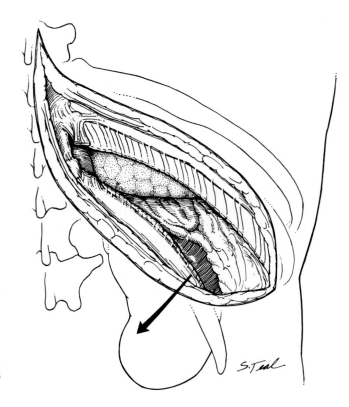

FIG. 2-3. The rib can be retracted inferiorly with ease once the costovertebral ligaments have been divided. This approach greatly widens the aperture necessary for good retraction and exposure.

The key to the dissection is thorough mobilization of the inferior vena cava and right renal venous structures so that the adrenal gland can be mobilized from the vena cava to obtain superior exposure. The vena cava can be retracted medially in this area using vein retractors. Clips and silk ligatures are useful in dividing fatty nerve or small arterial structures surrounding the gland. Ligatures on the proximal glandular side assist in gentle traction, and the cava can be retracted medially to expose the common right adrenal vein. In larger tumors, exposure of the common right adrenal vein may require dissection of the caudate lobe of the liver. Deep Harrington retractors are useful in this hepatic retraction when necessary.

The left adrenal is more accessible when approached through the abdomen. One approach is to incise the mesentery of the transverse colon to the left of the middle colic artery and then to expose the left renal vein just below this (Fig. 2-7). This procedure is useful if the patient is thin and the tumor in not large. However, in larger patients or in those with big tumors, if one is working transabdominally, it is better either to reflect the colon, spleen, and pancreas medially (Fig. 2-8) or to simply incise the gastrocolic ligament and enter the lesser peritoneal sac. The posterior peritoneum is then incised exposing the adrenal directly below. The adrenal vasculature can then be easily divided between clips or ligatures as the gland is displaced laterally and medially. If the gastrocolic approach is used, the stomach and pancreas must be retracted

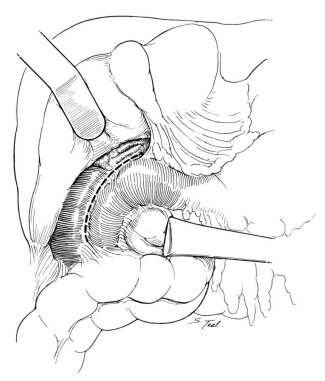

FIG. 2-5. The line of incision for the Kocher maneuver is lateral to the duodenum. The hepatic flexure of the colon is first retracted medially to demonstrate the first and second portions of the duodenum. The posterior incision begins at the foramen of Winslow and is carried down to the turn of the duodenum in its third portion.

medially and cephalad, the duodenum medially, and the colon laterally and inferiorly. For larger tumors it is safer if the mesocolon and lineophrenic ligaments are divided all the way around, sometimes even as high and medial as the gastroesophageal hiatus. This approach allows the spleen, colon, and pancreas to be reflected medially and anteriorly off Gerota's fascia to expose any large tumor below. In addition, this approach gives excellent exposure of the upper abdominal aorta, the medial diaphragm, the celiac and superior mesenteric vessels, and the crus of the diaphragm. Vascular control is more secure with this technique.

Thoracoabdominal approach. Another approach to the adrenal tumor is the lumbar extraperitoneal or thoracoabdominal incision (Fig. 2-9). An incision is made at the level of the eleventh or twelfth rib and the diaphragm and pleura are incised. On the left side, the spleen and colon are mobilized medially in their peritoneal envelope using blunt and sharp dissection. Then Gerota's fascia is exposed and the renal vein is identified. On the left, the common adrenal vein can usually be secured early and the tumor mobilized between clips or ligatures off the kidney and medial aspect of the diaphragm (Fig. 2-10). Various crural attachments and the inferior phrenic vascular supply are easily mobilized and divided. Some direct aortic or renal arterial communications are also encountered, but these are usually small and well visualized in advance provided the usual care is taken with exposure. After removal, the area is

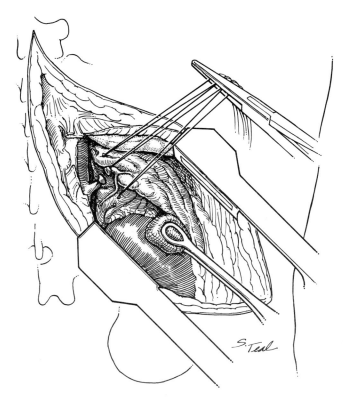

FIG. 2-4. After placement of a self-retaining retractor, the kidney is retracted caudad with a sponge stick. Ties can be placed on the medial, i.e., adrenal, aspect and cut and divided on the great vessel side of the dissection. This is a useful method for manipulation of the gland through this small incision.

FIG. 2-6. The Kocher maneuver permits mobilization of the duodenum and the head of the pancreas (pictured in retractor) medially. This exposes the vena cava and the hilar aspect of the kidney and adrenal.

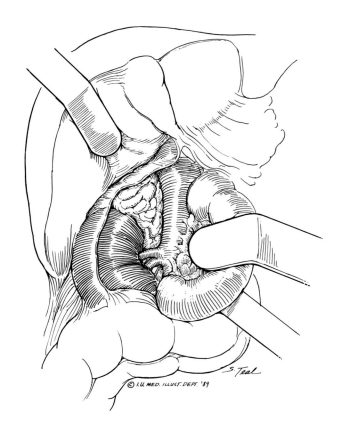

irrigated thoroughly and the peritoneal sac is simply dropped over the kidney, which has been allowed to resume its normal position. The wound is usually closed in layers with interrupted nonabsorbable suture material. On the right side the same principles apply. However, retraction of the liver off the anterior aspect of Gerota's fascia below may require more careful sharp and blunt dissection. Usually we prefer to enter the abdomen rather than to remain extraperitoneal in right adrenal surgery simply because this approach facilitates the exposure of the high vena cava and posterior venous vascular contributions of the adrenal gland itself. The location of the adrenal on each side is more central than lateral. Therefore, there is little reason to try to remain extraperitoneal, particularly on the right side.

Surgery for Virilizing Tumors

Before any operative procedure for a virilizing adrenal tumor, the differential diagnostic steps to rule out idiopathic and/or

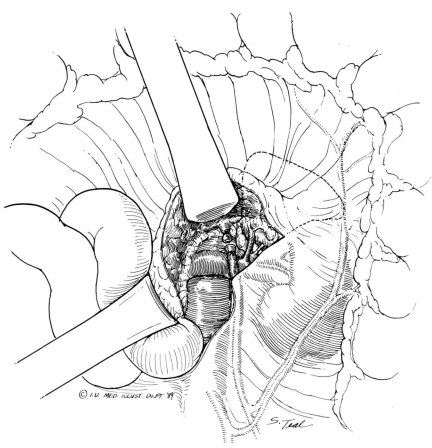

FIG. 2-7. Approach through the root of the small bowel with division of the inferior mesenteric vein to better expose the left renal hilum and adrenal vessels. This technique has long been used to facilitate supra-hilar dissection in retroperitoneal lymphadenectomies done through the anterior approach.

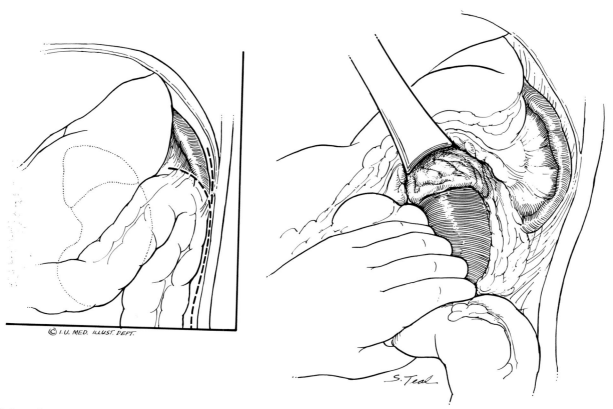

FIG. 2-8. Lateral approach to the left adrenal and the lines of paracolic incision, including lineocolic and lineophrenic attachments (see inset). This approach permits retraction of the colon medially and retraction of the pancreas medially and cephalad to expose the underlying adrenal.

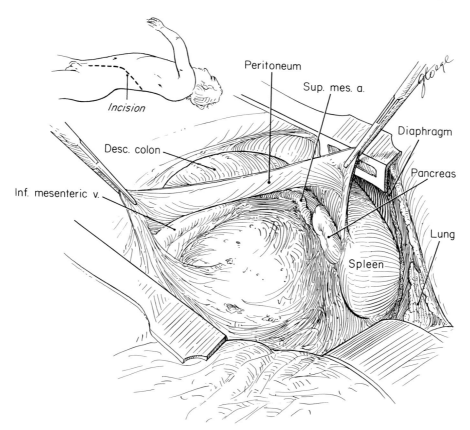

FIG. 2-9. Mobilization of the peritoneum off the underlying Gerota's fascia. The relationship of the inferior mesenteric artery, pancreas, and spleen is also shown. This approach is viewed from the left flank incision (see inset).

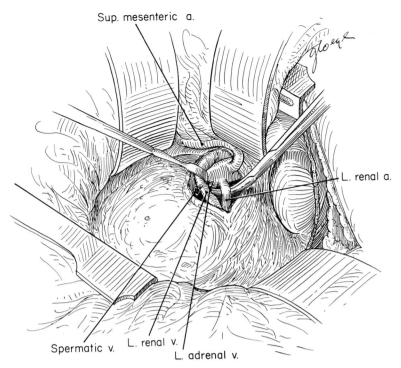

Sup. mesenteric a.

L. renal a.

Spermatic v.　L. renal v.　L. adrenal v.

FIG. 2-10. After the peritoneum and pancreas are retracted medially, the renal and adrenal vessels are mobilized by dividing Gerota's fascia, which overlies them.

iatrogenic cause must be taken (see p. 10). A good medical and family history is essential. Then differential chemistries and imaging studies can be done to rule out an ovarian cause as noted earlier. If the only lesion is an adrenal tumor, unilateral adrenalectomy is indicated.

The surgical approach to these tumors is the same as for the adrenal tumor causing Cushing's disease. Smaller tumors can be approached dorsally or by the lumbar routes. Larger tumors are best approached with large upper transverse incisions. Care must be taken to obtain central vascular exposure utilizing transabdominal techniques as noted earlier.

Surgery for Pheochromocytoma

PREPARATION FOR SURGERY. Within the operating room, a team approach consisting of internist, surgeon, and anesthesiologist is required. Preoperative treatment with phenoxybenzamine dampens or may even abolish the hypertensive episodes that can be associated primarily with induction of anesthesia and with handling of the tumor.

The adrenergic blockade created by phenoxybenzamine relieves the vasoconstrictor state produced by the excessive secretion of catecholamines and provides time prior to surgery for expansion of the vascular space.

Thus, the profound hypotension that may immediately follow removal of the pheochromocytoma is, for the most part, prevented. The management of the pheochromocytoma patient from the stage of tumor localization and throughout the perioperative period is not simple. It is our strong recommen-

dation that these procedures be performed in hospitals where several such cases are handled annually.

SURGICAL APPROACH. *The transabdominal approach.* Our preference is a high abdominal transverse incision, the so-called chevron incision, extending from the tip of the twelfth rib bilaterally up along the costal margins. Most bilateral adrenal exposures together with paravertebral examination are obtained with this approach.

To expose the right adrenal, the liver and gallbladder are retracted cephalad and the stomach and duodenum are drawn medially, after incision of the posterior peritoneum and development of the Kocher maneuver (see Figs. 2-2, 2-3). It is important to gently draw the kidney caudad and to develop and retract the inferior cava medially to obtain control of the right adrenal vein. It is also useful to identify and clip the small right adrenal arterial vessels as they arise from the origin of the right renal artery below the cava or directly from the aorta in this area.

The left adrenal gland may be exposed in the event of a small tumor by incising the posterior peritoneum and ligament of Treitz and ligating the inferior mesenteric vein and dividing it. This approach allows cephalad retraction of the body of the pancreas in a deep Harrington retractor. The adrenal is easily visualized just lateral to the superior mesenteric artery and medial to the upper pole of the left kidney. The left adrenal vein is easily secured, in most instances, through this approach (see Fig. 2-7, incision of the root of the small bowel and mobilization of the pancreas). If the left adrenal tumor is large, most prefer to incise the mesocolon and to divide the lineocolic and lineorenal attachments and again to mobilize the pancreas cephalad (see Fig. 2-8). If the left adrenal tumor is quite large, it is sometimes best to continue the incision of the mesocolon cephalad to include the lineophrenic attachments. Furthermore, exposure is facilitated by continuing the posterior peritoneal incision above the spleen to the gastroesophageal hiatus. Then the spleen and pancreas can be mobilized in continuity cephalad and medially, thus exposing the entire upper retroperitoneal space. Occasionally, division of the short gastric vessels may be necessary to mobilize the adrenal completely out of the left upper quadrant (see Figs. 2-7, 2-8).

Once exposed, the tumor is removed, with great care devoted to minimal manual pressure on the tumor itself. Ligatures and clips are preferred if possible, with gentle traction on proximal ligatures providing elevation of the tumor mass. With preoperative alpha blockade using phenoxybenzamine (Dibenzyline), this is somewhat less critical than it formerly was; nonetheless, it is an important consideration, even today, to ensure stable blood pressure throughout the operation. Every effort is made to tie the adrenal vein first. Opportunities to clip and divide small adrenal artery branches early in the angle between the crus of the diaphragm and the renal artery should be encouraged. Once the essential vascular tributaries are divided and ligated, the tumor is gently elevated out of the wound. One should attempt to stay wide around the tumor capsule, even taking adjacent nodes and fat to a moderate degree. Because 10% of these lesions are malignant, we feel wide excision is better than capsular or subcapsular enucleation.

Closure of the wound is generally with 0 nonabsorbable suture material. We prefer running sutures to the peritoneum and transversalis and the posterior rectus sheath, which is included. Several interrupted 0 sutures are placed at the midline in figure-eight fashion. The anterior rectus sheath is closed with interrupted 0 nonabsorbable sutures as is the internal oblique and external oblique. The subcutaneous tissue is closed with interrupted 3-0 chromic catgut and the skin with vertical interrupted skin staples.

Postoperative considerations include careful monitoring of the central venous pressure. We prefer a Swan-ganz catheter for optimal central wedge pressure. We also use intra-arterial lines from the moment of surgical induction to one or two days postoperatively. Hypotension is an exceedingly rare occurrence because these patients are generally well blocked for two weeks preoperatively with phenoxybenzamine. Some surgeons avoid preoperative blockade, preferring to transfuse patients postoperatively following tumor removal with whole blood and colloid to manage the pressure drops in the unblocked patients. Their rationale is that the palpation for other tumors is more effective in the unblocked patient. Because this is only a 10% factor and CT scanning is highly effective in localizing retroperitoneal tumors, we have avoided the uncertainties of this approach with its attendant risk of hepatitis and pressure swings.

Finally, a team approach cannot be overemphasized. Internists, anesthesiologists, and urologic surgeons, all with an endocrine background and experience, are the ideal combination for patient management, preoperatively and postoperatively.

REFERENCES

1. DONOHUE, J. P. Primary aldosteronism. In: *Current Urologic Therapy.* 2nd Ed. Edited by J. J. Kaufman, Philadelphia, W. B. Saunders Co., 1986, p. 5.

2. WEINBERGER, M. H., et al. Primary aldosteronism: Diagnosis, localization and treatment. Ann. Intern. Med., *90:*386, 1979.

3. HUNT, T. K., SCHAMBELAN, M., and BIGLIERI, E. G. Selection of patients and operative approach in primary aldosteronism. Ann. Surg., *182:*353, 1975.

4. NELSON, D. H. The adrenal cortex: Physiological function and disease. In: *Major Problems in Internal Medicine.* Edited by L. H. Smith, Jr. Cushing's Syndrome, Philadelphia, W. B. Saunders Co., 1980, p. 153.

5. GLENN, J. F., PETERSON, R. E., and MANNIX, H., JR. Cushing's disease. In: *Surgery of the Adrenal Gland.* New York, MacMillan, 1968.

6. RHAMY, R. K. Cushing's syndrome. In: *Urologic Surgery.* 3rd Ed. Edited by J. F. Glenn, Philadelphia, J. B. Lippincott, 1983, pp. 27–46.

7. CUSHING, H. *The Pituitary Body and its Disorders.* Philadelphia, J. B. Lippincott, Co., 1912.

8. HUTTER, A. M., and KAYHOE, D. E. Adrenal cortical carcinoma. Clinical features of 138 patients. Am. J. Med., *41:*572, 1966.

9. NEVILLE, A. M., and MACKAY, A. M. The structure of the human adrenal cortex in health and disease. Clin. Endocrinol. Metab., *1:*361, 1972.

10. LEWINSKY, B. S., GRIGOR, K. M., and SYMPINGTON, T. The clinical and pathologic featues of "non-hormonal" adrenocortical tumors. Cancer, *33:*778, 1975.

11. SINGER, W., et al. Ectopic ACTH syndrome: Clinicopathological correlations. J. Clin. Pathol., *31:*591, 1978.

12. EGDAHL, R. H. Surgery of the adrenal gland. N. Engl. J. Med., *278:*939, 1968.

13. LIDDLE, G. W. Tests of pituitary-adrenal suppressibility in the diagnosis of Cushing's syndrome. J. Clin. Endocrinol. Metab., *20:*1539, 1960.

14. JUBIZ, W., et al. Single dose metyrapone test. Arch. Intern. Med., *125:*472, 1970.

15. NEVILLE, A. M. The nodular adrenal. Invest. Cell Pathol., *1:*99, 1978.

16. SCOTT, H. W., JR., et al. Surgical experience with Cushing's disease. Ann. Surg., *185:*524, 1977.

17. GIVENS, J. R. Hirsutism and hyperandrogenism. Adv. Intern. Med., *21:*221, 1976.

18. FREITAS, J. E., BEIERWALTES, W. H., and NISHIYAMA, R. H. Adrenal hyperandrogenism: Detection by adrenal scintigraphy. J. Endocrinol. Invest., *1:*59, 1978.

19. FRANKEL, F. Ein Fall von Doppelseitigem, vollig latent verlaufenen Nebennieren-tumor und gleichzeitiger Nephritis mit veranderungen und Circulations apparat und retinitis. Arch. Pathol. Anat. Phys., *103:*244, 1886.

20. Mayo, C. Paroxysmal hypertension with tumor of retroperitoneal nerve. J.A.M.A., *89:*1047, 1927.

21. Pincoffs, M. C. A case of paroxysmal hypertension associated with suprarenal tumor. Trans. Assoc. Am. Physicians, *44:*295, 1929.

22. Shipley, A. M. Paroxysmal hypertension associated with tumor of the suprarenal. Ann. Surg., *90:*742, 1929.

23. Hume, D. M. Pheochromocytoma and hypertension: An analysis of 207 cases. Int. Abstr. Surg., *99:*458, 1960.

24. Stackpole, R. H., Melicow, M. M., and Uson, A. C. Pheochromocytoma in children. J. Pediat., *66:*315, 1963.

25. Ganguly, A., et al. Diagnosis and localization of Pheochromocytoma. Am. J. Med., *67:*21, 1979.

26. Sisson, J. C., et al. Scintigraphic localization of pheochromocytoma. N. Engl. J. Med., *305:*12, 1981.

27. Yazaki, T., et al. Usefulness of scintigraphic imaging using 131 iodine-metaiodobenzylguanidine in localization of asymptomatic pheochromocytoma. J. Urol., *134:*107, 1985.

28. Bravo, E. L., et al. Clonidine-suppression test. N. Engl. J. Med., *305:*623, 1981.

29. Conn, J. W.: Presidential address: Painting background; primary aldosteronism, a new clinical syndrome. J. Lab. Clin. Med., *45:*3, 1955.

30. Bodie, B., et al. Cleveland Clinic experience with adrenal cortical carcinoma. J. Urol., *141:*257, 1989.

RENAL
CELL
CARCINOMA

CHAPTER
3

Primary Renal Cell Carcinoma: An Overview

Sakti Das

The total incidence of primary renal cell carcinoma has increased slowly but perceptibly during the last decade. Approximately 23,000 patients are expected to be diagnosed with renal cell carcinoma in 1989, and an estimated 10,000 patients will succumb to this neoplasm.[1] The trend in overall survival has remained unchanged in the last decade with a relative 5-year survival of about half the patients diagnosed.

Primary renal cell carcinoma accounts for about 86% of all the primary malignant tumors of the kidney. Men are affected about 1.8 times more commonly than women.[2] The highest incidence of renal cell carcinoma is during the sixth and seventh decades of life.[3] The tumor has also been reported in adolescents and, rarely, in children.[4,5]

PATHOGENESIS AND HISTOPATHOLOGY

Grawitz's hypothesis in 1883[6] about the origin of renal adenocarcinomas from the adrenal rests and subsequent nomenclature of hypernephroma based upon a similar misconception is better abandoned in the light of now established data proving the genesis of renal cell carcinomas from the proximal tubular cells. Electron-microscopic studies by Oberling and associates revealed a striking similarity of the microvilli forming a brush border appearance in the cells of renal cell carcinomas and the proximal convoluted tubule cells.[7] Further immunologic studies using antibodies to the microvilli antigen proved that the renal cell carcinoma cells reacted exclusively to these brush border antibodies of the proximal convoluted tubules and not with antibodies derived from other areas of the nephron.[8] It is still unclear whether renal cell carcinoma evolves as a neoplastic transformation of renal tubular hyperplasia or from the renal cortical adenomas.[9] The overwhelming similarity between renal cortical adenoma and renal cell carcinoma in their histogenesis, light and electron-microscopic appearances, histochemical features, and frequent coexistence in the same organ supports the theory that cortical adenomas are small renal cell carcinomas that have not yet manifested invasion or metastasis.[10,11]

Renal cell carcinomas are histologically characterized by a mixture of clear, granular, or spindle-like sarcomatoid cells arranged in solid, cystic, tubular, or papillary patterns. The individual cells are fairly uniform with delicate cytoplasmic membrane, moderate cellular and nuclear pleomorphism, and rare mitotic figures. Neoplasms with features like papillary architecture, predominantly clear cell composition, and low grade based on nuclear morphology have been reported to have better prognosis.[12,13] An aneuploid DNA pattern on flow cytometry of renal cell carcinoma indicates high-grade tumor with worse prognosis.[14] Heterogeneity of histologic appearance in different areas of the same tumor is, however, common in renal cell carcinoma.

CLINICAL PRESENTATION

Renal cell carcinoma can present with a myriad of clinical manifestations ranging from the classic triad of hematuria, pain, and abdominal mass to the more obscure symptoms of pyrexia, anemia, weight loss, erythrocytosis, acute varicocele, hypercalcemia, hepatosplenomegaly, hypertension, and protein-losing enteropathy. Of the classic triad, gross or microscopic hematuria is the presenting feature is about two thirds of the patients.[15]

About 7 to 20% of patients develop pyrexia due to the production of endogeneous pyrogen.[15-18] Anemia secondary to unexplained bone marrow depression with low serum iron and low total iron-binding capacity is found in 20 to 30% of the patients.[18,19] Interestingly, 1 to 5% of the patients manifest erythrocytosis due to secretion of erythropoietin by the carcinoma cells.[15,19] Up to 40% of the patients with renal cell carcinoma develop renin-mediated hypertension.[20,21] Hypercalcemia, often refractory to medical management, has been attributed to ectopic parahormone secretion, prostaglandin release by the tumor, or multiple bony metastases.[22,23] In the absence of metastatic disease, these symptoms are expected to abate following removal of the renal cell carcinoma.

Sudden appearance of scrotal varicocele, especially on the right side, must prompt a search for possible renal cell carcinoma.[24] It often indicates tumor thrombus permeation in the left renal vein or vena caval thrombus in the case of right-sided varicocele.

Probably the most interesting paraneoplastic syndrome is the hepatic dysfunction with hepatosplenomegaly in renal cell carcinoma that was described originally by Creevy[25] and subsequently by Stauffer.[26] The abnormal hepatic functions occur in the absence of liver metastasis and appear to carry dire prognostic stigmata.[27] Other rare syndromes include protein-losing enteropathy,[28] immune-complex glomerulopathy,[29,30] and amyloidosis leading to renal failure.[30,31] Persistence of these symptoms or their reappearance after initial reversal following nephrectomy indicates metastatic or recurrent disease.[32]

More recently, about 18% of patients have been reported to be diagnosed incidentally as a result of investigation prompted by nonurologic symptoms. These serendipitously detected tumors are generally of low stage and are associated with improved survival.[33]

DIAGNOSTIC IMAGING

Excretory urography with nephrotomography is usually the initial study whereby space-occupying lesions in the kidneys are suspected. Ultrasonography is utilized as the next evaluation to determine whether the lesion is solid or cystic unless the urography already provides a high index of suspicion for a neoplasm. Solid, complex cystic and equivocal swellings are evaluated by computed tomography (CT). We do not utilize angiography as a routine diagnostic procedure for renal cell carcinoma. CT characteristics of renal cell carcinomas include: (1) a mass with an ill-defined margin and a heterogeneous core, (2) density of the mass often similar to that of the adjacent renal parenchyma and further enhanced following intravenous contrast administration to a lesser degree than normal renal parenchyma, (3) areas of necrosis or hemorrhage, and (4) areas of punctate or peripheral calcification. Several studies have claimed the superiority of CT over angiography in diagnostic accuracy, reduced morbidity, and cost effectiveness.[34-38] For the purpose of staging, CT is fairly accurate in diagnosing contiguous spread, renal vein and vena caval extension, and lymph node metastases. Postoperatively, CT is invaluable as a follow-up study for detection of any local recurrence in the renal fossa.[39]

Renal angiography is used only under special circumstances in the evaluation of renal cell carcinoma. In tumors involving solitary kidneys, angiography is necessary to delineate the renal vascular architecture before a parenchyma-sparing partial nephrectomy is undertaken. Equivocal lesions on CT may require further substantiation by angiography. Angiography is probably more efficacious than CT in discovering small contralateral neoplasms.[40]

Magnetic resonance imaging (MRI) is showing great potential as a noninvasive study for the diagnosis and staging of renal cell carcinoma.[41] Compared to CT, MRI has the advantage of multiplanar imaging and better soft tissue contrast. Sagittal or coronal imaging allows more critical assessment of the polar areas of the kidneys. Differentiation of renal tumor from adjacent neoplasms arising from the adrenals or retroperitoneum is also facilitated by MRI.[42] In the overall staging of renal cell carcinoma, the accuracy of MRI is equivalent to that of CT (91%), but it is potentially more accurate in determining vascular extension (see Chap. 8) and contiguous spread to the adjacent organs[43] (Fig. 3-1).

STAGING AND PROGNOSTIC CONSIDERATIONS

Pathologic staging of renal cell carcinomas aims at determining the prognosis and influence of treatment on the extent of the disease. The staging system of Flocks and Kadesky,[44] modified by Robson and associates,[45] is most commonly used and can be summarized as follows:

Stage I or A—the tumor is confined within the renal capsule.
Stage II or B—the tumor invades through the capsule into the perinephric space, but is still contained within the Gerota's fascia.
Stage III or C—the tumor involves the regional lymph nodes and/or renal vein and vena cava.
Stage IV or D—the tumor involves adjacent organs and/or distant metastases are present.

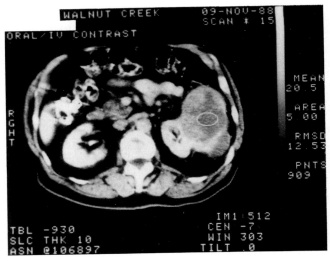 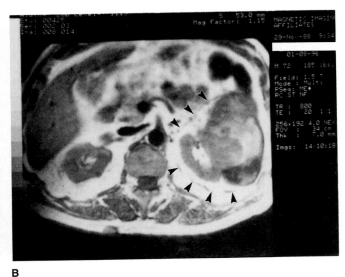

A   B

FIG. 3-1. CT scan (A) and MRI (B) of large left renal cell carcinoma. Arrow indicates Gerota's fascia on MRI.

The drawback of this staging system results from inappropriate assignment of several prognostic factors in stage III or C. In several series,[46,47] the survival of patients in stage III or C with renal vein or vena caval extension, not associated with lymph node involvement, was similar to that for patients with tumors contained in the kidney. It is now evident that lymphatic spread of renal cell carcinoma indicates a worse prognosis than what has been implicated previously.

The American Joint Committee for cancer staging and end results reporting[48] has proposed the TNM system whereby the lymph node involvement and venous permeation are separated and quantitated into different stages (Table 3-1). This all-encompassing staging system is comprehensive as well as complicated. We would welcome a further modification of Robson's staging system with lymph node metastases placed in a higher stage with a dire prognosis.

Prognosis of renal cell carcinoma is influenced by the pathologic stage, histologic type and grade, and the surgical procedure employed. Comparison of the survival statistics among different series is therefore difficult and is further compounded by the various staging systems used. The approximate 5-year survival following radical nephrectomy ranges from 60 to 82% for stage I or A, 47 to 80% for stage II or B, and 35 to 51% for stage III or C renal cell carcinoma. Patients with metastatic renal cell carcinoma have virtually no chance of surviving 5 years.[40]

TREATMENT OF LOCALIZED RENAL CELL CARCINOMA

The only effective treatment of localized renal cell carcinoma is its complete excision with adequate surgical margins. This excision is accomplished by radical nephrectomy whereby the Gerota's fascia with its contents (kidney, adrenal and perinephric fat) intact is removed with regional lymph node dissection. This procedure allows a better surgical clearance, especially for stage II lesions invading the perinephric fat, and removes the adrenal gland, renal vein, perirenal lymphatic channels, and hilar lymph nodes which may harbor tumor metastases. The results of radical nephrectomy are markedly superior to those of simple nephrectomy practiced in the early half of this century. Although such a comparison is debatable in the absence of a contemporaneous randomization, the distinct possibility of leaving behind tumor in the Gerota's compartment would create ethical problems in subjecting any renal cell carcinoma to simple nephrectomy. Radical nephrectomy is therefore at present the standard therapy for renal cell carcinoma.

Regional lymph node dissection as an integral part of radical nephrectomy remains controversial. Robson attributed increased survival to extended lymphadenectomy,[49] whereas Hulten and associates reported no survivors following lymphadenectomy of involved nodes.[50] In the absence of statistical data gathered from prospective studies comparing radical nephrectomy with and without lymphadenectomy, any claim of its utility or futility is conjectural. It is reasonable to presume that the initial metastasis lodges mostly in the hilar lymph nodes and the adjacent lymphatic field. Therefore these primary echelons of lymph drainage may be encompassed by regional lymph node dissection. Additionally, such dissection provides valuable staging information about the extent of the disease. There is, however, no proven improvement in survival with extended lymphadenectomy in patients with positive or negative lymph nodes.[51] The technique and the extent of regional lymph node dissection for renal cell carcinoma are detailed in the following chapter.

Local Excision

In recent years, several workers have made a plea for renal parenchyma sparing local excision of small renal cell carcinomas in patients with a normal contralateral kidney.[52-54] The proponents claim: (1) With the advanced imaging techniques, many tumors are often diagnosed serendipitously at an earlier stage. These small and incidentally diagnosed tumors have a lower grade and stage. (2) Incidence of local recurrence has been low after enucleation, local excision, polar resection, or partial nephrectomy. (3) Local excisional surgery for T1 and T2 tumors has yielded a survival rate similar to that of radical nephrectomy in the presence of a normal contralateral kidney.[52]

The prudence of conservative surgery of renal cell carcinoma has been questioned by others with the arguments that: (1) even the advanced imaging techniques are not capable of absolutely defining pathologic grade and stage;[55] (2) 20% of kidneys contain incidental small renal cell carcinomas accompanying the clinically overt tumor;[56] (3) size of the lesion may not determine the grade or malignant potential as there are reports of metastases from very small tumors;[57] (4) experimental ex situ surgery on carefully selected kidneys proved the futility of a local excisional approach in 42% of cases because of residual tumor, venous invasion, capsular penetration, and multifocal tumors.[58]

The advisability of conservative surgery of renal cell carcinoma in the presence of a normal contralateral kidney is under close scrutiny; at present this procedure is not recommended as routine management. The possibility that advances in imaging technology may enable selection of patients for such surgical conservatism in the future is thought-provoking.

TREATMENT OF RENAL CELL CARCINOMA IN THE SOLITARY KIDNEY AND BILATERAL RENAL CELL CARCINOMA

Renal cell carcinoma involving a solitary kidney, both the kidneys simultaneously, or a kidney with significant contralateral renal impairment, poses difficult situations. A rational balance must be maintained between adequate surgical excision of the tumor and preservation of functioning renal parenchyma to sustain life, preferably without chronic dialysis. Critical assessment of the extent of the tumor involvement, as well as angiographic study of the vascular architecture of the kidney and the tumor, is essential for planning the surgical strategy for complete tumor excision. Enucleation or excavation of tumor

TABLE 3-1. *TNM Classification of Primary Renal Cell Carcinoma*[48]

PRIMARY TUMOR

TX	Primary tumor cannot be assessed
T0	No evidence of primary tumor
T1	Tumor 2.5 cm or less in greatest dimension limited to the kidney
T2	Tumor more than 2.5 cm in greatest dimension limited to the kidney
T3	Tumor extends into major veins or invades adrenal gland or perinephric tissues but not beyond Gerota's fascia
	T3a Tumor invades adrenal gland or perinephric tissues but not beyond Gerota's fascia
	T3b Tumor grossly extends into renal vein(s) or vena cava
T4	Tumor invades beyond Gerota's fascia

REGIONAL LYMPH NODES (N)

NX	Regional lymph nodes cannot be assessed
N0	No regional lymph node metastasis
N1	Metastasis in a single lymph node, 2 cm or less in greatest dimension
N2	Metastasis in a single lymph node, more than 2 cm but not more than 5 cm in greatest dimension, or multiple lymph nodes, none more than 5 cm in greatest dimension
N3	Metastasis in a lymph node more than 5 cm in greatest dimension

DISTANT METASTASIS (M)

MX	Presence of distant metastasis cannot be assessed
M0	No distant metastasis
M1	Distant metastasis

STAGE GROUPING

Stage I	T1	N0	M0
Stage II	T2	N0	M0
Stage III	T1	N1	M0
	T2	N1	M0
	T3a	N0, N1	M0
	T3b	N0, N1	M0
Stage IV	T4	Any N	M0
	Any T	N2, N3	M0
	Any T	Any N	M1

HISTOPATHOLOGIC TYPE

The histopathologic types are:

Renal cell carcinoma
  Adenocarcinoma
  Renal papillary adenocarcinoma
  Tubular carcinoma
  Granular cell carcinoma
  Clear cell carcinoma (hypernephroma)

The predominant cancer is adenocarcinoma; subtypes are clear-cell and granular-cell carcinoma. A grading system as below is recommended when feasible. The staging system does not apply to sarcomas of the kidney. A separate classification is published for nephroblastomas.

HISTOPATHOLOGIC GRADE (G)

GX	Grade cannot be assessed
G1	Well differentiated
G2	Moderately well differentiated
G3-4	Poorly differentiated/undifferentiated

often leads to incomplete removal with residual tumor in the bed and is therefore not recommended. Even in multiple lesions, excision with the rim of adjacent uninvolved renal tissue is preferred.

For simultaneous bilateral tumors, we first approach the side with the smaller lesion that is more amenable to partial nephrectomy. After a recovery period of 4 to 6 weeks, when postoperative nuclear scan reveals adequate function on the operated side, contralateral radical nephrectomy can be performed. This allows one to prepare for a parenchyma-preserving operation in case the initially operated kidney reveals gross impairment of renal function. Occasionally, when the tumor on one side has been small and peripherally located, we have carried out synchronous bilateral surgery under the same anesthetic. The sophisticated surgical techniques of in vivo partial nephrectomy under regional hypothermia are discussed in Chapter 7. Ex vivo tumor excision and auto-transplantation may become necessary under special circumstances. In selected cases where renal parenchymal sparing is not anatomically feasible, radical nephrectomy of solitary or bilateral tumors and chronic dialysis may have to be considered. Renal transplantation should not be considered until at least one year after bilateral nephrectomy because of the possibility of metastases or appearance of a second malignant tumor perpetuated by necessary immunosuppression.

Wickham reported that 75% of patients with bilateral renal cell carcinomas who were not operated upon died within 24 months and, more selectively, patients with bilateral simultaneous tumors without surgical intervention did not survive beyond 5 months.[59] The dismal survival without an operation, and lack of any appreciable benefit from radiation therapy, chemotherapy, or immunotherapy, makes a strong case for every effort at surgical extirpation of these tumors. Reports indicate encouraging 5-year survival in about 70% of the operated patients.[60] The stage of the disease, cellular differentiation, and completeness of tumor removal are the most important prognostic determinants.[61]

TREATMENT OF METASTATIC RENAL CELL CARCINOMA

Nearly 30% of the renal cell carcinoma patients have evidence of metastasis at the time of their initial diagnosis. The accumulated data in these patients have dampened the original enthusiasm about postnephrectomy spontaneous regression of the metastases from renal cell carcinoma. It is true that such spontaneous regression does happen in fewer than 1% of the patients,[62,63] but whether this phenomenon is prompted or promoted by nephrectomy is not known. Therefore, we do not recommend palliative nephrectomy in anticipation of spontaneous regression of metastatic renal cell carcinoma.

Nephrectomy for the palliation of occasional unrelenting symptoms like hemorrhage, pain, fever, hepatopathy, erythrocytosis, or hypercalcemia may become necessary. One, however, should inform the patient and the family that only about 10% of such patients survive for one year, and the average survival is only 4 months.[64] Quite often vigorous medical measures, and sometimes angioinfarction, can offer the same palliation, obviating the need for a major surgical procedure.

Nephrectomy with excision of solitary or limited-volume metastasis has offered 5-year survival in up to 35% of selected patients.[65,66] All these series are small in number and retrospective in nature casting doubt on the statistical significance as well as the confidence limits of the diagnostic modalities used at that time to detect metastases. Whether such survival is biologically predetermined and might have happened without extensive surgery is not known. In relatively healthy young patients with resectable primary lesions and small volume metastases, however, extirpative surgery may be justified with the hope of significant palliation and prolongation of life.

Delayed nephrectomy after percutaneous angiographic embolization of the renal cell carcinoma was advocated by Swanson and associates as a form of putative immunotherapy stimulating the host-immune response.[67] As of 1986, 145 treated patients were analyzed.[68] Postoperatively 117 patients (81%) received medroxyprogesterone acetate (Depo-Provera). Their 6.89% complete response rate and 6.2% partial response rate were higher than the expected spontaneous regression rate reported in the literature. Patient selection, however, was biased toward inclusion of only those who were most likely to respond. Physicians recommend this therapy only to patients with parenchymal pulmonary metastases who most commonly respond to any form of therapy and are also most prone to undergo spontaneous regression. The role of Depo-Provera in the reported results is unclear. The median survival was not better than that for adjuvant nephrectomy alone. With an estimated operative mortality of up to 6% in this group of patients, we have not favored this treatment modality. A subsequent randomized Southwest Oncology Group study has failed to show any advantage of infarction-nephrectomy for metastatic renal cell carcinoma.[69]

Hormonal manipulation using estrogen antagonists in the form of progesterone or androgen has yielded objective responses in 7 to 25% of the patients with metastatic renal cell carcinoma.[70] Subsequent trials with the newer estrogen antagonist tamoxifen have not provided any better results.[71] Despite the infrequent responses, this form of hormonal therapy has only rare minimal side effects and is worth considering for such dismal disease, especially in the absence of more effective agents.

The prognostic outlook for metastatic renal cell carcinoma is grave, especially because of lack of effective adjuvant therapy. Several experimental protocols such as immunotherapy using aggregated soluble fraction of the autologous tumor,[72] alpha-interferon therapy,[73] and combination of coumarin with cimetidine[74] and interleukin[75] deserve mention. Adjuvant nephrectomy as an integral part of these protocols is indicated and should be offered to the patients as experimental therapeutic alternatives.

The overall results of radiation therapy, chemotherapy, hormonal therapy, and immunotherapy have been less than impressive and are further discussed in the appropriate sections of this book. Only a small percentage of patients have shown responses to any of these modalities.

REFERENCES

1. SILVERBERG, E., and LUBERA, J. A. Cancer statistics 1989. CA, *39:*3, 1989.

2. BENNINGTON, J. L., and BECKWITH, J. B. Tumors of the kidney, renal pelvis, and ureter. In: *Atlas of Tumor Pathology.* 2nd series, Fasc 12. Washington, D.C., Armed Forces Institute of Pathology, 1975.

3. KANTOR, A. F. Current concepts in the epidemiology and etiology of primary renal cell carcinoma. J. Urol., *117:*415, 1977.

4. LOVE, L., NEUMAN, H. A., SZANTO, P. B., and NOVAK, G. M. Malignant renal tumors in adolescence. Radiology, *92:*855, 1969.

5. BJELKE, E. Malignant neoplasms of the kidney in children. Cancer, *17:*318, 1964.

6. GRAWITZ, P. A. Die sogenannten Lipome de Niere. Virchows Arch. (Pathol. Anat.), *93:*39, 1883.

7. OBERLING, C., RIVIERE, M., and HAGNENAU, F. Ultrastructure of the clear cells in renal carcinomas and its importance for the demonstration of their renal origin. Nature, *186:*402, 1960.

8. WALLACE, A. C., and NAIRN, R. C. Renal tubular antigens in kidney tumors. Cancer, *29:*977, 1972.

9. COOPER, P. H., and WAISMAN, J. Tubular differentiation and basement membrane production in a renal adenoma: ultrastructural features. J. Pathol., *109:*113, 1971.

10. CRISTOL, D. S., McDONALD, J. R., and EMMETT, J. L. Renal adenomas in hypernephromatous kidneys: A study of their incidence, nature and relationship. J. Urol., *55:*18, 1946.

11. FISHER, E. R., and HORVAT, B. Comparative ultrastructural study of so called renal adenoma and carcinoma. J. Urol., *108:*382, 1972.

12. MANCILLA-JIMENEZ, R., STANLEY, R. J., and BLATH, R. A. Papillary renal cell carcinoma: A clinical, radiologic, and pathologic study of 34 cases. Cancer, *38:*2469, 1976.

13. PRITCHETT, T. R., LIESKOVSKY, G., and SKINNER, D. G. Clinical manifestations and treatment of renal parenchymal tumors. In: *Diagnosis and Management of Genitourinary Cancer.* Edited by D. G. Skinner and G. Hieskovsky. Philadelphia, W. B. Saunders Co., 1988, p. 337.

14. OTTO, U., BARSCH, H., HULAND, H., and KLOPPEL, G. Tumor cell deoxyribonucleic acid content and prognosis in human renal cell carcinoma. J. Urol., *132:*237, 1984.

15. SKINNER, D. G., et al. Diagnosis and management of renal cell carcinoma: A clinical and pathologic study of 309 cases. Cancer, *28:*1165, 1971.

16. CHISHOLM, G. D. Nephrogenic ridge tumors and their syndromes. Ann. N.Y. Acad. Sci., *230:*403, 1974.

17. CHERUKURI, S. V., JOHENNING, P. W., and RAM, M. D. Systemic effects of hypernephroma. Urology, *10:*93, 1977.

18. CLARKE, B. G., and GOADE, W. J., JR. Fever and anemia in renal cancer. N. Engl. J. Med., *254:*107, 1956.

19. GIBBONS, R. P., MONTIE, J. E., CORREA, R. J., and MASON J. T. Manifestations of renal cell carcinoma. Urology, *8:*201, 1976.

20. HOLLIFIED, J. W., et al. Renin-secreting clear cell carcinoma of the kidney. Arch. Intern. Med., *135:*859, 1975.

21. SUFRIN, G., et al. Hormones in renal cancer. J. Urol., *117:*433, 1977.

22. GOLDBERG, R. S., PILCHER, D. B., and YATES, J. W. The aggressive surgical management of hypercalcemia due to ectopic parathormone production. Cancer, *45:*2652, 1980.

23. CUMMINGS, K. B., and ROBERTSON, R. P. Prostaglandin: Increased production by renal cell carcinoma. J. Urol., *118:*720, 1977.

24. BENNINGTON, J. L., and KRADJIAN, R. M. *Renal Carcinoma.* Philadelphia, W. B. Saunders Co., 1967.

25. CREEVY, C. D. Confusing clinical manifestations of malignant renal neoplasms. Arch. Intern. Med., *55:*895, 1935.

26. STAUFFER, M. H. Nephrogenic hepatosplenomegaly (abstract). Gastroenterology, *40:*694, 1961.

27. BOXER, R. J., et al. Nonmetastatic hepatic dysfunction associated with renal cell carcinoma. J. Urol., *119:*468, 1978.

28. GLEESON, M. H., et al. An endocrine tumor in kidney affecting small bowel structure, motility and function. Gut, *11:*1060, 1970.

29. BARBAGELATTA, M., and CHOMETTE, G. Renal immunopathology in renal cell carcinoma. Virchows Arch., *404:*87, 1984.

30. CRONIN, R. E., et al. Renal cell carcinoma: Unusual systematic manifestations. Medicine, *55:*291, 1976.

31. ROBSON, C. J. The natural history of renal cell carcinoma. Prog. Clin. Biol. Res., *100:*447, 1982.

32. HANASH, K. A. The nonmetastatic hepatic dysfunction syndrome associated with renal cell carcinoma (hypernephroma): Stauffer's syndrome. Prog. Clin. Biol. Res., *100:*301, 1982.

33. THOMPSON, I. M., and PECK, M. Improvement in survival of patients with renal cell carcinoma—role of serendipitously detected tumor. J. Urol., *140:*487, 1988.

34. KOLHARI, K., et al. Preoperative radiographic evaluaton of hypernephroma. J. Comput. Assist. Tomogr., *5:*702, 1981.

35. JASCHKE, W., et al. Accuracy of computed tomography in staging of kidney tumors. Acta Radiol. (Diagn.), *23:*593, 1982.

36. PROBST, P., et al. Computerized tomography versus angiography in the staging of malignant renal neoplasm. Br. J. Radiol., *54:*744, 1981.

37. RICHIE, J. P., et al. Computerized tomography scan for diagnosis and staging of renal cell carcinoma. J. Urol., *129:*1114, 1983.

38. LANG, E. K. Angio-computed tomography and dynamic computed tomography in staging of renal cell carcinoma. Radiology, *151:*149, 1984.

39. BERNARDINO, M. E., et al. Computed tomography in the evaluation of post nephrectomy patients. Radiology, *130:*183, 1979.

40. DEKERNION, J. B. Renal tumors. In: *Campbell's Urology.* 5th Ed. Vol. 2. Edited by P. C. Walsh, R. E. Gittes, A. D. Perlmutter, and T. A. Stamey. Philadelphia, W. B. Saunders Co., 1986, pp. 1294–1342.

41. HRICAK, H., et al. Magnetic resonance imaging in the diagnosis and staging of renal and perirenal neoplasms. Radiology, *154:*709, 1985.

42. MEHTA, S. D., et al. Kidneys and retroperitoneum. In: *Magnetic Resonance Imaging.* 2nd Ed. Vol. 1. Edited by C. L. Partain, R. R. Price, J. A. Patton, M. D. Kulkarni, and A. E. James. Philadelphia, W. B. Saunders Co., 1988, pp. 503–523.

43. DEMAS, B. E., STAFFORD, S. A., and HRICAK, H. Kidneys. In: *Magnetic Resonance Imaging.* Edited by D. D. Stark, and W. G. Bradley. St. Louis, C. V. Mosby Co., 1988, pp. 1187–1232.

44. FLOCKS, R. H., and KADESKY, M. C. Malignant neoplasms of the kidney: An analysis of 353 patients followed five years or more. J. Urol., *79:*196, 1958.

45. ROBSON, C. J., CHURCHILL, B. M., and ANDERSON, W. The results of radical nephrectomy for renal cell carcinoma. Trans Am. Assoc. Genitourin. Surg., *60:*122, 1968.

46. SKINNER, D. G., PFISTER, R. F., and COLVIN, R. B. Extension of renal cell carcinoma into the vena cava: The rationale for aggressive surgical management. J. Urol., *107:*711, 1972.

47. SELLI, C., et al. Stratification of risk factors in renal cell carcinoma. Cancer, *52:*899, 1983.

48. BEAHRS, D. H., et al. Kidney. In: *Manual for Staging of Cancer.* Philadelphia, J. B. Lippincott Co., 1988, p. 200.

49. ROBSON, C. J.: Radical nephrectomy for renal cell carcinoma. J. Urol., *89:*37, 1963.

50. HULTEN, L., et al. Occurrence and localization of lymph node metastases in renal carcinoma. Scand. J. Urol. Nephrol., *3*:129, 1969.

51. SIMINOVITCH, J. P., MONTIE, J. E., and STRAFFON, R. A. Lymphadenectomy in renal adenocarcinoma. J. Urol., *127*:1090, 1982.

52. MARBERGER, M. Conservative surgery for renal adenocarcinoma. In: *International Perspectives in Urology.* Vol. 13. *Tumors of the Kidney.* Edited by J. B. deKernion and M. Pavone-Macaluso. Baltimore, Williams & Wilkins, 1986, pp. 157–172.

53. LIEBER, M. M. Renal cell carcinoma: New Developments (editorial). Mayo Clin. Proc., *60;*715, 1985.

54. CARINI, M., et al. Conservative surgical treatment of renal cell carcinoma: Clinical experience and reappraisal of indications. J. Urol., *140:*725, 1988.

55. SKINNER, D. G. Editorial comments on Carini, M., et al. J. Urol., *140:*730, 1988.

56. MUKAMEL, E., et al. Incidental small renal tumors accompanying clinically overt renal cell carcinoma. J. Urol., *140:*22, 1988.

57. TALAMO, T. S., and SHONNARD, J. W. Small renal adenocarcinoma with metastasis. J. Urol., *124:*132, 1980.

58. BLACKLEY, S. K., et al. Ex situ study of the effectiveness of enucleation in patients with renal cell carcinoma. J. Urol., *140:*6, 1988.

59. WICKHAM, J. E. A. Conservative renal surgery for adenocarcinoma. The place of bench surgery. Br. J. Urol., *47:*25, 1975.

60. TOPLEY, M., NOVICK, A. C., and MONTIE, J. E. Long term results following partial nephrectomy for localized renal adenocarcinoma. Presented at American Urological Association Annual Meeting, Las Vegas, 1983.

61. SMITH, R. B., et al. Bilateral renal cell carcinoma and renal carcinoma in the solitary kidney. J. Urol., *132:*450, 1986.

62. BLOOM, H. J. G. Hormone-induced and spontaneous regression of metastatic renal cancer. Cancer, *32:*1066, 1973.

63. MONTIE, J. E., et al. The role of adjunctive nephrectomy in patients with metastatic renal cell carcinoma. J. Urol., *117:*272, 1977.

64. DEKERNION, J. B., RAMMING, K. P., and SMITH, R. B. Natural history of metastatic renal cell carcinoma: A computer analysis. J. Urol., *120:*148, 1978.

65. O'DEA, M. J., et al. The treatment of renal cell carcinoma with solitary metastasis. J. Urol., *120:*540, 1978.

66. TOLIA, B. M., and WHITMORE, W. F., JR. Solitary metastasis from renal cell carcinoma. J. Urol., *114:*836, 1975.

67. SWANSON, D. A., et al. Angioinfarction plus nephrectomy for metastatic renal cell carcinoma—an update. J. Urol., *130:*449, 1983.

68. SWANSON, D. A., and WALLACE, S. Surgery of metastatic renal cell carcinoma and use of renal infarction. Semin. Surg. Oncol., *4:*124, 1988.

69. GOTTESMAN, J. E., et al. Infarction nephrectomy for metastatic renal carcinoma: Southwest Oncology Group study. Urology, *25:*248, 1985.

70. BLOOM, H. J. G. Medroxyprogesterone acetate (Provera) in treatment of metastatic renal cancer. Br. J. Cancer, *25:*250, 1971.

71. LANTERI, V. J., et al. High dose tamoxifen in metastatic renal cell carcinoma. Urology, *19:*623, 1982.

72. TYKKA, H. Active specific immunotherapy with supportive measures in the treatment of advanced palliatively nephrectomized renal adenocarcinoma. A controlled clinical study. Scand. J. Urol. Nephrol. (Suppl.), *63:*1, 1981.

73. DEKERNION, J. B., et al. The treatement of metastatic renal cell carcinoma with a human leukocyte interferon. Proceedings of the 19th Congress of Societe Internationale d'Urologie. J. Urol., *130:*1063, 1983.

74. MARSHALL, M. E., et al. Treatment of metastatic renal cell carcinoma with coumarin (1,2-benzpyrone) and cimetidine: A pilot study. J. Clin. Oncol., *5:*862, 1987.

75. ROSENBERG, S. A., et al. A progress report on the treatment of 157 patients with advanced cancer using lymphokine-activated killer cells and interleukine-2 or high-dose interleukine-2 alone. N. Engl. J. Med., *316:*889, 1987.

CHAPTER
4

Radical Nephrectomy: Thoracoabdominal Extrapleural Approach

"Diseases desperate grown
By desperate appliance are relieved,
Or not at all."
  WILLIAM SHAKESPEARE (Hamlet, Act IV, Scene III, 1.9).

Sakti Das

HISTORICAL PERSPECTIVES

Erastus Wolcott of Milwaukee performed the first reported nephrectomy in 1861 which was chronicled in brilliant detail by Charles Stoddard.[1] This serendipitous nephrectomy, of what was presumed preoperatively to be a hepatic cyst, was accomplished through an anterior transperitoneal approach.

Because of their deep thoracoabdominal location, the kidneys have been approached through a variety of incisions. The lumbar approach of Gustav Simon, for the first deliberately planned nephrectomy in 1869, had a significant limitation of exposure.[2] In 1876, Kocher advocated the anterior transperitoneal route to remove a "sarcomatous" kidney.[3] The transperitoneal approach, although providing better access to the pedicle and allowing examination of the contralateral kidney (of utmost importance in the period before pyelography), nonetheless became unpopular because of the increased mortality from peritonitis and shock.

The oblique flank incision described by Kuster in 1883 pioneered the development of a number of variations and modifications in the flank approach, allowing better access to the kidney without violation of the pleura or the peritoneum.[4] In 1926, Bernard Fey reported his extrapleural abdominothoracic incision along the eleventh rib, which continued downward and medially toward the epigastrium, with resection or downward displacement of the eleventh rib.[5] Use of this incision has had sporadic resurgence, with more recent modifications by Presman, Turner-Warwick, and others.[6–8]

SURGICAL OBJECTIVES AND RATIONALE

Ideal extirpative surgery for renal cell carcinoma is accomplished by (1) early ligation of the renal pedicle before any manipulation or mobilization of the neoplasm, (2) removal of the renal neoplasm with intact surrounding Gerota's fascia, and (3) regional lymphadenectomy. The incision or approach used should also allow an adequate intraperitoneal exploration for intra-abdominal metastases.

Advocates of the anterior transperitoneal and the thoracoabdominal intrapleural approaches have claimed that these incisions provide better access to the renal pedicle and the suprahilar regions, respectively, compared to the conventional flank incision. However, use of the tenth-intercostal-space or the eleventh-rib supracostal extrapleural transperitoneal approach makes feasible the early control of the renal pedicle, a thorough laparotomy, and excellent exposure of the suprahilar retroperitoneum. When exploration of the thoracic cavity is not needed, the supracostal incision can provide adequate exposure, while preventing the additional morbidity of thoracotomy.

The preference of radical nephrectomy over simple nephrectomy for the management of renal carcinoma has been championed by Robson.[9] Despite the lack of prospective studies comparing the two modalities, improved results of radical nephrectomy compared to those reported earlier reaffirm the importance of removing the intact Gerota's fascia with its contents, the kidney, and the adrenal gland. Many of these tumors, especially large or peripherally located ones, spread through the capsule into the perinephric fat, enhancing the chances of local recurrence as well as dissemination if Gerota's fascia is not excised.

The therapeutic value of lymphadenectomy for renal cell carcinoma, however, has not been unequivocally established. Rarely, a patient with micrometastases to one or two proximal nodes may be cured by lymphadenectomy, but involvement of the lymph nodes is usually an important prognostic determinant indicating disseminated disease. Lymphadenectomy is at present considered mainly an important staging procedure that allows the selection of patients who may need adjuvant therapy.[10]

An extensive bilateral retroperitoneal lymphadenectomy, similar to that performed for testicular tumors, is not warranted for renal cell carcinoma. To reduce the morbidity from such a procedure while accomplishing the objectives of lymphadenectomy, we limit regional lymphadenectomy to the clearing of the nodal tissues of the aortocaval area and the area around the ipsilateral great vessel (the aorta in the case of a tumor on the left side, and the vena cava for a tumor on the right side), from the level of the diaphragmatic crus above to the inferior mesenteric artery at the distal limit. The contralateral renal hilar region and the posterolateral aspect of the contralateral great vessel are not dissected.

INDICATIONS AND CONTRAINDICATIONS

Most radical nephrectomies can be conveniently performed through the modified high-flank or extrapleural thoracoabdominal approach. The location or the size of the tumor is not a contraindication.

The following situations, however, make alternative incisions more pragmatically desirable: (1) a few patients cannot be placed in the flank position because of a spinothoracic deformity or because they have circulatory decompensation in the lateral position; (2) if bilateral renal surgery is contemplated, an anterior transperitoneal incision is ideal; (3) in the case of tumors in a solitary kidney, either in situ or ex vivo (bench surgery) excision of the neoplasm is necessary. Ex vivo surgery is performed through the anterior approach; otherwise, the patient must be repositioned in the supine position to obtain better access to the hypogastric artery or the iliac vessels for autotransplantation; (4) if thrombus extraction from the renal vein or vena cava is contemplated for renal carcinoma on the left side, an anterior approach is again preferred, because adequate control of the inferior vena cava is difficult to achieve through a left flank incision; (5) an intrapleural thoracoabdominal incision may be necessary for diagnostic exploration of pulmonary metastasis or for therapeutic excision of the metastasis with radical nephrectomy; and (6) thoracotomy is also mandatory when better access to the proximal portion of the inferior vena cava or the right atrium is necessary to extract a tumor thrombus.

SURGICAL PROCEDURE

The patient is placed about midway between the full lateral and supine positions. This position is often achieved by placing the patient in the true lateral position; the upper torso is then allowed to roll backward. A small sandbag is placed near the scapula. The ipsilateral lower extremity is extended over the flexed opposite leg with a pillow between. The table is flexed, and wide adhesive tapes are applied across the iliac crest to the table to stabilize the patient (Fig. 4-1). The position of the eleventh rib is indelibly marked before skin preparation. An 18 French Foley catheter is inserted for intraoperative and postoperative monitoring of urine output. We prefer to stand on the right side of the patient for both right and left radical nephrectomy.

Incision

The incision begins near the angle of the eleventh rib at the posterior axillary line and continues along the upper costal margin toward the epigastrium. The anterior rectus sheath, the external oblique, latissimus dorsi and, more posteriorly, part of the serratus posterior inferior muscles are divided with cutting diathermy. The rectus abdominis muscle is transected, and the internal oblique and transversus abdominis are divided up to the tip of the eleventh rib (Fig. 4-2A).

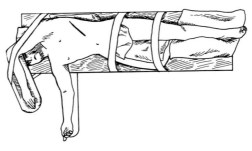

FIG. 4-1. Patient is positioned midway between supine and true lateral decubitus. Incision is made from angle of eleventh rib along its upper border toward epigastrium across midline (left-sided position).

The intercostal muscles of the tenth interspace are exposed and carefully dissected off the upper margin of the eleventh rib, and the underlying diaphragm is thereby exposed (Fig. 4-2B). This part of the dissection requires caution because the thin linear margin of the pleural reflection becomes apparent near the middle of the interspace.

Identification of the pleura is aided and its integrity confirmed when the anesthetist expands the lung, whereby the inferior pulmonary margin descends to occupy the pleural space. By blunt finger dissection, the pleura is pushed away from the inner surface of the lower rib (Fig. 4-2C). The pleura, if opened inadvertently, can be closed with mattress or continuous sutures of 3-0 chromic catgut, taking bites through the adjacent diaphragm for a secure hold. The suture is tied while the anesthetist expels the pneumothorax by positive pressure ventilation.

Further posteriorly, the sharp margin of the costovertebral ligament is encountered at the upper edge of the rib. The overlying latissimus dorsi and erector spinae muscles are strongly retracted, and the ligament is divided, allowing the rib to be hinged downward.

The exposed diaphragm is now incised parallel to the rib about 2 cm below the pleural reflection. The incised upper edge of the diaphragm is wrapped around the upper (tenth) rib and sutured to the serratus posterior inferior and, more anteriorly, to the deeper fibers of the latissimus dorsi (Fig. 4-2D). This modification by Witherington deters inadvertent pleural injury from retraction at later stages of the dissection.[8]

Anteromedially, the posterior rectus sheath and the peritoneum are opened widely, and a careful laparotomy is performed to detect any metastases or other associated disease. A self-retaining retractor is applied between the ribs in the posterior aspect of the wound.

Left Radical Nephrectomy

The descending colon is held up, and the peritoneum of the lateral paracolic gutter is incised (Fig. 4-3). Superiorly, this incision is carried through the anterior lamella of the splenocolic ligament, thereby allowing inferomedial mobilization of the splenic flexure. Care must be taken not to injure the inferior pole of the spleen at this stage. The splenic flexure

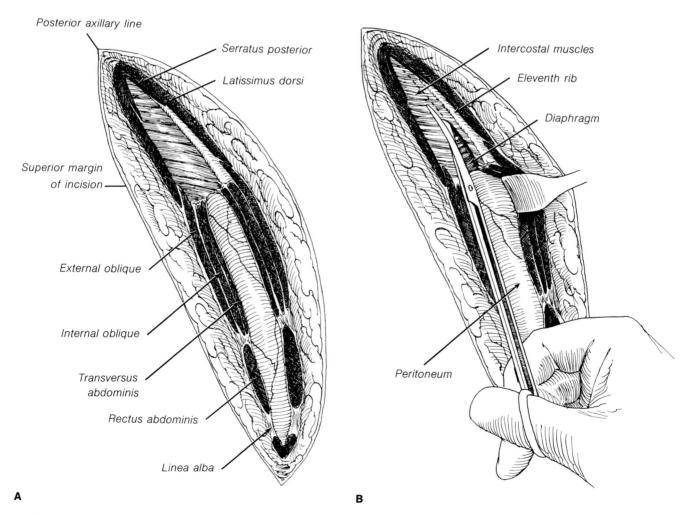

A

Posterior axillary line

Serratus posterior

Latissimus dorsi

Superior margin of incision

External oblique

Internal oblique

Transversus abdominis

Rectus abdominis

Linea alba

B

Intercostal muscles

Eleventh rib

Diaphragm

Peritoneum

FIG. 4-2. *A*, Division of parietal muscle layers, exposing intercostal muscles of tenth interspace (view of left-sided incision from patient's right side). *B*, Division of intercostal muscles, exposing underlying diaphragm.

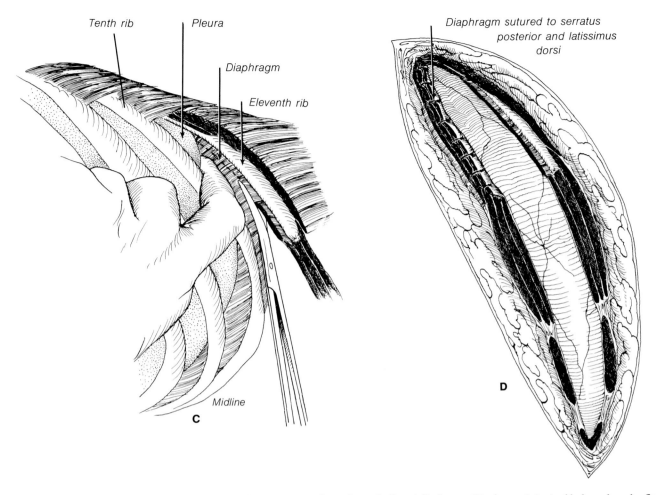

Tenth rib   Pleura

Diaphragm

Eleventh rib

Midline

C

Diaphragm sutured to serratus
posterior and latissimus
dorsi

D

FIG. 4-2. *C*, Pleura is reflected superiorly by blunt dissection away from eleventh rib and diaphragm. Diaphragm is incised below pleural reflection (view of left-sided incision from patient's right side). *D*, Superior edge of incised diaphragm is wrapped around tenth rib and sutured to serratus posterior inferior and latissimus dorsi.

and the descending colon, with their mesentery, are bluntly mobilized from the underlying Gerota's fascia and retroperitoneum. The hand inside the abdomen, lifting the colon with its peritoneal attachment and blood supply, is an excellent guide to the proper plane anterior to the Gerota's fascia. Generous mobilization of this posterior peritoneum and wide exposure of the retroperitoneum make subsequent dissection easy to perform. At this stage, the anteromedial aspect of the vena cava should be visible medially, as well as the origin of the superior mesenteric artery superiorly, and the posterior surface of the pancreas with the splenic vessels anterosuperiorly.

If the mesentery of the descending colon adheres to the tumor, the area in doubt should be circumscribed and left with the Gerota's fascia for en bloc removal. Ischemic injury to the colon is unlikely as long as its marginal arcades are preserved. The tumor must not be manipulated during this stage.

The large left renal vein coursing medially across the aorta is now easily identified (Fig. 4-4). As the diaphanous medial extension of the Gerota's fascia over the renal vein is dissected, the left adrenal vein is seen near the renal hilum. The adrenal vein is divided between ligatures of 2-0 silk to avoid tearing while retracting the renal vein. The renal artery lies

directly posterosuperior to the renal vein. The renal vein is retracted downward, allowing palpation and dissection of the renal artery.

The superior mesenteric artery and the renal artery must be identified as separate entities before any attempt at arterial ligation is made. The grave error of ligating the superior mesenteric artery has been known to occur, especially with large and medially encroaching tumors. The renal artery is ligated in continuity with 1-0 silk (Fig. 4-5*A*) and is not divided at this stage. Accessory renal arteries are palpated for at this stage and ligated similarly if detected. The renal vein is ligated and divided where it terminates at the inferior vena cava. The distal stump of the divided renal vein is held up by its ligature, and any lumbar vein must be sought entering the renal vein from behind (Fig. 4-5*B*). Such a lumbar vein must be divided between ligatures in case it tears and retracts into the paravertebral muscles, causing troublesome hemorrhage. The renal artery already ligated is now further dissected up to its origin, where it is doubly ligated and divided (Fig. 4-5*C*).

Starting below the divided renal vessels, the surgeon pushes the Gerota's fascia laterally away from the psoas major. At the lower extent of the wound, the ureter is divided be-

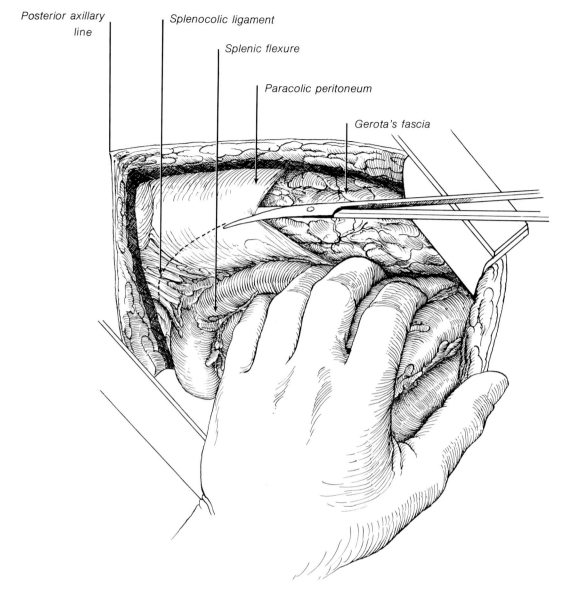

Posterior axillary line

Splenocolic ligament

Splenic flexure

Paracolic peritoneum

Gerota's fascia

FIG. 4-3. Incision of lateral paracolic peritoneum is carried above and medially through splenocolic ligament.

tween ligatures of 1-0 chromic catgut near the pelvic brim. The gonadal vessels are ligated with 2-0 silk and divided at about the same level (Fig. 4-6A). The kidney, ensheathed by Gerota's fascia, is now held medially and separated from the psoas major and quadratus lumborum muscles on its postero-lateral aspect (Fig. 4-6B). A few large collateral vessels require ligature and division.

Dissection is continued superiorly, stripping the thin layer of Gerota's fascia around the adrenal gland from the inferior surface of the diaphragm. Medially and above, the small adrenal branches from the aorta and phrenic arteries are divided between hemostatic clips (Fig. 4-7). The kidney harboring the tumor and the adrenal gland with the covering Gerota's fascia are removed en bloc.

Regional lymphadenectomy is now carried out, unless the nephrectomy is being performed as a palliative measure or the patient's age and general condition preclude further extensive

surgery. Dissection is begun at the suprahilar region, bringing down the tissues in front of the diaphragmatic crus lateral to the aorta. The node-bearing fibrofatty tissue is pushed medially over the aorta. As dissection continues along the subadventitial plane, the tissues in front of the aorta are brought downward, skirting the origins of the celiac and superior mesenteric artery up to below the origins of the renal arteries (Fig. 4-8A).

Similar dissection up and down the anteromedial surface of the vena cava separates the aortocaval nodal tissues away from the vena cava (Fig. 4-8B). A few lumbar veins require ligature and division. The adventitia in front of the aorta is split down to the origin of the inferior mesenteric artery. The medial leaf of adventitia with the aortocaval tissues is separated from the aorta dividing the lumbar arteries (Fig. 4-8C). The lateral aspect of the aorta is then dissected away from the para-aortic nodal tissue on the left side (Fig. 4-8D). As the lumbar arteries

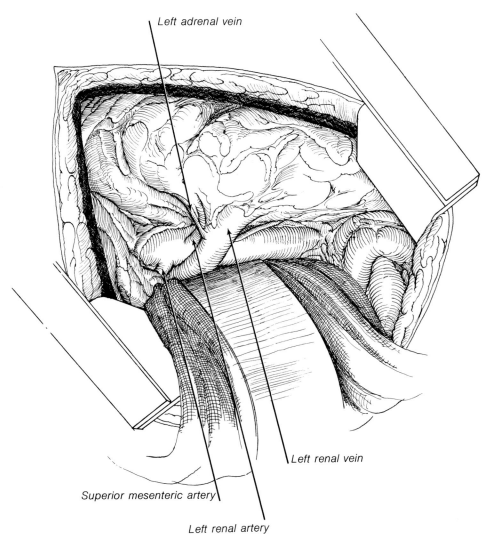

Left adrenal vein

Left renal vein

Superior mesenteric artery

Left renal artery

Fig. 4-4. Medial reflection of descending colon, exposing retroperitoneal structures.

in this area are divided, the aorta can be held up on vein retractors.

The lateral para-aortic nodal envelope is now grasped with the fingers. As it is pulled out, the dissected aortocaval nodal tissues are pushed behind the aorta and removed in continuity, exposing the anterior spinal ligaments (Fig. 4-8*E*).

Hemostatic clips must be used generously throughout the procedure to prevent postoperative lymph leakage or collection. The wound is copiously irrigated with distilled water. General hemostasis and, in particular, the integrity of the spleen are checked. Most of the inadvertent splenic tears can be managed by applying microfibrillar purified bovine corium collagen (Avitene), and splenectomy is rarely necessary. The wound is closed in layers without drains.

Right Radical Nephrectomy

On the right side, the inferior margin of the right lobe of the liver often encroaches on the posterior part of the wound after

the eleventh-rib supracostal incision. The avascular right triangular ligament is divided, and the inferior surface of the liver is carefully retracted upward. The incision of the lateral paracolic peritoneum is continued upward and medially to the front of the vena cava above the duodenum (Fig. 4-9). The second part of the duodenum is reflected medially to expose the entire width of the inferior vena cava.

The thin adventitial layer in front of the vena cava is dissected to expose the termination of the renal veins. The left renal vein and the medial margin of the vena cava are retracted to expose the right renal artery in a more posterior plane. The right renal artery is ligated in continuity at this site between the aorta and the vena cava (Fig. 4-10). The right renal vein is ligated and divided. The artery is then religated twice and is divided between the proximal two and distal single ligature.

On the right side, there are usually several adrenal veins with a short, direct course into the vena cava. They must be sought carefully along the lateral aspect of the vena cava behind the right lobe of the liver and divided between ligatures.

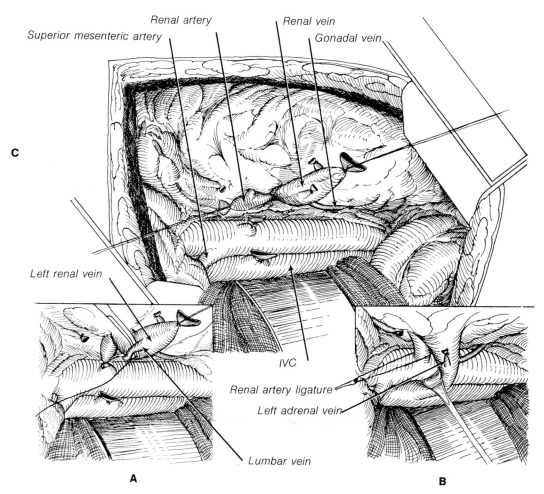

Superior mesenteric artery
Renal artery
Renal vein
Gonadal vein
Left renal vein
IVC
Renal artery ligature
Left adrenal vein
Lumbar vein

C

A

B

FIG. 4-5. *A*, Left renal vein is retracted downward after division of left adrenal vein. Renal artery is ligated in continuity. *B*, Distal stump of left renal vein is held up, and any lumbar vein entering from behind is sought. *C*, Left renal vein and artery have been doubly ligated and divided.

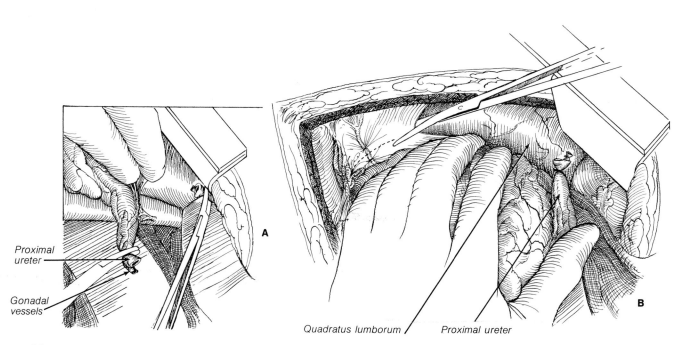

Proximal ureter
Gonadal vessels
A
Quadratus lumborum
Proximal ureter
B

FIG. 4-6. *A*, Ureter and gonadal vessels are ligated and divided near pelvic brim. *B*, Kidney enclosed by Gerota's fascia is dissected away from quadratus lumborum and psoas major muscles on posterolateral aspect.

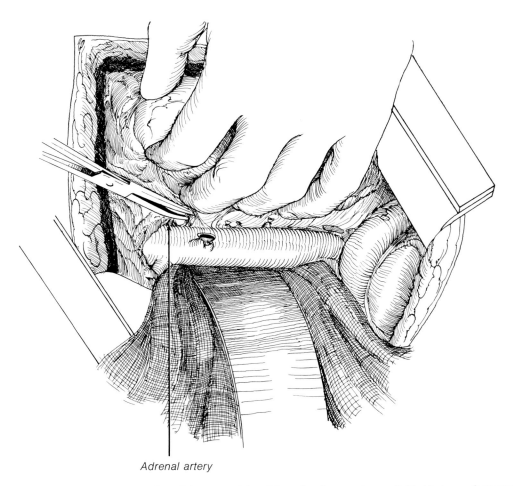

Adrenal artery

FIG. 4-7. Dissection is continued on superior and medial aspects. Adrenal branches from aorta are divided between hemostatic clips.

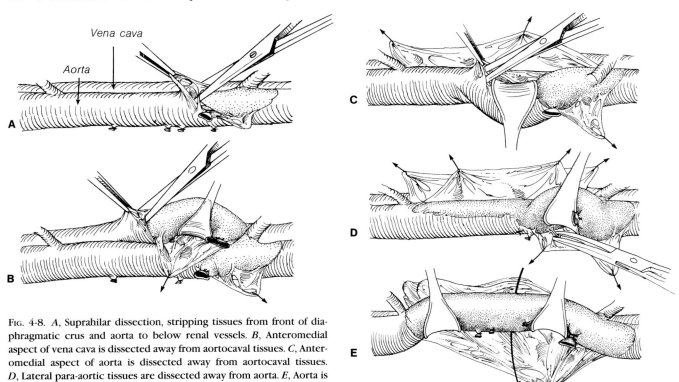

FIG. 4-8. *A,* Suprahilar dissection, stripping tissues from front of diaphragmatic crus and aorta to below renal vessels. *B,* Anteromedial aspect of vena cava is dissected away from aortocaval tissues. *C,* Anteromedial aspect of aorta is dissected away from aortocaval tissues. *D,* Lateral para-aortic tissues are dissected away from aorta. *E,* Aorta is held up on retractors; lateral para-aortic and aortocaval tissues are pulled out en bloc behind aorta.

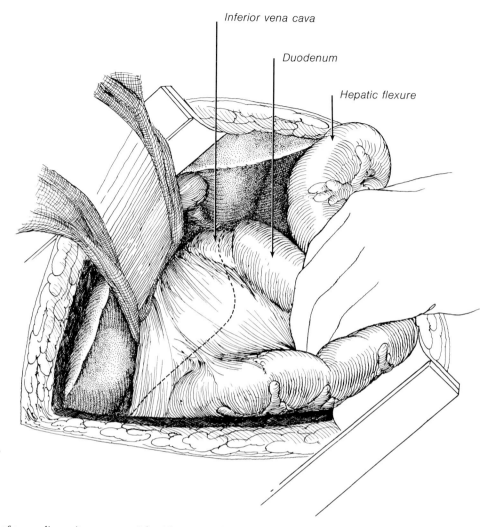

Inferior vena cava

Duodenum

Hepatic flexure

FIG. 4-9. Incision of paracolic peritoneum on right side is carried across front of inferior vena cava above duodenum.

The remainder of the procedure is similar to that described for the left side.

Regional lymphadenectomy is then carried out. The surgeon dissects the node-bearing tissues around the vena cava and the aortocaval area down to the level of the inferior mesenteric artery.

POSTOPERATIVE CARE

A chest roentgenogram is obtained routinely in the recovery room. Management of any inadvertent pleural injuries that escaped notice during the surgical procedure depends upon the degree of the resultant pneumothorax. Minor pneumothorax (less than 10%) is absorbed within a few days and does not require intervention. Major pneumothorax must be immediately drained via a needle introduced into the second intercostal space in the midclavicular line. The needle is connected to an underwater-sealed container and is removed as soon as no further air bubbles are expelled. Prompt expansion of the underlying lung is confirmed by a repeated chest roentgenogram.

Nasogastric suction is continued until postoperative ileus is resolved and intestinal peristalsis is resumed. Parenteral fluid replacement must take into account the large protein-rich transudate loss from the renal fossa and retroperitoneum. Partial colloid replacement with plasma or albumin is often necessary for the first few days. Vigorous pulmonary care and early ambulation are mandatory.

REFERENCES

1. STODDARD, C. L. Case of encephaloid disease of the kidney, removal. Med. Surg. Reporter, 7:126, 1861.

2. SIMON, G. Uber die Zulassigkeit der einseitigen Nephrotomie bei Harnleiterbauchfisteln: (Vortrag, gehalten im Operationssaal der

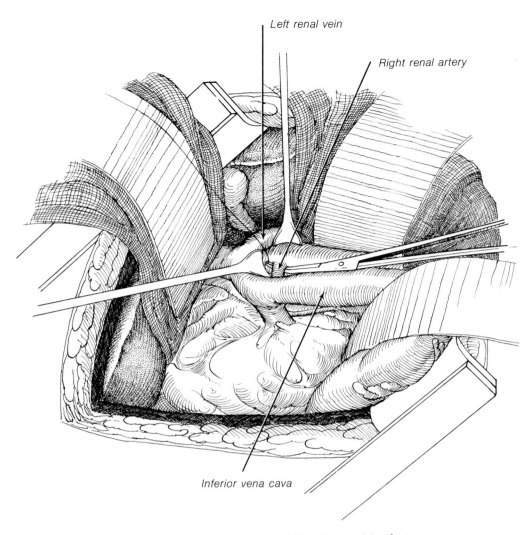

Left renal vein

Right renal artery

Inferior vena cava

Fig. 4-10. Right renal artery is dissected between vena cava and aorta and ligated near origin of artery.

chirurgischen Klinik unmittelbar border Operation.) In: *Chirurgie der Nieren.* Vol. I. Erlangen, Ferdinand Enke, 1871.

3. Kocher, T. Eine Nephrotomie wegen Nierensarkom. Dtsch. Z. Chir., *9:* 312, 1878.

4. Kuster, E. Uber einen Fall von Nierenextirpation mit Demonstration. (Wird in extenso verkoffentlicht werden.) Discussion. Berl. Klin. Wschr., *20:*604, 1883.

5. Fey, B. L'abord du rein par la voie thoraco-abdominale. Arch. Urol. Clin. Necker, *5:*169, 1926.

6. Presman, D. Eleventh intercostal space incision for renal surgery. J. Urol., *74:*578, 1955.

7. Turner-Warwick, R. T. The supracostal approach to the renal area. Br. J. Urol., *37:*671, 1965.

8. Witherington, R. Improving the supracostal loin incisions. J. Urol., *124:*73, 1980.

9. Robson, C. J. Radical nephrectomy for renal cell carcinoma. J. Urol., *89:*37, 1963.

10. DeKernion, J. B. Radical nephrectomy. In: *Modern Technics in Surgery (Urologic Surgery).* Edited by R. M. Ehrlich. New York, Futura, 1980.

C H A P T E R
5

Radical Nephrectomy: Thoracoabdominal Intrapleural Approach

Richard K. Heppe
E. David Crawford

Renal cell carcinoma has been poorly responsive to treatment with radiation, chemotherapy, and immunotherapy. The only chance for successful management of this disease is complete surgical extirpation. To this end, removal of the kidney with its investing Gerota's fascia and the adrenal gland has become the preferred treatment.

Radical nephrectomy may be accomplished through a variety of approaches. The intrapleural thoracoabdominal approach is one that we have found most useful. Because this method ensures wide exposure of the kidney, renal vessels, aorta, and vena cava, this incision is ideal for use with large or upper pole lesions, adrenal tumors, large retroperitoneal masses, and for retroperitoneal lymph node dissection. In addition, this approach may be used to advantage in renal transplantation, donor nephrectomy, partial nephrectomy, and nephroureterectomy for renal pelvic and ureteral tumors. When one is performing the operation for renal cell carcinoma, the intrapleural approach allows for palpation of the ipsilateral lung for metastases and, on the right side, for control of the vena cava in the chest in the event of a caval thrombus.

HISTORICAL PERSPECTIVES

One of the first descriptions of renal cell carcinoma was made in 1613, when Daniel Sennert described a "hard tumor" of a kidney and felt that it was an incurable disease resulting in cachexia or dropsy.[1] Confusion existed in the late 1800s concerning the origin of these tumors. Grawitz observed that tumors of the kidney had a histologic structure similar to that of adrenal tissue and contended that these tumors developed from aberrant adrenal rests.[2] The term "hypernephroma" was used in an attempt to describe the adrenal origin of these tumors.

The first tumor nephrectomy was performed accidentally in 1861 by Walcott, who thought the mass removed was a cyst of the liver.[3] However, it was found to be a renal neoplasm. Simon performed the first planned nephrectomy in 1869 on a 46-year-old woman whose left ureter had been damaged during a partial hysterectomy, resulting in urinary fistulas with drainage from the vagina and the abdominal scar.[4] The operation was successful and the fistulas were cured.

In the early period following Simon's operation, the mortality rate was high, but subsequent improvements in the surgical technique significantly reduced the postoperative complications. Most of the early nephrectomies were performed via the lumbar extraperitoneal or transperitoneal route. The need for improved exposure eventually led to the introduction of incisions through the lower thoracic cage. Fey first described the thoracoabdominal incision in 1926.[5] Marshall in 1946 found a tenth-rib thoracoabdominal incision valuable in the surgical repair of war injuries and envisioned the possibility of its use in civilian cases as well.[6] This approach incorporated many of the advantages of the transperitoneal and rib-resecting flank approaches.

SELECTION OF PATIENTS

Renal cell carcinoma is often referred to as the "internists' tumor" because of the bizarre pattern of metastases; therefore, a detailed history should be obtained and a careful physical examination performed to detect any unusual metastases. Patients considered for radical nephrectomy should have localized disease (stage A, B, or C). Preoperative evaluation should encompass those areas most commonly involved with metastases. Chest roentgenograms, chest CT scans, bone scans with spot films of abnormal areas, angiograms with selective and flush studies, liver function studies, hematologic parameters including clotting profile, and renal function tests are often part of the standard evaluation.

Vena caval studies should be performed in selected patients. Ultrasound is useful in detecting and defining the extent of vena caval thrombi.[7] We do not routinely employ angioinfarction of the renal artery. When one is confronted with metastatic disease, it is unrealistic to remove the primary tumor in the hope that the metastases will regress. Distant metastases are already present at the time of diagnosis in about one third of patients with renal cell carcinoma. Palliative nephrectomy may be justified in patients with a reasonable life expectancy who have severe symptoms secondary to a primary lesion, such as local pain, hemorrhage, or endocrinopathy. However, these symptoms are rarely severe enough to require nephrectomy and can usually be controlled by other means. An occasional patient with one or two isolated metastases amenable to surgical resection may undergo nephrectomy. Palliative nephrectomy may also be considered in a patient who has responded to a chemotherapeutic drug or other modality, such as immunotherapy. Angioinfarction followed by nephrectomy may lead to regression of metastasis in a small number of patients. A study by the Southwest Oncology group, however, found no benefit to this treatment in 30 patients with metastatic renal cell carcinoma.[8]

PREOPERATIVE PREPARATION

Preoperative preparation for radical nephrectomy is standard to most other major operative procedures. An intravenous infusion of Ringer's lactate is begun the evening prior to surgery to ensure adequate preoperative hydration. Patients who have large tumors or evidence of contiguous organ involvement should also undergo a standard bowel preparation.

The role of preoperative percutaneous transaortic occlusion of the renal artery remains uncertain, but one of the main advantages of this procedure is that it allows division of the renal vein without the need to first dissect out and divide the artery. Further delay of surgery after infarction allows for shrinkage of caval tumor thrombus, resolution of arteriovenous shunting, and improvement of the patient's nutritional status.[9] However, infarction may also induce severe pain, fever, and nausea and may compromise the patient's ability to tolerate an extensive operation. In patients who have a vena caval thrombus, this procedure may be helpful in minimizing disturbance of the tumor thrombus while the surgeon is attempting to obtain arterial control. However, we have not found infarction particularly useful in large tumors when attempting to decrease the amount of operative hemorrhage, since there is generally collateral circulation to the kidney.

SURGICAL PROCEDURE

After adequate presurgical preparation, the patient is brought to the operative suite, and general endotracheal anesthesia is employed. A central venous line is placed in most patients, especially in those who represent a high operative risk. An indwelling catheter is inserted in the bladder.

Position

One of the crucial initial aspects of the operation is the patient's position, which should be supervised by the operating surgeon. The patient is moved to the ipsilateral side of the operating table, and a large towel or sandbag is positioned under the back (Fig. 5-1). The break in the operative table should be located just above the iliac crest. The leg in contact with the operative table is flexed 90° and the pelvis is nearly supine. The ipsilateral shoulder is positioned approximately 30° off the horizontal, and the arm is brought across the chest and placed on a Mayo stand or an adjustable armrest. An axillary pad is positioned, and the patient is secured to the operative table with wide adhesive tape placed over the shoulders and hips. In the final position, the pelvis is nearly horizontal to the operative table.

Incision

The choice of a rib for resection depends on the nature of the primary renal tumor. In general, lower-pole tumors may be approached through a tenth-rib incision. However, in patients with large upper-pole tumors or with right-sided tumors and vena caval thrombi, the best approach is through an eighth- or ninth-rib incision. The incision is begun at the midaxillary line, is extended across the costochondral junction, and is curved slightly downward onto the abdominal wall in order to avoid injury to the intercostal nerves.

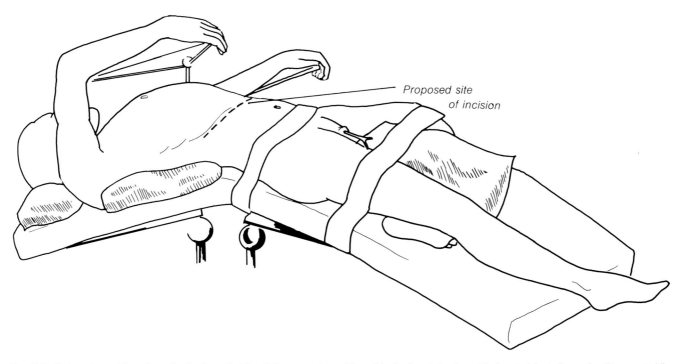

Proposed site
of incision

FIG. 5-1. Patient is positioned on the ipsilateral side of the operating table, with the break in the table located just above the iliac crest. The ipsilateral shoulder is positioned approximately 30° off the horizontal, and the arm is extended across the chest and placed on a Mayo stand or adjustable armrest.

The medial extent of the incision is determined by the extent of the tumor and the size of the patient; if necessary, it may even be extended across the epigastrium to the contralateral side. For extremely large tumors, the incision may be in a "T" form and may be carried inferiorly as a midline incision. (Figure 5-2 is an 8-week postoperative photograph of a 41-year-old woman who had an 8-pound renal tumor removed from such an incision.) The latissimus dorsi muscle is divided, and after division of the overlying muscle, the distal two thirds of the rib are resected subperiosteally (Fig. 5-3). The incision is carried medially and the anterior rectus sheath is incised.

Technique

An army-navy retractor is passed under the rectus abdominis, and the muscle itself is divided with the electrocautery unit (Fig. 5-4). The superior epigastric vessels encountered are either fulgurated or ligated with 3-0 chromic catgut sutures. The costochondral junction is divided sharply with Mayo scissors. The peritoneal cavity is entered after incising the posterior rectus sheath. The pleural cavity is entered through the posterior periosteum, and the diaphragm is divided for a distance of 10 to 15 cm dorsolaterally in the direction of its fibers; the lower edge of the lung must be protected while the diaphragmatic pleura and diaphragm are being incised. A Finochietto retractor is placed in the wound and positioned between the divided costal cartilages (Fig. 5-5).

The retractor is spread as widely as possible; because of the patient's position, the abdominal contents will fall to the contralateral side. The remainder of the procedure for radical nephrectomy is described in Chapter 4.

After en bloc removal of the kidney, the wound is carefully inspected for any bleeding, but the incision is not drained unless postoperative bleeding is a concern. We have not found it necessary to close the lateral paracolic incisions, but the

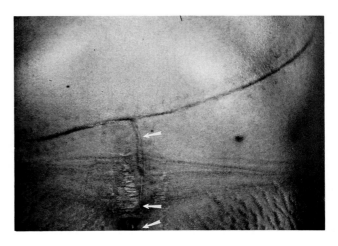

FIG. 5-2. Postoperative photograph of a left thoracoabdominal incision showing "T" dropped as a perpendicular in the midline (arrows). An 8-pound renal tumor was removed via this incision.

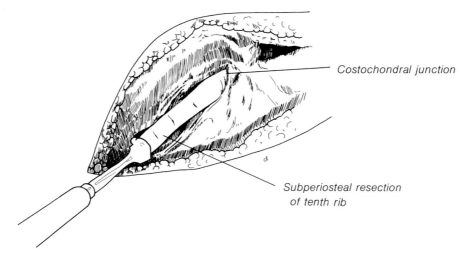

Costochondral junction

Subperiosteal resection
of tenth rib

FIG. 5-3. Tenth rib is resected in a subperiosteal fashion. Posterior to the rib is the periosteum and pleura, which is sharply incised to enter the pleural cavity. Care should be exercised not to damage the lung during this maneuver.

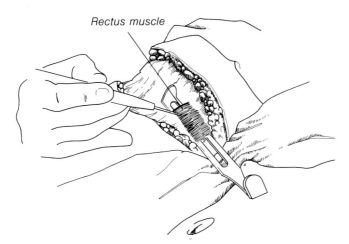

Rectus muscle

FIG. 5-4. An army-navy retractor is passed under the rectus muscle, and the muscle is divided with the electrocautery unit. After the costochondral junction is divided, the peritoneal cavity is entered.

omentum should be pulled over the loops of intestine whenever possible to prevent the formation of any adhesions. A No. 32 chest tube is positioned in the pleural cavity through a separate stab wound at the posterior axillary line and is secured with a No. 1 braided silk suture (Fig. 5-6).

We have found it helpful at the conclusion of the procedure to inject 5 ml of 0.75% solution of bupivacaine hydrochloride into the intercostal space of the incision and two interspaces above and below, as well as into the chest tube site.[10] The percutaneous injection is performed by placing a finger within the thorax to ensure proper needle placement. The syringe should be aspirated prior to each injection to prevent an inadvertent intravascular injection. The use of this solution reduces the postoperative analgesic requirement.

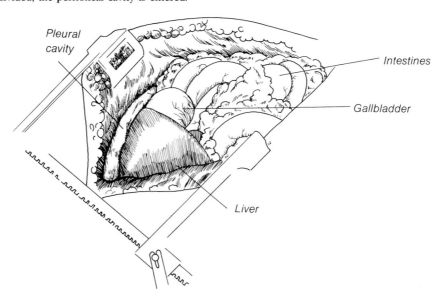

Pleural cavity

Intestines

Gallbladder

Liver

FIG. 5-5. Finochietto retractor is placed in the wound between the divided costal cartilage, exposing the abdominal contents.

POSTOPERATIVE CARE AND COMPLICATIONS

Postoperative care for radical nephrectomy is similar to that for most extensive surgical procedures. We observe the patient in the intensive care unit for at least 24 hours after the surgical procedure. The chest tube is connected to suction drainage for 24 hours or until significant drainage ceases and there is no evidence of an air leak. The tube is then connected to a water seal for four hours. An expiratory chest roentgenogram is obtained, and if there is no evidence of a pneumothorax the chest tube may be removed. If a possible air leak is still a significant concern after four hours of water seal, despite a negative chest roentgenogram, the tube may be clamped proximal to any connectors. Another chest roentgenogram should be taken in four hours. Under these circumstances, with a negative expiratory chest roentgenogram, one can be certain of a completely expanded lung with no air leak. As mentioned, postoperative pain can be significantly reduced by the routine employment of an intercostal nerve block. A nasogastric tube is left in place, and fluid intake is withheld until adequate bowel sounds are present and flatus is passed.

Some of the postoperative complications that may occur include secondary hemorrhage, pneumothorax, wound dehiscence, and intercostal neuralgia. Other less common complications include cerebral vascular accidents, precipitation of congestive heart failure, myocardial infarction, pulmonary embolus, atelectasis, and pneumonia. Proper selection of patients, adequate preoperative preparation, and good postoperative care and ambulation will prevent many of these problems.

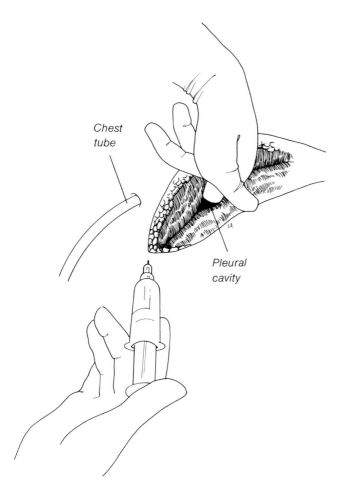

FIG. 5-6. Percutaneous injection of bupivacaine hydrochloride into the neurovascular bundle of the resected rib. Two interspaces above and below, as well as the chest tube site, are injected. The index finger is placed into the chest cavity to direct the position of the needle.

Closure

The diaphragm is closed in two layers (Fig. 5-7), the first layer consisting of interrupted 2-0 polyglactin (Vicryl) sutures, placed so that the knots are tied on the posterior surface of the diaphragm. A running 2-0 Vicryl suture is used on the pleural surface. The thoracic part of the incision is closed with interrupted figure-of-eight No. 1 Vicryl sutures through all the muscular layers of the chest wall (Fig. 5-8). It is important to include the diaphragm medially in the last one or two sutures. The sutures are then tied, starting with the most posterior stitch. The posterior rectus fascia and muscle layers are approximated with No. 0 Vicryl sutures. The previously placed thoracic sutures are secured and the subcutaneous tissue is approximated with 2-0 Vicryl sutures. The method of skin closure depends on the surgeon's preference.

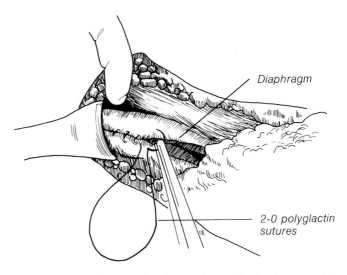

FIG. 5-7. The diaphragm is closed in two layers. The first layer consists of interrupted 2-0 polyglactin (Vicryl) sutures placed so that the knots are tied on the posterior surface of the diaphragm. A running 2-0 Vicryl suture is used on the pleural surface.

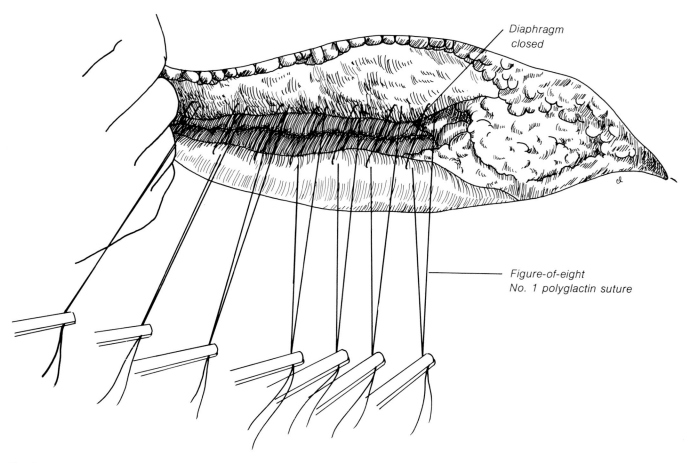

Diaphragm
closed

Figure-of-eight
No. 1 polyglactin suture

FIG. 5-8. Figure-of-eight No. 1 Vicryl sutures are placed through all muscular layers of the chest wall. It is important to include the diaphragm medially in the last one or two sutures. The sutures are not tied until all have been placed.

REFERENCES

1. SENNERT, D. *Medicinae Practicae.* Vol. 1. Venice, 1641.

2. GRAWITZ, P. A. Die Entstehung von Nierentumoren aus Nebennierengewebe, Verh, Disch. Ges. Chir., *13:*28, 1884.

3. MURPHY, L. J. T. Renal tumors. In: *The History of Urology.* Edited by L. J. T. Murphy. Springfield, Ill., Charles C Thomas, 1972.

4. SIMON, G. Exstirpation eine Niere an Menschen. Dtsch. Klin., *22:*137, 1870.

5. FEY, B. L'abord du rein par la voie thoraco-abdominale. Arch. Urol. Clin. Necker., *5:*169, 1926.

6. MARSHALL, D. F. Urogenital wounds in an evacuation hospital, J. Urol., *55:*119, 1946.

7. CRAWFORD, E. D., ROGERS, H. C., METTLER, F. A., and KLIMACH, W. Ultrasonic detection of renal tubular carcinoma extending into the inferior vena cava. J. Urol., *124:*538, 1980.

8. GOTTESMAN, J. E., CRAWFORD, E. D., GROSSMAN, H. B., et al. Infarction-nephrectomy for metastatic renal carcinoma. Southwest Oncology group study. Urology, *25:*248, 1985.

9. WETTLAUFER, J. N., KUMPE, D. A., and REDMOND, P. L. Preoperative ethanol renal embolization and planned delayed nephrectomy in select patients with poor risk renal cell carcinoma. Abstract No. 386. 84th Annual meeting of AUA, Dallas, May, 1989.

10. CRAWFORD, E. D., SKINNER, D. G., and CAPPARELL, D. B. Intercostal nerve block with thoracoabdominal incision. J. Urol., *121:*290, 1979.

CHAPTER
6

Radical Nephrectomy: Anterior Transabdominal Approach

Paul C. Peters

Radical nephrectomy is defined as the removal of the kidney and adrenal with surrounding Gerota's fascia intact, accompanied by removal of the ureter and ipsilateral gonadal vein to the level of the common iliac artery. In addition, we perform a regional lymphadenectomy from the crus of the diaphragm to the bifurcation of the common iliac artery on the ipsilateral side. Nodes anterior to the aorta and cava are removed at the level of the renal hilum.

PREPARATION OF THE PATIENT

Preparatory tests include cardiorespiratory evaluation, renal and liver function tests, and bone scan, and a preoperative detailed discussion with the patient of the variables that may be encountered within the abdomen, including the possibility of postoperative dialysis support when a solitary kidney is tumor-bearing. An abdominal CT is helpful to exclude metastatic disease, and magnetic resonance imaging and sonography are of particular help in evaluating extension into the venous system. Preoperative baseline electrolyte and blood gas determinations, hemogram, bleeding and clotting times, partial thromboplastin time, prothrombin time, platelet count, and bleeding time are also valuable. Typing and cross-matching for six units of blood should be completed prior to the surgical procedure.

We prefer to use angioinfarction prior to operation only in those patients in whom the tumor is large and crosses the midline. Until evidence from control studies demonstrates that angioinfarction performed several days before the procedure will enhance the immune response, we recommend performance of angioinfarction only a few hours prior to the procedure by the transfemoral approach.

The colon should be completely empty before the operation. This allows more room in the operative field, decreases the need for enemas and laxatives in the immediate postoperative period, and allows considerable flexibility in displacement of the colon for additional exposure needs. Evacuation of the colon may be accomplished by administration of a clear liquid diet for three days prior to operation or by the use of a one-hour cleaning technique described by Clayton.[1] Recently we have been using Colyte, which is a polyethylene glycol/sodium/potassium/salt solution containing the following ingredients:

polyethylene glycol 3350	227.1 g
sodium chloride	5.53 g
potassium chloride	2.82 g

sodium bicarbonate	6.63 g
sodium sulfate (anhydrous)	21.5 g

This solution is mixed to a volume of one gallon (3.785 liters) and the patient is instructed to drink it in 1½ hours. This amount completely cleanses the colon. For those individuals who cannot drink this volume in that short period of time, the material may be given by means of a nasogastric tube passed to the stomach. Antibiotic sterilization of the bowel with neomycin (1 g q. 1 hr × 4 and then 1 q. 4 hrs until n.p.o. for the surgical procedure), accompanied by erythromycin (1 g q. 6 hrs 24 hrs prior to operation) is a practical measure. Recently, we have switched to a protocol of 1 g of neomycin administered at 6:30 and 11:30 P.M., accompanied by 1 g of metronidazole (Flagyl) administered also at 6:30 and 11:30 P.M. (preferably after the colon has been cleansed by Colyte so that the antibiotic is not washed out with the voluminous amount of fluid in transit through the bowel).

SURGICAL PROCEDURE

The choice of incision for a transabdominal nephrectomy is determined by the patient's body habitus and by the position and mobility of the involved kidney. A vertical incision is preferred for the patient with a narrow subcostal arch. We usually use a transverse or chevron incision. An abdominal incision is employed for the patient who cannot tolerate the exaggerated flank position, and currently most of our radical nephrectomies are performed by a subcostal anterior transabdominal approach.

Incision

VERTICAL INCISION (Fig. 6-1). The patient is placed on the operating table in the supine position with the table slightly flexed to elevate the spine. The head of the table is elevated about 10° to encourage descent of the kidney. A vertical incision is made from the xiphoid to as far below the umbilicus as necessary, depending on the size and location of the neoplasm. The cranial portion of the incision may be extended lateral to the xiphoid to avoid injury to the internal mammary artery and to ensure adequate exposure of the kidney. The peritoneal cavity is entered in the midline in the upper part of the incision between the umbilicus and xiphoid, and the incision is extended with the intestines protected by an abdominal hand of the operator. The underlying liver is protected to prevent inadvertent injury of the gallbladder or intestinal contents. The ligamentum teres is identified, clamped, and divided before exploration of the peritoneal cavity, whether a vertical or transverse incision is used.

TRANSVERSE INCISION (Fig. 6-2). A transverse incision begins at the tip of the eleventh rib and is carried transversely, angling toward the xiphoid, across the abdomen, and into the rectus sheath of the opposite side for a distance of approximately 2 cm. The rectus muscles are divided and the peritoneal cavity is entered after division of the ligamentum teres. A thorough exploration of the abdominal cavity for metastatic disease is carried out at this time with palpation of the colon, liver, both kidneys, gallbladder, prostate, internal genitalia of the female, including ovaries and uterus, and colon. If no other disease is found, the operation proceeds forthwith.

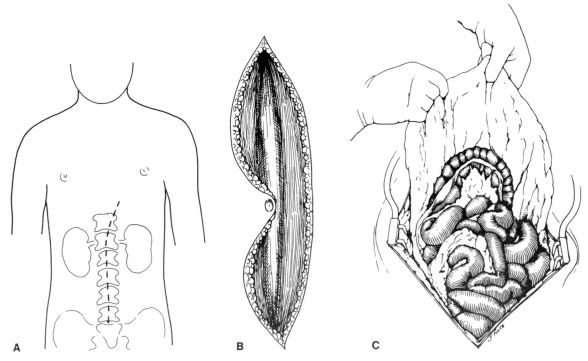

A   **B**   **C**

FIG. 6-1. *A*, Vertical midline approach showing the relationship of the incision to the kidneys. The cranial portion of the incision should be curved laterally to avoid injury to the internal mammary artery. *B*, Completed incision. *C*, Exposure of peritoneal contents.

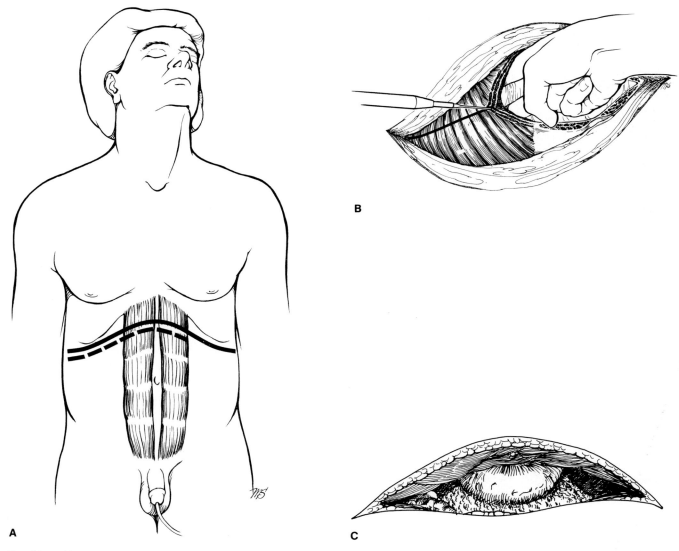

Fig. 6-2. *A,* Transverse abdominal incision between the tips of the eleventh ribs. *B,* Division of the external and internal oblique muscles with electrocautery. *C,* Exposure of the abdominal contents through a transverse incision.

Technique

A few points are emphasized in our technique for radical nephrectomy. Use of the Bookwalter retractor has negated the need for more than one assistant in most circumstances, has allowed the inclusion of retractors as needed to give excellent exposure, and has replaced the former use of multiple retractors and large superior retractors requiring great effort by an assistant. The Bookwalter retractor is also adjustable and may be changed in position. Retractors may be added or removed as needed during the procedure.

On the left side (Fig. 6-3), the posterior parietal peritoneal incision, made lateral to the colon after the abdomen is opened, is carried well above the splenic flexure. On large upper pole tumors, the incision may be carried around the splenic pedicles and superiorly and medially to the aorta near

its diaphragmatic hiatus. This allows safe medial retraction of the spleen and tail of the pancreas and gives excellent exposure for dissection of the renal artery and left adrenal gland.

Variables, such as the size of the tumor or extensive vascular invasion, may influence the method of handling the pedicle. Preoperative angioinfarction may help considerably by decreasing the volume of collateral circulation around the tumor, particularly in tumors that are large enough to cross the midline. It also offers the advantage of allowing the surgeon to ligate the renal vein before exposing the artery immediately beneath it, particularly when the renal vein is large and filled with tumor.

When the tumor has extended into the vena cava, control is obtained of all venous tributaries in the area, as well as the vena cava proximally and distally, prior to extraction of the tumor thrombus. The cava is mobilized proximally and distally

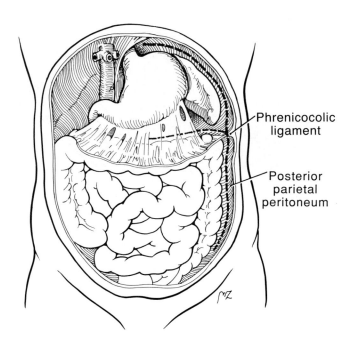

Phrenicocolic
ligament

Posterior
parietal
peritoneum

FIG. 6-3. Dotted line shows the extent of the incision in the posterior parietal peritoneum circumferentially around the splenic pedicle and continuing around the fundus of the stomach to a point near the esophageal hiatus.

to place vascular tapes around it so that angled vascular clamps may be used for temporary occlusion proximal and distal to the tumor thrombus. The entry point of the left renal vein must also be mobilized so that it can be temporarily occluded if a cavotomy is necessary.

In addition, the right gonadal vein should be divided between ligatures in right-sided tumors. On the right side, in addition, a large lumbar tributary commonly enters the cava posteriorly near the orifice of the renal vein. This tributary is ligated preferably at the time of proximal and distal mobilization of the inferior vena cava. By elevating the vascular tapes, one can reduce flow in the cava temporarily and can gently palpate the tumor thrombus to determine its extent. One can often milk it back into the renal vein so that a partial occlusion of the vena cava by a curved Satinsky or DeBakey vascular clamp will suffice to allow removal of the specimen with the thrombus included. The cava can be inspected to be certain there is no thrombus adherent to or invading the caval wall and can then be closed with a running 4-0 and 5-0 nonabsorbable polypropylene suture. In other circumstances, the tumor can be milked back below the diaphragm and removed via cavotomy with the cava and renal tributaries temporarily occluded as described earlier.

When the tumor extends into the heart, cardiac surgery consultants provide cardiac bypass or intrapericardial occlusion of the inferior vena cava, if necessary, for complete removal of tumor thrombus. This is dramatic surgery and does not often result in long-term survival. We advise thoracic sur-

gery consultation in such cases and recommend strongly that the operation be carried out in the room usually used for open heart surgery so that equipment needed by the thoracic surgeon in an urgent manner is readily available. When the inferior vena cava is extensively involved above and below the renal vein, it may be removed. On the left side, one may safely ligate the left renal vein in the case of a right-sided tumor, relying on established collateral branches and the gonadal and adrenal veins to effectively drain the left kidney. If the tumor has been obstructing the cava return for some time, good collateral drainage is usually present. When the right kidney is the one to be saved, autotransplantation or renal-portal anastomosis is suggested if the entire cava must be removed. One could consider an end-to-end superior anastomosis of the renal vein to the caval stump at the level of resection. Venous substitution prostheses are not recommended, as they tend to thrombose.

After one has controlled the artery and it has been divided between 0-silk ligatures and a suture ligature of 3-0 silk has been placed distal to the ligature on the artery, the vein can be treated in a similar manner if it has not been previously divided. The ureter is divided between 2-0 silk ligatures at the point where it crosses the common iliac artery. Gerota's fascia is then dissected. Clips and silk ligatures are used as necessary as one frees the superior attachments of Gerota's fascia from the diaphragm and from the posterior muscles of the abdomen and also as one clips or ligates any small adrenal branches that may be encountered. The kidney is then removed en bloc and nodes along the renal pedicle are dissected from the interaortocaval area from the crus of the diaphragm to the bifurcation of the common iliac artery on the ipsilateral side.

The therapeutic advantage of lymphadenectomy has yet to be demonstrated in a prospective randomized study. In a series of 352 cases from the Dallas hospitals, 16% of the patients having lymphadenectomy were classified as having stage C disease by the finding of positive nodes. These tumors would have been understaged had the lymphadenectomy not been performed. Six percent of those having the lymphadenectomy had microscopic nodal involvement only and these surely would have been missed. In addition, our data show a 25% 5-year survival for those who had positive nodes and a lymphadenectomy and only a 9% 5-year survival for those who had positive nodes without lymphadenectomy. We prefer to remove the gonadal vein as well on the ipsilateral side, although one infrequently finds microscopic involvement of this vessel.

On the left side, cases of renal cell carcinoma have been reported in which the tumor extended retrograde along the gonadal vein, manifest clinically by vaginal bleeding due to involvement of the apex of the vagina by metastatic disease. Figure 6-4 shows the extension of the incision in the posterior parietal peritoneum to the aortic hiatus of the diaphragm to allow one to mobilize the spleen and pancreas medially. The plane between Gerota's fascia and the peritoneum is easily defined in these cases to expose the pedicle prior to manipulation of the mass, as described previously.

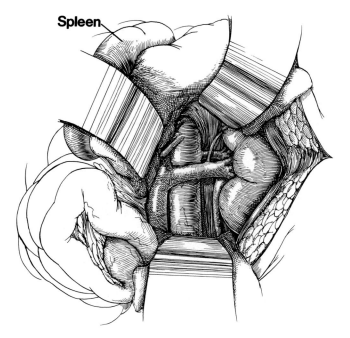

Spleen

Fig. 6-4. Exposure of the left kidney. Note the medial retraction of the spleen and tail of the pancreas. (Courtesy of William J. Fry, M.D.)

We do not utilize copious irrigation of the tumor bed. An effort has been made to reperitonealize the posterior parietal peritoneum in each case with a running 2-0 chromic gut suture, with care taken to place the sutures approximately 1 cm apart to prevent herniation of the bowel through the posterior parietal peritoneum in the postoperative course. No drains are used. A layered closure is completed with nonabsorbable sutures after hemostasis is secured by cautery and by ligation with silk sutures. Nasogastric suction and parenteral fluids are used until the passage of flatus is observed postoperatively.

REFERENCE

1. Clayton, R. S. A clean colon in one hour. Appl. Radiol., 9:69, 1980.

CHAPTER 7

Partial Nephrectomy, Extracorporeal Surgery, and Autotransplantation for Renal Cell Carcinoma

Steven M. Bernstein
Martin A. Koyle
Ruben F. Gittes

In the United States, approximately 20,000 new cases of renal cell carcinoma are diagnosed annually.[1] This frequency approximates that of ovarian, gastric, and pancreatic cancer, or all of the cases of leukemia combined.[1] For over two decades, radical nephrectomy has proved to be an efficacious therapy for localized renal cell carcinomas.[1] The early and often incidental diagnosis of this tumor is now possible because of the increased utilization and improvements in noninvasive imaging techniques.[2] Although radical nephrectomy remains the gold standard of therapy for most cases of renal cell carcinoma, the role of conservative therapy, that is partial nephrectomy, is presently evolving.

HISTORICAL PERSPECTIVE

The first partial nephrectomy was performed in 1884, by Wells, for removal of a perirenal fibrolipoma.[3] Although there was initial enthusiasm for this procedure in the late nineteenth century, the high complication and mortality rates limited its application.

Three subsequent contributions were particularly instrumental in the development of renal conserving therapy: renal angiography, renal allotransplantation, and renal preservation. In the middle of this century, Semb[4] and Puigvert[5] followed the original work of Seldinger and further clarified the selection factors and potential benefits of segmental nephrectomy. Although the fundamental techniques of renal transplantation and vascular surgery were initially described at the turn of the century by Alexis Carrel,[6] widespread practical use of such techniques awaited the first successful reports of renal allotransplantation from Boston and Paris in 1954. Autotransplantation and the concept of "bench surgery" for vascular and ureteral pathology were introduced 25 years ago for cases involving ureteral trauma.[7,8] Its use was later extended to include difficult cases involving renal stones and tumors, usually in the setting of a patient with a solitary kidney.[9]

INDICATIONS FOR PARTIAL NEPHRECTOMY

Renal Cell Carcinoma Involving Bilaterally or in a Solitary Kidney

In an effort to preserve as much functioning renal tissue as possible, partial nephrectomy is indicated for selected cases of renal cell carcinoma, specifically those with bilateral disease or those with tumor in a solitary kidney (Fig. 7-1). Many

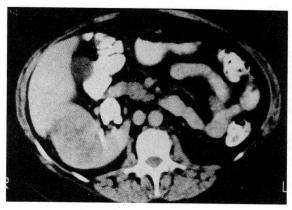

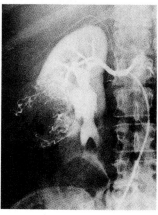

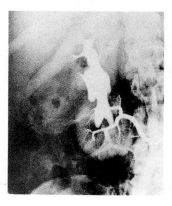

FIG. 7-1. A 63-year-old woman who previously had her left kidney removed for benign disease (infection) presented for evaluation of fevers. A CT scan demonstrated a large mass in the midportion of her solitary right kidney (A). Angiography (B&C) demonstrated separate major renal arteries to the upper and lower poles, suggesting that partial nephrectomy was feasible. (CT scans and angiograms courtesy of LTI Medica® and Bristol-Myers Company. Copyright 1986 by Learning Technology Incorporated.)

groups have shown that stage-I disease can be surgically well controlled in patients with solitary kidneys, with a local recurrence rate of about 10%.[10–19] Smith from UCLA and Zincke from the Mayo Clinic have reported 5-year survivals of 72% and greater than 85% respectively, in patients surgically treated for bilateral renal cell carcinoma or tumor in a solitary kidney when non-renal causes of death were excluded.[15,19]

Renal cell carcinoma is bilateral in 1 to 2% of cases, and this occurrence is divided equally between synchronous and asynchronous lesions. It was once thought that the presence of synchronous bilateral tumors inferred a worse prognosis. In 1980, however, Jacobs showed that these patients did as well as those with unilateral disease when patients with equivalent stages were compared.[11] The Mayo Clinic and the Cleveland Clinic have both reported 5-year survival rates of close to 80% in patients with synchronous bilateral renal cell carcinomas.[17,18] Of patients with Von Hippel-Lindau disease, 35 to 40% will develop renal cell carcinoma and the majority of these will have bilateral, recurrent tumors. Because many of these tumors occur within the wall of an otherwise benign-appearing renal cyst, there is no way to determine their identity other than by surgical excision and histopathologic examination. Therefore, all patients with von Hippel-Lindau disease who undergo partial nephrectomy or enucleation for renal cell carcinoma should also have all other solid and cystic renal lesions excised in order to ensure complete tumor extirpation. Partial nephrectomy is often technically demanding in these patients but the net results are clearly superior to earlier procedures which often entailed bilateral radical nephrectomy with subsequent dialysis and allotransplantation.[20]

We recommend approaching bilateral partial nephrectomy with staged procedures.[21] Staging allows one partial nephrectomy to be performed first and, after a satisfactory surgical result is assured, the contralateral kidney may be approached more safely. (Fig. 7-2). This approach minimizes the potential need for temporary dialysis should acute tubular necrosis occur if both kidneys were treated at one sitting. If one of the involved kidneys is extensively replaced by tumor, a radical nephrectomy on that side with contralateral partial nephrectomy is indicated. Conversely, if one of the kidneys contains only a very small tumor burden, both kidneys may be safely approached and bilateral procedures performed at the same procedure.[21]

Renal Cell Carcinoma in Patients with a Compromised Contralateral Kidney

This group includes patients with contralateral kidneys compromised by calculus disease, diabetes, glomerulonephritis, pyelonephritis, significant atrophy, ureteropelvic junction obstruction, hydronephrosis, and renal arterial disease. These processes may be progressive and result in chronic renal failure. In practice, it would therefore seem logical to make every effort to preserve as many nephrons as possible in an attempt

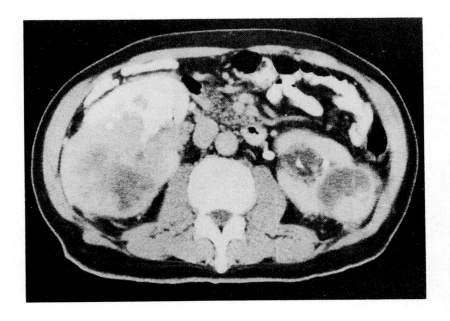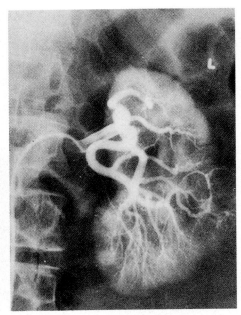

Fig. 7-2. A 68-year-old man developed right flank and upper quadrant pain, weight loss, and anorexia. The CT scan (A) revealed a large right renal tumor and a smaller tumor on the left. A right radical nephrectomy was performed. Selective angiography of the left kidney confirmed a midportion 5 cm tumor, amenable to renal-sparing surgery. (CT scans and angiograms courtesy of LTI Medica® and Bristol-Myers Company. Copyright 1986 by Learning Technology Incorporated.)

to delay or prevent dialysis and transplantation without jeopardizing the effectiveness of the cancer operation.

Transitional Cell Tumors of the Kidney

For almost all patients with transitional cell carcinoma of the upper urinary tract, radical nephroureterectomy with excision of a bladder cuff is the preferred treatment. Newer information, however, has shown that urothelial tumors have widely varying biologic behavior. Favorable results have subsequently been reported after more conservative management of certain carefully selected ureteral and renal pelvic tumors.[22,23,69–71]

Most authors presently recommend conservative surgery in patients with transitional cell tumors in the ureter or renal pelvis in the case of a solitary kidney, in patients with unilateral tumors and renal insufficiency, in those with bilateral upper tract tumors, and in patients with tumors associated with Balkan nephropathy.[24] The controversy exists over proper treatment of the unilateral, low-grade, low-stage urothelial tumors in the presence of a normal contralateral kidney. The Mayo Clinic has reported that the location of the tumor may play an important role in the success of conservative therapy, as patients with ureteral tumors did significantly better than those with renal pelvic tumors.[25] With continued refinements in imaging, cytodiagnostics, chemotherapy, and particularly in endourology, patients at lower risk for disease recurrence may be identified and treated conservatively in a manner analogous to bladder cancer.

Wilms' Tumor

Unlike renal cell and transitional cell carcinomas. Wilms' tumor is exquisitely sensitive to chemotherapy, particularly in those cases of favorable histology. Bilateral lesions, in particular, have proved to be amenable to secondary partial nephrectomy after initial biopsies and the institution of appropriate chemotherapy.

Partial nephrectomy might also be indicated for selected cases of unilateral Wilms' tumor after successful chemotherapy.[26] The theoretical advantage of leaving more functioning nephrons and minimizing the potential impairment of renal function must be weighed against the possibility of leaving islets of neoplastic tissue in the remaining parenchyma. This approach might be most feasible in cases where a small tumor is localized to a single pole, where there is sharp demarcation between the neoplastic and normal parenchyma, and where the capsule, vessels, and nodes are not grossly involved. To date, however, the question of chemotherapy combined with partial nephrectomy has not been addressed by the National Wilms' Tumor Study. Until a large body of experience reports success for this "conservative" surgery, nephrectomy remains the therapy of choice in cases of unilateral disease.

Polar Mass of Uncertain Nature

When all standard imaging modalities have failed to elucidate the nature of a renal mass, a tentative partial nephrectomy may

be indicated for the purpose of excisional biopsy and frozen-section evaluation. Because carcinoma remains a more common diagnostic entity than other mass lesions (oncocytoma, multilocular cyst, and angiomyolipoma), even the smallest suggestion of carcinoma usually leads to more radical extirpation.

Progress in the area of noninvasive imaging (ultrasonography, computed tomography, and MRI) has had a profound impact upon the diagnosis of renal cell carcinoma and other solid renal mass lesions. Small, solid renal tumors are now commonly identified incidentally during diagnostic examinations performed for nonrenal complaints.[2] These asymptomatic lesions represent a new, distinct therapeutic challenge. Usually of low grade and stage, these tumors may be associated with a much more favorable prognosis than those tumors found during evaluation of renal complaints. It has yet to be determined if a procedure less aggressive than radical nephrectomy will result in equally good survival.[10]

Lieber has reported that oncocytomas, once considered a rare entity, indeed represent 3 to 5% of renal cell carcinomas.[72] The preoperative diagnosis of oncocytoma is often difficult and may require fine-needle aspiration, particularly in the case of bilateral, large, asymptomatic lesions. Even though they may present as multifocal, bilateral lesions, they virtually always behave in a benign fashion and parenchymal-sparing surgery is therefore indicated.

Non-cancer Indications

Renal-sparing surgery is occasionally indicated in the absence of cancer. This includes congenital anomalies such as duplication, atrophy secondary to obstruction, granulomatous disease with localized scarring, excision of benign renin-secreting tumors, localized renal infarction secondary to trauma, localized chronic inflammatory processes such as an abscess with an organized wall, solitary renal stone in a scarred renal pole, and the rare unilateral essential hematuria where an identifiable cause is responsible for episodic hemorrhage.

THE CONTROVERSIES

Renal Cell Carcinoma in Patients with a Normal Contralateral Kidney

Since 1960, radical nephrectomy has been accepted as the treatment of choice for patients with unilateral localized renal cell carcinoma and a normal contralateral kidney.[1] This approach has recently been challenged based on the results of partial nephrectomy in bilateral disease and in patients with solitary kidneys.[10–19] The premise for this approach is that renal cell carcinoma is a localized process and that the uninvolved renal tissue should be spared if surgically possible. The benefit of sparing nephrons is presently being weighed against the risks of increased operative time, increased surgical risk, and the risk of leaving behind residual disease. The suggestion

that the loss of a critical mass of renal tissue is associated with albuminuria, hypertension, and progressive renal dysfunction in the animal model has yet to be proven in humans and therefore cannot be considered an indication for nephron-sparing surgery at present.[27,28]

In favor of partial nephrectomy for renal cell carcinoma, several studies have reported results comparable to those treated with radical nephrectomy. The European Intrarenal Surgical Society reported a 5-year survival rate of 78% for patients with unilateral disease.[12] The Cleveland Clinic has reported an overall survival rate of 60%.[17] Their experience of 23 patients included no operative deaths, the development of urinary fistulae in 3 patients, and acute tubular necrosis necessitating interim dialysis in 2 patients. In a later followup to this early experience, the Cleveland group conceded that the long-term benefits of nephron-sparing surgery have yet to be convincingly proven.[13] They concluded that partial nephrectomy should presently be limited to patients in whom preservation of functioning renal parenchyma is a "relevant clinical consideration," such as those listed earlier, and that radical nephrectomy should be considered the standard of care for all other cases of renal cell carcinoma.

Mukamel et al. have argued against the practice of partial nephrectomy for small, localized lesions.[29] This is based on a study that demonstrated the multifocal nature of renal cell carcinoma. Of 66 kidneys with small, well-defined renal cell carcinoma, 20% were found to contain small nodules of carcinoma that were not contiguous with the primary lesion. These incidental lesions ranged in size from 1 to 15 mm, however, and their clinical significance is therefore questionable. It is possible that some of these lesions, particularly the larger ones, might harbor malignant potential if left behind by partial nephrectomy.

At the present time, radical nephrectomy remains the standard therapy for unilateral renal cell carcinoma in face of a normal contralateral kidney, until sufficient series documenting the long-term results of partial versus radical nephrectomy for similarly matched patients with unilateral renal cell carcinomas are reported.

Does Enucleation Have a Role in Renal Cell Carcinoma?

Despite recent reports condoning enucleation for small, low grade, round lesions in order to minimize blood loss and maximize remaining renal tissue,[18,30–33] the reliability of enucleation has not been proven. Smith reported three cases of local recurrence after enucleation and attributes them to microinvasion of tumor cells into the tumor capsule.[15] Careful microscopic examination by Marshall and others have also shown that enucleation would fail to allow an adequate margin to eliminate the tumor in many cases.[34] Novick's results with 100 patients from the Cleveland Clinic strongly supports this concept by showing that only 2 of 9 patients with local recurrence were alive with renal function and cancer free. An exception to this rule is the patient with von Hippel-Lindau disease, in whom the tumors tend to be bilateral, recurrent and particularly well-circumscribed. Simple enucleation has been performed with excellent results in this select group of patients.[35,36] Marberger has suggested that enucleation can be safely performed in any patient with tumors less than 7 cm in diameter, with partial nephrectomy reserved for larger tumors. Thus, the role of enucleation continues to remain a controversial issue.

PREOPERATIVE PREPARATION

The extent of tumor burden must be determined as precisely as possible before the operation can be planned. Accurate staging may be performed using information gleaned from a combination of CT scanning, MRI scanning, and ultrasound. Angiograms, including oblique views, are essential to the planning of partial nephrectomy in all but the simplest of cases. These studies facilitate dissection of the renal arterial tree and tumor removal and minimize operative blood loss and damage to the adjacent parenchyma. Digital subraction angiography is not felt to provide sufficient information to warrant its routine substitution for selective renal angiography at the present time.[21]

In addition to the usual preoperative care, the patient should receive aggressive preoperative hydration in order to assure appropriate renal perfusion. Five percent dextrose in half normal saline should be infused at a rate between 100 and 200 ml per hour for at least 12 hours prior to the induction of anesthesia.[37] Once the patient is anesthetized, a Foley catheter is placed to avoid overdistention of the bladder, to prevent back-pressure in the collecting system, and to facilitate postoperative fluid management. A central venous pressure line is placed in most patients, except those with cardiopulmonary compromise for whom a Swan-Ganz catheter is preferable. Consideration should also be given to arterial access for accurate pressure monitoring throughout the procedure and into the postoperative period. An appropriate prophylactic antimicrobial is administered prior to the skin incision.

INTRAOPERATIVE PROTECTION AGAINST ISCHEMIA

Maintenance of stable blood pressure throughout the case is requisite to optimal perfusion of the renal bed. Renal arterial spasm associated with dissection is potentiated by hypovolemia and hypotension. Blood pressure should be maintained primarily by the instillation of volume and secondarily with the judicious use of renal enhancing doses of pressor agents such as dopamine, when necessary.

Although controversy exists as to the benefit of anticoagulation, the general consensus condones its use in adults to help prevent the occasional disaster of intravascular thrombosis following inadvertent intimal injury.[37] Heparin is administered intravenously as a 5000 unit bolus prior to clamping the pedicle and is generally not reversed, thereby extending its effect

throughout the operation. Although this practice may result in some additional bleeding, its use is currently felt to be justified in the adult patient. Because of the smaller potential benefit in children and young adults, however, heparin is not routinely used in these patients.

Intraoperative diuretics are also routinely used just prior to clamping the renal vessels, as their protective effect against the acute tubular necrosis of ischemia and pigment nephritis has been clearly demonstrated. Mannitol is given intravenously as a 12.5 to 25 gm bolus to increase renal plasma flow, reduce interstitial edema after clamping, and possibly to protect against intratubular protein-plugging.

RENAL PRESERVATION

History of Renal Preservation

When surgery requires arterial occlusion for longer than 30 minutes, protection from ischemic renal injury is necessary in order to prevent permanent damage. The simplest and most practical methods of preservation are based on principles of local hypothermia to minimize cellular metabolic activity and ischemic damage.

Fifty years ago, Bickford was able to show that hypothermia induced by surface cooling exerted a protective effect against relatively short periods of renal ischemia.[38] Lyman subsequently demonstrated that hypothermia of 4 to 6°C in the hibernating hamster greatly reduced oxygen consumption.[39] More recently, Ward has shown that 15°C is the optimal temperature for preserving renal function during short periods of ischemia.[40] This degree of hypothermia also increases the oxygen solubility, thereby reducing the net oxygen requirement and allowing the use of an asanguineous perfusate. A side-effect of this severe hypothermia, however, is inactivation of the cell-wall sodium-potassium pump. This allows an influx of sodium into the cells with cellular swelling and the efflux of potassium. Perfusate solutions containing hyperosmotic concentrations of potassium and magnesium have been developed to help prevent this intracellular potassium loss. Osmotic agents, including glucose and mannitol, have also been added to these preparations to attempt to minimize pump inactivation and cellular swelling.

Renal cortical levels of adenosine triphosphate (ATP) have been shown to drop precipitously within 1 minute of renal artery cross-clamping.[73] Cortical energy delivery after 1 minute of ischemia has been shown to be on the order of one-half that of pre-ischemic levels.[41] When this marked energy loss is combined with the large obligatory loss incurred during the period of warm ischemia, the importance of energy preservation can be appreciated.

Initial perfusion solutions were based on the composition of blood products. In 1963, Humphries successfully preserved the canine kidney for 24 hours using extracorporeal hypothermic perfusion with a dilute serum preparation.[42] Subsequently, Belzer was able to preserve the canine kidney for 72 hours using a hypothermic pulsatile perfusion apparatus and cryoprecipitated plasma.[43] This development allowed for the consistently successful long-term (>24 hours) preservation of human kidneys for allotransplantation. Subsequent perfusates included other blood-like products including plasma protein fraction.[44,45]

Attention has also been turned to surface cooling, which offers the potential advantages of technical simplicity and cost-effectiveness. Early flushing solutions contained electrolyte compositions similar to extracellular fluid and allowed reliable preservation for up to 5 hours. After the nature of sodium-potassium pump inactivation was understood, Collins introduced a flushing solution containing an electrolyte composition more similar to that of intracellular fluid and was able to preserve the canine kidney for 24 hours.[46] The composition of Collins' solution and others based on the electrolyte composition of intracellular fluids, such as Sach's solution, have undergone continuing refinement.

Physiology of Renal Ischemia

The initiating event that leads to cellular destruction is inactivation of the sodium-potassium pump. This decreases the membrane electrical potential, causing increased membrane permeability.[42] Calcium has been shown to rapidly cross these "debilitated" membranes and manifest its toxic effects in two significant ways. Excess intracellular calcium inactivates the cell wall phospholipases, which contributes to the destruction of the cell wall and further increases its permeability. As the intracellular levels continue to increase, calcium begins to diffuse into the mitochondria, where it causes disruption of respiration with an attendant decrease in cellular energy production and an increase in free radical production. The free radicals then act in conjunction with the excess calcium to further the mitochondrial injury and reduce cellular respiration.[48]

Recent work has suggested the importance of oxygen toxicity as a major limiting factor in organ preservation.[49,50] This toxicity appears to act by irreversibly modifying protein structures and lipid components as well as contributing to mitochondrial injury and inhibiting cellular energy production. Reducing agents, such as reduced glutathione, have been added to some perfusate solutions in an attempt to alter the oxidation-reduction potential and thereby minimize oxidative injury. Jellinek has attempted to more carefully characterize the role of the oxidation-reduction potential by subjecting the isolated, in vivo canine kidney to perfusion solutions with a range of redox potentials.[50] The redox potential was monitored by an electrochemical cell and adjusted by the addition of an equimolar mixture of ascorbic acid and glutathione. Animal survival and renal function (based on serum creatinine) were evaluated over time. Perfusion solutions balanced to a redox potential of −17.0 mV had superior function, with function deteriorating as variance increased from this point. This suggests that more careful control of the redox potential may allow for improved short-term survival as well as prolonging the period of organ viability.

The area of reperfusion injury has also become more fully understood, and free radicals are again implicated as potential toxic mediators. During periods of ischemia, ATP regeneration is limited and hypoxanthine accumulates. Upon reperfusion or when oxygen is supplied the enzyme xanthine oxidase is activated. Once activated, this enzyme converts hypoxanthine to xanthine and an oxygen free radical is generated. The restoration of blood flow is therefore potentially injurious in a manner quite similar to that of ischemia. Although both processes result in the production of oxygen free radicals, they are produced via different paths; ischemia acts primarily by disruption of the mitochondrial respiratory mechanism, and reperfusion acts through the degradation of high energy phosphate compounds. The oxygen-free radicals then appear to directly attack the cellular membrane, resulting in eventual cellular demise.[51]

Pharmacologic Management of Renal Ischemia

Mannitol has been shown to have a protective effect in renal ischemia.[52] This effect appears to act through a myriad of mechanisms, including its properties as a free hydroxyl scavenger and its ability to prevent cell swelling, flush the tubule of cellular debris, preserve renal blood flow, and arrest mitochondrial calcium accumulation.[52]

Because free radicals are generated during reperfusion by the conversion of hypoxanthine to xanthine, it seems reasonable that inhibition of this process would result in a decrease in free-radical production and improved post-ischemic renal function. Allopurinol, a xanthine oxidase inhibitor, has been shown to improve renal blood flow after ischemia in some settings.[53] Rats receiving allopurinol prior to renal ischemia have been shown to experience a smaller increase in serum creatinine and a more rapid return to normal renal function than control rats.[54]

Naturally-occurring, free-radical scavengers such as glutathione, are also being evaluated. Although an effective scavenger, glutathione appears to be overwhelmed and unable to protect the animal during periods of excess free-radical production. Superoxide dismutase is another effective free-radical scavenger and has also been shown to afford ischemic protection. When administered after the ischemic event, animals treated with superoxide dismutase have been shown to experience a significantly attenuated rise in serum creatinine and a more rapid return to baseline renal function.[54]

Calcium channel blockers are known to impede the entry of calcium into the cell by interfering with the voltage-dependent calcium channel transport mechanism and have, therefore, been considered in an attempt to limit the calcium influx into the ischemic renal cell. In particular, verapamil has been shown to elicit significant vasodilatation and diuresis when infused into the renal artery.[55-57] This ability to inhibit smooth muscle vascular spasm and establish a diuresis in the ischemic kidney appears to be similar to that of mannitol and has been shown to be equally effective in some cases.[58] Further work is presently needed to more precisely delineate the mechanism of action and the therapeutic role of calcium channel blockers in renal ischemia.

Energy-providing compounds have been studied in an attempt to diminish the effects of warm ischemia on the kidney. Of these, the most promising appears to be ATP-magnesium chloride. Although its mechanism has not been fully elucidated, it may act via vasodilator prostaglandins and by decreasing the metabolism of adenine, which reduces adenosine, a vasoconstrictor. Animals treated with this compound have been shown to recover renal function much more rapidly than control animals or those given dopamine or phenoxybenzamine.[59,60] As our understanding of the physiology of renal ischemia continues to improve, so does the potential of improving renal preservation.

In Situ Preservation

Surface cooling is usually adequate for partial nephrectomy. In 1975, Boyce described a simple and safe technique that allows successful preservation up to 120 minutes. Mannitol is administered prior to dissecting the renal vasculature. After the kidney is mobilized and isolated with a plastic sheet of Lahey bag, 5000 units of heparin is administered and the renal artery is clamped. A supercooled solution of normal saline or lactated Ringer's solution is then poured around the isolated kidney. Covering the kidney with ice slush for ten minutes after renal artery occlusion ensures that the kidney will be adequately cooled to 15°C (Fig. 7-3). Precooling in this manner affords important protection during the unavoidable periods when it must be temporarily lifted out of the ice slush. The deleterious effects of rapid rewarming and subsequent ischemic renal injury must be stressed and every effort should be made to keep all renal tissue submerged in the ice slush as much as possible throughout the procedure.

Iced solution is repeatedly poured to replace the melted solution and care is taken to minimize the amount of slush that enters the body cavity by keeping a pool suction tube in the plastic sheet or Lahey bag at all times. Dangerous cardiac dysrythmias have resulted from the sudden cooling of venous return and from transmural direct cooling of the heart across the pericardium. This straightforward technique has been widely accepted and obviates the need for continuous monitoring of renal core temperature and heat exchange coils. Intermittent unclamping of the renal artery for short periods of recirculation should be avoided, as it has been shown to be more damaging than beneficial.[61] In cases requiring renal ischemia for prolonged periods (>90 minutes), a Swan-Ganz catheter may be introduced into the renal artery to allow for more reliable intraparenchymal cooling. A venotomy is then made to allow for the egress of fluid. Other, more complex methods of in situ renal hypothermia involve plastic pouch perfusion and the use of advanced cooling coils. Although these systems also allow preservation of up to 3 hours, they are considerably more complex to use and in most cases their use is not necessary.

Extracorporeal Preservation

When extracorporeal partial nephrectomy was first performed, the preservation techniques were adapted from those used for renal allotransplantation. This utilized continuous pulsitile perfusion with two separate batches of cryoprecipitated, filtered plasma (one before, and one after excision of tumor cells) and a cumbersome workbench. It also required cannulation of the artery or vein, which can be potentially dangerous. Preservation can be more simply accomplished by flushing the kidney with cold Collins' solution and maintaining hypothermia by immersing the kidney in a bowl of iced saline. This combination of renal flushing followed by surface cooling is presently used by most transplant surgeons and has been shown to provide ex vivo protection for greater than 48 hours.

In the operating room, the flushing solution is prepared no more than 20 minutes prior to use. This is connected to standard sterile intravenous tubing which will subsequently be used to cannulate the kidney. The radical nephrectomy is then performed except that an attempt is made to keep the ureter intact. A small Heifitz or non-crushing Bulldog clamp is placed on the ureter to prevent retrograde flow into the kidney. After the excised kidney is placed in a basin of iced saline, the renal artery is cannulated with the IV tubing or with a smaller adaptor in the case of multiple renal arteries. The kidney is then flushed under gravity flow until the venous effluent is clear and the entire kidney is pale and cold. Gentle massage of the renal surface during flushing facilitates this process. Resection

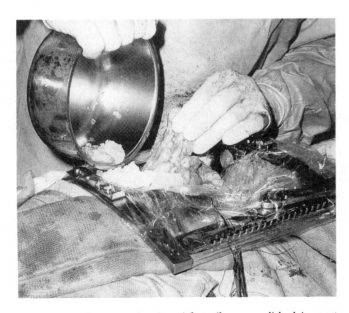

FIG. 7-3. Renal preservation is satisfactorily accomplished in most cases of partial nephrectomy using surface cooling methods. After the kidney is mobilized, it is wrapped in a Lahey bag and covered with iced slush. (Surgical photography by Lester V. Bergman courtesy LTI Medica® and Bristol-Myers Company. Copyright 1986 by Learning Technology Incorporated.)

of the tumor is begun once the kidney is uniformly pale. Reflushing can later be used to distend the vessels to facilitate both vascular dissection and hemostasis at the termination of the procedure.

OPERATIVE APPROACH

In Situ versus Extracorporeal Resection

Partial nephrectomy can be performed in situ in virtually all cases. Extracorporeal tumor resection, "Bench Surgery," followed by autotransplantation, is reserved for the rare, large, hypervascular, centrally placed tumors, including those involving the hilar structures. Novick reported a significantly higher incidence of acute tubular necrosis and the need for temporary dialysis in those patients undergoing bench surgery compared to those treated with in situ partial extirpation.[13] They attribute this not only to the profound ischemic insult but also to the fact that a larger mass of tissue is usually removed. This finding amplifies the fact that appropriate dialysis and monitoring should be available in centers where patients undergo such surgery. Of particular note in Novick's experience are the similar rates of survival and tumor recurrence observed in the ex vivo and in vivo treated groups.

The surgical approach to patients with bilateral lesions is less well-defined. Bilateral synchronous tumors may be treated with bilateral partial nephrectomies or radical nephrectomy and contralateral partial nephrectomy. At exploration, some patients will be found to have more extensive disease than anticipated and partial nephrectomy will thus be technically unfeasible. Thus, all patients should be advised that they may require bilateral radical nephrectomies and may be placed on dialysis. If these patients survive a minimum of 12 months (preferably 24 months) without evidence of metastatic disease, they may be considered candidates for renal transplantation. In limited worldwide experience with transplantation after bilateral nephrectomies for renal cell carcinoma, survival appears to be better in the setting of synchronous tumors.[20,62]

IN SITU PARTIAL NEPHRECTOMY

Surgical principles for in situ partial nephrectomy for renal adenocarcinoma include excision of all Gerota's fascia with perinephric fat, resection of regional lymphatics and lymph nodes, wound exclusion with a barrier, and wound irrigation with distilled water (Fig. 7-4). Especially small, well-encapsulated peripheral lesions may occasionally be excised in less than 30 minutes and vascular occlusion and hypothermia may, therefore, not be necessary in these exceptional cases. For larger, less accessible tumors requiring longer operative time, the renal pedicle must be occluded, and renal cooling is employed. The procedure itself may be divided into four sequential steps: exposure and vascular control, renal preservation, tumor resection, and renal reconstruction. As in other exten-

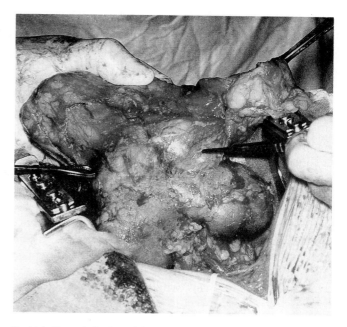

FIG. 7-4. Gerota's fascia and the perinephric fat have been dissected off the normal renal portion but will be removed with the segmental nephrectomy specimen. (Surgical photography by Lester V. Bergman courtesy of LTI Medica® and Bristol-Myers Company. Copyright 1986 by Learning Technology Incorporated.)

sive surgical procedures, exposure and vascular control are the mainstays of a successful operation.

Incision

The incision to be used should take several factors into account. The patients' body habitus, history of prior renal surgery, and tumor location are important considerations, as is the surgeon's personal preference and experience. The thoracoabdominal incision offers excellent exposure of the upper pole as well as allowing the possibility of simultaneous lung biopsy if necessary. Because it is time-consuming to open and close, however, it is best reserved for large upper pole tumors. The anterior transperitoneal approach may be preferable for patients who require bilateral renal surgery, who have had previous renal surgery through the flank, or who may need radical nephrectomy with extracorporeal surgery and autotransplantation. The anterior subcostal transperitoneal incision offers good exposure of the kidney and its vasculature, and may be easily extended as a chevron when necessary to expose tumors found on the contralateral side. The eleventh rib may be used as a landmark and generous anterior extension may be achieved to obtain excellent exposure. Some surgeons avoid the anterior incision in obese patients, however, suggesting that the kidney is often too deep in the wound to allow adequate exposure and access. Such an incision is useful in the patient who will require bench surgery. A second hockey-stick incision is made in the ipsilateral lower quadrant for autotransplantation. In most cases, we advocate an extraperitoneal or transperitoneal flank incision through the bed of the eleventh rib. An incision at this level allows the surgeon to operate on the mobilized kidney virtually at skin level and provides excellent exposure of the peripheral renal vessels.

Exposure

In partial nephrectomy, unlike radical nephrectomy, the kidney must be seperated from Gerota's fascia except for the area directly over the tumor. This is necessary to accurately determine the line of resection and to inspect the renal surface for palpable tumor spread. Gerota's fascia is then incised in the midlateral plane of the kidney, beginning at the superior pole and proceeding inferiorly. The perirenal fat around the tumor is left undisturbed. Hemostasis of the small vessels may be achieved with vascular clips. Mobilization is also started at the upper pole and blunt dissection is used to completely free up the kidney and deliver it through the wound.

The ipsilateral renal vessels and ureter are isolated with vascular tape. The great vessels are then controlled in a similar fashion. At this time, the surgeon must confirm his preoperative findings and elect to proceed with the most appropriate surgical plan. Vasospasm may be reduced by returning the kidney to its bed and optimizing systemic blood pressure. Topical papaverine or lidocaine may also be of some use when such vasospasm is encountered. The need to clamp the renal pedicle or artery must be carefully considered at this point. Although the pedicle must always be mobilized and accessible for immediate control, the requirement for clamping depends on the resection to be performed. For peripheral lesions, such as the tip of the upper or lower pole, occlusion of the pedicle is not always necessary. Identification of the branch vessels on preoperative angiogram allows the accurate control of main feeder vessels and may obviate the need to clamp the main renal artery.

If the renal artery is to be clamped, extreme care should be exercised to minimize the risk of vascular injury, particularly to the delicate intima. A long bulldog clamp with vascular teeth or a full-length clamp of the Satinsky type may be chosen. The clamp selected should first be tested by clamping the thenar web to estimate the degree of occlusion. Two gentle clamps in series are better than one single clamp applied too tightly. Clamping the renal artery together with the vein will further help to cushion the jaws, although we prefer to control the renal vein separately with a Rummel tourniquet (Fig. 7-5).

The optimum material for hemostasis within the kidney is another matter of discussion. Some surgeons prefer to use silk or metal clips to control intraparenchymal vessels, others prefer absorbable suture material.[63] The argument against nonabsorbable material is based on the knowledge that some degree of urinary extravasation frequently occurs and that permanent material can serve as a nidus for infection and stone formation or lead to the development of a urocutaneous fistula.

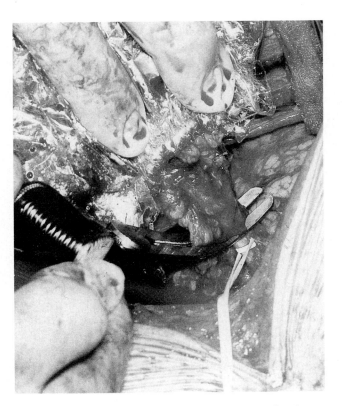

FIG. 7-5. A noncrushing vascular bulldog clamp has been placed across both renal artery and vein. (Surgical photography by Lester V. Bergman courtesy of LTI Medica® and Bristol-Myers Company. Copyright 1986 by Learning Technology Incorporated.)

Urine output should be continuously monitored as an index of effective renal perfusion. Mannitol is given as an intravenous bolus to promote a brisk diuresis prior to mobilization of the vessels. Once the diuresis has begun, the renal entry may be safely clamped. The kidney is brought up into the operative field and surrounded by a sterile sheet of plastic or a Lahey bag. The ice slush is then poured.

Excision of Polar Lesions

Several important points regarding polar lesions should be kept in mind. Preoperative arteriography must be obtained and studied in these cases because of the frequent occurrence of a main arterial branch that arches upward into the renal hilum before descending into the middle or lower parts of the kidney. In the best of circumstances, a segmental artery branch supplying the tumor can be identified preoperatively by angiography. Intraoperatively, this branch can then be isolated and injected with indigo carmine in order to stain the corresponding renal segment blue (Fig. 7-6). If the tumor is indeed located within such a segment, the vessel may be safely sacrificed. This maneuver avoids the necessity of clamping the main renal artery and rendering the entire kidney ischemic.

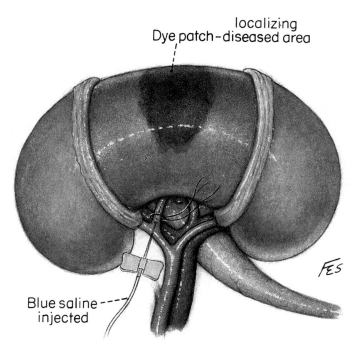

localizing
Dye patch-diseased area

Blue saline
injected

F̄ES

FIG. 7-6. The injection of a segmental vessel with dilute indigo carmine stains the corresponding renal segment and allows vessels to be sacrificed appropriately and safely. (From Gittes, R. F. In *Reconstructive Urologic Surgery: Pediatric and Adult.* Edited by E. J. Libertino and L. A. Zinman. Baltimore, Williams & Wilkins, 1977.)

Some polar lesions located in an extreme peripheral location and lacking involvement of the collecting system may be excised using a variety of techniques not requiring total renal ischemia. In some cases, simple compression of the kidney between an assistants' fingers may afford enough segmental ischemia to allow that portion of the kidney to be incised with minimal bleeding. Alternatively, partial nephrectomy clamps and tourniquets have been designed to provide more reliable and less physically tiring vascular control.[64,65] A 2-cm margin should be observed around all tumors. For lower pole lesions, the upper pole is separated from the adrenal gland leaving the gland in its fatty bed. For upper pole lesions, the peripheral margin should not be compromised by efforts to save the ipsilateral adrenal gland.

Polar lesions can be excised in one of two manners, by wedge resection or guillotine amputation. In either case, the kidney and the ureter are mobilized and the vessels are isolated in the usual manner. In the wedge resection, Gerota's fascia is then incised over the pole opposite the lesion and rolled back toward the lesion. The wedge can then be incised and the lesion is removed. In a guillotine amputation, the capsule is left intact and incised superficially at least 2 cm away from the lesion. The plane between capsule and renal parenchyma is best developed bluntly with the fingertip and the cortex can be transected superficially with a sharp knife. Once through the cortex, blunt dissection with the knife handle is preferred to allow for early identification of vessels and collecting system components that may be identified and se-

cured. If a main polar segmental vessel is encountered, it is controlled separately and can be injected distally with a dilute solution of indigo carmine as previously described.

Once the specimen has been removed, pressure may be intermittently released to facilitate the identification of small pulsating vessels at the corticomedullary junction. These arteries may then be controlled with shallow figure-of-eight sutures of 4-0 catgut (Fig. 7-7). Open veins require minimal suturing if the pedicle is unobstructed. After the tumor has been completely removed, the margins should be examined by frozen section to confirm the absence of residual disease.

Final reconstruction after polar resection must then take into account the extent of the resection, consistency of the kidney, and the availability of renal capsule. The wedge defect can be closed with horizontal mattress sutures of 3-0 chromic passed through the capsule, across the defect, and secured to the opposing capsule (Fig. 7-8). The capsule is rolled back to its initial position and, if it completely covers the defect, it may be simply sutured in place with horizontal mattress sutures. If the capsule is insufficient to cover the defect or if the kidney is particularly broad and stiff, a patch of peritoneum, dura, perinephric fat, or transversalis fascia may be used. In this case, the patch is used to reapproximate the original capsule. Bolsters of retroperitoneal fat can be placed between the parenchyma and capsule to minimize the tearing effect of the sutures on the tissue. This parenchymal approximation helps to minimize vascular oozing. After a guillotine amputation, hemostasis of the defect bed must first be meticulously controlled before

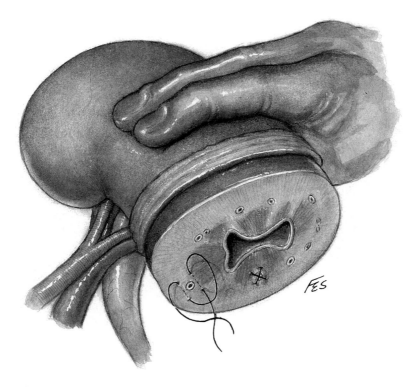

FIG. 7-7. In partial nephrectomy, individual vessels are identified and ligated using a figure-of-eight suture of 4-0 chromic catgut or PGA. (From Gittes, R. F. In *Reconstructive Urologic Surgery: Pediatric and Adult.* Edited by E. J. Libertino and L. A. Zinman. Baltimore, Williams & Wilkins, 1977.)

reconstruction is performed. Refractory venous oozing may be treated with oxycellulose or similar material used in a topical fashion. If the collecting system was opened, it may be closed with interrupted sutures of 5-0 catgut. The renal pelvis is then injected with a dilute indigo carmine solution using a 23-gauge butterfly (or through a nephrostomy tube if one has been placed) to confirm watertight integrity, as suggested by Gittes (Fig. 7-9).[37] Internal stents and nephrostomy tubes are useful in cases involving extensive dissection of the collecting system (Fig. 7-10).

Excision of Midportion Lesions

This procedure is significantly more complex and difficult than partial polar nephrectomy. Conceptually, it is dependent on the complete definition of the renal arteries by arteriography.

The incision and approach are as previously outlined for polar lesions. Once the kidney is mobilized with its perinephric fat intact and the adrenal has been isolated to be left in vivo, the renal artery is controlled with a vessel loop. The perinephric fat is sharply dissected circumferentially to the foothills of the tumor mound. This fat, still attached to the outer surface of the tumor capsule, can be grasped to apply traction for the sharp excision that follows. The renal pelvis is dissected free both anteriorly and posteriorly. Exposure for this portion of the procedure may be facilitated with a Gil-Vernet retractor.

The renal sinus is opened and vessel loops are placed around the renal pelvis and the neck of each infundibulum, as well as the hilar veins and the segmental arteries. At this point, the surgeon should place an index finger inside the renal sinus and bimanually palpate the entire renal cortex (Fig. 7-11). The edges of the bulky tumor are readily defined and the extent of inner protrusion of the tumor is determined directly by the fingertip. The primary and secondary arterial branches to the involved parenchyma should be circumscribed with silk suture to allow for loose traction during the dissection and their eventual ligation. Any secondary artery thought to supply the affected parenchyma may be positively identified by injecting a dilute solution of indigo carmine. The dye is injected distally into the isolated vessel and the corresponding parenchyma is observed for color change. The appropriate venous branches are then identified and doubly ligated, followed by the involved calcyceal infundibulum. Unnecessary dissection of the individual renal arteries or veins should be avoided.

Mannitol and heparin are injected systemically, the artery and the vein are clamped, and external cooling is initiated. The renal capsule is circumscribed around the tumor, allowing for a 2-cm margin. This may be accomplished in two steps by inscribing the margin with a thin cut followed by a deeper cut through the cortex on a slant parallel to the tumor's buried portion. If necessary, the capsule may be carefully peeled back on each side to expose the involved parenchyma. Gentle traction can be applied with the gauze pad on the fat covering the

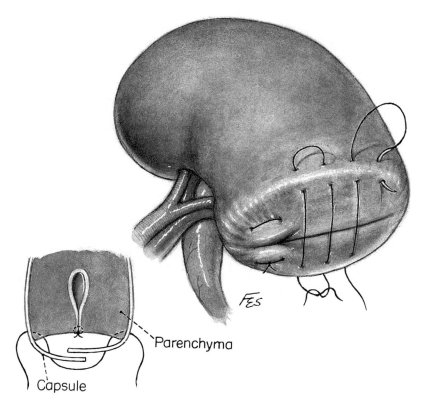

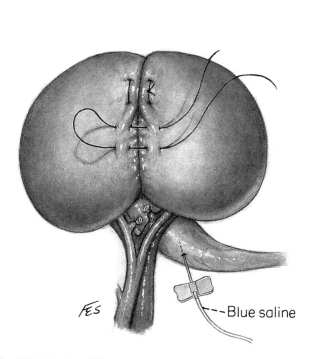

FIG. 7-8. If there is any available capsule after partial nephrectomy, it can be used to cover the raw parenchyma. It is secured with horizontal mattress sutures of 2-0 or 3-0 absorbable suture. (From Gittes, R. F. In *Reconstructive Urology Surgery: Pediatric and Adult.* Edited by E. J. Libertino and L. A. Zinman. Baltimore, Williams & Wilkins, 1977.)

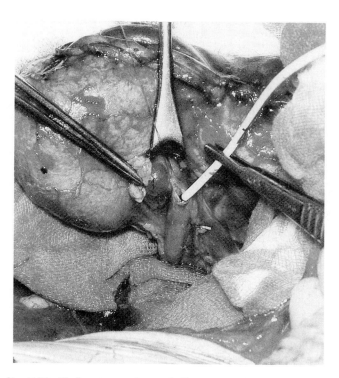

FIG. 7-9. Injection of blue saline to confirm watertight integrity of the collecting system. (From Gittes, R. F. In *Reconstructive Urologic Surgery: Pediatric and Adult.* Edited by E. J. Libertino and L. A. Zinman. Baltimore, Williams & Wilkins, 1977.)

FIG. 7-10. Nephrostomy tubes and silastic internal stents are often helpful in cases requiring extensive dissection of the collecting system. (Surgical photography by Lester V. Bergman courtesy of LTI Medica® and Bristol-Myers Company. Copyright 1986 by Learning Technology Incorporated.)

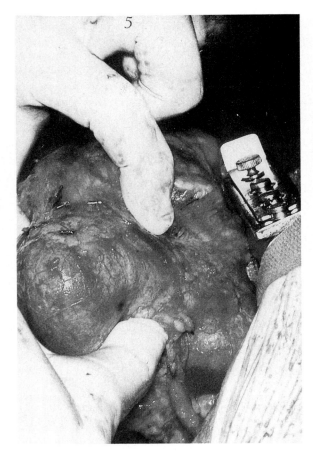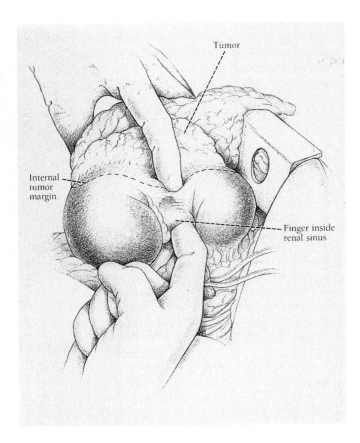

Fig. 7-11. Bimanual palpation of the kidney allows more accurate definition of the extent of tumor involvement. (Surgical photograph by Lester V. Bergman and drawing by William B. Westwood courtesy LTI Medica® and Bristol-Myers Company. Copyright 1986 by Learning Technology Incorporated.)

tumor in order to afford better visualization of the affected tissue.

Excision of the lesion may be facilitated and the hilar vessels protected by replacement of the index finger into the involved renal sinus. A full-thickness central wedge is excised. Large, deep tumors may lead the sharp dissection into the renal sinus where some calices may require transection in order to leave involved papillae with the specimen. All bleeding must be carefully controlled throughout the dissection, as a blood-free field permits ligation of any residual arterial or venous twigs tethering the specimen to the hilar vessels. Excision is completed by division of tertiary vascular branches and the corresponding infundibulum.

The specimen is examined at this point to ensure that an adequate margin of normal tissue has been excised. This should be accompanied by formal frozen-section evaluation by the pathologist to confirm negative margins, including the portion of renal capsule and perinephric fat submitted en bloc with the specimen.

After the tumor excision is complete the negative margins are confirmed, hemostasis and watertight closure of the collecting system are obtained as described for polar lesions. The central defect is then filled with retroperitoneal fat, muscle,

and/or a coagulating material (i.e.: Gelfoam, Surgicel) to initiate reconstruction. The decision must then be made to reapproximate the renal poles over the defect or to simply cover the denuded surface. Although more difficult to perform, reapproximation of the renal poles is considered the first-line approach as it affords better hemostasis and covers the exposed collecting system with renal parenchyma (Fig. 7-12). This affords protection against excessive postoperative blood loss and the formation of fistulae. A double pad of hemostatic woven oxycellulose (Surgicel) may be tucked into the crease and horizontal mattress sutures of 3-0 chromic are placed to include the edge of the residual capsule. If there is no capsule, a tuft of Surgicel or loose fat can buttress the suture.

The secondary approach of simply covering the renal defect may be utilized if the residual band of renal cortex is particularly rigid and fails to allow the flexion necessary to approximate the renal poles. In this case, a free patch of peritoneum is harvested and secured to the capsule and cortical edge of each pole. Horizontal mattress sutures of 3-0 chromic may be used to effectively secure this layer. Alternatively, a piece of perinephric fat may be imbricated over the denuded area. A double leaf of Surgicel gauze tucked under the patch aids in venous hemostasis. Other large defects can be closed

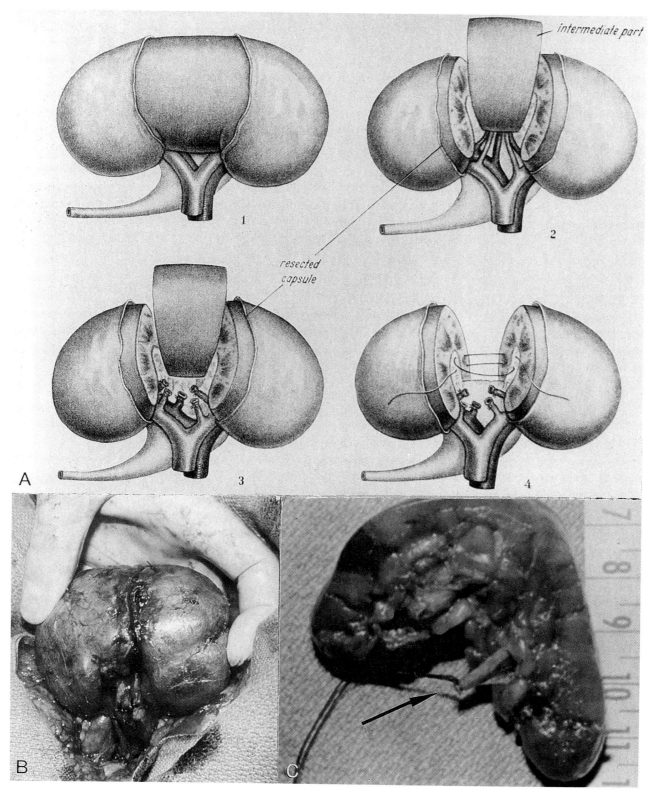

FIG. 7-12. *A,* Technique for excision and closure of midportion lesions. *B,* Anastomosis of upper and lower poles has been performed after midportion nephrectomy. *C,* The arrow identifies a ligated calyx containing a cortical rest. (From Gittes, R. F., and Elliot, M. L. J. Urol., *109:*14, 1973.)

with free patches of transversalis muscle and fascia or lower lumbodorsal fascia.

A third reconstruction option is used only for the uncommon case of multiple cortical craters. The craters are packed with a free lump of perinephric fat and battened down with a crisscrossing pair of horizontal mattress sutures of 2-0 or 3-0 chromic catgut.

Placement of a double-J ureteral stent is advisable when extensive repair of the collecting system has been performed, particularly when the overlying material is only nonviable Surgicel and an avascular peritoneal patch. The stent may be placed via a small pylotomy and threaded down into the bladder.[63] We recommend leaving the stent in place for one month to optimize healing.

Closure

After renal reconstruction, the patient's volume status should be carefully re-evaluated and necessary blood should be replaced prior to releasing the arterial clamp. Once the clamp is removed, the kidney should promptly resume function. Any new bleeding areas are immediately controlled. Copious postoperative urinary output is essential to dilute any minor bleeding into the collecting system and prevent the formation of clots. Attention to fluid balance in the operating room is of primary importance in the prevention of postoperative oliguria.

The need for drainage and the type employed is the subject of some controversy. The theoretical risk of seeding tumor along the drain line must be weighed against the risk of a urine leak that is a potential complication after extensive resection of the collecting system. We recommend the use of suction drainage in such circumstances to minimize the risks of urinoma although others prefer Penrose drains. The muscle, fascia, and skin are closed in the usual manner.

EXTRACORPOREAL PARTIAL NEPHRECTOMY AND AUTOTRANSPLANTATION

General Considerations

The first autotransplantation after partial nephrectomy for a renal tumor was performed by Calne in 1971.[66] This procedure is more technically challenging than in-situ surgery and should be reserved for a select group of patients.

The advantages of ex-vivo surgery include better visualization and access to the tumor in a bloodless surgical field. This affords more complete excision of regional lymph nodes and lymphatics and reduces the possibility of tumor spill. Extracorporeal partial nephrectomy also enables the removal of complex renal tumors previously considered inoperable. Although it has been suggested that extracorporeal partial nephrectomy might reduce the risk of tumor recurrence,[11,17] this has not been proven.[13] The disadvantages of ex-vivo surgery include increased risk of ischemic renal damage, prolonged operating time, and increased complexity of technique

with the need for arterial and venous anastomoses and their attendant complications.[15]

In addition to the renal angiography, the pelvic vessel anatomy should also be imaged as part of the preoperative evaluation. Significant vascular disease is common in the tumor age group and arteriography allows the surgeon to pre-select the least-impaired vessels for autotransplantation.[74]

The cooled preservation solution and sterile intravenous tubing for kidney perfusion must be prepared before the incision is made. The workbench must also be prepared and may consist of a Mayo stand with waterproof sterile covering and a shallow dish for the kidney. The bench should be placed adjacent to the open wound to allow surgery to be performed on the kidney while the ureter remains attached to the bladder. An intestinal suction catheter can be placed under the cloth towels covering the Mayo stand to remove irrigation fluid.

Technique of Extracorporeal Tumor Excision

Extracorporeal partial nephrectomy and renal autotransplantation are generally performed through either a single midline incision or via separate ipsilateral subcostal and Gibson incisions. A traditional radical nephrectomy is then performed with two exceptions; mobilization is completed prior to the final ligation of the vessels, and the ureter is left intact distally if possible. As with in-situ partial nephrectomy, mannitol and heparin are administered just prior to the final ligation of the vessels.

Immediately after the renal vessels are divided, the kidney is removed and flushed with 500 to 1000 cc of chilled preservation solution until the venous effluent is clear. The kidney is then immediately submerged in a basin of iced slush saline in order to maintain hypothermia. This simple technique obviates the need for the more cumbersome pump oxygenator in the vast majority of cases. In the unusual circumstances where deterioration of the patient's condition requires rapid closure without time to complete the autotransplant, or when there is uncertainty by the pathologist concerning tumor margins by frozen section, the kidney may be cold-stored or placed on the pump for more prolonged periods of preservation.

If a pump-oxygenator is used, it can be attached to the renal artery with long silicone tubes and cannulas will allow the perfusion to flow while the bench surgery is in progress. Because the pump reuses the perfusate several times, it is at least theoretically possible to recirculate tumor cells from the tumor portion into the normal portion of the kidney. This potential problem may be avoided by starting pump perfusion only after the tumor has been excised. An alternative would be to use an in-line millipore filter to attempt to strain tumor cells out of the recirculating fluid. The pump allows the surgeon to identify potential sites of troublesome bleeding after the tumor is removed and hemostasis may thus be maintained prior to the autotransplantation.

It is preferable to leave the ureter attached to the bladder, if at all possible, to maximize perservation of the vascular supply.[74] This is particularly important in the case of larger hilar or lower pole tumors in which complete tumor excision may unavoidably result in devascularization of a portion of the renal pelvis or proximal ureter. When the ureter is successfully preserved the extracorporeal operation can be performed in its entirety on the patient's abdominal wall. The ureter should be temporarily occluded while the kidney is outside the body in order to prevent retrograde blood flow into the kidney. If the surgeon finds that he is unable to comfortably perform the operation on the abdominal wall, the ureter should be divided distally and the kidney placed in the slush basin on a separate workbench. This will allow increased exposure to the kidney and simultaneous access to the iliac fossa by a second surgical team to prepare for autotransplantation.

Tumor excision and reconstruction in bench surgery follows the principles of hilar dissection presented earlier for in-situ polar and midportion partial nephrectomy. Because time is not critical, both hemostasis and the dissection itself should be carried out in a meticulous fashion. When tumor is present, frozen section of the margins of residual parenchyma, hilar fat, and lymph nodes should be sent for pathologic review. Once the tumor is resected, it is important to replace the basin holding the kidney with a new one in order to remove any extraneous tumor cells from the operative field.

Technique of Autotransplantation

We prefer performing this aspect of the procedure through a separate ipsilateal extraperitoneal Gibson or hockey-stick incision. A self-retaining Balfour or ring retractor allows adequate exposure in virtually all cases. Alternatively, if a midline inci-

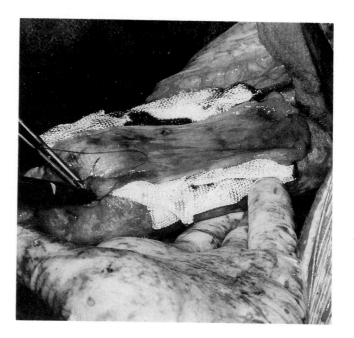

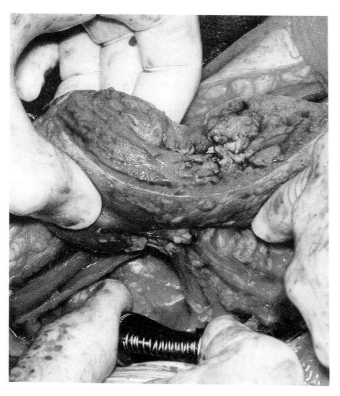

FIG. 7-13. Pole-to-pole closure may not be feasible in some cases after excision of a midportion lesion. This is because of the intrinsic bend of some residual renal cortical tissue. (Surgical photography by Lester V. Bergman courtesy of LTI Medica® and Bristol-Myers Company. Copyright 1986 by Learning Technology Incorporated.)

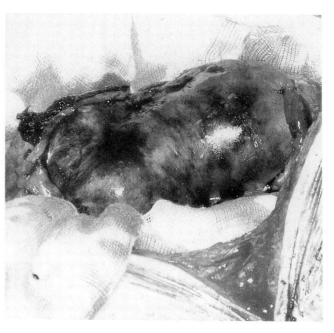

FIG. 7-14. *A,* A free patch of peritoneum, transversalis muscle or fascia, or lumbodorsal fascia may be used to cover defects such as those seen in Figure 13. Here a double leaf of Surgicell is covered with a patch of peritoneum, which is secured to the capsule with horizontal mattress sutures of 3-0 chromic. *B,* This demonstrates the reconstructed kidney. (Surgical photography by Lester V. Bergman courtesy of LTI Medica® and Bristol-Myers Company. Copyright 1986 by Learning Technology Incorporated.)

sion has been used for the nephrectomy, the incision may be extended caudally to allow adequate access to the groin vessels. The ipsilateral external iliac artery and vein are mobilized and controlled with vascular or umbilical tapes. The kidney is kept wrapped in an ice-containing sponge in order to minimize transient rewarm ischemia during handling of the kidney.

When the ureter is left intact in its native position the autotransplantation may be easily accomplished by the flip-over technique or by allowing the kidney to lie in its normal situation with the vessels lying anteriorly. The flip-over involves turning the reconstructed kidney over back to front in order to have the vessels posterior with the renal pelvis and looping ureter lying anteriorly (Fig. 7-15).

Control of the external iliac vein is accomplished with a Satinsky clamp or by applying Rummel tourniquets proximally and distally from the site of the intended venotomy. A small ellipse is then made in the recipient vein to allow for a wide anastomosis with the graft vein. Heparinized saline is flushed into the venotomy to remove residual blood. The venous anastomosis is secured with 5-0 nonabsorbable vascular sutures using two separate continuous running sutures along the front and back walls respectively. In a deep pelvis, where visibility

may be restricted, the vein may be triangulated with a Carrel stitch in order to prevent the inadvert placement of a suture through the back wall. The recipient vein is left occluded until the arterial anastomosis is completed. If the patency of the anastomosis is in question, however, a bulldog clamp can be placed distally on the renal vein and the clamps removed from the external iliac vein. This maneuver provides adequate assessment of the venous anastomosis while preventing retrograde rewarming of the kidney.

The artery is then clamped proximally and distally with bulldogs or a Satinsky. An arteriotomy is made with a knife and extended with tenotomy or Pott's scissors. We usually perform the arterial anastomosis in an end-to-side fashion to the external iliac artery using interrupted or running 5-0 or 6-0 sutures. Alternatively, the hypogastric artery may be used. The surgeon must be prepared to deal with recipient vessel problems such as endarterectomy if severe plaque is encountered.

After the anastomoses are completed, the vascular clamps are slowly released in a sequential fashion. The venous clamps are released first, followed by the distal and then the proximal arterial clamps. Any bleeding points on the kidney are controlled. Pressure will frequently stop any parenchymal oozing. In cases requiring ureteral transection, continuity of the urinary tract can be re-established by performing a ureteroneocystostomy. We have found the extravesical approach to ureteroneocystostomy to be reliable and easily performed.

COMPLICATIONS AND SPECIAL POSTOPERATIVE PROBLEMS

Of 309 partial nephrectomies performed at the Mayo Clinc for various pathologic entities, only one death occurred in the immediate postoperative period. Secondary hemorrhage and delayed nephrectomy were reported in two (0.6%) and eight (2.6%) patients, respectively. The majority of complications (three urinomas and seven fistulae) occurred after wedge resection, not guillotine amputation. Conservative, nonoperative therapy, with or without ureteral stent placement, was shown to be successful in most cases in the absence of distal obstruction.[67]

Temporary urinary fistulas have been noted in several series with an incidence as high as 20%. Established cutaneous fistulae and secondary perinephric urinoma are rare, fearsome, and largely preventable with meticulous technique. Several causes of postoperative fistulae have been identified. Stewart has discussed the danger of leaving an undrained renal pyramid on the cut surface of the kidney.[68] Obstruction of the collecting system by blood clot can also lead to fistula formation if not relieved. After several days of persistence of the fistula, retrograde studies should be performed to determine the point of obstruction. The decision must then be made to intervene by repairing the obstruction itself or to simply decompress the system with stents. Placement of ureteral stents is often adequate with resolution of the fistula shortly after decompression.

Vascular thrombosis may be caused by cross-clamping the renal pedicle or by undetected intimal injury from the perfu-

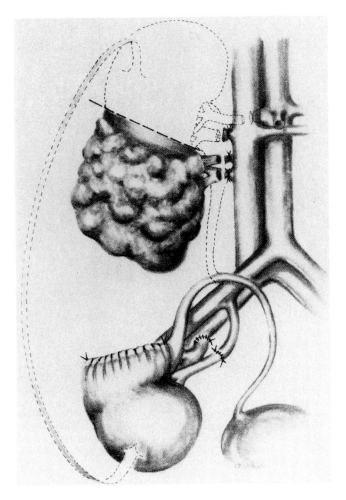

FIG. 7-15. The flip-over technique. (From Gittes, R. F., and McCullough, D. L. J. Urol., *113*:12, 1975.)

sion cannula during the extracorporeal procedure. Thrombosis may result in renal loss and amplifies the importance of gentle, meticulous vascular technique.

Although some temporary impairment in renal function is to be expected, oliguria should be evaluated on the first postoperative day with renal perfusion and ultrasound scans in order to provide baseline images for comparison. Serum creatinine levels rise to a maximum at 48 to 72 hours postoperatively, but will usually return to normal by day 10. Only rarely do patients require temporary dialysis for acute tubular necrosis.[17] Patients at increased risk are often identifiable and include those with advanced age diabetes, pre-existing renal disease, and those who have received nephrotoxic agents in the perioperative period. Most important prophylactic steps relate to the maintenance of adequate renal perfusion throughout the case by minimizing ischemia time and promoting diuresis. Ultrasound can be used to document the size and ultrasonic density of the kidney, and Doppler ultrasound and nuclear scan can demonstrate the adequacy of renal perfusion, an important factor in patients who have undergone autotransplantation. Once the diagnosis is made, therapy consists of a trial of diuretics followed by supportive care and observation with supplemental hemodialysis as necessary. Fortunately, most patients will recover from this insult with minimal attenuation of renal function.

CONCLUSION

The increased sophistication of noninvasive imaging and the popularity of "screening" studies will continue to uncover an expanding pool of asymptomatic renal mass lesions of uncertain biologic significance. Moreover, as the fields of chemotherapy, tissue, and molecular biology continue to advance, we may soon be able to accurately predict the malignant potential of these lesions and treat them adjuvantly. This progress should allow the urologic pendulum to continue to swing away from total extirpation for all suspicious renal mass lesions toward a more selective and renal-sparing approach.

REFERENCES

1. LIEBER, M. M. Renal cell carcinoma: New developments. Mayo Clin. Proc., 60:715, 1985.
2. KOHNAK, J. W., and GROSSMAN, H. B. Renal cell carcinoma as an incidental finding. J. Urol., 134:1094, 1985.
3. WELLS, S. Successful removal of two solid circumrenal tumors. Br. Med. J., 1:758, 1884.
4. SEMB, C. Partial resection of the kidney: Operative technique. Acta. Chir. Scand., 109:360, 1955.
5. PUIGVERT, A. Partial nephrectomy for renal lithiasis. Experience with 208 cases. Int. Surg., 461:555, 1966.
6. CARREL, A., and GUTHRIE, C. C. Successful transplantation of both kidneys from a dog into a bitch with removal of both normal kidneys from the latter. Science, 23:394, 1906.
7. HARDY, J. D. High ureteral injuries—Management by autotransplantation of the kidney. JAMA, 184:97, 1963.
8. SERRALLACH-MILA, N., et al. Renal autotransplantation. Lancet, 2:1130, 1965.
9. GELIN, L. E., et al. Total bloodlessness for extracorporeal renal organ repair. Rev. Surg., 28:305, 1971.
10. BAZEED, M. A., et al. Synchronous bilateral renal cell carcinoma: Total surgical excision. Eur. Urol., 12:238, 1986.
11. JACOBS, S. C., BERG, S. I., and LAWSON, R. D. Synchronous bilateral renal cell carcinoma: Total surgical excision. Cancer, 46:2341, 1980.
12. MARBERGER, M., et al. Conservative surgery of renal carcinoma: The EIRSS experience. Br. J. Urol., 53:528, 1981.
13. NOVICK, A. C., STREAM, S., and MONTIE, J. E. Conservative surgery for renal cell carcinoma: a single center experience with 100 patients. J. Urol., 141:835, 1989.
14. SCHIFF, M., JR., BAGLEY, D. H., and LYTTON, B. Treatment of solitary and bilateral renal carcinomas. J. Urol., 121:581, 1979.
15. SMITH, R. B., et al. Bilateral renal cell carcinoma and renal cell carcinoma in the solitary kidney. J. Urol., 132:450, 1984.
16. TOPLEY, M. Partial nephrectomy for kidney tumors. Yrbk. Urol. Nsltr. 1:1, 1983.
17. TOPLEY, M., NOVICK, A. C., and MONTIE, J. E. Long-term results following partial nephrectomy for localized renal adenocarcinoma J. Urol., 131:1050, 1984.
18. ZINCKE, H., and SWANSON, S. K. Bilateral renal cell carcinoma: influence of synchronous and asynchronous occurrence on patient survival. J. Urol., 128:913, 1982.
19. ZINCKE, H., ENGEN, D. E., HENNING, K. M., and McDONALD, M. W. Treatment of renal cell carcinoma by in situ partial nephrectomy and extracorporeal operation with autotransplantation. Mayo Clin. Proc., 60:651, 1985.
20. SPECS, E. K., et al. Transplantation in patients with a history of renal cell carcinoma: Long-term results and clinical considerations. Surgery, 91:282, 1982.
21. NOVICK, A. C. Partial nephrectomy for renal cell carcinoma. Urol. Clin. North Am., 14:419, 1987.
22. MARSHALL, F. F. The in situ surgical management of renal cell carcinoma and transitional cell carcinoma of the kidney. World J. Urol., 2:130, 1984.
23. WALLACE, D. M. A., et al. The late results of conservative surgery for upper tract urothelial carcinomas Br. J. Urol., 47:537, 1981.
24. LIEBER, M. M., and GOLDWASSER, B. Z. Role of partial nephrectomy in management of renal tumors, including surgical technique. In *Diagnosis and Therapy of Genitourinary Tumors.* Edited by D. G. Skinner and G. Lieskovsky. Philadelphia, W. B. Saunders Co., 1988, pp: 704–720.
25. ZINCKE, H., and NEVES, R. J. Feasibility of conservative surgery for transitional cell carcinoma of the upper urinary tract. Urol. Clin. North Am., 11:717, 1984.
26. VERGA, G., and PARIGI, G. B. Partial nephrectomy for Wilm's tumor. J. Urol., 135:981, 1986.
27. ANDERSON, S., MEYER, T. W., and DeGRAPHENREID, R. L. Control of glomerular hypertension preserves glomerular structure and function in rats with renal ablation. Clin. Res., 32:564A, 1984.
28. BRENNER, B. M., et al. Dietery protein intake and the progressive nature of kidney disease: the role of hemodynamically mediated glomerular injury in the pathogenesis of progressive glomerular sclerosis in aging, renal ablation and intrinsic renal disease. N. Engl. J. Med., 307:652, 1982.
29. MUKAMEL, E., et al. Incidental small renal tumors accompanying clinically overt renal cell carcinoma. J. Urol., 140:22, 1988.

30. CARINI, M., et al. Conservative surgery for renal cell carcinoma. Eur. Urol., 7:19, 1981.

31. GRAHAM, S. D., JR., and GLEN, J. F. Enucleation surgery for renal malignancy. J. Urol., 122:546, 1979.

32. JAEGER, N., WEISSBACH, J., and VAHLENSIECK, W. Value of enucleation of tumor in solitary kidneys. Eur. Urol., 11:369, 1985.

33. NOVICK, A. C., et al. Surgical enucleation for renal cell carcinoma. J. Urol., 135:235, 1986.

34. MARSHALL, F. F., et al. The feasibility of surgical enucleation for renal cell carcinoma. J. Urol., 135:213, 1986.

35. LOUGHLIN, K. R., and GITTES, R. F. Urological management of patients with von Hippel-Lindau's disease. J. Urol., 136:789, 1986.

36. SPENCER, W. F., et al. Surgical treatment of localized renal cell carcinoma in von Hippel-Lindau disease. J. Urol., 139:507, 1988.

37. GITTES, R. F. Partial nephrectomy. In situ or extracorporeal. In: *Campbell's Urology.* 5th Edition. Vol. 3. Edited by P. C. Walsh, R. F. Gittes, A. D. Perlmutter, and T. A. Stamey. Philadelphia, W. B. Saunders Co. 1986, pp. 2454–2477.

38. BICKFORD, R. G., and WINSTON, F. R. The influence of temperature on the isolated kidney of the dog. J. Physiol. 89:198, 1937.

39. LYMAN, C. P. The oxygen consumption and temperature regulation of hibernating hamsters. J. Exp. Zool., 109:55, 1948.

40. WARD, J. P. Determination of the optimum temperature for regional renal hypothermia during temporary renal ischemia. Br. J. Urol., 47:17, 1975.

41. COLLSTE, H., et al. ATP in cortex of canine kidneys undergoing hypothermic storage. Life Sci., 10:1201, 1971.

42. HUMPHRIES, A. L., et al. Successful reimplantation of canine kidney after 24-hr. storage. Surgery, 54:136, 1963.

43. BELZER, F. O., ASHBY, B. S., and DUMPHY, J. E. Twenty-four hour and 72-hour preservation of canine kidneys. Lancet, 2:536, 1967.

44. CLAES, G., et al. Albumin as perfusate in continuous perfusion for renal preservation. Fourth International Transplant Conference. New York, Grune and Stratton, 1972, p. 46.

45. JOHNSON, R. W. G., et al. Evaluation of a new perfusion solution for kidney preservation. Transplantation, 13:270, 1972.

46. COLLINS, G. M., BRAVO-SHUGARMAN, M., and TERASAKI, P. I. Kidney preservation of transplantation. Lancet, 2:1219, 1969.

47. SHIRES, G. T., et al. Alterations in cellular membrane function during hemorrhagic shock in primates. Ann. Surg., 176:288, 1972.

48. ARNOLD, P. E., et al. In vitro versus in vivo mitochondrial calcium loading in ischemic acute renal failure. Am. J. Physiol., 248:F845, 1985.

49. COFF, J. E., et al. Redox maintenance and organ preservation. Transplant Proc., 9:1569, 1977.

50. JELLINEK, M., et al. Oxidation-reduction maintenance in organ preservation. Arch. Surg., 120:439, 1985.

51. MCDOUGAL, W. S. Renal perfusion/reperfusion injuries. J. Urol., 140:1325, 1988.

52. SCHRIER, R. W., et al. Protection of mitochondrial function by mannitol in ischemic acute renal failure. Am. J. Physiol., 247:F365, 1984.

53. HANSSON, R., et al. Effect of xanthine oxidase inhibition on renal circulation after ischemia. Transplant Proc., 14:51, 1982.

54. PALLER, M. S., HOIDAL, J. R., and FERRIS, T. F. Oxygen free radicals in ischemic acute renal failure in the rat. J. Clin. Invest., 74:1156, 1984.

55. ICHIKAWA, I., MIELE, J. F., and BRENNER, B. M. Reversal of renal cortical actions of angiotensin II by verapamil and manganese. Kidney Int., 16:137, 1979.

56. MCCROREY, H. L., et al. Effect of calcium transport inhibitors on renal hemodynamics and electrolyte excretion in the dog. In *Hormonal Regulation of Sodium Excretion.* Edited by B. Lichardus, R. W. Schrier, and J. Ponce. New York, Elsevier/North Holland Biomechanical Press, 1980, pp. 113–120.

57. WAIT, R. B., WHITE G., and DAVIS, J. H. Beneficial effects of verapamil on postischemic renal failure. Surgery, 94:276, 1983.

58. MALIS, C. D., et al. Effects of verapamil in models of ischemic acute renal failure in the rat. Am. J. Physiol., 245: F735, 1983.

59. OSIAS, M. B., et al. Postischemic renal failure: accelerated recovery with adenosine triphosphate-magnesium chloride infusion. Arch. Surg., 112:729, 1977.

60. SIEGEL, N. J., et al. Enhanced recovery from acute renal failure by the postischemic infusion of adenine nucleotides and magnesium chloride in rats. Kidney Int., 17:338, 1980.

61. NOVICK, A. C. Hypothermia: In vivo and ex vivo. Urol. Clin. North Am., 10:637, 1983.

62. PENN, I. Transplantation in patients with primary malignancies. Transplantation, 24:424, 1977.

63. GITTES, R. F., and MARSHALL, F. F. Urologic surgery, midportion partial nephrectomy for tumor of solitary kidney. Bristol Laboratories Monograph, 1986.

64. GOLDWASSER, B., et al. Partial nephrectomy using a new dissecting instrument. J. Urol., 136:54, 1986.

65. STORM, F. K., KAUFMANN, J. J., and LONGMIRE, W. P. Kidney resection clamp: New instrument. Urology, 6:494, 1975.

66. CALNE, R. Y. Tumour in a single kidney: Nephrectomy, excision and autotransplantation. Lancet, 2:761, 1971.

67. LEACH, G., LIEBER, M. M. Partial nephrectomy: Mayo Clinic experience 1957–1977. Urology, 15:219, 1980.

68. STEWART, H. H. Partial nephrectomy in treatment of renal calculi. Hunterian Lecture. Ann. Roy. Coll. Surgeons England, 11:32, 1952.

69. GITTES, R. F. Management of transitional cell carcinoma of the upper tract-Case for conservative local excision. Urol. Clin. North Am., 7:559, 1980.

70. MARSHALL, F. F., and WALSH, P. C. In situ management of renal tumors: renal cell carcinoma and transitional cell carcinoma. J. Urol., 131:1045, 1984.

71. MONTIE, J. E., and NOVICK, A. C. Partial nephrectomy for renal cell carcinoma (Editorial). J. Urol., 140:129, 1988.

72. LIEBER, M. M., TOMERA, K. M., FARROW, G. M. Renal oncocytoma. J. Urol., 125:481, 1981.

73. FOKER, J. D., et al. Adenosine triphosphate levels in perfused canine kidneys. Eur. Surg. Res., 4:275, 1972.

74. GITTES, R. F., and MCCULLOUGH, D. L. Bench surgery for tumor in a solitary kidney. J. Urol., 113:12, 1975.

CHAPTER
8

Surgical Management of Renal Cell Carcinoma with Vena Caval Extension

Kenneth B. Cummings

The intraoperative management of renal cell carcinoma (RCC) with intraluminal inferior vena caval extension demands well-conceived exacting surgery. RCC is predominantly a hypervascular tumor deriving its blood supply from the renal artery. Invasion of the intrarenal veins is a common event, with tumor extension into the renal veins occurring in 30% of cases.[1,2] Tumor propagation in the renal vein is by direct extension, with the tumor thrombus carrying its own blood supply parasitized from the renal artery. The incidence of intraluminal inferior vena caval extension ranges from 4 to 10%.[3,4] This event is frequently noted at the time of selective renal arteriography, as previously reported by Kahn, and represents the radiographic appearance of tumor vessels within the tumor thrombus (Fig. 8-1A,B).[5] Propagation of tumor growth within the lumen of the inferior vena cava is in the direction of venous flow. Because of the relative shortness of the right renal vein, inferior vena caval tumor thrombi occur more frequently with right-sided tumors.[6] The reported incidence of extension of inferior vena caval tumor thrombi to the right atrium ranges from 14 to 41%.[4,6,7] Kerney, reporting on 24 cases of inferior vena caval tumor thrombi managed surgically, delineated the level of caval extension, noting that 16% were supradiaphragmatic, 46% attained the level of the hepatic veins, and 38% were subhepatic.[8] The insidious natural history of intraluminal growth may be appreciated from Kaufman's report of the value of inferior vena cavograms in which he noted that 50% of patients with complete caval occlusion had no associated symptoms.[9] The growth rate in these cases obviously permitted the development of sufficient collateral venous return to the heart from the lower torso via the lumbar and azygos system to obviate symptoms referable to caval obstruction.

RATIONALE FOR AGGRESSIVE SURGICAL EXTIRPATION

Initial reports of inferior vena caval extension from RCC reflected a uniformly poor prognosis.[6,10,11] Marshall, in 1970, reported 11 such patients, 8 of whom were dead or dying 1 year postoperatively.[3] Skinner reported a 55% 5-year survival (6 of 11 patients) and a 43% 10-year survival (4 of 11 patients).[12] It is noteworthy that none of the 6 survivors had lymph node involvement or preoperative evidence of meta-

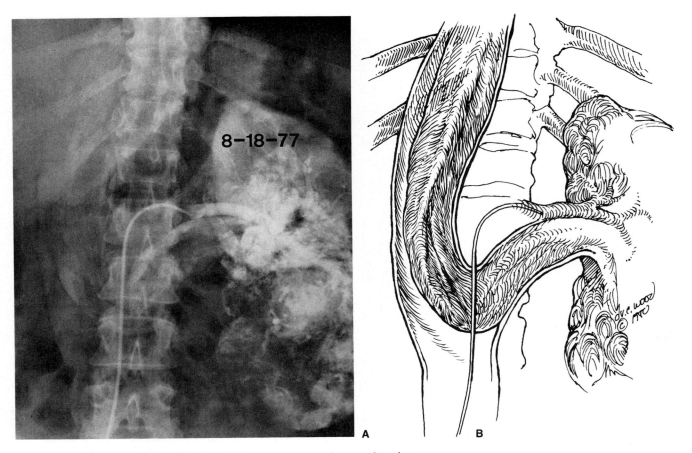

FIG. 8-1A,B, Selective renal arteriography demonstrating arterialized tumor thrombus.

static disease.[13] When applied to other series, this observation provides the general guidelines for operative intervention. Schefft and associates reviewed 21 patients who underwent surgical extirpation for RCC extending into the inferior vena cava.[14] Six of the 12 patients (50%) with no evidence of metastatic disease preoperatively had complete removal of all apparent tumor and survived 1 to 10 years postoperatively. Cherrie and associates reviewed the UCLA experience in 27 patients with intraluminal vena caval extension of RCC.[15] They did not find that intraluminal extension in itself portended a poor survival and reported a 53% 5-year survival in such patients (median of 81 months). By contrast, in this group of patients, the presence of perinephric fat extension or regional lymph node involvement adversely affected survival, with 35% of such patients surviving 2 years and no patient surviving 5 years. DeKernion's review of the natural history of metastatic RCC in 86 patients revealed a dismal prognosis for those patients who had evidence of metastatic disease at the time of diagnosis (41 patients).[16] One-year survival for this group was less than 10%, with most patients dead within 6 months. Several similar reports failed to support aggressive surgical intervention when systemic disease is evident at the time of diagnosis.[17,18]

Regional lymph node or contiguous organ involvement is

acknowledged to significantly shorten survival. Skinner reported no survivors when the renal vein as well as regional nodes were involved.[13] This finding suggests that such tumors are biologically different, having achieved direct vascular extension as well as invasion of lymphatics with metastases to regional nodes. There are no hard data stating that involvement of the regional nodes and inferior vena cava at the time of nephrectomy portends as dismal a prognosis as the presence of distant metastases.

Technologic advances, including cardiopulmonary bypass and circulatory arrest of the lower torso, have permitted operative intervention with acceptable surgical risk even in patients with supradiaphragmatic inferior vena caval tumor extensions. The reported operative mortality for radical nephrectomy and extirpation of inferior vena caval tumor thrombi ranges from 4 to 15%.[3,14] Intraluminal inferior vena caval extensions from RCC, regardless of its distal extent, should not contraindicate aggressive surgical extirpation. However, preoperative evidence of distant metastases would preclude patients from surgical consideration. Additionally, the presence of grossly positive regional lymph nodes or contiguous organ involvement noted at the time of surgical exploration suggests that an aggressive extirpative surgical procedure does not have merit.

CLASSIFICATION OF INFERIOR VENA CAVAL TUMOR THROMBI AND DIAGNOSTIC IMAGING

Detailed imaging studies are necessary to define the limits of vena caval tumor thrombi and are central in the planning of surgical extirpation. Computerized tomography (CT) scans have become fundamental in the evaluation of renal tumors.[19] The definition of the presence of caval extension is excellent[20] (Fig. 8-2A,B). However, definition of the cephalad extent and magnitude of collateral circulation is inadequate. Magnetic resonance imaging (MRI) has shown significant promise.[21] This imaging modality has several advantages: 1) it is not invasive, 2) it does not require employment of iodinated contrast agents, and 3) it provides coronal as well as transverse images. This modality in coronal sections usually defines the apical extension of the tumor and may permit visualization of the magnitude of collateralization via the azygos system (Figs. 8-3, 8-4A,B). Additionally, the main renal artery supplying the involved kidney may be defined (Fig. 8-5).

The quality of MRI evaluation of intraluminal tumor extensions and the magnitude of caval and collateral blood flow are likely to be improved with newly available flow-compensation software.[22] The signal void created by flowing blood on spin-echo magnetic resonance (MR) images has enabled investigators to evaluate noninvasively the patency of the vessels.[23] Unfortunately, various flow-related phenomena can produce intraluminal signals that may mimic those of thrombus.[24] New MR pulse sequences with short repetition times include FLASH (flat low-angle shot) and GRASS (gradient-recalled acquisition in a steady state).[22,25] In these pulse sequences, flowing blood appears bright because fully magnetized protons continually enter the selected section, while protons in adjacent tissues (thrombus) become partially saturated, lowering their relative signal intensity.[26] The magnitude of vascularization of the thrombus is therefore an important factor in this imaging modality.

Real time ultrasound (US) is useful despite its tendency to be "user-dependent." It is capable of defining flow and intra-

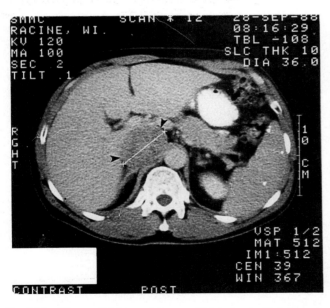

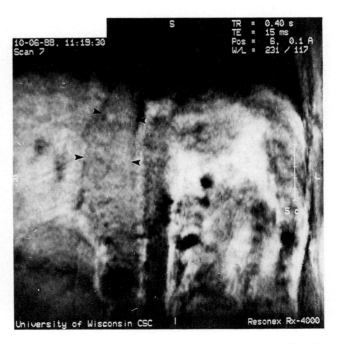

FIG. 8-2A. CT scan of right renal tumor with intraluminal inferior vena caval (IVC) extension. B, CT scan through midportion of the liver demonstrates low-density region where the IVC is expected. This region represents a surgically confirmed tumor thrombus extending superiorly within the IVC.

FIG. 8-3. MRI, coronal image, of a large intraluminal tumor thrombus extension within the IVC with the apex confirmed surgically to be within the right atrium.

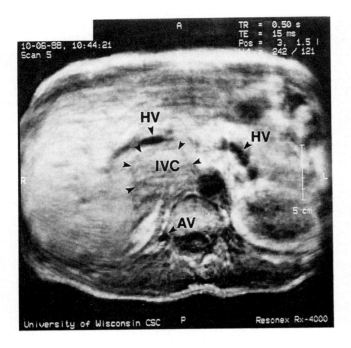

(above the hepatic veins or supradiaphragmatic), a right-heart catheterization is necessary (Fig. 8-7A,B).

The details of the surgical approach are dependent on the level of intracaval extension. Involvement of the right heart requires employment of cardiopulmonary bypass. Supradiaphragmatic-intrapericardial, and infradiaphragmatic-retrohepatic thrombi require intrapericardial control of the inferior vena cava. If collateral venous return is insufficient to permit an adequate cardiac output, the circulating blood volume can be effectively divided by cross-clamping the aorta at the diaphragmatic hiatus, permitting temporary circulatory arrest of the lower torso with normal perfusion of the upper torso. Infrahepatic and limited caval extension from the renal vein are managed with control of the vena cava above the tumor thrombus.

The intraluminal caval extension can be classified according to the level of the involvement and the surgical approach necessary (Fig. 8-8).

SURGICAL CONSIDERATIONS

Systemic vascular control is essential to the prevention of intraoperative complications (tumor embolization to the lungs, uncontrolled hemorrhage, and failure to perform a complete tumor thrombectomy). The facts gleaned from imaging studies both classify the intracaval thrombi with respect to the location and provide information regarding the collateral venous return. These studies permit anticipation of patient tolerance of proximal caval occlusion. The absence of significant collateral venous return predicts the need for achieving circulatory arrest of the lower torso by cross-clamping the aorta or

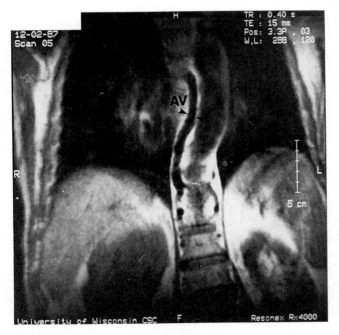

FIG. 8-4A. MRI, transverse image, through the liver demonstrating intraluminal hepatic inferior vena caval (IVC) extension (arrows). Blood flow in the hepatic vein (HV) and azygos vein (AV) is illustrated. B, MRI, coronal image, illustrating significant collateral blood flow in the azygos vein (AV).

luminal mass.[27] This ability is of particular value in evaluating flow in the contralateral renal vein and hepatic veins in the presence of total caval occlusion.

However, at present, inferior vena cavography remains the most accurate method of defining the limits of an intracaval thrombus and of demonstrating the magnitude of collateral venous return (Fig. 8-6A,B). In cases of complete obstruction of the vena cava or a questionable level of proximal extension

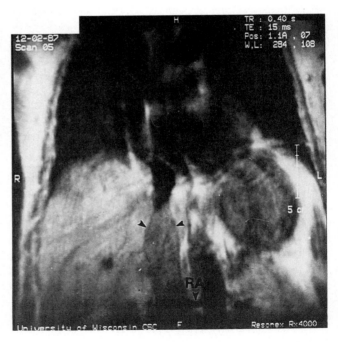

FIG. 8-5. MRI, coronal image, demonstrating the aorta and renal artery (RA) (arrows) to the involved kidney in a patient with intraluminal tumor extension causing complete caval occlusion.

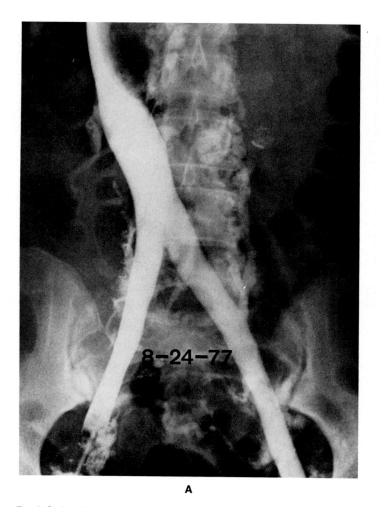
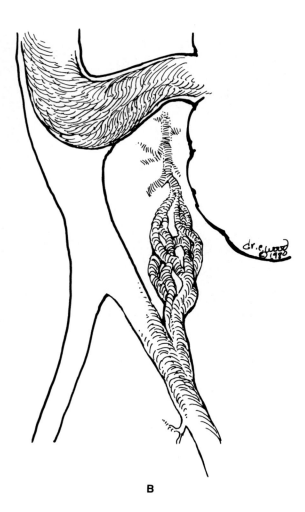

| A | B |

FIG. 8-6A,B. Inferior vena cavogram showing tumor thrombus.

alternatively by placing the patient on cardiopulmonary by-pass. A description of the principles of surgical procedure and technical considerations in extirpation of caval thrombi is best approached on the basis of the established classification.

SUPRADIAPHRAGMATIC-INTRAPERICARDIAL (IB) AND INFRADIAPHRAGMATIC-RETROHEPATIC (IIA) EXTENSION

A tumor thrombus that extends intraluminally in the vena cava to the level of the hepatic veins (retrohepatic) or is supradiaphragmatic but does not extend into the heart requires a similar surgical approach. It is necessary to gain caval control intrapericardially above the apex of the tumor thrombus. Technical variation is dictated by the kidney involved and the magnitude of the collateral venous return. Patients who do not have complete caval obstruction either by tumor thrombus or by "bland" thrombus, which forms below the tumor thrombus (infrarenally), rarely develop significant venous collateral. In such patients, intrapericardial interruption of the inferior vena caval return results in significant diminution of venous return and cardiac output and also results in profound

hypotension. This condition can be prevented by temporary circulatory arrest to the lower torso, which effectively divides the circulating blood volume with resulting perfusion of the upper torso at normal pressure and flow.[28]

Caval thrombi emanating from a left renal tumor are best approached through a midline incision with the patient supine (Fig. 8-9A). Caval thrombi emanating from a right-sided tumor may alternatively be approached through a high (eighth to ninth rib) thoracoabdominal incision with the patient in the modified flank position with torque of the lower torso[29] (Fig. 8-9B). With the patient in a supine position, we use a midline abdominal incision with a median sternotomy to permit supradiaphragmatic intrapericardial vascular control of the inferior vena cava.

The sites and sequence of vascular interruption for a IB intracaval right renal tumor thrombus are shown in Figure 8-10.

Surgical Technique

An intra-arterial and Swan-Ganz catheter are placed before exploratory laparotomy. The abdomen is explored and a care-

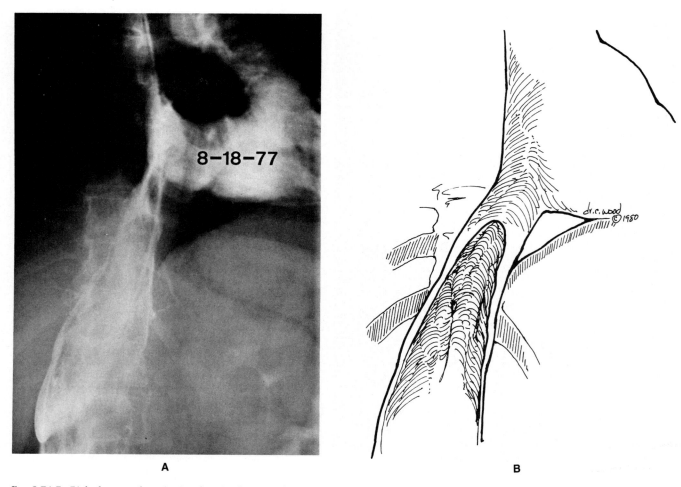

A

B

FIG. 8-7*A,B.* Right heart catheterization for visualization of the apex of the tumor thrombus.

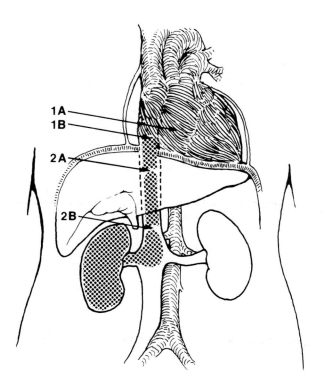

ful examination for evidence of metastatic disease is completed. The right and transverse colon, small bowel mesentery, and duodenum are mobilized to the left (Fig. 8-11) with interruption of the inferior mesenteric vein if this structure impedes adequate mobilization. The bowel is then placed in a Lahey bag and retracted in a cephalad direction to expose the retroperitoneum, right renal tumor, and retroperitoneal vessels (Fig. 8-12). The renal hilum is then explored carefully. Any suspicious nodes are excised and submitted for frozen section. If the patient is considered to be a suitable surgical candidate, the renal artery is ligated employing 2 ligatures of 0 silk. Ligation of the renal artery may result in shrinkage of the tumor thrombus.

The abdominal incision is extended in a cephalad direction with a median sternotomy. Bone wax is applied to the incised

1. Supradiaphragmatic	2. Infradiaphragmatic
A. Intracardiac	A. Retrohepatic
B. Intrapericardial	B. Infrahepatic

FIG. 8-8. Vena caval tumor thrombus classification.

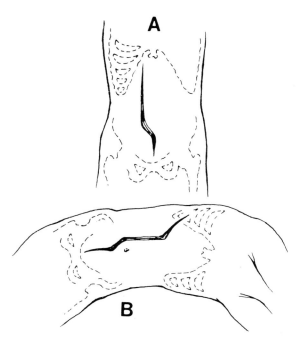

FIG. 8-9. Options for surgical incisions. *A,* Midline incision with the patient in a supine position. *B,* High thoracoabdominal incision with the patient in a modified flank position.

surface of the sternum to control bleeding. The pericardium is opened and its edges are secured to the drapes at the wound margins with interrupted 2-0 silk sutures. Palpation of the intrapericardial inferior vena cava reveals the apex of the tumor thrombus. A cardiac tourniquet loop is employed to secure the inferior vena cava proximal to the thrombus (Fig. 8-13).

Temporary occlusion of the inferior vena cava is performed and the vital signs are observed. When collateral circulation is not adequate as evidenced by a significant drop in systemic blood pressure, it is necessary to cross-clamp the aorta at the diaphragmatic hiatus above the celiac axis (Fig. 8-14).

When this decision has been made, attention is returned to the abdomen, and the operative field is prepared for execution of thrombectomy from the inferior vena cava and radical nephrectomy. The liver is next delivered free of its diaphragmatic attachments (coronary and triangular ligaments) by incising these and exposing the bare area of the diaphragm (Figs. 8-15, 8-16).[30] This exposure is further facilitated by the previously performed median sternotomy. The liver is now rotated medially to expose the retrohepatic vena cava. Caudad to the main hepatic veins there are usually several small hepatic veins that are best interrupted, thus providing better exposure and facilitating tumor thrombectomy.

The proximal lumbar veins are identified and interrupted with care to prevent disruption in the continuity of the intraluminal caval thrombus. When caval obstruction by tumor thrombus is complete, lumbar veins may serve to communicate via the azygos and hemiazygos systems with the remaining patent inferior vena cava. Under such circumstances, lumbar veins may approach the size of the external iliac veins and are best occluded with a Rummel tourniquet rather than sacrificed. The inferior vena cava is then further exposed and a Rummel tourniquet is passed around the distal vena cava just above the bifurcation (Fig. 8-17). Prior palpation will define the presence of a distal "bland" thrombus and its extent. When a "bland" thrombus extends below the bifurcation of the vena cava into the iliac veins, it is necessary to gain venous control

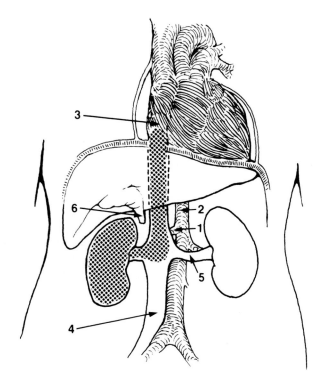

1. Right renal artery
2. Proximal aorta
3. Proximal I.V.C.
4. Distal I.V.C.
5. Left renal vein
6. Porta hepatis

FIG. 8-10. Sequence of vascular interruption for a IB intracaval right renal tumor.

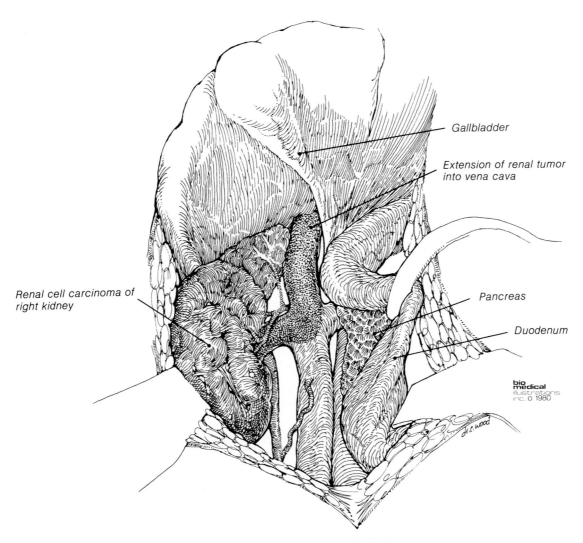

Gallbladder

Extension of renal tumor
into vena cava

Renal cell carcinoma of
right kidney

Pancreas

Duodenum

bio
medical
illustrations
inc. © 1980

FIG. 8-11. Retroperitoneal mobilization in preparation of the surgical field for a right-sided tumor.

distal to the limits of the "bland" thrombus. A Rummel tourniquet is then placed around the left renal vein and left loosely in position (Fig. 8-17). If it is not necessary to cross-clamp the aorta, it is advisable to place a vascular tape around the left renal artery. This tape may be employed to secure the renal artery in the event that collateral venous drainage (left adrenal and left gonadal) is inadequate to prevent venous engorgement of the left kidney when the main left renal vein is occluded.

It has been estimated that 25% of the inferior vena caval return is from the hepatic veins and, despite aortic cross-clamping, venous bleeding from the portal vascular bed via the hepatics will impair adequate visualization of the interior of the vena cava at the time of thrombectomy.[31] This can be markedly reduced by employing Pringel's maneuver (cross-clamping the porta hepatis) (Fig. 8-18).[32] At the foramen of Winslow, the porta hepatis is easily defined between the index finger and thumb. An alternative to cross-clamping the porta hepatis in its entirety is to dissect out the vascular structures (portal vein and hepatic artery) and to secure these with vascular tapes. This method has a theoretical advantage of pre-

venting crush injury to the common bile duct, but we consider it an unnecessary additional step. The aorta is then exposed at the diaphragmatic hiatus above the celiac axis sufficiently to permit occlusion with an aneurysm clamp under direct vision (Fig. 8-14).

Prior to vascular isolation of the inferior vena cava from the right atrium to the pelvis, it is advisable to administer 25 g of mannitol intravenously and to give a single dose of heparin. This protects against renal and hepatic injury as well as thrombotic phenomena in the lower torso should circulatory arrest be prolonged due to extended cross-clamping.

The patient is then placed in a 20° Trendelenburg position. The aorta is cross-clamped. When the pulmonary wedge pressure increases to 15 mm Hg and systolic blood pressure is 120 mm Hg, the intrapericardial inferior vena cava is occluded. Occlusion of the abdominal aorta and the intrapericardial inferior vena cava effectively divides the circulating blood volume in half. Attention to the systemic arterial and left ventricular filling pressures allows precise sequential clamping of the aorta and vena cava to avoid upper torso hyper- or hypovolemia. Venous return from the lower extremities constitutes

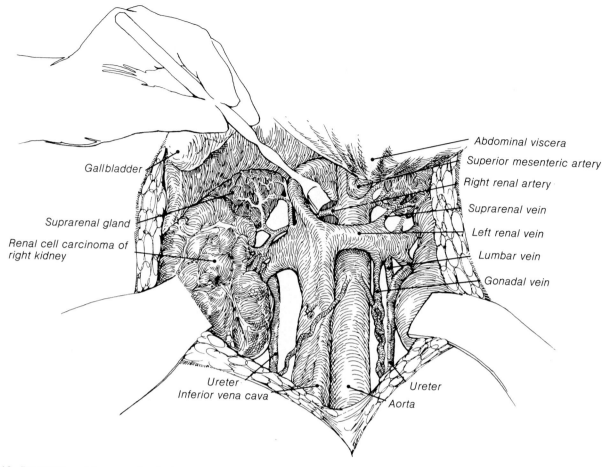

Labels on figure (clockwise from top-right):
Abdominal viscera
Superior mesenteric artery
Right renal artery
Suprarenal vein
Left renal vein
Lumbar vein
Gonadal vein
Ureter
Aorta
Inferior vena cava
Ureter
Renal cell carcinoma of right kidney
Suprarenal gland
Gallbladder

FIG. 8-12. Preparation of the operative bed for surgical extirpation.

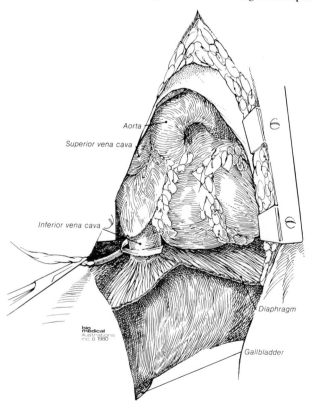

Labels on figure:
Aorta
Superior vena cava
Inferior vena cava
Diaphragm
Gallbladder

bio medical illustrations inc. © 1980

FIG. 8-13. Intrapericardial control of the inferior vena cava.

a major source of blood loss at the time of cavotomy and is eliminated next by distal caval occlusion (Fig. 8-17). An atraumatic occlusive clamp is then applied to the porta hepatis (Fig. 8-18), and the remaining Rummel tourniquet on the left renal vein is occluded (Fig. 8-17).

The incision in the vena cava is initiated with a scimitar (No. 12 blade) and is continued with Pott-Smith scissors proximally to a level just below the hepatic veins (see Fig. 8-17). A No. 20 Foley catheter with a 30 ml balloon is used for tumor thrombus extraction and is found to be less traumatic than a Fogarty catheter.[28,33] The catheter is advanced through the cavotomy until its tip can be palpated above the apex of the tumor thrombus within the pericardium. The tumor thrombus is usually delivered intact with gentle downward traction on the catheter and manual caval compression (Figs. 8-19, 8-20).

Bleeding from the cavotomy results from the uncontrolled lumbar veins and blood remaining in the liver draining via the hepatic veins. Ordinary disposable suction allows for clear visualization of the inferior vena cava and thereby permits precise rapid removal of the thrombus. The tumor thrombus often adheres loosely to the intima of the vena cava, and actual mural invasion of the caval wall is a rare event.[34] Kitner dissection of the thrombus from the intima of the cava may be necessary. In case the thrombus appears more densely adherent, insertion of the index finger into the cavotomy below the hepatic veins enables most surgeons to reach the level of the

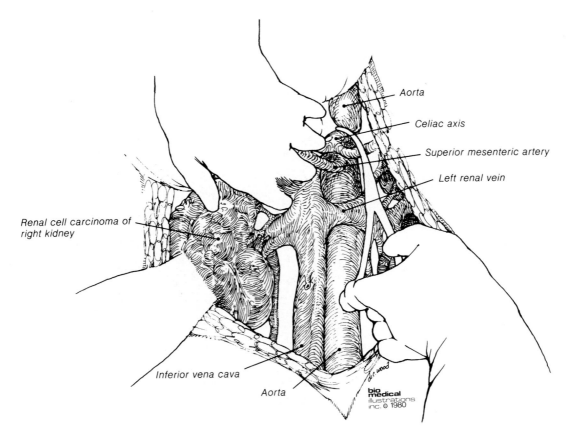

Fig. 8-14. Aortic cross-clamp at the diaphragmatic hiatus.

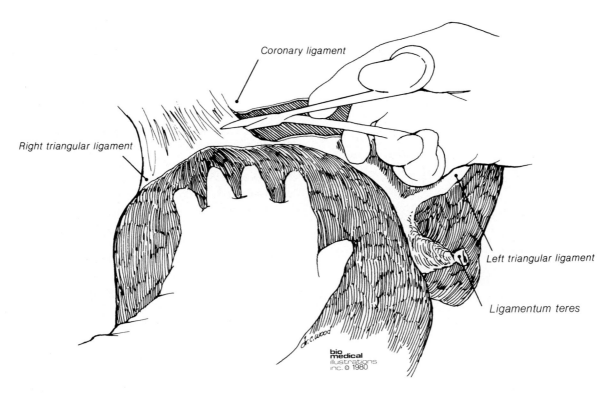

Fig. 8-15. Mobilization of the liver.

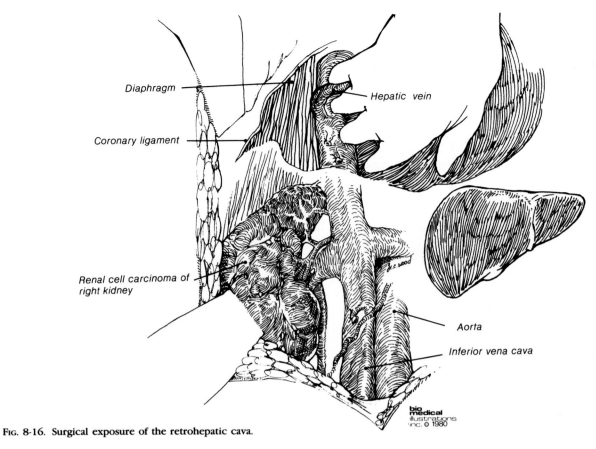

Diaphragm

Coronary ligament

Renal cell carcinoma of
right kidney

Hepatic vein

Aorta

Inferior vena cava

FIG. 8-16. Surgical exposure of the retrohepatic cava.

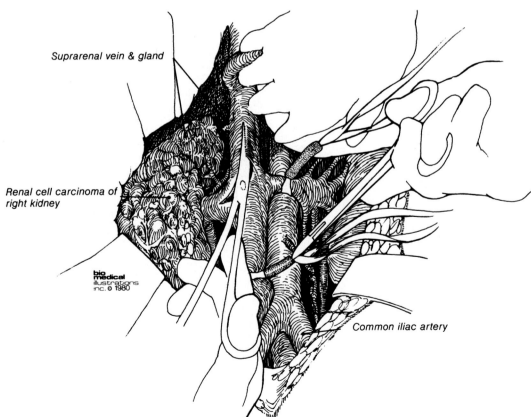

Suprarenal vein & gland

Renal cell carcinoma of
right kidney

Common iliac artery

FIG. 8-17. Completed vascular isolation of the inferior vena cava and initiation of cavotomy.

right atrium and to free any attached thrombi fragments. The inferior vena cava is next flushed vigorously with sterile water. Rarely we have employed an endarterectomy curette to detach any visible "presumed tumor" remaining within the vena cava. However, on subsequent pathologic analysis no viable tumor was detected in this material. A Satinsky clamp is then placed across the cavotomy. The remaining posterior wall of the renal vein is transected and its proximal end is secured (Fig. 8-21). The sequence of removal of the various vascular clamps is important to allow evacuation of air and debris before systemic circulation is restored and to avoid hypotension (Fig. 8-22). The left renal vein tourniquet is released first followed by removal of the clamp on the porta hepatis. The Satinsky clamp is briefly vented with the caval edges secured with Allis clamps to insure adequate replacement of the clamp subsequent to the escape of entrapped air. The position of the patient (20° Trendelenburg) protects against air embolization and promotes egress through the cavotomy as the isolated cava fills with blood. The aortic cross-clamp is then released followed by the occlusive tourniquets at the distal and proximal ends of the vena cava. The cavotomy is closed with a running suture of 5-0 polypropylene, which is then oversewn to provide a two-layer caval closure.

Radical nephrectomy and regional lymphadenectomy are then performed. In patients with significant collateral circulation via the azygos and phrenic veins, care must be taken during mobilization of the posterior and subphrenic portions of the kidney. Accessory venous tributaries from the involved kidney frequently communicate with this venous network and may be transected. After delivery of the kidney, the renal bed should be carefully explored for venous bleeding. These veins in the retroperitoneum and beneath the diaphragm may bleed vigorously and are best secured with carefully placed figure-of-eight ligatures (Fig. 8-23).

Infradiaphragmatic-retrohepatic tumor thrombi (IIA) should be approached in the same fashion because it is impossible in adults to gain proximal caval control above the hepatic veins extrapericardially (Fig. 8-24).[35]

Cross-clamping times have ranged from 14 to 30 minutes and have not been associated with hepatic or renal injury.

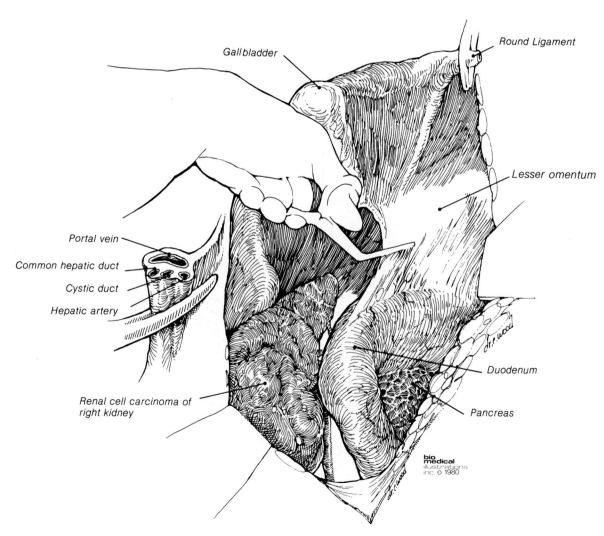

FIG. 8-18. Vascular control of the porta hepatis.

Normothermic vascular isolation of the liver during hepatic resection is tolerated for up to 30 minutes.[35,36] If collateral venous return is sufficient to obviate the need for cross-clamping the aorta, consideration must be given to the prevention of venous engorgement of the normal kidney and viscera. When the left kidney is involved with tumor, it is best to secure the right renal artery with a vascular tape during the period of right renal venous occlusion (Fig. 8-25). Marshall reported a case in which renal failure lasted for 24 days following occlusion of the left renal vein for only 30 minutes.[3] Other authors have advocated the occlusion of the superior mesenteric artery at the time of venous occlusion of the porta hepatis (Pringel's maneuver) to prevent vascular engorgement of the

bowel.[34] This technique is appropriate when the aorta is not cross-clamped.

Rarely thrombus extension into the hepatic veins has occurred with an associated Budd-Chiari syndrome. The normal venous effluent from the hepatic veins probably accounts for the rarity of this event. However, should intraluminal extension into the hepatic veins pose difficulty in complete extirpation of the tumor thrombus, the occlusive clamp on the porta hepatis should be released. Venous hemorrhage with this maneuver is brisk and should aid in removal of residual intraluminal tumor thrombi within the hepatic veins. Employment of a dental mirror to aid visualization has permitted the successful use of an endarterectomy curette.

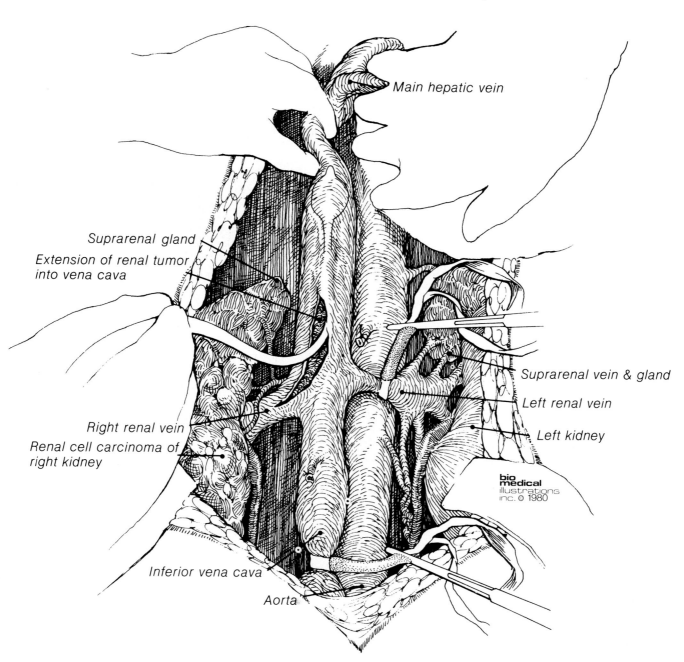

FIG. 8-19. Technique for extraction of a tumor thrombus from the inferior vena cava.

Alternative Techniques for IA and IIB Extension

In elderly patients and in patients with recognized atherosclerosis of the aorta, it may be inappropriate to cross-clamp the aorta. It has been our recent policy to routinely include a member from the cardiac surgery department in our operative team. The midline abdominal incision with median sternotomy is employed. When the intrapericardial inferior vena cava is occluded, the patient is observed to determine if collateral venous return will provide an adequate cardiac output. In the event that cardiac output falls and systemic blood pressure drops, the patient is placed on cardiac bypass. The systemic administration of heparin required for such a procedure contributes significantly to the ultimate blood loss, but is unavoidable. Those aspects previously described in detail for the management of supradiaphragmatic-intrapericardial tumor thrombi (other than aortic cross-clamping) of necessity are followed. Important variations include: (1) distal caval control (Fig. 8-17) prior to initiating bypass and (2) consideration of occlusion of the superior mesenteric artery. The first is necessary because one component of cardiac bypass includes cannulation of the iliac vein. When bypass is initiated, the risk of retrograde tumor flow is real. The second prevents vascular congestion of the bowel during the period of portal venous occlusion.

In the event that the required cavotomy is of such length to preclude occlusion with a Satinsky clamp, it may be sewn from cephalad to caudad after flushing. Prior to final caval closure, an occlusive clamp is placed, caval in-flow is restored, the cava is vented, and final closure is completed.

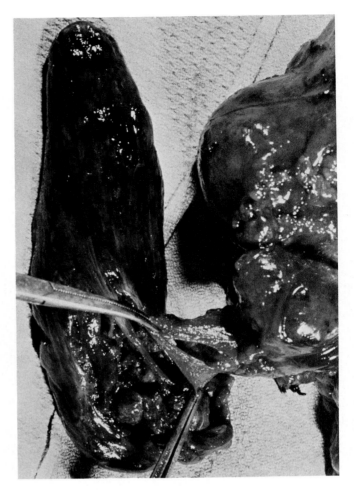

FIG. 8-20. Extracted intact tumor thrombus.

INFRADIAPHRAGMATIC-INFRAHEPATIC (IIB) EXTENSION

Incision

We prefer a thoracoabdominal incision for intraluminal caval thrombi extension at this level. The intraluminal caval extension here is less apt to obstruct the vena cava, and in this clinical situation the vena cava may be controlled below the hepatic veins. Venous return via the hepatic veins is estimated to represent 25% of the total inferior vena caval cardiac return and is sufficient to sustain adequate cardiac output in most patients.[31] With significant hypotension, the aorta may be cross-clamped.

Technique

The sequence of vascular control for this level of involvement is illustrated in Figure 8-26. When proximal caval exposure is inadequate to permit its occlusion by placement of a vascular tourniquet, the liver is best mobilized as previously described (Figs. 8-15, 8-16). Interruption of the lumbar veins reduces blood loss and improves visualization at the time of cavotomy. Alternatively, a vena cava clip may be placed just above the tumor thrombus. However, because this approach prevents only gross embolization of tumor thrombi, we prefer the former approach.

The sequence of vascular control for right-sided tumors is as follows: (1) right renal artery, (2) subhepatic vena cava, (3) distal vena cava above the bifurcation, and (4) left renal vein (Fig. 8-26). If collateral venous drainage of the left kidney is not sufficient to prevent venous engorgement, the left renal artery may be secured with the previously placed vascular tape. Cavotomy and thrombus extraction are carried out as previously described.

Cavectomy has been advocated by certain authors and can be safely performed.[30] For right renal tumors, this procedure can be performed without significantly jeopardizing the remaining left kidney, but cavectomy for left renal tumors requires management of the venous drainage from the right kidney. An end-to-side renal protal vein anastomosis has been employed with success.[8,30] Cavectomy should rarely be employed because of the rarity with which direct caval invasion occurs.[26] Furthermore, in those cases in which caval invasion has been documented, the dismal survival rates have not been improved with cavectomy.[8,30]

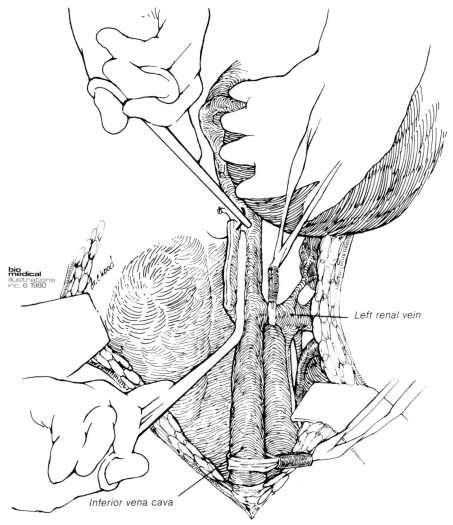

FIG. 8-21. Vena caval closure.

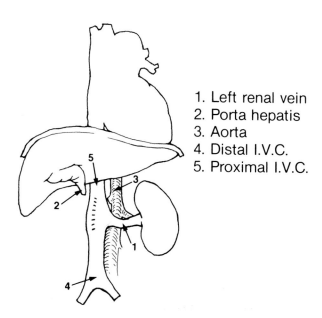

1. Left renal vein
2. Porta hepatis
3. Aorta
4. Distal I.V.C.
5. Proximal I.V.C.

FIG. 8-22. Sequence of vascular restoration.

SUPRADIAPHRAGMATIC-INTRACARDIAC (IA) EXTENSION

Tumor thrombi that have reached this level require cardiopulmonary bypass or, alternatively, hypothermia and cardiac arrest. When the right atrial extension is modest, it is reasonable to displace the tumor apex manually into the intrapericardial inferior vena cava or to provide occlusion above this level. In such circumstances, the remainder of the procedure is performed as previously described with cardiac bypass.

In the event that cardiac extension is significant, the heart is opened and the tumor extracted. In patients with extensive intrathoracic tumor extension or demonstrable obstruction of the hepatic veins on ultrasound, the technique reported by Marshall and associates is appropriate.[37] Such patients are initially placed on bypass with the skull packed in ice. Core body temperature is reduced to 19.5°C and the circulation is arrested. The operation is then performed as indicated in a bloodless field. After closure of the vena cavotomy, the cardio-

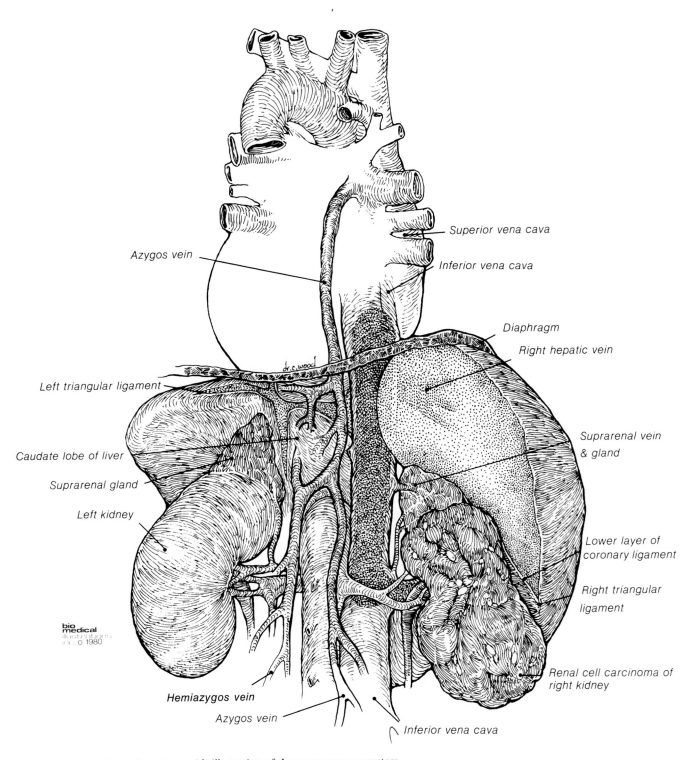

Azygos vein

Superior vena cava

Inferior vena cava

Diaphragm

Right hepatic vein

Left triangular ligament

Caudate lobe of liver

Suprarenal gland

Left kidney

Suprarenal vein & gland

Lower layer of coronary ligament

Right triangular ligament

Renal cell carcinoma of right kidney

Hemiazygos vein

Azygos vein

Inferior vena cava

FIG. 8-23. Retroperitoneal anatomy with illustration of the azygos venous system.

pulmonary bypass circulation is reinstituted and the heart defibrillated when core temperature is warmed to 36°C. The reported patient on whom this procedure was performed was young and presumably free from associated atherosclerotic disease of the coronary and cerebral vessels. Whether such a technique would be suitable in older patients is debatable.

CONCLUSION

Current surgical techniques have made surgical extirpation of intraluminal caval extension from RCC relatively safe. Because of the variability in vascularization of the tumor thrombi, a neat extraction as depicted in Figure 8-20 is not always possi-

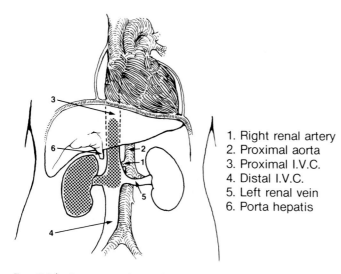

FIG. 8-24. Sequence of vascular interruption for a IIA infradia-phragmatic-retrohepatic tumor.

1. Right renal artery
2. Proximal aorta
3. Proximal I.V.C.
4. Distal I.V.C.
5. Left renal vein
6. Porta hepatis

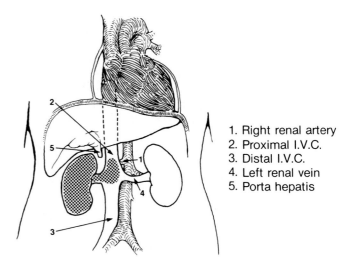

FIG. 8-26. Sequence of vascular interruption for a IIB infradia-phragmatic-infrahepatic tumor thrombus.

1. Right renal artery
2. Proximal I.V.C.
3. Distal I.V.C.
4. Left renal vein
5. Porta hepatis

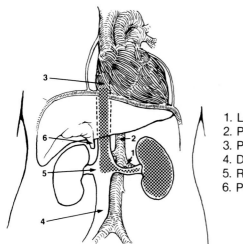

1. Left renal artery
2. Proximal aorta
3. Proximal I.V.C.
4. Distal I.V.C.
5. Right renal vein
6. Porta hepatis

FIG. 8-25. Sequence of vascular interruption for a IB left renal tumor.

ble. Tumor thrombi that have lost their vascular supply vary in appearance from a "gritty yellow and friable" to "necrotic curd." The intraluminal tumor extraction in these situations is technically more difficult, is time-consuming, and is often performed "piecemeal."

In those cases in which the girth of the extrahepatic vena cava has been dramatically increased, we have excised an appropriate longitudinal strip of caval wall, performing "cavaplasty" at the time of caval closure.

When resection of the intraluminal extension is complete and performed as outlined without dissemination, prognosis is dependent on known factors related to tumor extension and nodal involvement. The procedure is not warranted in patients with gross nodal disease or known metastatic disease.

REFERENCES

1. ANGERVALL, L., CARLSTROM, E., WAHLQVIST, L., and AHREN, C. H. Effects of clinical and morphological variables on spread of renal carcinoma in an operative series. Scand. J. Urol. Nephrol., 3:124–140, 1969.
2. ROBSON, C. L., CHURCHILL, B. N., and ANDERSON, W. The results of radical nephrectomy for renal cell carcinoma. J. Urol., 101:297–301, 1969.
3. MARSHALL, V. F., MIDDLETON, R. D., HALLSWAY, G. R., and GOLDSMITH, E. I. Surgery for renal cell carcinoma in the vena cava. J. Urol., 103:414, 1970.
4. SVENE, S. Tumor thrombus of the inferior vena cava resulting from renal cell carcinoma. Scand. J. Urol. Nephrol., 3:245, 1969.
5. KAHN, P. C. The epinephrine effect in selected renal angiography. Radiology, 85:301, 1965.
6. NEY, C. Thrombosis of the inferior vena cava associated with malignant renal tumors. J. Urol., 55:583, 1946.
7. ARKLESS, R. Renal carcinoma: How it metastasizes. Radiology, 84:496, 1965.
8. KERNEY, G. P., et al. Results of inferior vena cava resection for renal cell carcinoma. J. Urol. (submitted for publication).
9. KAUFMAN, J. J., BURKE, D. E., and GOODWIN, W. E. Abdominal venography in urological disease. J. Urol., 75:160, 1956.
10. RICHES, E. W., GRIFFITHS, I. H., and THACKRAY, A. C. New growths of the kidney and ureter. Br. J. Urol., 23:297, 1951.
11. MYERS, G. H., JR., FEHRENBAKER, L. G., and KELALIS, P. P. Prognostic significance of renal vein invasion by hypernephroma. J. Urol., 100:420, 1968.
12. SKINNER, D. G., PFISTER, R. F., and COLVIN, R. Extension of renal cell carcinoma into the vena cava: The rationale for aggressive surgical management. J. Urol., 107:711, 1972.
13. SKINNER, D. G., VERMILLION, C. D., and COLVIN, R. B. The surgical management of renal cell carcinoma. J. Urol., 107:705, 1972.

14. Schefft, P., Novick, A. C., Straffon, R. A., and Steward, B. H. Surgery for renal cell carcinoma extending into the inferior vena cava. J. Urol., *120:*28, 1977.

15. Cherrie, R. J., Goldman, D. G., Lindner, A., and DeKernion, J. B. Prognostic implications of vena caval extension of renal cell carcinoma. J. Urol., *128:*910–912, 1982.

16. DeKernion, J. B. Ramming, K. P., and Smith, R. B. The natural history of metastatic renal cell carcinoma: A computer analysis. J. Urol., *120:*148, 1978.

17. Middleton, R. G. Surgery for metastatic renal cell carcinoma. J. Urol., *97:*973, 1978.

18. Katz, S. A., and Davis, J. E. Renal adenocarcinoma: Prognostics and treatment reflected by survival. Urology, *10:*10, 1977.

19. Marks, W. N., Korobkin, M., Callen, P. W., and Kaiser, J. A. CT diagnosis of tumor thrombus of the renal vein and inferior vena cava. A.J.R., *131:*843–846, 1978.

20. Levine, E., Lee, K. R., and Weigel, J. Preoperative determination of abdominal extent of renal cell carcinoma by computed tomography. Radiology, *132:*395–398, 1979.

21. Hricak, H., et al. Magnetic resonance imaging in the diagnosis and staging of renal and perirenal neoplasms. Radiology, *154:*709–715, 1985.

22. Bradley, W. G. When should GRASS be used. Radiology, *169:*574–575, 1988.

23. Hricak, H., et al. Abdominal venous system: Assessment using MR. Radiology, *156:*415–422, 1985.

24. Axel, L. Blood flow effect in magnetic resonance imaging. A.J.R., *143:*1157–1166, 1984.

25. Haase, A., et al. FLASH imaging: Rapid NMR imaging using low flip angle pulses. J. Magn. Reson., *67:*258–266, 1986.

26. Wehrli, F. W. Introduction to fast-scan magnetic resonance. Milwaukee General Electric, 1–12, 1986.

27. Green, D., and Steinbach, H. L. Ultrasound diagnosis of hypernephroma extending into the inferior vena cava. Radiology, *115:*679–680, 1975.

28. Cummings, K. B., et al. Intraoperative management of renal cell carcinoma with supradiaphragmatic caval extension. J. Urol., *122:*829, 1979.

29. Goodwin, W. E. Ileal ureter. In: *The Craft of Surgery.* Edited by P. Cooper. Boston, Little, Brown and Company 1971.

30. McCullough, D. L., and Gittes, R. F. Vena cava resection for renal cell carcinoma. J. Urol., *112:*162, 1974.

31. Leiter, E. Inferior vena caval thrombosis in malignant renal tumors. J.A.M.A., *198:*1167, 1966.

32. Pringel, J. H. Notes on the arrest of hepatic hemorrhage due to trauma. Ann. Surg., *48:*541, 1908.

33. Freed, S. Z., and Gliedman, N. R. The removal of renal cell carcinoma thrombus extending into the right atrium. J. Urol., *113:*163, 1975.

34. Skinner, D. G., and DeKernion, J. B. Clinical manifestations and treatment of renal parenchymal tumors. In: *Genitourinary Cancer.* Edited by D. G. Skinner and J. B. DeKernion. Philadelphia, W. B. Saunders Co., 1978.

35. Heaney, J. P., et al. An improved technique for vascular isolation of the liver: Experimental study and case reports. Ann. Surg., *163:*237, 1966.

36. Albo, D., Jr., Christianson, C., and Rasmussen, B. L. Massive liver trauma involving the suprarenal vena cava. Am. J. Surg., *118:*1960, 1969.

37. Marshall, F. F., Reitz, B. A., and Diamond, D. A. A new technique for management of renal cell carcinoma involving the right atrium: Hypothermia and cardiac arrest. J. Urol., *131:*103–107, 1984.

CARCINOMA OF THE RENAL PELVIS AND URETER

CHAPTER 9

Primary Carcinoma of the Upper Urinary Tract Urothelium: An Overview

Richard J. Babaian

CARCINOMA OF THE RENAL PELVIS

Malignant tumors of the renal pelvis make up 7 to 8% of all renal neoplasms but represent less than 1% of all genitourinary tumors. They are more frequent in men than in women, at a sex ratio approximating 3:1. Their peak incidence is in the seventh decade, with 80% occurring between 40 and 70 years of age. Almost one third of these patients have an associated lesion in the ipsilateral ureter or bladder at the time of diagnosis, and 40 to 50% ultimately demonstrate urothelial tumors at other sites.[1]

Causes

Exposure to those environmental substances that have been associated with the development of bladder cancer has also been incriminated in the development of renal pelvic carcinoma. The occupational carcinogens that have been identified include beta-naphthylamine, 4-aminobiphenyl, 4-nitrobi-

phenyl, and 4,4'-diaminobiphenyl.[2] These agents are found in the dye, textile, printing, plastic, rubber, and cable industries. In addition, benzidine, used by laboratory technicians to detect occult blood, is a carcinogen. Schmauz and Cole have postulated that only at high-level exposure are the carcinogens active in the upper urinary tract.[3]

Nonoccupational factors that have been incriminated in the development of urothelial neoplasms include dietary additives (nitrosamine), abnormal tryptophan metabolism, and tobacco smoking.[2] A significant odds ratio (76.5:5.8, males to females) has been observed for cigarette smokers, as has a significant positive trend related to pack years. An index combining intensity and duration shows the highest risk among the heaviest smokers and evidence of risk reduction for those who quit smoking.[4] Phenacetin, an aniline derivative, has also been identified as a carcinogen of the upper urothelium as well as of the urinary bladder. It has been postulated that one of the N-hydroxylation byproducts of phenacetin metabolism is carcinogenic.[5]

Clinical Presentation

The most common symptom of patients with renal pelvic tumors is hematuria, which occurs in more than 80% of patients.[6] Flank pain has been described by 24 to 37% of patients, and 5 to 20% complain of symptoms of bladder irritation.[6] Physical findings are frequently absent; however, a flank mass secondary to the tumor or to an associated hydronephrosis is present in one fifth of the patients. It is important to remember that the symptoms secondary to pelvic tumors may be masked by the concomitant manifestations of bladder and/or ureteral tumors, reported to occur in 33% of patients.

Diagnosis

Excretory urographic results of almost all patients with renal pelvic carcinoma are abnormal. The most common pyelographic finding is a filling defect in the renal pelvis, demonstrated in 50 to 75% of all patients. Other radiographic findings may include ureteropelvic or infundibular stenosis, hydronephrosis, a splaying of the calyces suggesting a renal mass and, occasionally, nonvisualization of the affected renal unit. Attempts to correlate the radiographic findings with either the stage or grade of the neoplasm have been unsuccessful. A retrograde pyelogram can be useful and is mandatory when the excretory urogram is inconclusive (Fig. 9-1). An antegrade pyelogram can be useful in selected patients whose renal unit is not visualized and in whom a retrograde urogram cannot be obtained.

Ultrasonography and computed tomography have not added appreciably to the accurate diagnosis of renal pelvic lesions.[7] Routine angiography is of little value because of the avascular nature of these epithelial tumors. However, the procedure may help to demonstrate other pathologic conditions, such as renal artery aneurysms and vascular impressions, which can cause a filling defect on a pyelogram and which at times suggest a renal pelvic neoplasm. In addition, angiography may provide information regarding parenchymal invasion, which can occur with this disease.

Routine voided or catheterized urinary cytologic studies are of limited value because reports are false-negative in at least 30% of cases[8] and can be false-positive when an unsuspected bladder cancer is present. The accuracy of a cytologic diagnosis increases with the degree of cellular anaplasia. In addition, collecting a barbotage specimen following selective ureteral catheterization increases the likelihood of an accurate diagnosis to 80%.[9] Leistenschneider and Nagel have reported a 50% detection rate for stage 0, grade I tumors; 80% for stage A, grade I to II; and 100% for higher stage and grade neoplasms.[9] Interestingly, these investigators had no false-positive diagnoses. Similar results can be achieved by using retrograde brushings (Fig. 9-2).[10]

The ureteroscope, making possible endoscopic visualization of the upper tracts, is a more recent addition to the urologist's diagnostic arsenal. The development from a rigid to a

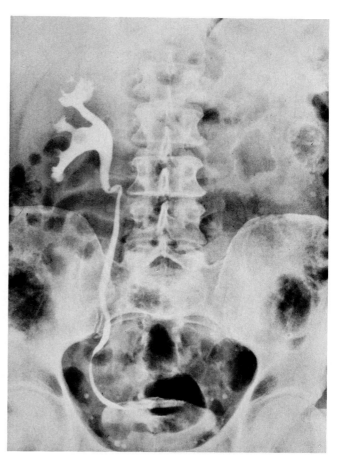

FIG. 9-1. A retrograde pyelogram demonstrating a filling defect in the renal pelvis caused by transitional cell carcinoma.

flexible ureteroscope with maneuvering and biopsy capabilities reflects continuing technologic advances.

Cystoscopic evaluation is a mandatory component of a complete evaluation because of the high incidence of other associated urothelial tumors. Additional studies useful in accurately assessing the extent of the disease include a chest roentgenogram, multichannel blood analysis (including liver and renal function tests), and abdominal computed tomography.

Pathologic Considerations

Three histologic types of carcinoma (transitional cell, squamous cell, and adenocarcinoma) may be recognized in renal pelvic carcinoma; the transitional cell type predominates, occurring in approximately 85% of patients. Squamous cell carcinoma, which occurs equally in men and women, accounts for 14% of the total number of renal pelvic carcinomas and is associated with calculus disease and chronic irritation. Only 1% of these neoplasms are adenocarcinomas, which occur predominantly in women and are associated with chronic infection or irritation.

In an attempt to reduce the variation in grade assessment from one observer to another and to increase the comparabil-

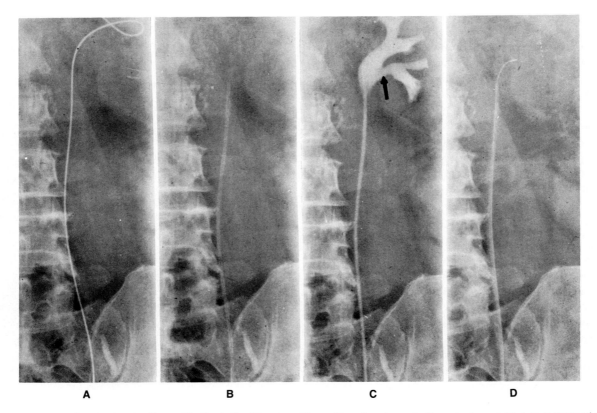

FIG. 9-2. Biopsy procedure depicted radiographically. *A,* Flexible wireguide positioned cystoscopically up to the renal pelvis. *B,* Ureteral catheter in place. *C,* Retrograde pyelogram demonstrating the location of the suspected tumor (arrow). *D,* After contrast material is removed, brush is inserted and directed to the site of lesion for biopsy. (From von Eschenbach, A. C. Retrograde brush biopsy in the diagnosis of renal pelvis and ureteral tumors. The Cancer Bulletin, *31:*17–20, 1979. Copyright Medical Arts Publishing Foundation, Houston.)

ity of cancer statistics between the different institutions, a three-grade system has been proposed by Mostofi and the World Health Organization.[11] In this system, grade I includes those tumors that display the least degree of cellular anaplasia compatible with the diagnosis of malignancy. Grade III tumors exhibit the most severe degrees of anaplasia, and grade II tumors demonstrate cellular changes intermediate between grades I and III. The clinical usefulness of this system is demonstrated by its ability to be correlated with survival rates.

Staging

The limited accuracy of the available staging procedures has precluded the development of a useful clinical staging system. Consequently, a pathologic staging system modified from the one Batata and associates developed for ureteral carcinoma has been proposed for carcinoma of the renal pelvis.[1] In this system, stage O neoplasms are confined to the mucosa, stage A tumors invade the lamina propria, stage B invades muscle, stage C extends into the peripelvic fat and/or renal parenchyma, and stage D demonstrates regional nodal involvement or other metastases (Fig. 9-3).

Although the specific red-cell adherence test has demonstrated little, if any, clinical applicability, it has provided interesting data. Investigators have reported its ability to segregate

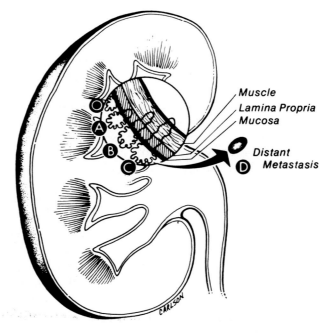

FIG. 9-3. Staging system modified from Batata and associates based on the extent of penetration applied to carcinoma of the renal pelvis. (From Babaian, R. J., and Johnson, D. E. Carcinoma of the renal pelvis. The Cancer Bulletin, *31:*21–25, 1979. Copyright Medical Arts Publishing Foundation, Houston.)

invasive from noninvasive lesions, to predict the clinical course of disease, and to suggest a potential method for selecting the optimal therapy for individual patients.[12-15]

Treatment

Although investigators agree that a conservative nephron-sparing procedure is indicated for patients who have renal insufficiency or bilateral synchronous tumors, controversy continues regarding the optimum management of renal pelvic carcinoma. The traditional treatment of choice has been nephrectomy with complete ureterectomy, including excising a cuff of bladder around the ureteral orifice. The technique of transvesical intussusception ureterectomy accomplishes this aspect of the surgical procedure simply and safely.[16] Several investigators, however, have recommended a universal conservative approach.[17-19] A review of these reports suggests that many of their patients were carefully selected and represent exceptional rather than the usual pathologic conditions. Table 9-1 presents a summary of conservative treatment results.

Previously we reported from The University of Texas M.D. Anderson Cancer Center that, since low-grade low-stage lesions did not occur frequently, subjecting patients to the hazard of a mistaken frozen-section diagnosis and the increased risk of wound seeding inherent in conservative therapy was not warranted.[25] However, today nephroureteroscopy has enhanced clinical staging and surveillance to the degree that a consideration of conservative treatment seems reasonable. Conservative therapy today offers several alternatives, including local excision, partial nephrectomy, and laser ablation combined with topical therapy via either the antegrade or retrograde route.[26-29] One report proclaims that conservative therapy is feasible for patients with superficial low-grade upper-tract tumors, based on the author's experience with nephrectomy and partial ureterectomy.[19] However, that procedure is not really conservative therapy, and therefore to extrapolate its results to nephron-sparing therapy does not seem justified. Nevertheless, this report does raise the issue of ureteral stump recurrence rates, unusually low in the group of patients described, which indirectly affects the feasibility of conservative therapy for renal pelvic tumors. Is it the low likelihood of associated urothelial abnormalities in these authors' patients, the removal of urothelial-urine contact, or some other undetermined event that accounts for their low incidence of ureteral stump recurrence? At a time when minimizing therapy while maintaining good results is in vogue, we must remember the potential ramifications and associated morbidity of a conservative approach to the treatment and follow-up of a surgically curable disease.

There is little doubt, based on urothelial mapping, that high-grade upper-tract disease is multifocal and not amenable to conservative therapy.[30-32] In addition, the usually high incidence of ureteral stump recurrence following nephrectomy and partial ureterectomy (25 to 30%), the low incidence of bilaterality (2%) or of the asynchronous development of

TABLE 9-1. *Results of Conservative Therapy*

| AUTHOR | NUMBER OF PATIENTS | TUMOR SITE | RECURRENCES | | FOLLOW-UP PERIOD |
			%	(No.)	
Gibson, 1967[17]	2	Renal pelvis	0		
	1	Junction mid and lower ureter	0		
Petkovic, 1972[20]	27	Renal pelvis	70	(19/27)	
	29	Ureteral	7	(2/29)	
Brown and Roumaini, 1974[18]	2	Distal ureter	0		
	1	Proximal ureter	0		
	1	Renal pelvis	0		
Mazeman, 1976[21]	44	Distal ureter	14	(6/44)	
	50	Proximal ureter	50	(25/50)	3 yrs.
	23	Renal pelvix	48	(11/23)	
Babaian and Johnson, 1979[1]	6	Distal ureter	17	(1/6)	±3.7 yrs.
Pagano, 1984[22]	4	Distal ureter	0		4–16 mos.
Bazeed et al., 1986[23]	6	Renal pelvis	50	(3/6)	8–53 mos.
	3	Ureter 1 proximal, 2 distal	0		5–65 mos.
Ziegelbaum et al., 1987[24]	14	Renal pelvis	39 1 operative death	(5/13)	0.5–5 yrs.

upper tract tumors, and the incidence of lymphatic permeation (20%) and renal parenchymal involvement (30%) suggest that complete nephroureterectomy remains the procedure of choice for both low-grade and high-grade disease.

The value of lymphadenectomy in the treatment of this disease is at present undetermined. Because it adds little to the operative time and morbidity and can be useful in determining the need for adjuvant chemotherapy, it is routinely performed. Because the presence of lymph node metastasis usually indicates a poor prognosis and generalized disease, with hematogenous metastasis becoming clinically evident within a short time, platinum-based chemotherapy is recommended postoperatively for these patients.

The role of neoadjuvant chemotherapy for patients with presumed stage C disease is currently under investigation.

Prognosis

The overall 5-year survival rate previously reported from the M.D. Anderson Cancer Center was 53% and was influenced by both the grade and the stage of the neoplasm (Fig. 9-4).[1] Patients with stages O and A disease have better survival rates than patients with stages B, C, and D (P = .005 and .009, respectively). The survival rate for patients with grade I neoplasms is statistically higher than that for patients with grade III tumors (P = .03), as is the survival rate for patients with grade II lesions as compared with that for patients with grade III tumors (P = .05). Only one patient with a grade I (stage A

or O) tumor has died. The expected median survival times of patients with grade II and III neoplasms are 144 and 35 months, respectively. Only 3 of 26 patients with superficial disease (O and A) have died. The expected survival times for patients with stages B, C, and D disease are 53 and 10 months, respectively. In addition, a history of metachronous or synchronous transitional cell carcinoma of the bladder is an adverse prognostic factor (50% mortality versus 21% for those without bladder involvement at 5 years).[33]

In 29 patients studied at the M.D. Anderson Cancer Center, metastases were found in the following order of frequency: lymphatic, 21%; lung, 18%; bone, 17%; liver, 17%; other sites, 27%.[1] Fifty percent of the patients in that study presented with (22%) or developed (28%) metastases, with 28% occurring at multiple sites. The median time interval from treatment to metastasis was 8.7 months; the mean survival time of these patients from metastasis to death was 7.5 months.

Because of the high likelihood of tumor subsequently developing within the urinary bladder, all patients should be routinely monitored with cystoscopic examination at 4-month intervals for the first 3 years, at 6-month intervals for the next 2 years, and then annually, provided no subsequent tumors are demonstrated. At each follow-up, a careful check for recurrent or metastatic disease should be performed. These evaluations should include, in addition to a history and physical examination, a chest roentgenogram, a urinalysis, urinary cytology, a serum multichannel blood analysis, and periodic intravenous pyelograms.

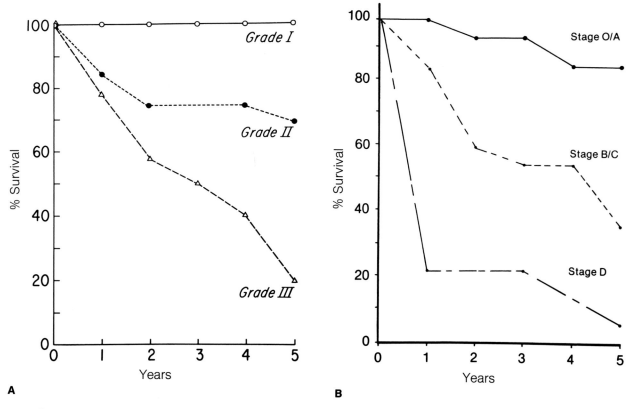

FIG. 9-4. *A,* Survival rates according to histologic grade of tumor. *B,* Survival rates according to stage of tumor.

CARCINOMA OF THE URETER

Although carcinoma of the ureter is an uncommon neoplasm accounting for less than 1% of all genitourinary malignant tumors, there has been a 30-fold increase in the number of reported cases since 1934. This greater incidence probably reflects improvements in the available diagnostic techniques and the higher survival rates of patients with bladder cancer, who have a greater chance than the general population of developing ureteral carcinoma.

Rayer, in 1841, was the first to describe primary ureteral carcinoma.[34] However, it was not until 1878 that Wising and Blix reported the first documented case of this neoplasm.[35] In 1902, Albarran made the first preoperative diagnosis of this disease,[36] and the first long-term survivor following nephroureterectomy was reported by Crance and Knickerbocker in 1924.[37]

Causes and Epidemiologic Factors

The etiologic factors previously discussed for carcinoma of the renal pelvis also apply to malignant ureteral tumors. The sex distribution of this disease is distinctly male-predominant. Most patients with ureteral neoplasms are in the sixth and seventh decades. The age range from two large series was 29 to 79 years, with a combined mean of 61.9 years.[38,39] There is no known predilection for one anatomic side over the other; however, the distal ureter has been reported as the primary site in 53 to 73% of patients.[38,39] The midureter is the second most common site, followed only infrequently by the proximal ureter.

Clinical Manifestations

The most common presenting symptom is hematuria, which occurs in 59 to 83% of patients.[38,39] Flank pain has been reported in 20 to 45% of patients, and symptoms of bladder irritation, a palpable abdominal mass, and malaise occur to a lesser degree.[38,39] A prior history of bladder cancer was found in 16% of patients with carcinoma of the ureter, and 9% of patients in this same group had concomitant bladder neoplasms.[39] Consequently, primary carcinoma of the ureter appears to be associated with other urothelial neoplasms.

Diagnosis

The intravenous pyelogram of almost all patients with carcinoma of the ureter is abnormal. Two common urographic findings are an intraluminal filling defect and hydronephrosis, with or without hydroureter. The affected renal unit is nonvisualized in 32 to 46% of patients.[39] A retrograde urogram can help to establish or confirm the diagnosis of ureteral carcinoma. It is mandatory when the pyelogram is inconclusive or when a renal unit is nonvisualized (Fig. 9-5). Bergman's sign, coiling of the ureteral catheter at the point of the lesion secondary to dilatation of the ureter immediately distal to the tumor, has

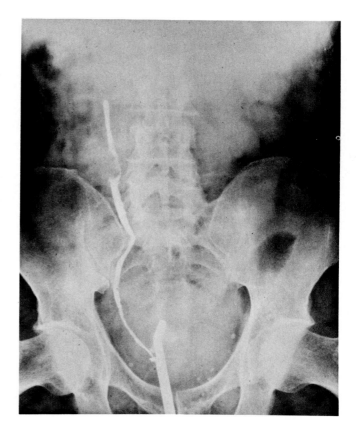

FIG. 9-5. A retrograde ureterogram demonstrating a filling defect in the right ureter secondary to primary transitional cell carcinoma.

been reported as pathognomonic for this neoplasm. Retrograde brushings as described by Gill et al. can also help establish the correct preoperative diagnosis.[40] Retrograde biopsy of the intraureteral tumor using a Dormia stone basket is another useful technique in the preoperative assessment of ureteral carcinoma.[41] As discussed previously, ureteroscopy has been added as a diagnostic tool and is helpful both to visualize and to obtain a biopsy of the upper tract.

Angiography is of little value because of the vascular nature of these epithelial tumors, but it may be useful in distinguishing primary from secondary neoplasms of the ureter.[42] Urinary cytologic studies in general have been of limited value, since false-negative interpretations have been reported for more than 30% of the patients studied. However, the true incidence of positive results from cytologic studies of voided urine samples increases as tumor anaplasia increases, varying from 11% for grade I lesions to 83% for grade IV neoplasms.[8] As previously noted, barbotage may also increase diagnostic accuracy. Because of the increased risk of other associated urothelial tumors in patients with ureteral lesions, cystoscopic examination is a mandatory component of the overall evaluation. Other studies that may be useful in accurately assessing the extent of disease include a chest roentgenogram, abdominal computed tomography, and a multiple-channel serum analysis (including both liver and renal function tests).

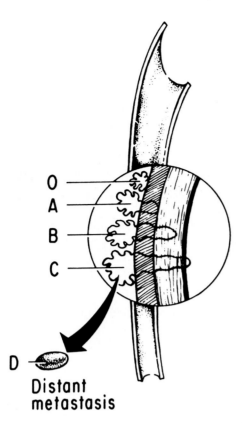

O
A
B
C

D
Distant
metastasis

FIG. 9-6. Staging system modified from Batata and associates for carcinoma of the ureter.

The histologic cell types and their frequencies and the grading and staging systems previously discussed for carcinoma of the renal pelvis also pertain to primary ureteral carcinoma (Fig. 9-6).

Treatment

Although the number of reported cases of this neoplasm has risen sharply, the paucity of patients seen by any one investigator or group has precluded unanimity of opinion as to the proper management of ureteral carcinoma. The traditional treatment for this neoplasm has been nephrectomy with total ureterectomy, including an excision of a cuff of bladder around the ureteral orifice. However, numerous pleas have been made for the conservative treatment of patients with superficial disease.[17,20] A more aggressive approach, including regional lymphadenectomy and radiotherapy, has been recommended for patients with invasive disease.[43]

As a result of the M.D. Anderson experience and in consideration of the collectively gained experience with this neoplasm reported in the literature, Johnson and I formulated a therapeutic plan based on both the grade and the stage of the disease.[44] All low-grade (I and II), low-stage (O and A) malignant lesions located in the distal third of the ureter are treated by distal ureterectomy and ureteroneocystostomy, using a psoas hitch procedure. We consider a neoplasm noninvasive if,

on radiography, the ureter appears pliable and unobstructed. If all other clinical staging parameters, including ureteroscopy and biopsy (if the latter is deemed necessary), support this diagnosis, a total distal ureterectomy is performed and the grade and stage of the neoplasm are confirmed by frozen-section examination. The results of this approach have been gratifying, and have confirmed the premise that conservative therapy is justified in selected cases.[21,44]

The uncommon occurrence of a low-grade ureteral neoplasm and the low incidence of a tumor occurring in the proximal two thirds of the ureter argue against routinely considering conservative therapy for lesions in this site. If ureteroscopy and biopsy confirm a low-grade solitary lesion, conservative therapy (local resection or laser ablation) can be considered for a patient with a normal contralateral kidney if the potential risks of radiologic and endoscopic follow-up seem warranted when a disease has such a high rate of curability with conventional therapy. Furthermore, previous experience suggests a high probability of a tumor developing distal to the original site after local resection or partial ureterectomy. For patients with high-grade (II to III) disease regardless of stage and patients with infiltrating disease, nephroureterectomy with excision of a bladder cuff remains the procedure of choice. The rationale for this approach is the rarity of bilateral tumors, the low incidence of asynchronous upper-tract tumors (5%), and the high risk of tumor recurrence in the ureter distal to the original neoplasm (30%).[39] In an attempt to improve the poor prognosis of patients with primary invasive ureteral carcinoma, postoperative irradiation should be considered when the patient either rejects or is not a candidate for chemotherapy.[45] Several studies have reported long-term survival after postoperative radiotherapy when surgical extirpation or complete removal was not possible.[38,46] Lymphadenectomy and chemotherapy are employed as described for renal pelvic tumors.

It is well known that an associated upper-tract tumor is rare in a patient who has either a superficial or invasive bladder cancer. Recently, however, a 29% incidence of recognizable ureteral carcinoma in situ has been reported in patients with multifocal carcinoma in situ of the bladder treated with intravesical bacille Calmette Guérin (BCG).[47] Most of the abnormalities were limited to the distal third of the ureter. All but one of these patients who had no associated renal pelvic tumors have been successfully treated conservatively with either distal ureterectomy or endoscopic resection; ipsilateral tumor has not recurred after a minimum follow-up of 3 years.

Clinically, when upper-tract cytologic studies are positive but bladder cytology and bladder and prostatic urethral biopsies are negative, ureteroscopy of the affected side is performed. If the ureteroscopic findings are abnormal, a biopsy is performed and therapy is then dictated by the pathologic grade and location of the lesion. If no endoscopic abnormality is seen or the biopsy is reported as negative for cancer, the cytology is repeated at 6 weeks and 3 months and endoscopy and retrograde pyelography are repeated at 3 months, regardless of the cytology report. If the cytologic result remains posi-

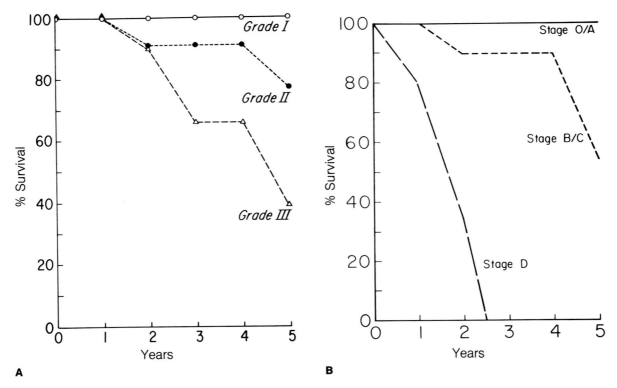

FIG. 9-7. *A*, Survival rates according to histologic grade of tumor. *B*, Survival rates according to stage of tumor. (From Babaian, R. J., and Johnson, D. E. Primary carcinoma of the ureter. J. Urol., *123:*357, 1980. Copyright 1980, Williams & Wilkins, Co., Baltimore.)

tive and nothing else is suspect, the patient is monitored for another 3 months before topical upper-tract therapy is considered. BCG is our agent of preference in such a situation, administered via either an antegrade or a retrograde approach.

Prognosis

The effect on survival rates of such factors as age, sex, and multiplicity of tumors is controversial. Function of the involved renal unit has a statistically significant effect on survival ($P = .003$). Patients whose intravenous pyelogram showed no demonstrable function tended to have neoplasms that were of a higher grade and stage. Their expected median survival was 21.1 months, as compared with 156 months for patients who demonstrated renal function on excretory urograms.

The overall 5-year survival rate of patients in the M.D. Anderson Cancer Center series was 67% and was influenced by both the grade and the stage of the lesions (Fig. 9-7). Patients with superficial disease had significantly higher survival rates than patients with invasive and metastatic disease ($P = .02$). No patient with stage O or A disease has died, whereas the median survival periods for patients with stages B, C, and D disease were 66, 56, and 20 months, respectively.

Metastatic disease developed in 15 patients (39%) 2 months to 16 years after therapy was administered to the primary lesion (median, 17 months), and 47% of metastases were evident within 12 months. The median survival period after metastatic disease developed was 15 months.

Because of the associated development of bladder cancer in more than 40% of patients with primary ureteral carcinoma and the high incidence of the subsequent development of metastatic disease (39%), routine periodic evaluation, including endoscopy, is imperative.

REFERENCES

1. BABAIAN, R. J., and JOHNSON, D. E. Carcinoma of the renal pelvis. Cancer Bull., *31:*21, 1979.
2. OTSSU, R., and HOPP, M. L. The etiology of cancer of the bladder. Surg. Gynecol. Obstet., *138:*97, 1974.
3. SCHMAUZ, R., and COLE, P. Epidemiology of cancer of the renal pelvis and ureter. I.N.C.I., *523:*1431, 1974.
4. MCLAUGHLIN, J. K., et al. Etiology of cancer of the renal pelvis. I.N.C.I., *71:*287, 1983.
5. JOHANSSON, S., et al. Uroepithelial tumors of the renal pelvis associated with abuse of phenacetin-containing analgesics. Cancer, *33:*743, 1974.
6. BATATA, M., and GRABSTALD, H. Upper urinary tract urothelial tumors. Urol. Clin. North Am., *3:*79, 1976.
7. MULHOLLAND, S. G., et al. Ultrasonic differentiation of renal pelvic filling defects. J. Urol., *122:*14, 1979.
8. ZINCKE, H., et al. Significance of urinary cytology in the early de-

tection of transitional cell cancer of the upper urinary tract. J. Urol., *116:*781, 1976.

9. LEISTENSCHNEIDER, W., and NAGEL, R. Lavage cytology of the renal pelvis and ureter with special reference to tumors. J. Urol., *124:*597, 1980.

10. VON ESCHENBACH, A. C. Retrograde brush biopsy in the diagnosis of renal pelvic and ureteral tumors. Cancer Bull., *31:*17, 1979.

11. MOSTOFI, F. K., SOBIN, L. H., and Torlini, H. *Histological Typing of Urinary Bladder Tumors.* Geneva, World Health Organization, 1973.

12. HALL, L., et al. The use of the red cell surface antigen to predict the malignant potential of transitional cell carcinoma of the ureter and renal pelvis. J. Urol., *127:*23, 1982.

13. LIPPERT, M., et al. Detection of cell surface antigen in cancer of renal pelvis and ureter. Urology, *22:*366, 1983.

14. KING, C. T., et al. A comparison of clinical course with blood group antigen testing by specific red cell adherence and immunoperoxidase in ureteral and renal pelvic tumors. J. Urol., *130:*871, 1983.

15. GHAZIZADEH, M., et al. Prognostic value of the specific red cell adherence test in upper urothelial tumors. Br. J. Urol., *55:*473, 1983.

16. JOHNSON, D. E., and BABAIAN, R. J. Transvesical intussusception ureterectomy. Urology, *13:*522, 1979.

17. GIBSON, T. E. Local excision in transitional cell tumors of the upper urinary tract. J. Urol., *97:*619, 1967.

18. BROWN, H. E., and ROUMAINI, G. K. Conservative surgical management of transitional cell carcinoma of the upper urinary tract. J. Urol., *112:*184, 1974.

19. MURPHY, D. M., ZINCKE, H., and FURLOW, W. L. Primary grade I transitional cell carcinoma of the renal pelvis and ureter. J. Urol., *123:*629, 1980.

20. PETKOVIC, S. D. Conservation of the kidney in operations for tumors of the renal calyces: A report of 25 cases. Br. J. Urol., *44:*1, 1972.

21. MAZEMAN, E. Tumors of the upper urinary tract calyces, renal pelvis and ureter. Eur. Urol., *2:*120, 1976.

22. PAGANO, F. Conservative treatment of lower ureteral tumor: Modified ureteroneocystostomy for upper urinary tract endoscopic control. J. Urol., *132:*555, 1984.

23. BAZEED, M. A., et al. Local excision of urothelial cancer of the upper urinary tract. Eur. Urol., *12:*89, 1986.

24. ZIEGELBAUM, M., et al. Conservative surgery for transitional cell carcinoma of the renal pelvis. J. Urol., *138:*1146, 1987.

25. JOHNSON, D. E., DE BERNARDINI, M., and AYALA, A. G. Transitional cell carcinoma of the renal pelvis: Radical or conservative treatment? South Med. J., *67:*1183, 1974.

26. HERR, H. W. Durable response of a carcinoma in situ of the renal pelvis to topical bacillus Calmette-Guerin. J. Urol., *134:*531, 1985.

27. DE KOCK, M. L. S., and BREYTENBACH, I. H. Local excision and topical thiotepa in the treatment of transitional cell carcinoma of the renal pelvis: A case report. J. Urol., *135:*566, 1986.

28. SMITH, A. D., ORIHUELA, E., and CROWLEY, A. R. Percutaneous management of renal pelvic tumors: A treatment option in selected cases. J. Urol., *137:*852, 1987.

29. HUFFMAN, J. L., et al. Endoscopic diagnosis and treatment of upper-tract urothelial tumors: A preliminary report. Cancer, *55:*1422, 1985.

30. MAHADEVIA, P. S., KARWA, G. L., and KOSS, L. G. Mapping of urothelium in carcinomas of the renal pelvis and ureter. Cancer, *61:*890, 1983.

31. HENEY, N. M., et al. Prognostic factors in carcinoma of the ureter. J. Urol., *125:*632, 1981.

32. NOCKS, B. N., et al. Transitional cell carcinoma of the renal pelvis. Urology, *14:*472, 1982.

33. REITELMAN, C., et al. Prognostic variables in patients with transitional cell carcinoma of the renal pelvis and proximal ureter. J. Urol., *138:*1144, 1987.

34. RAYER, P. F. O. Traite' des Maladies des Reins. Paris, J. B. Baillere, *3:*699, 1841.

35. WISING, P. J., and BLIX, C. Cancer of the ureters and secondarily of the mesentery. Hygeia, *40:*468, 1878.

36. ALBARRAN, M. J., 1902, cited by Melicow, M. M., and Findlay, H. V. Primary benign tumors of the ureter: Review of literature and report of a case. Surg. Gynecol. Obstet., *54:*680, 1932.

37. CRANCE, A. M., and KNICKERBOCKER, H. T. Primary carcinoma of the ureter: Report of a case living over twenty-five years following nephroureterectomy. J. Urol., *64:*300, 1950.

38. BATATA, M. A., et al. Primary carcinoma of the ureter: A prognostic study. Cancer, *35:*1626, 1975.

39. BABAIAN, R. J., and JOHNSON, D. E. Primary carcinoma of the ureter. J. Urol., *123:*357, 1980.

40. GILL, W. B., LU, C. T., and THOMSEN, S. Retrograde brushing: A new technique for obtaining histologic and cytologic material from ureteral renal pelvic and renal calyceal lesions. J. Urol., *109:*573, 1978.

41. KISIRJAMA, T., JIRONAHA, H., and FUKUDA, K. Six years of experience with retrograde biopsy of intraureteral carcinoma using the Dormia stone basket. J. Urol., *116:*308, 1976.

42. LANG, E. K. The arteriographic diagnosis of primary and secondary tumors of the ureter and renal pelvis. Radiology, *93:*799, 1969.

43. SKINNER, D. G. The technique of nephroureterectomy with regional lymph node dissection. Urol. Clin. North Am., *5:*253, 1978.

44. JOHNSON, D. E., and BABAIAN, R. J. Conservative surgical management of noninvasive distal ureteral carcinoma. Urology, *13:*365, 1979.

45. BABAIAN, R. J., JOHNSON, D. E., and CHAN, R. C. Combination nephroureterectomy and postoperative radiotherapy for infiltrative ureteral carcinoma. Int. J. Radiat. Oncol. Biol. Phys., *6:*1229, 1980.

46. BRADY, L. W., et al. Radiation therapy: A valuable adjunct in the management of carcinoma of the ureter. J.A.M.A., *206:*2871, 1968.

47. HERR, H. W., and WHITMORE, W. F., Jr. Ureteral carcinoma in situ after successful intravesical therapy for superficial bladder tumors: Incidence, possible pathogenesis and management. J. Urol., *138:*292, 1987.

CHAPTER
10

Radical Nephro-ureterectomy For Carcinoma of the Renal Pelvis and Ureter

Robert E. Donohue

Transitional cell carcinoma of the renal pelvis and ureter is thought to arise from an interaction between carcinogens in the urine and the urothelial lining of the upper tract. The bladder, because of its reservoir function, has its urothelium continuously exposed to the carcinogens, whereas contact between carcinogens and the upper urinary tract is limited by peristaltic activity.

Renal pelvic and ureteral tumors are relatively rare in the United States and Great Britain compared with transitional cell carcinoma of the bladder (Table 10-1).[1,2]

Approximately 50% of patients with these tumors of the upper urinary tract had antecedent tumors of the urothelium or concurrent tumors, or subsequently developed other transitional cell tumors in the residual urothelium following treatment of the pelvic or ureteral tumors.[1,2]

Ideal surgical treatment for this tumor consists of radical nephrectomy, adrenalectomy, and complete removal of the ureter, ureteral orifice, and a cuff of bladder mucosa surrounding the ureteral orifice. There are several exceptions to this rule: a more conservative approach is indicated in patients with transitional cell carcinoma in a solitary kidney, in patients

TABLE 10-1. *Comparison of Incidence of Renal Pelvic, Ureteral, and Bladder Tumors*

	NUMBER OF PATIENTS	
TUMOR SITE	MEMORIAL SLOAN-KETTERING[1] HOSPITAL (UNITED STATES)	BRISTOL TUMOR REGISTRY[2] (GREAT BRITAIN)
Renal pelvis	89	43
Ureter	77	54
Bladder	3,269	2,770

with low-grade tumors, in patients who present with bilateral simultaneous tumors, in patients with tumors associated with the Balkan nephropathy, and in patients with tumors associated with analgesic abuse.[3–5]

These tumors are manifestations of a diffuse multifocal epithelial change, and careful monitoring of the remaining urothelial lining by excretory urography, endoscopy, and cytology is required for the life of the patient.

Rayer first described these tumors in 1840 and demonstrated the multifocal nature of the urothelial change in the case of a 58-year-old woman found at autopsy to have renal pelvic, ureteral, and bladder tumors.[6] Reynes in 1902 recommended nephroureterectomy and bladder cuff removal for the treatment of this multifocal disease.[7] Thomas was one of the first surgeons to complete this operation. In 1920, he performed a nephroureterectomy and resection of the trigone for a lesion of the left renal pelvis and a bladder papilloma of the left ureteral orifice.[8]

Fraley has popularized opening the empty bladder to facilitate complete removal of the ureter and the mucosa surrounding the orifice.[9] He described opening the bladder, previously filled with nitrofurazone (Furacin) and subsequently emptied before surgical cystotomy. This approach permits direct and complete removal of the ipsilateral ureteral orifice and cuff of bladder mucosa, while protecting the remaining orifice and lessening the risk of wound implantation by exfoliated tumor cells. Thiotepa and sterile water have also been similarly employed as preoperative instillation therapy.

Johansson and Wahlqvist in 1979 reviewed their experience with radical nephroureterectomy.[10] Their operation, a complete radical nephroureterectomy and resection of a cuff of bladder, ipsilateral adrenalectomy, and retroperitoneal lymph node dissection, had a 5-year survival rate of 84%.

We use an eleventh-rib, extrapleural, extraperitoneal approach for the radical nephrectomy and upper ureterectomy. A node dissection can also be completed at that time. The specimen is passed down into the pelvis. Thiotepa is instilled into the bladder for 30 minutes while the first incision is being closed. The Thiotepa is drained from the bladder. Through a separate lower abdominal transverse incision, the bladder is opened. Under direct vision, the ipsilateral ureteral orifice is circumscribed and dissected with a cuff of bladder mucosa. After adequate intravesical mobilization of the ureter, the distal portion of the ureter is passed extravesically, and the removal of the lower third of the ureter is completed in the pelvis.

Strong reported a series of 9 patients of nephroureterectomy with excision of the ureteral orifice and cuff of bladder mucosa done via the extravesical tenting technique.[11] This study showed that while the intramural ureter and orifice were thought to have been excised, subsequent cystoscopic examination[5] and retrograde pyelogram[5] revealed that the orifice and the intramural ureter remained intact in all 9 patients.

Strong also stated that an additional 12 patients underwent a partial ureterectomy in which total excision was not attempted; 5 of these 12 patients had recurrences, 3 had an orifice recurrence treated by transurethral resection, 1 required a segmental resection of the bladder, and 1 was unresectable at exploration. Thus, 24% of patients with partial or incomplete nephroureterectomy developed a recurrence in the ureteral stump. In this same series, 23 patients had a complete nephroureterectomy, done in one or two stages. There was no local recurrence in this last group of patients.

PREOPERATIVE PREPARATION

Several preoperative guidelines should be followed to facilitate the patient's treatment:

1. maximization of pulmonary function
2. avoidance of preoperative antiplatelet drugs
3. mechanical bowel preparation: a chemical preparation is added if extension to the GI tract is suspected or damage to the GI tract is anticipated
4. intraoperative compression stockings

SURGICAL PROCEDURE

After the patient has been anesthetized, he is turned so that the side with the tumor is elevated, and sandbags are placed beneath the shoulder and upper pelvis to achieve an angle of 30 to 45° (Fig. 10-1). An axillary pad is placed inside the opposite axilla to avoid brachial plexus injury, and another pad is placed beneath the opposite elbow to prevent ulnar nerve injury.

Eleventh-Rib Incision

The patient's skin is shaved, and the lower chest and abdomen are scrubbed with providone-iodine scrub for 10 minutes. This scrub is removed, povidone solution is applied, and sterile drapes are placed.

An incision is made over the eleventh rib and carried down inferiorly toward the umbilicus, lateral to the ipsilateral rectus muscle. The muscle layers are incised over the rib posteriorly with the electrocautery unit. The periosteum in the midline of the eleventh rib is incised and elevated off the rib. The "up the down side" and "down the up side" rule for mobilization of the periosteum from the underlying rib allows for safer subperiosteal removal of the rib.

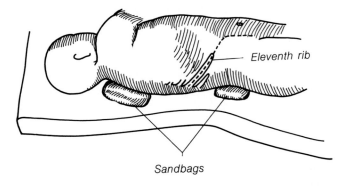

FIG. 10-1. The patient is placed at a 30 to 45° angle with sandbags beneath the shoulder and upper pelvis. An incision is made over the eleventh rib and extended caudad, lateral to the ipsilateral rectus muscle.

The Alexander elevator is used to open a plane in the periosteum in the anterior midline of the rib. The periosteum is swept cleanly, both superiorly and inferiorly. The Doyen elevator is passed under the rib, but anterior to the underlying posterior periosteum so that Sharpey's fibers can be separated and the underlying tissues protected. The rib is easily lifted from its periosteal bed (Figs. 10-2, 10-3), and care is taken not to injure the neurovascular bundle running beneath it.

The rib is resected subperiosteally with the right-angle rib resector. The excursion of the lung is noted and an incision is made in the base of the periosteum to avoid both the pleural space and the peritoneal cavity (Fig. 10-4). If either or both are entered, they should be left open until the surgical procedure is completed.

The external and internal oblique muscles are incised medially for the full extent of the wound. The transversus muscle is separated bluntly after the peritoneum has been reflected off its inferior surface, and the lumbodorsal fascia is incised and separated. The edges of the wound are freed in all layers, and the Finochietto retractor is inserted. Gerota's fascia is identified, the kidney is located within the fascia, and the renal pedicle is dissected. Early ligation is planned, if feasible.

Renal Pedicle

On the right side, the renal vein is identified and, with a right-angle clamp, the vein is isolated from its surrounding tissues circumferentially for a distance of 2 to 3 cm, ending medially at its junction with the inferior vena cava (Fig. 10-5). A right-angle clamp is passed behind the vein and two No. 1 silk sutures are delivered into the jaws of the right-angle clamp. The clamp is carefully removed from behind the vein with the sutures.

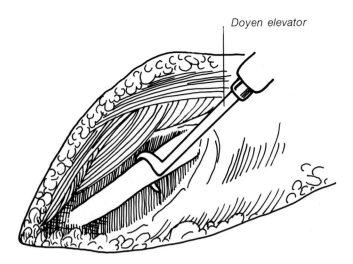

FIG. 10-3. The Doyen elevator is used to separate the rib from the periosteum posteriorly.

The two sutures are separated a distance of 2 to 3 cm. The medial suture is placed at the junction of the renal vein and the inferior vena cava. The other suture is drawn several centimeters laterally. Neither is tied at this time.

A vein retractor is carefully placed behind the vein, and the vein is lifted superiorly. The right renal artery is identified visually or by palpation behind and inferior to the right renal vein. It is isolated circumferentially from its surrounding fascia for a distance of two centimeters. The artery enters the field from behind the inferior vena cava.

A right-angle clamp is placed behind the isolated artery, and two sutures of No. 1 silk are carried around the artery (Fig.

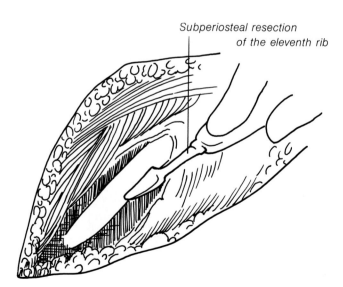

FIG. 10-2. After the periosteum is incised in the midline of the eleventh rib, the Alexander elevator sweeps the periosteum off the anterior rib surface, both superiorly and inferiorly. The technique for direction is "up the down side" and "down the up side."

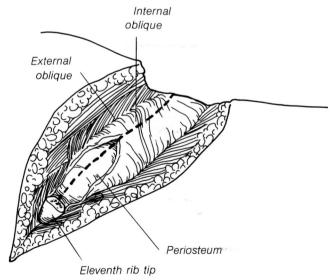

FIG. 10-4. The eleventh rib is resected sharply. The bed of the periosteum that remains is the site of the deeper incision (dotted line); care is taken to insure that the pleura is not entered. The medial aspect of the incision is made sharply through the external and internal oblique muscles, while the transversus muscle is separated bluntly.

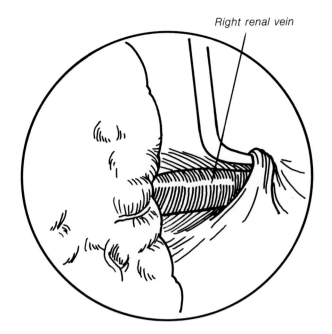

Right renal vein

FIG. 10-5. The tissue overlying the renal vein is elevated with a right angle clamp to allow mobilization of the vein and passage of ligatures.

10-6). The sutures are separated for a distance of approximately 2 cm, and the medial suture is tied first. The lateral suture is tied and the artery is transected between the two ligatures. Care is taken to allow a medial cuff of 1 to 1 ½ cm on the artery (Fig. 10-7). The edge of this cuff is closed with a running 5-0 cardiovascular silk suture.

The renal vein sutures are separated for a distance of 2 to 3 cm. The medial suture, placed at the junction of the renal

vein and the inferior vena cava, is tied. The lateral suture is tied and the renal vein is transected. Again, a cuff of 1 to 1½ cm on the vena caval or medial side of the renal vein should remain. This cuff is closed with a running 5-0 cardiovascular silk suture.

If tumor is thought to extend into the renal vein or the vena cava, careful palpation of the medial renal vein and the vena cava to determine its presence is mandated. If the tumor cannot be teased from the vena cava and the junction of the renal vein with the vena cava and withdrawn into the renal vein laterally so that the vein can be ligated, a Satinsky clamp may be employed with opening of the lateral wall of the inferior vena cava. The wall of the inferior vena cava is closed using two layers of running cardiovascular silk suture.

On the left side, the left renal vein is identified. The vein and its three major tributaries are isolated circumferentially from the surrounding tissues. The inferior tributaries of the left renal vein are the gonadal vein laterally and the lumbar vein medially. The superior tributary is the left adrenal vein (Fig. 10-8).

Sutures are placed around each of these three tributaries by the previously described technique. These sutures are tied and the veins interrupted.

The left renal vein, which has been previously cleared circumferentially from its surrounding fascia, has two No. 1 silk sutures passed around it. One of these sutures is placed at the junction of the renal vein with the inferior vena cava, and the other is placed toward the renal hilum. Neither is tied.

A renal vein retractor is carefully placed around the left renal vein. The vein is elevated and drawn inferiorly. The left renal artery can be palpated superiorly behind the vein. This artery is isolated circumferentially, as described previously,

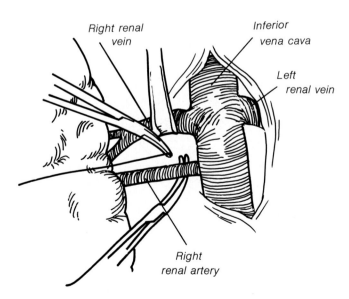

Right renal vein

Inferior vena cava

Left renal vein

Right renal artery

FIG. 10-6. The right renal artery is identified by palpation beneath the vein. After identification, with a right-angle clamp, the artery is cleaned in the same manner as the vein. With a right-angle clamp beneath the artery, a suture is passed on a tonsil clamp to the mouth of the right-angle clamp and the suture is passed around the artery.

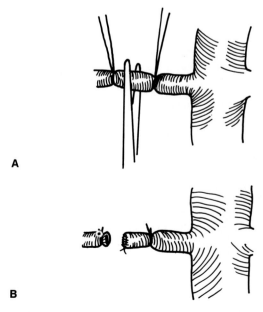

A

B

FIG. 10-7. *A,* The artery is doubly ligated, proximally and distally, and then *(B)* the proximal end is oversewn with a 5-0 cardiovascular silk suture.

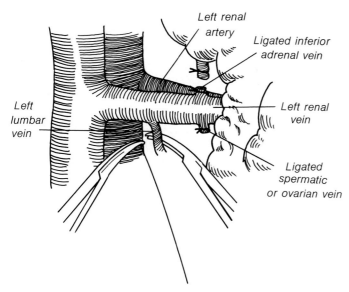

FIG. 10-8. The same technique for ligation is employed on the left side. A suture is passed around the lumbar vein proximally and distally after the vein has been cleaned and ligated. Sutures are passed around the main renal vein but are not tied until after the branches have been ligated. The artery is identified above the vein and cleaned, isolated, and ligated, and the proximal end is sutured with a 5-0 cardiovascular silk suture.

for a distance of 2 to 3 cm. The left renal artery is ligated and divided in a manner similar to that described for the right side. The renal vein sutures are then similarly tied and the renal vein is transected.

An alternative technique is to identify the vein, isolate and elevate it, palpate and isolate the artery, and pass a silk suture around the artery proximally. The artery is tied with silk. After the arterial inflow has been stopped, the vein can be isolated, cleaned, tied medially and laterally, and transected. The artery is then isolated lateral to the first tie and transected. The proximal portion is suture-ligated with a cardiovascular silk suture. This isolation of the renal artery and the renal vein should be accomplished by careful dissection with a right-angle clamp and ligatures passed on a tonsil clamp.

Nephrectomy, Adrenalectomy, and Upper Ureterectomy

To complete the removal of the kidney and adrenal, dissection is carried out carefully along the lateral aspect of the vena cava or the aorta, and metal clips (Ligaclips) are used on small vessels and lymphatics. As the cephalic portion of the specimen is approached on the right side, care must be taken to identify, isolate, and ligate the middle adrenal vein. On the left side, the inferior adrenal vein draining into the left renal vein has already been ligated.

After medial dissection of the kidney, still within Gerota's fascia, has been completed, the fascia is bluntly dissected from the surrounding retroperitoneal structures. On the right side, the gonadal vein entering the vena cava inferior to the renal

vein should be identified, cleaned, ligated, and interrupted to prevent injury to the vein during ureteral mobilization. The ureter is identified and dissected into the pelvis as far as possible. The specimen, consisting of the kidney and adrenal gland with Gerota's fascia and the upper ureter, should be placed as far down as possible into the pelvis.

Any suspicious nodal tissue from the renal hilar area can now be easily removed, and a staging node dissection can be performed, if planned. The wound should be irrigated and checked for hemostasis. If the pleural space has been entered, the appropriate chest tube should be employed and the pleural space closed, but no retroperitoneal drain should be used. The peritoneum, if opened, should be closed. The muscles are closed in layers, with continuous 2-0 polyglycolic acid sutures used for the two inner layers and a continuous or interrupted suture for the external oblique, depending upon the surgeon's preference. The skin is closed in the usual manner. All drapes are removed, the sandbags are taken away, and the patient is positioned supine on the table.

Approach to the Distal Ureter

The patient's pubic hair is shaved in the operating room, and the skin of the abdomen, groin, and genital area is scrubbed and prepped. A Foley catheter is inserted into the bladder and the urine is drained. The bladder is irrigated with saline solution. A solution of 60 mg of Thiotepa in 15 ml of saline solution is inserted and the catheter is clamped. The abdomen is freshly draped, and a Pfannenstiel (transverse lower abdominal) incision is made (Fig. 10-9). The patient may be draped to allow

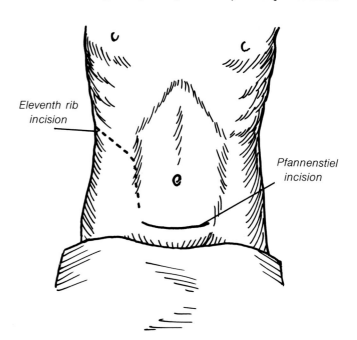

FIG. 10-9. After the patient is redraped and reprepared, a catheter is inserted, thiotepa instilled through the catheter, and the catheter clamped. A transverse lower abdominal incision is made. The preparation and draping are done so that an extension on the ipsilateral side can be made without difficulty.

extension toward the side of the nephroureterectomy if needed.

The fascia is cut transversely and freed cephalad and caudad. The rectus muscles are retracted laterally and the bladder is freed digitally. The superficial fat behind the rectus muscle is separated from the deep fatty tissue and retracted with the rectus muscle. The inferior epigastric vessels located behind the rectus muscle can be more adequately protected from the retractor blades by this technique. This approach also allows easy access to the extravesical space, where the final stage of the radical nephroureterectomy is completed.

The bladder wall is grasped with Babcock clamps and opened in the midline. With instillation of chemotherapy for 30 minutes and subsequent bladder drainage prior to this incision, spillage and implantation of viable tumor cells are minimized. The clamps are replaced with figure-of-eight chromic traction sutures. A Dennis-Browne adult retractor is placed around the incision, and the appropriate small retractor arms are inserted.

Both ureteral orifices should be identified and the orifice draining the normal renal unit should be observed for urine excretion. By careful identification of the orifices, injury to the remaining orifice can be avoided during the following dissection (Fig. 10-10). A No. 5 pediatric feeding tube should be passed up the orifice on the side of the nephroureterectomy and the ureteral orifice sutured closed around the tube. Placing slight traction on the pediatric feeding tube, the surgeon elevates the mucosa of the ureteral orifice and, beginning on the inferomedial aspect, carefully incises around the entire circumference of the orifice to achieve an adequate cuff. The inferior and medial muscle layers of the trigone should be incised with scissors.

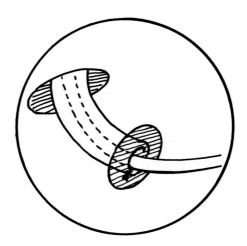

Fig. 10-11. The ureter is pulled into the bladder as mobilization progresses. This is the same technique as that employed in intravesical ureteral reimplantation.

Dissection of the Ureter

After the circumferential incision, with traction maintained, is completed, the ureter is dissected and freed from the surrounding bladder muscle by the technique employed in intravesical ureteral mobilization for ureteral reimplantation (Fig. 10-11). As the plane between the ureter and bladder is clearly identified, the ureter can be easily mobilized throughout its length in the bladder tunnel. The ureteral muscle is stripped throughout from the bladder muscle, and the ureter and pediatric feeding tube are passed out into the ipsilateral extravesical space (Fig. 10-12).

The vas deferens may prevent adequate exposure of this space, and a segment should be removed. The vas is identified, isolated for a distance of 7 to 9 cm, and interrupted medially and laterally with Ligaclips. With 7 to 9 cm of vas excised, wide access to the extravesical area and the sacral portion of the ureter is allowed. If adequate exposure is still not obtained, the Pfannenstiel incision can be extended upward toward the ipsilateral anterior superior iliac spine.

Specimen Removal and Closure

The peritoneum should be swept superiorly with blunt dissection. The pelvic mass containing the kidney and ureter is delivered into this pelvic area, and the remainder of the ureter is bluntly separated from the surrounding tissues. The specimen is removed and the wound irrigated with water. The bladder wall defect from the ureteral mobilization is repaired in two layers with interrupted 4-0 chromic sutures; the deep muscle layer is closed initially from inside the bladder, and then the mucosal layer is closed. Biopsy of pelvic lymph nodes or a formal node dissection can now be carried out.

The bladder itself is closed in two layers. The first layer approximates mucosa and muscle in a continuous layer with 2-0 chromic sutures. The second layer is also closed with 2-0

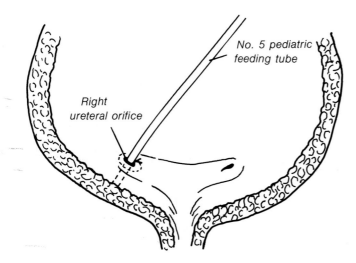

No. 5 pediatric feeding tube

Right ureteral orifice

Fig. 10-10. The trigone is exposed, and a No. 5 pediatric feeding tube is passed up the orifice to be resected and sutured in place. Incision into the bladder mucosa is started in the inferomedial aspect of the bladder mucosa, allowing an appropriate cuff to be circumcised.

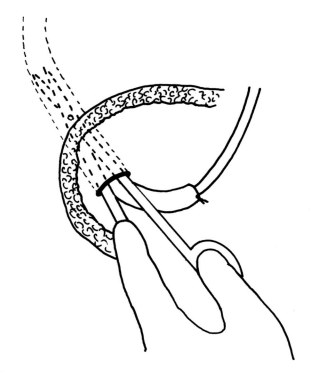

FIG. 10-12. After adequate ureteral mobilization, scissors are used to complete the tunnel to the extravesical pelvis.

chromic sutures, which can be either figure-of-eight interrupted sutures or continuous sutures. A drain is placed down to the ipsilateral perivesical space, and another drain is left in the supravesical space, both exiting through a separate drain site below the Pfannenstiel incision.

A catheter is inserted in the urethra to drain the bladder; a suprapubic tube is not necessary. The rectus muscle is approximated with 2-0 chromic sutures and the rectus sheath is closed with continuous or interrupted 2-0 chromic sutures. The subcutaneous tissue is approximated with 4-0 chromic sutures and the skin is closed with nylon sutures or skin staples.

POSTOPERATIVE CARE

The catheter should be left in place for 7 days, particularly in older male patients with prostatism. The drains can be mobilized on the third day and should be removed by the fifth day, provided that satisfactory healing is in progress and there is no gross leakage.

Serum creatinine, electrolytes, blood gases, central venous pressures, and pulmonary wedge pressures are monitored as necessary during the postoperative period.

Follow-up examinations include frequent cytologic studies of voided urine samples, excretory urography, and periodic endoscopic examinations.

Resection of new or recurrent lesions, biopsy of suspicious areas using the cold-cup biopsy forceps, random bladder biopsy of the vesical mucosa, and upper tract brushing of any filling defect are performed as indicated.

REFERENCES

1. BATATA, M., and GRABSTALD, H. Upper urinary tract urothelial tumors. Urol. Clin. North Am., 3:70, 1976.
2. WILLIAMS, C., and MITCHELL, J. Carcinoma of the renal pelvis—A review of 43 cases. Br. J. Urol., 45:370, 1973.
3. PETKOVIC, S. Conservation of the kidney in operations for tumors of pelvis and calyces: A report of 26 cases. Br. J. Urol., 44:1, 1972.
4. JOHANSSON, S., et al. Uroepithelial tumors of the renal pelvis associated with abuse of Phenacitin containing analgesic. Cancer, 33:743, 1974.
5. ZINCKE, H., and NEVES, R. Feasibility of conservative surgery for transitional cell cancer of the upper urinary tract. Urol. Clin. North Am., 11:717, 1984.
6. RAYER, P. F. O. Traite des maladies des reins. Paris, J. B. Baillere, 3:699, 1841.
7. STRICKER, O. Papillomatous tumors of the renal pelvis. Arch. Klin. Chir., 140:663, 1926.
8. THOMAS, G., and REGNIER, E. Tumors of the kidney and pelvis. J. Urol., 11:205, 1924.
9. FRALEY, E. E. Cancer of the renal pelvis. In: Genitourinary Cancer. Edited by D. G. Skinner and J. B. deKernion. Philadelphia, W. B. Saunders Co., 1978.
10. JOHANSSON, S., and WAHLQVIST, T. A prognostic study of urothelial renal pelvic tumors. Cancer, 43:2525, 1979.
11. STRONG, D., et al. The ureteral stump after nephroureterectomy. J. Urol., 115:654, 1976.

Distal Ureterectomy

Ian M. Thompson

Transitional cell carcinoma of the ureter is an unusual neoplasm, constituting 2 to 5% of all uroepithelial tumors.[1,2] Possibly due to a function of its low surface area, tumors of the ureter are 2½ times less common than their counterparts in the renal pelvis.[3] Over the past several decades, the management of this tumor swung from local excision only to dogmatic acceptance of nephroureterectomy alone. Critical review of accumulating evidence suggests that in properly selected cases, renal preservation can be achieved with no compromise in cancer control. Distal ureterectomy has been the best-accepted procedure for these cases of transitional cell carcinoma of the distal ureter.

PATHOGENESIS

A variety of conditions and agents have been epidemiologically linked with transitional cell carcinoma of the ureter. Like its uroepithelial analogue in the bladder, cigarette smoking carries with it a relative risk of 2.5 for transitional cell carcinoma of the ureter.[4] Phenacetin abuse is well-documented to be associated with transitional cell carcinoma of the renal pelvis and ureter.[4] A lower risk to the bladder may be caused by

the degradation of the aniline-like byproducts of phenacetin when exposed to urine. Chronic inflammation and stone disease as well as cyclophosphamide therapy may all lead to urothelial dysplasia and subsequent tumor formation.[5,6] An unusual type of endemic nephropathy has been described in the Balkan countries of Yugoslavia, Romania, and Bulgaria.[7] Although the etiology remains unknown, it is associated with a 100 to 200-fold increase incidence of transitional cell carcinoma of the upper tract and ureter and 10% incidence of bilaterality. In conservatively treated patients, intervening renal failure, not ureteral cancer, is the usual cause of death. Several series have suggested a genetic predilection to transitional cell carcinoma of the ureter although the association is distinctly unusual.[8,9]

PATHOLOGY

Although almost every tumor histologic type has been described in the ureter, transitional cell carcinoma constitutes

---

The opinions or assertions contained herein are the private views of the authors and are not to be construed as reflecting the views of the Department of the Army or the Department of Defense.

over 90% of all primary tumors.[10] Other, unusual tumor types include adenocarcinoma and leiomyosarcoma, both representing less than 1% of all primary ureteral tumors.[11,12] Benign polyps can radiographically mimic neoplasms but are more commonly detected in the proximal-third ureter.[13] Like their vesical counterpart, inverted papillomas of the ureter behave in a uniformly-benign fashion.[14] Metastatic tumors to the ureter are most frequently of breast, colorectal, cervical, prostatic, or bladder origin.[15]

PRESENTATION

Ureteral tumors, by their growth characteristics and location within a narrow conduit, tend to eventually lead to ureteral obstruction with its concomitant symptoms. However, patients with transitional cell carcinoma of the ureter will usually present with one of four complaints: hematuria, obstruction, symptoms of metastatic disease, or asymptomatic (serendipitously-detected) (Table 11-1). Of presenting complaints, hematuria or the lack of symptoms are usually associated with the best prognosis as obstruction or a palpable mass are more often associated with a higher stage tumor. Despite an increasing public awareness of health concerns, delay in presentation remains the rule with a range of 1 day to 9 years delay reported and an average delay in diagnosis of 7 months from initial symptoms.[16,17]

NATURAL HISTORY AND STAGING

Figure 11-1 depicts what is felt to be the progression from normal uroepithelium to development of transitional cell carcinoma of the ureter. The concept of polychronotropism or a 'field change' phenomenon is difficult to separate from the distal 'seeding' concept. Both theories explain the high incidence of subsequent bladder tumors (10 to 55%) in patients following resection of ureteral tumors, but the former best accounts for the 2 to 10% incidence of contralateral, metachronous ureteral tumors.[7,19,20] Data derived from patients with carcinoma in situ and treated with BCG tend to support

TABLE 11-1. *Clinical Presentation of Ureteral Tumors*

PRESENTING COMPLAINT	PERCENT OF CASES
Gross Hematuria	60–80
Pain	15–40
Irritative Voiding Symptoms	10
Asymptomatic/Microhematuria	10–15

the possibility of pagetoid spread of transitional cell carcinoma from the bladder into the distal ureter.[21] It is important to recognize that transitional cell carcinoma of the ureter most commonly occurs in the distal-third ureter (Table 11-2).

This stepwise progression of uroepithelial tumors has led to the development of various staging schemes. The most commonly-applied form is the modification of Jewett's bladder tumor staging system.[23] Only recently has the American Joint Committee on Cancer developed a TNM system for tumors of the ureter and renal pelvis.[24] Table 11-3 displays both systems as well as estimated five-year survivals by stage.

DIAGNOSIS

When prompted by symptoms suggestive of urologic disease, the diagnosis of transitional cell carcinoma of the ureter is usually made radiographically. Excretory urography (IVP) will usually reveal, either obstruction or nonvisualization or a filling defect (Table 11-4). Unilateral nonvisualization and hydronephrosis without a distinct cutoff require further investigation with retrograde pyelography, although the characteristics of filling defects on IVP can assist in rendering the correct diagnosis. Radiolucent ureteral calculi, blood clots, or sloughed papillae can mimic ureteral tumors. Calculi can be confirmed with CT scanning, by noting shadowing on ultrasound or by repeat pyelography following a trial of alkalinization. Papillae and clots, under appropriate clinical circum-

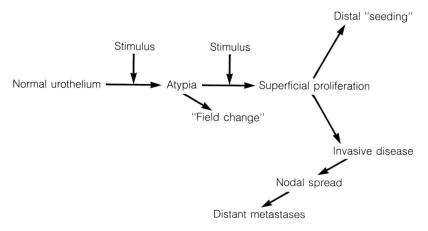

FIG. 11-1. Theoretical mechanism of development of bladder cancer.

TABLE 11-2. *Location of Primary Ureteral Tumors*[10,18,22]

LOCATION	PRECENT OF ALL TUMORS
Upper third	3-25
Middle third	6-24
Lower third	66-73

stances, can be observed, the pyelogram repeated in 10 to 14 days, and confirmed by their disappearance. Characteristics of ureteral tumors include the "chalice sign" (contrast filling a distended ureter above a rounded-ureteral tumor) or the feather-like appearance of contrast material highlighting the ragged, papillary fronds of an exophytic ureteral tumor.

Retrograde pyelography with cytologic collection is a mainstay in the diagnosis of ureteral tumors. Retrograde studies are over 90% accurate in establishing the diagnosis and are essential to completely evaluate the entire ureter and renal pelvis. If conservative surgery is contemplated, the importance is even more acute as 35% of patients with ureteral tumors will have coexisting urothelial tumors and half of these will be in the renal pelvis.[2] In addition to the further characterization of the filling defect, retrograde pyelography gives some insight into the local stage of the tumor as periureteral spread can lead to narrowing and inelasticity of the adjacent ureter.

At the time of retrograde pyelography, placement of a ureteral catheter in proximity to the filling defect allows cytologic confirmation of transitional cell carcinoma. Several authors have suggested that this should be performed before contrast studies because of cytologic changes induced by exposure to contrast. However, in our experience, this has not been a concern.[26] Barbottage collection under furosemide diuresis will double diagnostic yield over voided cytology.[27] Retrograde brushing of the lesion can improve the diagnostic accuracy to over 80% by the collection of large aggregates of tumor cells.[26] With the advent of ureteroscopy, most ureteral tumors will now be visually confirmed if cytologic methods prove unsuccessful. Small, flexible ureteroscopes can allow for rapid confirmation of the diagnosis and survey of the adjacent urothelium.

TREATMENT OPTIONS

Since the early reports of Kimball and Ferris in 1934 and Scott in 1943, nephroureterectomy has been the standard treatment of upper tract uroepithelial neoplasms.[29,30] The high recurrence rate in ureteral stumps following incomplete nephroureterectomy, the low contralateral recurrence rate, and the cost and "inconvenience" of prolonged surveillance of the ipsilateral ureter have all been used to justify this procedure.

Although Petkovic credits Albarran (1903) as the first to perform a kidney-preserving operation for transitional cell carcinoma of the ureter, Vest (1945) is credited with providing

TABLE 11-3. *Staging Systems and Survival*[2,10,23–25]

MODIFIED JEWETT SYSTEM			AJCC TNM SYSTEM	
STAGE	DESCRIPTION	FIVE-YEAR SURVIVAL	STAGE	DESCRIPTION
			TX	Primary tumor cannot be assessed
			TO	No evidence of primary tumor
			TIS	Carcinoma in situ
O	Confined to mucosa	100%	Ta	Papillary noninvasive carcinoma
A	Involvement through lamina propria	80–95%	T1	Tumor invades subepithelial connective tissue
B	Into muscular wall	40–80%	T2	Tumor invades muscularis
C	Periureteral spread	15–33%	T3	Tumor invades beyond muscularis into periureteric or peripelvic fat or renal parenchyma
D	Metastatic disease	0%	T4	Tumor invades adjacent organs or through the kidney into perinephric fat
			NX	Regional lymph nodes cannot be assessed
			NO	No regional lymph node metastases
			N1	Metastasis in a single lymph node, 2 cm or less in greatest dimension
			N2	Metastasis in a single lymph node, more than 2 cm but not more than 5 cm in greatest dimension, or multiple lymph nodes, none more than 5 cm in greatest dimension
			N3	Metastasis in a lymph node more than 5 cm in greatest dimension
			MX	Presence of distant metastasis cannot be assessed
			MO	No distant metastasis
			M1	Distant metastasis

TABLE 11-4. *Pyelographic Appearance of Ureteral Tumors*[2,10,16,17]

APPEARANCE	PERCENT OF TUMORS
Filling Defect	40–55
Non-Visualization	20–30
Hydronephrosis	11–17
Mass	4–8
Normal	6

evidence of the efficacy of such a procedure.[31,32] Bloom's data (1970), suggesting that the stage and the grade of the tumor had a more profound effect on survival than the choice of surgery, further popularized renal-conserving procedures.[33] Of all such surgical procedures, the best justified by clinical data is *distal ureterectomy for low grade, low stage, distal ureteral tumors.* The rationale for this procedure is as follows:

1. *The stage of the primary tumor, not the treatment selected, is the primary determinant of the result.* Many series have demonstrated survival to be independent of treatment selected. Heney et al. found 5-year survivals to be virtually identical, stage-for-stage, when comparing nephroureterectomy and segmental resection.[25] This finding was confirmed by Bloom.[33] Two other series have confirmed this finding with one caveat: complete nephroureterectomy can provide a rare long-term survivor for deep infiltrating tumors, whereas this did not occur with partial ureteral resection.[2,23]

2. *When biopsy or cytologic washings suggest a low-grade neoplasm, it is usually of a low-stage.* Murphy et al. have demonstrated that 95% of grade-I tumors are pathologically noninvasive.[16]

3. *When the lesion is of low-grade, ipsilateral recurrence is unlikely.* Grossman reported one case of ipsilateral tumor recurrence following segmental ureterectomy for grade-I transitional cell carcinoma of the ureter. However, in his review of 26 such cases from the literature, he was unable to find another case of recurrence.[34] Murphy has suggested that recurrence rate is independent of the surgical procedure.[16] One factor that may explain this low recurrence rate is the status of the adjacent urothelium. Although 80% of patients with grade-III lesions will have adjacent urothelial changes, *no patient* in one series with a grade-I lesion had adjacent urothelial abnormalities.[25]

4. *Distal ureterectomy for low-grade, low-stage ureteral carcinoma has excellent long-term survival rates.* Several series have reported 100% 5-year survival for distal ureterectomy for grade-I, stage-I transitional cell carcinoma of the ureter.[10,23,25,35] Petkovic's series of 44 patients with ureteral tumors at high risk of recurrence or renal failure caused by endemic nephropathy, illustrated the clear superiority of distal ureterectomy over other methods of conservative treatment of ureteral tumors.[31]

Several other factors make distal ureterectomy an attractive treatment alternative. Many ureteral tumors will be amenable

to distal ureterectomy as most stage I tumors occur in the distal-third ureter.[10,18,22] Several authors have reported distal ureterectomy to have a lower morbidity rate than nephroureterectomy.[33] Finally, although most series have reported contralateral ureteral recurrence rates of 2%, some have noted recurrence rates of up to 8 to 10%.[7,36] This clinical circumstance makes a previously "spared" contralateral renal unit an attractive asset.

Other renal sparing methods of treatment for ureteral tumors include segmental resection with ureteroureterostomy, autotransplantation, ileal interposition, or cutaneous ureterostomy.[34,37,39] Although segmental resection may occasionally be effective, these options have largely been abandoned because of associated morbidity and poor results. One new, potentially effective treatment alternative is transurethral resection/fulguration. Huffman et al. reported on 14 patients treated in this manner.[40] The efficacy of this treatment will await larger series of patients and longer follow-up.

PATIENT SELECTION AND PREOPERATIVE EVALUATION

The criteria for patient selection for distal ureterectomy have been presented above. Absolute indications include bilateral tumors, solitary kidney, or renal insufficiency. The primary relative indication is a low-grade, low-stage ureteral tumor in the distal ureter. It is imperative that the urologist use all his clinical tools to assure himself of this diagnosis. This includes the use of retrograde pyelography to evaluate the entirety of the ureter and renal pelvis to exclude other ureteral lesions. Barbottage cytology, brush biopsy, or ureteroscopy should be used to provide a preoperative cellular or tissue diagnosis. Finally, as bilateral tumors can occur synchronously, the contralateral ureter and renal pelvis should be completely visualized on radiographic studies.

Preoperative medical evaluation is essential because the average age of patients with ureteral tumors is 65 and because most will have concomitant medical problems. Cardiovascular evaluation should ensure adequate exercise tolerance, a normal electrocardiogram, and optimal blood pressure control if the patient is hypertensive. Smoking patients should be encouraged to stop several weeks before surgery and spirometric pulmonary function tests with and without bronchodilators may assist in planning perioperative and postoperative pulmonary management. All patients should have blood coagulation parameters checked preoperatively and all platelet-inhibiting drugs should be stopped at least 2 weeks in advance with a bleeding time obtained the day before surgery in such a patient. Serum creatinine should be obtained preoperatively and, if abnormal, creatinine clearance may be necessary to establish baseline renal function. Preoperative urine culture must be sterile and a single intravenous dose of a cephalosporin is administered 1 hour preoperatively. Sequential compression leg stockings are placed intraoperatively and are kept in place until the patient is ambulatory, to decrease the risk of thromboembolic phenomena.

DISTAL URETERECTOMY

Anatomy of the Ureter

The ureter courses toward the pelvis, lying in its upper third upon the anterior surface of the psoas major muscle. After crossing the iliac vessels at the level of the bifurcation of the common iliac artery, it courses laterally and posterior then medially to pass behind the bladder, thus entering its intramural portion. During its course above the pelvis, the ureter is often adherent to the posterior peritoneum and can be most easily located using this relation. In the male, after crossing the iliac vessels, the ureter lies in proximity to the hypogastric artery and passes posterior to the vas deferens and, more distally, posterior to the superior vesical artery. After coursing retrovesically, the ureter enters its muscular hiatus at the cranial aspect of the seminal vesicle. In the female, the ureter lies behind the round ligament and makes a steeper course into the pelvis, lying posterior to the uterine and superior vesical arteries. During this course, the ureter receives arterial tributaries from the uterine, vesical, and hypogastric arteries.

Surgical Technique

The patient is placed upon the operating table in the supine position. Either general or spinal anesthesia can be used with the understanding that, if intraoperative assessment suggests the need for nephroureterectomy, the patient with a regional block may require intubation. An 18- or 20-French Foley catheter with a 5 cc balloon is placed and the bladder is filled to capacity, by gravity, with sterile water.

Incision

Several incisions can be used to approach the distal ureter. These include Gibson, midline, Pfannensteil, and paramedian. The paramedian has the advantage of allowing access to both sides of the bladder for mobilization if a hitch procedure is required and is more conveniently extended toward the flank if nephroureterectomy is deemed appropriate (Fig. 11-2).

The incision is made 2 cm lateral to the midline, from the level of the pubis to 2 to 3 cm above the umbilicus. The rectus sheath is exposed and incised and the belly of the rectus muscle is mobilized and retracted laterally. Perforating vessels may require electrocautery or ligation. It is usually unnecessary to divide the inferior epigastric vessels, however, the friability of the vein may make this necessary. The posterior rectus sheath and the transversalis fascia are divided, exposing the extraperitoneal space adjacent to the bladder (Fig. 11-3).

The exposure of the ureter is facilitated by first exposing the obturator fossa. This is often best accomplished bluntly, either with finger dissection or employing Singley forceps or a sponge-stick. As an extraperitoneal approach is preferable, the peritoneum may be mobilized medially to expose the distal ureter. The vas deferens or round ligament are then dissected free and the peritoneal attachments laterally are divided.

The ureter is best identified as it crosses the iliac vessels but is often retracted anteromedially along with the perito-

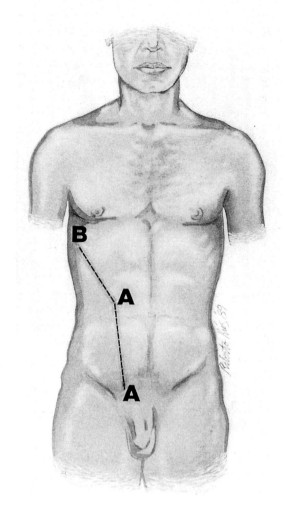

Fig. 11-2. A paramedian incision (A-A) is preferred for distal ureterectomy. If more extensive disease necessitating nephroureterectomy is encountered, it may be extended to (B), at the tip of the 12th rib.

neum. A vessel loop is then placed around the ureter and the ureter is dissected as far as possible to the intramural hiatus. Several small ureteral vessels are encountered. These are to be clipped with small metal clips and divided. The area of the ureteral tumor is examined grossly for evidence of extraureteral disease. If the ureteral wall appears nodular or fibrotic and if extraureteral disease is detected, consideration should be given to frozen section analysis and nephroureterectomy. A formal pelvic lymphadenectomy is not performed but the nodal regions in the obturator fossa and about the hypogastric and iliac vessels are palpated and sampled if there is evidence of gross nodal disease.

A midline cystotomy incision is made with the electrocautery. The bladder is then emptied (Fig. 11-4A). A wide Deaver retractor is placed to retract the bladder superiorly. Both ureteral orifices are identified and the ipsilateral orifice is grasped with a long Allis clamp (Fig. 11-4B). A circumferential incision is made through the mucosa around the orifice with the electrocautery or scissors, while gentle traction is placed on the Allis clamp. The orifice is then oversewn with a long tag left on the suture for traction. The intramural ureter is further mobi-

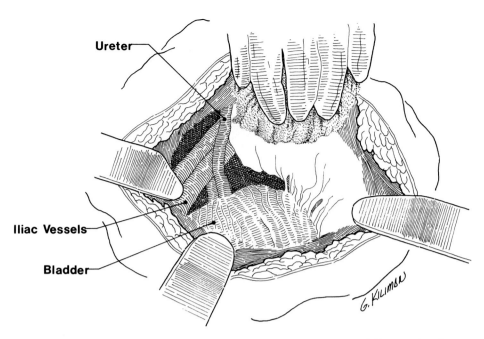

Ureter

Iliac Vessels

Bladder

G. KILIMAN

FIG. 11-3. The incision is carried through the posterior rectus fascia. The peritoneum is swept cranially, exposing the course of the distal ureter.

lized with Metzenbaum scissors until the ureter is completely free (Fig. 11-4C). The ureter is then brought out into the paravesical space and a right angle clamp applied 1 cm above the palpable tumor. A large metal clip is placed above the clamp and the ureter is divided (Fig. 11-5). The distal ureter is then divided above the clip and the segment of the ureter is sent for frozen section to exclude the presence of urothelial disease at the margin of resection. The positions of the clips are noted to allow proper orientation of the specimen by the pathologist. The distal ureter and tumor are then inspected on the back table and opened. Should inspection suggest the presence of extraureteral disease, pathologic confirmation should be obtained and consideration must be given to nephroureterectomy. The ureteral hiatus is closed in two layers, first closing the muscle layer extravesically with interrupted 2-0 chromic sutures, then closing the mucosa with interrupted 3-0 chromic sutures.

URETERAL REIMPLANTATION

Ureteroneocystostomy

With adequate mobilization, direct reimplantation of the ureter is often possible following removal of tumors involving the distal ureter. It must be emphasized that compulsive preservation of the periureteral blood supply (coursing in the adventitia) is mandatory to prevent postoperative ischemia, stricture, obstruction, or necrosis with subsequent urine leak. A site is selected lateral and superior to the native orifice and a tonsil clamp is passed from within the bladder through the bladder wall (Fig. 11-6A). This maneuver can often be performed bluntly but, on occasion, a stab incision will facilitate passing

the clamp through the bladder wall. With a spreading motion, the neohiatus is widened. A tag suture of 3-0 chromic is placed in the distal ureteral wall, grasped with the tonsil clamp, and the ureter is gently pulled into the bladder. Using either a right angle or a long tonsil clamp, a 2 to 3 cm submucosal tunnel is created in the direction of the bladder neck (Fig. 11-6B). A stab incision is made at the lower limit of the tunnel and a second clamp passed retrograde through the tunnel, the ureteral tag suture grasped, and the ureter passed gently through the tunnel (Fig. 11-6C). The ureter is spatulated and anastomosed to the bladder with interrupted 5-0 chromic sutures. Two distal sutures of 4-0 chromic are placed deeply into the detrusor muscle to adequately secure the ureter and prevent retraction (Fig. 11-6D). The mucosa overlying the new ureteral hiatus is closed with interrupted 5-0 chromic sutures.

Although ureteral stenting is not required, edema commonly leads to transient obstruction. For this reason, a 7-French, double-J ureteral stent is placed to be removed cystoscopically 2 to 3 weeks postoperatively. A 26-French Malecot suprapubic catheter is placed through a separate incision into the bladder and brought out medial to the wound. A large Penrose drain is placed lateral to the bladder and brought out a separate stab skin incision.

Psoas Hitch

For ureteral lesions in the upper pelvic ureter, a psoas hitch is required to ensure a tension-free anastomosis. This allows up to an additional 4 cm of length. The surgeon's fingers are inserted into the bladder incision and a horn of bladder pulled craniolaterally toward the tendon of the psoas muscle. If additional length is required, the peritoneum may be swept off the

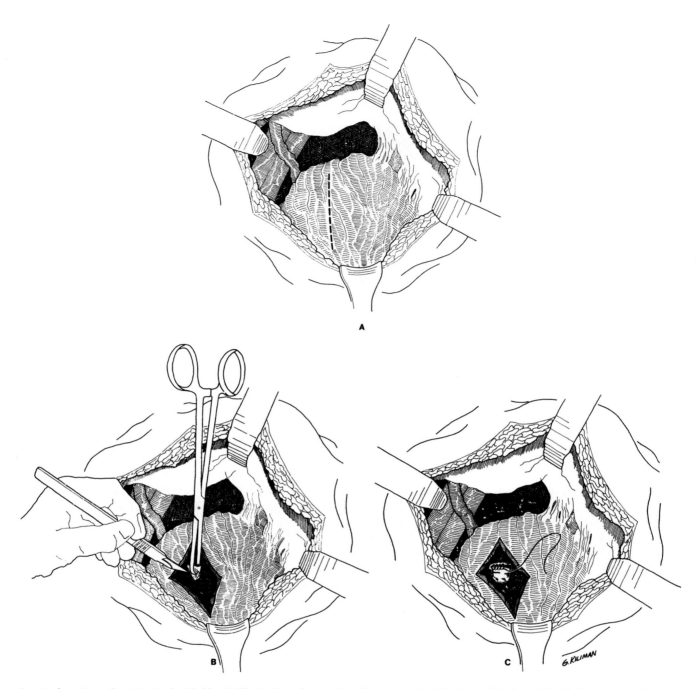

Fig. 11-4. *A*, Line of incision in the bladder. *B*, The ipsilateral ureteral orifice is grasped with a long Allis clamp. The bladder mucosa about the ureteral orifice is incised. *C*, With traction on the oversewn orifice, the intramural ureter is dissected through the bladder.

superior aspect of the bladder and the superior portion of the contralateral vesical pedicle divided for improved mobility.

A row of 2-0 chromic sutures are placed from the apex of the bladder horn into the tendon of the psoas muscle, lateral to the iliac vessels with care taken to avoid incorporation of the genitofemoral nerve (Fig. 11-7A). The sutures are placed but not tied until the ureteral reimplantation has been accomplished. Ureteral reimplantation is then performed as discussed above (Fig. 11-7B). As before, a suprapubic catheter penrose drain and ureteral stent are placed at the time of closure.

Boari Flap

For ureteral tumors above the iliac vessels for which distal ureterectomy is contemplated, a Boari flap can be used to 'span the gap'. However, if this is contemplated, the cystostomy incision must be made accordingly. Before the bladder is opened, the peritoneum is swept off the bladder dome and a flap with a base placed posteriorly is created. The ureteral defect is first measured and the flap of bladder is marked on the anterior surface of the bladder (Fig. 11-8A). It is often helpful to make the bladder flap 4 or 5 cm longer than the

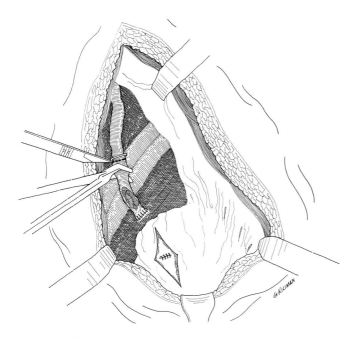

FIG. 11-5. The ureter is passed through the ureteral hiatus and dissected free of its attachments to several centimeters above the tumor. A right angled clamp is placed 2 cm above the tumor and a clip is placed proximal to the clamp. The ureter is then divided between the two.

ureteral defect and at least 4 cm in width at its base. The flap is then created with electrocautery and stay sutures are placed at the corners of its apex to facilitate mobilization (Fig. 11-8B). A submucosal ureteroneocystostomy is accomplished at the apex of the flap (Fig. 11-8C). On occasion, it may be necessary to place a line of chromic sutures through the posterior surface of the flap to 'hitch' it to the psoas muscle to assure a tension-free anastomosis. The ureteral stent is placed and the suprapubic tube placed at a location distant from the ureteroneocystostomy. The bladder closure is begun with interrupted 2-0 chromic sutures in two layers (Fig. 11-8D). The flap is then tubularized and the mucosal surface first closed with interrupted 3-0 chromic sutures followed by interrupted 2-0 chromic sutures for the detrusor component of the flap. An additional row of 4-0 chromic sutures are placed from the ureteral wall to the adjacent detrusor muscle, to prevent subsequent ureteral retraction.

Closure

Before closure is accomplished, the Penrose drain and suprapubic catheter are brought out through separate stab incisions

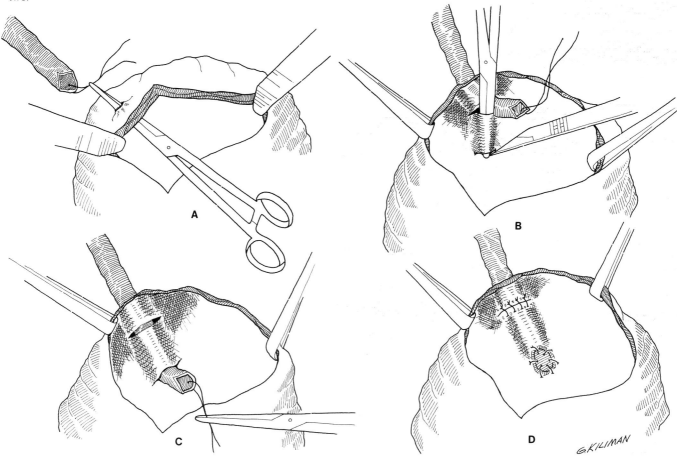

FIG. 11-6. A, A long tonsil clamp is passed through the bladder wall and the neohiatus widened. The ureteral traction suture is grasped and the ureter is pulled into the bladder. B, A submucosal tunnel has been created inferomedially from the new ureteral hiatus. C, With the traction suture, the ureter is gently advanced through the tunnel. D, The new ureteral orifice is created with interrupted sutures of 5-0 chromic catgut. Two 4-0 chromic sutures are placed distally to minimize the risk of retraction.

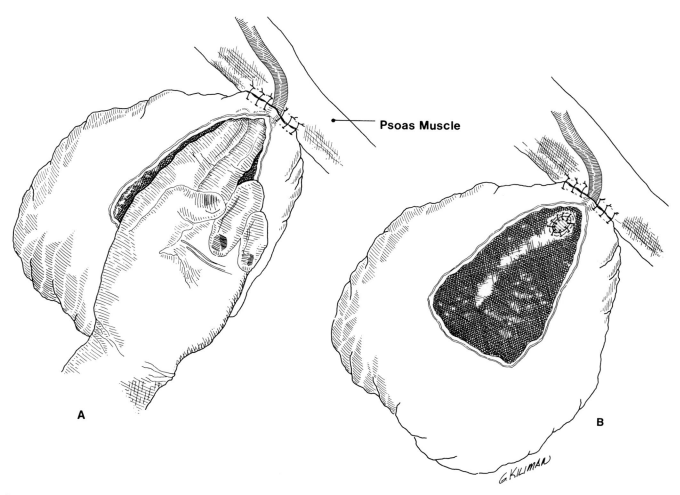

Psoas Muscle

G.KILIMAN

Fɪɢ. 11-7. *A*, The surgeon's hand is used to elevate the bladder to the ipsilateral psoas muscle. Several 2-0 chromic sutures are placed between the bladder and the psoas fascia. *B*, The ureter is brought into the submucous tunnel and anastomosed to the new site of implantation.

and secured with silk sutures (2-0 or 0). Care should be taken to ensure that the tip of the suprapubic tube is not resting upon the posterior bladder wall or ureteral anastomosis as the former can lead to disabling bladder spasms and the latter to anastomotic disruption. The rectus fascia are closed using interrupted figure-of-eight stitches with absorbable sutures. The skin is closed with staples. An elastic abdominal fishnet is placed above the gauze dressings and facilitates frequent dressing changes without the skin irritation associated with tape.

Postoperative Care

In the immediate postoperative period, urine output is recorded every 2 hours and the suprapubic catheter is checked and, if necessary, irrigated to ensure unobstructed drainage. Ambulation is begun no later than the first postoperative day. Oral feedings are withheld until active bowel sounds are heard and the patient is passing flatus. Earlier feeding, despite an extraperitoneal approach, often leads to nausea or an ileus. Electrolytes and serum creatinine are followed during hospital convalescence. Bleeding that is sufficient to require transfusion is quite uncommon with this procedure.

The suprapubic catheter is removed on postoperative day five and, if no increased drainage is noted, the Penrose drain is removed on day six. The double-J stent is removed 2 to 3 weeks after surgery, at the time of the postop office check. An excretory urogram is obtained at that time. Mild hydroureteronephrosis is often noted because of residual edema.

Complications

With adherence to proper technique, complications with this procedure should be infrequent. Significant bleeding is unusual but even minimal postoperative bleeding can clot off the suprapubic tube. Infections are minimized by assurance of sterile preoperative urine cultures, perioperative antibiotics, and adequate wound drainage. Late ureteral stenosis can occur and is usually because of overzealous ureteral skeletonization, stripping the ureter of its blood supply with subsequent distal ischemia. Preservation of the ureteral adventitia and avoidance of direct handling of the ureteral mucosa with forceps should prevent this complication. Ureteral obstruction may also be caused by kinking of the ureter at the anastomosis. It is imperative that the ureter follow a gentle curve as it courses into the bladder. This can often be checked at the time of stent place-

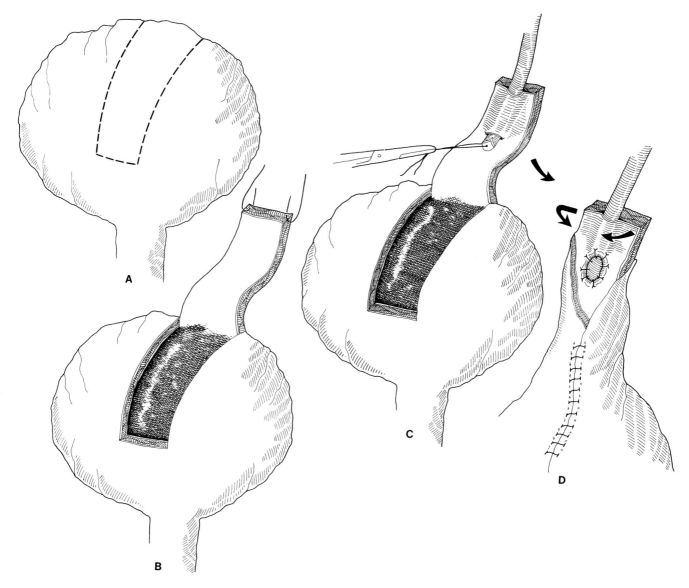

Fig. 11-8. *A*, A posteriorly based flap is marked to prepare the Boari flap. Although depicted here as rectangular, additional length can be obtained using an oblique or curved flap. *B*, The Boari flap has been fashioned and elevated. Traction sutures at the corners of the flap assist in manipulation during ureteral reimplantation. *C*, The ureter is brought through the submucosal tunnel in the flap. *D*, Ureteral implantation is completed. The Boari flap is closed along with the bladder using two layers of interrupted chromic catgut sutures.

ment. If acute angles are encountered, it is best to take down and repair the anastomosis. Vesicoureteral reflux can occur following ureteral reimplantation but is probably of no consequence to the patient. In some cases, reflux may be beneficial, allowing easier ureteroscopic upper tract access or reflux of chemotherapeutic agents placed intravesically.

Follow-up

As bladder tumors can occur in up to half of patients with a history of transitional cell carcinoma of the ureter, surveillance cystoscopy is mandatory for these patients.[19] Excretory urograms are repeated at 6 months, one year, and yearly thereafter. Voided urinary cytology should be obtained at the time of each office visit.

Adjuvant Therapy

For low-grade, low-stage ureteral tumors, excision alone is sufficient therapy. If permanent pathologic interpretation finds T3 disease, the patient is at high risk of local recurrence. Radiation therapy has been anecdotally effective in this circumstance and Brookland's series suggests radiation therapy may reduce local recurrences.[38,41] However, the metastatic disease rate was unchanged and patient selection was uncontrolled. Intraureteral instillation of thiotepa, Mitomycin C, and BCG have all been reported, but this therapy is not often necessary.[40,42,43] Platinum-based chemotherapy (MVAC) may be effective for patients with upper tract urothelial tumors, but is usually reserved for disease that is measurable by imaging studies.[44]

REFERENCES

1. KHAN, A. U., et al. Primary carcinoma in situ of the ureter and renal pelvis. J. Urol., 121:681, 1979.
2. MILLS, C., and VAUGHAN, E. D. Carcinoma of the ureter: Natural history, management and 5-year survival. J. Urol., 129:275, 1983.
3. STRONG, D. W., PEARSE, H. D., TANK, E. S., and HODGES, C. V. The ureteral stump after nephrourecterectomy. J. Urol., 115:654, 1976.
4. McCREDIE, M., STEWART, J. H., and FORD, J. M. Analgesics and tobacco as risk factors for cancer of the ureter and renal pelvis. J. Urol., 130:28, 1983.
5. MOLONEY, P. J., FENSTER, H. N., and McLOUGHLIN, M. C. Carcinoma in the defunctionalized urinary tract. J. Urol., 126:260, 1981.
6. SCHIFF, H. I., FINKEL, M., and SHAPIRA, H. E. Transitional cell carcinoma of the ureter associated with cyclophosphamide therapy for benign disease: A case report. J. Urol., 128:1023, 1982.
7. PETKOVIC, S. D. Epidemiology and treatment of renal pelvic and ureteral tumors. J. Urol., 114:858, 1975.
8. MAHBOUBI, A. O., AHLVIN, R. C., and MAHBOUBI, E. O. Familial aggregation of urothelial carcinoma. J. Urol., 126:691, 1981.
9. MARCHETTO, D., LI, F. P., and HENSON, D. E. Familial carcinoma of ureters and other genitourinary organs. J. Urol., 130:772, 1983.
10. BABAIAN, R. J., and JOHNSON, D. E. Primary carcinoma of the ureter. J. Urol., 123:357, 1980.
11. RAY, P., and LINGARD, W. F. Primary adenocarcinoma of ureter: A case report. J. Urol., 106:655, 1971.
12. WERNER, J. R., KLINGENSMITH, W., and DENKO, J. V. Leiomyosarcoma of the ureter: Case report and review of literature. J. Urol., 82:68, 1959.
13. FIORELLI, C., et al. Ureteral intussusception by a fibroepithelial polyp. J. Urol., 126:110, 1981.
14. FROMOWITZ, F. B., et al. Inverted papilloma of the ureter. J. Urol., 126:113, 1981.
15. RICHIE, J. P., WITHERS, G., and EHRLICH, R. M. Ureteral obstruction secondary to metastatic tumors. Surg. Gynecol. Obstet., 148:355, 1979.
16. MURPHY, D. M., ZINCKE, H., and FURLOW, W. L. Primary grade 1 transitional cell carcinoma of the renal pelvis and ureter. J. Urol., 123:629, 1980.
17. MURPHY, D. M., ZINCKE, H., and FURLOW, W. L. Management of high grade transitional cell carcinoma of the upper urinary tract. J. Urol., 125:25, 1981.
18. KIM, K. H., LEITER, E., and BRENDLER, H. Primary tumors of the ureter. J. Urol., 107:955, 1972.
19. KAKIZOE, T., et al. Transitional cell carcinoma of the bladder in patients with renal pelvic and ureteral cancer. J. Urol., 124:17, 1980.
20. CLAYMAN, R. V., LANGE, P. H., and FRALEY, E. E. Cancer of the upper urinary tract. In *Principles and Management of Urologic Cancer*, 2nd Edition. Edited by N. Javadpour. Baltimore, Williams and Wilkins, 1983, pp. 544–559.
21. HERR, H. W., and WHITMORE, W. F. Ureteral carcinoma in situ after successful intravesical therapy for superficial bladder tumors: Incidence, possible pathogenesis and management. J. Urol., 138:292, 1987.
22. WERTH, D. D., WEIGEL, J. W., and MEBUST, W. K. Primary neoplasms of the ureter. J. Urol., 125:628, 1981.
23. BATATA, M., and GRABSTALD, H. Upper urinary tract urothelial tumors. Urol. Clin. North. Am., 3:79, 1976.
24. American Joint Committee on Cancer. Renal pelvis and ureter. In *Manual for Staging of Cancer,* 3rd Edition. Philadelphia, J. B. Lippincott Co., 1988, pp. 205–207.
25. HENEY, N. M., et al. Prognostic factors in carcinoma of the ureter. J. Urol., 125:632, 1981.
26. BLUTE, R. D., GITTES, R. R., and GITTES, R. F. Renal brush biopsy: Survey of indications, techniques and results. J. Urol., 126:146, 1981.
27. ZINCKE, H., et al. Significance of urinary cytology in the early detection of transitional cell cancer of the upper urinary tract. J. Urol., 116:781, 1976.
28. LEISTENSCHNEIDER, W., and NAGEL, R. Lavage cytology of the renal pelvis and ureter with special reference to tumors. J. Urol., 124:597, 1980.
29. KIMBALL, F. N., and FERRIS, H. W. Papillomatous tumor of the renal pelvis associated with similar tumors of the ureter and bladder. J. Urol., 31:257, 1934.
30. SCOTT, W. W. A review of primary carcinoma of the ureter. J. Urol., 50:45, 1943.
31. PETKOVIC, S. D. A plea for conservative operation for ureteral tumors. J. Urol., 107:220, 1972.
32. VEST, S. A. Conservative surgery in certain benign tumors of the ureter. J. Urol., 153:97, 1945.
33. BLOOM, N. A., VIDONE, R. A., and LYTTON, B. Primary carcinoma of the ureter: A report of 102 new cases. J. Urol., 103:590, 1970.
34. GROSSMAN, H. B. The late recurrence of grade 1 transitional cell carcinoma of the ureter after conservative therapy. J. Urol., 120:251, 1978.
35. KJAER, T. B., JORGENSEN, T. M., FREDERIKSEN, P., and GENSTER, H. G. Transitional cell tumours of the upper urinary tract. Radical or conservative treatment? Scand. J. Urol. Nephrol., 15:235, 1981.
36. JOHNSON, D. E., DeBERARDINIS, M., and AYALA, A. G. Transitional cell carcinoma of the renal pelvis: Radical or conservative surgical treatment? South. Med. J., 67:1183, 1974.
37. THOMPSON, I. M., and ROSS, G. An analysis of 50 skin flap cutaneous ureterostomies. J. Urol., 105:649, 1971.
38. LIEBER, M. M., and LUPU, A. M. High grade invasive ureteral transitional cell carcinoma with a congenital solitary kidney: Long-term survival after urecterectomy and radiation therapy. J. Urol., 120:368, 1978.
39. VAN CANGH, P. J., et al. Renal autotransplantation for widespread uretereal lesions. J. Urol., 113:16, 1975.
40. HUFFMAN, J. L., MORSE, M. J., HERR, H. W., and WHITMORE, W. F. Consideration for treatment of upper urinary tract tumors with topical therapy. Urology, 26 (Suppl.):47, 1985.
41. BROOKLAND, R. K., and RICHTER, M. P. The postoperative irradiation of transitional cell carcinoma of the renal pelvis and ureter. J. Urol., 133:952, 1985.
42. SMITH, A. Y., VITALE, P. J., LOWE, B. A., and WOODSIDE, J. R. Treatment of superficial papillary transitional cell carcinoma of the ureter by vesicoureteral reflux of mitomycin C. J. Urol., 138:1231, 1987.
43. POWDER, J. R., et al. Bilateral primary carcinoma of the ureter: Topical intraureteral thiotepa. J. Urol., 132:349, 1984.
44. SCHER, H. I., et al. Neoadjuvant MVAC (Methotrexate, Vinblastine, Doxorubicin and Cisplatin) for extravesicular urinary tract tumors. J. Urol., 139:475, 1988.

Endourologic Diagnosis and Management of Upper Tract Urothelial Carcinoma

Jeffrey A. Snyder
Arthur D. Smith

The diagnosis, staging, and treatment of primary transitional cell carcinoma of the upper urinary tract often present challenging therapeutic dilemmas. The advent of endourologic techniques has facilitated access to the urinary tract by means of a "controlled" approach that obviates the need for opening the urinary tract. Nonetheless, potential exists for tumor spillage and subsequent spread to surrounding tissues. Technically, the skills required to perform these procedures are an extension of standard cystoscopic and endoscopic evaluations, already familiar to urologists.

The endourologic method of investigation and treatment seems most suited for patients with any of the following criteria: a solitary kidney, evidence of a filling defect in the urinary tract on contrast film, painless hematuria without radiologic evidence of a filling defect in the urinary tract, positive urinary cytology with no evident cause in the lower urinary tract, or the need for surveillance of previously treated urothelial carcinoma. Where ureteroscopic investigation is unsuccessful,

percutaneous nephroscopy may be helpful.[1] However, this treatment modality should not be advocated in patients with bilateral renal units. An exception to this rule may be patients with evidence of bilateral urothelial transitional cell carcinoma of low grade and low stage. All of this investigation has been facilitated by the invention of the flexible, deflectable fiberoptic instruments that complement the pre-existing, rigid ureteroscopes.

Although enthusiasm for the endourologic modality has been good, long-term results of therapy by this renal-sparing technique have yet to be ascertained. This is not the first time that conservative "parenchyma"-sparing surgery has been advocated.[2–4]

Obvious questions that remain to be answered are the effect of urinary tract perforation and subsequent tumor spillage on the natural history of the disease, the accuracy in staging and curing of low-grade, low-stage disease, and the necessity of special expertise and instrumentation in treating patients in this manner, thereby creating specialty referral clinics.

EPIDEMIOLOGY

Transitional cell carcinomas of the renal pelvis account for approximately 5 to 7% of all kidney tumors. Though most urothelial tumors are found within the bladder (90%) and the urethra (6 to 8%), tumors of the renal pelvis and ureter account for 2–4% of all urothelial neoplasms.

If a solitary focus of upper tract transitional cell carcinoma is found, there may be up to a 50% incidence of future development of a histologically similar bladder tumor. With tumors affecting both the renal pelvis and the ureter simultaneously, that probability would increase to greater than 75%. There is also a 2 to 4% incidence of developing a transitional cell carcinoma in the contralateral kidney. This is in contradistinction to those patients whose primary tumor source is within the bladder. They have a 2 to 3% incidence of future development of upper tract tumors of the same histologic type.

There is a 3 to 1 male-to-female predominance with this disease, except in those patients with an etiology suggestive of analgesic abuse. In these cases, the incidence is approximately equal in men and women.[5,6]

ETIOLOGIC CONSIDERATIONS

In 1895, Rehn made the observation that there was an increased incidence of transitional cell carcinoma of the bladder in dye workers.[7] The same observation was made related to tumors of the renal pelvis and ureter occurring among dye workers in England.[8,9] Although originally ascribed to aniline dyes, it was later found that the carcinogenic agents in contact with the urinary tract were, in fact, alpha-naphthylamine, beta-naphthylamine, and benzidine. A latency period of 10 years was usually found between the point of exposure to these carcinogens and the development and diagnosis of the urothelial tumor(s).[9]

Various retrospective and prospective analyses have been reported dealing with the relationship between chronic phenacetin abuse, papillary necrosis, and the development of transitional cell carcinoma of the renal pelvis. Armstrong, et al., observed that there was no significant difference in analgesic consumption patterns between patients with renal cell carcinomas and control groups.[10] Conversely, McCrede et al., reported cancers of the renal pelvis in association with chronic analgesic abuse whether or not they contained phenacetin as the main ingredient.[11] Subsequently, the same group reported that carcinoma of the renal pelvis was associated with use of phenacetin-containing substances.[12] MacLaughlin, however, found no significant increase in the risk of developing renal pelvic carcinoma, whether his study population utilized phenacetin or acetaminophen on a long-term basis.[13] Obviously, much has yet to be appreciated regarding the etiology of transitional cell carcinoma of the upper urinary tract.

Despite various other studies,[14,18] long-term, high-doses (more than 2,000 grams) of phenacetin appear to be associated with an increased risk of developing renal pelvic carcinoma and, possibly, carcinoma of the bladder.[14–19]

Other etiologic agents have been proposed, including chemical Balkan nephropathy,[20,21] cigarette smoking,[22,23] and chronic inflammation and infection.[24,25] Although rarely seen now, two dozen cases of renal pelvic carcinoma following exposure to Thorotrast have been reported.[26] Chronic stones in the renal pelvis may be associated with the development of squamous cell carcinoma as opposed to transitional cell carcinomas.

PATHOLOGY OVERVIEW

Urine Cytology

High-grade transitional cell carcinomas of the upper urinary tract are more frequently associated with positive urinary cytologies than are low-grade neoplasms.[27] When there is distal obstruction within the urinary tract, cytologic evidence may prove falsely negative because of the inability of the cells to be collected distal to the point of obstruction. Urine cytology, in conjunction with brush biopsies and tissue biopsies, help to confirm the diagnosis. Flow cytometry is another potentially useful diagnostic tool, for identifying transitional cell carcinoma in voided urine specimens.

Gross Characteristics

The majority of renal pelvic transitional cell carcinomas appear as exophytic papillary lesions. Infiltrative lesions associated with necrosis and ulceration are much less common, with an intermediate group being both exophytic and infiltrative. Microscopically, the low-grade neoplasms tend to be exophytic in nature, whereas high-grade lesions tend to be predominantly infiltrating. This is often helpful during ureteroscopy when differentiating those patients whose disease is amenable to local resection and fulguration as opposed to those with infiltrating disease that requires radical extirpation.

Microscopic Features

Moderately differentiated, papillary, transitional cell carcinomas are the most common carcinomas, followed by fewer cases of low-grade, well-differentiated carcinoma and finally, poorly differentiated high-grade tumors. Knocks et al., demonstrated the correlation between tumor grade and tumor stage.[27] The majority of the tumors they studied were found to be low grade (1-2), with minimal or no evidence of invasion. Most high-grade tumors are found to be advanced stage disease at the time of diagnosis.

Carcinoma-in-situ has also been observed in association with, and in the absence of, papillary transitional cell carcinomas.[28–30] Patients with carcinoma-in-situ of the renal pelvis or ureter usually present with microscopic hematuria, and positive urine cytologies. Radiographic evidence of demonstrable neoplasms is usually absent.

It is not uncommon to find tumor invasion of the renal collecting system extending into the renal parenchyma and peripelvic fat and retroperitoneum. However, it is uncommon for transitional cell carcinomas to differentiate with squamoid changes. This is most commonly seen with high-grade lesions.

Vascular lymphatic invasion may be present, with involvement of renal hilar lymph nodes. Between 30 and 60% of patients will have extension beyond the wall of the renal pelvis at the time of diagnosis.

Staging of renal pelvic and ureteral carcinomas may be done by one of the following methods:

U.I.C.C.	STAGE	JEWETT	PATHOLOGIC DESCRIPTION
pTa	I	O	Confined to mucosa
pT$_1$	II	A	Confined to lamina propria
pT$_2$, pT$_{3a}$	III	B$_1$, B$_2$	Confined to muscularis
pT$_{3b}$, pT^4, N+	IV	C, D	Gross invasion of peripelvic tissue and/or lymph nodes

Essentially, the critical determinants for appropriate management of upper urothelial tumors are tumor stage, tumor grade, the multicentricity of the lesion on the same side, or contralateral renal involvement.

Bilateral renal pelvic neoplasms have been reported in approximately 42 cases in the literature. Eleven of these were synchronous and 19 were metachronous. The interval of diagnosis of the subsequent tumor was anywhere from 6 months to 19 years following the initial tumor diagnosis. There were also associated ureteral and bladder tumors in 26% of these patients.

Synchronous lesions of the ureter have been reported in approximately 20% of cases, whereas simultaneous bladder tumors were diagnosed in 13% of patients with renal pelvic tumors. Ureteral stump carcinoma in the residual distal ureter developed in approximately 10 to 12% of cases that were treated by radical nephrectomy and partial ureterectomy only.

Squamous cell carcinoma of the renal pelvis is the second most common urothelial malignancy seen. It is found most frequently in men during the sixth and seventh decade of life. Bilateral disease is uncommon. There have been several cases that have occurred in horseshoe kidneys.[31,32] Renal lithiasis is often an etiologic factor in the development of squamous cell carcinoma of the upper tract.

Patients with squamous cell carcinoma often present with a papular mass (75%), hematuria, and flank pain. There may also be associated hypercalcemia.[32,33] At the time of diagnosis, it is not uncommon to find peripelvic infiltration with areas of necrosis in the tumor. Histologically, these tumors are moderately to poorly differentiated squamous cell carcinomas. They are often times multifocal.

Adenocarcinoma of the renal pelvis is a relatively uncommon entity.[34] These usually occur with a peak incidence in the sixth to seventh decade in about half of the patients and a mean age of 60 years old. Hematuria is a less frequent complaint. Approximately half of the patients complain of flank discomfort, whereas only one-third present with a papular mass.

Various other mesenchymal neoplasms such as hemangiomas,[35] leiomyomas,[36-38] leiomyosarcomas,[39-41] and mixed neoplasias like carcinosarcoma,[42,43] have been rarely reported.

DIAGNOSIS OF TRANSITIONAL CELL CARCINOMA

The most common presentation of transitional cell carcinoma of the urinary tract is gross, painless hematuria. This has been found in approximately 90% of cases.[44-49] Flank pain is the presenting complaint in approximately 20% of patients, and the combination of flank pain and hematuria is found in another 20% of patients.[50-55] A palpable mass is present in only 10% of cases of transitional cell carcinoma of the proximal ureter and renal pelvis.[56] Renal pelvic filling defects are usually detected in the workup of hematuria on intravenous urography (IVU). Only 10% of patients will have simultaneous diagnoses of urolithiasis in association with transitional cell carcinoma of the renal pelvis.[57-59]

The demonstration of a radiolucent filling defect on intravenous urography or retrograde ureteral pyelography is the most common radiologic finding, and is suggestive of transitional cell carcinoma of the upper tracts (Fig. 12-1). This represents an excellent initial screening modality in conjunction with renal tomography. For better visualization of the ureters, a compression belt should be placed around the abdomen, or the patient may be placed in the prone position to distend the ureters and upper urinary tracts.

The differential diagnoses that must be entertained should include all malignant lesions, a radiolucent calculus, blood clots, benign tumors such as papillomas, inflammatory processes (ureteritis cystica), sloughed papillae, artifacts, or overlying intestinal gas.

Patients with transitional cell carcinoma of the upper tracts rarely present with distant metastases, hypercalcemia, and possible peripheral nerve involvement.[60-63]

Urinary cytology has been helpful in the demonstration of transitional cell carcinoma of the renal pelvis. Positive cytology is more commonly encountered in high-grade transitional cell carcinomas than in low-grade lesions.[27] Retrograde pyelography is a useful adjunct for confirming the presence of a filling defect of the renal pelvis and ureter. This may be combined with aspiration or barbotage of the ureter to obtain urine for cytologic examination with brush biopsies.[64-68] Retrograde brush biopsies, thin-needle biopsies, and direct-vision biopsies by ureteroscopic methods will confirm the location and extent of disease.

Ultrasonography is helpful in differentiating radiolucent filling defects caused by non-opaque renal calculi from neoplasms. Stones have a characteristic shadowing on ultrasound, whereas soft tissue masses causing a filling defect will not shadow in the same manner. The usefulness of ultrasound is limited within the renal pelvis and is difficult to utilize within the ureter.

Computerized tomography (CT) scanning is useful for visualizing filling defects of the upper urinary tract, especially

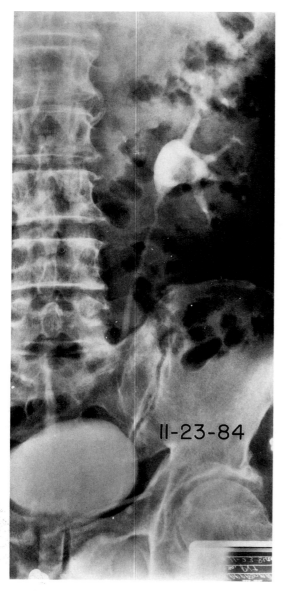

Fig. 12-1. Filling defect in the left renal pelvis, on intravenous urogram (IVU).

with local infiltration through the collecting system walls. It is most useful for preoperative staging and can demonstrate advanced or aggressive disease of the upper urinary tract.[69]

Renal angiography may show hypertrophy of the renal arterial segment going to the renal pelvis, or may demonstrate a tumor blush in certain circumstances. However, the yield in upper tract transitional cell carcinoma is not as great as with renal cell carcinoma, and its usefulness is limited.[53]

URETEROSCOPY OF THE UPPER URINARY TRACT

Technologic improvements in the development of rigid and flexible ureteroscopes have facilitated the safe examination of the upper urinary tract. Ureteroscopy is especially useful in the diagnostic evaluation of upper tract hematuria with otherwise normal radiologic imaging tests. Tumors of the urinary tract may be diagnosed, biopsied, and treated by resection, electrocoagulation, or laser ablation. It is also possible to follow these patients by periodic ureteroscopic examination in conjunction with urine cytologic examination.

Ureteroscopy is also helpful in differentiating filling defects of the renal pelvis and ureter. These may be blood clots, tumors, or radiolucent stones, or benign lesions such as papillomas, cystitis, pyelitis/ureteritis cystica, or other lesions.

Often, in the workup of gross hematuria, imaging techniques are not able to illustrate the site or the cause of the bleeding. Ureteroscopy is helpful at the time of active bleeding in detecting the cause and treating it by coagulation or laser fulguration.

Ureteroscopic management of upper urothelial tumors is especially useful for low-grade tumors in patients with solitary kidneys and in poor-risk patients who could not otherwise tolerate an open operative procedure.

In 1929, Hugh Young was able to insert a pediatric endoscope into a dilated ureter, and pass it up to the level of the renal pelvis in a child with posterior urethral valves.[70] Subsequently, Rupel was able to place a panendoscope into the renal pelvis by means of an open operative procedure and extract a calculus that was causing anuria.[71] Several other accounts were published reporting successful visualization of the interior of the renal collecting system by means of a nephrostomy tract created via an open operative procedure.[72, 73]

Numerous instruments were designed to visualize the lower urinary tract, especially the distal ureter. In 1978, Lyon reported on his experience of endoscoping the distal ureter.[76] Two years later, Perez-Castro and Martinez-Pinerio described their experience in ureteroscopy, whereby visualization was attained up to the level of the renal pelvis in both men and women.[75]

It was not until 1969 that a 9-French, flexible fiberoptic ureteroscope was utilized to visualize the ureter in a retrograde fashion.[76] In 1980, Perez-Castro reported a case of ureteroscopic stone removal utilizing an 11-French rigid endoscope. It was then realized that rigid and flexible instruments could be passed through a cystoscopic approach up a dilated ureter, so that diagnostic as well as therapeutic procedures could be performed.

Modern technology has permitted the development of short, rigid ureteroscopes, both short and long barrel, and actively and passively deflectable, flexible, fiberoptic nephroureteroscopes. Therefore, retrograde ureteroscopic evaluation can now be performed on the dilated or nondilated ureter.

Instrumentation

First-generation ureteroscopes were developed with the goal of visualizing the distal portion of the ureter. The standard lengths of these instruments measured approximately 20 cm and were generally available with diameters of 13- and 14.5-

French. As indications were extended into the mid and proximal ureter and renal pelvis, working lengths increased to approximately 40 cm and outer diameters decreased to approximately 11.5-French. The major concern was to develop an instrument that was small enough to negotiate the narrow ureter yet still maintaining a large enough working port to allow the passage of working elements such as biopsy forceps, cauterizing electrodes, or stone baskets. One of the major setbacks in reducing the working outer diameter of these ureteroscopes is that the working port did not permit adequate water flow, especially when utilizing working element accessories. The 11.5-French ureteroscopes will allow 5-French flexible accessories to be utilized, however, irrigation flow is greatly diminished with these instruments in the working channel. There are more than two dozen models of rigid ureteroscopes on the market, ranging from a diameter of approximately 10-French to a maximum diameter of 14-French. Variation in beak shape, eye piece location, accessory channel, and working length make the permutations of the various instrument specifications almost endless. A good working knowledge of all available instruments is essential when dealing with these challenging endoscopic cases.

Intraoperative Management

The indications for ureteroscopic intervention with ureteric or renal pelvic tumors has been discussed previously. Proper patient selection is important to achieve adequate treatment and good postoperative results.

Ureteroscopy should not, in the opinion of the author, be performed by the inexperienced endourologist. Variations in anatomy as well as tortuosity of the ureter may make negotiation of the urinary tract difficult. Therefore, there is a steep learning curve that must be achieved before attempting one of these challenging cases. With the exception of the small diameter flexible ureteroscopes, it is most often necessary to dilate the intramural ureter prior to insertion of the ureteroscope. Various dilators, both rigid and inflatable, have been employed in the past. These may include metallic, radio-opaque, bead, bougies, Amplatz fascial dilators, or high-pressure balloon dilators. Slow, progressive dilatation may be accomplished, however, a rapid sequence ureteral dilatation may also be performed.[79]

Most recently, an instrument called the Ureteromat has found favor by many endourologists in dilating the ureter and avoiding trauma.[78] This device is an electric irrigation device that pumps fluid through the ureteroscope and simultaneously measures intraureteric pressure to avoid ureteral injury.

The technique for using this instrument involves advancement of the ureteroscope into the ureteral orifice. The Ureteromat is set at a maximum pressure of 200 mm. of mercury and a flow rate of 400 ml per minute. This provides excellent visualization. The pressure and flow rate are useful for dilating the intramural ureter, but are certainly more useful once this portion of the ureter is bypassed. Upon advancing

the ureteroscope, the pressure is reduced, usually to 100 mm of mercury and a flow rate of 200 ml per minute. One can then proceed toward the renal pelvis without much difficulty. Pressure and flow rates can be subsequently reduced for the treatment of neoplasms.

The experience utilizing this instrument has been quite favorable and has been primarily responsible for the significant reduction in complications during and following ureteroscopic manipulation. This tool has made ureteroscopic evaluation easier, quicker, and less traumatic. Visualization of the pathologic lesion is also much easier with the increased pressure and increased flow rates developed, especially in the face of hematuria.

Although concern has been expressed about the high intraureteric pressure,[79] with the reduced elapsed time of instrumentation, this procedure has not proven to be harmful.

Technique of Ureteroscopy

Following the selection of the appropriate ureteroscope, the instrument is introduced into the bladder and advanced up the intramural ureter. A guidewire is then advanced up the ureter, or the same guidewire used for dilatation may be used. This will straighten the course of the ureter and reduce the majority of the ureteric kinks that may be present. The ureteroscope is advanced under direct vision, avoiding rapid lunges and uncontrolled passage of the instrument.

Once beyond the intramural ureter, the ureteroscope is advanced in a posterolateral direction. The ureter passes anteromedial to the psoas muscle and bends both medially and anteriorly along its course.[80] Once the renal pelvis is negotiated, the 70° lens may be inserted and inspection of the entire collecting system can be accomplished.

At this point, various accessories may be utilized to biopsy, resect, or fulgurate the neoplasm(s). Diagnosis may be accomplished by means of brush biopsies or biopsy forceps. The tumor resection may be accomplished with the ureteroscopic resectoscope, or the tumor may be ablated utilizing the Nd.:YAG laser. This can all be done under direct vision, thereby facilitating tumor removal.

Once the tumor is visualized, it can be resected utilizing the ureteroscopic loop resectoscope. (Fig. 12-2) Bleeding points can be fulgurated with the loop, a bugby electrode or a laser fiber, to achieve hemostasis. Tumor fragments may be removed from the ureteroscope and the bladder. Because of the delicate nature of the ureter, cautery and resection should be gingerly practiced to avoid ureteral or renal pelvic perforation.

Successful ureteroscopic management of superficial, low-grade transitional cell carcinomas within the urinary tract has thus far been satisfactory.[81,82] Surprisingly, the recurrence rates have been similar to the results obtained by open surgical excision, approximating 17%. Similar results have been obtained by Smith et al. for the percutaneous management of renal pelvic tumors.[83]

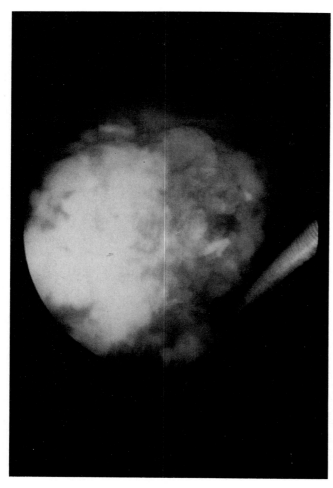

Fig. 12-2. Papillary transitional cell carcinoma of the proximal ureter. The safety guidewire is visualized through UPJ.

Although not a mainstay for the treatment of transitional cell carcinoma of the ureter and renal pelvis, ureteroscopy certainly represents an interesting avenue of exploration. Further, well-controlled prospective studies will be necessary before this becomes an established mode of treatment.

Postoperative Care

Following endourologic management of these tumors, it is important to stent the ureter to protect it during the period of mucosal regeneration. The authors have generally utilized double-J, indwelling stents or open-ended, ureteral stents draining to the outside for a period of 24 to 48 hours in the uncomplicated cases. Where ureteral injury has occurred, stents are left in situ until radiographic evidence of healing has occurred. This is usually documented postoperatively by means of an intravenous urogram.

Additional intrarenal administration of Bacillus Calmette-Guerin (BCG) has also been advocated for the treatment of transitional cell carcinoma of the upper tracts.[84]

A second-look procedure is suggested in the management of patients following endourologic resection of urothelial tumors. Routine cytologic samples can be collected at standard intervals and confirmation of positive cytologic examination with direct vision endoscopy is advisable.

ANTEGRADE PERCUTANEOUS MANAGEMENT OF UPPER TRACT UROTHELIAL TUMORS

Ever since the first percutaneous nephrostomy tube was inserted into an obstructed kidney in 1955,[85] the field of endourology has flourished. Within this specialized area, surgical procedures have evolved which enable us to view the collecting system of kidneys and ureters (nephroureteroscopy), to extract renal calculi (nephrostolithotomy), to treat caliceal diverticula, to relieve ureteropelvic junction stenosis (endopyelotomy), and to treat transitional cell carcinomas of the renal pelvis (percutaneous tumor extraction).

Indications

Similar indications for percutaneous tumor extraction apply as with ureteroscopic tumor extraction. The location of the suspected tumor is typically within the renal pelvis and within easy access of the percutaneous nephroscope. Patient selection must be specific to those patients having a solitary renal unit, poor-risk patients that would not tolerate an open procedure, or those patients whose cytologic examination is positive and radiologic imaging fails to demonstrate a tumor source.

Smith et al., in 1986, reported on nine patients with transitional cell carcinomas of the renal pelvis that were resected percutaneously.[83] Three patients had tumor within a solitary kidney, one had bilateral synchronous disease, one had renal insufficiency, two were poor-risk surgical candidates, and two patients had solitary, low-grade, superficial tumors.

Surgical Technique

Following detection of a tumor within the renal pelvis, a contrast study defining the renal anatomy is necessary. Proper selection of a nephrostomy tube insertion site is important to gain easy access to the suspected tumor. A standard antegrade approach under fluoroscopic control may be easily obtained utilizing the technique described by Castaneda-Zuniga.[86]

Once a 34-French, Amplatz sheath is placed within the renal collecting system, nephroscopy is performed. Antegrade flexible ureteroscopy may also be utilized to inspect the ureter down toward the bladder. Tissue diagnosis should be confirmed with biopsies of the tumor, as well as random biopsies of the renal pelvis.

Once tissue diagnosis is confirmed, a standard resectoscope may be utilized to remove all visible tumor (Fig. 12-3). Often, the transitional cell carcinomas of the renal pelvis are flimsy and are not amenable to resection with the loop. When larger volumes of tumor are encountered, we have found it efficacious to utilize the cold-cup biopsy forceps to remove all visible signs of tumor. The base of the tumor is then fulgurated with electrocautery or laser fulguration (Fig. 12-4). A large bore, 24-French re-entry nephrostomy tube is left within the renal pelvis and the ureteral catheter segment is placed down the ureter (Fig. 12-5).

The nephrostomy tube is left in place during the postoperative period, and a second-look procedure is performed after one month. At that time, nephroscopy will confirm any evidence of residual disease within the renal pelvis. Because the nephrostomy tube tract has already been established, it is easy to perform this under local anesthesia. Random biopsies are again performed within the renal pelvis, and any suspicious areas may be either resected or fulgerated with the Nd:YAG laser. Within the renal pelvis, the power setting should be reduced to approximately a maximum pulse of 15 to 20 watts for 20 seconds. In a study by Orihuela, one patient received intrarenal mitomycin C 20 mg in 50 ml of sterile water, and six patients received BCG on a weekly basis.[83] This was administered via an infusion pump over 1 hour to increase contact time within the renal pelvis.

The nephrostomy tube is usually removed following a completed course of BCG therapy. Follow-up included serial cytologic examinations every 3 months, as well as contrast radiologic studies.

Woodhouse et al. reported insertion of radioactive iridium wire (^{192}Ir) into the nephrostomy tract in order to prevent tumor seeding along the tract site.[87] Of the six patients treated, one developed wide-spread multifocal disease throughout the urinary tract, and subsequently died of uremia. Three patients showed no recurrence of the disease with a maximum of 36 months follow-up, and two developed recurrences either in the bladder or the ureter. However, no seeding was observed within the nephrostomy tube tract site.

Complications to these procedures are related more to the insertion of the nephrostomy tube and are similar to the complications of bleeding and perforations seen with percutaneous stone extractions. Patients found to have invasive tumors through the renal pelvic wall, who have extension of disease outside the kidney, or who have evidence of disease spread to the regional lymph nodes, are treated by radical nephroureterectomy.

Future Perspectives

In patients demonstrating spread of disease to localized lymph nodes, local extension beyond the renal pelvis (Fig. 12-6), or who have metastatic disease elsewhere and present with hematuria or obstruction, percutaneous techniques may be useful for local control and relief of symptoms. Following local control and debulking, chemotherapy regimens can be tried.

These percutaneous procedures can be utilized in selected patients who have unilateral renal involvement with low-grade, papillary, transitional cell carcinomas of the renal pelvis. Follow-up is easily performed by means of urine cytology, random biopsy, and CT scan surveillance. Further experience

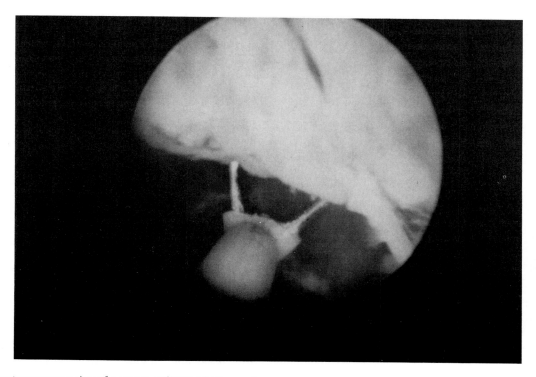

FIG. 12-3. Percutaneous resection of a tumor, utilizing a loop resectoscope.

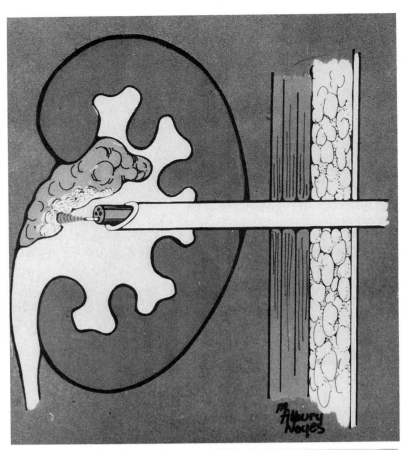

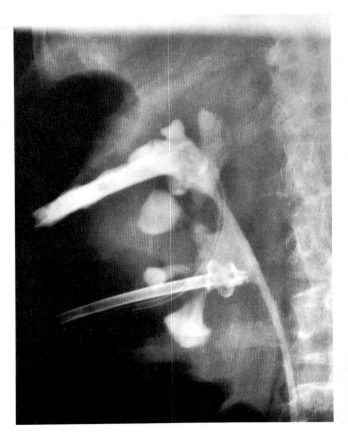

FIG. 12-5. At the termination of the surgical procedure, a percutaneous 24-French re-entry nephrostomy tube is placed in the upper pole, with a ureteral stent attachment inserted down the ureter. A 14-French nephrostomy tube is placed in the lower pole. A circle nephrostomy tube is placed for postoperative chemotherapy.

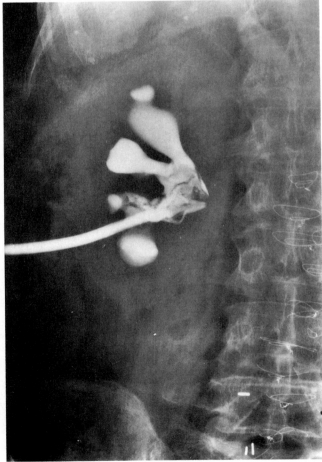

FIG. 12-6. "Moth-eaten" nephrostogram of invasive TCC of the renal pelvis.

is warranted prior to endorsing this as a standard treatment in our armamentarium.

CONCLUSION

Not only can diagnostic dilemmas be solved by means of ureteroscopy, but treatment regimens can be designed that permit adequate management of low-grade, low-stage transitional cell carcinomas. Proper patient selection and accurate preoperative staging is mandatory for determining who can be best managed by this procedure. Careful postoperative follow-up examination is essential and should be stringent at this early stage of development of this technique.

Long-term results have yet to be clearly established. Therefore, this surgical technique should still be considered experimental.

Even patients staged with positive lymph nodes or metastatic disease may be treated with this technique with the hope of debulking gross tumor and thereby facilitating future chemotherapeutic regimens to control the disease process.

Closed, controlled endoscopic visualization of the interior of the urinary tract has permitted improved access for diagnosis and treatment of urinary tract tumors in carefully selected patients. In experienced hands, the success rate for this select group of patients can be expected to further improve with the rapidly developing advancements of both flexible and rigid instruments used in the field of endourology.

REFERENCES

1. ORIHUELA, E., and SMITH, A. D. Percutaneous treatment of transitional cell carcinoma of the upper urinary tract. Urol. Clin. North Am., 15:425, 1988.
2. McCARRON, J. P., MILLS, C., and VAUGHN, E. D., JR. Tumors of the renal pelvis and ureter: Current concepts in management. Semin. Urol., 1:75, 1983.
3. MURPHY, D. M., ZINCKE, H., and FURLOW, W. L. Primary grade 1 transitional cell carcinoma of the renal pelvis and ureter. J. Urol., 123:629, 1980.
4. ZINCKE, H., and NEUES, R. J. Feasibility of conservative surgery for transitional cell cancer of the upper urinary tract. Urol. Clin. North Am., 11:717, 1984.
5. BABAIAN, R. J., and JOHNSON, D. E. Primary carcinoma of the ureter. J. Urol., 123:357, 1980.
6. SCHELLHAMER, P. F., and WHITMORE, W. F., JR. Transitional cell carcinoma of the urethra in men having cystectomy for bladder cancer. J. Urol., 115:56, 1976.
7. REHN, L. Uber basentumoren bei fuchsinarbeitern. Arch. Klin. Chir., 50:588, 1895.
8. MacALPINE, J. B. Papilloma of the renal pelvis in dye workers. Two cases, one of which shows bilateral growths. Br. J. Surg., 35:137, 1947.
9. POOLE-WILSON, D. B. Occupational tumors of the renal pelvis and ureter in the dye making industry. J. Proc. Royal Soc. Med., 62:93, 1969.
10. ARMSTRONG, B., GARROD, A., and DOLL, R. A retrospective study of renal cancer with special reference to coffee and animal protein consumption. Br. J. Cancer, 33:127, 1976.
11. McCREDE, M., et al. Analgesics and cancer of the renal pelvis in New South Wales. Cancer, 49:2617, 1982.
12. McCREDE, M., STEWART, J. H., and FORD, J. M. Analgesics and tobacco as risk factors for cancer of the ureter and renal pelvis. J. Urol., 130:28, 1983.
13. McCREDE, M., et al. Phenacetin-containing analgesics and cancer of the bladder and renal pelvis in women. Br. J. Urol., 55:220, 1983.
14. McLAUGHLIN, J. K., et al. Etiology of cancer of the renal pelvis. J. Natl. Cancer Inst., 71:287, 1983.
15. FOKKENS, W. Phenacetin abuse related to bladder cancer. Environ. Res., 20:192, 1979.
16. HULTEGREN, N., LAGERGREN, C., and LJUNGQUIST, A. Carcinoma of the renal pelvis and renal papillary necrosis. Acta Surg. Chir. Scand. 130:314, 1965.
17. HOYBYE, G., and NIELSEN, O. E. Renal pelvis carcinoma in phenacetin abusers. Scand. J. Urol. Nephrol., 5:190, 1971.
18. ADAM, W. R., et al. Anaplastic transitional cell carcinoma of the renal pelvis in association with analgesic abuse. Med. J. Aust. 1:1108, 1970.
19. MAHONEY, J. R., et al. Analgesic abuse, renal parenchymal disease, and carcinoma of the kidney and ureter. Aust. N. Z. J. Med., 7:463, 1977.
20. PETKOVIL, S. D. A plea for conservative operation for ureteral tumors. J. Urol., 107:220, 1987.
21. PETKOVIL, S. D., et al. Tumors of the renal pelvis and ureter: Clinical and etiological studies. J. Urol. (Paris), 77:429, 1971.
22. CLAYMAN, R. V., LANGE, P. H., and FRALEY, E. G. Cancer of the upper urinary tract. In Principles of Management of Urologic Cancer. Edited by N. Javadpour. Baltimore, Williams & Wilkins, 1983.
23. MORRISON, A. S., and COLE, P. Urinary tract. In Cancer Epidemiology and Prevention. Edited by D. Scholtenfield and J. F. Fraumenie Jr. Philadelphia, W. B. Saunders Co., 1982, p. 925.
24. POOLE-WILSON, D. B. Occupational tumors of the renal pelvis and ureter in the dye making industry. Proc. Royal Soc. Med., 62:93, 1969.
25. BOOTH, C. M., CAMERON, K. M., and PUGH, R. C. B. Urothelial carcinoma of the kidney and ureter. Br. J. Urol., 52:430, 1980.
26. GRAMPA, G. Radiation injury with particular reference to Thorotrast. Pathol. Annu., 6:147, 1971.
27. KNOCKS, B. N., et al. Transitional cell carcinoma of the renal pelvis. Urology, 19:472, 1982.
28. SARNACKI, C. T., et al. Urinary cytology and the clinical diagnosis of urinary tract malignancy: A clinicopathic study of 1,400 patients. J. Urol., 106:761, 1971.
29. MURPHY, W. M., VON BUEDINGEN, R. P., and POLEY, R. W. Primary carcinoma-in-situ of renal pelvis and ureter. Cancer, 34:1126, 1974.
30. STRAGIER, M., et al. Primary carcinoma-in-situ of the renal pelvis and ureter. Br. J. Urol. 52:401, 1980.

31. THOMPSON, I. M., SCHNEIDER, J., and KAVAN, L. C., Bilateral squamous cell carcinoma of the kidneys. J. Urol., 79:807, 1958.

32. DEAN, A. C. B., LAMBIE, A. T., and SHIVAS, A. A. Hypercalcemic crisis in squamous cell carcinoma of the renal pelvis. Br. J. Urol., 56:375, 1969.

33. DEAN, A. C. B., et al. Squamous cell carcinoma of the renal pelvis presenting with hypercalcemia. J. Urol., 119:126, 1978.

34. ACKERMAN, L. V. Mucinous adenocarcinoma of the pelvis of the kidney. J. Urol., 55:36, 1946.

35. ANDERSON, J. B., et al. Hemangioma of the kidney pelvis. J. Urol., 70:869, 1953.

36. LITZKY, G. M., SEIDEL, R. F., and O'BRIEN, J. E. Leiomyoma of the renal pelvis. J. Urol., 105:171, 1971.

37. BELIS, J. A., et al. Genitourinary leiomyomas. Urology, 13:424, 1979.

38. UCHIDA, M., et al. Leiomyoma of the renal pelvis. J. Urol., 125:572, 1981.

39. CROSBIE, A. H., and PINKERTON, H. Malignant leiomyoma of the kidney. J. Urol., 27:27, 1932.

40. DOCKERTY, M. B., and PRIESTLEY, J. T. Sarcoma of the kidney. J. Urol., 50:564, 1943.

41. TOLIA, B. N., HAJDU, S. I., and WHITMORE, W. F., JR. Leiomyosarcoma of the renal pelvis. J. Urol., 109:974, 1973.

42. FAUCI, P. A., JR., THERHAG, H. G., and DAVIS, J. G. Carcinosarcoma of the renal pelvis. J. Urol., 85:897, 1961.

43. RIDOLFI, R. L., and EGGLESTON, J. C. Carcinosarcoma of the renal pelvis. J. Urol., 119:569, 1978.

44. RICHES, E. W., GRIFFITHS, I. H., and THACKRAY, A. C. New growths of the kidney and ureter. Br. J. Urol., 23:297, 1951.

45. TAYLOR, W. N. Tumors of the kidney pelvis. J. Urol., 82:452, 1959.

46. NEWMAN, D. M., et al. Transitional cell carcinoma of the upper urinary tract. J. Urol., 98:322, 1967.

47. GRACE, D. A., et al. Carcinoma of the renal pelvis: A 15-year review. J. Urol., 98:566, 1968.

48. DONNELLY, J. D., and KOONTZ, W. W. Carcinoma of the renal pelvis: A 10-year review. South Med. J., 68:943, 1975.

49. HALL, L. et al. The use of the red cell surface antigen to predict the malignant potential of transitional cell carcinoma of the ureter and renal pelvis. J. Urol., 125:23, 1982.

50. WILLIAMS, C. B., and MITCHELL, J. P. Carcinoma of the renal pelvis: A review of 43 cases. Br. J. Urol., 45:370, 1973.

51. WAGLE, D. G., MOORE, R. H., and MURPHY, G. P. Primary carcinoma of the renal pelvis. Cancer, 33:1642, 1974.

52. SAY, C. C., and HORI, J. M. Transitional cell carcinoma of the renal pelvis: experience from 1940 and 1972 in literature review. J. Urol., 112:438, 1974.

53. CUMMINGS, K. B., et al. Renal pelvic tumors. J. Urol., 113:158, 1975.

54. STRAGIER, M., et al. Primary carcinoma-in-situ of renal pelvis and ureter. Br. J. Urol., 52:401, 1980.

55. MAHADEVIA, P. S., KARWA, G. L., and KOSS, L. G. Mapping of urothelium in carcinomas of the renal pelvis and ureter. Cancer, 51:890, 1983.

56. WILLIAMS, C. B., and MITCHELL, J. P. Carcinoma of the renal pelvis: A review of 43 cases. Br. J. Urol., 45:370, 1973.

57. McDONALD, J. R., and PRIESTLEY, J. T. Carcinoma of the renal pelvis: Histopathologic study of 75 cases with special reference to prognosis. J. Urol., 51:245, 1944.

58. GRABSTALD, H., WHITMORE, W. F., and MELAMED, M. R. Renal pelvic tumors. JAMA, 281:845, 1971.

59. LEONG, C. H., et al. Carcinoma of the renal pelvis: Analyses of the diagnostic problems in 23 cases. Br. J. Urol., 63:102, 1976.

60. SARNACKI, C. T., et al. Urinary cytology and the clinical diagnosis of urinary tract malignancy: A clinicopathic study of 1,400 patients. J. Urol., 106:761, 1971.

61. FAWCETT, D. P., and McBRIEN, M. P. Transitional cell carcinoma of the renal pelvis presenting with peripheral neuropathy. Br. J. Urol., 49:202, 1977.

62. MANDELL, J., MAGEE, M. C., and FREED, F. A. Hypercalcemia associated with uroepithelial neoplasms. J. Urol., 119:844, 1978.

63. RUBENSTEIN, M. A., WALZ, B. J., and BUCY, J. G. Transitional cell carcinoma of the kidney: 25 year experience. J. Urol., 119:594, 1978.

64. McCARRON, J. P., JR., CHASKO, S. B., and GRAY, G. F., JR. Systemic mapping of nephroureterectomy specimens removed for urothelial cancer, pathologic findings, and clinical correlations. J. Urol., 128:243, 1982.

65. STRONG, D. S., and PEARSE, H. D. Recurrent urothelial tumors following surgery for transitional cell carcinoma of the upper urinary tract. Cancer, 38:2173, 1976.

66. RICHIE, J. P. Management of ureteral tumors. In Genitourinary Cancer. Edited by D. G. Skinner and J. B. deKernion. Philadelphia, W. B. Saunders Co., 1978, p. 150.

67. BERGMAN, H., FRIDENBERG, R. M., and SAYEGH, V. New roentgenologic signs of carcinoma of the ureter. Am. J. Roent., 86:707, 1961.

68. GITTES, R. F. Retrograde brushing and nephroscopy in the diagnosis of upper tract urothelial cancer. Urol. Clin. North Am., 11:617, 1984.

69. BARON, R. L., et al. Computed tomography of transitional cell carcinoma of the renal pelvis and ureter. Radiology, 144:125, 1982.

70. YOUNG, H. H., and McKAY, R. W. Congenital valvular obstruction prostatic urethra. Surg. Gynecol. Obstet., 48:509, 1929.

71. RUPEL, E., and BROWN, R. Nephroscopy with removal of stone following nephrostomy for obstructive calculus anuria. J. Urol., 46:172, 1941.

72. TRATTNER, H. R. Instrumental visualization of the renal pelvis and its communications: Proposal of a new method: Preliminary report. J. Urol., 60:817, 1948.

73. LEADBETTER, W. F. Instrumental visualization of the renal pelvis at operation as an aid to diagnosis: Presentation of a new instrument. J. Urol., 63:1006, 1950.

74. LYON, E. S., BANNO, J. J., and SCHOENBERG, H. W. Transurethral ureteroscopy in men using juvenile cystoscopy equipment. J. Urol., 122:152, 1979.

75. PEREZ-CASTRO E. E., and MARTINEZ-PINERIO, J. A. Transurethral ureteroscopy-apparent urological procedure. Arch. Esp. Urol. 33:445, 1983.

76. MARSHALL, V. F. Fiber optics in urology. J. Urol., 91:110, 1964.

77. SMITH, A. D. Rapid dilatation of ureteral orifice for ureteroscopy. Urology, 26:407, 1985.

78. PEREZ-CASTRO, E. Ureteromat: Method to facilitate ureterorenoscopy and avoid dilatation. Urol. Clin. North Am., 15:315, 1988.

79. VAZQUEZ, G., STEIN, B., and SURYA, B. V. Rapid hydrodistention of ureter. Urology, 29:319, 1987.

80. SNYDER, J. A., and SMITH, A. D. Anatomy of the ureter. In Endourology Principles and Practice. Edited by Smith, Castaneda-Zuniga, and Bronson. New York, Thieme, Inc., 1986.

81. HUFFMAN, J. L. Ureteropyeloscopic approach to upper tract urothelial tumors. World J. Urol., 3:58, 1985.

82. HUFFMAN, J. L., et al. Endoscopic diagnosis and treatment of upper tract urothelial tumors: A preliminary report. Cancer, 55:1422, 1985.

83. Smith, A. D., Orihuela, E., and Crowley, A. R. Percutaneous management of renal pelvic tumors: A treatment option in selected cases. J. Urol., *137*:852, 1987.

84. Orihuela, E., Herr, H. W., and Pirsky, O. M. Toxicity of intravesical BCG and its management with superficial bladder tumors. Cancer, *60*:326, 1987.

85. Goodwin, W. E., Cassey, W. C., and Woolf, W. Percutaneous trocar (needle) nephrostomy in hydronephrosis. JAMA, *157*:891, 1955.

86. Castaneda-Zuniga, W. R., et al. Percutaneous nephrostomy: Basic approach of fluoroscopic techniques. In *Endourology: Principles and Practice.* Edited by Smith, Castaneda-Zuniga, and Bronson. New York, Thieme, Inc., 1986.

87. Woodhouse, C. R. J., Kellett, M. J., and Bloom, H. J. G. Percutaneous renal surgery and local radiotherapy in the management of renal pelvic transitional cell carcinoma. Br. J. Urol., *58*:245, 1986.

RETROPERITONEAL TUMORS

Surgical Management of Retroperitoneal Tumors

Robert B. Smith

Retroperitoneal tumors comprise a diffuse group of tumors, of which metastatic carcinoma of the testicle is the most common. Primary retroperitoneal tumors are a group of rare tumors that originate from the various tissues of the retroperitoneum such as fat, muscle, vessels (arterial, lymphatic, or venous), fibrous tissue or vestigial embryonic remnants. The retroperitoneal tumors covered in this chapter will deal with lesions arising from the various tissues mentioned in the retroperitoneum. Tumors occurring primarily from the kidney, ureter, liver, pancreas, adrenal, spleen, duodenum, or metastatic tumors with primary sites other than the retroperitoneal space, will not be included in this discussion. It appears that these tumors develop de novo and not by dedifferentiation from pre-existing lesions. Retroperitoneal tumors have been reported to develop after tissue injuries or following radiation injury.[1,2] Retroperitoneal sarcomas have also been reported arising after chemotherapy for primary testicular tumors. Sarcomatous degeneration of teratomas from the testicle have been reported.[3] More than 80% of primary retroperitoneal tumors are malignant. With the exception of lymphomatous tumors, curability depends on completeness of resection,[4] or the availability of adjuvant chemotherapeutic agent. The majority of these lesions are relatively radioresistant. From review of the literature, high percentages of these tumors have been found unresectable upon initial exploration. A high mortality rate is also associated with the resection of such lesions.[5–12]

Classification

Primary tumors are best classified according to the tissue of origin. The terminology for malignant tumors is complicated. Over 50 different types of soft tissue sarcoma have been described. All tumors are derived from mesenchymal cells or neural crest tissues. Tumors of mesodermal origin include those arising from adipose tissue (lipoma and liposarcoma), smooth muscle (leiomyoma and leiomyosarcoma), skeletal muscle (rhabdomyoma and rhabdomyosarcoma), connective tissue (fibroma and fibrosarcoma), blood vessels (hemangioma, hemangiosarcoma, hemangiopericytoma, and leiomyomas and leiomyosarcomas of venous structures), lymphatic vessels (lymphangioma or lymphangiosarcoma) and lymph nodes (lymphoma, Hodgkin's disease, and lymphosarcoma). Many portions of a single tumor may be well differentiated, whereas other portions may be totally undifferentiated. Thus, a small biopsy may not give a proper assessment of the malignant potential of the entire lesion.

Tumors of neural origin include neurilemoma, Schwannoma (sheath origin), ganglioneuroma, symphathicoblastoma, and neuroblastoma (sympathetic origin) and tumors of chromaffin tissue including paraganglioma, malignant periganglioma, and pheochromocytoma. Tumors arising from embryonic remnants include urogenital ridge tumors, chordoma, and benign and malignant primary retroperitoneal teratomas.

Tumors of lymphatic origin are the most common (40%), with lymphosarcoma representing half of these tumors. Reticulum cell sarcoma and Hodgkin's disease account for most of the remaining tumors. These tumors are treated as a systemic illness. Because surgical removal of the retroperitoneal portion of the malignancy is not the primary treatment for these lymphatic tumors, these tumors will not be discussed any further in this chapter. Liposarcoma (15%), leiomyosarcoma (10%), and rhabdomyosarcoma (8%) are the most common remaining tumors of the retroperitoneum. Tumors such as fibrosarcoma, extra-adrenal neuroblastoma, hemangiopericytoma, extra-gonadal germ cell tumors, malignant undifferentiated tumors, malignant histiocytoma, and other sarcomas are more rare.

Benign retroperitoneal tumors comprise only 15 to 20% of the total and include lipoma, leiomyoma, lymphangioma, xanthogranuloma, ganglioneuroma, neurofibroma, and extra-adrenal pheochromocytoma, in addition to rare retroperitoneal cysts arising from remnants of the urogenital ridge. It is often difficult to differentiate between a benign and malignant lipoma, leiomyoma, fibroma, or hemangiopericytoma. In addition, as mentioned previously, there is tremendous histologic variation within portions of a single tumor.[13] One area may be well differentiated, whereas other portions may be totally undifferentiated, making classification according to the primary cell of origin difficult when only small tissue samples are available. There is also evidence that these tumors have the potential to dedifferentiate into any other soft tissue elements. Local recurrence is a common sequelae, even with the so-called benign lesions. Complete radical resection is necessary for all of the lesions because of the high probability of local recurrence, as well as the possibility of sarcomatous degeneration of many of these "benign lesions." Previously mentioned sarcomatous degeneration may reflect only the variability in the initial lesion, with the selective growth of the more undifferentiated components. Many pathologic studies of soft tissue sarcomas have indicated that there is rarely a true tumor capsule, even though the tumors appear to be grossly encapsulated. The pseudocapsule consists of compressed surrounding cells that almost certainly have been violated by microscopic malignant cells.[14]

Signs and Symptoms

Retroperitoneal tumors rarely produce early symptoms. They usually attain a large size before symptoms are noted. Abdominal pain is the most common presenting symptom, followed by abdominal enlargement. Systemic symptoms such as weight loss, weakness, fever, nausea, vomiting, and decreased appetite are frequently associated symptoms but often occur relatively late in the course of the disease. Swelling of the lower extremities, back pain, leg pain, and lower extremity paresthesia or weakness are usually signs of advanced disease.

An abdominal mass is the most consistent finding on physical examination. The mass generally does not move with respiration. On occasion, flank or abdominal tenderness may be present. Ascites may be present but is more common in patients with a lymphomatous lesion. Peripheral neuropathy involving the femoral nerve can also occur with a retroperitoneal pelvic mass. Surprisingly, early complaints referrable to the genitourinary tract are rare, despite the proximity of these tumors to the kidney, ureter, and bladder (Fig. 13-1).

Diagnosis

Diagnostic evaluation of these patients should include an intravenous pyelogram, barium enema, upper GI series, and CT and/or MRI scan. The improved quality of CT and MRI scanning have made the other tests less essential in every case. A lymphangiogram or Gallium scan may be indicated for evaluation of possible lymphomatous disease. In selected cases in which the diagnosis of metastatic testicular tumor or pheochromocytoma is likely, the levels of the following substances should be measured: urinary catecholamines, vanylmandelic acid (VMA), and the testis tumor markers, beta HCG and alpha fetoprotein. In cases suggestive of lymphoma, fine-needle aspiration biopsy may provide the diagnosis of the lesion, obviating the need for exploratory laparotomy and biopsy.

An inferior vena cavagram should be performed in all cases of large retroperitoneal masses to aid in surgical planning, unless the MRI scan has given this important information. An angiogram is essential in the evaluation of retroperitoneal tumors, not only to assess the vascularity of the lesions, but also to aid in surgical planning. Hypervascular lesions such as hemangiopericytoma can be extremely dangerous to remove, because of the risk of associated blood loss. Preoperative embolization can enable resection of even highly vascularized lesions. Figure 13-2 demonstrates the potential usefulness of this technique in the large hypervascular retroperitoneal hemangiopericytoma.[15] Angiosarcomas, rhabdoymosarcomas, and metastatic non-seminomatous testis tumors, in addition to hemangiopericytoma, may have a hypervascular pattern. Most retroperitoneal tumors, however, are hypovascular (Fig. 13-3). Under normal circumstances, the four-paired lumbar arteries do not contribute significant blood supply to normal retroperitoneal structures. The hypogastric artery provides the main supply to the retroperitoneum, with significant contribution from gonadal, adrenal, or renal arteries. Branches from the

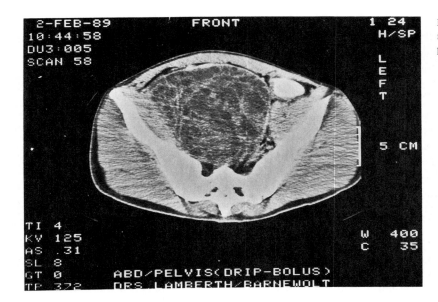

FIG. 13-1. A huge retroperitoneal teratoma with significant distortion and displacement of the bladder. The patient denied having any voiding symptoms.

superior, inferior mesenteric artery and celiac axis may also contribute, in addition to the intercostal, inferior phrenic arteries. Often hypertrophy in one of these arteries, including enlargement of a lumbar artery, may be the only indication that a retroperitoneal tumor exists.[16]

Fine-needle aspiration can be considered in non-lymphomatous tumor. The physician must be cognizant of the tremendous variability of the histologic pattern within a given tumor (Fig. 13-4).[13] The success of management of these tumors depends upon complete local excision and, because many of these tumors are unresectable when the original diagnosis is made, a preoperative tissue diagnosis is essential for determining whether the lesion is radiosensitive and whether an available chemotherapy agent may be effective. Preoperative radiation therapy, with or without intra-arterial chemotherapy, may improve the chance of resecting such a lesion.[7] In patients in whom a fine-needle aspiration is not successful in obtaining an adequate tissue specimen, peritoneoscopy with biopsy should be utilized. Whereas it is relatively safe to use fine-needle aspiration in any tumor, peritoneoscopy with direct needle biopsy should be used in only those patients with hypovascular lesions on angiography.

There is often a disagreement among pathologists regarding the tissue origin in some of these tumors. It appears, however, that this is much less important than the histologic grade of the tumor (the number of mitotic figures per high powered field). The American Joint Committee on Cancer has recommended a staging system where groups of patients are categorized regarding their probable therapeutic outcome (Table 13-1). Survival rate can be directly correlated to these clinical groupings.[17] This system obviates the need for exact histologic classification of the tumor.

Standard metastatic evaluation should be carried out as indicated by the nature of the primary lesion before definitive therapy is undertaken. Lung is a primary site of spread for these retroperitoneal malignant sarcomas.

TABLE 13-1. *Stage Grouping For Soft-Tissue Sarcomas**

	STAGE I
IA:	G_1, T_1, N_0, M_0 Grade-1 tumor less than 5 cm in diameter with no regional lymph node or distant metastases
IB:	G_1, T_2, N_0, M_0 Grade-1 tumor 5 cm or greater in diameter with no regional lymph node or distant metastases

	STAGE II
IIA:	G_2, T_1, N_0, M_0 Grade-2 tumor less than 5 cm in diameter with no regional lymph node or distant metastases
IIB:	G_2, T_2, N_0, M_0 Grade-2 tumor 5 cm or greater in diameter with no regional lymph node or distant metastases

	STAGE III
IIIA:	G_3, T_1, N_0, M_0 Grade-3 tumor less than 5 cm in diameter with no regional lymph node or distant metastases
IIIB:	G_3, T_2, N_0, M_0 Grade-3 tumor 5 cm or greater in diameter with no regional lymph node or distant metastases
IIIC:	Any G, T_1, or T_2, N_1, M_0 Tumor of any histologic grade or size (no invasion) with regional lymph node metastases but without distant metastases

	STAGE IV
IVA:	Any G, T_3, any N, M_0 Tumor of any histologic grade or malignancy that grossly invades bone, major vessels, or major nerves with or without regional lymph node metastases but without distant metastases
IVB:	Any G, any T, any N, M_1 Tumor with distant metastases

*From American Joint Committee on Cancer. *Manual for Staging of Cancer.* 2nd Edition. Edited by O. H. Beahrs and M. H. Myers. Philadelphia, J. B. Lippincott Co., 1983, p. 111.

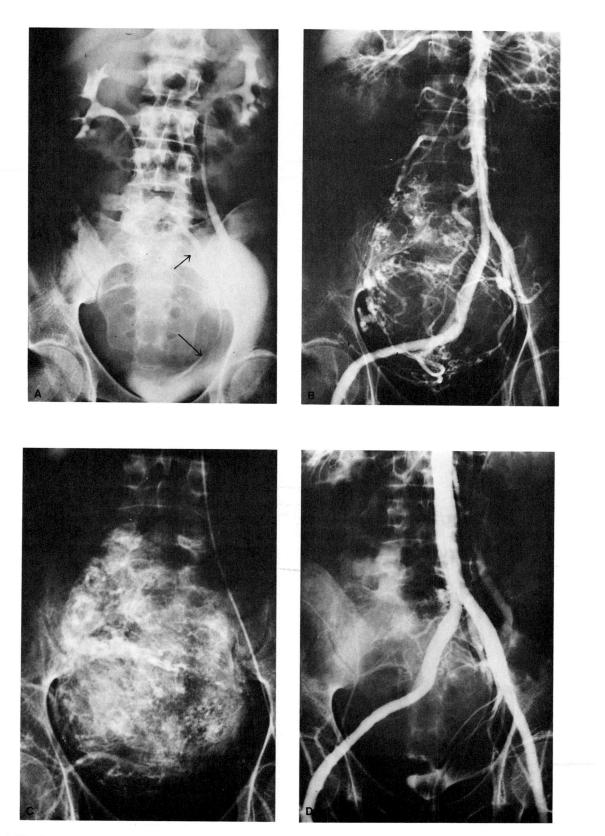

Fig. 13-2. *A,* IVP of a retroperitoneal pelvic hemangiopericytoma. Note the medial deviation of the bladder and right ureter (arrow). *B,* Angiogram. Note the hypervascularity with the blood supply from the third and fourth lumbar arteries, both hypogastric arteries, and right lateral femoral circumflex artery. *C,* The late angiogram phase showing diffuse hypervascularity of this hemangiopericytoma. *D,* Angiogram after gelatin sponge (Gelfoam) embolization (compare with B). (From Smith, R. B., et al. Preoperative vascular embolization as an adjunct to successful resection of a large retroperitoneal hemangiopericytoma. J. Urol., *115:*206, 1976. Copyright 1976, The Williams and Wilkins Co., Baltimore. Reprinted by permission of publisher).

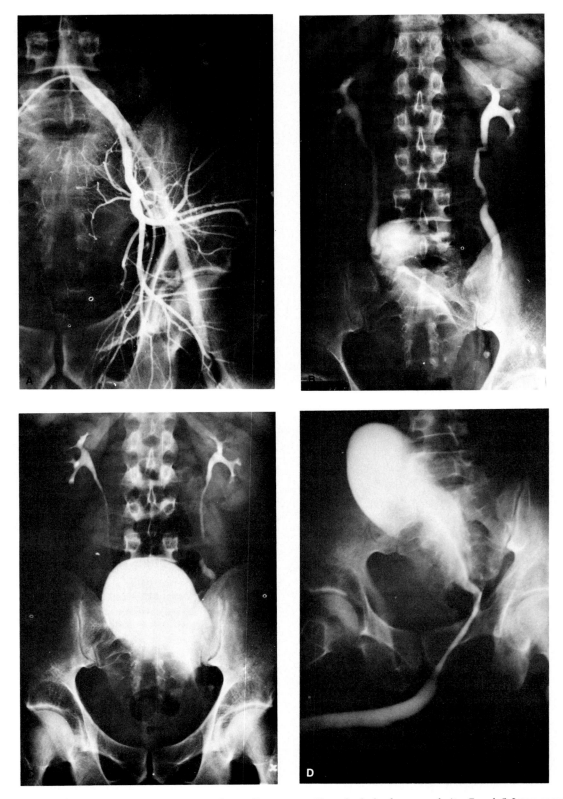

FIG. 13-3. *A,* Pelvic angiogram of a large retroperitoneal myxoliposarcoma. Note the lack of neovascularity. *B* and *C,* Intravenous pyelogram. *D,* Voiding cystourethrogram. This lesion was excised completely, leaving the bladder, prostate, and rectum intact.

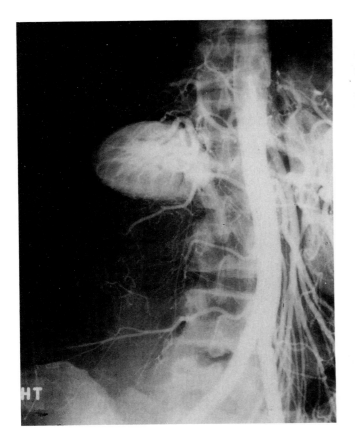

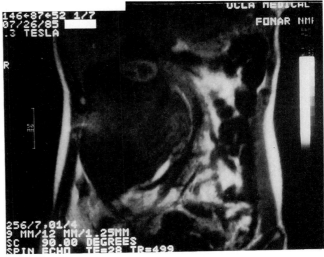

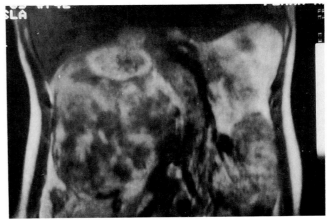

Fig. 13-4. A large retroperitoneal liposarcoma. *A,* Angiogram demonstrating upward displacement of kidney. *B,* MRI T-1 weighted image. *C,* MRI T-2 weighted image demonstrating the great variability in the tumor.

Treatment

The treatment of choice for these lesions is wide, local excision. It must be understood that these tumors often extend well beyond their so-called pseudocapsule. Microscopic extension tends to occur along fascial planes and maybe as far as 6 to 7 cm beyond all gross disease.[18,19] Metastasis to regional lymph nodes is an uncommon event.

To maximize the possibility of a successful resection, appropriate preoperative systemic chemotherapy, radiation therapy, or infusional chemotherapy may decrease the size of these primary lesions, increasing the chance of resectability. Also, some of these tumors may develop a dense capsule following chemotherapy, which can aid in the resection. Another advantage to preoperative therapy is the theoretical decrease in the likelihood of tumor embolization during the manipulation of the tumor at the time of resection. The surgical treatment of retroperitoneal sarcomas includes a wide resection of the tumor including wide normal margins. Removal of adjacent organs or vessels may be necessary to achieve complete surgical resection. Besides some responses to chemotherapy

and radiation therapy recently, a wide surgical excision is still the accepted primary means of treatment. Best results have been achieved in those tumors where a margin greater than 3 cm can be obtained. If this is not feasible, preoperative adjuvant chemotherapy or radiation therapy should be given.

Preoperative Preparation

Adequate preoperative preparation is essential. Intra-arterial lines and Swan-Ganz catheters are helpful in monitoring these potentially extensive procedures. Adequate blood should be ordered preoperatively, because blood loss can be considerable in these cases. Although it is rarely necessary to type and cross for more than 6 units, the blood bank should be warned of the potential magnitude of blood loss to assure that enough units of specific blood are available.

Consent of the patient should be obtained to allow removal of contiguous structures that may be involved by the primary lesion. In cases involving the high retroperitoneum, en bloc resection of the kidney, vena cava, or ureter may be necessary.

In cases of retroperitoneal pelvic tumors, consent should be obtained for anterior or posterior exenteration or both, along with the appropriate urinary or fecal diversion.

Complete bowel preparation (mechanical and antibiotic) is essential should bowel injury occur or should bowel resection become necessary. The patient should be well hydrated with intravenous fluids the night before surgery. The use of hypotensive anesthesia, with controlled use of nitroprusside, may lessen intraoperative blood loss in high-risk patients.

SURGICAL PROCEDURE

Tumors Above the Pelvis: Thoracoabdominal Incision

It is essential that the patient be positioned properly before the incision is made. The torque flank position is ideal, with the shoulders at a 40 to 45 degree angle and the pelvis in as supine a position as possible. The patient should be placed as close as possible to the operating surgeon, with the table fully hyperextended (Fig. 13-5). The use of the thoracoabdominal approach for lesions above the true pelvis maximizes the chance for a complete resection. The superior exposure afforded by this approach and the access to all retroperitoneal vessels, including the ipsilateral great vessels (inferior vena cava or aorta), above the diaphragm makes this the incision of choice. The thoracoabdominal incision also allows palpation of the mediastinal area and the ipsilateral lung parenchyma.

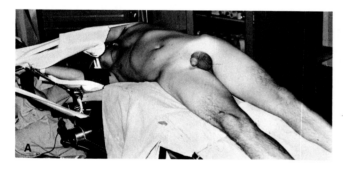

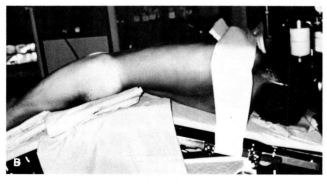

FIG. 13-5. A, Operative position (torque flank position). Note the shoulder angle 40 to 45° to the horizontal. The table is fully hyperextended. B, The pelvis is nearly in the supine position. The patient is as close as possible to the surgeon's side of the table.

The level of the thoracoabdominal incision depends on the size and location of the tumor. Most commonly, it is made in the 8th, 9th, or 10th interspace, and should extend at least to the midaxiliary line posteriorly. It is my experience that resection of a rib is not necessary to facilitate exposure, but may be used at the discretion of the surgeon. The larger the mass, the higher should be the incision. The incision crosses over to the midline, transecting the rectus muscle in the epigastrium, which prevents denervation of the rectus muscle. The incision can then be extended inferiorly as midline or paramedian incision toward the pubis. For large tumors, a T incision is made anteriorly or posteriorly to the main thoracoabdominal incision (Fig. 13-6).

No attempt is made to remain outside the peritoneum in operations for large retroperitoneal lesions. The peritoneum should be entered promptly to save time and to facilitate exposure. The transverse colon, descending or ascending colon, small bowel, duodenum, and pancreas are completely mobilized to gain access. For left-sided tumors, the peritoneal incision is made down the left lateral peritoneal reflection from the splenic flexure around the sigmoid colon to the pelvic brim. A medial incision is also made in the colon mesentery maintaining the integrity of the marginal artery (Fig. 13-7). Ligation of the inferior mesenteric artery aids in mobilization of the descending colon and should be performed for large left-sided lesions.

Right-sided lesions are exposed by incising the posterior peritoneum from the hepatic flexure down the ascending colon and around the cecum. The incision is then carried superiorly to the ligament of Treitz (Fig. 13-8). This allows complete mobility of the right colon, small bowel, duodenum, and pancreas on the superior mesenteric artery pedicle. Care should be taken not to occlude the superior mesenteric artery by extensive tension. All bowel contents are then placed in a Lahey bag. For left-sided tumors that are large or cross over the midline, this peritoneal incision can be combined with the left lateral peritoneal incision as in Figure 13-7. If the abdominal contents have been mobilized on the superior mesenteric artery pedicle, it is important to check from time to time to make sure that the blood flow via the superior mesenteric artery has not been occluded because of a kink or excessive tension on the pedicle. As mentioned previously, ligation of the inferior mesenteric artery aids in mobilization of the descending colon and should be performed for large, left-sided lesions. The marginal artery must remain intact, however. In older patients, diarrhea or cramping abdominal pain may result from inferior mesenteric artery ligation, but this is rare in young individuals and only occasionally presents serious problems in any age group. Although it has not occurred in our series at UCLA, ischemic damage to the colon may occur. If ischemic damage is noted, the ischemic portion of the colon should be resected primarily and the colon reanastomosed. The decision to protect the anastomosis by a proximal diverting colostomy depends on the surgeon's preference, the success of the preoperative bowel preparation, and the technical quality of the anastomosis.

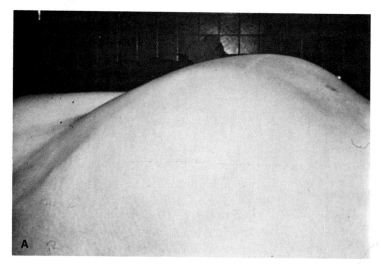

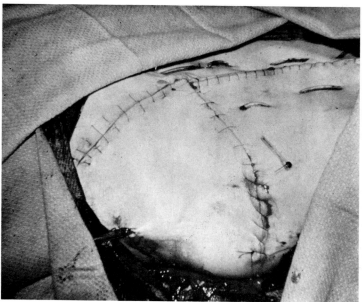

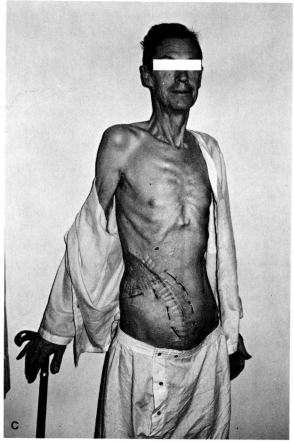

FIG. 13-6. *A,* A huge retroperitoneal tumor obvious on inspection. *B,* The thoracoabdominal incision via the 8th interspace was not sufficient to gain adequate posterior exposure. A posterior T-extension of the incision was made. *C,* Postoperative appearance of the incision.

After proper mobilization of the aforementioned structures, an attempt should be made to secure control of the feeding vessels as determined by a preoperative angiogram. In the case of hypervascular tumors, preoperative embolization is a valuable adjunct to the surgical procedure in lessening the amount of intraoperative blood loss. The ipsilateral great vessel, and on occasion, the contralateral great vessel, should be mobilized by ligating the lumbar vessels below the level of the renal pedicle. Ischemic damage to the spinal cord should not occur, as the spinal cord ends at the level of the first lumbar vertebra. Extensive experience in surgical procedures for aortic aneurysms has confirmed the safety of this maneuver.[20] Reports still exist, however, of spinal ischemia following this maneuver, but these are rare,[21] and are probably related to prolonged periods of hypotension associated with aneurysm resections.

In rare cases, these retroperitoneal lesions have been noted to invade or encase the aorta or iliac artery. In these cases, the aorta or iliac artery should be resected and then replaced with a Dacron bypass graft. There are usually four pairs of lumbar arteries found distal to the main renal artery, these arteries should be individually ligated with 3-0 or 4-0 silk ties proximally, and hemostatic clips on the distal portion of the vessels. The use of hemoclips in the proximal portion is dangerous and may be a source of serious intraoperative or postoperative hemorrhage if a clip becomes dislodged.

Vena caval obstruction by invasion or encasement by a tumor occurs more commonly (Fig. 13-9). The vena cava can be resected en bloc with the tumors, especially if the tumor has obstructed the vena cava preoperatively. In these instances, collateral venous channels are established mainly via paraspinus venous plexus, but retroperitoneal venous collat-

LAHEY BAG
(Bowel on SMA pedicle)

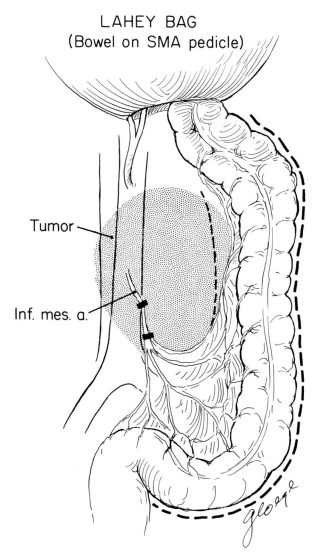

FIG. 13-7. A peritoneal incision for left-sided tumors. The incision is made down the left lateral peritoneal reflection from the splenic flexure, around the sigmoid colon, to the pelvic brim. A medial incision is also made in the colon mesentery, maintaining the integrity of the marginal artery. Ligation of the inferior mesenteric artery aids in mobilization of the ascending colon and should be performed for large left-sided lesions. This can be combined with the maneuver depicted in Figure 13-7 for large lesions.

eral vessels may also be present and troublesome at the time of tumor resection. If necessary, these may be ligated to allow exposure or to ensure complete removal of the lesion.

It is dangerous to ligate the vena cava above the level of the renal veins, especially if only the right kidney remains. In these cases, all attempts should be made to maintain the integrity of the vena cava or to perform some form of venous drainage procedure to the right renal vein via the splenic or portal vein. Even ligation of the left renal vein at its insertion in the vena cava is not without risk, despite well-documented potential collateral flow via the left adrenal, lumbar, and gonadal veins. Cases of significant morbidity with prolonged acute tubular necrosis have been reported,[22] and have also been seen in our series. En bloc resection of contiguous structures invaded by

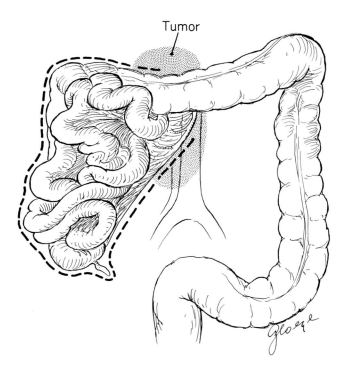

FIG. 13-8. The posterior peritoneum is incised from the hepatic flexure down the ascending colon and around the cecum. The incision is then carried superiorly to the ligament of Treitz. This allows complete mobility of the right colon, small bowel, duodenum, and pancreas on a superior mesenteric artery pedicle. Care should be taken not to occlude the superior mesenteric artery by intensive tension. All bowel contents are placed in a Lahey bag.

direct extension should be performed if technically feasible. Resection of the posterior body wall musculature is often necessary to obtain clear margins.

Both ureters should be identified and protected. Stripping of ureteral adventitia should be avoided if at all possible. Major lymphatic vessels should be occluded with hemaclips to lessen the likelihood of lymphocele or chylous ascites. Care should be taken not to injure the cisterna chyli, which is in the area of the crus of the diaphragm, usually behind the right renal artery. If encountered and opened, it should be ligated or controlled with a suture or hemaclip.

If technically feasible, one or both of the sympathetic chains should be preserved to prevent ejaculatory failure. Unnecessary dissection over the anterior aspect of the lower portion of the aorta near its bifurcation could also cause ejaculatory failure. In cases of large retroperitoneal tumors, and particularly in bulky metastatic testicular tumors, it is often necessary to sacrifice both sympathetic trunks. The patient should be forewarned of this possibility and encouraged to deposit semen in a sperm bank preoperatively if future children are desired.

Reperitonealization is not necessary but may be done. Drains are not routinely left in place unless a specific indication exists (i.e. pancreatic injury or resection). A large chest tube is left indwelling until chest drainage ceases. The thoracoabdominal incision is closed in a standard manner, taking care to resect extra rib cartilage at the costal margin, as this

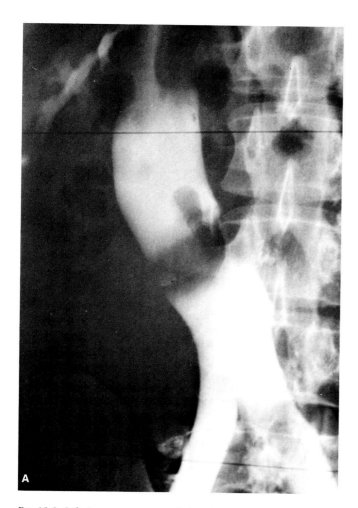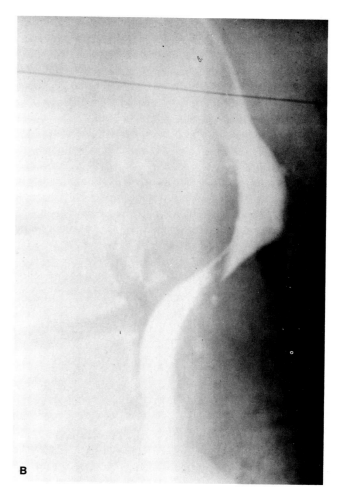

FIG. 13-9. Inferior vena cavagram. *A,* Anterior posterior view. Note the lateral deviation of the vena cava with intraluminal filling defects. *B,* Lateral view. Note the anterior displacement of the vena cava with intraluminal invasion.

may be a cause of painful postoperative wound if cartilage is allowed to override. The injection of bupivacain hydrochloride (Marcaine) (5 cc of 0.75 solution) may decrease postoperative pain.[23]

Tumors of the True Pelvis

A lesion in the true pelvis is best approached through a midline lower abdominal intra or extraperitoneal incision, although a transverse or unilateral Gibson incision can be used depending upon the surgeon's preference. The superior exposure afforded by the midline incision and the possibility of an intraperitoneal approach makes it ideal. On occasion, the extent of pelvic retroperitoneal tumors is underestimated, especially in regard to their upward extension. A low transverse or unilateral extraperitoneal incision may seriously compromise the surgeon's operative exposure. It is often possible to excise these pelvic masses without performing cystectomy or proctectomy. Figure 13-3 demonstrates a large retroperitoneal myxoliposarcoma that was removed without removal of the bladder, prostate, or rectum. However, the surgeon must carefully prepare these patients both medically and emotionally for possible exenteration.

POSTOPERATIVE CARE AND COMPLICATIONS

Postoperative care is standard as with any major surgical procedure. A large, third-space fluid loss occurs with these procedures, and replacement of this loss with colloid is essential in the early postoperative period (usually 50 to 75 cc/hour for 36 to 48 hours). The chest tube is connected to a three-bottle suction device (Pleurovac) until significant drainage ceases. It is then usually connected to water/seal drainage for an additional 24 hours prior to removal, to lessen the likelihood of subsequent hydro- or hemothorax. Nasogastric drainage is generally maintained until postoperative ileus abates. Monitoring with a Swan-Ganz catheter is utilized if medically indicated. I do not favor prophylactic anticoagulation in these cases because complications from this therapy, in my experience, exceeded the benefit. Pulsatile pneumatic stockings, however, have been shown to lessen the likelihood of deep venous thrombosis in the extremities and should be utilized.[24]

Devascularization of the spinal cord has not occurred in our series. Lymphoceles can be a problem, as can chylous ascites or chylothorax. These complications, on occasion, may require operation.[25] Extraperitoneal lymphoceles can be treated with external drainage or the creation of an intraperitoneal window. Lymphoceles rarely occur when a primary intraperitoneal approach is used. Chylous ascites is almost always caused by damage to the cisterna chyli. Spontaneous resolution usually occurs unless proximal obstruction of the thoracic duct is present. Patients with significant lymphocele or chylous ascites should be placed on a medium-chain fatty acid diet to decrease lymphatic outflow. On occasion, reoperation may be necessary to ligate the lymphatic leaks. Chylothorax usually responds to prolonged chest tube drainage and a medium-chain fatty acid diet.

Ureteral injuries, when seen, must be managed with great care, because the extensive retroperitoneal mobilization necessary may devascularize a ureter. Ureteral lesions in the lower or middle third should be managed by ureteral reimplantation, or implantation with a psoas hitch, a Boari flap or a combination of these techniques. Primary reanastomosis is dangerous because of precarious blood supply, especially in the middle or upper third injuries to the ureter and in cases where preoperative radiation therapy or chemotherapy have been employed. Autotransplantation, ileal ureter replacement, and even nephrectomy are treatment options in upper-third injuries. Ischemic injury to the bowel should be managed by resection of the ischemic segment. Late bowel fistulas are best managed by incision and drainage and the placement of the bowel at prolonged rest, with the institution of parenteral hyperalimentation.

On occasion, a polar renal artery can be damaged, and reanastomosis should be attempted if feasible. If this is not technically feasible, simple ligation usually suffices. In cases where a unilateral sympathectomy has been performed, temperature difference in the lower extremity should be expected in the postoperative period.

Radiation Therapy

Radiation therapy as a definitive treatment modality for retroperitoneal sarcomas has little use. High local recurrence rates of up to 80 to 85% have been reported as well as survival rates of less than 10%.[26-29] Radiation therapy may have a place in sarcomas of the extremities, but the intraabdominal and retroperitoneal organs make tumoricidal doses very difficult to deliver. Radiation therapy, however, may be useful as an adjunct to complete surgical excision for soft tissue retroperitoneal sarcomas.[30] This is based on the hypothesis that microscopic disease that still persists following radical local excision is more sensitive to radiation therapy than is the gross tumor itself. It is difficult to find series with significant improvement from this combination of therapy because of the dose limitations secondary to the intra-abdominal structures. Several institutions[31,32] have been working with a technique of intraoperative radiotherapy which has the advantage of selectively radiating the tumor bed, lessening the radiation dose given to adjacent organs. In a pilot study published in 1988, 35 patients were randomized to receive adjuvant external beam radiation therapy or experimental intraoperative radiation therapy.[32]

There did not seem to be a significant difference, however, in the actual disease-free survival and overall survival of the two experimental groups. The intraoperative radiation group, however, tended to show an improvement regarding local recurrence of the disease. Whether this is translated in superior patient survival will depend on further followup.

Chemotherapy

Doxorubicin (Adriamycin) is the only single chemotherapeutic agent with any significant activity in patients with disseminated soft tissue sarcoma. There is approximately a 40% response rate in patients with disseminated disease.[33-35] Some patients achieving complete responses had long-term disease-free survival in excess of 5 years. These responses indeed may be durable. Complete response rates, however, in this population are rare and the majority of patients are not cured by the Adriamycin therapy. Numerous studies have been put forth combining Adriamycin with other drugs such as cyclophosphamide, vincristine, dacarbazine, methyl CCNU and high-dose methotrexate with leucovorin rescue. There is no study, however, that demonstrates that any combination is better than Adriamycin alone. The standard dose of Doxorubicin is 70 mg/m^2 intravenously every 3 weeks. Work by Haskell and associates showed that intra-arterial chemotherapy may have some benefit in retroperitoneal sarcomas.[36] A clear benefit has been demonstrated in extremity sarcomas, however, the arterial supply is generally more defined in those tumors. It is often difficult to completely perfuse a retroperitoneal sarcoma by the arterial route as many of these tumors are hypovascular. Eilber and co-workers have described the use of preoperative doxorubicin, given by the intraarterial route, combined with rapid fraction radiation followed by complete en bloc resection of the tumor.[37,38] The local recurrence rate with extremity sarcomas has been exceedingly low with a high 5-year survival projected to be 75%. Similar responses in retroperitoneal sarcomas have not been obtained, but more time is needed to follow these patients as the numbers are small. Once again, the radiation dose is somewhat limited by the adjacent organs.

In summary, retroperitoneal sarcomas are best managed by obtaining a preoperative angiogram to determine the vascularity of the tumor. If feeding vessel or vessels are found that significantly supply the tumor with blood, then consideration should be given to treating the patient with preoperative intra-arterial doxorubicin. Radiation therapy cannot be given in meaningful amounts in the preoperative setting because of the adjacent organs. Complete radical excision of the retroperitoneal sarcoma should be carried out in all cases where technically possible. The combined role of surgery and intraoperative radiation therapy has yet to be determined.

Statistical analysis is difficult because of the rarity of these tumors and the diffuse histologic character of the retroperitoneal sarcomas and the cellular variability within each given tumor.

REFERENCES

1. PACK, G. T., and BRAUND, R. R. The development of sarcoma in myositis ossificans. JAMA, *119:*776, 1942.
2. PETTIT, V. D., CHAMNES, J. T., and ACKERMAN, L. V. Fibromatosis and fibrosarcoma following irradiation therapy. Cancer, 7:149, 1954.
3. ULBRIGHT, T. M., et al. The development of non-germ cell malignancies within germ cell tumors. A clinical pathological study of 11 cases. Cancer, *54:*1824, 1984.
4. KINNE, D. W., et al. Treatment of primary and recurrent retroperitoneal liposarcomas: 25 years experience at Memorial Hospital. Cancer, *31:*53, 1973.
5. DEWEERD, J. H., and DOCKERT, M. B. Lipomatous retroperitoneal tumors. Am. J. Surg., *84:*397, 1952.
6. BEK, V. Primary retroperitoneal tumors. Neoplasia, *17:*253, 1970.
7. WILEY, A. L., et al. Clinical and theoretical aspects of treatment of surgically unresectable retroperitoneal malignancies with combined intraarterial Actinomycin D and radiation therapy. Cancer, *36:*107, 1975.
8. RHAMY, R. K. Retroperitoneal tumors. In *Urologic Surgery.* 2nd Edition. Edited by J. Glenn. Hagerstown, Harper & Row, 1975, p. 859.
9. MCGRATH, P. C., et al. Improved survival following complete excision of retroperitoneal sarcomas. Ann. Surg., *200:*200, 1984.
10. BENGMARK, S., et al. Retroperitoneal sarcoma treated by surgery. J. Surg. Oncol., *14:*307, 1980.
11. SOLLA, J. A., and REED, K. Primary retroperitoneal sarcomas. Am. J. Surg., *152:*496, 1986.
12. SALVADORI, B., et al. Surgical treatment of 43 retroperitoneal sarcomas. Eur. J. Surg. Oncol., *12:*29, 1986.
13. SNOVER, D. C., et al. Variability of histologic pattern in recurrent soft tissue sarcomas originally diagnosed as liposarcoma. Cancer, *49:*1005, 1982.
14. BOWDEN, L., and BOOKER, R. J. The principles and technique of resection of soft parts for sarcoma. Surgery, *44:*963, 1958.
15. SMITH, R. B., et al. Preoperative vascular embolization as an adjunct to successful resection of a large retroperitoneal hemangiopericytoma. J. Urol., *115:*206, 1976.
16. LOWMAN, R. M., et al. The angiographic patterns of the primary retroperitoneal tumors. Radiology, *104:*259, 1972.
17. American Joint Committee on Cancer. *Manual for Staging of Cancer.* 2nd Edition. Edited by O. H. Beahrs and M. H. Myers. Philadelphia, J. B. Lippincott Co., 1983.
18. KREMENTZ, E. T., and SHAVER, J. C. Behavior and treatment of soft tissue sarcomas. Ann. Surg., *157:*770, 1963.
19. GERNER, R. E., and MOORE, G. E. Synovial sarcoma. Ann. Surg., *181:*22, 1975.
20. DEBAKEY, M. E., et al. Aneurysms of the abdominal aorta: Analysis of results of graft replacement therapy one to eleven years after operation. Ann. Surg., *160:*622, 1964.
21. FERGUSON, L. R. J., et al. Spinal ischemia following abdominal aortic surgery. Ann. Surg., *181:*267, 1975.
22. MCCULLOUGH, D. L., and GITTES, R. F. Ligation of the renal vein in the solitary kidney: Effects on renal function. J. Urol., *113:*295, 1975.
23. CRAWFORD, E. D., et al. Intercostal nerve block with thoracoabdominal incision. J. Urol., *121:*290, 1978.
24. COE, M. P., et al. Prevention of deep vein thrombosis in urologic patients: A controlled, randomized trial of low-dose heparin in external pneumatic compression boots. Surgery, *83:*230, 1978.
25. LIVINGSTON, W. D., CONFER, D. J., and SMITH, R. B. Large lymphocele resulting from retroperitoneal lymphadenectomy. J. Urol., *124:*543, 1980.
26. MCNEER, G. P., et al. Effectiveness of radiation therapy in the management of sarcoma of soft somatic tissues. Cancer, *22:*391, 1968.
27. GILBERT, H. A., et al. Soft tissue sarcomas of the extremities. J. Surg. Oncol., *7:*303, 1975.
28. WINDEYER, B., et al. The place of radiotherapy in the management fibrosarcoma of the soft tissues. Clin. Radiol., *17:*32, 1966.
29. HARRISON, L. B., GUTIERREZ, E. and FISCHER, J. J. Retroperitoneal sarcomas: The Yale experience and a review of the literature. J. Surg. Oncol., *32:*159, 1986.
30. TEPPER, J. E., et al. Radiation therapy of retroperitoneal soft tissue sarcomas. Int. J. Radiat. Oncol. Biol. Phys., *10:*825, 1984.
31. SANDELAR, W. F., et al. Experimental and clinical studies of intraoperative radiotherapy. Surg. Gynecol. Obstet., *157:*205, 1983.
32. KINSELLA, T. J., et al. Preliminary results of a randomized study of adjuvant radiation therapy in resectable adult retroperitoneal soft tissue sarcoma. J. Clin. Oncol., *6:*18, 1988.
33. GOTTLIEB, J. A., et al. Chemotherapy of sarcoma with combination of Adriamycin and dimethyltrizoneimidazolecarboxamide. Cancer, *30:*1632, 1972.
34. POON, M. C., et al. Inflammatory fibrous histious cytoma: An important variant of malignant and fibrious histious cytoma—highly responsive to chemotherapy. Ann. Intern. Med., *97:*858, 1982.
35. TAN, C., et al. Adriamycin-An antitumor antibiotic in the treatment of neoplastic diseases. Cancer, *32:*9, 1973.
36. HASKELL, C. M., et al. Adriamycin (NSC-123127) by arterial infusion. Cancer Chemother. Rep. (Part 3), *6:*187, 1975.
37. EILBER, F. R., et al. A clinicopathologic study: Preoperative Intraarterial Adriamycin and radiation therapy for extremity soft-tissue sarcoma. In *Management of Primary Bone and Soft Tissue Tumors.* Chicago, Yearbook Medical Publishers, 1977, p. 411.
38. EILBER, F. R., et al. Limb salvage for skeletal and soft tissue sarcomas—Multidisciplinary preoperative chemotherapy. Cancer, *53:*2579, 1984.

An Anatomic Approach to the Pelvis

John F. Redman

As described in the chapter on the anatomic approach to the kidneys and retroperitoneum, a knowledge of the retroperitoneal connective tissue is a basic element in the understanding of the potential planes for dissection in the pelvis.

RETROPERITONEAL CONNECTIVE TISSUE OF THE PELVIS

Three primary visceral structures are located in the pelvis: the bladder with associated prostate in the male, the uterus and vagina in the female, and the rectum. The anatomic relationships are easier to understand if one imagines that these structures have dropped through the floor of the peritoneal cavity into the pelvis, carrying the retroperitoneal connective tissue with them and that, in addition, an isthmus of peritoneum extended at one time between these structures. With growth of the pelvic viscera, the leaves of peritoneum adhered together, leaving a fusion fascia with an obliteration of the peritoneum itself.

The terminology used by Tobin to describe the retroperitoneal connective tissues is useful in maintaining clarity (Fig. 14-1).[1] In the pelvis, the outer stratum of retroperitoneal connective tissue is the ventral intrinsic fascia of the iliacus, obturator internus, and levator ani muscle, collectively termed the transversalis fascia. The inner stratum is the supporting connective tissue of the peritoneum per se and also forms the fascia covering the vessels and nerves of the rectum, the so-called rectal fascia. The intermediate stratum surrounds the bladder, prostate, and vagina. In more obese individuals, this stratum may be laminated both dorsally and ventrally, creating potential fascial spaces.

The term "endopelvis fascia" is used frequently in describing the anatomy of the pelvis, but it can be confusing. In some references, the term endopelvic fascia is given only to the overlaying of the transversalis fascia onto the retroperitoneal connective tissue covering the pelvic viscera, or is used interchangeably with the term transversalis fascia in the pelvis (Fig. 14-2). However, in other references, the outermost layer of the intermediate retroperitoneal connective tissue covering the pelvic viscera is termed the endopelvic fascia. A helpful terminology for a surgically important aspect of the endopelvic fascia might be that used by Tobin in describing "fascial collars," which apppear to be formed from the outer stratum

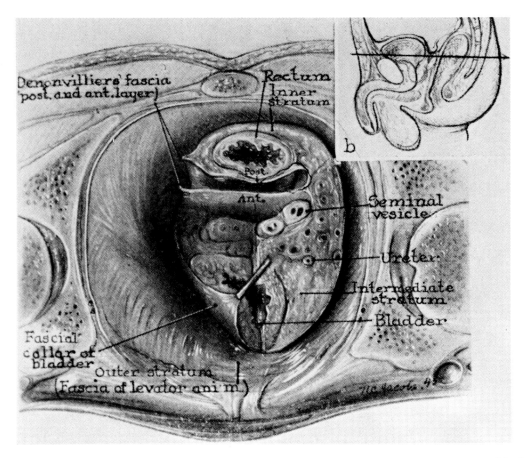

FIG. 14-1. Strata of the retroperitoneal connective tissue. (From Tobin, C. E., Benjamin, J. A., and Wells, J. C.: Continuity of the fasciae lining the abdomen, pelvis and spermatic cord. Surg. Gynecol. Obstet., *83*:575, 1946. By permission of Surgery, Gynecology & Obstetrics.)

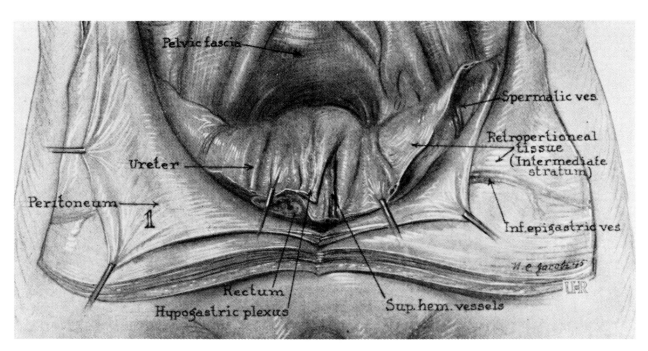

FIG. 14-2. Pelvic fascia and associated retroperitoneal tissue. (From Tobin, C. E., Benjamin, J. A., and Wells, J. C.: Continuity of the fasciae lining the abdomen, pelvis and spermatic cord. Surg. Gynecol. Obstet., *83*:575, 1946. By permission of Surgery, Gynecology & Obstetrics.)

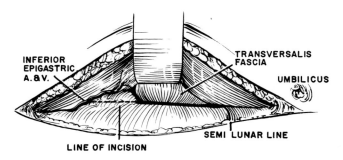

INFERIOR EPIGASTRIC A. & V.

TRANSVERSALIS FASCIA

UMBILICUS

SEMI LUNAR LINE

LINE OF INCISION

FIG. 14-3. Location of the transversalis fascia in relation to the semilunar line of Douglas, as evident upon midline incision.

(transversalis fascia) around the prostate and the lower part of the rectum and vagina.[1]

There is also some confusion in the literature regarding the existence of a transversalis fascia over the lower abdominal wall. McVay and Anson feel that the rectus abdominis muscle is separated from the retroperitoneal connective tissue (subserosal layer) only by its own intrinsic fascia below the level of the arcuate line, although the position of the arcuate line can be variable.[2] In the region of the midline, it is difficult to secure a plane between the dorsal investing fascia of the rectus and the subserosal covering of the bladder.

Whether or not a "transversalis fascia" exists caudal to the semilunar line of Douglas, when the rectus abdominis muscles are dissected free from the underlying connective tissue, a relatively dense fascial-like structure is identified. After being incised some distance laterally from the midline, it is found on dissection to be contiguous with the transversalis fascia of the pelvic side wall (Fig. 14-3).

Regarding a further controversial point in the anatomy of the pelvis, the nature and position of Denonvilliers' fascia,[3,4] Tobin and Benjamin present a surgically useful viewpoint (Fig. 14-4).[4] The posterior layer of Denonvilliers' fascia is the ventral aspect of the retroperitoneal connective tissue (inner stratum) that surrounds the rectum. The anterior layer of Denonvilliers' fascia is the dorsal aspect of the fusion fascia produced by the obliteration of the peritoneal cul-de-sac, which existed between the bladder and prostate and the rectum. This fusion fascia seems to end at approximately the midportion of the prostate. In addition to a narrow wedge of this fascia caudal to the midportion of the prostate, Denonvilliers' fascia is represented by the dorsal aspect of the retroperitoneal connective tissue covering the prostate. A fusion fascia also exists between the seminal vesicles and the base of the bladder.

Two other anatomic aspects of the pelvis bear mentioning (Fig. 14-5). One is the obliterated umbilical artery, which is known as the lateral umbilical ligament. This extends from the hypogastric artery to the umbilicus and is embedded in the lateral aspects of the retroperitoneal connective tissue surrounding the bladder. In cases of a single umbilical artery, the ligament will obviously exist only on one side. The dome of

the bladder is connected also to the umbilicus by a midline cord, the median umbilical ligament, and is adherent to the peritoneum dorsally and to the exraperitoneal connective tissue ventrally.

SURGICAL APPROACHES TO THE PELVIS

Lateral Retroperitoneal Approach

Following incision of the transversus abdominis, the transversalis fascia may be incised to create a cleavage plane between the transversalis fascia and retroperitoneal connective tissue. The ureter and spermatic vessels are contained in the retroperitoneal connective tissue (subserosal layer) (Fig. 14-6). Freeing of the ureter or spermatic vessels requires incision into the subserosal layer. The lateral umbilical ligament is vital to the maintenance of this plane, in that the pelvic viscera are medial to the lateral umbilical ligament. The lateral umbilical ligament is also a key to identifying the hypogastric artery, from which it is derived.

The loose fat attached to this glistening layer of retroperitoneal connective tissue belongs more appropriately to the fat and connective tissue accompanying the iliac vessels (dorsal lamina of the intermediate stratum). This yellowish fat is also found in a large quantity around the obturator nerve and along the lateral aspect of the rectum deep in the pelvis. It can be easily teased away from the extraperitoneal connective tissue surrounding the rectum and bladder and from the transversalis fascia lining the pelvic floor and side walls.

The peritoneum is held deep in the pelvis at the level of the internal ring. Freeing of the peritoneum from the pelvis requires sharp incision of the attachment of the peritoneum at the internal ring. At times, a patent processus vaginalis peritonei is present, but whether it is or not, the fibrous cord that persists will require division. To accomplish this division, an incision is made into the subserosal layer to mobilize the peritoneum, the spermatic vessels and the vas in the male, and the round ligament in the female.

Regardless of how far medially the peritoneum is reflected even over the bifurcation of the great vessels, the ureter remains with the peritoneum because it is encased in the subserosal layer. If the ureter is dissected free from the peritoneum by incision of the subserosal layer, it will be noted in the pelvis that the ureter lies under the lateral umbilical ligament and the leash of vessels that proceed from the hypogastric medially to the bladder, the so-called lateral vesical pedicle. Access to the ureterovesical hiatus requires division of at least some of these vessels encased in subserosal tissue (the cranial portion of the lateral vesical pedicle).

Transverse and Midline Retroperitoneal Pelvic Approach

Regardless of whether the initial incision is a transverse incision or a midline incision in the lower aspect of the abdomen,

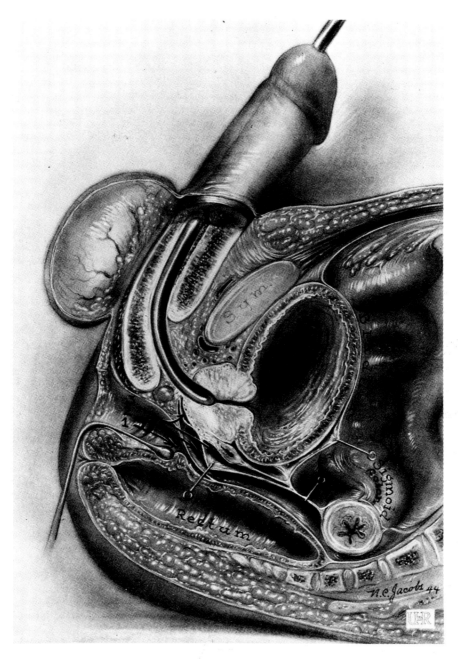

Fig. 14-4. Potential planes of dissection (1) between rectal musculature and the inner stratum of retroperitoneal connective tissue (posterior layer of Denonvilliers' fascia), (2) between the posterior layer of Denonvilliers' fascia and the dorsal aspect of fusion fascia (anterior layer of Denonvilliers' fascia), and (3) between the anterior layer of Denonvilliers' fascia and the capsule of prostate and seminal vesicles. (From Tobin, C. E., and Benjamin, J. A.: Anatomical and surgical restudy of Denonvilliers' fascia. Surg. Gynecol. Obstet., *80:*373, 1945. By permission of Surgery, Gynecology & Obstetrics.)

it essentially becomes a midline incision upon separation of the rectus abdominis muscles. Maintenance of the correct tissue plane requires some care at this stage of the dissection. The retroperitoneal connective tissue, transversalis fascia, and intrinsic fascia of the rectus abdominis and pyramidalis muscles are all represented in the midline.

In the adult, it is generally easier to laterally reflect the rectus abdominis muscles ventral to their intrinsic fascia, which is adherent to transversalis fascia. It is difficult to obtain a plane of cleavage near the midline because the peritoneum and retroperitoneal connective tissue are adherent to the transversalis fascia. We prefer to reflect the rectus until the lateral rectus border can be visualized just lateral to the inferior epigastric vessels.

The underlying transversalis fascia is suffused with whitish aponeurotic fibers, which can be seen emanating from the

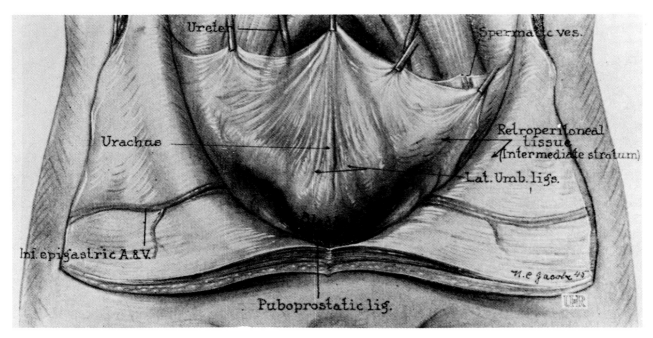

FIG. 14-5. Lateral umbilical ligament. (From Tobin, C. E., Benjamin, J. A., and Wells, J. C.: Continuity of the fasciae lining the abdomen, pelvis and spermatic cord. Surg. Gynecol. Obstet., *83*:575, 1946. By permission of Surgery, Gynecology & Obstetrics.)

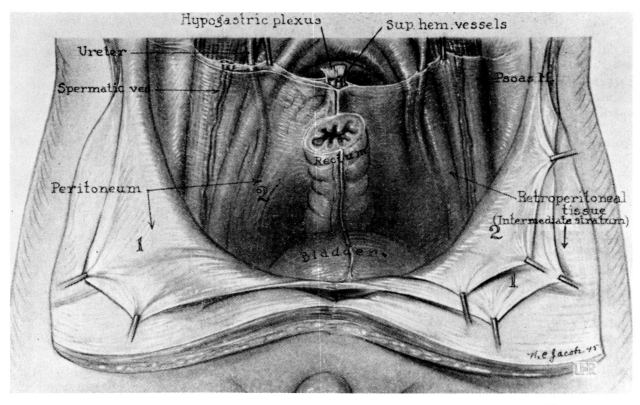

FIG. 14-6. Ureter and spermatic vessels are shown contained in the retroperitoneal tissue. (From Tobin, C. E., Benjamin, J. A., and Wells, J. C.: Continuity of the fasciae lining the abdomen, pelvis and spermatic cord. Surg. Gynecol. Obstet., *83*:575, 1946. By permission of Surgery, Gynecology & Obstetrics.)

aponeurosis of the transversus abdominis muscle. With insinuation of a retractor, such as a Richardson retractor, under the belly of the rectus abdominis, the transversalis fascia can be incised between pickups, exposing the fat of the subserosal layer. With dissection of retroperitoneal connective tissue (subserosal layer) from the transversalis fascia, the incision in the transversalis fascia can be increased. It is best to incise caudally to develop a plane and then to progress cranially. A retractor is slipped laterally under the lateral aspect of the transversalis fascia as it is opened, and the retroperitoneal tissue (subserosal layer) is swept medially.

The peritoneal envelope contained within the retroperitoneal connective tissue can be swept medially as the dissection proceeds cranially, until the adherence of the transversalis fascia with the posterior rectus sheath is encountered. The transversalis fascia can be incised by moving cranially through the semilunar line of Douglas. Laterally, at the level of the iliac crest, the retroperitoneal connective tissue is somewhat adherent to the transversalis fascia, and at times a sharp incision or two with scissors is necessary to maintain the plane of dissection. The peritoneal envelope can be freed from the dorsal muscular wall all the way to the midline and over the midline as the dissection proceeds across the iliac vessels and the aorta or vena cava.

The peritoneum seems to be adherent to the level of the internal ring, and indeed it is, being held by either a frank patent processus vaginalis or by the cord that represents the obliterated patent processus vaginalis. With incision of the subserosal layer, the obliterated processus can be incised sharply and the peritoneum freed away from the pelvic floor and from the vas and the spermatic cord. In the female, the round ligament may be cut. This dissection frees all of the peritoneal envelope away from the pelvic side wall and exposes the extraperitoneal tissue surrounding the pelvic viscera.

Deep in the pelvis, along the neck of the bladder in the female and the prostate in the male, the levator ani muscle and the aponeurotic tissue of the endopelvic fascia approximating these structures (fascial collar) will be noted. Large veins are found immediately under the limiting membrane of the retroperitoneal connective tissue, embedded in the fat surrounding the capsule of the prostate. With the freeing of the endopelvic fascia from the retroperitoneal tissue, the plane of dissection can be carried around the dorsal aspect of the prostate. Generally, there is a midline adherence, which takes some force to break through to extend this cleavage plane to the contralateral side.

On the ventral aspect of the prostate near its apex, the endopelvic fascia appears to be thickened on either side of the midline. These are the so-called puboprostatic ligaments, and although no vessels are contained within this tissue, the dorsal vein of the penis, which is located just under the pubic arch, moves cranially through the arch and then trifurcates, sending a branch over the ventrum of the prostate and lateral branches

along the inner aspect of the pubis. It is difficult to obtain a plane between the pubis and the retroperitoneal connective tissue with its veins over the prostate without some tearing of the veins.

To return to the level of the umbilicus, a plane can be developed around the umbilicus between the transversalis fascia and the retroperitoneal connective tissue. If this plane is developed circumferentially around the umbilicus, the peritoneum of the umbilicus can be divided sharply, totally freeing the peritoneal envelope from the anterior abdominal wall. If the peritoneum extends to the umbilicus per se, a small defect in the peritoneum is created, which can be closed if the dissection is to be done through a totally retroperitoneal approach.

Generally, there is little retroperitoneal connective tissue between the peritoneum and the musculature of the bladder. Practically, the peritoneum is adherent to the musculature of the bladder at the bladder dome. This adherence extends from the umbilicus along the median umbilical ligament over the upper fifth of the posterior aspect of the bladder wall.

A plane of cleavage can be developed extraperitoneally between the retroperitoneal connective tissue of the bladder and the obliterated peritoneum of the cul-de-sac of Douglas, or between the extraperitoneal connective tissue of the rectum and the obliterated peritoneum of the cul-de-sac of Douglas (anterior layer of Denonvilliers' fascia). The development of this plane is usually begun intraperitoneally, as in the case of a cystectomy or in the freeing of the bladder to create a psoas hitch. To obtain this plane, an incision is made in the peritoneum deep in the cul-de-sac of Douglas, between the rectum and bladder or between the rectum and the vagina. With incision of the peritoneum only, a cleavage plane can be developed between the bladder and the rectum.

When the incision is made in the peritoneum, much of the retroperitoneal tissue seems to stay with the bladder. If the surgeon does not dip into this fat and allows it to remain with the bladder, the cleavage plane is more easily identified, particularly as the rectum itself is approached. The plane is between the vesical fascia and the ventral aspect of the anterior Denonvilliers' fascia.

This plane of dissection can be carried dorsal to the seminal vesicles in most instances, to meet the dissection that was begun below with the lateral reflection of the endopelvic fascia from the prostate. If the plane of dissection is started closer to the rectum, a similar plane is started between the retroperitoneal connective tissue covering the rectum (posterior layer of Denonvilliers' fascia) and the obliterated cul-de-sac of Douglas (dorsal aspect of anterior Denonvilliers' fascia).

The lateral vesical pedicles and the lateral prostatic pedicles are essentially the same structure and are actually the vasculature of the bladder and the prostate contained within the retroperitoneal connective tissue. These broad bands of tissue also contain the ureter and the vas. However, the vessels per se are located ventral to the vas and ureter.

The retroperitoneal connective tissue surrounding the bladder and prostate or bladder and vagina and rectum appears almost sheet-like and presents a definite plane separate from the loose "packing material" fat found along the iliac vessels, around the obturator vessels and nerves and the perirectal fossa, and in the deep recess adjacent to the rectum on either side.

Perineal Approach

The incisions into the perineum provide a rather limited exposure to the pelvis, but at times this exposure may be quite useful in gaining access to the dorsal aspect of the prostate or seminal vesicles. With incision of the skin and the superficial fascia of the perineum, the fat of the ischiorectal fossa is noted. Laterally, the ischiorectal fossa is bounded by the obturator internus muscle and medially by the levator ani.

In the midline lies the central tendon of the perineum, the key to the development of the incision. Central tendon represents the fusion of the rectal fascia (retroperitoneal connective tissue of the rectum) and the fascia of the retroperitoneal connective tissue surrounding the prostate with the intrinsic fascia of the striated muscles of the urinary and anal sphincters. If the incision in the central tendon is made dorsally, the plane will be obtained between the rectal musculature per se and the retroperitoneal connective tissue of the rectum. An incision made ventrally gains a plane directly between the prostatic capsule and the extraperitoneal connective tissue over the prostate. The "correct" cleavage plane theoretically would be between the retroperitoneal connective tissue of the rectum and prostate and, more cranially, between the fusion fascia of the cul-de-sac of Douglas and the rectal fascia, i.e., between the anterior and posterior layers of Denonvilliers' fascia respectively. Access to the seminal vesicles requires an incision into the anterior layer of Denonvilliers' fascia and its underlying retroperitoneal connective tissue.

REFERENCES

1. TOBIN, C. E., BENJAMIN, J. A., and WELLS, J. C. Continuity of the fasciae lining the abdomen, pelvis and spermatic cord. Surg. Gynecol. Obstet., 83:575, 1946.
2. McVAY, C. B., and ANSON, B. J. Composition of the rectus sheath. Anat. Rec. 77:213, 1940.
3. UHLENHUTH, E., WOLFE, W. M., SMITH, E. M., and MIDDLETON, E. B. The rectogenital septum. Surg. Gynecol. Obstet., 86:148, 1948.
4. TOBIN, C. E., and BENJAMIN, J. A. Anatomical and surgical restudy of Denonvilliers' fascia. Surg. Gynecol. Obstet., 80:373, 1945.

SECTION
V

CARCINOMA OF THE PROSTATE

Prostatic Carcinoma: An Overview

Joseph R. Drago
Robert A. Badalament

EPIDEMIOLOGIC FACTORS

In the United States, prostate cancer is the most common male cancer and the third leading cause of cancer deaths. In 1989, the American Cancer Society estimates that there will be 103,000 new cases of prostate cancer and 28,500 deaths.[1] Epidemiologic factors associated with the development of prostate cancer have been identified and form the basis for hypotheses concerning possible etiologic mechanisms.

Fewer than 1% of patients with clinically detectable prostate cancer are less than 50 years old; thereafter the incidence and mortality rates continually increase with age.[2] Cumulative data from consecutive autopsy series of men 80 years or older have demonstrated the incidence of carcinoma detected by routine and step-section microscopic examination to be 34% and 53%, respectively.[3] Although the impression of many physicians is that prostate cancer in younger men has a more aggressive biologic potential, on a stage-for-stage basis this belief cannot be substantiated. However, younger men have a higher incidence of metastatic disease at presentation than do older patients.[3] Furthermore, because longevity would otherwise be greater in younger men, a higher likelihood of the prostate cancer producing a significant clinical impact may be anticipated.

The international incidence of prostate cancer varies markedly. Black Americans have the highest reported incidence, Japanese men the lowest.[4,5] The observation that immigrants from low-risk countries, such as those going from Japan to the United States have incidence figures between those of the country of origin and those of the United States implies that in addition to race alone, environmental factors may play an etiologic role.[5,6] In the United States, the relative incidence of prostate cancer in black, white, and immigrant Japanese men is approximately 4:2:1.[5,7] In addition to race and environmental factors, genetic predisposition may also be a factor; the mortality from prostate cancer has been reported to be up to three times more frequent in relatives of patients with prostate cancer than in those of control subjects.[8–10]

Both prostate cancer and benign prostatic hyperplasia (BPH) are common in older men and may be found concurrently. However, the relationship between prostatic hyperplasia and carcinoma remains controversial and undefined. The two most frequently quoted studies have produced contrasting results. Greenwald and associates followed 838 cases of BPH and 802 age-matched control subjects for 10 years but failed to identify any difference in prostate cancer incidence between the two groups.[11] Armenian and coworkers reported a 3.7 to 5.1 times higher age-adjusted death rate from prostatic carcinoma among patients with BPH compared to age-matched controls.[12] Carcinoma usually arises from the peripheral part of the prostate and BPH from the inner portion of the gland.[13,14] Additionally, studies of small-volume prostate cancers have concluded that prostate cancer originates in nonhypertrophied senile tissue and compressed atrophic glands (sclerotic atrophy) outside the expanding nodules of hypertrophy.[11,15] Thus, the histologic data suggest that the etiologic factors for prostate cancer and BPH are unrelated.

Several studies have documented that sexually hyperactive and promiscuous men have a higher incidence of prostate cancer than control subjects.[8,9,16,17] Although the possible role of coital frequency or number of sexual partners in the development of prostate cancer remains uncertain, a sexually transmitted infectious agent has been postulated. An increased incidence of prostate cancer reported among men whose sexual partners had cervical cancer supports this theory.[18] However, studies of celibate men, such as Catholic priests, show a reportedly higher incidence of prostate cancer than amongst a control population.[19] Although epidemiologic support for the sexually transmitted agent hypothesis is sparse, laboratory studies support this theory. Cytomegalovirus (CMV-Mj) isolated from prepubertal prostate and herpes virus type II isolated from prostate carcinoma cause in vitro transformation of human prostate cell lines and hampster cells, respectively.[20,21] Additionally, antibody titers specific to these viruses are higher in prostate cancer than in control subjects.[9,20] RNA viruses have also been implicated in the etiology of prostate cancer by the finding of reverse transcriptase activity, RNA virus-like particles, and RNA tumor virus core protein in human prostate cancer tissues.[22–24]

As discussed previously, prostate cancer is a disease of the elderly; its incidence continually increases with age. Because the changes of advancing age are associated with changes in the hormonal milieu, sex hormones have been implicated in the etiology of prostate cancer. Further evidence favoring a hormonal role includes the presence of steroid hormone receptors in the prostate, the requirement of sex hormones for the normal growth and development of the prostate, the failure of prostate cancer to develop in castrated men, the response of patients with prostate cancer to estrogen administration or androgen deprivation, and the lower incidence of latent prostate cancer in cirrhotics who tend to have hyperestrogenism.[25–27] Noble demonstrated that prostate cancer can be induced in experimental animals by prolonged administration of male sex hormones.[28] Several studies have demonstrated that levels of testosterone and its metabolite, dihydrotestosterone, are higher in carcinomatous than in normal prostatic tissue. Testosterone levels were higher in carcinomatous than in hyperplastic tissue, whereas dihydrotestosterone levels were higher in hyperplastic tissue.[29–31]

Epidemiologic studies comparing total plasma hormone levels of patients with prostate cancer with the levels of controls have reported conflicting data.[29,32–35] However, total plasma testosterone and dihydrotestosterone do not reflect the biologically active fraction of hormone, which is the portion not bound to serum hormone-binding globulin. This may explain the conflicting results. In contrast, serum prolactin levels have provided more consistent findings. Of seven studies, five have demonstrated that serum prolactin levels were higher in patients with prostate cancer than in patients with BPH or normal prostate.[32,35–38] No difference was noted in two studies.[39,40] Further, prolactin increases prostatic uptake and metabolism of testosterone. Thus, elevated prolactin levels may result in an enhanced uptake of testosterone into the prostate, its accelerated conversion into dihydrotestosterone, and therefore an increased risk of prostate cancer.

ANATOMIC CONSIDERATIONS

Classic concepts of prostate anatomy, initially described by Lowsley[41] and later by Franks,[42] have been extensively modified. McNeal has proposed a new classification based on his studies of serial sections through the prostate in different carefully selected planes.[43] In his model, the prostate has been divided into four major regions: peripheral zone, central zone, transitional zone, and the periurethral gland region. The spatial orientation of these regions is illustrated in Figure 15-1.

The peripheral zone and the central zone comprise approximately 70% and 20% of the glandular prostate, respectively. The acini of the peripheral zone are small, rounded, and uniform. In contrast, the acini of the central zone are large and irregular. The transitional zone accounts for about 5 to 10% of the glandular prostate, and the periurethral gland region about 1%. On transrectal prostatic ultrasonography, it is difficult to identify the periurethral gland region; however, the other zonal regions are usually quite distinct.

The peripheral zone, transitional zone, and periurethral glands are histologically identical because of their common origin from the urogenital sinus. In contrast, the central zone has histologic characteristics that suggest Wolffian duct origin. Approximately 70% of cancers develop in the peripheral zone, 20% in the transitional zone, and 10% in the central zone. Thus, relative to its volume, the central zone is resistant to the development of carcinoma. Benign prostatic hyperplasia occurs in the transitional zone and periurethral gland region. Hyperplasia of the transitional zone is primarily glandular, whereas in the periurethral glandular region stromal hyperplasia predominates.

PATHOLOGIC CONSIDERATIONS

McNeal has recently identified duct-acinar dysplasia as a premalignant lesion characterized by nuclear and cytoplasmic abnormalities in the cells lining preexisting ducts and acini.[44] The spectrum of dysplastic abnormalities ranges from mild (grade 1), characterized by variably enlarged nuclei, cell

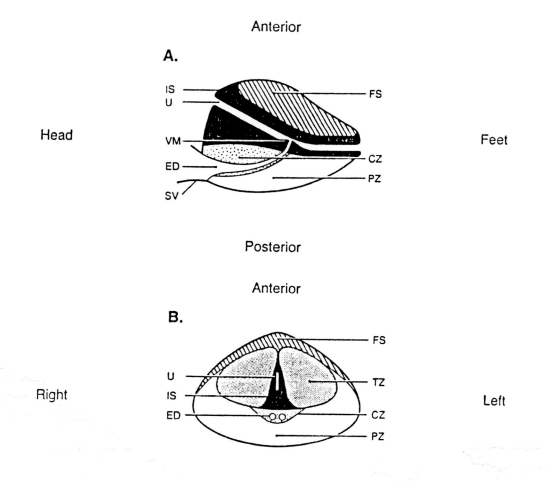

Anterior

A.

Head   Feet

IS
U
VM
ED
SV

FS
CZ
PZ

Posterior

Anterior

B.

Right   Left

U
IS
ED

FS
TZ
CZ
PZ

Posterior

FIG. 15-1. Prostate anatomy. A, Sagittal midline projection. B, Axial midline projection. CZ, central zone; ED, ejaculation duct; FS, fibromuscular stroma; IS, internal sphincter; PZ, peripheral zone; TZ, transitional zone; U, urethra; VM, verumontanum. (Used with permission of Radiology Department, St. Joseph Mercy Hospital, Ann Arbor, MI.)

crowding, irregular spacing, and increased density of cytoplasmic staining, to severe (grade 3), where cells have prominent nuclear enlargement, hyperchromasia, and numerous large nucleoli. Duct-acinar dysplasia has been discovered in approximately 80% of prostates with invasive carcinoma and 40% of prostates without carcinoma. Additionally, foci of invasive carcinoma have been identified at their points of origin from dysplastic ducts. Immunohistochemical studies have shown a loss of differentiation antigens proportional to the severity of dysplasia. The clinical implications of finding dysplasia on prostatic biopsy in the absence of frank carcinoma remain to be defined.

Adenocarcinoma constitutes 98% of all prostatic carcinomas.[3] The characteristic features of prostatic adenocarcinoma are based primarily on glandular architecture and secondarily on cytologic features. Although multiple classifications for the histologic grading of prostate cancer have been proposed, the Gleason grading system is most frequently utilized.[45] This grading system is based upon the degree of glandular differentiation and growth pattern of the tumor in relation to the pros-

tatic stroma; individual cellular characteristics are not considered. The pattern may vary from a well-differentiated grade 1 tumor to a poorly differentiated grade 5 tumor. The Gleason system assigns a histologic grade to both the primary and secondary patterns, with the Gleason score representing the sum of the two. As a result, the Gleason score ranges between 2 and 10. Thus, the Gleason staging system is unique in that histologic grade is based on the majority of the specimen and not the most undifferentiated portion.

Recently, the value of prostatic specific antigen (PSA) in the management of patients with prostate cancer has been established. Identified in 1979, this antigen is produced exclusively by normal and neoplastic prostatic ductal epithelium and is secreted into the glandular lumen.[46] The half-life is 2.2 days and its serum concentration is proportional to the total prostatic mass. Pathologists have taken advantage of the specificity of PSA for prostate by using PSA and prostatic acid phosphatase immunochemical stains to investigate metastatic tumors for possible prostatic origin.[47,48] Although, the reported sensitivity of serum PSA in the detection of prostate cancer is

73 to 96%,[49-53] PSA may also be elevated in 55 to 83%[52,53] of patients with BPH. Thus, its lack of specificity to differentiate BPH from cancer makes PSA an ineffective screening modality for early-state prostate cancer. Prostatic specific antigen is particularly useful in monitoring patients following radical prostatectomy. Stamey and associates have suggested that patients with PSA elevations following radical prostatectomy receive 6,000 rads to the pelvis.[53] Hormonal therapy alone or in combination with radiotherapy is an alternative option.

Prostatic adenocarcinoma spreads by direct extension into the seminal vesicles, bladder, membranous urethra, and pelvic sidewalls. Prostatic carcinoma invading the rectum is relatively uncommon owing to protection afforded it by Denonvilliers' fascia. Regional and distant metastases may also occur by lymphatic and hematogenous routes. Surgical staging series have demonstrated that the obturator lymph node group is the primary landing site for pelvic nodal metastases.[54,55] Subsequent lymphatic invasion involves the iliac and para-aortic lymph nodes.[54,55] Lung metastases result from either further lymphatic spread via the thoracic duct or hematogenous dissemination from the prostatic venous plexus. Bone metastases most frequently involve the vertebral column, ribs, and pelvic bones.[56] The bone lesion is unique in that it appears radiographically as an osteoblastic lesion, not an osteolytic one. This increased radiographic density is not produced by an increase in calcium deposition, but by an increase in noncalcified osteoid, which replaces the air spaces within the bone, producing the paradoxic appearance of increased bone density in areas of calcium loss.

CLINICAL PRESENTATION AND DIAGNOSIS

Sixty-four percent of patients with adenocarcinoma of the prostate present with localized disease.[1] Most of these patients either are asymptomatic or have bladder outlet obstructive symptoms. Patients may also present with severe irritative bladder symptoms in the absence of infection, but isolated hematuria or hematospermia is rare. A minority may be diagnosed in prostate cancer screening clinics.

Patients with metastatic disease most often complain of bone pain. Frequently, the disease is erroneously attributed to degenerative arthritis, and pathologic fracture or spinal cord compression may occur. Occasionally, palpable peripheral lymphadenopathy or lower extremity edema due to pelvic adenopathy is the presenting symptom. Renal failure due to bilateral ureteral obstruction, visceral metastases, anemia, and cachexia may also be the initial signs of prostate cancer.

Localized prostate cancer is best detected by digital rectal examination. Digital guided biopsy of a palpable nodule reveals carcinoma in approximately 50% of cases.[57] With the recent advent of higher-frequency transducers, transrectal ultrasonography has improved the ability to define internal prostatic anatomy and pathology. The utilization of a thin-needle, spring-driven biopsy gun under ultrasonic guidance permits the outpatient acquisition of multiple biopsy specimens. At the Ohio State University, ultrasonic guidance is the preferred method to obtain prostate biopsies in patients with clinically

localized cancer. Prior to biopsy, patients are administered a Fleet's enema and a single 400-mg tablet of norfloxacin as recommended by Stamey.[58] In over 1,000 biopsies, only one patient required hospitalization for infection and one for hematuria. Although fine-needle aspiration cytology may also be obtained under ultrasonic guidance, in our experience it offers no particular advantage over biopsy obtained from a fine-needle, spring-driven biopsy gun.[59]

The use of transrectal ultrasound in the screening of asymptomatic patients for prostate cancer remains controversial. Both the National Prostate Cancer Detection Program and the Southwest Oncology Group have ongoing protocols that will attempt to better define the role of transrectal ultrasound in this setting. Utilizing digital rectal examination alone as a screening modality, Chodak and associates have reported a prostate cancer detection rate of 1.4%.[60] At the Ohio State University, 320 patients have been evaluated in a double-blind comparison of digital rectal examination and transrectal prostatic ultrasound. Of the 320 patients evaluated, 13 (4.1%) had palpable nodules; all these patients also had ultrasonic evidence of carcinoma. Additionally, 10 (3.2%) patients with no evidence of carcinoma on digital rectal examination had carcinoma discovered by means of ultrasonography.[61] The biologic potential and thus the appropriate treatment of this latter group of patients remain uncertain.

STAGING

Selection of treatment in prostatic adenocarcinoma is based on the extent of disease. Multiple staging systems have been proposed; they are all similar in that they designate the disease as either being confined to the prostate, having local spread involving either regional or distant lymph nodes, or involving bone or other parenchymal sites. Although the tumor, node, metastasis (TNM) system of staging prostate cancers has been adopted by the American Joint Committee for Cancer Staging and End Results Reporting,[62] the A, B, C, D system proposed by Whitmore[63] and later modified by Jewett[64] is more commonly used in the United States (Tables 15-1, 15-2). In the Whitmore-Jewett classification, there is no universal agreement on definitions of stage A1 versus A2 disease. Stage A1 disease has been arbitrarily defined as well-differentiated carcinoma involving three or less of the prostatic chips following transurethral resection[65] or, alternatively, less than 5% of total gland volume.[66] Lee and associates have introduced a modification of the A, B, C, D classification system based on the ultrasound staging of prostate cancer.[67] Although this classification is currently used on a limited basis, with increasing utilization of transrectal prostatic ultrasound, it may be more commonly applied.

Transrectal prostatic ultrasound appears to be an invaluable staging tool in the evaluation of prostate cancer.[58,68] Not only does it permit detection of nonpalpable tumors, but it also allows visualization of capsular penetration and seminal vesicle invasion. Additionally, transrectal ultrasound also provides volumetric estimates of tumor and hyperplastic tissue. Because serum PSA concentrations are directly related to pros-

TABLE 15-1. *TNM Classification of Prostatic Carcinoma*

PRIMARY TUMOR (T)

TX   Minimum requirements cannot be met

T0   No tumor palpable; includes incidental findings of cancer in a biopsy or operative specimen. Assign all such cases a G, N, or M category

T1   Tumor intracapsular surrounded by normal gland

T2   Tumor confined to gland, deforming contour, and invading capsule, but lateral sulci and seminal vesicles are not involved

T3   Tumor extends beyond capsule with or without involvement of lateral sulci and/or seminal vesicles

T4   Tumor fixed or involving neighboring structures. Add suffix (m) after "T" to indicate multiple tumors (e.g., T2m)

NODAL INVOLVEMENT (N)

NX   Minimum requirements cannot be met

N0   No involvement of regional lymph nodes

N1   Involvement of a single regional lymph node

N2   Involvement of multiple regional lymph nodes

N3   Free space between tumor and fixed pelvic wall mass

N4   Involvement of juxtaregional nodes

Note: If N category is determined by lymphangiography or isotope scans, insert "1" or "i" between "N" and appropriate number (e.g., N12 or Ni2). If nodes are histologically positive after surgery, add "+"; if negative, add "−."

DISTANT METASTASIS (M)

MX   Not assessed

M0   No (known) distant metastasis

M1   Distant metastasis present (specify)
Specify sites according to the following notations:

PUL (Pulmonary)	MAR (Bone marrow)
OSS (Osseous)	PLE (Pleura)
HEP (Hepatic)	SKI (Skin)
BRA (Brain)	EYE (Eye)
LYM (Lymph nodes)	OTH (Other)

Note: Add "+" to the abbreviated notation to indicate that the pathology (*p*) is proved.

---

tatic volume, we consider PSA elevation that is disproportionate to prostatic volume to be an indication for biopsy. Patients should not only have biopsies of suspicious or equivocal lesions, but also should have random biopsies of each zonal region on both right and left prostatic sides. Furthermore, the posterior biopsies should include tissue from the prostatic-seminal vesicle junction. Owing to the higher incidence of carcinoma associated with dysplasia, we consider this condition to be an indication for repeat biopsy.

Although serum PSA is an ineffective screening modality, it is useful in the staging of prostatic cancers. A PSA value greater than 40 ng/ml has been associated with microscopic capsular penetration, seminal vesicle invasion, and microscopic invasion of pelvic lymph nodes.[53] Additionally, markedly elevated PSA levels have been correlated with a high incidence of distant metastases. When compared to prostatic acid phosphatase, PSA is more sensitive but less specific in the detection of prostate cancer. Furthermore, the use of PSA and prostatic acid phosphatase jointly has not enhanced the clinical utility of PSA alone.[49]

The pelvic lymph nodes are typically the first site of metastatic spread in prostate cancer. Donohue and associates reported that the incidence of positive pelvic lymph nodes was 2% for clinical stage A1, 26% for stage A2, 10% for stage B1, 25% for stage B2, and 46% for stage C.[69] Lymphangiography, computerized tomography, and magnetic resonance imaging have been utilized in the evaluation of pelvic nodal status. Lymphangiography is of limited value because the hypogastric and obturator lymph nodes that are frequently involved with metastatic disease are inconsistently visualized, resulting in

false positive rates of 10 to 17%, and false-negative rates of 22 to 40%.[70,71] Computerized tomography and magnetic resonance imaging are limited by their inability to identify microscopic disease. Despite these limitations, these tests are useful when employed in conjunction with fine-needle aspiration to histologically confirm a positive study.[72] However, a negative cytology does not exclude metastases and is an indication for a pelvic lymph node dissection. Thus, in general, radiographic techniques are unreliable in the evaluation of pelvic lymphatics for metastatic disease.

TABLE 15-2. *Whitmore-Jewett Staging Classification of Prostate Cancer*

Stage A: Clinically unrecognized
A1   <5% of prostatic tissue neoplastic
A2   >5% of prostatic tissue neoplastic, all high-grade tumors

Stage B: Clinically intracapsular
B1   nodule <2 cm surrounded by palpably normal tissue
B2   nodule >2 cm, or multiple nodules

Stage C: Clinically extracapsular, localized to periprostatic area
C1   minimal extracapsular extension
C2   large tumors involving seminal vesicles and/or adjacent structures

Stage D: Metastatic disease
D1   pelvic lymph node metastases, or ureteral obstruction causing hydronephrosis
D2   distant metastases to bone, viscera, or other soft tissue structures

Because of the failure of noninvasive techniques to accurately evaluate the pelvic lymph nodes, pelvic lymphadenectomy has been used for staging purposes in patients with clinically localized adenocarcinoma of the prostate. The limits of staging lymph node dissection vary. Some surgeons carry the dissection to the level of the aortic bifurcation, and others remove the presacral and presciatic lymph nodal groups, along with the external iliac, obturator, and hypogastric nodes.[70,73–77] We favor limiting the dissection to the triangle bounded by the inferior margin of the external iliac vein, the endopelvic fascia, and the hypogastric vessels, including the obturator lymph node group (Fig. 15-2). Several observations support the practice of a more limited dissection. First, the therapeutic value of lymph node dissection remains unproven. Secondly, few patients have periaortic, presacral, presciatic, or common iliac lymph node metastases in the absence of external iliac, hypogastric, or obturator lymph node involvement. Golimbu and associates identified nodal extension in only 2 of 30 patients who had presacral and presciatic dissection when the external iliac, hypogastric, and obturator nodes did not also have metastases.[78] Additionally, Spellman and colleagues reported that periaortic metastases occur only when pelvic lymph nodes are involved.[79] Finally, more extensive lymph node dissection is associated with higher morbidity, especially delayed lower extremity and genital lymphedema.

A chest radiograph and radionuclide bone scan are indicated to detect the presence of distant metastatic disease. Paget's disease, degenerative arthritis, and trauma may cause increased radionuclide uptake and therefore false-positive studies. Radiographs, computerized tomography, magnetic resonance imaging, or bone biopsy may be useful in evaluating equivocal bone scans. Diffuse symmetrical metastatic uptake (superscan) may be falsely interpreted as normal. The findings of minimal soft tissue visualization and absence of renal excretion of radionuclide should raise the suspicion of a falsely negative superscan.[70,80]

Repeat circumferential transurethral resection has been advocated to surgically restage patients with occult focal (stage A1) adenocarcinoma of the prostate. Cumulative data from five series, which included 229 patients with stage A1 adenocarcinoma, revealed that a second transurethral resection demonstrated significant residual tumor in 24% of patients and produced upstaging in 7%.[81–85] Transperineal biopsy is a relatively inaccurate method to detect residual carcinoma.[84,85] Epstein and Walsh have reported that among 50 men with untreated stage A1 disease, followed for a minimum of 8 years, 8 (16%) have progressed. Furthermore, 6 of the 8 men who progressed died from prostate cancer.[86] In 16 men with stage A1 adenocarcinoma of the prostate treated by radical prostatectomy, only 2 had no tumor in the prostatectomy specimen. Among the 14 patients with residual tumor, most would not have had tumor identified on repeat transurethral resection. Thus, the Johns Hopkins experience would support the finding that, especially in younger patients, repeat transurethral resection is not necessary since definitive therapy should be offered for stage A1 disease.

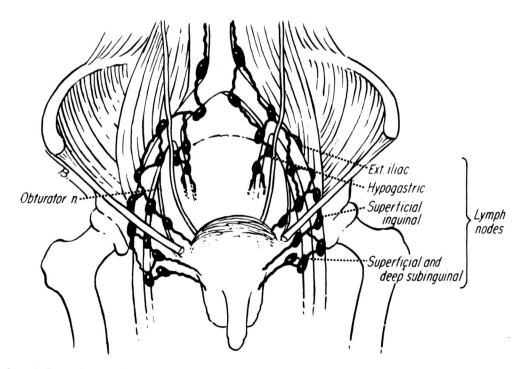

FIG. 15-2. Shaded area indicates the area of limited pelvic lymph node dissection for staging of prostate cancer. (From Paulson, D. F. The prostate. In: *Genitourinary Surgery.* Edited by D. F. Paulson. New York: Churchill Livingstone, 1984.)

Although not a routine part of staging for prostate carcinoma, flow cytometry may be applied as a supplemental parameter to predict tumor progression. Several investigators have shown that there is a steplike relationship between tumor grade and stage to diploid, tetraploid, and aneuploid DNA content.[87-89] Additionally, the proportion of multiple aneuploid stemlines also increases with grade. Preliminary reports suggest that flow cytometry may be able to predict response to hormonal therapy. Zetterberg and Esposti demonstrated that, in general, responders had diploid or tetraploid DNA content, whereas nonresponders had aneuploid tumors.[90] Another study noted a change from aneuploid to diploid DNA content with estrogen therapy.[91] The Memorial Sloan-Kettering Cancer Center group performed flow cytometric analysis of metastatic nodal tissue from 82 patients with prostate cancer treated by ^{125}I seed implants.[92] Cox regression analysis demonstrated that ploidy was the strongest predictor of survival. The median survival of the patients with diploid tumors and aneuploid tumors was 8.8 and 5.0 years, respectively. A recent report from the Mayo Clinic correlated DNA ploidy to survival in 91 patients with stage D1 adenocarcinoma of the prostate.[93] Survival was significantly better in the patients with diploid tumors than in the patients with tetraploid or aneuploid tumors. These findings were substantiated in a similar study from Duke University that examined 88 patients with pathologic stage B and C disease.[94] Thus, flow cytometry appears to significantly enhance prognostic stratification; its exact role, however, remains to be defined by prospective studies.

TREATMENT

The optimal management of men with localized prostatic carcinoma remains controversial. No treatment with close surveillance is a viable option in select patients, such as patients with stage A1 disease, very advanced age, or poor medical status.[95] Treatment options include radical prostatectomy, external beam or interstitial radiotherapy, and hormonal therapy (Table 15-3). The selection of treatment is based on projected survival of the patient, as well as on patient and physician preferences.

Radical prostatectomy has a long history as the definitive treatment for localized prostate cancer. There is no evidence that any other treatment modality produces better control of the primary lesion and of distant metastases than does total excision of the prostate.[96] Radical prostatectomy can be performed via a perineal or a retropubic approach. The advantages of a perineal prostatectomy include a relatively avascular field for dissection, good exposure for reconstruction of the vesicourethral anastomosis, and dependent postoperative drainage. The major disadvantage of this approach is that it does not allow for lymph nodal evaluation with this incision. The retropubic approach is favored by many surgeons because they have increased familiarity with pelvic structures and because simultaneous pelvic lymphadenectomy may be performed.

Despite the therapeutic advantages of radical prostatectomy, alternative forms of treatment were sought because of the significant morbidity of the procedure. The two most significant complications included stress urinary incontinence and erectile impotency. Approximately 5% of patients had complete incontinence and another 15 to 20% experienced mild to moderate stress incontinence.[97,98] The incidence of impotency after radical prostatectomy exceeded 90%.[57,99] Improvements in the surgical technique introduced by Walsh have reduced the morbidity of radical prostatectomy.[100-102] The use of epidural anesthesia, bulldog clamps on the hypogastric arteries, and improved control of the dorsal vein complex has permitted surgery to be performed in a relatively bloodless field. At the Ohio State University, we prefer to obtain early control of the hypogastric vessels by retracting elastic vessel loops that have been passed around each vessel twice. Among our last 30 patients undergoing radical prostatectomy, 22 did not require blood transfusion, 4 received one autologous unit of blood, 2 received 2 units of blood, and 2 received 3 units of blood. In this group the average blood loss was 456 ml.[103] These modifications have permitted identification and preservation of branches of the pelvic plexus that innervate the corpora cavernosa resulting in a postoperative potency rate of approximately 50 to 70%.[96,103,104] Additionally, the incontinence rate now approaches zero because the urogenital diaphragm is not violated and more precise placement of vesicourethral anastomotic sutures is possible. Thus, radical prostatectomy has become a more acceptable therapeutic option.

Radical prostatectomy performed in patients with carcinoma clinically confined to the prostate has been shown to produce 15-year cancer-free survival comparable to that of an age-matched control population.[105] Earlier series have reported 15-year cancer-free survivals in the range of 30.8 to 39.3%.[106-108] More current series report better 15-year cancer-free survival ranging from 48 to 51% in a cumulative total of 344 patients.[109-111] In the study by Gibbons and associates, the actual survival observed in the prostatectomy group was better than that expected for the general population of the same age.[111] Although the reasons for differences in survival between the earlier and more current studies are uncertain, improved staging accuracy is a plausible explanation.[110]

The modern era of irradiation therapy for prostate cancer coincides with the development of cobalt 60 radiation sources and the linear accelerator. These devices permitted the delivery of tumoricidal doses of irradiation with improved tolerance of normal tissues. Currently most patients are treated with a 4- or 10-Mev linear accelerator employing a four-field technique with the isocenter localized to treat the prostate with a dose of approximately 7,000 rads and the regional pelvic lymph nodes with a dose of 4,500 to 5,000 rads delivered over 7 weeks.[112,113] Complications of external radiotherapy include chronic symptomatic cystitis in 10% (bladder augmentation or supravesical urinary diversion required in 1 to 2%), urethral stricture and/or urinary incontinence in 5 to 8%, chronic radiation enteritis in 10% (colostomy required in

TABLE 15-3. *Curative Therapy for Localized Prostate Cancer*

RADICAL PROSTATECTOMY	5-YR SURVIVAL NO. PATIENTS (%)	10-YR SURVIVAL NO. PATIENTS (%)	15-YR SURVIVAL NO. PATIENTS (%)
Culp and Meyer[109] (1973)			
Stages A and B*	—	83/115 (72)	40/ 74 (54)
Stages A and B†	—	66/115 (57)	36/ 74 (48)
Hodges et al.[108] (1979)			
Stages A and B*	156/195 (80)	107/195 (54)	23/195 (27)
Walsh and Jewett[110] (1980)			
Stage B1*	—	—	29/ 57 (51)
Gibbons et al.[111] (1984)			
Stage B*	92/ 97 (95)	40/ 54 (74)	16/ 29 (55)
Stage B†	87/ 92 (90)	36/ 54 (67)	14/ 29 (48)
External Beam Radiotherapy			
Bagshaw[113] (1988)			
DLP (Stages A and B)‡	265/327 (81)	89/151 (59)	15/ 42 (36)
ECE (Stage C)‡	130/210 (62)	28/ 78 (36)	4/ 24 (18)
[125]I Seed Irradiation§			
Whitmore et al.[129] (1987)			
Stages B1−2 (node +/−)†	—	25/ 76 (33)	—
Stages B1−2 (node −)†	—	25/ 59 (42)	—
Stages B1−2 (node −)*	—	46/ 59 (78)	—
Combined [198]AU Seeds and External Irradiation			
Carlton and Scardino[131] (1988)			
Stages A2 and B (node +/−)‡	329/382 (86)	122/207 (59)	43/155 (28)
Stages A2 and B (node −)‡	221/243 (91)	73/111 (66)	32/ 91 (35)
Stages A2 and B (node −)†	187/243 (77)	61/111 (55)	46/ 91 (50)

*Actual survival.
†NED survival.
‡Actuarial survival.
§Memorial Sloan-Kettering Cancer Center Staging System utilized. Stages B1−2 include all nodules confined to one lobe.
Abbreviations: Node +/−, pelvic lymph node status positive or negative; Node −, pelvic lymph node status negative.

1%), and impotence in 41%.[113–117] Severe genital and/or lower extremity lymphedema is an uncommon complication of external radiotherapy. However, an incidence of more than 40% has been reported in patients who have had prior pelvic lymphadenectomy.[118,119]

Recently, Bagshaw has updated the Stanford experience of definitive external irradiation in 879 patients with adenocarcinoma of the prostate.[113] Acid phosphatase and pelvic lymph node status were not utilized in clinical staging. Patients were divided into two categories: 477 patients with disease limited to the prostate (DLP) and 402 patients with extracapsular extension (ECE). Among patients with DLP, stages A and B, the actuarial survival was 81%, 59%, and 36% at 5, 10, and 15 years, respectively. Of patients with ECE, stage C, the actuarial survival was 62%, 36%, and 18%.

Optimal treatment selection in patients with organ-confined disease remains undefined. The effectiveness of radi-

otherapy must be questioned in light of a positive postirradiation biopsy rate of 24 to 74%.[112] Although a positive postirradiation biopsy may not prove that a particular tumor has biologic significance,[120] several authors have shown that it does predict an accelerated rate of disease progression.[121–123] It is difficult to use the results of nonrandomized single institutional studies to compare the effectiveness of radical prostatectomy versus that of external-beam radiotherapy. Variables such as different radiation delivery techniques and doses, staging studies, and patient selection criteria invalidate such an approach. The only randomized prospective study comparing radical prostatectomy and external beam radiotherapy was reported in 1982 by the Uro-oncology Research Group and has been updated.[124,125] In this study, 98 patients with clinical stage A2 or stage B (T1−2N0M0) adenocarcinoma of the prostate, normal serum acid phosphatase levels, negative bone scans, and no pelvic nodal metastasis as determined by staging pelvic lymphadenectomy were randomized into two treatment groups: 55 patients were treated with external beam radiotherapy and 43 had radical prostatectomy. Patients were followed for a minimum of 80 months. When the first evidence of treatment failure was used as the end point, radical prostatectomy was significantly more effective in establishing disease control.

Interstitial radiotherapy has also been used as curative treatment for organ-confined adenocarcinoma of the prostate. Interstitial ^{125}I implantation therapy for prostate cancer was developed at Memorial Sloan-Kettering Cancer Center.[126] Patients with stage A tumors diagnosed following transurethral prostatectomy were not offered interstitial therapy, since the remaining prostatic tissue would not hold the required 30 to 35 seeds properly. Thus, candidates for this form of therapy were mainly limited to patients with stage B or limited stage C disease. Approximately 25,000 rads were delivered to the center of the prostate and 18,000 rads to the periphery over a 12-month period a dose biologically equivalent to 7,000 rads of external beam irradiation.[127] The advantages of interstitial ^{125}I implantation include simultaneous staging pelvic lymphadenectomy and implantation, a technically easier operation, preservation of potency in over 90% of patients, and maintenance of continence.[128] Disadvantages include the possibility of geographic misses and treatment failures due to inhomogeneous distribution of seeds and variability of radiation emitted from each seed.

Whitmore and associates have reported on the first 164 patients treated with interstitial ^{125}I implantation, all with a minimum follow-up of 10 years.[129] Among the 99 patients with stage B disease, 28 (28%) were disease-free at 10 years. Twenty-seven of the 71 (37%) patients with stage B disease and negative lymph node status and 1 of the 28 (4%) stage B lymph node-positive patients were disease-free at 10 years. Only 5 of 64 (8%) of stage C patients were disease-free at 10 years; however, these 5 patients were among the 26 (19%) with negative lymph node status. Despite a relatively low 10-year disease-free survival, overall 10-year survival for stage B and C patients was approximately 50% and 15%, respectively. The most favorable group included patients with stage B1 (small nodule) and stage B2 (<1 lobe) node-negative disease. Ten-year overall and disease-free survival was 78% and 38%, respectively.

Carlton and associates developed definitive therapy with interstitial [198]Au and external beam irradiation used in combination.[130] The advantage of this form of therapy over interstitial ^{125}I implants is that a uniform dose of radiation may be more easily delivered because the higher energy of [198]Au makes geometric seed placement less critical. Furthermore, because only about 6 to 10 seeds are implanted, patients having undergone prior transurethral prostatectomy are not excluded from implantation. Thus, the biologic equivalent of 3,000 to 3,500 rads of external beam radiotherapy is delivered to the prostate and seminal vesicles.[127] The dose of supplemental external beam irradiation has been dependent on pelvic lymph node state. If modified pelvic lymphadenectomy is

negative, 4,500 rads have been given to the prostate and periprostatic tissue. If pelvic lymph node status is positive, then 5,500 rads have been delivered to the whole pelvis and prostate.

Thus far, 510 patients have been treated with combined [198]Au seed implantation and external beam radiotherapy.[131] Hormonal therapy was not administered until recurrence of tumor was documented, and the mean follow-up was 8.6 years. Among patients with clinical stages A2 and B prostate cancer, the actuarial disease-free survival rates at 5, 10, and 15 years were $86 \pm 4\%$, $59 \pm 6\%$, and $28 \pm 13\%$, respectively. For patients with clinical stage C prostate cancer, the actuarial disease-free survival rates at 5, 10, and 15 years were $74 \pm 8\%$, $34 \pm 12\%$, and $17 \pm 13\%$, respectively.

The actuarial survival rates for the subset of patients with negative pelvic lymph nodes were superior to those for patients with positive pelvic lymph nodes. Among patients with pathologic stages A2 and B (node-negative) prostate cancer, the actuarial 5- 10- and 15-year disease-free survival rates were $91 \pm 3\%$, $66 \pm 7\%$, and $35 \pm 16\%$, respectively. For patients with pathologic stage C (node-negative) prostate cancer, the actuarial 5- 10- and 15-year disease-free survival rates were $86 \pm 9\%$, $44 \pm 16\%$, and $30 \pm 20\%$, respectively.

Of the 510 patients, 147 without any clinical evidence of local or distant recurrence were subjected to follow-up biopsy 1 to 3 years following treatment. Results of the biopsy were positive in 50 patients (34%), and 38 of these patients (76%) subsequently developed recurrent disease. Results of the post-irradiation biopsy were negative on 96 patients (66%), and of these patients 33 (34%) subsequently developed disease recurrence. Thus, postirradiation biopsy was shown to be a powerful predictor of disease recurrence.

Although hormonal therapy may be used in select patients with organ-confined prostate cancer, it is generally reserved for the treatment of metastatic disease. Bilateral scrotal orchiectomy appears to be the simplest and most reliable way of reducing serum androgens and avoiding cardiovascular complications associated with other forms of endocrine therapy.[132] Alternative forms of hormonal manipulation, such as estrogens,[133,134] progestational agents,[134,135] antiandrogens,[136–141] and LHRH agonists,[142–145] appear to have no therapeutic advantage over orchiectomy. Furthermore, there is no convincing evidence that total androgen ablation as first-line hormonal therapy is superior to orchiectomy.[145–147] The timing of endocrine therapy has not been shown to affect response duration or survival of patients with metastatic prostate cancer.[148–150] Thus, most clinicians prefer to reserve hormonal therapy for symptomatic disease progression. Following initiation of hormonal therapy in patients with symptomatic metastatic disease, 50% of patients will relapse within 3 years.[150,151] Medical or surgical adrenalectomy or hypophysectomy in patients relapsing after primary hormonal therapy is associated with a subjective response in most patients, but objective responses have been uncommon.[152,153]

Because additional endocrine manipulations are rarely beneficial after primary hormonal therapy has been instituted, the use of chemotherapy may be considered at this time. If chemotherapy is to be utilized, first-line hormonal therapy should be continued to prevent normalization of serum testosterone levels and subsequent tumor stimulation. In general, the results of cytotoxic chemotherapy have been disappointing. Eisenberger and associates have recently summarized the results of single-agent phase II trials in hormone-resistant prostatic carcinoma.[154] Among a total of 1162 evaluable patients, 86 (7.5%) had an objective response (complete response (CR) + partial response (PR)). The most frequently used single agents include cyclophosphamide,[155] 5-fluorouracil,[156,157] doxorubicin,[158,159] estramustine phosphate,[160,161] methotrexate,[162] and cisplatin.[163,164] Multiple-drug regimens have failed to demonstrate significant superiority over single agents in controlled phase III clinical trials.[154,165–167] Despite response to chemotherapy, the median survival with hormone-refractory prostate cancer is less than 40 weeks and is not significantly longer than survival of patients treated with standard palliative measures.[168]

It is evident from the poor response of traditional chemotherapy regimens that new therapeutic approaches are needed. One such approach involves the combination of androgen priming and chemotherapy. The rationale is that androgens stimulate prostate cancer growth and that chemotherapy may be more effective against rapidly proliferating cells. In a prospective randomized controlled study of 85 patients with prostate cancer refractory to orchiectomy, Manni and colleagues concluded that androgen priming did not potentiate the efficacy of chemotherapy (cyclophosphamide, doxorubicin, and 5-fluorouracil).[169] Current investigation with androgen priming in hormone-sensitive patients with stage D disease is now underway.[170] Another approach being examined has been to treat with chemotherapy first followed by endocrine therapy at the time of progression.[171]

Quality of life, cost, and toxicity are important issues that need to be discussed with patients prior to initiation of chemotherapy. Because chemotherapy offers no survival benefit, patients undergoing potentially toxic regimens should be limited to participants of clinical trials. For the individual patient with hormone-resistant cancer, a trial with a single agent, in an outpatient setting, that is associated with minimal morbidity and reasonable cost appears to be justifiable.[165,172]

REFERENCES

1. SILVERBERG, E., and LUBERA, J. A. Cancer statistics. Ca-A, *39*:3, 1989.
2. MURPHY, G. P., et al. The national survey of prostate cancer in the United States by the American College of Surgeons. J. Urol., *127*:928, 1982.
3. PETERSEN, R. O. Prostate. Neoplastic disorders. In: *Urologic Pathology.* Edited by R. O. Petersen. Philadelphia, Lippincott, Co., 1986.
4. PAGANINI-HILL, A., ROSS, R. K., and HENDERSON, B. E. Epidemiology of prostatic cancer. In: *Diagnosis and Management of Genitourinary Cancer.* Edited by D. G. Skinner and G. Lieskovsky. Philadelphia, W. B. Saunders Co., 1988.
5. HAENSZEL, W., and KURIHARA, M. Studies of Japanese migrants. I. Mortality from cancer and other diseases among Japanese in the United States. J. N. C. I., *40*:43, 1968.
6. STASZEWSKI, J., and HAENSEL, W. Cancer mortality among the Polish-born in the U.S. J. N. C. I., *35*:291, 1965.
7. HIGGENSSON, J., and OETTLE, A. G. Cancer incidence in the Bantu and "Cape Colored" races of South Africa: Report of a cancer survey in the Transvaal (1953–1955). J. N. C. I., *24*:589, 1960.
8. STEELE, R., et al. Sexual factors in the epidemiology of cancer of the prostate. J. Chronic Dis., *24*:29, 1971.
9. SCHUMAN, L. M., et al. Epidemiology study of prostatic cancer: Preliminary report. Cancer Treat. Rep., *61*:181, 1977.
10. WOOLF, C. M. An investigation of the familial aspect of carcinoma of the prostate. Cancer, *13*:739, 1960.
11. GREENWALD, P., et al. Cancer of the prostate among men with benign prostatic hyperplasia. J. N. C. I., *53*:335, 1974.
12. ARMENIAN, H. K., et al. Lancet, *2*:115, 1974.
13. FRANKS, L. M. The incidence of carcinoma of the prostate: An epidemiological study. Recent results. Cancer Res. *39*:149, 1972.
14. BRESLOW, N., et al. Latent carcinoma of the prostate at autopsy in seven areas. Int. J. Cancer, *20*:680, 1977.
15. FRANKS, L. M. Latent carcinoma of the prostate. J. Pathol. Bacteriol., *68*:603, 1954.
16. KRAIN, L. S. Some epidemiologic variables in prostatic carcinoma in California. Prev. Med., *3*:154, 1974.
17. ROTKIN, I. D. Studies in the epidemiology of prostatic cancer; expanded sampling. Cancer Treat. Rep., *61*:173, 1977.
18. FEMINELLA, J. G., and LATTIMER, J. K. An apparent increase in genital carcinomas among wives of men with prostatic carcinomas: An epidemiologic survey. Pirquet Bull. Clin. Med., *20*:3, 1973.
19. ROSS, R. P., et al. A cohort study of mortality from cancer of the prostate in Catholic priests. Br. J. Cancer, *43*:233, 1981.
20. SANFORD, E. L., et al. Evidence for the association of cytomegalovirus with carcinoma of the prostate. J. Urol., *118*:789, 1977.
21. CENTIFANO, Y. M., et al. Herpesvirus particles in prostate carcinoma cells. J. Virol., *12*:1608, 1973.
22. FARNSWORTH, W. E. Human prostatic reverse transcriptase and RNA-virus. Urol. Res., *1*:106, 1973.
23. OHTSUKI, Y., et al. Brief communication: Virus-like particles in a case of human prostate carcinoma. J. N. C. I., *58*:1493, 1977.
24. McCOMBS, R. M. Role of oncornaviruses in carcinoma of the prostate. Cancer Treat. Rep., *61*:131, 1977.
25. SANFORD, E. J., RHONER, T. J., and RAPP, F. Virology of prostate cancer. Cancer Chemother. Rep., *59*:33, 1975.
26. SANFORD, E. J., et al. Lymphocyte reactivity against virally-transformed cells in patients with urologic carcinoma. J. Urol., *118*:809, 1977.
27. GEDER, L., et al. Cytomegalovirus in carcinoma of the prostate: In vitro transformation of human cells. Cancer Treat. Rep., *61*:139, 1977.
28. NOBLE, K. L. The development of prostate adenocarcinoma in the Nb rat following prolonged sex hormone administration. Cancer Res. *37*:1929, 1977.

29. Habib, E. K., et al. Androgen levels in the plasma and prostate tissue of patients with benign hypertrophy and carcinoma of the prostate. J. Endocrinol., 71:99, 1976.

30. Geller, J. et al. Dihydrotestosterone concentration in prostate cancer tissue as a predictor of tumor differentiation and hormonal dependency. Cancer Res., 38:4349, 1978.

31. Kreig, M., Bartsch, W., and Voigt, K. D. Binding, metabolism and tissue level of androgens in human prostatic, benign prostatic hyperplasia and normal prostate. Exerpta Med. ICS, 494:102, 1980.

32. Bartsh, W., Steins, P., and Becker, H. Hormone blood levels in patients with prostatic carcinoma and their relation to the type of carcinoma growth differentiation. Eur. Urol., 7:129, 1977.

33. Hammond, G. L. Endogenous steroid levels in human prostate from birth to old age: A comparison of normal and diseased tissues. J. Endocrinol., 78:7, 1978.

34. Ghanadian, R., Puah, C. M., and O'Donoghue, E. P. N. Serum testosterone and dihydrotestosterone in carcinoma of the prostate. Br. J. Cancer, 39:696, 1979.

35. Saroff, J., Kirdani, Y., and Ming Chu, T. Measurements of prolactin and androgens in patients with prostatic diseases. Oncology, 37:46, 1980.

36. Harper, M. E., et al. Plasma steroid and protein hormone concentrations in patients with prostatic carcinoma, before and after oestrogen therapy. Acta Endocrinol., 81:409, 1976.

37. Griffiths, K., et al. Protein hormones and prostate cancer. Prog. Cancer Res. Ther., 144:185–192, 1980.

38. Rolandi, E., et al. Evaluation of LH, FSH, TSH, Prl and GH secretion in patients suffering from prostatic neoplasms. Acta Endocrinol., 95:23, 1980.

39. Hammond, G. I., et al. Serum FSH, LH and prolactin in normal males and patients with prostatic diseases. Clin. Endocrinol., 7:129, 1977.

40. Jacobi, G. H., Rathgen, G.H., and Altwein, J. E. Serum prolactin and tumors of the prostate: Unchanged basal levels and lack of correlation to serum testosterone. J. Endocrinol. Invest., 3:15, 1980.

41. Lowsley, O. S. The development of the human prostate gland with reference to the development of other structures at the neck of the bladder. Am. J. Anat., 13:299, 1912.

42. Franks, L. M. Benign nodular hyperplasia of the prostate: A review. Ann R. C., Surg., 14:92, 1954.

43. McNeal, J. E. The prostate gland: Morphology and pathobiology. Monogr. Urol., 9:36, 1988.

44. McNeal, J. E. Significance of duct-acinar dysplasia in prostatic carcinogenesis. Prostate, 13:91, 1988.

45. Gleason, D. F. Classification of prostatic carcinomas. Cancer Chemother. Rep., 50:125, 1966.

46. Wang, M. C., et al. Purification of a human prostatic specific antigen. Invest. Urol., 17:159, 1979.

47. Feiner, H. D., and Gonzalea, R. Carcinoma of the prostate with atypical immunohistologic features: Clinical and histologic correlates. Am. J. Surg. Pathol., 10:765.

48. Allhoff, E. P., et al. Evaluation of prostate specific acid phosphatase and prostate specific antigen in identification of prostatic cancer. J. Urol., 129:315, 1983.

49. Drago, J. R., et al. The relative value of prostatic-specific antigen and prostatic acid phosphatase in the diagnosis and management of adenocarcinoma of the prostate: The Ohio State University experience. Urology, 34:187, 1989.

50. Ferro, M. A., et al. Tumour markers in prostatic carcinoma. A comparison of prostate-specific antigen with acid phosphatase. Br. J. Urol., 60:69, 1987.

51. Myrtle, J. F., et al. Clinical utility of prostate specific antigen (PSA) in the management of prostate cancer. Adv. Cancer Diagnos. 1:1, 1986.

52. Seamonds, B., et al. Evaluation of prostatic-specific antigen and prostatic acid phosphatase as prostate cancer markers. Urology, 28:472, 1986.

53. Stamey, T. A., et al. Prostate specific antigen as a serum marker for adenocarcinoma of the prostate. N. Engl. J. Med., 317:909, 1987.

54. Barzell, W., et al. Prostatic adenocarcinoma: Relationship of grade and local extent to the pattern of metastases. J. Urol., 118:278, 1977.

55. McLaughlin, A. P., et al. Prostatic carcinoma: Incidence and location of unsuspected lymphatic metastases. J. Urol., 115:89, 1976.

56. Dodds, P. R., Caride, V. J., and Lytton, B. The role of vertebral veins in the dissemination of prostatic carcinoma. J. Urol., 126:753, 1981.

57. Jewett, H. J., Significance of the palpable prostatic nodule. J.A.M.A., 160:838, 1956.

58. Stamey, T. A., and Hodge, K. K. Ultrasound visualization of prostate anatomy and pathology. Monogr. Urol., 9:53, 1988.

59. Geraniotis, E., et al. Transrectal fine-needle aspiration of the prostate: A comparison with core biopsy techniques in the diagnosis of carcinoma. J. Urol., in press, 1990.

60. Chodak, G. W., et al. Comparison of digital rectal examination and transrectal ultrasonography for diagnosis of prostate cancer. J. Urol., 135:951, 1986.

61. Drago, J. R., Nesbitt, J. A., and Badalament, R. A. Transrectal ultrasound: Use in detection of prostatic carcinoma. Urology, 34:120, 1989.

62. Wallace, D. M., Chisholm, G. D., and Hendry, W. F. TNM classification for urological tumors (UICC)–1974. Br. J. Urol., 47:1, 1975.

63. Whitmore, W. F., Jr. Hormone therapy in prostate cancer. Am. J. Med., 21:697, 1956.

64. Jewett, H. J. The present status of radical prostatectomy for stages A and B prostatic cancer. Urol. Clin. N. Am., 2:105, 1975.

65. Boxer, R. J. Adenocarcinoma of the prostate gland. Urol. Survey, 27:75, 1977.

66. Bartsch, G., et al. Incidental carcinoma of the prostate—grading and tumor volume in relation to survival rate. World J. Urol., 1:24, 1983.

67. Lee, F., et al. Needle aspiration and core biopsy of prostate cancer: Comparative evaluation with biplanar transrectal US guidance. Radiology, 163:515, 1987.

68. Drago, J. R., et al. Localized prostate carcinoma: Comparison of transrectal ultrasound and magnetic resonance imaging. Urology, in press, 1990.

69. Donohue, R. E., et al. Pelvic lymph node dissection: Guide to patient management in clinical locally confined adenocarcinoma of the prostate. Urology, 20:559, 1982.

70. Paulson, D. E., and the Uro-Oncology Research Group: Impact of current staging procedures in assessing disease extent of prostatic carcinoma. J. Urol., 121:300, 1979.

71. Smith, M. J. V. The lymphatics of the prostate. Invest. Urol., 3:439, 1966.

72. Wajsman, Z., et al. Transabdominal fine-needle aspiration of retroperitoneal lymph nodes in staging of genitourinary tract cancer: Correlation with lymphography and lymph node dissection findings. J. Urol., 128:1238, 1982.

73. FLOCKS, R. H., CULP, D., and PROTO, R. Lymphatic spread from prostatic cancer. J. Urol., *81:*194, 1975.

74. FREIHA, F. S., PISTENMA, D. A., and BAGSHAW, M. A. Pelvic lymphadenectomy for staging prostatic carcinoma: Is it always necessary? J. Urol., *122:*176, 1979.

75. MCLAUGHLIN, A. P., et al. Prostate and lymphatic metastases. J. Urol., *115:*89, 1976.

76. MCCULLOUGH, D. L., PROUT, G. R., and DALY, J. J. Carcinoma of the prostate and lymphatic metastases. J. Urol., *111:*65, 1974.

77. WILSON, C. S., DAHL, D. S., and MIDDLETON, R. G. Pelvic lymphadenectomy for the staging of apparently localized carcinoma of the prostate. J. Urol., *117:*197, 1977.

78. GOLIMBU, M., MORALES, P., AL-ASKARI, S., and BROWN, J. Extended pelvic lymphadenectomy for prostatic cancer. J. Urol., *121:*617, 1979.

79. SPELLMAN, M. C., et al. An evaluation of lymphangiography in localized carcinoma of the prostate. Radiology, *125:*737, 1977.

80. SMITH, J. A., and DATZ, F. L. Interpretation of the equivocal bone scan in patients with prostate cancer. Probl. Urol., Probl. Pros. Cancer Cont., *1:*124, 1987.

81. PARFITT, H. E., JR., et al. Accuracy of staging in A₁ carcinoma of the prostate. Cancer, *51:*2346, 1983.

82. BRIDGES, C. H., et al. Stage A prostatic carcinoma and repeat transurethral resection: A reappraisal 5 years later. J. Urol., *129:*307, 1983.

83. SONDA, L. P., et al. Incidental adenocarcinoma of the prostate: The role of repeat transurethral resection in staging. Prostate, *5:*141, 1984.

84. KOPPER, B., et al. Staging of incidental carcinoma of the prostate by diagnostic secondary transurethral resection (abstract 550), J. Urol., part 2, *131:*241A, 1984.

85. CARROLL, P. R., et al. Incidental carcinoma of the prostate: Significance of staging transurethral resection. J. Urol., *133:*811, 1985.

86. EPSTEIN, J. I., and WALSH, P. C. Stage A prostate cancer is incidental but not insignificant: Data to support radical prostatectomy for young men with stage A₁ disease. Probl. Urol., Probl. Pros. Cancer Cont., *1:*34, 1987.

87. FRANKFURT, O. S., et al. Relationship between DNA ploidy, glandular differentiation, and tumor spread in human prostate cancer. Cancer Res., *45:*1418, 1985.

88. RONSTROM, L., TRIBUKAIT, B., and ESPOSTI, P. L. DNA pattern and cytologic findings in fine needle aspirates of untreated prostatic tumors: A flow-cytofluorometric study. Prostate, *2:*79, 1981.

89. TRIBUKAIT, B., RONSTRUM, L., and ESPOSTI, P. L. Quantitative and qualitative aspects of flow DNA measurements related to the cytologic grade in prostatic carcinoma. Anat. Quant. Cytol., *5:*107, 1983.

90. ZETTERBERG, A., and ESPOSTI, P. L. Prognostic significance of nuclear DNA levels in prostatic carcinoma. Scand. J. Urol. Nephrol. (Suppl.), *55:*53, 1980.

91. LEISTENSCHNEIDER, W., and NAGEL, R. Cytological and DNA-cytophotometric monitoring of the effect of therapy in conservatively treated prostatic carcinoma. Scand. J. Urol. Nephrol. (Suppl.), *55:*197, 1980.

92. STEPHENSON, R. A., et al. Flow cytometry of prostate cancer: Relationship of DNA content to survival. Cancer Res., *47:*2504, 1987.

93. WINKLER, H. Z., et al. Stage D₁ prostatic adenocarcinoma: Significance of nuclear DNA ploidy patterns studied by flow cytometry. Mayo Clin. Proc., *63:*103, 1988.

94. LEE, S. F., et al. Flow cytometric determination of ploidy in prostatic adenocarcinoma: A comparison with seminal vesicle involvement and histopathological grading as a predictor of clinical recurrence. J. Urol., *140:*769, 1988.

95. WHITMORE, W. E., JR. Natural history and staging of prostate cancer. Urol. Clin. N. Am., *11:*205, 1984.

96. WALSH, P. C., AND LEPOR, H. The role of radical prostatectomy in the management of prostatic cancer. Cancer, *60:*526, 1987.

97. SMITH, J. A., and MIDDLETON, R. G. Radical prostatectomy for stage B₂ prostatic cancer. J. Urol., *127:*702, 1982.

98. BOXER, R. J., KAUFMAN, J. J., and GOODWIN, W. E. Radical prostatectomy for carcinoma of the prostate, 1951−1976: A review of 329 patients. J. Urol., *117:*208, 1977.

99. CULP, O. S. Radical prostatectomy: its past, present, and possible future. J. Urol., *98:*618, 1968.

100. WALSH, P. C., LEPOR, H., and EGGLESTON, J. C. Radical prostatectomy with preservation of sexual function: Anatomic and pathologic considerations. Prostate, *4:*473, 1983.

101. REINER, W. G., and WALSH, P. C. An anatomic approach to the surgical management of the dorsal vein and Santorini's plexus during radical retropubic surgery. J. Urol., *121:*198, 1979.

102. PETERS, C. A., and Walsh, P. C. Blood transfusion and anesthetic practices in radical retropubic prostatectomy. J. Urol., *134:*81, 1985.

103. DRAGO, J. R., NESBITT, J. A., and BADALAMENT, R. A. Radical nerve-sparing prostatectomy: The first 30 patients treated with epidural anesthesia. J. Surg. Oncol., *40:*182, 1989.

104. CATALONA, W. J., and DRESNER, S. M. Nerve-sparing radical prostatectomy: Extraprostatic tumor extension and preservation of erectile function. J. Urol., *134:*1149, 1985.

105. Consensus conference: The management of clinically localized prostate cancer. J.A.M.A., *258:*2727, 1987.

106. JEWETT, H. J. et al. The palpable nodule of prostatic cancer: Results 15 years after radical excision. J.A.M.A., *203:*403, 1968.

107. SCHROEDER, F. H., and BELT, E. P. Carcinoma of the prostate: A study of 213 patients with stage C tumors treated by total perineal prostatectomy. J. Urol., *114:*257, 1975.

108. HODGES, C. V., PEARCE, H. D., and STILLE, L. Radical prostatectomy for carcinoma: 30-year experience and 15-year survivals. J. Urol., *122:*180, 1979.

109. CULP, O. S., and MEYER, J. J. Radical prostatectomy in the treatment of prostatic cancer. Cancer, *32:*1113, 1973.

110. WALSH, P. C., and JEWETT, H. J. Radical surgery for prostatic cancer. Cancer, *45:*1906, 1980.

111. GIBBONS, R. P., et al. Total prostatectomy for localized proatatic cancer. J. Urol., *131:*73, 1984.

112. HAFERMANN, M. D. External radiotherapy, Urology, *17*(Suppl.):15, 1981.

113. BAGSHAW, M. A., Radiation therapy for cancer of the prostate. In: *Diagnosis and Management of Genitourinary Cancer,* Edited by D. G. Skinner and G. Lieskovsky. Philadelphia, W. B. Saunders, Co., 1988.

114. RAY, G. R., CASSADY, R., and BAGSHAW, M. A. Definitive radiation therapy of carcinoma of the prostate: A report on 15 years experience. Radiology, *106:*407, 1973.

115. MCGOWAN, D. G. Radiation therapy in the management of localized carcinoma of the prostate. Cancer, *39:*98, 1977.

116. PEREZ, C. A., et al. Radiation therapy in the definitive treatment of localized carcinoma of the prostate. Cancer, *40:*1425, 1977.

117. LOH, E. S., BROWN, H. E., and BEILER, D. D. Radiotherapy of carcinoma of the prostate: A preliminary report. J. Urol., *106:*906, 1971.

118. HILL, D. R., CREWS, Q. E., and WALSH, P. C. Prostate carcinoma:

Radiation treatment of the primary and regional lymphatics. Cancer, *34*:156, 1974.

119. PISTENMA, D. A., BAGSHAW, M. A., and FREIHA, F. S. Extended field radiation therapy for prostatic carcinoma: Status report of a limited prospective trial. In: *Cancer of the Genitourinary Tract.* Edited by D. E. Johnson and M. L. Samuels. New York, Raven Press, 1979.

120. HERR, W. H., and WHITMORE, W. F., JR. Significance of prostatic biopsies after radiation therapy for carcinoma of the prostate. Prostate, *3*:339, 1982.

121. FREIHA, F. S., and BAGSHAW, M. A. Carcinoma of the prostate: Results of post-irradiation biopsy. Prostate, *5*:19, 1984.

122. SCARDINO, P. T., et al. The prognostic significance of post-irradiation biopsy results in patients with prostatic cancer. J. Urol., *135*:510, 1986.

123. LYTTON, B., et al. Results of biopsy after early prostatic cancer treatment by implantation of ^{125}I seeds. J. Urol., *121*:306, 1979.

124. PAULSON, D. F., et al. Radical surgery vs. radiotherapy for stage A_2 and stage B ($T_{1-2}N_0M_0$) adenocarcinoma of the prostate. J. Urol., *128*:502, 1982.

125. PAULSON, D. F. Treatment selection in organ-confined disease. Probl. Urol., Probl. Pros. Cancer Cont., *1*:53, 1987.

126. WHITMORE, W. F., JR. HILARIS, B., and GRABSTALD, H. Retropubic implantation of iodine 125 in the treatment of prostate cancer. J. Urol., *108*:918, 1972.

127. SCARDINO, P. T., GUERRIERO, W. G., and CARLTON, C. E. *Surgical Staging and Combined Therapy with 198-AU Grain Implantation and External Irradiation.* Edited by D. E. Johnson and M. A. Boileau. New York, Grune and Stratton, 1982.

128. GROSSMAN, H. B., et al. 125-I implantation for carcinoma of the prostate: Further follow-up of first 100 cases. Urology, *20*:591, 1982.

129. WHITMORE, W. F., JR., et al. Interstitial irradiation using I-125 seeds. In: *Prostate Cancer.* Part B: *Imaging Techniques, Radiotherapy, Chemotherapy, and Management Issues.* New York, Alan R. Liss, 1987.

130. CARLTON, C. E., JR., et al. Irradiation treatment of carcinoma of the prostate: A preliminary report based on 8 years of experience. J. Urol., *108*:924, 1972.

131. CARLTON, C. E., and SCARDINO, P. T. Long-term results after combined radioactive gold seed implantation and external radiotherapy for localized prostatic cancer. In: *A Multidisciplinary Analysis of Controversies in the Management of Prostate Cancer.* Edited by D. S. Coffey, M. I. Resnick, F. A. Dorr, and J. P. Karr. New York, Plenum Press, 1988.

132. GRAYHACK, J. T., KELLER, T. C., and KOZLOWSKI, J. M. Carcinoma of the prostate: Hormonal therapy. Cancer, *60*:589, 1987.

133. NESBITT, R. M., and BAUM, W. C. Endocrine control of prostatic carcinoma. Clinical and statistical survey of 1818 cases. J. A. M. A., *143*:1317, 1950.

134. BLACKARD, C. E. The Veterans Administration Cooperative Urological Research Group studies of carcinoma of the prostate: A review. Cancer Chemother. Rep., *59*:225, 1975.

135. GELLER, J., ALBERT, J., and YEN, S. S. C. Treatment of advanced cancer of prostate with megestrol acetate. Urology, *12*:537, 1978.

136. SOGANI, P. C., and WHITMORE, W. F., JR. Experience with flutamide in previously untreated patients with advanced prostatic cancer. J. Urol., *122*:640, 1979.

137. MACFARLANE, J. R., and TOLLEY, D. A. Flutamide therapy for advanced prostatic cancer: A phase II study. Br. J. Urol., *57*:172, 1985.

138. SMITH, R. B., WALSH, P. C., and GOODWIN, W. E.: Cyproterone acetate in the treatment of advanced carcinoma of the prostate. J. Urol., *110*:106, 1973.

139. WEIN, A. J., and MURPHY, J. J.: Experience in the treatment of prostatic carcinoma with cyproterone acetate. J. Urol., *109*:68, 1973.

140. TRACHTENBERG, J. Ketoconazole therapy in advanced prostatic cancer. J. Urol., *132*:61, 1984.

141. BAMBERGER, M. H., and LOWE, F. C. Ketoconazole in initial management and treatment of metastatic prostate cancer to spine. Urology, *32*:301, 1988.

142. The Leuprolide Study Group: Leuprolide versus diethylstilbestrol for metastatic prostate cancer. N. Engl. J. Med., *311*:1281, 1984.

143. DEBRUYNE, F. M., et al. Long-term therapy with a depot luteinizing hormone-releasing hormone analogue (Zoladex) in patients with advanced prostatic carcinoma. J. Urol., *140*:775, 1988.

144. PRESANT, C. A., SOLOWAY, M. S., and KLIOZE, S. S., et al. Buserelin as primary therapy in advanced prostatic carcinoma. Cancer, *56*:2416, 1985.

145. SCHROEDER, F. H., et al. Metastatic cancer of the prostate managed with buserelin versus buserelin plus cyproterone acetate. J. Urol., *137*:912, 1987.

146. BELAND, G. Comparison of total androgen blockade and orchiectomy in metastatic cancer of prostate. In: *A Multidisciplinary Analysis of Controversies in the Management of Prostate Cancer.* Edited by D.S. Coffey, M.I. Resnick, F.A. Dorr, and J.P. Karr. New York, Plenum Press, 1988.

147. SCHULZE, H., ISAACS, J., and SENGE T. Inability of complete androgen blockade to increase survival of patients with advanced prostatic cancer as compared to standard hormonal therapy, J. Urol., *137*:909, 1987.

148. GROSSMAN, H. B., Hormonal therapy of prostatic carcinoma: Is there a rationale for delayed treatment? A review article. Urology, *27*:199, 1986.

149. ISAACS, J. G., The timing of androgen ablation therapy and/or chemotherapy in the treatment of prostatic cancer. Prostate, *5*:1, 1984.

150. LEPOR, H., ROSS, A., and WALSH, P. C.: The influence of hormonal therapy on survival of men with advanced prostatic cancer. J. Urol., *128*:335, 1982.

151. VEST, S. A., and FRAZIER, T. H. Survival following castration for prostatic cancer. J. Urol., *56*:97, 1946.

152. BRENDLER, H. Adrenalectomy and hypophysectomy for prostatic cancer. Urology, *2*:99, 1973.

153. WORGUL, T. J., et al. Clinical and biochemical effect of aminoglutethimide in the treatment of advanced prostatic carcinoma. J. Urol., *129*:51, 1983.

154. EISENBERGER, M. A., BEZERDJIAN, L., and KALASH, S. A critical assessment of the role of chemotherapy for endocrine resistant prostatic carcinoma. AUA Update Series, *7*:217, 1988.

155. CARTER, S. K., and WASSERMAN, T. H. The chemotherapy of urologic cancer. Cancer, *36*:729, 1975.

156. MOORE, G. E., BROSS, I. D., and AUSMAN, R. Effects of 5 fluorouracil (NCS-19893) in 389 patients with cancer. Eastern Clinical Drug Evaluation Program. Cancer Chemother. Rep., Part I, *52*(6):641, 1968.

157. ANSFIELD, F. J., SCHROEDER, J., and CURRERI, A. R. Five years clinical experience with 5 fluorouracil. J.A.M.A., *181*:295, 1962.

158. BLUM, R. H. An overview of studies with Adriamycin (Nsc-123127) in the United States. Cancer Chemother. Rep., Part III, 6(2):247, 1975.

159. Scher, H., et al. Phase II trial of doxorubicin in bidimensionally measurable prostatic adenocarcinoma. J. Urol., *131:*1099, 1984.

160. Jonsson, G., Hogberg, B., and Nilsson, T.: Treatment of advanced prostatic carcinoma with estramustine phosphate (Estracyt). Scand. J. Urol. Nephrol., *11:*231, 1977.

161. Nilsson, T. Estracyt—clinical experiences. Scand. J. Urol. Nephrol., *55*(Suppl.):135, 1980.

162. Loening, S. A., Beckley, S., and Brady, M. F.: Comparison of estramustine phosphate, methotrexate, and cis-platinum in patients with advanced, hormone refractory prostate cancer. J. Urol., *129:*1001, 1983.

163. Yagoda, A., Watson, R. C., and Natale, R. B.: A critical analysis of response criteria in patients with prostatic cancer treated with cis-diaminedichloride platinum II. Cancer, *144:*1553, 1979.

164. Merrin, C. E.: Treatment of genitourinary tumors with cis-dichloro diammine platinum II. Experience in 250 patients. Cancer Treat. Rep., *63*(9–10):1579, 1979.

165. Gibbons, R. P.: Prostate cancer. Chemotherapy. Cancer, *60:*586–588, 1987.

166. Catalona, W. J.: Chemotherapy. In: *Prostate Cancer.* Edited by W. J. Catalona. Orlando, Grune & Stratton, 1984.

167. Tannock, I. F. Is there evidence that chemotherapy is of benefit to patients with carcinoma of the prostate? J. Clin. Oncol., *3:*1013, 1985.

168. Scher, H. I., and Sternberg, C. N. Chemotherapy of urologic malignancies. Semin. Urol., *3:*239, 1985.

169. Manni, A., et al. Androgen priming and chemotherapy in advanced prostate cancer: Evaluation of determinants of clinical outcome. J. Clin. Oncol., *6:*1456, 1988.

170. Manni, A., and Drago, J. R.: Personnel communication, 1989.

171. Seifter, E. J., Bunn, P. A., and Cohen, M. H. A trial of combination chemotherapy followed by hormonal therapy for previously untreated metastatic carcinoma of the prostate. J. Clin. Oncol., *4:*1365, 1986.

172. Gibbons, R. P.: Editorial comments. In: A critical assessment of the role of chemotherapy for endocrine resistant prostate cancer. AUA Update Series, *7:*217, 1988.

Pelvic Lymphadenectomy

William R. Morgan
Michael M. Lieber

For many decades pelvic lymphadenectomy has played an important role in the management of various gynecologic malignant tumors.[1] Most gynecologic oncologists would agree that removal of the pelvic lymph nodes and sometimes the periaortic lymph nodes as well is important in the management of patients with certain stages of cervical, endometrial, ovarian, and vulvar carcinoma. The value of pelvic lymphadenectomy for male patients with malignant genitourinary tumors has been recognized by most urologic oncologists only within the past 10 to 15 years. Even 10 years ago, many patients with invasive bladder carcinoma or apparently localized adenocarcinoma of the prostate did not undergo a pelvic lymphadenectomy as part of their surgical treatment. However, at present, few such patients who are reasonable risks for such an operation are treated without a pelvic lymphadenectomy at leading urologic centers. With an increasing role for adjuvant polychemotherapy treatments for patients with transitional cell carcinoma of the bladder, it has become most important to determine whether such patients have metastatic deposits in the pelvic lymph nodes at the time of radical cystectomy. Such patients with positive nodes now commonly receive postoper-

ative chemotherapy with a combination regimen such as M-VAC. The increasingly widespread use of nerve-sparing, potency-preserving radical prostatectomy has given a fresh new impetus to the retropubic surgical approach to radical prostatectomy with a concurrent pelvic lymphadenectomy through the single incision. Moreover, pelvic lymphadenectomy is widely accepted as important for patients with certain stages of penile and urethral carcinoma for whom surgical treatment is a consideration. Urologists treating these pelvic malignancies surgically must be able to carry out pelvic lymphadenectomy based on a sound theoretical, anatomical, and technical basis.

ROLE OF PELVIC LYMPHADENECTOMY IN STAGING AND PROGNOSIS: PROSTATE CARCINOMA

Multiple published studies over the past decade have demonstrated that the presence of metastatic deposits in the pelvic lymph nodes in patients who appear to have localized disease is important prognostically for patients with adenocarcinoma of the prostate. The presence of positive pelvic lymph nodes historically has been an accurate indicator of eventual systemic disease progression, usually osseous metastases. After reviewing the first 100 patients who underwent interstitial iodine-125 implantations for prostate carcinoma, Grossman and colleagues found that the presence of lymph node metastases was the most significant indicator of subsequent disease progression, more so than local stage or grade.[2] Smith and associates described 64 patients with pelvic nodal metastases treated with radiation therapy or expectantly. At 5 years follow-up, 70% had developed recurrent disease and 39% were dead from prostate cancer.[3] Forty-four similar stage D-1 patients were treated by Kramer and associates with either radical surgery, external beam radiation, or delayed hormonal therapy. For these patients with stage D-1 prostate adenocarcinoma, median survival was only 39.5 months and the median time to first disease progression was less than 2 years.[4] Prout and associates described 32 cases of stage D-1 prostate cancer treated in a similar way. The probability of surviving 5 years with no evidence of disease for this group of patients was only 34%.[5]

As these and other clinical investigators have shown, a high percentage of patients with nodal metastases go on to develop disease progression and many eventually die of their disease. By contrast, those patients who undergo pelvic lymphadenectomy and do not have metastatic deposits in the pelvic lymph nodes generally have a favorable long-term response to local treatment. For example, in a study carried out at Stanford University, pelvic lymphadenectomy was performed before definitive external beam radiotherapy for localized prostate cancer.[6] Among 57 patients in this study with no pelvic lymph node involvement at the time of exploration, only one patient went on to die from disseminated disease. This contrasted with a high progression and high death rate for prostate cancer for patients who were found to have lymph node metastases. In addition, a large surgical series from the Mayo Clinic, in which the primary treatment for localized prostate carcinoma was radical retropubic prostatectomy, demonstrated that for patients with disease limited to the prostate and with no pelvic lymph node involvement, postoperative survival expectation up to 10 years was equal or superior to that of an age-matched control group.[7]

Additional data from the Mayo Clinic and other institutions suggest that patients with metastatic deposits in the pelvic lymph nodes benefit in terms of time to first disease progression from early endocrine therapy.[8,9] The beneficial effect of early endocrine therapy is particularly significant for the 40 to 45% of patients with DNA diploid primary tumors.[10] Because early endocrine therapy is so helpful in this group of patients, determining the status of their pelvic lymph nodes is quite important at the time of surgery.

NONINVASIVE ALTERNATIVES TO PELVIC LYMPHADENECTOMY

Non-invasive techniques to assess the status of pelvic lymph nodes for patients with pelvic urologic malignancies have been studied extensively. These techniques include computed tomography (CT),[11,12] magnetic resonance imaging (MRI),[13] and pedal lymphangiography.[14–16] To date, all these modalities have been somewhat disappointing and none has been successful in identifying metastatic nodal disease with an accuracy comparable to formal pelvic lymphadenectomy. CT scanning detects macroscopic nodal disease when lymph nodes are greater than 1.2 to 1.5 cm in diameter. Nodes of this size are often amenable to percutaneous needle biopsy which, if positive, may obviate the need for surgery. CT scanning cannot, however, detect microscopic and small macroscopic nodal deposits,[11] and has been associated with a high false-negative rate (7 of 23 scans in one series) when compared with pelvic lymphadenectomy.[12] Data evaluating the efficacy of MRI in the detection of pelvic nodal metastases are limited. Mukamel correlated MRI and pathologic findings in 21 patients prospectively. In this series, MRI was unable to detect grossly involved lymph nodes found at the time of surgery.[13] Lymphangiography has also been studied extensively. Two large series reported sensitivities of 35 and 56%, and specificity of 82 and 95%.[14–15] Many believe that the so-called obturator nodes, the medial chain of the external iliac nodes, are not routinely opacified by lymphangiography. This is probably not the case.[16] However, the internal iliac lymph nodes, which are also part of the first echelon of lymphatic drainage from the prostate, are opacified in only about 50% of cases.[14,17]

LYMPHATIC ANATOMY

The study of the anatomy of prostatic lymphatics is clouded by a lack of uniformity in the terms used to describe pelvic lymphatic structures. However, a general understanding of the lymphatic anatomy of the pelvis is important for the accurate performance of pelvic lymphadenectomy. This lymphatic anatomy was described by Cuneo and Marcille at the turn of the century. Their results, along with studies by other anatomists from the earlier part of the twentieth century, were summarized by Rouviere in 1938.[18] More recently, lymphographic studies performed by radiologists have substantiated the earlier observations of the gross anatomists. An excellent description of the lymphographic anatomy of the pelvis can be found in Clouse's recent text.[19] Excluding the small periprostatic and perivesical lymph nodes, the first echelon of lymphatic drainage from the prostate courses through four major pathways ending in three nodal groups—the external iliac nodes, the hypogastric (or internal iliac) nodes, and the nodes of the sacral promontory (Figs. 16-1 and 16-2).[18,19]

External Iliac Nodes

The external iliac lymphatics are made up of three chains: lateral, intermediate, and medial chains. The lateral chain consists of one to three lymph vessels that run along the lateral aspect of the external iliac artery. The intermediate chain is the least important of the three and runs between the external iliac artery and vein. The medial or internal lymph chain is the most important and contains the greatest number of lymph

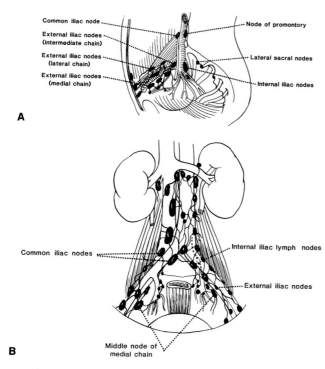

A

B

Fig. 16-1. Lymphatic anatomy of the pelvis. Iliopelvic lymph nodes: external iliac group, internal iliac group, and common iliac group. These are the lymphatics that must be removed during the performance of a systematic pelvic lymphadenectomy. *A,* lateral view; *B,* anterior view. (After Rouviere.)

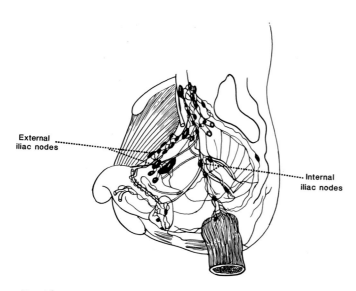

Fig. 16-2. Lymphatic drainage of the prostate gland. Disregarding the small periprostatic lymph nodes, the first echelon of lymph node drainage from the prostate is to the iliopelvic nodes, particularly those along the external and internal iliac vessels. Accurate staging of prostatic adenocarcinoma requires excisional biopsy of these lymph nodes. (After Rouviere.)

vessels and nodes. This chain is located medial and posterior to the external iliac vein and superior to the obturator nerve. Its most inferior node often represents a continuation of the lymph node of Cloquet or the other deep inguinal nodes. Cephalad to the medial retrocrural node is the middle node of the medial chain. This is a large and constant node, which appears to "look into" the pelvic cavity. This particular node, the middle node of the medial external iliac chain, is important as an early metastatic site for pelvic malignancies and is the node most urologic surgeons are likely to identify as the obturator node in the course of pelvic lymphadenectomy. The term "obturator node" is lost in a mist of confusion. It does not correspond to any standard anatomic description and probably should be used merely as shorthand to identify the middle node of the medial chain of the external iliac lymphatic group.[18,19]

Internal Iliac Nodes

The internal iliac or hypogastric group of nodes, usually four to eight in number, are located along the internal iliac artery and its branches. This group of nodes has been poorly defined by the anatomists. Moreover, because it is rarely visualized on pedal lymphograms, more modern studies of the anatomy of the internal iliac group have been limited.[19] However, these nodes are often involved in the early spread of prostatic carcinoma, so that the fibrofatty tissue along the course of the internal iliac artery and its branches should be excised during the course of pelvic lymphadenectomy.

Included in the internal iliac group are the lateral sacral nodes (presciatic nodes), two or three in number, which are found along the lateral sacral arteries opposite the second and third sacral foramina. These nodes have been reported to harbor solitary metastatic deposits of prostatic carcinoma.[19,20]

The Nodes of the Sacral Promontory

This group of nodes, also known as the medial group of the common iliac nodes,[18] consists of two to four nodes located near the L-5, S-1 intervertebral disc. Although these nodes are not removed routinely during lymphadenectomy, some investigators have advocated their inclusion.[20]

WHAT MARGINS CONSTITUTE AN ADEQUATE PELVIC LYMPHADENECTOMY FOR PROSTATE ADENOCARCINOMA?

From series in which the external iliac and hypogastric nodes were consistently sampled during pelvic lymphadenectomy for prostate cancer, we can learn the frequency of lymph node metastasis in various locations. In reviewing these series, one must bear in mind that the medial chain of the external iliac node group is commonly referred to by surgeons as the "obturator nodes" because of its proximity to the obturator nerve and vessels. The term "external iliac nodes" generally refers to only the lateral and intermediate chains that are located directly lateral to and overlying the external iliac artery (lateral chain) and between the external iliac artery and vein (intermediate chain).

Pistenma reported the incidence of lymph node metastasis by location in 93 patients as follows: obturator 31%, internal iliac 24%, external iliac 22%, common iliac 17%, and para-aortic 18%.[21] Patients with common iliac or para-aortic disease rarely do not also have involvement of the external and internal iliac nodes as prostate cancer rarely "leap frogs" over the first echelon of lymphatic drainage.[14,17,22,23] McLaughlin found that of patients with metastatic lymph node disease, 87% had disease in the obturator and hypogastric nodes alone or in combination with other nodal groups, 9% had disease located only in the external iliac nodes, and 4% had disease only in the common iliac nodes.[22] Fowler and Whitmore reported the results of 115 patients with metastatic nodal disease. Forty percent had disease localized in the obturator and hypogastric areas, 37% were in the obturator, hypogastric, and external iliac areas, and 23% were in the external iliac area alone. Of 35 patients with solitary nodal metastases, 61% were located in the obturator and hypogastric areas and 39% were located in the external iliac area.[24]

Historically, a "standard" pelvic lymphadenectomy involved removal of the external iliac nodes (lateral, intermediate, and medial chains), as well as the internal iliac nodes lateral to and overlying the hypogastric artery.[5,17,24,25] This did not include the presciatic group of internal iliac nodes nor the nodes of the sacral promontory. Hence, the margins of the dissection were: laterally, the genitofemoral nerve; medially, the bladder wall and ureter; posteriorly, the obturator nerve and vessels; and distally, the superficial circumflex iliac vessels and Cooper's ligament. Superiorly, the dissection was carried up to the bifurcation of the common iliac artery (some advocated extending a variable distance up onto the common iliac artery[5,17,25]) and brought down the hypogastric artery to the level of the obturator vessels.[24] Most studies of the nodal distribution in metastatic prostate cancer were based on a dissection of this type. Sampling of all the nodal groups that are involved in the first order of prostatic lymphatic drainage would require excision of the entire external iliac, hypogastric, and sacral promontory lymph nodes (presacral nodes). Standard pelvic lymphadenectomy traditionally did not include removal of the deeper presacral and presciatic nodes. However, this has been advocated by Golimbu and associates and has been termed extended pelvic lymphadenectomy.[20] These investigators found the presacral group to be involved with metastatic prostate cancer in 8 of 15 patients (53%). In one case, it was the only area involved. Presciatic nodes were involved in 47% of cases and in one case, they were the only site of metastatic disease. The routine inclusion of these deeper nodal groups in lymphadenectomy has not been widely accepted and further analysis is required to establish the usefulness of this technique.

In 1978, Whitmore began modifying his lymphadenectomy by omitting the dissection of the nodal tissues surrounding and lateral to the external iliac artery, making the lateral limit of the dissection the lateral margin of the external iliac vein rather than the genitofemoral nerve.[26] With this technique

(termed the modified pelvic lymphadenectomy), he found no change in the incidence of positive nodes when compared to the standard technique. However, review of his earlier reports of metastatic nodal distribution suggests that a limited dissection that does not include the "external iliac nodes" (lateral and intermediate chains) will not detect up to 23% of cases with multiple nodal metastases and 39% with a solitary metastasis.[24] Benefits of the modified technique included a shortened operating time and decreased postoperative lymphedema. Standard lymphadenectomy had been associated with prepubic, groin, and genital edema in about 50% of patients as well as occasional severe lower extremity edema. This was essentially eliminated by the modified technique.[26] Others have also found less lymphedema and a similar rate of nodal metastasis as compared with the standard procedure.[27] Most investigators who initially advocated a standard lymphadenectomy have now adopted the modified technique.[25,26,28]

PELVIC LYMPHADENECTOMY IN TRANSITIONAL CELL CARCINOMA OF THE BLADDER

The pattern of lymphatic spread of bladder cancer parallels that of prostate cancer. In a series reported by Smith and Whitmore, the most common nodal groups involved with metastases were the obturator (74%) and the external iliac (65%), followed by the common iliac (19%), hypogastric (17%), and perivesical (16%). Involvement of nodes proximal to the bifurcation of the common iliac artery was not found without concomitant distal involvement.[29] Because of this stepwise spread of disease, a therapeutic effect of pelvic lymphadenectomy for patients with limited nodal metastases has been suggested, particularly when a meticulous complete dissection is performed. Lieskovsky and Skinner projected a 36% 5-year survival for patients with metastatic nodal disease treated in this fashion.[30] A similar series from our institution found only a slight benefit in survival (not statistically significant) for patients with a single metastatic node treated with a complete pelvic node dissection compared with a partial pelvic node dissection.[31] A large series from Memorial Sloan-Kettering suggested that pelvic lymphadenectomy adds only 1 to 2% to the 5-year survival of patients with bladder cancer treated with cystectomy (7% of the 20% incidence of nodal involvement).[32] Regardless of the therapeutic effect, pelvic lymphadenectomy is justifiable for two other reasons. First, it identifies tumors that are unlikely to respond to radiotherapy. In a series of 77 node-positive patients treated with preoperative radiotherapy followed by cystectomy, only 3 responded to treatment.[33] Second, pelvic lymphadenectomy identifies patients at risk for eventual progression who may benefit from adjuvant systemic cytotoxic chemotherapy. The M.D. Anderson group has used CISCA (Cisplatin, Cytoxan, and Adriamycin) chemotherapy in 24 patients at high risk for recurrence after cystectomy. A significantly superior disease-free survival was seen (p<0.02) compared with a similar untreated group.[34] Similarly, M-VAC (Methotrexate, Vinblastine, Adriamycin, and Cis-platinum) chemotherapy has been shown to produce a 69% complete and partial remission rate in 83 adequately treated transitional cell cancer patients with advanced stages (N+MO and NOM+).[35]

WHAT CONSTITUTES AN ADEQUATE PELVIC LYMPHADENECTOMY FOR BLADDER CANCER?

Those who support a therapeutic benefit of pelvic lymphadenectomy in patients with limited nodal metastases favor a meticulous lymphadenectomy that includes the tissue removed during a standard lymphadenectomy for prostate cancer (see earlier description) with extension of the dissection proximally to the level of the aortic bifurcation.[36] Because the group of patients who would potentially benefit from this approach is small, many feel lymphadenectomy serves chiefly as a prognostic tool that aids in the selection of those who may require adjuvant therapy. Therefore, the lower risk of postoperative lymphedema and the shorter operating time associated with a modified lymphadenectomy may outweigh the small potential benefit gained by the more extensive dissection.

PREOPERATIVE PREPARATION

Pelvic lymphadenectomy requires no special preoperative preparation. If the procedure is to be used concomitantly with radical retropubic prostatectomy or radical cystectomy, many surgeons might then use a combined mechanical and antibiotic bowel preparation prior to the operation to reduce the risk of sepsis in case an injury to the rectum occurs. Since the pelvic veins, if injured, have the potential for generating substantial blood loss, typing and cross-matching several units of blood is appropriate before pelvic lymphadenectomy, when performed with radical retropubic prostatectomy or radical cystectomy.

Many surgeons use mini-dose heparin therapy or other forms of perioperative anticoagulation to reduce the incidence of thrombophlebitis and pulmonary emboli in the postoperative period. Such thromboembolic complications often constitute the most common major problem in series of pelvic lymphadenectomies performed in the course of either radical retropubic prostatectomy or radical cystectomy. No definite conclusion can be drawn at this time as to the value of perioperative anticoagulation in this setting. There are strong proponents of the technique as well as others who have found an increased incidence of postoperative complications, such as pelvic lymphoceles. Certainly, perioperative mini-dose heparin should be considered in the patient with a history of thrombophlebitis of the lower extremities. Moreover, because they seem to constitute little risk, intermittent pneumatic compression stockings seem appropriate for patients undergoing radical pelvic cancer surgery.

SURGICAL PROCEDURE

The patient is positioned supine on the operating table. The sacrum is positioned over the break in the operating table so that extension of the table at this point will tend to open up the pelvis to improve visualization. The lower position of the head also encourages the intraperitoneal viscera to retreat cephalad out of the operating field. After the abdominal skin is prepared and disinfected in the usual manner, a urethral catheter is positioned in the bladder. This keeps the bladder decompressed during the course of the pelvic operation and allows monitoring of urine output.

Incision

We generally use a lower midline abdominal incision, extending from just above the umbilicus to well down over the anterior surface of the pubis near the base of the penis (Fig. 16-3). Bilateral inguinal incisions have been recommended by certain authors.[37] For patients with clinically localized adenocarcinoma of the prostate, bilateral extraperitonal pelvic lymphadenectomy is performed. There is evidence that such an extraperitoneal approach to the pelvic lymph nodes (compared to intraperitoneal dissection) reduces the risk of intestinal complications if such patients subsequently require radiotherapy administered to the pelvis.[38] Whether or not an extraperitoneal approach is important for patients who are not going to receive subsequent radiotherapy is unclear. Nevertheless, most currently use an extraperitoneal approach for patients with prostate carcinoma. An intraperitoneal technique is often employed for pelvic lymphadenectomy performed preliminary to radical cystectomy.

The Pfannenstiel incision also provides excellent exposure for bilateral extraperitoneal pelvic lymphadenectomy (Fig. 16-3). This incision is particularly useful for patients with an obese abdominal wall. The subcutaneous abdominal fat pad often thins out as it approaches the pelvis, and a properly placed Pfannenstiel incision is often below this thick subcutaneous fat, which can then be retracted superiorly.

The skin incision is carried sharply through the subcutaneous fat. Usually, there are numerous small veins in the subcutaneous fat, especially at the caudal end of a midline wound. These are coagulated with diathermy. The fascia of the anterior abdominal wall is then sharply divided, the midline is identified, and the rectus muscles are retracted laterally. To obtain the best possible exposure of the retropubic area in patients who are to have radical retropubic prostatectomy, it is important to extend the incision of the anterior fascia far enough caudally, to the surface of the pubis.

The prevesical space is entered and with a gentle sweep of both forefingers, the anterior surface of the bladder and iliac vessels are exposed. Gentle blunt and sharp dissection is then required to move the peritoneum with its intestinal contents superiorly, out of the pelvis so that pelvic lymphadenectomy can be performed conveniently. Some sharp dissection is often required laterally to free the peritoneum from its attachment to the anterior abdominal wall and iliopsoas region.

At this point, the spermatic cord is readily identified as it courses from behind the peritoneum to the inguinal canal. Penrose drains are placed around each spermatic cord and the cords are retracted laterally out of the field during pelvic lym-

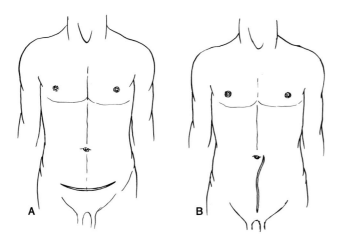

Fig. 16-3. Incisions for pelvic lymphadenectomy. Extraperitoneal pelvic lymphadenectomy can be readily accomplished either through a Pfannestiel incision (A) or a lower midline incision (B).

phadenectomy. If fertility is of no concern, retraction of the spermatic cord is facilitated by division of the vas deferens after ligation with either hemostatic metal clips or suture.

Technique

We perform pelvic lymphadenectomy on one side of the pelvis and then the other. The procedure can be performed in a careful, systematic fashion in approximately 10 to 15 minutes for each side, depending in part on the patient's body habitus. With the aid of a deep Harrington retractor, the bladder is retracted medially. Using a medium-width Deaver retractor,

the colon and the peritoneal envelope are retracted superiorly. Usually a third, smaller retractor, such as a rake, Israel, or large Richardson retractor, is necessary to retract and elevate the abdominal wall in the area where the iliac vessels approach the femoral canal. This placement of retractors allows adequate exposure of the surgical field for pelvic lymphadenectomy in almost all patients except those who are obese or who have an unusually deep pelvis.

MODIFIED PELVIC LYMPHADENECTOMY

The modified pelvic lymphadenectomy involves the en bloc excision of the fibrofatty tissues surrounding the external iliac vein, with the nodal tissue lying in the space beneath the vein between the pelvic sidewall and the bladder to the level of the obturator vessels. The margins of the dissection are the junction between the external iliac artery and vein laterally, the femoral canal and the bony pelvis inferiorly, the obturator nerve and vessels posteriorly, and the hypogastric artery up to the level of its origin from the common iliac artery superiorly (Fig. 16-4). An incision is made in the fibroareolar tissues overlying the external iliac vein from the level of the hypogastric artery proximally to the femoral canal distally. The incision lies parallel to the direction of the lymphatic channels, therefore, ligation of these tissues is not usually necessary. A plane of dissection is established on the surface of the external iliac vein and the overlying tissues are swept medially and inferiorly. With the aid of a vein retractor, this plane of dissection is continued until the smooth surface of the obturator internus muscle is encountered beneath the external iliac vein. At this point, the dissection is carried distally to the area

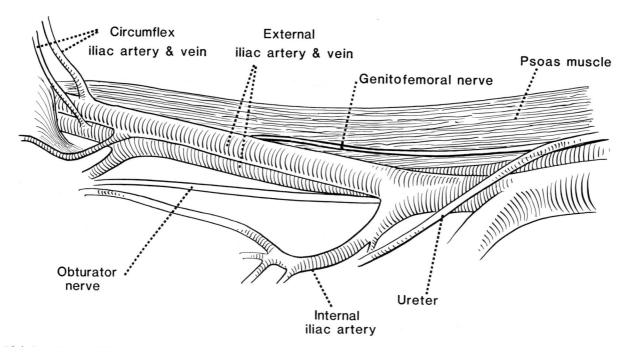

Fig. 16-4. Lateral view of the right pelvis. At the termination of pelvic lymphadenectomy, the major structures in the region should be sharply delineated. All the fat and node-laden connective tissue should have been removed from around the distal common iliac artery, the internal iliac artery and its major branches, the external iliac vessels, and the obturator fossa. (After Skinner.)

where the vein enters the femoral canal. The circumflex iliac vein is often identified arising from the external iliac vein as it emerges from the femoral canal. This vessel can be seen coursing laterally with a similarly named artery arising from the external iliac artery. These small vessels at the level of the femoral canal mark the distal margin of the dissection. The large lymph node of Cloquet (the most inferior node of the medial chain of the external iliac nodes) is found here and should be included in the specimen. Usually several large lymph channels from the lower extremities can be seen entering the pelvis. To prevent a postoperative lymph collection, it is important to ligate these carefully, either with fine sutures or, more conveniently, with metal hemostatic clips of different sizes. An abnormal or accessory obturator vein is often found in this vicinity draining into the external iliac vein from below after traversing the obturator foramen. As this vessel is fragile and easily torn, it is usually best controlled by dividing the vein between silk ligatures. The nodal tissue is then detached from the bony pelvis and Cooper's ligament distally, again securing any bridging lymphatics with small metal clips. The specimen is now free from the external iliac vein anteriorly, the pelvic sidewall laterally, and the femoral canal and Cooper's ligament distally. The obturator nerve and vessels are now readily visible and the nodal package can often be bluntly swept superiorly away from these structures. Preservation of the obturator artery may play a role in the prevention of post-

operative sexual dysfunction as the internal pudendal artery occasionally arises from this vessel. Therefore, if a potency-sparing procedure is planned, attempts should be made to preserve this vessel.[39] All the fibrofatty tissue posterior to the obturator nerve is then systematically cleaned out. Few nodes are encountered in this area. The ooze from the small vessels in the floor of the obturator fossa can be controlled by temporarily packing a small gauze sponge in this area at the termination of this part of the procedure. The dissection then proceeds proximally to the angle between the external iliac vein and the hypogastric artery. Attention is directed toward removal of as much of the fibrofatty tissue as possible from around the internal iliac artery and its branches in the pelvis. This part of the operation is sometimes difficult to do en bloc with the previous portion of the procedure. In certain instances, ligation and division of the obliterated umbilical artery will make it easier to manipulate the internal iliac artery. We have not made an extensive dissection behind the internal iliac artery in order to avoid injury to the internal iliac vein. Once the nodal package is freed from this region, it can be delivered as an en bloc specimen. The dissection is not carried proximally onto the common iliac artery.

At the termination of the dissection, all the fibrofatty tissue within the margins of the dissection should have been removed. The external iliac vein should be completely bare and the tissues overlying the external iliac artery have been left

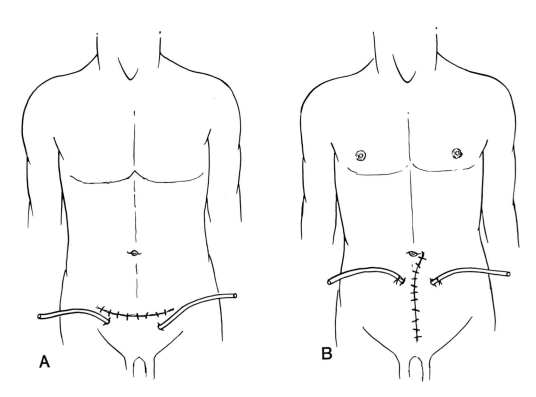

Fig. 16-5. At the termination of the operation, large Hemovac drains are left in each side of the pelvis to remove any blood or lymph that might collect. The muscle layers are closed with interrupted figure-of-eight, absorbable sutures such as polyglycolic acid (No. 0 Dexon) or polyglactin (No. 0 Vicryl). Sutures of 3-0 chromic are used to approximate the subcutaneous fascia, and staples are used as illustrated to approximate the skin edges. Pelvic drains may be removed when no more fluid is obtained.

undisturbed. The white obturator nerve should hang freely suspended across the obturator fossa which has been dissected cleanly. All bleeding should be controlled at this point. If radical prostatectomy is contemplated, the superior surface of the endopelvic fascia is already exposed and radical prostatectomy can begin immediately.

Large, closed-suction drains are left in the obturator fossa on each side to prevent postoperative collection of blood or lymph. These drains are removed several days postoperatively when negligible fluid is collected.

Closure

The Hemovac drains are brought out through separate stab incisions on each side of the abdominal wound avoiding the inferior epigastric vessels. The anterior rectus fascia is closed with interrupted figure-of-eight heavy, absorbable sutures. Fine catgut sutures may be used in the subcutaneous tissue, and skin staples are used to close the skin. These staples are removed approximately 7 days postoperatively (Fig. 16-5).

COMPLICATIONS OF PELVIC LYMPHADENECTOMY

Wound complications (infection, dehiscence, hematoma, and seroma) occur with a frequency of 3 to 24%.[28,40] Thromboembolic events are perhaps the most serious of all complications related to this procedure. Most large series report at least one pulmonary embolus with rates between 0.7 and 4.6%.[27,28,40–42] This potentially lethal, albeit infrequent, event has lead to the use of routine pre- and postoperative anticoagulation by some surgeons, with favorable results. Others argue that anticoagulation leads to an increase in the rate of lymphocele formation and prolonged lymph leak. Sogani and associates reported a 5% incidence of prolonged lymph leak, lymphocele, or hematoma in 276 patients undergoing pelvic lymphadenectomy without anticoagulation. This is contrasted with a rate of 8.4% in 95 patients receiving prophylactic mini-dose heparin.[43] This same association has been confirmed by others in smaller series.[42,44] Lymphocele, if asymptomatic, can be managed conservatively and followed with serial ultrasound or CT examinations.[43] However, once symptomatic, these collections must be drained, either percutaneously or surgically, to prevent further complications such as abscess, sepsis, ureteral obstruction, or venous obstruction (with resultant lower extremity thrombosis and pulmonary emboli).

Chronic lower extremity and genital lymphedema has been associated with standard pelvic lymphadenectomy in as many as 12% of cases,[28] and is present temporarily in 50% of patients.[26] This complication is, however, reported to be much less frequent when the modified technique is used.[26,27] Other reported complications of pelvic lymphadenectomy that are unusual include: severe bleeding related to intraoperative vascular injury, obturator nerve injury, and ureteral injury.[41] These problems should be avoidable if a careful, deliberate surgical technique is employed.

REFERENCES

1. Nelson, J. H., *Atlas of Radical Pelvic Surgery.* 2nd Edition. New York, Appleton-Century Crofts, 1977.
2. Grossman, H. B., Batata, M., Hilaris, B., and Whitmore, W. F., Jr. 125-I implantation for carcinoma of prostate: Further follow-up of first 100 cases. Urology, *20:*591, 1982.
3. Smith, J. A. Jr., Haynes, T. H., and Middleton, R. G. Impact of external irradiation on local symptoms and survival free of disease in patients with pelvic lymph node metastasis from adenocarcinoma of the prostate. J. Urol., *131:*705, 1984.
4. Kramer, S. A., et al. Prognosis of patients with stage D1 prostatic adenocarcinoma. J. Urol., *125:*817, 1981.
5. Prout, G. R., Jr., et al. Nodal involvement as a prognostic indicator in patients with prostatic carcinoma. J. Urol., *124:*226, 1980.
6. Bagshaw, M. A. Perspectives in the radiation treatment of prostatic cancer: History and current focus. In *Prostatic Cancer.* Edited by G. Murphy. Littleton, PSG Publishing, 1979.
7. Zincke, H., et al. Radical retropubic prostatectomy and pelvic lymphadenectomy for high-stage cancer of the prostate. Cancer, *47:*1901, 1981.
8. Neuwirth, H., et al. Stage D1 carcinoma of the prostate: Radical prostatectomy with early endocrine therapy improves survival. Abstract 563, 84th Annual Meeting of the American Urological Association, Dallas, Texas, 1989.
9. Kramolowsky, E. V. The value of testosterone deprivation in stage D1 carcinoma of the prostate. J. Urol., *139:*1242, 1988.
10. Winkler, H. Z., et al. Stage D1 prostatic adenocarcinoma: Significance of nuclear DNA ploidy patterns studied by flow cytometry. Mayo Clin. Proc., *63:*103, 1988.
11. Levine, M. S., et al. Detecting lymphatic metastases from prostatic carcinoma: Superiority of CT. Am. J. Roentgenol., *137:*207, 1981.
12. Benson, K. H., et al. The value of computerized tomography in evaluation of pelvic lymph nodes. J. Urol., *126:*63, 1981.
13. Mukamel, E., et al. The value of computerized tomography scan and magnetic resonance imaging in staging prostatic carcinoma: Comparison with the clinical and histological staging. J. Urol., *136:*1231, 1986.
14. Liebner, E. J., and Stefani, S. Uro-Oncology Research Group: An evaluation of lymphography with nodal biopsy in localized carcinoma of the prostate. Cancer, *45:*728, 1980.
15. Hilaris, B., et al. Radiation therapy and pelvic node dissection in the management of cancer of the prostate. Am. J. Roentgenol., *121:*832, 1974.
16. Merrin, C., et al. The clinical value of lymphangiography: Are the nodes surrounding the obturator nerve visualized? J. Urol., *117:*762, 1977.
17. Johnson, D. E., and von Eschenbach, A. C. Roles of lymphangiography and pelvic lymphadenectomy in staging prostate cancer. Urology, *17*(Suppl):66, 1981.
18. Rouviere, H. *Anatomy of the Human Lymphatic System.* Ann Arbor, Edwards Brothers, Inc., 1938.
19. *Lymphatic Imaging Lymphography, Computer Tomography and Scintigraphy,* 2nd Edition. Edited by M. E. Clouse and S. Wallace.

Baltimore, Williams & Wilkins, 1985.

20. GOLIMBU, M., et al. Extended pelvic lymphadenectomy for prostatic cancer. J. Urol., *121:*617, 1979.

21. PISTENMA, D. A., BAGSHAW, M. A., and FREIHA, F. S. Extended-field radiation therapy for prostatic adenocarcinoma: Status report of a limited prospective trial. In *Cancer of the Genitourinary Tract.* 23rd Edition. Edited by D. E. Johnson and M. L. Samuels. New York, Raven Press, 1979, pp. 229–247.

22. MCLAUGHLIN, A. P., et al. Prostatic carcinoma: Incidence and location of unsuspected lymphatic metastases. J. Urol., *115:*89, 1976.

23. FLOCKS, R. H., CULP, D., and PORTO, R. Lymphatic spread from prostatic cancer. J. Urol., *81:*194, 1959.

24. FOWLER, J. E., JR., and WHITMORE, W. F., JR. The incidence and extent of pelvic lymph node metastases in apparently localized prostatic cancer. Cancer, *47:*2941, 1981.

25. SMITH, J. A., JR., et al. Pelvic lymph node metastasis from prostatic cancer: Influence of tumor grade and stage in 452 consecutive patients. J. Urol., *130:*290, 1983.

26. HERR, H. W. Pelvic lymphadenectomy and iodine-125 implantation. In *Genitourinary Tumors: Fundamental Principles and Surgical Techniques.* Edited by D. E. Johnson and M. A. Boileau. New York, Grune and Stratton, 1982, pp. 63–73.

27. BRENDLER, C. B., et al. Staging pelvic lymphadenectomy for carcinoma of the prostate: Risk versus benefit. J. Urol., *124:*849, 1980.

28. LIESKOVSKY, G., SKINNER, D. G., and WEISENBURGER, T. Pelvic lymphadenectomy in the management of carcinoma of the prostate. J. Urol., *124:*635, 1980.

29. SMITH, J. A., JR., and WHITMORE, W. F., JR. Regional lymph node metastasis from bladder cancer. J. Urol., *126:*591, 1981.

30. LIESKOVSKY, G., and SKINNER, D. G. Role of lymphadenectomy in the treatment of bladder cancer. Urol. Clin. North Am., *11:*709, 1984.

31. ZINCKE, H., et al. Pelvic lymphadenectomy and radical cystectomy for transitional cell carcinoma of the bladder with pelvic nodal disease. Br. J. Urol., *57:*156, 1985.

32. HERR, H. W. Bladder cancer: Pelvic lymphadenectomy revisited. J. Surg. Oncol., *37:*242, 1988.

33. WHITMORE, W. F., and BATATA, M. Status of integrated irradiation and cystectomy for bladder cancer. Urol. Clin. North Am., *11:*681, 1984.

34. LOGOTHETIS, C., et al. Adjuvant chemotherapy for invasive bladder carcinoma: A preliminary report. Abstract C-421. In: Proc. Am. Soc. Clin. Oncol. *4:*108, 1985.

35. STERNBERG, C. N., et al. M-VAC (Methotrexate, Vinblastine, Doxorubicin, and Cis-platin) for advanced transitional cell carcinoma of the urothelium. J. Urol., *139:*461, 1988.

36. LIESKOVSKY, G. Pelvic lymphadenectomy. In *Urologic Surgery.* 3rd Edition. Edited by JF Glenn. Philadelphia, J. B. Lippincott Co., 1983, pp. 939–947.

37. DAHL, D. S., et al. Pelvic lymphadenectomy for staging localized prostatic cancer. J. Urol., *112:*245, 1974.

38. BAGSHAW, M. A. Perspectives in the radiation treatment of prostatic cancer: History and current focus. In *Prostatic Cancer.* Edited by G. Murphy. Littleton, PSG Publishing, 1979.

39. EPSTEIN, J. I., et al. Frozen section detection of lymph node metastases in prostatic carcinoma: Accuracy in grossly uninvolved pelvic lymphadenectomy specimens. J. Urol., *136:*1234, 1986.

40. BABCOCK, J. R., and GRAYHACK, J. T. Morbidity of pelvic lymphadenectomy. Urology, *13:*483, 1979.

41. PAUL, D. B., et al. Morbidity from pelvic lymphadenectomy in staging carcinoma of the prostate. J. Urol., *129:*1141, 1983.

42. KOONCE, J., SELIKOWITZ, S., and MCDOUGAL, W. S. Complications of low-dose heparin prophylaxis following pelvic lymphadenectomy. Urology, *28:*21, 1986.

43. SOGANI, P. C., WATSON, R. C., and WHITMORE, W. F., JR. Lymphocele after pelvic lymphadenectomy for urologic cancer. Urology, *17:*39, 1981.

44. CATALONA, W. J., KADMON, D., and CRANE, D. B. Effect of mini-dose heparin on lymphocele formation following extraperitoneal pelvic lymphadenectomy. J. Urol., *123:*890, 1980.

Nerve-Sparing Radical Prostatectomy

Perinchery Narayan

Until recently, impotence was a common complication and a major deterrent to the performance of radical prostatectomy. In 1982, Walsh and Donker studied the surgical anatomy of the cavernous nerves and, by elegant anatomic dissections, described a technique to avoid their injury during pelvic surgery.[1] The operation of "nerve-sparing" radical prostatectomy was thus conceived. Since 1982, the technique has been refined to include successful nerve sparing in radical prostatectomy as well as cystoprostatectomy.[2,3]

Surgical injury to the cavernous nerves may occur at several sites during radical prostatectomy. Injury may occur at the time of urethral transsection, during mobilization of the apex of the prostate, during dissection of the lateral and inferior surfaces of the prostate, during ligation of the prostatic vascular pedicles, and during mobilization of the seminal vesicles. In order to understand the mechanisms for potential injury of the cavernous nerves, one needs to have a clear understanding of the location of the pelvic autonomic plexus, the pathways of the "nervi erigentes" that provide innervation to the corpora, and the relationship of these nerves to the prostate, bladder, and seminal vesicles. Further, a knowledge of the vascular supply of the prostate and its interrelationships to the cavernous nerves is important in preventing inadvertent injury to the nerves during ligation of these vessels. This chapter will address the indications for nerve-sparing prostatectomy, the neural and surgical anatomy of cavernous nerves, potential sites of nerve injury, and technique of prevention of injury during radical prostatectomy. Results of nerve-sparing radical prostatectomy, limitations of the technique, and methods to enhance the results will also be discussed.

INDICATIONS

Radical prostatectomy, like other cancer surgery, is best performed in patients with early localized disease. In the past, this operation had a poor reputation because of two major considerations: (1) the morbidity and mortality of the surgical procedure, and (2) the inability to decide which patients with prostate cancer were likely to progress and therefore need therapy. Current refinements in surgical techniques, an improved understanding of continence mechanisms,[4] improved anesthetic techniques,[5] use of autologous transfusions, and prophylaxis for embolic complications, have greatly reduced the morbidity and mortality of radical prostatectomy. The variable biologic behaviour of prostatic cancer is still poorly understood. However, refinements in diagnostic techniques such as ultrasonography[6,7] and serum prostate-specific antigen,[8] as well as recent knowledge that even low-grade, low-stage cancers will metastasize if patients live long enough,[9] make it possible to more confidently offer a larger number of younger patients with smaller tumors the options of surgical therapy. It is important, therefore, for urologists to become familiar with this technique so that more patients have the surgical option.

NEUROPHYSIOLOGY OF ERECTION

Erectile function is governed by somatic, sympathetic, and parasympathetic nerves.[10] The parasympathetic nerves are the most important component of this triad in maintaining erectile function. These nerve fibers arise from sacral second through fourth nerve roots and synapse in the inferior hypogastric (pelvic) plexus (Fig. 17-1). Post-ganglionic fibers of the parasympathetic nerves form the cavernous nerves that travel on either side of the prostate. The parasympathetic nerves are largely responsible for initiating the arterial and sinusoidal relaxation that begins tumescence. The sympathetic fibers arise from the thoracolumbar sympathetic ganglia ($T_{11,12}$, L_1-L_3). Fibers from these ganglia course laterally downward between

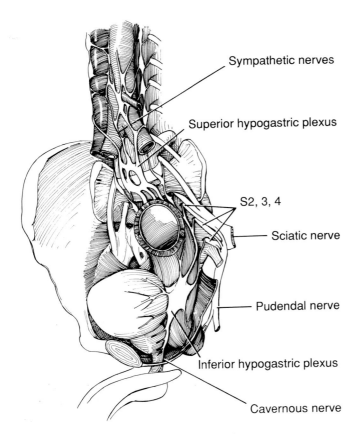

FIG. 17-1. Neuro-anatomy of pelvic autonomic nerves.

Sympathetic nerves

Superior hypogastric plexus

S2, 3, 4

Sciatic nerve

Pudendal nerve

Inferior hypogastric plexus

Cavernous nerve

the aorta and the inferior vena cava. They arborize in the superior and inferior hypogastric plexus and travel via the pudendal and cavernous nerves to supply the urogenital system. The sympathetic fibers are responsible in part for mediating the detumescence phase of penile erection. Unlike other visceral functions, the sympathetic and parasympathetic divisions of the autonomic nervous system do not necessarily release antagonistic neurotransmitters in mediating erectile function. It is now recognized that not only can both systems elicit synergistic effects, both systems can also synthesize, store, and release cholinergic as well as adrenergic neurotransmitters. The somatic nerve fibers arise from the sacral second, third, and fourth segments, and travel via the pudendal nerve. These fibers are responsible for carrying tactile sensation from the surface of the penis. The pudendal nerve courses in the pudendal canal in the lateral pelvic wall and is not subject to injury during radical prostatectomy.

SURGICAL ANATOMY OF CAVERNOUS NERVES

Anatomically, the inferior hypogastric plexus is located on the surface of the bodies of the sacral second, third, and fourth vertebrae behind the seminal vesicle and bladder neck areas (Fig. 17-1). From this plexus, a group of nerve fibers coalesce to form the right and left cavernous nerves. Branches of the inferior hypogastric plexus provide innervation to the bladder, prostate, seminal vesicles, vas deferens, proximal urethra, and corpora cavernosa. Nerve fibers to these organs arise from the plexus both directly and from smaller branches along the course of the cavernous nerves (Fig. 17-1). Autonomic nerve fibers to the penis travel upward from the hypogastric plexus and, at the level of the base of the prostate, form the right and left cavernous nerves. They then travel on either side of the prostate in the lateral pelvic fascia outside the prostatic capsule and Denonvilliers' fascia. Normally, the cavernous nerves course along a path 0.5 to 1 cm away from the prostatic capsule. However, when there is prostatic enlargement, there is compression of the lateral fascia and the nerves may be closer to the prostatic surface.

ARTERIAL AND VENOUS ANATOMY OF THE PROSTATE

A relatively bloodless field facilitates nerve-sparing surgery. An intimate knowledge of the rich vascular supply of the prostate and appropriate measures to control blood loss are essential to the performance of adequate nerve preservation during radical pelvic surgery. The majority of the arterial supply of the prostate arises from branches of the inferior vesical artery (Figs. 17-2 and 17-3). The prostatic branch is usually given off at the level of the prostate around the 5- and 7-o'clock positions (right and left), in the groove between the prostate and the bladder neck. Perforating branches from this artery penetrate the prostatic capsule and then divide, supplying both the prostatic tissue and the prostatic urethra (Fig. 17-3). The terminal portion of the inferior vesical artery courses downward,

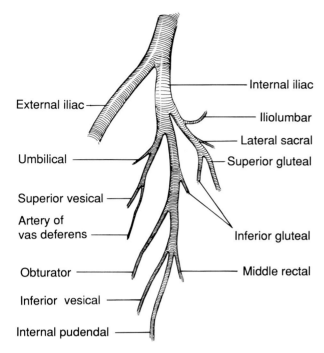

External iliac —

Umbilical —

Superior vesical —

Artery of
vas deferens —

Obturator —

Inferior vesical —

Internal pudendal —

— Internal iliac

— Iliolumbar

— Lateral sacral

— Superior gluteal

— Inferior gluteal

— Middle rectal

FIG. 17-2. Branches of the internal iliac (hypogastric) artery.

along with the cavernous nerve (Fig. 17-3), as part of the "neurovascular bundle." Branches from these vessels form additional capsular arteries of the prostate.

The arterial supply of the penis normally comes from the terminal branches of the internal pudendal artery (Fig. 17-2). These terminal branches include the perineal artery, the bulbourethral artery, and the cavernous (deep) and dorsal (superficial) arteries of the penis. Variations in arterial supply may result in an accessory internal pudendal artery forming an additional or sole blood supply to either side of the penis.[11-13] The significance of this variation lies in the fact that the accessory pudendal artery may arise from the obturator, inferior, or superior vesical arteries. All of these latter vessels are subject to complete or partial injury during radical prostatectomy and cystoprostatectomy. Thus, there are vascular and neural components for impotence following radical prostatectomy.

The venous blood supply of the prostate is formed by the dorsal vein and the plexus of veins surrounding the prostate anteriorly and laterally (Santorini's plexus). The deep dorsal vein is part of the intermediate venous system draining the penis. After the deep dorsal vein penetrates the urogenital diaphragm, it divides into an anterior branch and several lateral branches (Figs. 17-4 and 17-5). Veins from the anterior surface of the prostate and bladder wall coalesce to join the superficial branch of the dorsal vein complex usually traversing between the two puboprostatic ligaments. The lateral branches of the

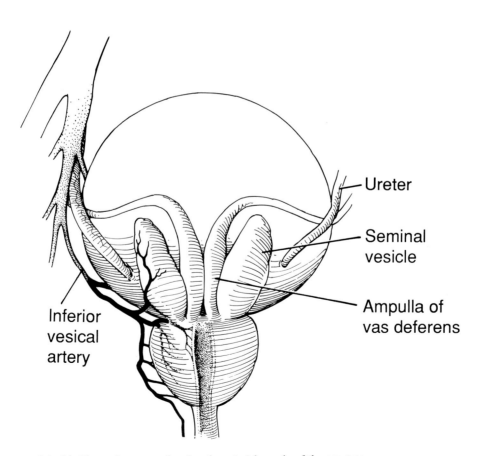

Inferior
vesical
artery

— Ureter

— Seminal
vesicle

— Ampulla of
vas deferens

FIG. 17-3. Posterior view of the bladder and prostate showing the arterial supply of the prostate.

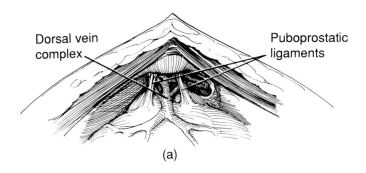

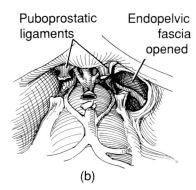

(b)

FIG. 17-4. (a) Dorsal vein complex and puboprostatic ligaments. (b) Dorsal vein complex with endopelvic fascia opened, superficial branches of the dorsal vein ligated, and puboprostatic ligaments incised.

dorsal vein complex travel on the lateral sides of the prostate and communicate with branches of the crural, obturator, and internal pudendal veins. Eventually they drain via the inferior vesical and hemorrhoidal veins into the internal iliac veins.

POTENTIAL SITES OF CAVERNOUS NERVE INJURY AND METHODS OF PREVENTION

The author performed nerve-sparing operations in over 100 patients (1985–1989) at UCSF and Veterans Administration Medical Center in San Francisco. The technique used was modified from that of Walsh and is described herein. An early important step in radical prostatectomy is the achievement of a relatively bloodless field by adequate ligation of the dorsal vein complex. Walsh recommends bilateral temporary occlusion of the hypogastric artery to minimize blood loss.[2] Temporary occlusion of the hypogastric artery is easily accomplished, using small ("bulldog") vascular clamps. We have used this technique on occasion, although not as a routine.

The first step in radical retropubic prostatectomy is to open the endopelvic fascia on each side (Fig. 17-4b). Next, the puboprostatic ligaments are identified and carefully incised. The puboprostatic ligaments are superficial and, during their incision, care must be taken not to injure branches of the dorsal vein complex directly behind them. The third step is to ligate the dorsal vein. Before ligating the main dorsal vein complex, the superficial branch is ligated and divided (Fig. 17-4). The main dorsal vein complex is ligated next, using two

to three ligatures of 0 Dexon. These sutures are passed using a long-nosed right angle clamp (Fig. 17-5). We prefer 0 Dexon to silk because silk sutures occasionally migrate into the vesicourethral anastomoses and may cause irritative voiding symptoms. The proximity of the prostate to the pubic bone

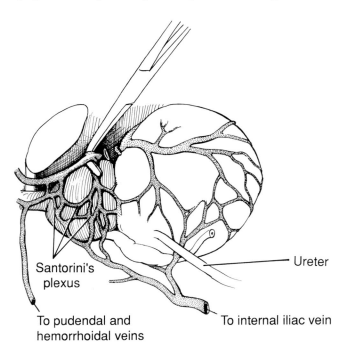

FIG. 17-5. Ligation of the dorsal vein complex.

does not allow two sets of ligatures to be placed on the dorsal vein complex for division of the complex between ligatures. Therefore, ligatures are placed only on one side, as close as possible to the pubic bone. The dorsal vein complex is incised below these ligatures. Incision of the dorsal vein complex is accomplished gradually and methodically to avoid slippage of the ligatures and to accomplish satisfactory suture ligation of backbleeding from the proximal veins on the prostatic surface. These proximal veins are suture-ligated as they are visualized, using 2-0 chromic catgut on a UR4 needle (semicircular needle) or a TT4 needle. If the ligatures on the dorsal vein slip during incision of the vein complex, the complex can be suture-ligated against the pelvic wall fascia using 2-0 chromic catgut. In situations when bleeding from the dorsal vein complex is brisk, either because of inadequate ligation or because of inadvertent injury of the veins, distal traction on the Foley catheter may be used to cause compression of the prostate against the dorsal vein complex and pubic bone. This may be used intermittently to provide temporary hemostasis during suture ligation of the dorsal vein complex. Following division of the puboprostatic ligaments and dorsal vein complex, the urethra is transected. This is done under direct vision by making a urethrotomy in the anterior urethra (Fig. 17-6). Next, the posterior urethral wall is carefully transected under direct vision, using the Foley catheter for traction (Fig. 17-7).

Studies of radical prostatectomy specimens and prostatic anatomy by ultrasonography, reveal that the prostatic apex is longer by 0.5 to 1 cm dorsally than ventrally. Care must be exercised during transection of the posterior urethral wall to ensure that this apical extension is not inadvertently incised. The apex is freed by incising the fibers of the rectourethralis (Fig. 17-7). Visualization of the apex is facilitated by traction

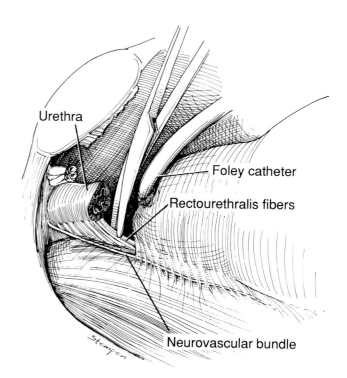

FIG. 17-7. Incision of the rectourethralis fibers to free the apex of the prostate.

on the catheter following division of the urethra. During dissection of the apex, care must be taken to confine the dissection to the midline during incision of the rectourethralis fibers, to avoid injury to the cavernous nerves. Once the apex is freed, the lateral attachments of the fascia along with any small vessels may be ligated with an absorbable ligature (we use 3-0 Dexon sutures on a T5 needle) and divided (Fig 17-8). Having

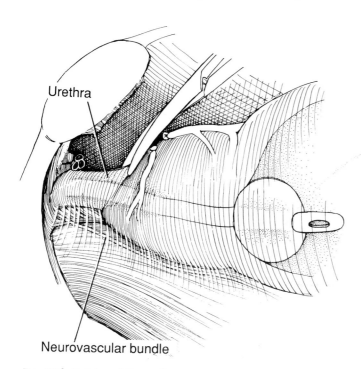

FIG. 17-6. Incision of the urethra.

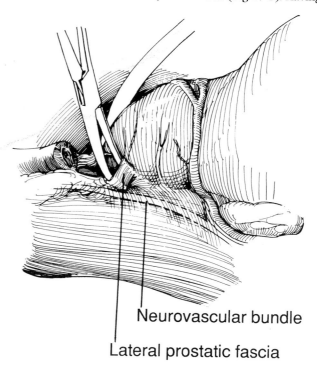

FIG. 17-8. Dissection of the lateral prostatic fascia.

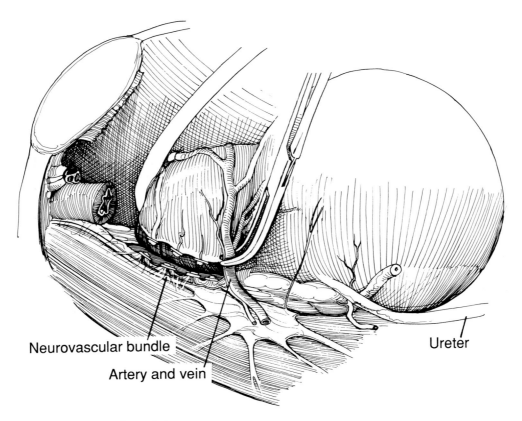

Neurovascular bundle

Artery and vein

Ureter

Fig. 17-9. Ligation of the prostatic vascular pedicle.

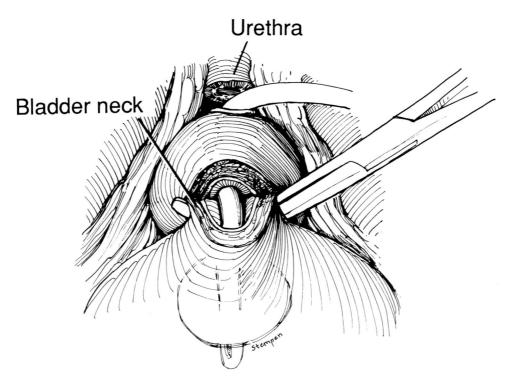

Urethra

Bladder neck

Fig. 17-10. Dissection of the bladder neck.

divided the lateral fascial attachments on either side, the prostate may be bluntly dissected off the rectum posteriorly. The next step is to ligate the vascular pedicles of the prostate. The key here is to ligate the vessels away from the cavernous nerves by staying as close to the prostate as possible (Fig. 17-9).

Following this, the bladder is incised anteriorly at the groove between the prostate and the bladder neck, and the prostate is dissected off the posterior bladder wall. Careful, meticulous dissection of the bladder neck will ensure preservation of the circular bladder neck fibers (Fig. 17-10). The ejaculatory ducts are identified and incised under large hemoclips. The concern for potential nerve injury here is during removal of the seminal vesicles. Injury to the autonomic nerve fibers is avoided by confining the dissection close to the seminal vesicles and by securing all bleeding as close to the seminal vesicles as possible. Once the prostate is removed, the bladder neck needs to be repaired. During dissection of the prostatic base from the bladder neck, careful incision of the bladder neck and dissection of it away from the prostate, will ensure a small, tight bladder neck. This will limit the extent of repair necessary (Fig. 17-10). Prior to bladder neck repair, we routinely perform 4-quadrant frozen-section biopsies from the bladder neck and distal urethra. Bladder neck repair may be performed using a standard racquet handle closure or, if the defect is minimal, by a "fish mouth" technique (Fig. 17-11). We use two layers of 4-0 Maxon sutures for this repair. To ensure adequate mucosal to mucosal approximation during vesicourethral anastomosis, we leave a small cuff of excess bladder mucosa on the posterior bladder neck during dissection of the prostate from bladder neck. This mucosa is incor-

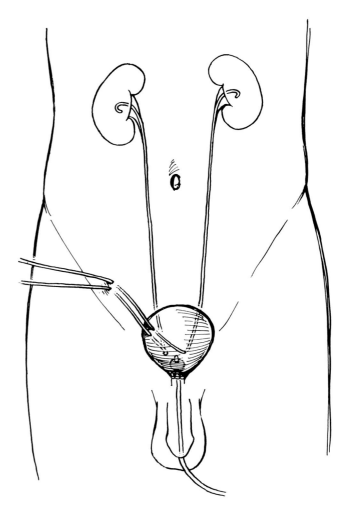

FIG. 17-12. Placement of single J, temporary diversion stents for extensively repaired bladder neck.

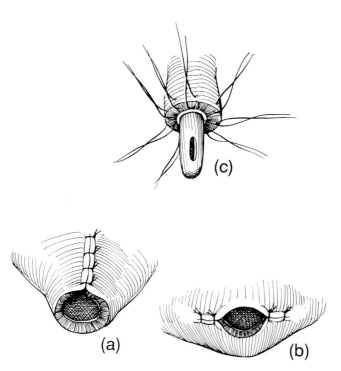

FIG. 17-11. Repair of bladder neck, (a) racquet handle technique, (b) fishmouth technique, and (c) urethral anastomosis.

porated in the anastomotic sutures to ensure mucosal to mucosal approximation of bladder neck and urethra. Alternatively, in large bladder neck defects, we use the technique of tethering the mucosa down to the bladder neck, as recommended by Walsh. These measures prevent problems of postoperative anastomotic contractures. In situations where there is a large intravesical component of prostate, or prior transurethral surgery has resulted in a large resected bladder neck, we temporarily divert the urine using bilateral single J-stents. These are placed intraoperatively prior to bladder neck repair, and exit out through the anterior bladder wall (Fig. 17-12). The stents are removed 7 to 10 days postoperatively. Use of these stents minimizes the anastomotic leak that may accompany extensive bladder neck repair and allows earlier removal of the Foley catheter. Additionally, it is possible that by reducing the anastomotic leak in the first few postoperative days, the degree of fibrosis at the bladder neck area is diminished. This may translate into better and earlier recovery of continence.

Anastomosis of the urethra to the bladder is achieved using 6 to 8 sutures of 3-0 Maxon. The anastomosis is performed

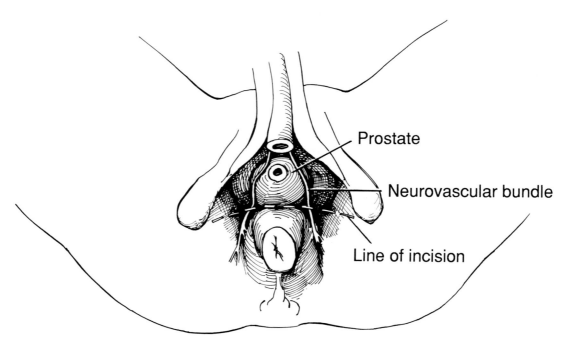

Fig. 17-13. View of the neurovascular bundle in radical perineal prostatectomy.

over a 20-French Silastic catheter. Initial positioning of the patient with the legs extended on splints (Kraus "airplane" splints) allows an assistant to place a sponge stick in the perineum to push the urethra in. This allows a gain of 1 to 2 cms in urethral length, making it easily accessible for placement of urethral anastomotic sutures, especially in patients with deep pelves. In heavy patients with deep pelves, a wedge pubectomy of the inner table of the pubic bone in the midline may be necessary both for visualization of the dorsal vein complex and for vesicourethral anastomoses.

NERVE-SPARING RADICAL PERINEAL PROSTATECTOMY

Radical perineal prostatectomy has two major advantages over radical retropubic prostatectomy. One is the ease of urethral visualization and the other is the reduced blood loss, because the dissection is performed below the dorsal vein complex. The major disadvantage is the need for two separate incisions and the need to reposition the patient following pelvic lymphadenectomy. Radical perineal prostatectomy can also incorporate the nerve-sparing modification by recognition and preservation of the lateral fascia of the prostate, which contains the neurovascular bundles (Fig. 17-13). Critical steps include limitation of dissection close to the urethra, preservation of the fascia lateral to the prostate, and ligation of the vascular pedicles close to the prostate. These steps are feasible and recent reports have discussed the successful use of this technique in nerve-sparing prostatectomy.[14,15]

RESULTS OF NERVE-SPARING RADICAL PROSTATECTOMY

Results of nerve sparing radical prostatectomy depend on a number of factors. They include the age of the patient, the degree of potency prior to surgery, the stage of the cancer, prior urologic surgery (especially transurethral resection prior to radical prostatectomy), medication history and presence of coexistent medical conditions such as diabetes, peripheral vascular disease, atherosclerosis, and hypertension. In our experience, best results are achieved in 70% of patients under age 65 who are in good health with minimal coexisting medical conditions, provided they have low stage cancer (A, B_1). Even in these patients, postoperative penile Doppler studies at 6 months indicate that often there is damage to the vascular supply of the penis, resulting in diminution of erectile function, though it may be adequate for vaginal penetration. Examples of vascular compromise that we have noted include partial fibrosis of one or both cavernous arteries and varying degrees of venous leakage not present preoperatively. Erectile function in these patients does improve with time, but often patients may not be willing to tolerate a partial erection for 12 to 24 months after surgery. In these patients, nonsurgical therapies such as use of vacuum suction devices, intracavernous injections of smooth muscle relaxants, (Papaverine hydrochloride or Prostaglandin E_1), and alpha blockers (Phentolamine) may be necessary to supplement natural potency.[16] Patients who have additional risk factors such as smoking, hypertension, peripheral vascular disease, and diabetes have only a 30 to 40% chance of preserving potency even though they have low-stage cancer and are under 65 years of age. In older patients, the ability to achieve erections is quite tenuous and any compromise in vascular supply of the penis or mild injury to the nerves, appears to cause lasting loss of erectile function. Early postoperative treatment with nonsurgical therapies may help some patients, and penile implant surgery may be necessary in others. Patients with large B_2 cancers seem to suffer more nerve damage during surgery, consistent with the removal of a larger gland that is compressing the nerves and often, in fact, planned resection of the neurovascular bundle on one side or both sides becomes necessary.[17] Patients who have had prior transurethral resection will often have fibrosis involving the periprostatic area, resulting in a more difficult dissection with increased risk of injury to the cavernous nerves.

DOES NERVE SPARING COMPROMISE CANCER CONTROL?

The cavernous nerves are located outside the prostatic capsule and the Denonvilliers' fascia. It would seem logical that as long as the cancer is confined within the prostatic capsule, cavernous nerve sparing should have no influence on cancer control. Other data in support of this argument are the long-term successes of radical perineal prostatectomies, where the dissection was confined within the lateral pelvic fascia.[18] Although this effort was made to avoid injury to the lateral venous plexus and dorsal veins, rather than for nerve-sparing, the anatomic approach was similar to nerve-sparing surgery. Walsh has also reported on pathologic studies of the first 100 consecutive patients who underwent nerve-sparing surgery. Despite capsular penetration occurring in 41 of these patients, only 7 had positive margins. All seven patients had extensive extracapsular extension, five had seminal vesicle involvement, and in none were the margins positive only at the site of the nerve sparing modification.[19] Finally, an intimate knowledge of the anatomic confines of the prostate and the location of the neurovascular bundle helps to perform more extensive resection of the periprostatic fascia and neurovascular bundle area in patients with large cancers (B_2) where extracapsular extension is suspected. Furthermore, in these patients the neurovascular bundle can be preserved on the opposite side if the cancer is present extensively only on one side. This approach has also resulted in preservation of potency in significant numbers of patients.[17]

SUMMARY

In summary, nerve-sparing radical prostatectomy is safe and effective in preserving potency in approximately 70% of patients under age 65 with good preoperative potency, low-stage prostatic cancers and minimal vascular and medical risk factors.

REFERENCES

1. WALSH, P. C., and DONKER, P. J. Impotence following radical prostatectomy: Insight into etiology and prevention. J. Urol., *128*:492, 1982.
2. WALSH, P. C., LEPOR, H., and EGGLESTON, J. C. Radical prostatectomy with preservation of sexual function: Anatomical and pathological considerations. Prostate, *4*:473, 1983.
3. SCHLEGEL, P. N., and WALSH, P. C. Neuroanatomical approach to radical cystectomy with preservation of sexual function. J. Urol., *138*:1402, 1987.
4. PRESTI, J. C., JR., et al. Pathophysiology of urinary incontinence after radical prostatectomy. J. Urol., (in press).
5. DRAGO, J. R., NESBITT, J. A., and BADALAMENT, R. A. Radical nerve-sparing prostatectomy. The first 30 patients treated with epidural anesthesia. J. Surg. Oncol., *40*:182, 1989.
6. LEE, F., et al. Transrectal ultrasound in the diagnosis of prostate cancer: Location, echogenicity, histopathology and staging. Prostate, *7*:117, 1985.
7. DAHNERT, W. F., et al. Prostatic evaluation by transrectal sonography with histopathologic correlation: The echopenic appearance of early carcinoma. Radiology, *158*:97, 1986.
8. STAMEY, T. A., et al. Prostatic specific antigen as a serum marker for adenocarcinoma of the prostate. N. Engl. J. Med., *317*:909, 1987.
9. EPSTEIN, J. I., et al. Prognosis of untreated stage A1 prostatic carcinoma: A study of 94 cases with extended followup. J. Urol., *136*:837, 1986.
10. deGROAT, W. C., and STEERS, W. D. Neuroanatomy and Neurophysiology of penile erection. In *Contemporary Management of Impotence and Infertility.* Edited by E. A. Tanagho, T. F. Lue, and R. D. McClure. Baltimore, Williams & Wilkins, 1988.
11. BREZA, J., et al. Detailed anatomy of penile neurovascular structures: Surgical significance. J. Urol., *141*:437, 1989.
12. TRAMIER, D., et al. Radiological anatomy of the internal pudendal artery (a. pudenda interna) in the male. Anat. Clin., *3*:195, 1981.
13. JUSKIEWENSKI, S., et al. A study of the arterial blood supply to the penis. Anat. Clin., *4*:101, 1982.
14. WELDON, V. E., and TAVEL, F. R. Potency-sparing radical perineal prostatectomy: Anatomy, surgical technique and initial results. J. Urol., *140*:559, 1988.
15. WEISS, J. P., et al. Preservation of periprostatic autonomic nerves during total perineal prostatectomy by intrafascial dissection. Urology, *26*:160, 1985.
16. LUE, T. F., and TANAGHO, E. A. Physiology of erection and pharmacological management of impotence. J. Urol., *137*:829, 1987.
17. WALSH, P. C., EPSTEIN, J. I., and LOWE, F. C. Potency following radical prostatectomy with wide unilateral excision of the neurovascular bundle. J. Urol., *138*:823, 1987.
18. EGGLESTON, J.C., and WALSH, P. C. Radical prostatectomy with preservation of sexual function: Pathological findings in the first 100 cases. J. Urol., *134*:1146, 1985.
19. WALSH, P. C. Radical prostatectomy, preservation of sexual function, cancer control: The controversy. Urol. Clin. North Am., *14*:663, 1987.

Radical Retropubic Prostatectomy; Antegrade Approach

E. David Crawford

Prostate cancer is the most common male neoplasm. Unfortunately, most patients present with disease that is either locally advanced or metastatic at the time of diagnosis. Physician and patient awareness of this cancer are resulting in discovery of increasing number of early cases that are confined to the prostate and are, therefore, amenable to cure. It is anticipated that with refinements in transrectal ultrasound, further evaluation of prostate specific antigen (PSA), and carefully conducted screening programs, even more patients will be diagnosed with potentially curable disease.

Radical surgical extirpation of the cancerous prostate remains the time-honored therapy for cancerous lesions confined to the gland. The procedure includes the en bloc removal of the prostate, ejaculatory ducts, seminal vesicles, and the investing Denonvilliers' fascia. Ideally, the procedure also involves division of the vascular and lymphatic supply prior to manipulation of the gland.

HISTORICAL PERSPECTIVES

Kuchler described the technique for radical perineal prostatectomy in 1858.[1] This report was followed in 1903 by Young's performance of the first radical prostatectomy in this country.[2] Young's selection of patients was apparently not as sophisticated as the current process because most of his patients ultimately succumbed to metastatic disease. However, to date there have been few changes in the surgical technique that he described in 1903.

The perineal approach to radical prostatectomy remained popular until 1947, when Millin introduced the retropubic method.[3] Early interest in Millin's approach stemmed from the urologists' familiarity with retropubic anatomy. The addition of staging pelvic lymphadenectomy has added a new dimension to our surgical methods and serves to strengthen the use of the retropubic approach. McLaughlin feels that the concept of radical prostatectomy has been extended to include an extraperitoneal pelvic lymphadenectomy.[4] This conclusion is based on the fact that 35% of patients who are assumed to have clinical disease confined to the prostate will be found to have unsuspected lymph node metastases at the time of lymphadenectomy.[4]

Our method for radical retropubic prostatectomy is a modification of the technique as first described by Ansell and later advocated by Campbell.[5,6] Dissatisfaction with Millin's classic retropubic approach prompted the development of Campbell's technique, which emphasizes dissection of the prostate from the base to the apex. Campbell reported less local contamination and manipulation during removal of the prostate, with a resultant decreased chance of disseminating cancer cells.

A successful cancer operation includes three basic principles: proper selection of patients, removal of all malignant tissues with acceptable tumor-free margins, and tissue dissection performed in the proper sequence to minimize iatrogenic lymphatic and hematogenous dissemination. This technique fulfills the latter two criteria; the first premise must be fulfilled by careful presurgical evaluation. In addition to meeting the requirements for a good cancer operation, I feel this technique offers a number of distinct advantages over the classic perineal or retropubic approaches to prostatectomy.

This approach initially allows for a predictable anatomic dissection. Common to both the classic approach and Campbell's retropubic approach is the opportunity to perform a staging pelvic lymphadenectomy and the advantage of the urologist's knowledge of retropubic anatomy. With Campbell's approach, however, there is less time-consuming hemorrhage early in the procedure because division of the dorsal vein of the penis and periurethral venous plexus is one of the final steps. Placement of the urethral sutures under direct vision at the time of anastomosis decreases the chance of incontinence as well.

SELECTION AND EVALUATION OF PATIENTS

Radical surgical procedures employed to cure prostate cancer are based on the premise that all cancer cells reside in the tissue removed. Therefore, proper selection of patients is mandatory. The selection of patients with prostatic adenocarcinoma amenable to surgical excision has been outlined (see Chapter 15). The need for total prostatic excision is based on the study by Byar and Mostofi.[7] They found, after evaluation of step sections of 208 prostates removed for early carcinoma, that tumor was present in both posterior lobes in 80% of cases, that is was multifocal in 85%, and it was present in one of the first two apical step sections in 75% of cases.

The propensity for dissemination increases with the size of the neoplasm. McNeal has reported that dissemination is usually limited to tumors over 1 ml in volume.[8] Therefore, patients with clinical stage-B1 disease represent the ideal candidates for radical prostatectomy. We also perform radical prostatectomy in patients with stage-A2 disease who have negative results from staging lymphadenectomy. We have not found that the operation performed after transurethral resection is compromised. Patients with stage-B2 disease are not ideal candidates for radical prostatectomy because the propensity for lymph node involvement is high (14 to 45%).[4,9,10] In fact, many patients who have stage-B2 disease are found to have pathologic stage-C disease.[10] At this time, we do not advocate a radical surgical procedure for patients with stage-C or stage-D1 disease. However, studies are in progress to assess the value of combining radical prostatectomy with some form of hormonal manipulation.

Evaluation of the grade of the tumor is important because the higher-grade tumors appear as more advanced disease.[12] The candidate for radical prostatectomy should have a thorough radiologic and laboratory evaluation, in addition to a diligently performed physical examination. Tests to detect distant spread of the disease include a bone scan, intravenous pyelogram, chest roentgenogram, PSA, and acid phosphatase and alkaline phosphatase determinations. In addition, a cystoscopic examination is important in evaluating the urethra for strictures and the bladder for concomitant neoplasms.

The psychologic aspects of the operation, including impotence, must be discussed in detail with the patient and his spouse during the initial and preoperative visits. In our early series of 150 patients undergoing radical prostatectomy, 50% of patients did not engage in regular sexual activity and 50% of those who did desired a penile prosthesis after the surgical procedure. Modification of the surgical technique can preserve potency in up to 75% of the potent patients under 70 years of age with B1 disease.

ANATOMIC CONSIDERATIONS

Knowledge of the anatomic features of the prostate, including its blood vessels and fascia, is imperative for the success of this surgical procedure, yet urologists remain confused as to the exact nature of Denonvilliers' fascia, the endopelvic fascia, and the puboprostatic ligaments.

Endopelvic Fascia

STRUCTURE. The endopelvic fascia represents a condensation of the pelvic fascia and a continuation of the transversalis fascia as it enters the pelvis. At the arcus tendinous or white line, the pelvic fascia reflects medially off the obturator internus muscle. From this white line, one leaf of the fascia sweeps medially and thickens to form a sheath covering the anterior and lateral surfaces of the prostate. This condensation is known as the endopelvic fascia. The puboprostatic ligaments represent its anterior reflection from the pubic bone, which supports the gland and blends with the prostatic capsule. These paired ligamentous structures are avascular.

The endopelvic fascia fuses with Denonvillier's fascia at the posterolateral margin of the prostate. The anatomic importance of the endopelvic fascia lies not only in its support of the prostate, but also in the fact that it contains, beneath its lateral reflections, much of the vascular and lymphatic supply of the gland. The anterior and lateral reflections of the endopelvic fascia must be divided in the course of a radical prostatectomy. We prefer early ligation of the lateral reflections prior to any manipulation of the gland. Our approach is to treat these lateral reflections as anatomic pedicles and to ligate them as such.

Profuse bleeding occurring during the division of the prostatomembranous urethra is often mistakenly thought to rise from the puboprostatic ligaments. However, microscopic studies by Albers and associates show these ligaments to be composed mostly of collagen and variable amounts of smooth muscle.[13] The ligaments are attached to the inferior border of the pubis, lateral to the cartilaginous symphysis, and on the prostatic side they blend with the lateral leaves of the endopelvic fascia at the prostatovesical junction. Sharp division of the puboprostatic ligaments results in their retraction because of the smooth muscle component.

VENOUS DRAINAGE. A rich system of venous drainage is located in the recess between the puboprostatic ligaments and also on the lateral aspects of the prostate. Our approach to this highly vascular area involves a vertical incision in the endopelvic fascia, approximately 1 cm lateral to its reflection onto the prostatic surface (Fig. 18-1). This incision allows for development of a plane between the prostate and the rectum, and also prevents inadvertent injury to the lateral prostatic venous plexus. An incision made in close proximity to the prostate risks laceration of this lateral plexus.

The puboprostatic ligaments are divided sharply, to establish a connection between the superior aspect of the previous incision in the endopelvic fascia, to expose the superficial branch of the dorsal vein in the penis (Fig. 18-2). The superior vein trifurcates at the prostatomembranous urethral junction and should be dissected from the undersurface of the pubis to expose this trifurcation (Fig. 18-2). The superficial vein is ligated with 2-0 chromic ligature, and a plane is established

between the ventral surface of the urethra and the posterior surface of the dorsal vein. The dorsal vein is then ligated with a 2-0 chromic ligature.

The deep dorsal vein on the bladder side of the chromic ligature is divided sharply. To expose the prostatomembranous junction, it is necessary to carefully dissect the surface of the stump from the anterior surface of the urethra. Blood loss is minimized with this careful anatomic approach. However, a precise execution of this maneuver is not always possible, in which case the veins are transected sharply prior to division of the urethra.

Denonvillier's Fascia

Anatomic descriptions of the nature and confines of Denonvillier's fascia remain confusing. In addition, anatomists employ a number of terms to describe it, including "prostato-peritoneal membrane," "rectal fascia," "anterior and posterior layers of Denonvilliers," and "pearly gates." The excellent review by Tobin contains an in-depth evaluation of Denonvillier's fascia, its origin, and its surgical importance.[14] Clinically, Denonvillier's fascia is not only an important anatomic landmark in the surgical approach to the prostate and seminal vesicles, but also an effective barrier in preventing extensions of pus, extravasation of urine, and spread of malignant tumors of the prostate, seminal vesicles, and rectum.

STRUCTURE. Compressed between the posterior surface of the seminal vesicles, prostate, bladder, and the anterior rectal wall are three distinct layers. Overlying the ventral rectal surface and intermingled with the external longitudinal musculature is a layer of areolar and fatty rectal fascia known as the posterior layer of Denonvillier's fascia. The remnant of the peritoneal cul-de-sac in the fetus is located anterior to the rectal fascia (Fig. 18-3).[14] This layer is known as the anterior layer of Denonvillier's fascia or the prostatoperitoneal membrane, and is in the form of a "V."

The apex of the "V" is attached to the superior layer of the urogenital diaphragm at the inferior border of the prostate (Fig. 18-4). The two limbs of the "V" extend dorsolaterally to cover the posterior surface of the seminal vesicles. More importantly, where the ampullae join the prostate, this fibrous membrane fuses with the prostatic capsule. Therefore, an attempt to establish a plane anterior to this layer often results in the disruption of the prostatic capsule, with the resultant risk of entering the tumor or leaving an involved capsule behind.

Anterior to this layer is a framework of connective tissue that is continuous around the prostate and seminal vesicles. This framework is believed to blend with the anterior layer of Denonvillier's fascia. There is a difference of opinion about whether this layer is a branching of the anterior layer of Denonvillier's or a separate anatomic layer.[14] Regardless of its origin, it appears that upon reaching the tips of the seminal vesicles, this anterior layer splits, and one leaf passes caudally over the posterior surface of the seminal vesicles, vasa, and

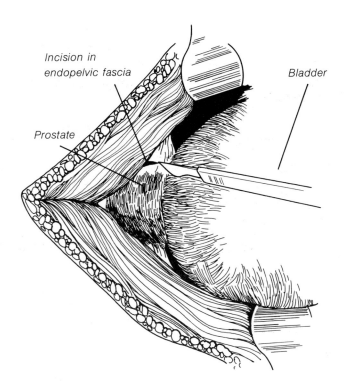

Incision in
endopelvic fascia

Prostate

Bladder

FIG. 18-1. Incision is made in the endopelvic fascia approximately 2 cm lateral to its reflection onto the prostatic surface.

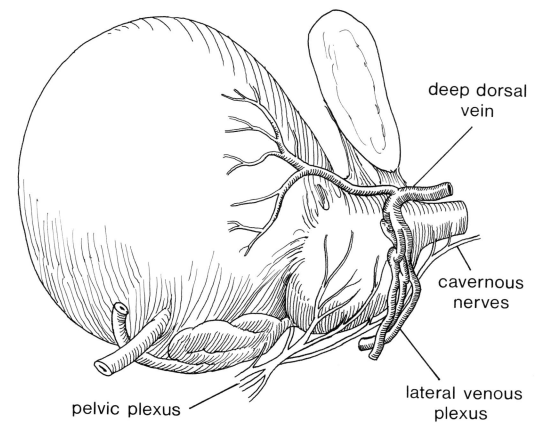

deep dorsal
vein

cavernous
nerves

lateral venous
plexus

pelvic plexus

Fig. 18-2. Anatomic depiction of deep dorsal vein and its tributaries behind the symphyses pubes and the cavernous nerves coursing posterolaterally close to the prostate and the membranous urethra.

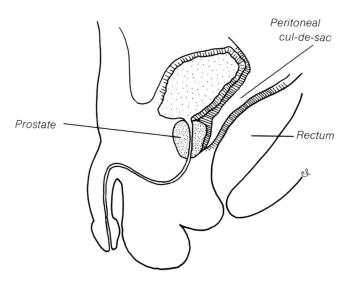

Peritoneal
cul-de-sac

Prostate

Rectum

Fig. 18-3. Median view from the pelvis of a full-term fetus demonstrating the peritoneal cul-de-sac extending between the seminal vesicles, prostate, and rectum.

prostatic capsule. It then extends to meet the anterior layer at the apex of the prostate.

The second leaf extends over the ventral surface of the seminal vesicles to the bladder base, where it reflects superiorly over the fundus of the bladder and then fuses with the first leaf. Between these leaves is located an anatomic compartment, which is the space entered when the prostate base, seminal vesicles, and vasa are freed from the bladder and rectum.

PLANES OF DISSECTION. The clinical importance of these three layers located between the rectum and prostate is obvious. There are three potential spaces that can be entered in an attempt to separate the prostate from the anterior rectal wall. One is between the longitudinal rectal musculature and the rectal fascia (posterior layer of Denonvillier's fascia). The second is between the rectal fascia and the prostatoperitoneal membrane (anterior layer of Denonvillier's fascia). The third is between the prostatoperitoneal membrane and the fibrous covering of the prostate and the seminal vesicles. The preferred plane is between the anterior and posterior layers of Denonvillier's fascia. This plane is also referred to as the posterior compartment of Denonvillier's fascia, or the space of Proust.

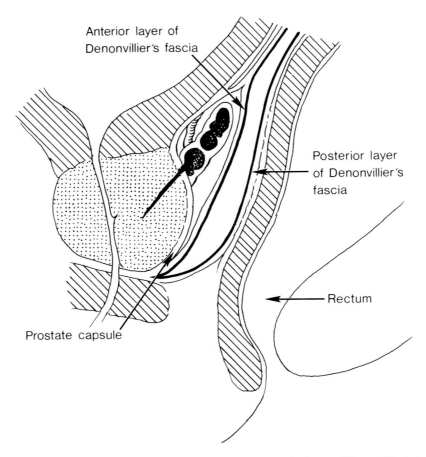

Anterior layer of
Denonvillier's fascia

Posterior layer
of Denonvillier's
fascia

Rectum

Prostate capsule

Fig. 18-4. Midline saggital view of the male pelvis showing the relationships between the layers of Denonvillier's fascia, rectum and prostate.

SURGICAL PROCEDURE

The evening prior to the operation, intravenous volume expanders are administered to ensure adequate hydration. A broad-spectrum antibiotic is given with the intravenous fluids. We have abandoned the routine employment of a bowel preparation. Mechanical preparation is employed consisting of cleansing enemas and ¼% neomycin retention enemas given at midnight and 6:00 A.M. Those not familiar with the procedure should employ a full bowel preparation in case of rectal injury.

The patient is placed in the supine position on the operating table. After adequate endotracheal anesthesia, the kidney rest is elevated under the lumbar spine area, providing slight hyperextension (Fig. 18-5). The entire abdomen, scrotum, penis, and inner thighs are prepared. The patient is draped in the usual manner with a sterile towel placed over the scrotum and under the penis. A sterile 22-French catheter is inserted and connected to a gravity drainage system. Another sterile towel is placed over the penis and preparation is made for the surgical incision.

Incision

A midline incision is made, beginning at the symphysis pubis and extending superiorly to the lateral side of the umbilicus

(Fig. 18-6). At this point, an electrocauterization unit is employed for the division of the subcutaneous tissues. The rectus fascia is identified and incised, the midline is identified, and the rectus muscles are retracted laterally. The layer immediately deep to the rectus muscles is the investing fascia of the rectus abdominis muscles, which is contiguous with the transversalis fascia (Fig. 18-7). This layer is entered sharply (expos-

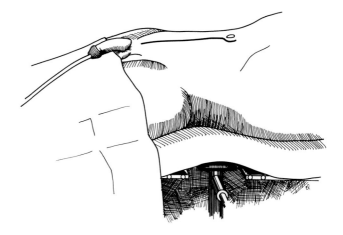

Fig. 18-5. Surgical position, demonstrating elevation of the kidney rest under the lumbar spine area, placement of urethral catheter, and proposed incision site.

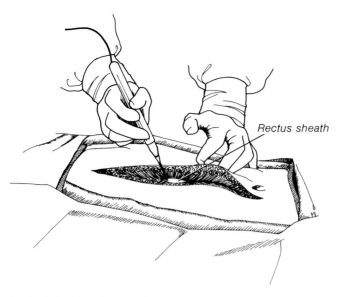

FIG. 18-6. Incision through subcutaneous tissues, exposing the rectus sheath.

ing the underlying retroperitoneal connective tissue), and dissection is carried inferiorly and laterally until the external iliac vessels are identified. Failure to remain deep to this plane often results in inadvertent injury to the inferior epigastric vessels and also creates difficulty in approaching the prostate and pelvic vessels.

The peritoneal reflection is identified, with the vas and spermatic vessels coursing in its medial aspect (Fig. 18-8). The spermatic vessels are dissected free and, with sharp dissection, the reflection is freed from the psoas muscle. The vas is sharply dissected free and divided between two medium-large Ligaclips (Fig. 18-9). The obliterated processus vaginalis will

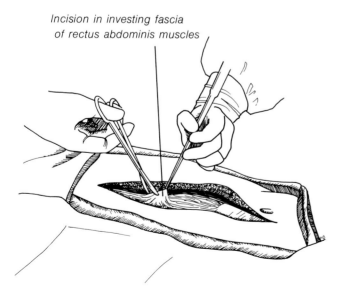

FIG. 18-7. The incision has been carried through the rectus fascia, and the rectus muscles have been retracted laterally. An incision is being made in the investing fascia of the rectus abdominis muscles, exposing the retroperitoneal connective tissue.

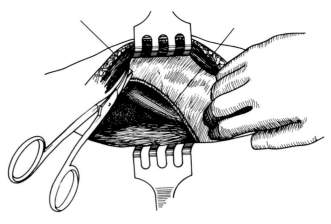

FIG. 18-8. Peritoneal reflection with the vas and spermatic vessels is identified, and an incision is made at the internal ring lateral to the spermatic vessels.

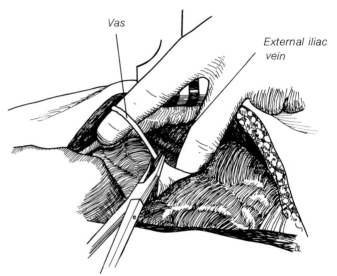

FIG. 18-9. The vas is divided between two medium-large Ligaclips.

be adherent to the internal ring and requires sharp dissection to mobilize the peritoneal reflection. This maneuver provides excellent exposure for the pelvic lymphadenectomy and prostatectomy.

TECHNIQUE

A bilateral pelvic lymphadenectomy is carried out as described in Chapter 16.

If the results of the frozen section analysis are negative for cancer, radical removal of the prostate is begun. The bladder is deflated and slight traction is placed on the urethral catheter.

The operator palpates the catheter balloon at the bladder neck and, with the other hand, makes a small incision with the electrocautery unit at the prostatovesical junction (Fig. 18-10). The cautery current is employed for the incision, and the superficial branch of the deep dorsal vein is usually encountered traversing the junction at the midline. The bladder is

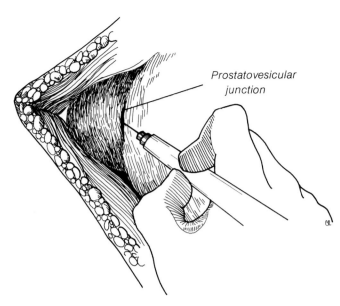

Fig. 18-10. Incision at the prostatovesical junction made with the electrocautery unit.

entered and the incision is carried laterally between the 3 and 9 o'clock positions. The catheter is removed from the bladder and advanced towards the symphysis pubis. The trigone and ureteral orifices are identified, and ureteral catheters are passed up each ureter. Indigo carmine may be injected intravenously to aid in the identification of the ureteral orifices. I rarely find this necessary.

The next step is the division of the trigonal floor from the prostate (Fig. 18-11). The first assistant places two fingers in the open bladder and provides cephalad traction. Two Allis clamps are placed on the lateral aspects of the bladder neck and are retracted laterally. This maneuver results in stretching of the junction of the trigone and prostate in a horizontal plane. Failure to execute this maneuver may result in a false plane leading into the thick posterior bladder wall and trigonal muscles. The incision should be approximately 2 cm in length and should be carried posteriorly until the ampullae of the vasa are visualized. There is little danger of injuring the rectum because the anterior compartment of Denonvillier's fascia with the vasa and seminal vesicles is interposed between the posterior bladder wall and the rectum (Fig. 18-4).

With Metzenbaum scissors, a plane is established over the anterior surface of the seminal vesicles and vasa (Fig. 18-12). The dissection will develop a pedicle containing the tissue between the initial and trigonal incisions. This pedicle is clamped and divided between Ligaclips. On the bladder side, it is important that the Ligaclips not be at the future anastomotic site since these may act as foreign bodies. The posterior bladder lip is dissected from the vasa and seminal vesicles with sharp dissection. The lip may be elevated with an Allis clamp, taking care not to apply excessive cephalad traction because the bladder musculature may tear easily.

The ampullae of the vasa are individually mobilized and clamped with Ligaclips (Fig. 18-13). The seminal vesicles are situated lateral to the ligated stumps. Further mobilization of the posterior bladder lip may be necessary to expose the tips of each seminal vesicle. Dissection under the posterior bladder lip must be performed with care because the ureters are in

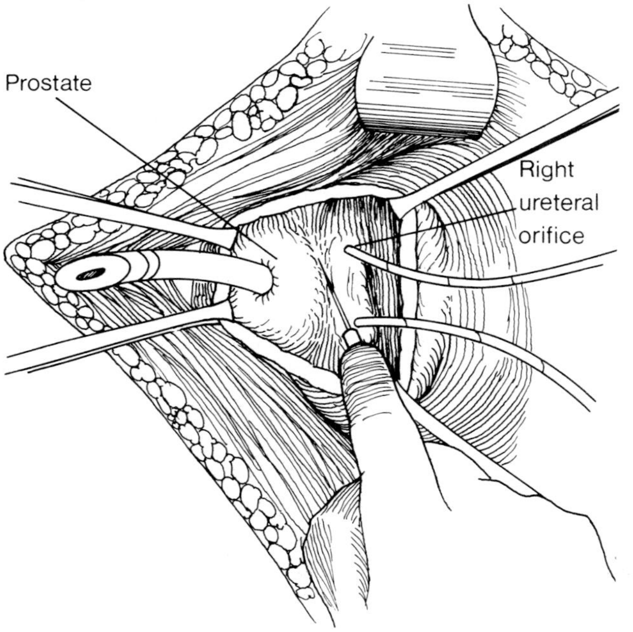

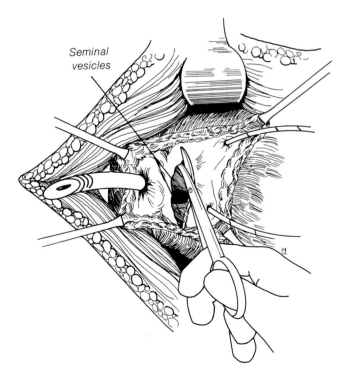

Fig. 18-11. Ureteral catheters are placed in both the ureteral orifices. Incision is made posteriorly in the trigone at the prostatovesical junction.

Fig. 18-12. The incision carried in a lateral direction, with Metzenbaum scissors establishing a plane over the anterior surface of the seminal vesicles and vasa.

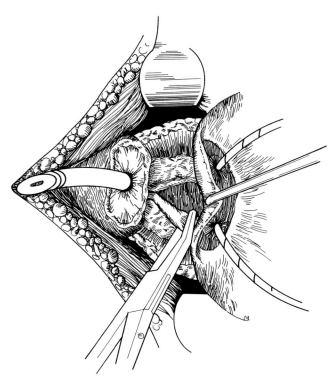

FIG. 18-13. The ampullae of the vasa are identified, dissected cranially, and divided between Ligaclips. The seminal vesicles are situated lateral to the ligated stumps.

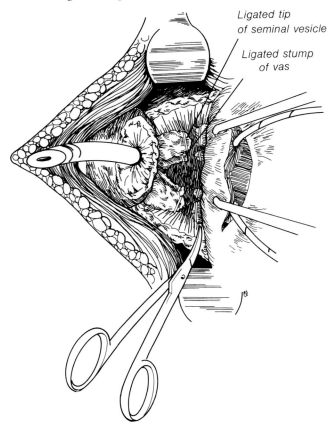

FIG. 18-14. Seminal vesicles and ampullae of the vasa have been divided. The dissection is carried dorsally, completely mobilizing the seminal vesicles and vasa from the rectum.

close proximity. The blood supply to the seminal vesicles enters the tip at the superior aspect; therefore, this area is carefully dissected and clipped (Fig. 18-14). The vascular supply is divided between the clips and the dissection is carried along the lateral and medial borders of each seminal vesicle until its attachment to the base of the prostate is identified. There is less blood loss and the removal is facilitated by dissecting deep to the areolar tissue surrounding the vasa and seminal vesicles.

The prostate is now free from the bladder and the seminal vesicles, and the vasa are free from the rectum. This maneuver has been performed within the anterior compartment of Denonvillier's fascia. The cranial portions of the lateral pedicles is carefully divided with Ligaclips (Fig. 18-15). The anterior layer of Denonvillier's fascia fuses with the prostatic capsule at the junction of the vasa with the prostate. Therefore, any attempt to proceed bluntly through this plane often results in laceration of the prostatic capsule with the resulting risk of tumor spill. The plane must be sharply entered proximal to the fusion with the prostatic capsule in order to proceed between the anterior and posterior layers of Denonvillier's fascia.

There are two ways to accomplish this. One can sharply enter the plane proximal to the point where the anterior layer fuses with the prostatic capsule, or one can proceed in a retrograde manner, freeing the rectum from the prostate and then dividing over the dissecting finger. I have found that it is easier to develop the plane in a retrograde manner. To accomplish this, a vertical incision is made in the endopelvic fascia approximately 1½ cm lateral to the prostate (Fig. 18-1). (This incision has been described in the section on the endopelvic fascia.)

With blunt finger dissection, a plane is established between the posterior surface of the prostate and the rectal wall. Superior and lateral to the plane will be the reflection of the en-

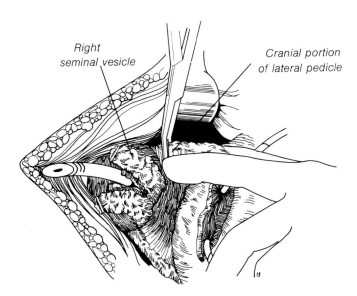

FIG. 18-15. Division of the cranial portion of the lateral pedicle of the prostate.

dopelvic fascia onto the prostate. The dissection is continued cranially and posteriorly to the fusion of the anterior layer of Denonvillier's fascia with the prostatic capsule. At this point, an incision is made over the dissecting finger. The prostate is now free from the anterior rectal wall. The lateral pedicle lying anterior to the index finger is held up with a small Penrose drain (Fig. 18-16).

Before dividing the lateral pedicles, it is advisable to use a sweeping motion with the index finger to further dissect the rectum from the lateral prostatic pedicles. Once these pedicles have been sufficiently dissected, they are ligated as far posteriorly as possible because they contain abundant lymphatic and vascular channels (Fig. 18-17). The dissection is carried caudally and connected with the previous incision in the endopelvic fascia. The only remaining attachments of the prostate are the urethra and the puboprostatic ligaments.

There should be minimal blood loss up to this point in the surgical procedure. Inadvertent injury to the lateral prostatic venous plexus during blunt dissection can be controlled with a laparotomy pack or a gauze sponge. The next step in the procedure is to fashion a new bladder neck in preparation for anastomosis to the urethra. The first assistant places his or her index finger in the bladder neck and elevates it superiorly (Fig. 18-18). The location of the ureteral orifices is noted and the bladder is closed vertically from the posterior region to the anterior region with interrupted 2-0 chromic catgut sutures. Care is taken to avoid the ureteral orifices in any of these sutures. The catheters are left in place for identification until the closure is complete. The bladder closure is continued anteri-

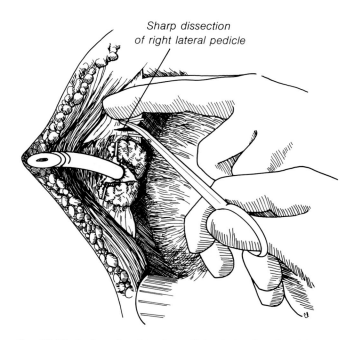

FIG. 18-17. A plane dorsal to the pedicles is developed and divided between Ligaclips.

orly until the opening fits snugly around the average index finger. If the opening is close to the ureteral orifices, we extend the incision through the anterior bladder wall. This ensures that the anastomotic stitches will be well away from the ureteral orifices. A second layer of running 2-0 chromic sutures is placed from the posterior to the anterior region. Again, extreme care must be exercised to avoid inadvertent suturing

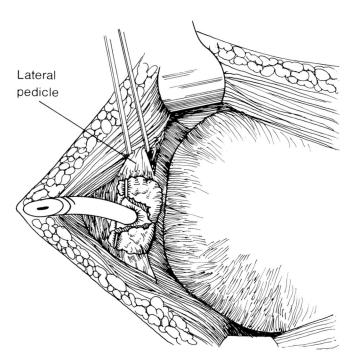

FIG. 18-16. A plane is established with blunt finger dissection between the dorsal surface of the prostate and the rectum. The lateral pedicle defined anterior to the finger is held up with a penrose drain.

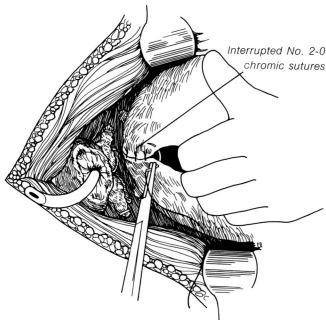

FIG. 18-18. The bladder neck is closed with interrupted 2-0 chromic sutures so that the final opening fits snugly around the average index finger.

of a ureteral orifice. A watertight closure is attained and the ureteral catheters are removed. The bladder mucosa of the new bladder neck is everted with 5-0 chromic sutures.

The puboprostatic ligaments are identified and an incision is made horizontally in the endopelvic fascia connecting the previous vertical incision to the puboprostatic ligaments. The ligaments are sharply divided and little bleeding is encountered because they are avascular structures. The venous system will be noted in the recess between the puboprostatic ligaments (see the section on endopelvic fascia). The dorsal vein trifurcates and is divided as outlined (Fig. 18-2).

There should be minimal bleeding. However, if troublesome hemorrhage arises, it can be controlled with fulguration or Ligaclips. An alternate method for controlling bleeding from the dorsal vein of the penis is to locate the vein at the base of the penis and ligate it. Aggressive attempts to control bleeding with Ligaclips or suture-ligatures frequently result in injury to the membranous urethra or the urogenital diaphragm. Therefore, the best course is to proceed rapidly with division of the urethra, which will control the bleeding.

The junction of the prostatic apex with the membranous urethra is palpated. The rectum should be completely free from the prostatic apex and membranous urethra before proceeding with division of the urethra. Any adherence may be bluntly dissected away with the index finger. Complete skeletonization of the membranous urethra should be avoided because the areolar tissues surrounding the urethra add strength to the subsequent anastomosis.

With a right-angled clamp under the membranous urethra, an incision is made anteriorly, exposing the catheter just distal to the prostatic apex (Fig. 18-19). We do not leave a section of

apical tissue on the urethral side. It is helpful to place the urethra on a mild stretch by applying traction posteriorly and cranially on the prostate. Once the urethra has been transected between the 11- and 1-o'clock positions, a full-thickness section of the urethra is transfixed at the 12-o'clock position with a 2-0 chromic catgut suture on a ⅝ in. circular needle (Fig. 18-20). This suture may be placed from inside out or from outside in. However, we find this first stitch is most easily placed by sliding the needle along the catheter into the urethra and out again. Because other sutures may be placed from outside in rather than from inside out, it is important to iden-

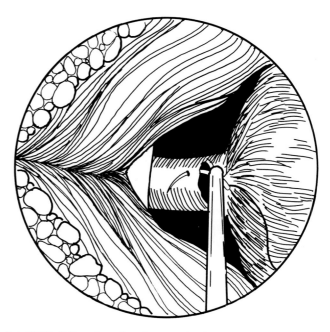

Fig. 18-20. Full section of urethra transfixed at the 12-o'clock position with a 2-0 chromic catgut suture.

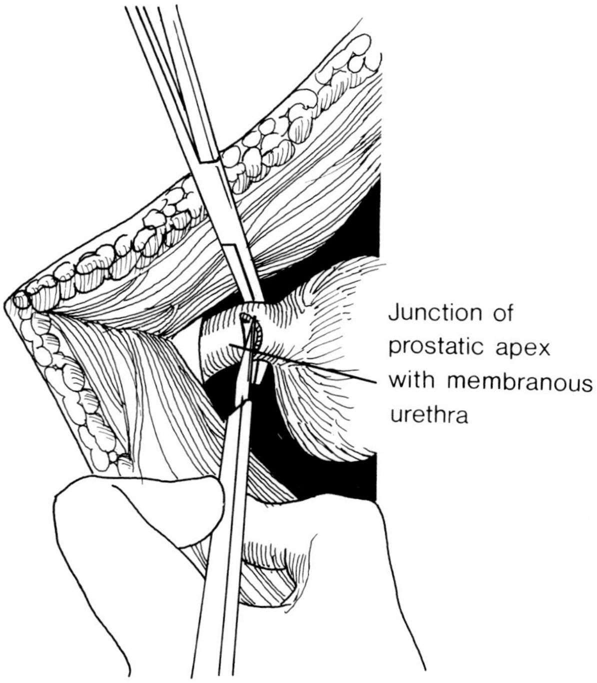

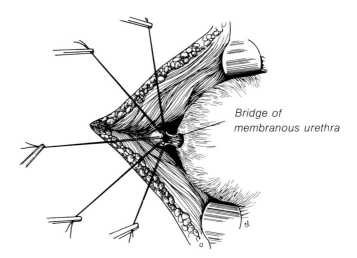

Fig. 18-19. An incision is made through the anterior circumference of the urethra lifted up by a right-angled clamp.

Junction of prostatic apex with membranous urethra

Bridge of membranous urethra

Fig. 18-21. Bridge of membranous urethra prior to final division and removal of the prostate.

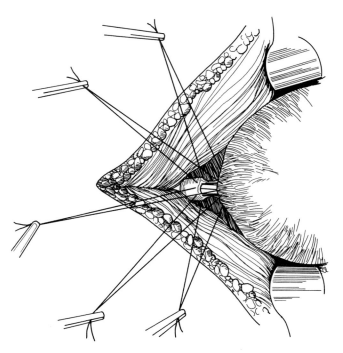

FIG. 18-22. All sutures have been placed through the bladder and are ready to tie.

tify which stitches will require placement of a tapered needle to complete the anastomosis with the bladder. We mark the sutures that will require a needle with a straight hemostat and the sutures placed from the outside in, which do not require placement of a needle with a Crile hemostat.

Approximately half of the circumference of the anterior urethra is sharply divided, and two more sutures are placed at the 2- and 10-o'clock positions. The urethra is further divided, and sutures are then placed at the 4- and 8-o'clock positions. The catheter is divided and removed from the urethra, leaving only the posterior portion of the membranous urethra intact (Fig. 18-21). At this time, one or two sutures are placed in the posterior position of the urethra and the remaining tissue is divided proximal to those sutures. These sutures should be placed prior to dividing the urethra because it will retract, making it difficult to identify.

Any remaining lateral attachments of the prostate are clamped and divided, and the specimen is removed from the operative field. Care must be taken to ensure proper orientation of the sutures. They should be arranged in the operative field in an orderly fashion so that they can be placed into the bladder neck in sequence.

CLOSURE

The bladder neck is placed in a position near the urethra, and the 6-o'clock suture is placed through the bladder opening. The 4- and 8-o'clock sutures are placed through the bladder neck. We find it helpful to cut the needle from each suture after it has been placed to avoid any confusion and to keep the sutures in proper order for later tying. A well-lubricated 22-French catheter with a 5 ml balloon is passed into the urethra and placed through the bladder neck. The balloon is inflated to 10 ml and left in position. The remaining sutures are placed, with the 12-o'clock suture being the final suture (Fig. 18-22). Those sutures that have been placed from inside out will require a tapered needle for proper placement. Gentle traction is placed on the catheter and the bladder neck is brought down to the urethra. The sutures are tied, beginning with the

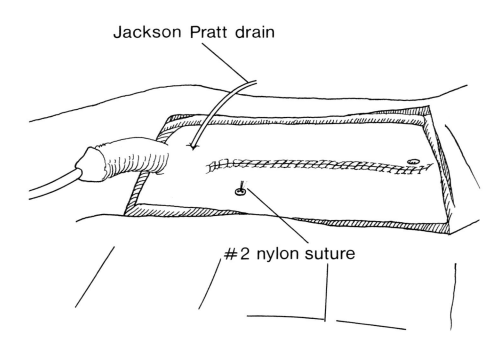

Jackson Pratt drain

#2 nylon suture

FIG. 18-23. Completed closure with the nylon "security stitch" anchoring the tip of the Foley catheter to the button on the abdominal wall.

6-o'clock stitch and with lateral alternation, until the 12-o'clock stitch is tied. At this point, the bladder is irrigated until clear. We have not found it necessary to place a suprapubic tube with this procedure.

A ½ in. Penrose or Jackson-Pratt drain is placed near the anastomotic site and brought through a separate stab wound, and the surgical incision is closed. If the rectus muscles have been divided from their tendinous insertion in the symphysis pubis, these are approximated. The rectus fascia is closed with figure-of-eight absorbable sutures, and the subcutaneous tissues are then reapproximated. The skin is closed in the usual fashion.

In addition to hemorrhage, the two major intraoperative problems that can occur are ureteral injury and rectal perforation. Major injuries to the ureter are best treated with a formal reimplantation. However, minor disruptions may be treated by leaving a ureteral catheter in place for 4 to 5 days postoperatively. An inadvertent rectal laceration may be closed primarily in two layers.[15] The rectum is dilated postoperatively and the patient is placed on a fast for 5 days. We perform a diverting colostomy in patients who have multiple or extensive rectal lacerations and in those who have had prior pelvic irradiation.

One major problem that can occur in the early postoperative period is rupture of the balloon, with subsequent removal of the catheter. We therefore place a "security stitch" by passing a No. 2 nylon suture through the catheter eye, the bladder, and the anterior abdominal wall, and secure it with a button to the skin (Fig. 18-23). The catheter is brought over the anterior abdominal wall and secured to mild traction for 48 hours. Because of the secure watertight anastomosis with this procedure, we do not use prolonged traction on the catheter.

NERVE-SPARING TECHNIQUE

The antegrade technique can be modified for potency preservation. The prostatic base, seminal vesicles, and ampullae of the vasa are dissected from the bladder neck. The vessels are dissected and ligated close to the prostatic capsule in order to preserve the neurovascular bundle (Fig. 18-24). The dissection then proceeds in an antegrade manner to the prostatourethral junction. Meticulous dissection of the plexus from the surface of the urethra is facilitated by the increased mobility of the gland. As described earlier, division of the dorsal vein and urethra at the conclusion of the procedure precludes troublesome hemorrhage early in the operation.

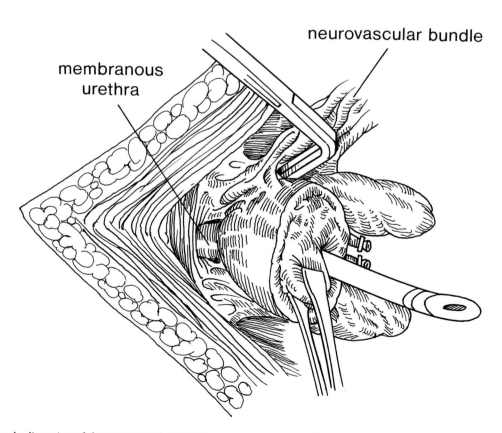

FIG. 18-24. Antegrade dissection of the neurovascular bundle in close proximity to the prostate.

Radical Retropubic Prostatectomy; Antegrade Approach / 191

POSTOPERATIVE MANAGEMENT

The patient may be observed in the surgical intensive care unit for 24 to 48 hours after the surgical procedure. It is important to carefully monitor the vital signs, including urinary output, and to ensure that no blood clots obstruct the catheter. In general, the urine remains clear throughout the postoperative recovery period. Because of the pelvic lymph node dissection, the majority of patients will experience a third-space fluid loss, requiring one unit of plasma protein fraction (Plasmanate) every 4 to 6 hours for the first 24 hours. The placement of a central venous pressure line in elderly patients, prior to the surgical procedure, is helpful in monitoring fluid replacement. The catheter is kept on mild traction over the anterior abdominal wall for 2 days and then released. A nasogastric tube connected to low suction is kept in place for approximately 36 hours or until the patient is passing flatus.

All patients are made ambulatory as soon as possible after the surgical procedure. The remainder of the postoperative care is common to all major surgical procedures. The catheter is left in place for 2 weeks. We begin advancing the drains as soon as the drainage ceases. The patient may be discharged on the fifth to seventh postoperative day, to return on the fourteenth day for removal of the catheter. Retrograde urethrogram is not routinely obtained unless the urethrovesical anastomosis has been difficult and urinary extravasation is suspected.

POSTOPERATIVE COMPLICATIONS

In our series of 350 consecutive patients undergoing this procedure for radical prostatectomy, there has been one postoperative mortality, 22 minor wound infections, 2 major dehiscenses requiring secondary closure, and 4 pulmonary emboli. With the routine intraoperative use of intermittent pneumatic compression stockings, the incidence of clinically evident deep venous thrombosis has been rather low. Those patients diagnosed as having this condition are treated with heparin as an anticoagulant. We do not employ low-dose heparin because it has not been proven effective in extensive pelvic operations and because its use increases the incidence of lymphoceles and hematuria.[16,17]

There was one rectal fistula in our series. Twenty patients developed what was thought to be excessive postoperative blood loss and required transfusions of 3 to 7 units of packed red blood cells. Postoperative stricture formation at the bladder outlet has been encountered in 4% of the patients. However, this has been an uncommon complication since we began everting the bladder mucosa. Osteitis pubis has not been observed in any patient. We have encountered one ureteral injury. The ureter was reimplanted.

There have been several unusual complications with the procedure. In one patient, symptoms of urinary obstruction occurred several months after the procedure. Upon cystoscopic examination, the patient was found to have a Ligaclip protruding into the urethra near the anastomosis. This was easily removed cystoscopically, but as a result, we have become aware of the fact that any Ligaclips in and about the anastomosis should be removed prior to finalizing the procedure. Three patients experienced anuria 24 hours after the procedure. Evaluation revealed this to be obstructive in origin, and it was thought to be secondary to edema of the ureteral orifices. Within 24 hours, the edema subsided and the patients had a normal postoperative course. Four postoperative lymphoceles occurred.

One of the more important functional results of the operation is postoperative urinary continence. In our series, 1.8% remained totally incontinent. Three cases followed a salvage prostatectomy after irradiation failure.

This technique for radical retropubic prostatectomy provides for a predictable and carefully anatomic prostatic removal. Once the anatomic planes and technique for the procedure are understood, the operative time for radical prostatectomy is between 1½ and 2 hours. Because of its anatomic design, the procedure is readily taught to the residents. The postoperative complications have been minimal and urinary incontinence has been negligible.

REFERENCES

1. KUCHLER, H. Uber prostatavergrosserungen. Deutsch. Klin., *18*:458, 1866.
2. YOUNG, H. H. The early diagnosis and radical cure of carcinoma of the prostate—Being a study of 40 cases and presentation of a radical operation which was carried out in four cases. Bull. Johns Hopkins Hosp., *16*:315, 1905.
3. MILLIN, T. *Retropubic Urinary Surgery.* Baltimore, Williams & Wilkins, 1947.
4. McLAUGHLIN, A. P., et al. Prostatic carcinoma: Incidence and location of unsuspected lymphatic metastases. J. Urol., *115*:89, 1976.
5. ANSELL, J. S. Radical transvesical prostatectomy: Preliminary report on an approach to surgical excision of localized prostatic malignancy. J. Urol., *83*:373, 1959.
6. CAMPBELL, E. W. Total prostatectomy with preliminary ligation of the vascular pedicles. J. Urol., *81*:464, 1959.
7. BYAR, D. P., and MOSTOFI, F. K. Carcinoma of the prostate: Prognostic evaluation of certain pathologic features in 208 radical prostatectomies. Cancer, *30*:5, 1972.
8. McNEAL, J. E. Origin and development of carcinoma in the prostate. Cancer, *23*:24, 1969.
9. RAY, G. R., et al. Operative staging of apparently localized adenocarcinoma of the prostate: Results in fifty unselected patients. Cancer, *38*:73, 1976.
10. WILSON, C. S., DAHL, D. S., and MIDDLETON, R. G. Pelvic lymphadenectomy for the staging of apparently localized prostatic cancer. J. Urol., *117*:197, 1977.
11. WALSH, P. C., and JEWETT, M. J. Radical surgery for prostatic cancer. Cancer, *45*:1906, 1980.
12. MURPHY, G. P., and WHITMORE, W. F., JR. A report of the workshops on the current status of the histologic grading of prostate cancer. Cancer, *44*:1895, 1979.

13. Albers, D. D., et al. Surgical anatomy of the pubovesical ligaments. J. Urol., *109:*388, 1973.

14. Tobin, C. E., and Benjamin, J. A. Anatomical and surgical restudy of Denonvillier's fascia. Surg. Gynecol. Obstet., *80:*373, 1945.

15. Goodwin, W. E. Complications of perineal prostatectomy. In *Complications of Urologic Surgery. Prevention and Management.* Edited by R. B. Smith and D. G. Skinner. Philadelphia, W. B. Saunders Co., 1976.

16. Catalona, W. J., Kadmon, D., and Crane, D. B. Effect of mini-dose heparin on lymphocele formation following extra-peritoneal pelvic lymphadenectomy. J. Urol., *123:*890, 1980.

17. Hindsley, J. P., Jr., et al. Mini-dose heparin therapy in pelvic lymphadenectomy and implantation for localized prostatic cancer. Urology, *15:*272, 1980.

CHAPTER
19

Total Perineal Prostatectomy

Joseph D. Schmidt

Total perineal prostatectomy (prostatoseminal-vesiculectomy) was first described for the treatment of prostatic cancer by Young in 1903.[1] Since that time, many of Young's disciples, among them Jewett and Culp, have made considerable contributions.[2–4] Much experience has also been amassed and reported by Belt, Schroeder, and Tomlinson and associates.[5–7]

RATIONALE

The advantages of performing total prostatectomy by the perineal route include excellent exposure for a direct vesicourethral anastomosis, better control of the vascular pedicles, a relatively short operating time, and decreased risk of cardiopulmonary complications, particularly in patients with concurrent disease in these areas. Most importantly, the procedure is ideal for the patient with the isolated prostatic nodule (clinical stage B1 or T1) in whom the incidence of pelvic lymph node involvement is 8 to 10%. Accurate staging by prior pelvic lymphadenectomy helps select those patients who will be best treated by extirpation of the primary cancer, i.e., patients with pathologic stages B1, B2, and C disease.

Disadvantages of the perineal route include the increased risk of prolonged urinary fistula or rectal injury, lack of expo-

sure for assessment of the regional lymph node status (unless prior lymphadenectomy is performed), and the need for the surgeon to have had special training in the surgical anatomy of the perineum.

The retropubic and perineal routes for prostatectomy can be combined in two ways. First, if the gross findings and frozen-section analysis reports at the time of pelvic lymphadenectomy indicate no evidence of regional nodal involvement, the retropubic incision can be closed and the patient turned to the exaggerated lithotomy position for concomitant total perineal prostatectomy. This combination utilizes the principles of the perineal approach for prostatectomy and allows the patient to undergo the entire procedure at one time. It may, however, be more time-consuming than the procedure done entirely by the retropubic route, and it does not eliminate the possibility of a false-negative report on the resected pelvic lymph nodes submitted for frozen-section analysis.

Alternatively, pelvic lymphadenectomy can be performed as a single procedure (first stage) and the patient returned to the operating room for a total perineal prostatectomy (second stage) 1 week or more later, depending on the permanent surgical pathologic report on the lymph nodes resected from the pelvis. This second combination is more costly and requires that the patient undergo anesthesia twice. On the other hand, because those patients who undergo total perineal prostatectomy after a negative staging pelvic lymphadenectomy are more carefully selected and often have less extensive local disease, the overall survival and disease-free survival rates after this procedure are relatively higher.

Subsequent to the nerve-sparing modifications of the retropubic prostatectomy by Walsh et al,[8–11] similar modifications of total perineal prostatectomy to maintain potency have appeared.[12,13] The common denominators for preservation of erectile function postprostatectomy appear to be (1) younger patients as surgical candidates and (2) small-volume, well-differentiated, and localized (organ-confined) prostate cancer enabling the urologist to adopt these nerve-sparing modifications.

SURGICAL PROCEDURE

The patient is placed in the exaggerated lithotomy position (Fig. 19-1). Adequate support and elevation of the hips and sacrum are afforded by folded sheets, blankets, or small pillows. The stirrups are manipulated cephalad and outward to open up the perineum.

Following preparation and draping of the skin, a modified rubber O'Conor rectal shield is sutured around the anal verge with interrupted 2-0 silk sutures (Fig. 19-2). The rectal shield allows for palpation of the prostate and manipulation of the anterior rectal wall as needed during the initial dissection and exposure. A curved Lowsley prostatic tractor is passed into the bladder, and the wings are opened fully, bringing the prostate closer to the perineum.

Incision

The curvilinear inverted U-incision is made between the ischial tuberosities and 2 to 3 cm anterior to the rectal shield margin. Sharp dissection is continued through the subcutaneous tissue and Colles' fascia. The ischiorectal fossae are developed first bluntly, then sharply down to the palpable tips of the Lowsley prostatic tractor wings. The central tendon of the perineum is divided sharply, and dissection continues outside or anterior to the anal sphincters (Fig. 19-3A).

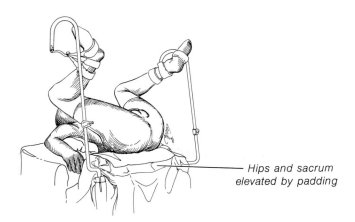

FIG. 19-1. Position for the operative procedure. The hips and sacrum are elevated by padding.

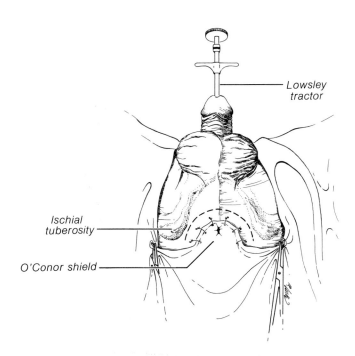

FIG. 19-2. O'Conor rectal shield is sutured in place. Lowsley prostatic tractor is passed into the bladder and the wings are opened fully, bringing the prostate closer to the perineum. Curvilinear U-incision is outlined.

The membranous urethra is easily located by palpation of the strut of the Lowsley tractor at the level of the urethral bulb. Careful rectal examination via the O'Conor shield will tent up the rectourethralis muscle attachments, which are divided sharply in a transverse direction (Fig. 19-3B). Partial lateral transection of the levator ani muscles is optional, depending upon exposure and the size of the prostate gland.

Technique

The posterior layer of Denonvillier's fascia (also known as the ventral rectal fascia) is incised transversely at the level of the distal prostate, either with a scalpel or with electrocautery (Fig. 19-4). The remainder of this layer is gently pushed posteriorly and cephalad, allowing placement of a padded Deaver retractor over the anterior rectal wall. This padded retractor protects the rectum throughout the remainder of the procedure. The base of the prostate is fully exposed, and the seminal vesicles can be palpated anterior to their fascial investments.

The distal leaf of the posterior layer of Denonvilliers' fascia is elevated, allowing exposure of the prostatic apex and proximal membranous urethra (Fig. 19-5). Using Metzenbaum scissors (standard or preferably a right-angled variety), the surgeon can dissect the urethra free from the prostatic apex and can thus better preserve it for later anastomosis to the bladder neck. The urethra is freed entirely with a right-angled clamp, entered sharply distal to the prostatic apex, and transected. The Lowsley tractor is closed and withdrawn; the straight Young prostatic tractor is placed through the prostatic urethra into the bladder, and the wings are fully expanded.

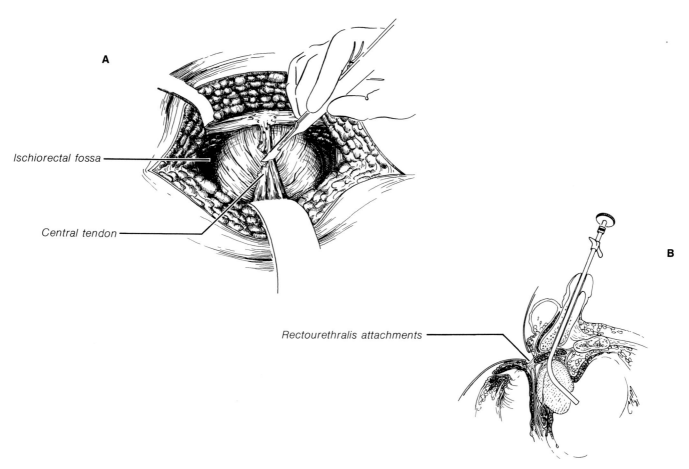

A

Ischiorectal fossa ——

Central tendon ——

B

Rectourethralis attachments ——

Fig. 19-3. *A*, Ischiorectal fossae are developed both bluntly and sharply down to the palpable tip of the Lowsley tractor. The central tendon of the perineum is sharply divided. *B*, Sagittal section identifies rectourethralis attachments that must be incised sharply to free the prostate from the rectum.

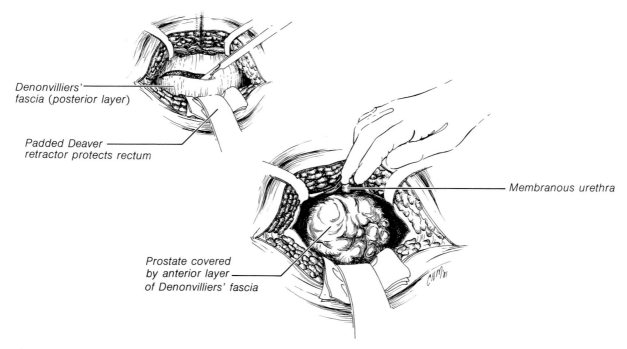

Denonvilliers' fascia (posterior layer) ——

Padded Deaver retractor protects rectum ——

Membranous urethra ——

Prostate covered by anterior layer of Denonvilliers' fascia ——

Fig. 19-4. The posterior layer of Denonvillier's fascia is incised and the urethra is identified.

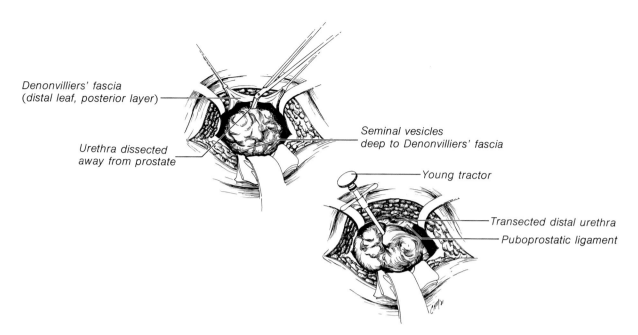

*Denonvilliers' fascia
(distal leaf, posterior layer)*

*Urethra dissected
away from prostate*

*Seminal vesicles
deep to Denonvilliers' fascia*

Young tractor

Transected distal urethra
Puboprostatic ligament

Fɪɢ. 19-5. The distal leaf of the posterior layer of Denonvillier's fascia is elevated, and the urethra is dissected free from the prostatic apex. The urethra is sharply divided and the Lowsley tractor is withdrawn. A straight Young prostatic tractor is placed, exposing the puboprostatic ligaments, which are divided.

Alternatively, the posterior layer at Denonvilliers' fascia (ventral rectal fascia) can be incised vertically in the midline from the prostatic base, then distally over the prostatomembranous urethral junction. This maneuver aids in avoiding the neurovascular bundles located posterolaterally as well as in allowing the clean dissection of the membranous urethra inside fascial planes, thus reducing the chance of injury to the adjacent cavernous nerves.

The anterior surface of the prostate can now be dissected bluntly to the level of the puboprostatic ligaments and vesicoprostatic junction. Control of the puboprostatic ligaments is best afforded by the use of large hemoclips and coagulation. Attempts to place hemostatic sutures often fail. Control of these structures allows good exposure of the anterior surface of the bladder, identification of which is made easier by gentle rotation of the Young prostatic tractor.

At this point, the prostatic substance can be literally peeled away from and off the funnelling bladder and bladder neck fibers by a combination of sharp and blunt dissection (Fig. 19-6). This maneuver should be continued at least until the urothelium at the bladder neck is identified, completely encircled, and divided, leaving only the posterior attachments of the prostate intact.

If needed for retraction, a Penrose drain can be inserted across the prostatic urethra and the straight Young prostatic tractor removed. The bladder neck and bladder are swept cephalad with a sponge stick, exposing the anterior investing fascia over the seminal vesicles (Fig. 19-7). The bladder neck, if intact, will remain continent until stretched or otherwise manipulated. A search for the ureteral orifices generally is not needed; instead, 5 ml of indigo carmine are administered intra-

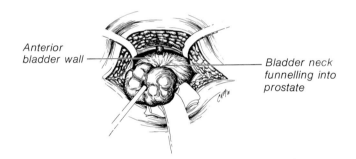

*Anterior
bladder wall*

*Bladder neck
funnelling into
prostate*

Fɪɢ. 19-6. The bladder neck is exposed after division of the puboprostatic ligaments.

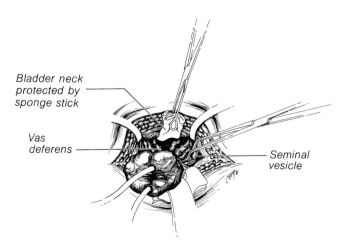

*Bladder neck
protected by
sponge stick*

*Vas
deferens*

*Seminal
vesicle*

Fɪɢ. 19-7. The seminal vesicles are exposed by sweeping the bladder neck cephalad.

venously at this point for later identification of an intact trigone and bladder neck.

The midline is entered sharply between the vasa deferentia and the seminal vesicles. Each vas deferens is exposed and isolated individually, and divided between hemoclips (Fig. 19-8). The fascia over the seminal vesicles is entered sharply as cephalad as possible, and the vascular pedicles are identified and controlled with hemoclips. Again, in an attempt to avoid injury to the neurovascular bundles and thus to maintain potency, the lateral vascular pedicles at the prostatic base should be divided as close to the prostate as possible. A wider, more lateral dissection and division of the pedicle may be required on the side of the obvious tumor. Because there should be no back-bleeding from the prostate at this point in the procedure, hemoclips are required only on the proximal portions of the vascular pedicles. The surgical specimen is removed.

Either an Emmett-type of Foley catheter (22 or 25 French) or a standard 30-ml balloon Foley catheter (22 or 24 French) is passed through the urethra to the level of the transected membranous urethra (Fig. 19-9). The continent, intact bladder neck is brought down with the help of Allis forceps. Direct anastomosis is carried out, with interrupted No. 0 or 2-0 chromic catgut sutures on a ⅝ curved needle, beginning anteriorly at the 12-o'clock position. Suturing is performed by bilateral advancement; all knots are tied outside the urinary tract.

Each suture is cut after being tied to avoid later confusion. An assistant's sliding of the urethral catheter in and out of the membranous urethra allows the surgeon to place the sutures

accurately. Each suture is passed in full-thickness fashion through the bladder neck and includes some adjacent Denonvillier's fascia and perineal striated muscle on the urethral side for improved support. Should a nerve-sparing modified prostatectomy be attempted, the sutures distally should include only the urethral wall and not the adjacent Denonvillier's fascia and skeletal muscle. This maneuver may avoid inadvertent injury to the cavernous nerves. Suturing of the anastomosis continues and ends posteriorly at the six-o'clock position, by which time a total of six to eight sutures has been required. In addition, at this point, the urethral catheter will slide directly into the bladder.

Reconstruction of the bladder neck, if needed, can be easily accomplished on the posterior aspect of that structure, eliminating trigonal injury, before the anastomotic sutures are placed. A conventional "tennis racket" repair (handle placed posteriorly, racket face anteriorly) is recommended for such a reconstruction if the bladder neck is too large for direct anastomosis. The catheter is irrigated to determine if the anastomosis is watertight (Fig. 19-10). Additional sutures can be placed as needed.

Thereafter, the catheter balloon is inflated to 30 ml, and is brought down snugly to the bladder neck. The wound is re-examined for hemostasis, and the anterior rectal wall is inspected to be sure that it is intact. Nonabsorbable sutures can be placed at this time if there is any indication of disruption of the rectal wall. A Penrose drain is placed down to the anastomosis and is brought out through a corner of the wound, where it is sutured to the skin with a 2-0 or 3-0 silk suture.

Closure

Wound closure is simple and rapid and requires interrupted 2-0 or No. 0 chromic catgut sutures for Colles' fascia, 3-0 or 4-0 chromic catgut sutures for the subcutaneous layers as needed, and interrupted 2-0 or 3-0 chromic catgut sutures for the skin layer. The O'Conor shield and its silk sutures are removed, and a modified compression dressing is placed over the wound. The patient's legs are carefully and slowly lowered. The urethral catheter is secured to the patient's abdomen and attached to straight drainage, with a side arm for intermittent irrigation as needed. The catheter is not generally sutured to the glans penis.

POSTOPERATIVE CARE AND COURSE

Because of the excellent hemostasis and good dependent drainage afforded by the perineal exposure, only rarely will a patient require observation in the intensive care unit after he leaves the recovery room. The need for catheter irrigation for bleeding and clots is unusual. Intravenous hydration is continued for 24 to 48 hours until the patient can assume full oral intake. There should be little paralytic ileus following the perineal procedure unless a pelvic lymphadenectomy has been performed concomitantly; then, as in other abdominal procedures, the patient is given nothing by mouth until normal in-

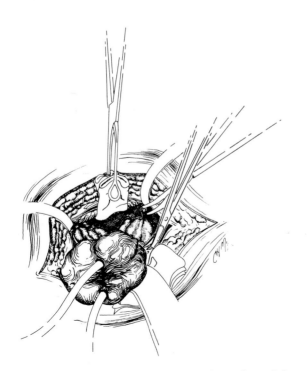

FIG. 19-8. The vasa, seminal vesicles, and lateral vascular pedicles are divided, and the specimen is removed.

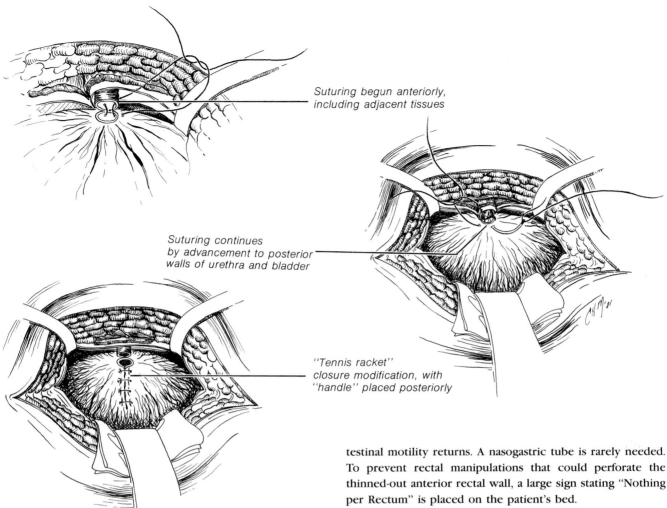

Suturing begun anteriorly, including adjacent tissues

Suturing continues by advancement to posterior walls of urethra and bladder

"Tennis racket" closure modification, with "handle" placed posteriorly

FIG. 19-9. Methods of vesicourethral anastomosis.

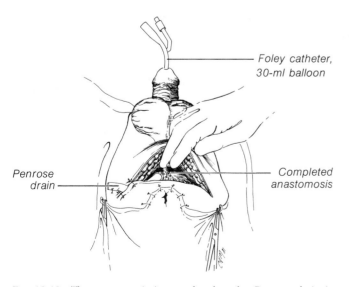

Foley catheter, 30-ml balloon

Penrose drain

Completed anastomosis

FIG. 19-10. The anastomosis is completed, and a Penrose drain is brought out the lateral aspect of the incision.

testinal motility returns. A nasogastric tube is rarely needed. To prevent rectal manipulations that could perforate the thinned-out anterior rectal wall, a large sign stating "Nothing per Rectum" is placed on the patient's bed.

The patient is allowed limited activity out of bed the day following the operation if his vital signs are stable and if there is no indication of bleeding. The dressing placed at operation is changed 24 to 48 hours following the procedure and thereafter as needed, according to the quantity of drainage from the Penrose drain. The drain is not manipulated until the fifth to seventh day, at which time it is removed. Because the perineal wound has been closed with absorbable chromic sutures, removal of sutures is rarely needed. The nursing staff and patient are instructed to cleanse the wound with soap and water and hydrogen peroxide and to apply a clean dressing after defecation.

The indwelling urethral catheter remains in place for a minimum of 3 weeks; this period may be longer if a perineal urinary fistula develops. Unless there has been complete disruption of the vesicourethral anastomosis, all perineal urinary fistulas will heal with continued urethral catheter drainage. The patient may be discharged from the hospital any time after the seventh day, to return later for removal of the urethral catheter and a voiding trial. Should there be any question of a perineal urinary fistula, either an indigo carmine test or a gravity retrograde cystogram is indicated. If results of either test are positive, the urethral catheter is left indwelling for a minimum of another week or until the test results are normal.

At the time of the voiding trial, each patient is instructed to expect some degree of urinary incontinence, whether it be due to stress, urgency, true incontinence, or some combination of these. Pharmacologic manipulations are postponed as long as possible to allow each patient to acquire urinary control on his own. Patients are instructed in perineal isometric exercises, as well as in voluntary interruption of the voided urinary stream.

If drug enhancement of the urinary sphincters is required, a combination of propantheline bromide (Pro-Banthine) 15 mg, three to four times daily or methantheline bromide (Banthine) 25 to 50 mg, three to four times daily and ephedrine sulfate 25 mg, three to four times daily is administered until urinary control is achieved. A minimum trial period of 6 months is required before any long-term pronouncements are made regarding the final degree of urinary control.

General physical activity is limited for the first 2 to 3 months postoperatively until the element of stress causing urinary incontinence has been eliminated. Counseling on the subject of penile prostheses for impotence is resumed 8 to 12 months following the operation unless spontaneous erectile activity has returned. Regular follow-up for prostatic cancer (both for local recurrence and for metastatic disease) is instituted at the first 3-month visit and continues as in any course of definitive therapy for localized prostatic cancer.

REFERENCES

1. YOUNG, H. H. The early diagnosis and radical cure of carcinoma of the prostate. Bull. Johns Hopkins Hosp., *16*:315, 1903.
2. JEWETT, H. J. The case for radical perineal prostatectomy. J. Urol., *103*:195, 1970.
3. CULP, O. S. Radical perineal prostatectomy: Its past, present and possible future. J. Urol., *98*:618, 1968.
4. JEWETT, H. J. The present status of radical prostatectomy for stages A and B prostatic cancer. Urol. Clin. North Am., *2*:105, 1975.
5. BELT, E. Radical perineal prostatectomy in early carcinoma of the prostate. J. Urol., *48*:287, 1942.
6. SCHROEDER, F. H., and BELT, E. Carcinoma of the prostate: A study of 213 patients with stage C tumors treated by total perineal prostatectomy. J. Urol., *114*:257, 1975.
7. TOMLINSON, R. L., CURRIE, D. P., and BOYCE, W. H. Radical prostatectomy: Palliation for stage C carcinoma of the prostate. J. Urol., *117*:85, 1977.
8. WALSH, P. C., and DONKER, P. J. Impotence following radical prostatectomy: Insight into etiology and prevention. J. Urol., *128*:492, 1982.
9. WALSH, P. C., LEPOR, H., and EGGLESTON, J. C. Radical prostatectomy with preservation of sexual function: Anatomical and pathological considerations. Prostate, *4*:473, 1983.
10. WALSH, P. C., and MOSTWIN, J. L. Radical prostatectomy and cystoprostatectomy with preservation of potency: Results using a new nerve-sparing technique. Br. J. Urol., *56*:694, 1984.
11. WALSH, P. C. Radical retropubic prostatectomy. In: *Campbell's Urology.* 5th ed. Vol. 3. Edited by P. C. Walsh, R. F. Gittes, A. D. Perlmutter, and T. A. Stamey. Philadelphia, W.B. Saunders Co., 1986, pp. 2765–2775.
12. WEISS, J. P., SCHLECKER, B. A., WEIN, A. J., and HANNO, P. M. Preservation of periprostatic autonomic nerves during total perineal prostatectomy by intrafascial dissection. Urology, *26*:160, 1985.
13. WELDON, V. E., and TAVEL, F. R. Potency-sparing radical perineal prostatectomy: Anatomy, surgical technique and initial results. J. Urol., *140*:559, 1988.

C H A P T E R
20

Interstitial Brachytherapy for Prostatic Carcinoma

Joseph T. Spaulding

Interstitial brachytherapy is a term used to describe the tissue implantation of radiotherapeutic sources. Brachy- is derived from the Greek root meaning short, and emphasizes the placement of the radioactive material *close* to the target tumor. This term distinguishes this method from teletherapy, the use of radioactive sources *far* from the tumor, such as external beam irradiation.

The interstitial placement of sources is not a new concept, either in radiotherapy or, more pertinently, in the management of prostatic cancer. Brachytherapy was first suggested in 1901 by Pierre Curie, 2 years before he and his wife Marie shared the Nobel Prize in physics with Antoine Henri Becquerel for the experiments that led to the discovery of radium.[1] At first, cumbersome tubes of radium were inserted into the tumor and then removed after an interval. Shortly thereafter, radium sulfate was incorporated into steel or platinum to form radium needles. Janeway, at Memorial Hospital in New York, developed a method in which radon gas was collected into small glass tubes, which were then left in tumors for an indefinite period of time, taking advantage of radon-222's short half-life.[2] The Memorial Hospital experience with these latter sources was reported in 1917.[3] The beta radiation from these radium-derived sources led to an intensive tissue necrosis. This was successfully filtered by Failla, who encapsulated the radon gas in gold capillary tubes, creating the first "gold seeds".[4,5] This term was a careless misnomer, not to be confused with gold-198, in common use today.

A set of rules for the distribution of sources within a tumor was developed in Manchester in the early 1930's, and helped therapists to deliver a uniform tumor dose.[6] Quimby, in New York, popularized a system of rules and tables from which the minimum dose on the surface of an implant, within which the sources are uniformly spaced, is derived.[7,8]

Despite good clinical results, enthusiasm for brachytherapy waned in the late 1940's because of concerns regarding radiation exposure, difficulties with source availability and manufacture, the tedious dose calculations required, and most importantly, the development of external beam teletherapy. Interest in brachytherapy resurged about a decade later, however, with the development of new radioactive sources and the computerization of dosimetry calculations.[9]

BRACHYTHERAPY FOR PROSTATE CANCER

Brachytherapy for prostatic carcinoma did not lag behind this evolution in interstitial therapy as a whole, but mirrored it. In 1909, Pasteau and Degrais were the first clinicians to attempt "close therapy" for cancer of the prostate by utilizing an intra-urethral radium capsule.[10] Barringer, at Memorial Hospital in 1915, described a transperineal technique of radium needle implantation in the prostate.[11] In 1941, he reported on two long-term survivors of the procedure who were disease free 6 and 7 years later.[12]

Early orthovoltage teletherapy supplanted interstitial treatment of prostate cancer, as it was a technique more widely available, but the use of radiotherapy for this condition fell into disfavor because of appreciable bladder and rectal toxicity. Simultaneously, the impressive report in 1941 by Huggins and Hodges of disease regression in response to hormonal maneuvers appeared.[13]

Rubin Flocks and coworkers, in 1951, began to inject radioactive colloidal gold into the prostate and involved nodes, later combining similar injections into the surgical bed with radical prostatectomy and aggressive local fulguration in the management of extensive extracapsular disease.[14] Despite the difficulty in documenting local failure after such intensive focal therapy, his 4% local failure rate after the combined treatment was distinctly lower than that commonly reported after surgery alone, in stage-C disease (25 to 30%).

As the solely palliative value of hormonal manipulation in prostatic carcinoma was becoming evident, Del Gato,[15] George,[16] and particularly Bagshaw[17] were generating impressive reports of supervoltage teletherapy with decreased pelvic toxicity, excellent clinical local control rates, and encouraging early survival figures. Pelvic lymphadenectomy preliminary to external beam radiotherapy or radical prostatectomy was incorporated in treatment plans with the growing awareness of the prognostic impact of nodal status. Evidence of long-term survival in patients with prostate cancer treated by external beam radiotherapy, autopsy documentation of eradication of the cancer in some cases so treated, the potential advantages of interstitial therapy in terms of treatment-related morbidity (incontinence, impotency, and proctitis) compared to either surgery or teletherapy, and a desire to expand the role of the surgeon beyond the most limited disease extent, led to the reintroduction of interstitial brachytherapy for prostatic carcinoma.

Carlton et al., in 1965, began a protocol in which prostatic carcinoma was implanted with gold-198 and supplemented with external beam irradiation.[18] Starting in 1970, Whitmore et el. placed iodine-125 seeds into localized prostatic carcinoma and to date has so treated over 1000 patients at Memorial Hospital in New York.[19] Both centers employed open exposure of the prostate after extraperitoneal pelvic lymphadenectomy. Many others have adopted these protocols without significant modification.

The next evolution in prostatic cancer brachytherapy was the use of temporary implants, with afterloading of sources following the transperineal template-guided introduction of hollow needles. As popularized by Syed et al., an isotope (iridium-192) with a slightly higher energy and a much longer half-life compared to radioactive gold was selected for this adaptation, which included pelvic node dissection and supplemental external beam treatment.[20] This trial was prompted by a dissatisfaction with the manual retropubic placement of these needles and a resultant inconsistency of implant quality. The depth of the transperineal needle insertion, particularly at the bladder base, was monitored through a retropubic exposure.

The most recent development in brachytherapy for prostatic carcinoma has been the use of transrectal ultrasound to monitor the template-guided positioning of the carrier needles and the placement of the sources. Holm et al. first introduced this application of ultrasound, and combined pelvioscopic examination of the pelvic nodes ipsilateral to the palpable tumor, thereby avoiding open lymphadenectomy.[21] In this country, this technique of brachytherapy is currently performed without any invasive lymph node evaluation, often on an outpatient or short-stay basis, with iodine-125 and, more recently, with palladium-103 as the implanted sources.[22] Although the initial reports are too preliminary for evaluation of the results of these modifications, the dosimetry curves and the gross symmetry of the implants are impressive.

ADVANTAGES OF BRACHYTHERAPY

Brachytherapy occupies a secure position in the radiotherapeutic management of cancer and is felt by many experienced therapists to be the ideal form of treatment whenever applicable. An implant can be custom tailored to an irregular target and the tumor localization is, of course, much more precise. A higher total-tumor dose can be delivered with an implant than by external beam therapy, while the surrounding tissues receive substantially less radiation and realize minimal acute complications and late damage. The high tumor doses are well tolerated because the volume irradiated is relatively small and closely approximates the tumor. This is compared to external beam treatment, where the irradiated volume includes all the tissue between the beam and the target.

For prostatic therapy, this may involve an eight- to twenty-fold difference in volumes receiving 50% of minimum tumor dose.[23] A linear accelerator with a 360° rotational technique will deliver the planned dose in about 6 weeks, and the rectum and bladder will receive 65 to 70% of the maximum dose delivered. With an interstitial implant of iodine-125, the dose will be delivered over the course of about a year and the bladder and rectal dose is only 30 to 40% of the minimal peripheral dose, with a much higher ration centrally. Tumor dose means *maximum* tumor dose for external beam treatment, while for brachytherapy, it designates the *minimum* tumor dose, that is, the dose at the periphery of the target.

DISADVANTAGES OF BRACHYTHERAPY

Interstitial radiotherapy involves a minor surgical procedure, requires a special technical expertise not universally available, and presents a radiation risk to all those involved in the treatment. Local failure because of radioresistant clones or underdosed "cold spots" is always a concern despite the high tumor doses attainable. And with these high-dose applications comes the risk of late radiation damage. Recent comparative experience of implant and external beam therapy in early stage prostatic carcinoma suggests that with equivalent tumor-free survival and excellent local control rates, come fewer and less severe side effects for brachytherapy patients.[24] Larger tumors with poorly defined margins are not so effectively treated. Compared to external radiotherapy, the regional lymphatics are never irradiated by the implant.

RADIOBIOLOGY OF BRACHYTHERAPY

The unique characteristics of brachytherapy that distinguish it from teletherapy are the *continuous* nature of the radiation and, depending on the source, the relatively *low dose rate* of emission. For cell death, a certain number of hits must be recorded during the cell cycle. Cells in the M and late G2 phases of the cell cycle are more radiosensitive, while S-phase cells are relatively radioresistant. Unless the target cells are exposed to sufficient irradiation per cell cycle, cell death will not exceed new cell formation, and the shorter the interval between treatment fractions, the less time for repair of sublethal cell damage. With continuous emission and an essentially infinite number of treatment fractions, treatment success would depend less on cell cycle duration than with fractionated telebeam therapy.

Continuous therapy is associated with a relatively rapid reduction in tumor volume, which sustains the initial dose rate as the individual sources approach closer with target shrinkage. In fact, a substantial portion of the tumor may be exposed to an increased dose rate (20%) as a result of this feature.

There is a therapeutic advantage realized with low dose rate emission, which is expressed as improved recovery of normal tissues from sublethal damage relative to target tumor cells. This concept is based on a comparison of tolerance studies of normal skin with lethal dose observations in skin cancer.[25]

The low rate of energy release characteristic of many implant isotopes does offer, in vitro, a better rate of hypoxic cell kill that is comparable to that seen with neutron beam therapy.[26] This may be an important clinical feature because telebeam treatment failure is often ascribed to the persistence and proliferation of a relatively radioresistant central tumor mass that is hypoxic, but not so hypoxic that repair of sublethal damage is inhibited.

As a rule, reduction in the dose rate results in reduced cell kill, yet the magnitude of this effect depends on the ability of the individual cell line to recover from the injury. The length of the individual cell cycle seems to impact the minimum effective dose rate. As the rate of energy release decreases from values above 200 cGy/hr, the target cell survival rate increases as the cells repair sublethal damage. With intermediate dose rates (10 to 100 cGy/hr), cell survival actually *decreases* as the dose rate initially declines, presumably the result of cell redistribution into radiosensitive phases of the cell cycle. Continued decrements in dose rate lead to less impact on cell sur-

vival; target cell proliferation begins to assert itself, and the tumor may actually grow, although at an impaired rate.

Recent radiobiologic studies have documented in vitro ineffectiveness of iodine-125 (low dose rate) implants in rapidly growing targets.[27] Mitchell was able to demonstrate that cells would accumulate in a radiosensitive (G2) phase of the cell cycle in response to a low dose rate range unless the rate was too low.[28] At that point, the cells would escape redistribution and cell division outstripped cell death. This implies that the selection of a specific implant isotope should be correlated with the tumor grade. Consistent with these laboratory observations, considerable clinical experience is accumulating that suggests that iodine-125, a very low dose rate isotope (~8 cGy/hr), is ineffective for moderate and high-grade prostate tumors, which manifest this insensitivity as a substantial rate of local failure.[29,30]

CURRENT BRACHYTHERAPEUTIC RADIONUCLIDES

Currently, implantation of prostatic carcinoma revolves around the use of four radioisotopes: gold-198, iodine-125, iridium-192, and palladium-103. Each source can be described in terms of half-life, dose rate, spectrum of radiation, and radiation strength (see Table 20-1). A long half-life is a practical attribute that allows the radioactive source to be usable for long periods of time. Gold-198 seeds decay so rapidly ($T\frac{1}{2} = 2.7$ d) that there is essentially no shelf life and unused seeds must be discarded. If utilized in a temporary implant, long half-life sources can be reused, a clear economic benefit. Conversely, a source with a long half-life may pose radioprotection problems for the patient and his family. At the time of implantation, the dose emitting from a source with a long half-life is, however, much less than that given off by a short half-life isotope, implanted to provide the same biologic effect.

The spectrum of energy presented by brachytherapy isotopes in common use may include alpha, beta, and gamma radiation. The encapsulation of the source filters all or nearly all of the alpha radiation and as much as possible of any beta energy as well. This reduces the common isotopes used in modern brachytherapy to sources of gamma radiation of distinct ranges of radiation strength that may be matched to the specific characteristics of the individual implant.

Gold-198 seeds are easily produced and inexpensive. The isotope has a short half-life (2.7 d) and a moderate gamma energy strength (0.41 MeV). With the resultant high dose rate, the effective range of radiation (half-value layer in tissue) of each source is approximately 4.5 cm and a given implant volume may require only a few sources (e.g., prostate: 6–10). These can be placed expeditiously, thereby limiting exposure to medical personnel. In prostatic carcinoma, gold-198 implantation is used primarily as a boost to planned postoperative external teletherapy, which can be initiated safely 3 weeks after the implant because, by that time, the implant sources are spent. More recently, this isotope has been utilized alone as definitive therapy.[31]

TABLE 20-1. *Radioisotopes for Brachytherapy**

ISOTOPE	HALF-LIFE	ENERGY			INITIAL DOSE RATE (cGy/hr)
		ALPHA	BETA	GAMMA (MeV)	
Radium-226	1604 years	+	+	0.18–2.20	
Iridium-192	74.2 days	–	+	0.30–0.61	70–90
Iodine-125	60.2 days	–	–	0.028–0.035	5–10
Gold-198	2.7 days	–	+	0.41	
Palladium-103	17 days	–	–	0.020–0.023	20

*modified from Hilaris[5]

Iridium-192 has a long half-life (74.2 d), a gamma energy similar to that of gold-198 (0.30 to 0.61 MeV), and an effective range in tissue of 6 cm. Most of the concomitant beta radiation is filtered by the encapsulation with stainless steel, and that which escapes is absorbed within the first millimeter of tissue. The sources are supplied with 1 cm spacing in a nylon carrier ribbon for afterloading of temporary implants.

Iodine-125 is a pure emitter of low-energy (0.28 MeV), gamma radiation, with a half-value layer in tissue of 2 cm. The long half-life ($T\frac{1}{2}$ = 60.2 d) of this isotope results in a very low dose rate of emission (8 cGy/hr). Radioactive iodine in two resin spheres together with a gold marker are incorporated within a titanium capsule and typically demonstrate individual seed activity of 0.4 to 0.6 mCi.

The newest radioisotope, palladium-103, has a gamma radiation energy (0.21 MeV) similar in strength to that of iodine-125, but exhibits a much shorter half-life ($T\frac{1}{2}$ = 17 d). This results in an initially high dose rate upon implantation of 40 cGy, which tapers to 20 cGy over the first month. Purified palladium-103 is electroplated onto the surface of two graphite cylinders that are then sealed in titanium tubes with dimensions identical to those of the iodine-125 seed.

LOCAL CONTROL IN PROSTATIC CANCER BRACHYTHERAPY

There are several critical issues involved in assuring the control of prostatic carcinoma on the local level: the choice of isotope, the accurate placement of the sources, the determination of adequate total dose, and the role of external beam supplemental therapy.

Choice of Isotope

Mature follow-up of large numbers of patients implanted with either gold-198 or iodine-125 has shown significant local failure rates in advanced stage and grade patients, which have translated into disease progression. Most brachytherapists now feel that the use of a very low dose rate source such as iodine-125 is effective only for well-differentiated and small-volume prostate tumors. Although the dose rate of gold-198 is much higher, the implant was, until recently, used primarily as a boost in conjunction with external beam therapy, and without any designed effort at source placement.

Iridium-192 transperineal and template-guided temporary implants, supplemented with external teletherapy, seem to have provided excellent control locally, irrespective of tumor grade, though long-term reports are lacking. Although the high dose rate of this isotope probably accounts for the trend toward better local control in high grade disease compared to the I-125 experience, it is likely that the effort to provide careful and uniform Ir-192 source distribution is the crucial factor when comparing the gold-198 results.

Palladium-103 has a low gamma strength radiation of magnitude similar to I-125, but it is being promoted for its comparably high dose rate. Although this feature may afford higher cell kill, careful source distribution with ultrasound monitoring and template guidance is the additional technical feature of Pd-103 protocols that generates confidence for improved local control compared to iodine-125 experience.

Minimum Tumor Dose

Determination of the dose necessary to ablate a given tumor is largely empiric and must take into account the tolerance of the surrounding tissues. The doses to achieve control with interstitial treatment for most tumors have been found to be equivalent to 7,000 rads in 7 days.[32] It is possible to estimate the total dose of a particular isotope necessary to achieve this standard, therefore, comparisons can be made between isotopes, within limits imposed by the individual time-dose factors.

When total dose calculations for prostatic implantations with iodine-125 at Memorial Hospital were in the range of 16,000 to 18,000 rads, the clinical local control was good. It fell off appreciably, however, when the calculated minimal tumor dose was less. The current planned minimum tumor dose for palladium-103 implants is 12,000 rads, which, because of the increased dose rate, is felt to be biologically equivalent to the standard 16,000 rad goal of I-125 implants. Whether this proves to be sufficient or excessive awaits long-term analysis.

Symmetrical Distribution of Sources

Implant experience with I-125 has graphically demonstrated the importance of uniform dose distribution covering the entire target. At Memorial Hospital, when the dose distribution covered the whole prostate, the local failure rate was only 5%, compared to 24% when the distribution was not uniform throughout the prostate.[33] The retropubic, manually guided placement of the hollow needles through which the sources are implanted is intrinsically operator dependent, requiring a high degree of experience and skill. This results in variable and inconsistent dose distribution as the technique is popularized to other centers.

Attempts at improved dose distribution began with the introduction of iridium-192 sources using a perineal template.[20] The depth of needle guide introduction was controlled manually through the open exposure for the lymphadenectomy. The needle guides could be introduced more deeply into the region of the seminal vesicles than heretofore possible retropubically.

Further control of the implant dosimetry evolved with the development of transrectal sonography. With this adjunct, an accurate volume determination of the prostate can be made and the details of the brachytherapy planned, including the spatial distribution and number of sources needed. The implant volume is calculated and the proposed distribution and number of sources is then determined, leaving the individual source strength as the only variable. This is then computed and specified when the sources are ordered. At the time of actual implantation, the perineal template-guided placement of needles and sources can be monitored by ultrasound.[21] This percutaneous technique results in a symmetrically implanted volume whose size is, on the average, about double that treated with the open technique. Utilizing this method, an accurate dose-related implant with homogeneous seed distribution has been achieved 93% of the time.[22]

A variable to be considered in local control and accurate dosimetry is seed migration and loss. Ninety percent of patients undergoing open insertion of iodine-125 seeds lost an average of 8% of the implanted sources.[34] Intraoperatively displaced sources, about one-third of the total, are usually retrieved in the suction. The seeds lost early postoperatively usually pass transurethrally, although later seed migration within the pelvis, in periprostatic fat or pelvic veins has been documented. Early experience with closed transperineal implantation of palladium-103 suggests no loss of seeds at 17 days. The late (over 30 days) loss of individual sources is uncommon and would have lesser impact on both local control and radioprotection with the higher dose rate isotopes.

External Beam Therapy

External beam teletherapy has been used widely in conjunction with interstitial therapy. Originally, therapy was administered postoperatively to supplement the effect of the gold-198 implant. The field size was determined by the results of the lymphadenectomy: if the nodes were negative, only the prostate was irradiated (4,000–4,500 rads); if the nodes were positive, both the prostate and pelvis were treated (5,000–5,500 rads).[35] Later, when teletherapy was added to an existing implant with a long half-life such as iodine-125 ($T\frac{1}{2} = 60$ d), an appreciable increase in complications ensued.[36] This was not seen when supplementing the temporary (iridium-192)[20,37] or short half-life (gold-198) implants,[38,39] unless very high (7500 rads) combined doses to the pelvis were chosen.[40] Postoperative therapy has the advantage of knowing both the nodal status, with its impact on prognosis, and the dosimetry of the implant, with the ability to adjust the dose to the pelvis.

Subsequent investigators employed preoperative therapy. For some, the intent was to diminish the risk of tumor spread by the trauma of the seed implantation.[41,42] Increased complications were seen when the implant was supplemented postoperatively with additional teletherapy.[40] More recently, preimplant external beam therapy is being utilized as an adjunct to shrink large primary tumors and to generate better dimensions for percutaneous ultrasonically monitored implantation.[43,44] To date, this has been well tolerated by patients, but whether this technique will result in improved local control awaits mature followup.

PATIENT SELECTION

Candidates for consideration of prostatic carcinoma brachytherapy should be demonstrated to have no evidence of distant metastasis by the usual means. The survival of patients with metastases would not routinely justify an aggressive management of the prostate primary, particularly because the effect of the systemic treatment has such impressive local impact.

Nodal disease that is diagnosable prior to invasive assessment should, in most cases, preclude intervention, because such sizable adenopathy correlates with poor prognosis and the proposed procedure would not impact on the overall course of the disease. Extensive nodal disease detected at preliminary lymphadenectomy should similarly lead to abandonment of treatment of the primary. If the adenopathy is limited to only a few nodes, a case can be made that the uncertainty of the time course to progression allows reasonable consideration of palliative treatment of the primary tumor.

In view of the current inaccuracies of the completely closed assessment of the nodes, the unselective adoption of such an approach would be a step backward in the modern and scientific management of prostatic cancer, irrespective of considerations of comfort, potential morbidity, and expense. Whether relatively less invasive techniques such as pelvioscopy will be as reliable and widely applicable as modified pelvic lymphadenectomy remains to be demonstrated.

Suitable patients should have at least a 5-year life expectancy, and be surgical candidates if an open technique is the method of choice. Advanced age is not felt to be a contraindication to the closed technique.[22] Patients with more limited life expectancy can be satisfactorily managed with observation and hormonal maneuvers.

Stage-A patients include those diagnosed solely by ultrasonically guided biopsy as well as those classified as A1 or A2 on the basis of prostatectomy for presumed benign disease. Only those patients in whom the size of the resection defect would inhibit implant symmetry or foster seed loss should be considered unsuitable for interstitial therapy. Potential underdosing of the target should be taken into account if the tumor abuts on the resection defect. Assessment of the potential impact of the defect and correlation with the residual gland volume is most accurate with transrectal ultrasonography. Stage-B patients would be considered suitable for implantation as would stage-C patients, whose tumors are easily definable on rectal examination.

Tumor size is an important factor in appropriate patient selection. The results of mature brachytherapy experiences suggest that small prostatic tumors that are well differentiated are most effectively treated. Whether recent modifications in the methodology such as high dose rate isotopes, supplemental external beam teletherapy, template-guided, and ultrasonically monitored source placement will salvage some portion of the larger, more poorly differentiated tumors, remains to be demonstrated. Judgment is of considerable importance with the larger tumors, particularly if the placement of the guide needles or sources is to be done blindly or with only manual guidance. In this circumstance, the likelihood of imperfect dosimetry and local failure is high. Transperineal needle guide positioning with large tumors can be impeded by the interposition of the pubic arch. The role of preimplantation external beam teletherapy (4500 rads) as a means of reducing the target size is being tested in an uncontrolled fashion for tumors judged to be clinically large (stages B2 and C) or by ultrasonic volumetry (over 3 cc).[43,44]

High Gleason grade by itself should not be a contraindication to interstitial management. High-grade limited volume (below stage B2 and less than 3 cc) disease can be handled routinely. Current protocols are exploring the impact of permanent implants with high dose-rate sources (palladium-103) on higher grade tumors (Gleason score above 6/10).[43,44]

The role of brachytherapy for treatment of patients locally failing external beam therapy is not well established as the experience is limited. There may be a significant increase in rectal complications and urinary incontinence.[45]

SPECIFIC IMPLANTATION TECHNIQUES

Gold-198 Implantation[33]

After routine pelvic lymphadenectomy, modified to clear the obturator space and the external iliac vessels medial to the midplane of the artery without skeletonizing them, the prostate is mobilized by incising the endopelvic fascia lateral to the gland. The radiotherapist is then able to measure the prostate and note sites of extracapsular extension. High-activity gold grains are then placed throughout the gland, but clustered in the area of clinical involvement. A planned dose of 3500r requires 6 to 10 grains, depending on the activity of the sources and the size of the gland. By use of a hollow guide needle with a stylet, the grains are implanted individually, without a guiding finger in the rectum to assist distribution. Within 10 minutes, the implantation boost is completed and the wound is checked for hemostasis and closed without drainage. The urinary catheter is removed the next day and alimentation is begun with resolution of ileus. Radiation precautions, necessitated by the high energy emissions of gold-198, include a private room and limitation of visitors. Although grain loss per urethra is rare, the urine and bed sheets are monitored.

The external beam therapy is begun 2 to 3 weeks postoperatively, at which time the grains are exhausted. If the nodes are negative, the prostate receives 4500 r through a rotational technique at 250 r/d, 4 days per week. When the nodes are involved, the pelvis is included in the portal to 5000 r given in a split course with a 2-week rest after the first 3 weeks of treatment with the same fractionation scheme. If there are signs of acute toxicity, the rest period is extended because acute toxicity has been associated with late complications. There are no complications unique to this implant protocol.

Iodine-125 Implantation[9]

As developed at Memorial Sloan Kettering Cancer Center in New York, the patient is positioned in low lithotomy to provide both abdominal and rectal access. Preliminary cystoscopy allows exclusion of patients with undetected involvement of the bladder neck, prostatic urethra, or trigone. An O'Connor drape is introduced into the rectum to facilitate digital monitoring of the needle placement.

Retropubic exposure is afforded through a lower midline incision and an extraperitoneal pelvic lymphadenectomy of the modified version is performed. The endopelvic fascia lateral to the prostate is incised and the gland is mobilized without division of the puboprostatic ligaments. The implantation is begun by placing hollow needles throughout the gland, parallel to each other, at 1-cm intervals, with avoidance of urethral penetration. The depth of each guide needle is digitally monitored per rectum. Specific adjustment is made for paraprostatic and seminal vesicle extension by placement of additional needles. Silver clips are then placed to mark the margins of the gland for postoperative dosimetry.

By using a nomogram, the number of seeds required, the spacing between seeds, and the spacing between needles are determined from an estimation of the treatment volume (entered as the average dimension) and the seed strength in millicuries. The number of seeds used is often 50 to 75, with an average individual activity of 0.45 to 0.65 millicuries. After the seeds are placed, the wound is irrigated and Penrose drainage is established. The drains are removed progressively over days 3 to 5 with discharge by days 7 to 9. No supplemental radiotherapy is administered. A pilot study in patients with positive nodes showed no impact of such treatment on the time course to progression or on the pattern of failure. It did however, increase the rate of complication.

Iridium-192 Implantation[20]

The patient is placed in a low lithotomy position and an O'Connor drape is placed. The Foley catheter balloon is inflated with contrast for localization. After bilateral lymphadenectomy, the prostate is exposed and its size is estimated. The perineal template is positioned by first fixing the gland with a guide needle at the anterior prostate border just beneath the symphysis pubis and extending above the bladder neck. It is located on the template at the 12-o'clock position and other needles are placed at the 6- and then 3- and 9-o'clock positions, which act to secure the gland. Depth and position of these needles is judged manually with the rectal finger and retropubic exposure. Subsequently, 14 additional needles are systematically passed through the template holes to the same depth as the fixation needles. The template is sutured to the perineal skin and the guide needles are fixed in place.

Preliminary computerized dosimetry is then performed with dummy seed implantation and AP and lateral images. In order to obtain a relatively homogeneous dose distribution, one can utilize central differential unloading of sources, half-strength sources, or a less dense template pattern (for smaller glands). The dose rate to the prostate is 70 to 80 cGy/hr, while the rectum is exposed to 30 to 40 cGy/hr. After the interstitial irradiation has been completed, the sources are extracted and the template and guide needles removed.

Adjunctive external teletherapy is begun 10 to 14 days postoperatively. Treatment to a prostate-only portal with a 4000 r dose over 4 to 5 weeks is given to node-negative patients. Demonstration of nodal spread generates 4000 r at the same fractionation to the prostate plus pelvis with an additional 1000 r to the pelvis with a prostate block.

Ultrasound Controlled Implantation[22]

The development of transrectal ultrasound as both a precise volumetric tool and as an intraoperative monitor has engendered a renewed interest in the potential role of interstitial brachytherapy as a major therapeutic option for localized prostatic carcinoma. The radionuclide most commonly used has been iodine-125, but palladium-103 has recently been promoted for the theoretical advantage of its comparatively high dose rate. Clinical experience with the latter isotope, which dates from June, 1986, has not yet been published, but the technique of implantation is identical to that of iodine-125 placed with template guidance and ultrasonic monitor.

Transrectal ultrasonic determination of the precise size and shape of the prostate is the initial procedure after clinical staging. With the aid of a stepping unit which secures the probe and moves it precisely, 5 mm axial sonographic cuts are obtained and the circumference of each is outlined and recorded with the template grid superimposed. The prostate volume can now be computed and displayed. The volume to be implanted is then drawn and may include some periprostatic tissue in order to cover large lesions that may border on the capsule.

In order to achieve a minimum peripheral dose of 160 to 180 Gy, which is matched to the target volume, one must know the number, spacing, and the individual strength of the seeds. The spacing of the needles is predetermined by the template at 5 or 10 mm and the seed-to-seed interval is standardized at 10 mm. Therefore, the number of seeds is established by the tumor shape and volume. The only remaining variable in the total dose calculation is the individual seed strength, and that is then nomogram derived. Using computer-generated, three-dimensional isodose curves, the nomogram's seed distribution plan is checked. After any adjustments (including boosting the visible tumor), the precise number of sources with a specified strength are ordered. This often results in the use of a large number of low-activity sources compared with open-needle placement, where a lesser number of high activity sources are commonly implanted.

It is possible to predetermine the number of seeds for each needle in the distribution and the depth of penetration of each needle. The individual needles can then be preloaded with active sources and catgut spacers, and precisely labeled for the implantation.

The implantation itself is done under spinal anesthesia with the patient in lithotomy. The rectal ultrasound probe is placed and secured to the stabilizer apparatus when images similar to those of the volumetric determination are obtained. The perineal template is positioned and stabilizing needles are placed in the lateral positions. The implantation is begun in the most cephalad plane, which is usually at the bladder neck. The loaded needles are inserted through their preallocated spots in the template, beginning anteriorly and working posteriorly, so that the ultrasound image will not be distorted by previously placed sources. After the individual needle tips have been introduced to the appropriate location (documented on template coordinates), the needles are withdrawn with a rotary motion, against a fixed obturator, which deposits the load of seeds and spacers as planned. Alternatively, the seeds can be placed with the Mick applicator, which deposits the sources from a cartridge at the tip of the needle as it is progressively withdrawn.

Having completed the implantation of the needles extending to the most cephalad plane (the central volume), the sonographic probe is withdrawn to position the needles that extend to the next plane and the process is repeated. Progressively, the more peripheral needles are introduced as the more caudal planes are scanned.

Needle bevel can lead to considerable deviation of the needle from the intended site. This can be corrected by rotating the bevel on reinsertion or avoided by using trocar needles. The pubic arch can interfere with placement of the needles into the most anterior portions of the gland especially if the target is large. This can be managed with manual placement of these needles or by preliminary power-drilling of the symphysis and routine template introduction of the guides.

A Foley catheter is placed overnight with retrieval of any lost sources and the patient is discharged the following morning. Perioperative antibiotics are given, as well as a broad-spectrum parenteral agent preoperatively and an oral agent for 1 week postoperatively.

A limited experience utilizing transperineal closed introduction of gold-198 sources with ultrasound guidance has recently been published.[31]

COMPLICATIONS

Complications of this treatment can be classified as operative, postoperative, and late.[47] Unless designated as unique to a given technique, the complications described are universal to the modality of brachytherapy.

Operative

Blood loss seems directly related to the number of guide needles introduced and the degree of mobilization and exposure of the prostate. It is unmeasurable and not clinically evident with closed techniques.[31,48] Retropubic iodine-125 implants are associated with more blood loss than are gold-198 implants using the same approach but fewer prostate punctures.

Postoperative

The surgical convalescence of any group of patients will be marred by an irreducible minimum number of cases of pulmonary embolus, myocardial infarction, cerebrovascular accident, and thrombophlebitis. Careful and expeditious surgery in good-risk patients are the most important factors in their avoidance.

Those techniques that employ lymphadenectomy are associated with the development of lymphocele, although the incidence of this complication has been minimized by the widely adopted modified (limited) dissection. Drain tract cellulitis is not uncommon and can be minimized by drain placement through a separate site rather than through the incision. Frequent and sterile dressing changes are also important as is progressive drain removal over postoperative days 4 to 6.

Urinary retention is an infrequent problem, but of some significance. Preoperative resection is to be avoided for reasons outlined above. Short-term catheterization, alpha adrenergic blocking medication, temporary estrogens, or massage may be of benefit. Longer-term catheterization, until there is gland shrinkage, while feasible with high dose rate isotopes, is less acceptable for iodine-125 implantations. Suprapubic catheterization is a consideration for these groups. Transurethral surgery following implantation may be possible with minimal resection of seed-bearing tissue. Alternatively, prostatotomy with incision of the bladder neck and prostatic urethra to the verumontanum may be sufficient.

Late

Irritative voiding symptoms are common in the acute phase and generally resolve with time, but may be palliated with sitz baths, anticholinergics, or anti-inflammatory medications. Rarely does incontinence complicate implantation of the prostate. This can be of the urgency or stress type, the latter occurring usually in the face of prior transurethral resection. Radiation changes in the prostatic urethra may occasionally lead to gross hematuria.

Damage to the rectum may manifest itself as discomfort, diarrhea, or urgency, and these symptoms are usually self-limited. Bleeding from radiation proctitis in the mucosa subjacent to the prostate may respond to steroid enemas. Late and severe rectal complications such as ulceration, stenosis, and fistula, while less frequent in implanted patients than with external beam teletherapy,[49] became more common when the interstitial therapy was combined with external beam treatment. This was particularly true if the external beam supplement was to the whole pelvis and given after lymphadenectomy or following a long half-life (iodine-125) implantation where the two dose rates are superimposed.[36,40]

Lymphedema of the genitals, common but transient after open iodine-125 implantation, has not been reported after closed techniques. Lower extremity edema only complicates prostate brachytherapy combined with lymphadenectomy, and especially with external irradiation.

The rate of sexual dysfunction after prostate implantation has been remarkably low, whether by open or closed techniques, low or high dose rate isotopes, with or without external beam supplement. Over 90% of patients potent pretreatment with iodine-125 (over 70% with gold-198 and 85% with iridium-192) have the ability to achieve and maintain an erection adequate for sexual intercourse preserved. Ejaculatory disturbance was common and included decreased or absent ejaculate volume, and minor discomfort with ejaculation.[47]

RESULTS

Comparison of results between series' of various implantation techniques is complicated by differences in case selection, stage classification and distribution, percentage node positivity, and definition of disease free status. Several of the reports involve small numbers of patients with limited followup, which preclude a valid analysis. Table 20-2 shows the disease-free survival at 5 and 10 years correlated with the percentage of nodal involvement and the clinical stage of disease for three mature brachytherapy series. Evident trends include increasing treatment failure with increasing stage, increasing treatment failure with longer followup, and increasing treatment failure with increasing nodal positivity. The last association frustrates comparisons regarding efficacy among the different techniques.

Biopsy documentation of local status is available to only a limited extent. The rate of positive biopsy increases with increasing clinical stage, grade, and nodal involvement. Clinical status is an inaccurate means of assessment with positive biopsy rates in clinically normal glands of 35% after gold-198 implantation and negative biopsies in abnormal prostates 29% of the time. Local recurrence was uncommon in patients with

TABLE 20-2. *Comparison of Interstitial Implantation Series*

| | | HERR ET AL.[50] | | | SCHELLHAMMER ET AL.[51] | | | CARLTON/SCARDINO[35] | | |
		NO.	%NED	(% + NODES)	NO.	%NED	(% + NODES)	NO.	%NED	(% + NODES)
5 YEAR										
Clinical										
Stage:	B-1	24	78	(8)	9	88	(11)	116	68	(18)
	B-2	75	57	(35)	65	77	(15)	65	57	(30)
	C	65	37	(60)	30	50	(40)	90	37	(44)
10 YEAR										
Clinical										
Stage:	B-1		54			88			41	
	B-2		20			48			13	
	C		8			14			17	

NED: No evidence of disease
+Nodes: Positive nodes

negative biopsy (9%),[52] but was projected to rise to 82% by 10 years of followup if any biopsy was positive.[35] Interval endocrine therapy for systemic failure would, of course, obscure previously undetected local recurrence.

FOLLOW-UP

After the postoperative convalescence and implant dosimetry, the patients should be monitored as they would be after any attempt at cure of prostatic cancer. Serial prostate specific antigen determination and periodic bone scanning are important measures to follow. The limited information available on the response of PSA to radiotherapy suggests that a fall to normalcy can be expected with a beneficial response to therapy, and that a subsequent progressive rise is strongly suggestive of disease persistence or progression. Three monthly PSA determinations would seem appropriate until stable, with 6 monthly determinations thereafter. Bone scanning can be deferred until bone symptoms or a sustained but unexplained rise in PSA ensues and demands restaging.

Assessment of the primary tumor by digital rectal examination is simple but not easily quantifiable. A more objective measure of local tumor response is provided by periodic transrectal ultrasound evaluation, which can judge the interval change in volume, detect areas of persistent or recurrent tumor, and guide biopsy assessment.[53]

CONCLUSION

Radical prostatectomy has been eagerly embraced by most urologists as the most appropriate treatment for patients with localized prostatic carcinoma. This enthusiasm has been fueled by the natural inclination of surgeons to their art but particularly by the evolution of specific techniques to limit morbidity (blood loss, incontinence, and impotence). These modifications do not demand an extensive period of training prior to application and their impact can be immediate, although full expression of the benefits may require ongoing experience. The convenient and wide transferability of surgical excision will maintain that treatment modality in the forefront of the armamentarium against localized prostate cancer.

Modern brachytherapy techniques, conversely, require the clinician to acquire special technical expertise, additional equipment, and the enthusiastic cooperation of specially trained radiotherapeutic colleagues. As a result, the effective and energetic application of brachytherapy to localized prostatic carcinoma may remain an alternative approach. This will be boosted considerably if the initial enthusiasm for transperineal template guided and ultrasonically monitored prostate implantation with iodine 125 and palladium 103 is followed by substantial improvement in local control and disease-free survival when compared with standard techniques.

Two features of interstitial therapy, however, will continue to enthuse specially motivated candidates for this modality: low morbidity, especially with closed techniques, and a high and reproducible rate of potency preservation. As increasing numbers of elderly patients are screened (digital rectal exam, PSA, and ultrasound) and early and subclinical disease detected, many will aggressively seek out low-risk treatment, which holds some promise for cure. While potency has been maintained at high rates (80 to 90%), in many brachytherapy centers utilizing different interstitial techniques, similar reports have not been forthcoming from more than a few protagonists of radical prostatectomy.

REFERENCES

1. HILARIS, B. S. Historical Review. In *Handbook of Interstitial Brachytherapy.* Edited by B. S. Hilaris. Acton, Publishing Sciences Group, 1975, p. 13.

2. FAILLA, G. The development of filtered radon implants. Am. J. Roentgen., *16:*507, 1926.

3. JANEWAY, H. H. In *Radium Therapy in Cancer at the Memorial Hospital New York.* New York, Paul B. Hoeber, 1917.

4. FAILLA, G. Radium technic at the Memorial Hospital, New York. Arch. Radiol. Electrother., *24:*3, 1920.

5. HILARIS, B. S., and HENSCHKE, U. K. General Principles and Techniques of Interstitial Brachytherapy. In *Handbook of Interstitial Brachytherapy.* Edited by B. S. Hilaris. Acton, Publishing Sciences Group, 1975, p. 66.

6. PATERSON, R., and PARKER, H. M. A dosage system for gamma ray therapy. Br. J. Radiol., *7:*592, 1934.

7. QUIMBY, E. Q. The grouping of radium tubes in packs on plaques to produce the desired distribution of radiation. Am. J. Roentgen., *27:*18, 1932.

8. QUIMBY, E. Q. Dosage tables for linear radium sources. Radiology, *43:*572, 1944.

9. HILARIS, B. S. Historical Review. In *Handbook of Interstitial Brachytherapy.* Edited by B. S. Hilaris. Acton, Publishing Sciences Group, 1975, p. 13.

10. PASTEAU, O., and DEGRAIS, P. The radium treatment of cancer of the prostate. Arch. Roentgen. Ray. (London), *18:*396, 1914.

11. BARRINGER, B. S. Radium in the treatment of carcinoma of the bladder and prostate. JAMA, *68:*1227, 1917.

12. BARRINGER, B. S. Prostatic carcinoma. J. Urol., *47:*306, 1942.

13. HUGGINS, C. B., and HODGES, C. V. Studies on prostatic cancer, I. The effect of castration, of estrogen, and of androgen injection on serum phosphatase in metastatic carcinoma of the prostate. Cancer Res. *1:*293, 1941.

14. FLOCKS, R. H., KERR, H. D., ELKINS, H. B., and CULP, D. Treatment of carcinoma of prostate by interstitial radiation with radioactive gold: Preliminary report. J. Urol., *68:*510, 1952.

15. DEL REGATO, J. A. Radiotherapy in the conservative treatment of operable and locally inoperable carcinoma of the prostate. Radiology, *88:*761, 1967.

16. GEORGE, F. W., CARLTON, C. E., DYKHUIZEN, R. F., and DILLON, J. R. Cobalt 60 teletherapy in definitive treatment of carcinoma of the prostate; a preliminary report. J. Urol., *93:*102, 1965.

17. BAGSHAW, M. A., KAPLAN, H. S., and SAGERMAN, R. H. Linear accelerator supervoltage radiotherapy: VII. Carcinoma of the prostate. Radiology, *85:*121, 1965.

18. CARLTON, C. E., JR., DAWOUD, F., HUDGINS, P. T., and SCOTT, R., JR. Irradiation treatment of carcinoma of the prostate: A preliminary report based on 8 years of experience. J. Urol., *108:*924, 1972.

19. WHITMORE, W. F., JR., HILARIS, B. S., and GRABSTALD, H. Retropubic implantation of iodine125 in the treatment of prostatic cancer. J. Urol., *108:*918, 1972.

20. SYED, A. M. N., et al. Management of prostate carcinoma. Radiology, *149:*829, 1983.

21. HOLM, H. H., et al. Transperineal 125iodine seed implantation in prostatic cancer guided by transrectal ultrasonograpy. J. Urol., *130:*283, 1983.

22. RAGDE, H., et al. Use of transrectal ultrasound in transperineal 125iodine seeding for prostate cancer methodology. J. Endourol. *3:*209, 1989.

23. HILARIS, B. S., WHITMORE, W. F., BATATA, M. A., and GRABSTALD, H. Cancer of the prostate. In *Handbook of Interstitial Brachytherapy.* Edited by B. S. Hilaris. Acton, Publishing Sciences Group, 1975, p. 221.

24. MORTON, J. D., and PESCHEL, R. E. Iodine-125 implants versus external beam therapy for stages A2, B, and C prostate cancer. Int. J. Rad. Oncol. Biol. Phys., *14:*1153, 1988.

25. COHEN, L. Clinical radiation dosage. III. Biological factor in radon and isotope dosage. Br. J. Radiol., *23:*25, 1950.

26. NIAS, A. H. W., HOWARD, A., GREENE, D., and MAJOR, D. Response of Chinese hamster cells to protracted irradiation from 252 Cf and 60 Co. Br. J. Radiol., *46:*991, 1973.

27. MARCHESE, M. J., HALL, E. J., and HILARIS, B. S. Encapsulated iodine-125 in radiation oncology: I. Study of the relative biological effectiveness (RBE) using low dose rate irradiation of mammalian cultures. Am. J. Clin. Oncol. (CCT) 7:607, 1984.

28. MITCHELL, J. B., BEDFORD, J. S., and BAILEY, S. M. Dose-rate effects on the cell cycle and survival of S3 Hela and V79 cells. Radiat. Res., *79:*520, 1979.

29. KUBAN, D. A., EL-MAHDI, A. M., and SCHELLHAMMER, P. F. I-125 interstitial implantation for prostate cancer. Cancer, *63:*2415, 1989.

30. WHITMORE, W. F., et al. Interstitial irradiation using I-125 seeds. Prog. Clin. Biol. Res., *243B:*177, 1987.

31. CRUSINBERRY, R. A., KRAMOLOWSKY, E. V., and LOENING, S. A. Percutaneous transperineal placement of gold198 seeds for treatment of carcinoma of the prostate. Prostate, *11:*59, 1987.

32. ELLIS, F. Radiation effect and tolerance. In *Handbook of Interstitial Brachytherapy.* Edited by B. S. Hilaris. Acton, Publishing Sciences Group, 1975, p. 46.

33. SOGANI, P. C., MONTIE, J., and WHITMORE, W. F. Carcinoma of the prostate: treatment with pelvic lymphadenectomy and iodine-125 implants. Clin. Bull., *9:*24, 1979.

34. SOMMERKAMP, H., RUPPRECHT, M., and WANNERMACHER, M. Seed loss in interstitial radiotherapy of prostatic carcinoma with I-125. Int. J. Radiol. Oncol. Biol. Phys., *14:*389, 1988.

35. CARLTON, C. E., JR., and SCARDINO, P. T. Combined interstitial and external irradiation for prostatic cancer. In *Prostate Cancer, Part B: Imaging Techniques, Radiotherapy, Chemotherapy, and Management Issues.* New York, Alan R. Liss, 1987, pp. 141–169.

36. ABADIR, R., ROSS, G., JR., and WEINSTEIN, S. H. Carcinoma of the prostate treated by pelvic node dissection, iodine-125 seed implant and external irradiation: a study of rectal complications. Clin. Radiol., *35:*359, 1984.

37. KLEIN, F. A., MOINUDDIN ALI, M., MARKS, S. E., and HACKLER, R. H. Bilateral pelvic lymphadenectomy, iridium 192 template and external beam therapy for localized prostatic carcinoma: Complications and results. South. Med. J., *81:*27, 1988.

38. BOILEAU, M. S., et al. Interstitial gold and external beam irradiation for prostate cancer. J. Urol., *139:*985, 1988.

39. GUTIERREZ, A. E., and MERINO, O. R. Adenocarcinoma of the prostate: Radioactive gold seed implant plus external irradiation. Int. J. Radiat. Oncol. Biol. Phys., *15:*1317, 1988.

40. BOSCH, P. C., et al. Preliminary observations on the results of combined temporary 192iridium implantation and external beam irradiation for carcinoma of the prostate. J. Urol., *135:*722, 1986.

41. FLANIGAN, R. C., et al. Complications associated with preoperative radiation therapy and iodine-125 brachytherapy for localized prostatic carcinoma. Urology, *22:*123, 1983.

42. CHARYULU, K. C., BLOCK, N., and SUDARSANAM, A. Preoperative extended field radiation with I-125 seed implant in prostatic cancer:

A preliminary report of a randomized study. Int. J. Radiat. Oncol. Biol. Phys., *5:*1857, 1979.

43. BLASKO, J. C. Seattle experience with 290 patients—early results. Presented at *Prostate Ultrasound: Diagnosis/Treatment* Atlanta, GA. July 29, 1989.

44. McDONALD, H. P. Atlanta experience with 60 patients—outpatient ultrasonically guided transperineal radioactive palladium seed implantation for prostatic cancer. Presented at *Prostate Ultrasound: Diagnosis/ Treatment* Atlanta, GA. July 29, 1989.

45. CUMES, D. M., GOFFINET, D. R., MARTINEZ, A., and STAMEY, T. A. Complications of iodine125 implantation and pelvic lymphadenectomy for prostatic cancer with special reference to patients who had failed external beam therapy as their initial mode of therapy. J. Urol., *126:*620, 1981.

46. SCARDINO, P. T., GUERIERO, W. G., and CARLTON, C. E. Surgical staging and combined therapy with radioactive gold grain implantation and external irradiation. In *Genitourinary Tumors: Fundamental Principles and Surgical Techniques,* Edited by D. E. Johnson and M. A. Boileau. New York, Grune and Stratton, 1982, pp. 75–90.

47. FOWLER, J. E., BARZELL, W., HILARIS, B. S., and WHITMORE, W. F., JR. Complications of iodine125 implantation and pelvic lym-phadenectomy in the treatment of prostatic cancer. J. Urol., *121:*447, 1979.

48. KUMAR, P. P., et al. Transperineal 125Iodine endocurietherapy of prostate cancer. Am. J. Clin. Oncol., *11:*479, 1988.

49. SCHELLHAMMER, P. F., and EL-MAHDI, A. M. Pelvic complications after definitive treatment of prostate cancer by interstitial or external beam radiation, Urology, *21:*451, 1983.

50. HERR, H. Interstitial radiation by I[125] implantation. In *The Prostate.* Edited by J. M. Fitzpatrick and R. J. Krane. New York. Churchill Livingstone, 1989,

51. SCHELLHAMMER, P. F., KUBAN, D. A., and EL-MAHDI, A.: Interstitial I[125] brachytherapy for cancer of the prostate. In *The Management of Prostate Cancer.* Edited by P. Altman. London, Chapman and Hall Ltd., 1989.

52. SCHELLHAMMER, P. F., et al. Prostate biopsy after definitive treatment by interstitial iodine125 implant or external beam radiation therapy. J. Urol., *137:*897, 1987.

53. LEE, F., et al. Transrectal ultrasound in the diagnosis and staging of local disease after I125 seed implantation for prostate cancer. Int. J. Radiat. Oncol. Biol. Phys., *15:*1453, 1988.

CARCINOMA OF THE BLADDER

Bladder Carcinoma: An Overview

Michael J. Droller

B ladder cancer comprises a spectrum of neoplastic diatheses. Of the 35,000 new cases of bladder cancer diagnosed annually, nearly 75% will be localized to the bladder.[1] Of the 75% of these that will recur, only 10 to 20% will ultimately progress.[2] A variety of staging systems have been developed based on the varying prognosis of the different forms of bladder cancer.[3,4] Although these have implied the occurrence of a sequence of changes that inexorably result in progressive disease, it has become clear over the years that many patients are never at risk from their disease while others at their initial clinical presentation have a form of bladder cancer that is likely to cause their death.[5]

Limitations in our understanding of the behavioral patterns of bladder cancer persist, and therapeutic interventions appropriate to a particular form of the disease therefore remain controversial. The critical question of whether a cancer will remain regionally confined or whether cancer cells will metastasize remains unanswered. Moreover, we are completely ignorant regarding the timing of these events in the overall course of a patient's disease. It is only within this context, however, that the efficacy of a particular treatment can be reasonably assessed.

In this section we will attempt to provide an overview of what has been observed of the biology of bladder cancer and the efficacy of various therapeutic approaches. Current concepts of the natural history, staging, methods of diagnosis, and treatment options of the various forms of bladder cancer will be reviewed with a focus on those tumor characteristics that may correlate with distinct behavioral patterns.

BIOLOGIC CHARACTERISTICS OF BLADDER CANCER

It has been hypothesized that neoplastic transformation of the normal urothelium reflects an interaction between events known as "initiation" and "promotion." The first is a process in which lesions that are irreversible are introduced into the nuclear deoxyribonucleic acid (DNA). If a cell's capacity for DNA repair is decreased or if cell replication is accelerated, the process of carcinogenesis may be enhanced by the stabilization of the damage that has occurred by this process.[6] "Promotion" is the process whereby stimulation of cells already "initiated" leads to their proliferation and thereby fixes the changes in DNA in place.[7] Although promotion in the absence

Hypothetical Events and Pathways in the Natural History of Bladder Cancer

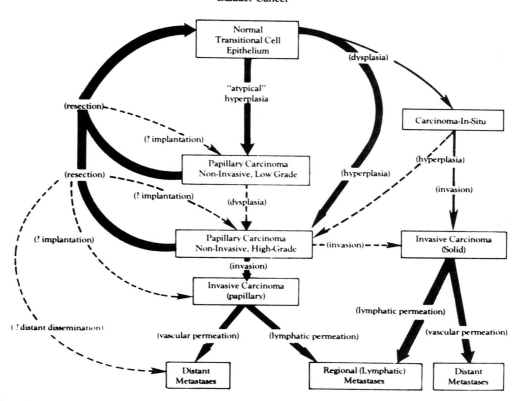

FIG. 21-1. Hypothetical pathways in the natural history of bladder cancer. (From Droller, M. J. Bladder cancer. Curr. Probl. Surg., *18*:209, 1981.)

of initiation may cause only cellular proliferation or hyperplasia, the stimulation of cells that have been initiated may lead to the phenotypic expression of a bladder cancer. This has been suggested to explain, at least in part, the apparent cumulative effects of the variety of carcinogens that have been implicated in the genesis of bladder cancer.[8] Promotion appears to require long periods of continued exposure to a particular agent and has been suggested to be reversible until a malignancy has actually appeared. Some have suggested that repetitive exposures of the transitional cell epithelium to both initiating and promoting agents may be necessary for the final development of a clinically recognizable cancer.

Numerous studies have identified a variety of agents as chemical carcinogens in the development of bladder cancer. These have included aromatic amines,[9] cigarette smoking,[10] artificial sweeteners,[11] and bladder irritants (e.g., schistosomiasis, bladder calculi, and urinary tract infections) in the presence of nitrosamines that may act as co-carcinogens.[12,13] Each has been associated with the possible stimulation of bladder cancer development. Although a genetic basis for bladder cancer has not been clearly defined, the presumed innate predisposition for or resistance against the development of a cancer may be important if environmental factors are to play an initiator or promoter role in the type of cancer that develops.[14]

The interaction of such substances with the uroepithelial cell is receiving renewed attention in the context of the chromosomal changes that are being observed in association with the putative roles of oncogenes and so-called antioncogenes in the genesis of neoplasia.[15,16] What accounts for the genesis of a neoplastic diathesis, that may either be manifest in the uncontrolled proliferation of cells or the development of the capacity to disseminate, is presently unclear. However, it is directly relevant to our understanding of the existence of different forms of bladder cancer as they present clinically and as they may dictate the types of therapy that may be most effective in controlling or eradicating a particular malignancy.

The suggestion that bladder cancer follows a pattern of sequential development is technically accurate. The occurrence of an initial transformational event by definition results in the formation of a malignancy in situ that produces a proliferative diathesis that may ultimately lead to an infiltrative diathesis and dissemination (Fig. 21-1). What is seen clinically, however, is a variety of bladder cancers in which the majority of patients present with a proliferative diathesis that is confined to the bladder. Only a small proportion of these actually progress to invasion. Of these, only a fraction present with muscle-infiltrative cancer. These varied presentations suggest the existence of variability in the developmental pathways of the different types of bladder cancer rather than a single and inexorable sequence of events.[17,18]

BIOLOGIC VARIABILITY OF BLADDER CANCER

Carcinoma in situ

After examining tumor-bearing bladders, Melicow described segments of flat epithelium characterized by the presence of neoplastic cells that were separate from the primary tumor. He used the term "carcinoma in situ" to describe these areas, and implied that they were a distinct cancer entity representing the earliest stage of bladder cancer.[19] Subsequent reports documented the development of infiltrative disease in as many as 75% of patients with diffuse carcinoma in situ, suggesting the potential aggressive nature of this diathesis.[20] Some forms of carcinoma in situ, however, did not lead to infiltrative disease.[21] Indeed, progression was often seen only in the context of the presence of superficially infiltrative cancers. In such instances, progression occurred in those patients in whom carcinoma in situ was at the margin of a superficial papillary cancer.[22] The fact that 30% of patients with presumed carcinoma in situ alone were found to have microscopic lamina propria infiltration, suggested that there might occur different forms of this diathesis.[23]

"Superficial" Transitional Cell Cancers

The term "superficial" was traditionally applied to those tumors that had not infiltrated the muscularis. It is now apparent, however, that the critical factor reflecting the biologic potential of a bladder cancer is manifested in the distinction between those tumors that are confined to the bladder mucosa and those that have penetrated the basement membrane and extended into the lamina propria.[24] Recent reports have suggested that penetration into the lamina propria reflects an enzymatic capability for invasiveness and possible metastasis that is not present in mucosally-confined tumors.[25] Therefore, although recurrence of disease is likely to be seen in 75% of patients with superficial cancers, patients presenting with mucosally-confined tumors are likely to recur with muscle infiltrative disease in only 3% of instances. Conversely, those with lamina propria infiltration will experience ultimate progression to muscle-infiltration in 25 to 30% of instances.[24]

The grade of disease has been correlated with the likelihood of progression. Only 1 to 2% of grade-1 patients, 11% of grade-2 patients, and 45% of grade-3 patients have been associated with the likelihood of progressive disease.[26] Correlation of tumor grade with the diffuseness of malignant transformation has been suggested in observations that 38% of grade-1 tumors, 55% of grade-2 tumors, and 66% of grade-3 tumors were associated with moderate or severe dysplasia in selected mucosal biopsies.[27]

Multiplicity of disease, however, has been associated with the likelihood of tumor recurrence rather than disease progression. In those patients who initially presented with multiple tumors, the likelihood of recurrence was 90%. In those patients who initially presented with a single tumor, the likelihood of recurrence was 65%.[24] However, when multiple tumors were found to be infiltrative of the lamina propria, con-comitant increased incidence of epithelial atypia and carcinoma in situ appeared to suggest a greater likelihood of progression.

Muscle-Infiltrative Cancers

Although the diagnosis of muscle-infiltrative transitional cell carcinoma has generally been viewed as having an ominous prognosis, these tumors are actually comprised of a variety of diatheses with differing biologic potentials. The most aggressive of these are found to have infiltrated deep muscle in a solid or nodular pattern with penetration occurring in a tentacular fashion by extension of clusters of tumor cells in finger-like projections between the muscle fascicles.[28] These contrast with those muscle-infiltrative cancers that have a more papillary appearance and that penetrate the bladder wall in an apparently more cohesive or "broad front" pattern, appearing not to penetrate the bladder wall as deeply.[28] The former have been found to involve the bladder wall vasculature (or lymphatics) twice as often as the latter.[29] That the latter have been found to have a papillary appearance in contrast to the more solid appearance demonstrated by the former, suggests different pathways of development, possibly akin to a predominantly "proliferative" rather than "dysplastic" process of development.[30]

50% of patients who present with muscle-infiltrative cancer develop metastases within 2 years of their initial diagnosis, despite radical therapy.[31] This implies that the process of metastasis may have occurred early in the development of these more aggressive tumors (possibly before they had become clinically manifest) and that the occurrence of muscle infiltration was simply the pathologic concomitant of the aggressive intrinsic nature of these cancer cells. However, it has also been observed that those muscle-infiltrative cancers that have a papillary appearance, that have infiltrated the musculature only superficially, and that may involve the bladder wall vasculature and lymphatics in only one-third of instances, appear to have an expected 5-year survival of 65 to 80%.[32] This stands in contrast to those tumors that have a more nodular architecture, deep muscle invasion, and involvement of the vasculature and lymphatics in two-thirds of instances, with a 5-year survival of less than 20%.[33] Taken together, it would appear that infiltrative cancers may follow separate developmental pathways in which infiltration of the bladder muscle may not necessarily reflect identical biologic potentials. The clinical course in the majority of muscle-infiltrative tumors may, therefore, possibly be determined by the type of transformation that characterizes the earliest events in tumor development.

STAGING OF BLADDER CANCER

The evolution of a staging system for bladder cancer has been derived from observations of the clinical course of different tumors in association with their depth of penetration through the bladder wall at their initial presentation. Corresponding differences in the biologic potential of the varying forms of bladder cancer, and the association of their pathologic appearance with their response to various types of therapy, have permitted further delineation and clarification of these distinctions.[3,4] Initial observations distinguished between superficial tumors (stage A; those that had only infiltrated superficially in the bladder wall), tumors that invade muscle (stage B), and tumors that invade the perivesical fat (stage C). This was later modified to take into account an apparent distinction between superficial invasion (stage B1) or deep invasion (stage B2) into the muscle. The superficial invasion appeared to have a more benign prognosis. The system was subsequently expanded to include a stage in which the lamina propria had not been invaded (stage 0) and stages in which metastasis either to pelvic lymph nodes (stage D1) or to distant lymph nodes and other organ systems (stage D2) were observed. The American Joint Committee and the UICC subsequently introduced a system that included a stage for carcinoma in situ (TIS), one for deep muscle invasion (T3A), and one for invasion into the perivesical fat (T3B). An additional modification subsequently proved necessary to distinguish between papillary tumors without lamina propria invasion (T_A) from those that had invaded the lamina propria (T_1). This is the accepted general staging system (Table 21-1).

Although a sequential progression of tumors might be suggested by such systems and would seem to account for the varying clinical presentations and pathologic appearances that are seen, behavioral differences even within these different stages of disease suggest that a variety of developmental pathways may account for the varying courses of tumors and their responses to standardized treatments.[34] It is likely that additional factors will ultimately be included in an overall staging system in order to more fully and precisely characterize a particular tumor in an individual patient, and to recognize its unique prognosis and its likelihood of being amenable to a particular form of therapy.

DIAGNOSIS

The majority of patients with bladder cancer present with either gross or microscopic hematuria.[35] Although the occurrence of hematuria in this setting is often referred to as "painless," bladder irritability (urgency, dysuria, or stangury) is likely to be present. This usually reflects the presence of diffuse carcinoma in situ or involvement by carcinoma in situ of the bladder neck or prostatic urethra.

The diagnostic steps indicated in a patient with hematuria are intravenous pyelography, cystoscopy, and urinary cytology. Pyelography allows visualization of the upper tracts, to help exclude a nonvesical source of the hematuria and to determine whether there is evidence of upper tract obstruction associated with a bladder lesion. The presence of hydronephrosis associated with bladder cancer generally indicates that the bladder cancer is infiltrative.[36]

Cystoscopy is used to verify the presence of a bladder tumor and to characterize its gross appearance. Cystoscopy also permits characterization of the urethral and bladder mucosa. Areas of erythema (especially with a "velvety" appearance) may represent carcinoma in situ. Evaluation of the efflux from each ureteral orifice may also be important to confirm the apparent absence of involvement of the upper tracts that may have been suggested by intravenous pyelography.

Once the cystoscopic diagnosis of bladder cancer is made, it may be appropriate to consider CT scan of the bladder to determine the degree of thickening of the bladder wall. Although the distinction between inflammation and tumor may not be possible if thickening is seen on CT scanning, the appearance of a thin wall in the presence of a "superficial" papillary lesion suggests that infiltration may not be present and may dictate the depth to which resection should extend. Correspondingly, thickening of the bladder wall in association with a more nodular tumor may reflect the likelihood of deeper infiltration and the extent to which resection is necessary.

TABLE 21-1. *Staging Systems of Bladder Cancer*

JEWETT 1946	JEWETT 1952	MARSHALL 1952	BLADDER CANCER STAGING (CLINICAL-PATHOLOGIC)		AMERICAN JOINT COMMITTEE UICC-1974 CLINICAL	PATHOLOGIC
		0	No tumor definitive specimen		T_0	P_0
A	A		Carcinoma in situ		TIS	PIS
			Papillary tumor—no invasion		T_A	P_A
		A	Papillary tumor-lamina propria invasion		T_1	P_1
B	B_1	B_1	Superficial	muscle invasion	T_2	P_2
	B_2	B_2	Deep		T_{3A}	
C	C	C	Invasion of perivesical fat		T_{3B}	P_3
		D_1	Invasion of contiguous viscera		T_4	P_4
			Involvement of pelvic nodes			N_{1-3}
		D_2	Involvement of juxtaregional nodes			N_4
			Distant metastases			M_1

From Droller, M. Bladder cancer. Curr. Probl. Surg., *18*:209, 1981.

Exfoliative cytology is an important adjunct in the diagnosis of bladder cancer. It can provide an indication regarding the presence of disease and may also help determine the extent of disease. When positive in the presence of a mucosally-confined papillary transitional cell cancer of low grade, it may indicate the presence of either carcinoma in situ or of another lesion elsewhere in the urinary tract. When persistently positive after resection of the presenting bladder lesion, it indicates the existence of disease at a location which has not yet been identified. The additional use of flow cytometry to determine the degree of ploidy of a barbotaged specimen may be useful in characterizing not only the nature of the presenting tumor diathesis, but also its malignant potential.[37]

Ultimately, diagnosis depends on transurethral resection of a visible lesion and mucosal biopsy of areas suspicious for in situ disease. Transurethral resection also allows staging and grading of disease, both of which permit assessment of prognosis. Both superficial and deep biopsy specimens should be obtained and these should be assessed separately. However, if a lesion appears to be superficial on endoscopic evaluation and CT scan has demonstrated a thin bladder wall, deep resection should be performed cautiously to avoid bladder perforation. Tumor architecture, cellular grade, pattern of infiltration, possible involvement of the vasculature and lymphatics in the bladder wall, and depth of penetration should each be assessed.

Multiple biopsies prior to formal tumor resection may assist in determining the extent of disease. Biopsies can be taken of the tumor itself, of the tumor margin, of regions near the ureteral orifices, of the bladder neck, and of the mucosa of the prostatic urethra. Such biopsies can be obtained with a cold-cup forceps.

TREATMENT

"Superficial" Bladder Cancer

Transurethral resection is generally curative in cases of superficial bladder cancer, especially if the presenting lesion is solitary and confined to the bladder mucosa. Cure in this instance is predicated on the assumption that the remainder of the urothelium is normal, even though there is a 75% likelihood that the patient will experience tumor recurrence. If this occurs, repeat transurethral resection or fulguration can be undertaken. Because progression in these instances is generally unlikely, this approach amounts to a cure of disease.

The presence of carcinoma in situ, at the margin of this type of tumor, may indicate a greater potential for the ultimate development of bladder wall infiltration.[22] Correspondingly, the presence of carcinoma in situ at other foci in the bladder may suggest the possibility of rapid recurrence, possibly with progressive disease. Such findings are generally more common in the presence of papillary tumors that have infiltrated the lamina propria.[24] This may signal the need for a more aggressive approach than simple transurethral resection. Moreover, because the possibility of progression of grade-3 stage T1 tumors is three times that of grade-1 stage T1 tumors (45% versus 15%),[2] grade of disease may also indicate the need for more aggressive therapy.

Intravesical chemotherapy in conjunction with transurethral resection has been suggested to prevent not only recurrence of disease but also potential progression of disease. Agents such as Thiotepa,[38] Adriamycin,[39] Mitomycin C,[40] and Bacillus Calmette-Guerin (BCG),[41] have each been used successfully for prophylaxis against tumor recurrence, approaching 30 to 50%.

Intravesical chemotherapy may be particularly important in treating either patients whose superficial tumors have infiltrated the lamina propria or patients who have diffuse carcinoma in situ. Because the risk of developing progressive disease in this setting is substantial, careful cystoscopic surveillance of such patients and accurate cytologic assessment are critical. Because ultimate progression in such instances, even with intensive intravesical chemotherapy, may be likely,[42] a deliberate decision as to whether to continue conservative therapy or to intervene with more aggressive treatment early in the course of disease often needs to be made.

The use of a neodymium-YAG laser in the fulguration of superficial tumors has gained some adherents because of its ability to treat recurrent superficial disease without requiring anesthesia.[43] Major disadvantages are the lack of accessibility of some tumors to treatment and the absence of tissue for pathologic assessment. The adjunctive use of photosensitizing agents such as hematoporphyrin derivatives to sensitize the cancer cells to the photodestructive effect of the laser has further encouraged investigation of the laser in the treatment of both multiple bladder tumors and of carcinoma in situ.[44]

Muscle-Infiltrative Transitional Cell Cancers

The standard approach to the treatment of muscle-infiltrative cancers has been radical cystectomy. The assumption in these instances is that the cancer is still confined to the bladder but has already penetrated too deeply to allow transurethral resection to eradicate all cancer cells from the bladder. However, notwithstanding various radiographic studies that suggest that such tumors are confined to the bladder, approximately 50% of such patients are found to develop distant metastases or regional pelvic recurrences within 2 years of cystectomy.[31]

The mutilative aspects of cystectomy, as well as its ineffectiveness in curing a large proportion of patients, prompted the use of radiation therapy as the sole treatment for muscle-infiltrative bladder cancer. This too, however, has been found to be ineffective in controlling regional disease or preventing ultimate tumor dissemination.[45] Therefore, a combined approach was taken using preoperative radiation therapy with radical cystectomy, on the assumption that radiation would sterilize cancer cells that conceivably were disseminated by surgical manipulation. Although initial observations supported the efficacy of this,[46] ultimate evaluations of survival and of the incidence of distant metastases and regional recurrence suggest that this approach is not particularly effective.[47]

In many instances, patients with deep muscle infiltrative disease actually had systemic disease at the time of their initial presentation. This has prompted the suggestion that combination chemotherapy might be useful in treating muscle-infiltrative bladder cancer. Several chemotherapeutic regimens have been found to have activity against metastatic disease. These include MVAC (methotrexate, vinblastine, adriamycin, and cisplatinum),[48] CMV (cisplatinum, methotrexate, and velban),[49] and CISCA (cisplatinum, cyclophosphlamide, and adriamycin).[50] In patients with measurable metastatic disease, combined partial and complete response rates for these regimens were initially claimed to be as high as 70%.[48] However, the only increases in survival seemed to occur in those patients who demonstrated a complete response, amounting to 10 to 15%.

These initially promising results led to the design of protocols in which chemotherapeutic regimens were given to patients prior to cystectomy. Some of these patients experienced eradication of tumor from their bladder on repeat pathologic evaluation.[51] However, these results were criticized for their staging inaccuracies both before treatment and after, for inadequacies in assessing treatment response, and for invalid comparisons between different patient groups. It should be remembered that muscle-infiltrative cancers comprise a spectrum of tumor diatheses, some of which may be more superficially infiltrative, less likely to be associated with vascular and lymphatic infiltration, and intrinsically likely to be associated with greater survival.

The development of these regimens has stimulated new enthusiasm for attempts to conserve the bladder. Clearly, neoadjuvant chemotherapy that might result in sterilization of the bladder might provide a cogent argument for conservative surveillance by repeated biopsy (or resection), allowing preservation of the bladder, normal voiding, and sexual function. Moreover, patients with only superficial muscle infiltrative disease might be managed either by segmental cystectomy or by deep transurethral resection, with careful follow-up cytology, resection, and CT scan to monitor any potential changes indicative of tumor recurrence and the need for chemotherapy (neoadjuvant, adjunctive, or "definitive"). The success of such approaches ultimately depends on their consistent therapeutic efficacy.

CONCLUSION

In our current understanding of bladder cancer, we recognize that the manifestation of this condition may take many forms. This may reflect not only those events that have led to the generation of a particular type of bladder cancer, but may also ultimately have bearing on the results of the particular treatment applied to the specific condition in the individual patient. Recognition and understanding of the pathways by which various forms of bladder cancer may develop may benefit the patient, either from more radical treatment earlier in the tumor's course, when it is still likely to be confined regionally, or from more conservative treatment if the tumor is likely to be controlled without the need for radical therapy. Taken together, the objective must be an attempt either to control or completely cure the disease while maintaining the full functional capabilities of the bladder cancer patient.

REFERENCES

1. American Cancer Society. Cancer statistics. Cancer, *39:*3, 1989.
2. CUTLER, S. J., HENRY, N. M., and FRIEDELL, G. H. Longitudinal study of patients with bladder cancer: Factors associated with disease recurrence and progression. In *Bladder Cancer*. Edited by W. W. Bonney and G. R. Prout. Williams & Wilkins, Baltimore, 1982, p. 35.
3. SKINNER, D. G. Current state of classification and staging of bladder cancer. Cancer Res., *37:*2838, 1977.
4. DROLLER, M. J. Bladder cancer. Curr. Probl. Surg., *28:*209, 1981.
5. KAYE, K. W., and LANGE, P. W. Mode of presentation of invasive bladder cancer: Reassessment of the problem. J. Urol., *128:*31, 1982.
6. WEINSTEIN, I. B., and TROLL, W. National Cancer Institute workshop on tumor promotion and cofactors in carcinogenesis. Cancer Res., *37:*3461, 1977.
7. COHEN, S. M. Urinary bladder carcinogenesis: Initiation-promotion. Semin. Oncol., *6:*157, 1979.
8. RYSER, H. J. Chemical carcinogenesis. N. Engl. J. Med., *285:*721, 1971.
9. MORRISON, A. S., and COLE, P. Epidemiology of bladder cancer. Urol. Clin. North Am., *3:*13, 1976.
10. MORGAN, R. W., and JAIN, M. G. Bladder cancer: Smoking, beverages and artificial sweeteners. Can. Med. Assoc. J., *111:*1067, 1974.
11. MORRISON, A. S., and BURING, J. E. Artificial sweeteners and cancer of the lower urinary tract. N. Engl. J. Med., *302:*537, 1980.
12. BRAND, K. G. Schistosomiasis-cancer: Etiologic considerations. A review. Acta Trop. (Basel), *36:*203, 1979.
13. EL-MENZABANI, M. M., EL-AASER, A. A., and ZAKHARY, N. I. A study on the aetiological factors of bilharzial bladder cancer in Egypt: I. Nitrosamines and their precursors in urine. Eur. J. Can., *15:*287, 1979.
14. LYNCH, H. T., and WALZAK, M. P. Genetics in urogenital cancer. Urol. Clin. North Am., 7:815, 1980.
15. SANTOS, E., et al. T24 human bladder carcinoma oncogene is an activated form of the normal human homologue of Balb- and Harvey-USV transforming genes. Nature, *298:*343, 1982.
16. PARADA, L., et al. Human EJ bladder carcinoma oncogene is homologue of Harvey sarcoma virus *yas* gene. Nature, *297:*474, 1982.
17. FRIEDELL, G. H. Carcinoma, carcinoma in situ, and "early lesions" of the uterine cervix and the urinary bladder: Introduction and definitions. Cancer Res., *36:*2482, 1976.
18. BROWN, P. N. The origin of invasive carcinoma of the bladder. Cancer, *50:*515, 1982.
19. MELICOW, M. M. Histological study of vesical urothelium intervening between gross neoplasm in total cystectomy. J. Urol., *68:*261, 1952.
20. UTZ, D. C., HANASH, K. A., and FARROW, G. M. The plight of the pa-

tient with carcinoma in situ of the bladder. J. Urol., *103*:160, 1970.

21. FARROW, G. M., et al. Clinical observations on 69 cases of in situ carcinoma of the urinary bladder. Cancer Res., *37*:2794, 1977.

22. ALTHAUSEN, A. F., PROUT, G. R., JR., and DALY, J. J. Noninvasive papillary carcinoma of the bladder associated with carcinoma in situ. J. Urol., *116*:575, 1976.

23. FARROW, G. M., UTZ, D. C., and RIFE, C. C. Morphological and clinical observations of patients with early bladder cancer treated with total cystectomy. Cancer Res., *36*:2495, 1976.

24. SMITH, G., et al. Prognostic significance of biopsy results of normal-looking mucosa in cases of superficial bladder cancer. Br. J. Urol., *55*:665, 1983.

25. GUIRGUIS, R., et al. Detection of autocrine motility factor in urine as a marker of bladder cancer. J. Natl. Cancer Inst., *80*:1203, 1988.

26. VARKARAKIS, M. J., et al. Superficial bladder tumor: Aspects of clinical progression. Urology, *4*:414, 1974.

27. HENEY, N. M., et al. Biopsy of apparently normal urothelium in patients with bladder carcinoma. J. Urol., *120*:559, 1978.

28. ANDERSON, C. K. Current topics on the pathology of bladder cancer. Proc. R. Soc. Med., *66*:283, 1973.

29. SOTO, E. A., FRIEDELL, G. H., and TILTMAN, A. J. Bladder cancer as seen in giant histologic sections. Cancer, *39*:447, 1977.

30. SJOLIN, K. E., NYHOLM, K., and TRAUTNER, K. Studies of transitional cell tumors of the bladder. Prognosis and causes of death. Acta Pathol. Microbiol. Scand., *84*:361, 1976.

31. PROUT, G. R., JR., GRIFFIN, P. P., and SHIPLEY, W. U. Bladder carcinoma as a systemic disease. Cancer, *43*:2532, 1979.

32. PRYOR, J. P. Factors influencing the survival of patients with transitional cell tumours of the urinary bladder. Br. J. Urol., *45*:586, 1973.

33. SKINNER, D. G., and LIESKOVSKY, G. Contemporary cystectomy with pelvic node dissection compared to preoperative radiation therapy plus cystectomy in management of invasive bladder cancer. J. Urol., *131*:1069, 1984.

34. DROLLER, M. J. Transitional cell cancer: Upper tracts and bladder. In *Campbell's Urology.* Edited by P. C. Walsh, R. F. Gittes, A. Permutter, and T. A. Stamey. Philadelphia, W. B. Saunders Co., 1986, p. 1343.

35. HENDRY, W. F. *Diagnosis and Management of Primary Bladder Cancer.* Edited by D. Raghavan. London, 1988, p. 69.

36. FRIEDLAND, G. W., et al. *Uroradiology: An Integrated Approach.* London, Churchill Livingstone, 1983.

37. MELAMED, M. R. Flow cytometry of the urinary bladder. Urol. Clin. North Am., *11*:599, 1984.

38. KOONTZ, W. W., et al. The use of intravesical thiotepa in the management of non-invasive carcinoma of the bladder. J. Urol., *125*:307, 1981.

39. EK, A., et al. Intravesical Adriamycin therapy in carcinoma-in-situ of the urinary bladder. Scand. J. Urol. Nephrol., *18*:131, 1984.

40. HULAND, H., et al. Long-term mitomycin C instillation after transurethral resection of superficial carcinoma: Influence on recurrence, progression and survival. J. Urol., *132*:27, 1984.

41. HERR, H., et al. Experience with intravesical bacillus Calmette-Guerin therapy of superficial bladder tumors. Urology, *25*:119, 1985.

42. DROLLER, M. J., and WALSH, P. C. Intensive intravesical chemotherapy in the treatment of flat carcinoma-in-situ. Is it safe? J. Urol., *134*:1115, 1985.

43. BENSON, R. C. Integral photoradiation therapy of multifocal bladder tumours. Eur. Urol., *12*(Suppl. 1):47, 1986.

44. BENSON, R. C., et al. Detection and localization of *in situ* carcinoma of the bladder with hematoporphyrin derivative. Mayo Clin. Proc., *57*:548, 1982.

45. GOSPODAROWICZ, M., et al. Definitive radiation therapy in the management of bladder cancer. Int. J. Radiat. Oncol. Biol. Phys., *10*:118, 1984.

46. WHITMORE, W. F., JR. Integrated irradiation and cystectomy for bladder cancer. Br. J. Urol., *52*:1, 1980.

47. DROLLER, M. J. The controversial role of radiation therapy as adjunctive treatment of bladder cancer. J. Urol., *129*:897, 1983.

48. STERNBERG, C. N., et al. Preliminary results of M-VAC (methotrexate, vinblastine, doxorubicin, and cisplatin) for transitional cell carcinoma of the urothelium. J. Urol., *133*:403, 1985.

49. HARKER, W. G., et al. Cisplatin, methotrexate, and vinblastine (CMV): An effective chemotherapy regimen for metastatic transitional cell carcinoma of the urinary tract: A Northern California Oncology Group study. J. Clin. Oncol., *3*:1463, 1985.

50. LOGOTHETIS, C. J., et al. Cyclophosphamide, doxorubicin, and cisplatin chemotherapy for patients with locally advanced urothelial tumors with or without nodal metastases. J. Urol., *134*:460, 1985.

51. RAGHAVAN, D. Neoadjuvant chemotherapy for invasive bladder cancer. Br. J. Urol., *61*:111, 1988.

Transurethral Resection of Bladder Tumors

Winston K. Mebust

Approximately 47,100 new cases of bladder carcinoma will be diagnosed this year.[1] Eighty percent of these will be superficial papillary lesions confined to the bladder. Melicow, in a large series, noted that 80% of these lesions occurred on the lateral or posterior walls.[2] However, other series have noted a tendency for their location to be near the ureteral orifices.[3] Approximately 70% of these superficial tumors are stage TA and 30% are stage T1.[4,5,6] Ninety-five percent of stage-TA lesions are usually low-grade, 60 to 70% of stage T1 are grade II, and 25 to 40% are grade III. Seventy percent of these superficial tumors will recur. Malmstrom et al. noted that progression to a higher T stage occurred in 15% of stage-TA lesions and in 29% of stage-T1 tumors.[7] In that series, the 5-year cancer mortality rate was 5% for TA lesions but 28% for T1. In another series of 172 patients who had initially Stage TA or T1 lesions, and were followed for a mean of 106 months, the 10-year survival rates were as follows: TA/GI (95%), TA/GII (89%), TA/GIII (84%), TI/GII (78%), and T1/GIII (50%).[8]

The management and prognosis of superficial bladder carcinoma is dictated by many factors. Recurrence and progression depends on the initial tumor stage, multiplicity, size, status of urinary cytology and DNA ploidy, and association of urothelial dysplasia or carcinoma in situ. Other etiologic risk factors, not as clearly defined, are smoking, dietary (e.g. artificial sweeteners), and occupational exposure to carcinogens.

Transurethral resection is the standard method for the initial staging and eradication of low-grade, non-invasive papillary carcinoma from the bladder. However, the urologist is also interested in preventing, or at least reducing, the recurrence of the carcinoma and the progression of the carcinoma to a higher T stage. Transurethral resection of a superficial bladder carcinoma can eradicate existing disease but cannot necessarily prevent recurrence or progression. With progression to a higher T stage, the risk of invasion and dissemination of the carcinoma obviously becomes greater and leads to a worse prognosis. Therefore, other therapeutic modalities (i.e. intravesical chemotherapy and immunotherapy) have been advocated as adjunctive therapy to transurethral resection of the bladder tumors. However, not all patients (30%) will develop recurrences and will not benefit by a prophylactic intravesical chemotherapy or an immunotherapy regimen.

This chapter will focus primarily on transurethral resection of superficial bladder cancer and, secondarily, will explore some of the factors contributing to recurrence and progression to determine which patients may benefit by the addition of intravesical chemotherapy.

PATIENT EVALUATION

Patients with carcinoma of the bladder usually present with the symptoms of intermittent, gross hematuria. Twenty percent may also present with bladder irritative symptoms such as dysuria and frequency, mimicking urinary tract infection. Carcinoma of the bladder has been found in 10% of patients with asymptomatic microhematuria. The patient is usually in his fifth decade and there is a 3:1 male-to-female preponderance.

The diagnosis is made by cystoscopy. The flexible cystoscopes are useful in that they seem to cause less patient discomfort than the rigid scope. Furthermore, they can be deflected retrograde, allowing better evaluation of the anterior bladder-neck area. Conversely, the standard, rigid, fiberoptic scopes have a wider and clearer field of vision.

At cystoscopy, bladder washings for cytology are obtained. If the lesion appears sessile rather than papillary, the urologist may wish to see if there is bladder-wall invasion by CT scan or ultrasound. This may alter the anticipated transurethral resection of the bladder tumor to simply a deep biopsy procedure, to determine the grade and stage of the tumor. Definitive therapy would then be some other modality rather than transurethral resection.

The upper urinary tracts should be evaluated by excretory urography to rule out an associated transitional cell carcinoma of the renal pelvis or ureter. Hydroureteronephrosis noted on the excretory urogram, in association with a bladder tumor, usually indicates that the bladder carcinoma is invasive. A superficial tumor rarely, if ever, causes ureteral obstruction and secondary hydronephrosis.

Engberg et al. have reported resecting superficial bladder carcinoma, under topical urethral anesthesia, with infiltration of the tumor base with a local anesthetic.[9] However, the majority of the patients will be operated on under a general or spinal anesthetic in either a hospital or an out-patient surgical center. Therefore, an evaluation of the patient's general health is warranted. Laboratory tests such as CBC, chemistry profile, urinalysis and culture, as well as an EKG and chest x-ray, would be included.

SURGICAL PROCEDURE

The use of prophylactic antibiotics in patients with sterile urine, who are undergoing transurethral surgery, is controversial. MacDermott et al. found these antibiotics to be useful in patients undergoing transurethral resection of bladder carcinoma,[10] and we routinely start the patient on an intravenous, first-generation cephalosporin just prior to the surgical procedure. After the patient is given an anesthetic, he is positioned in the dorsal lithotomy position. The genitalia are washed with a germicidal soap and the patient is draped. Water is used for bladder irrigation during the procedure because it can cause lysis of the free-floating tumor cells and hopefully reduce tumor implantation.

The cystoscopy is repeated. A careful bimanual pelvic examination is done next, to determine the presence of a palpable mass or fixation that would suggest a higher-stage carcinoma that may be better handled by other therapeutic modalities than transurethral resection. Random biopsies are obtained with cold-cup biopsy forceps and submitted separately to pathology. The finding of carcinoma in situ, or even dysplasia, has a significant effect on the patient's prognosis and subsequent therapy.[11] Either a constant flow (e.g. Iglesias) or an intermittent-flow resectoscope may be used. The constant flow has the advantage because the bladder remains stable at a fixed volume. The bladder wall thickness is not changed by filling, therefore, the chance of bladder perforation is reduced. It also allows uninterrupted resection, permitting quicker surgery and less fluid absorption, especially in cases of large-volume tumors.

Papillary Lesions

The majority of papillary transitional cell carcinomas are approximately 1 to 3 cm in size. They are usually located on the lateral or posterior wall of the bladder and are readily amenable to transurethral resection. If the lesion is near the bladder-neck or ureteral orifice, the location may complicate the surgical removal. This issue will be discussed in a later section.

Resection is usually begun at the superior portion of the tumor by moving the loop backward and forward, similar to transurethral resection of a benign prostatic adenoma (Fig. 22-1). However, a point will be reached where it may be more advisable to extend the resectoscope loop and, with a rocking motion similar to scraping a wall, the loop is brought down and the lesion is further removed (Fig. 22-2).

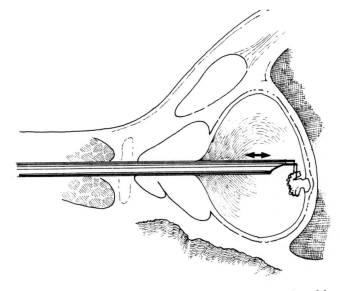

FIG. 22-1. Transurethral resection begun at the superior portion of the tumor.

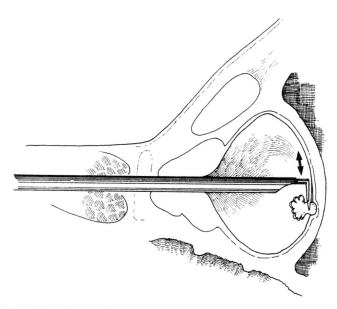

FIG. 22-2. Transurethral resection completed with rocking type of motion.

Bleeding should be well controlled as the resection proceeds, particularly with the larger lesions, so that the surgeon does not become disoriented because of poor visibility caused by excessive bleeding. Resection is usually begun at the top of the lesion so that as the blood flows down, it will not obscure the operator's lens. Eventually, the base of the lesion is reached and resected.

The base should be resected as a separate entity so that the proper depth of invasion may be determined. It is submitted as a separate specimen. An area approximately 1 cm around the base of the lesion should be resected and this area, including the base, is thoroughly fulgurated. The National Cooperative Study, in their review of transurethral resection of bladder tumors, noted that 41% of the tumors recurred at the site of the original resection, suggesting an inadequate initial resection fulguration.[12]

Multiple Papillary Lesions

Treatment of multiple papillary lesions with transurethral resection depends on the tumor's location and size, and on the surgeon's skill. In general, we found that it is advisable to remove the smaller lesions initially and to start at the dome of the bladder. This way, any bleeding goes toward the bladder base and does not obscure the surgeon's vision. The larger lesions are then resected in the manner similar to the technique described above.

In the case of a patient with large, bulky, intravesical tumors that do not permit an easy or complete transurethral resection, a number of procedures have been recommended. Tumor control may be obtained in some of these patients

using an open cystotomy with electroresection (Fig. 22-3). However, this is usually associated with significant bleeding and the risk of spilling tumor cells in the open wound, causing tumor implantation.

Other therapeutic modalities include intravesical chemotherapy, the increasing of intravesical pressure with the Helmstein balloon, mucosal stripping, and intercavitary irradiation. Bracken et al. have suggested that cystectomy be considered in such cases.[13] Soto et al. found a number of these patients, who had a simple cystectomy, to have areas of frank invasion into the bladder wall.[14] Bulky intravesical disease is usually evident at initial presentation or as Bracken et al. have noted, by the time of the second cystoscopy.[13] Fortunately, such problems are quite rare. However, in those patients where the tumor cannot be removed by standard transurethral resection, we would definitely consider a cystectomy.

Sessile Lesions

The finding of a sessile lesion is usually associated with a higher-grade, infiltrating bladder lesion as compared to the papillary type. If bladder invasion is documented by transurethral ultrasound of the bladder or CT scan, the surgeon may simply wish to biopsy the lesion and use another therapeutic modality. Only rarely may transurethral resection encompass a superficially invasive, sessile lesion.

Barnes reported that the 5-year survival rate for stage-B lesions, treated by transurethral resection, was 31%. However, he did not divide them into Stage B1 or B2.[15] Wolf et al., in a series of 52 patients, used transurethral resection as a primary mode of therapy in 22 patients (42%).[16] Of that group, 36%

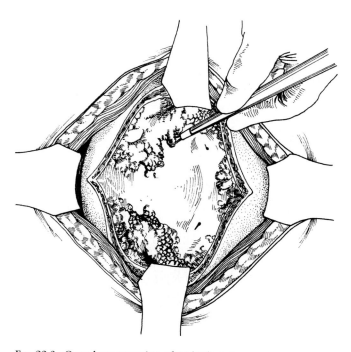

FIG. 22-3. Open-loop resection of multiple tumors.

had no recurrence at 5 years. Therefore, in selected cases, transurethral resection may be a definitive mode of therapy in patients with stage-T2 transitional cell carcinoma.

The resection is begun at the superior aspect of the lesion and bleeding is controlled, as the procedure continues, to avoid blocking the surgeon's vision (Fig. 22-4). It may be necessary to remove the bulk of the tumor and then to resect the tumor base and the bladder wall immediately adjacent. If this is to be the definitive procedure, the bladder muscle should appear clean and, in some instances, small areas of perivesical fat may be observed (Fig. 22-5A and B). A wider margin of adjacent bladder, approximately 2 cm, should be obtained rather than the small margin removed while resecting a superficial papillary tumor. The resected tumor fragments should be removed periodically during the procedure because their presence in the bladder may make it difficult to determine what tissue has been resected and what remains unresected.

As the base is approached, bleeding should be well under control and the pressure of the irrigating fluid should be just

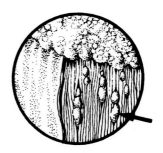

Fig. 22-5B. Deep resection of bladder wall with small areas of fat indicated by the arrow protruding through the muscle free of apparent tumor.

sufficient to allow good visualization, while reducing possible extravasation of the irrigating fluid. Undoubtedly, minimal extravasation does occur and if there is uninfected urine and the patient is asymptomatic, simple catheter drainage may be sufficient. However, if the patient develops pain and rigidity of the abdominal wall, perivesical drainage may be necessary.

CARCINOMA IN SITU

Patients with carcinoma in situ often present with symptoms of urinary urgency and frequency and are found to have microscopic hematuria. Cystoscopic examination of the bladder may reveal erythematous patches that, on biopsy, show carcinoma in situ. These may be single or multiple.

These lesions may be resected or fulgurated. However, Prout et al. pointed out, in 52 patients they reviewed, that transurethral resection by itself was not definitive therapy.[17] Herr and Laudone have reported that intravesical BCG was the effective adjuvant chemotherapy.[18]

POSTOPERATIVE CARE

Following resection of the tumor, hemostasis must be meticulous. Soloway and Masters suggested that intravesical chemotherapy, given at the time of resection, may reduce recurrent carcinoma.[19] We usually instill an agent such as thiotepa into the bladder, to be retained for approximately 1 hour. Therefore, hemostasis must be meticulous so that there is no subsequent clot retention.

Unless the resection is quite small, an indwelling catheter is left in place. The catheter may be connected to gravity drainage or to a continuous irrigation system. The catheter is left in place for 1 or 2 days until the urine is visibly clear, and antibiotics are given until the catheter is removed.

The patient is followed with periodic cystoscopy and bladder washings for cytology. These are usually done in the office, under local anesthesia, at 3-month intervals for the first year and 6-month intervals for the next 2 years. If the patient is cystoscopically clear, with negative cytologies, he is then cystoscoped on a yearly basis. Some advocate simply following

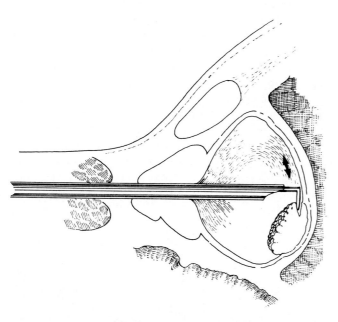

Fig. 22-4. Resection of sessile tumor with the rocking or scraping motion of the resectoscope loop.

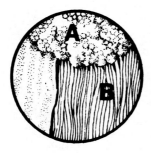

Fig. 22-5A. Endoscopic view of partially resected bladder tumor with the clean muscle fibers demonstrated (B) as compared to muscle wall with residual granular tumor (A).

the patient with cytology only. We feel that the average urologist does not have an expert in urinary cytology immediately available and, therefore, we recommend periodic cystoscopy.

Many factors influence the natural history of the disease. However, of the factors that contribute to the recurrence and progression of the disease, there are none whose presence or absence would clearly indicate which patients do not need to have continued cystoscopy surveillance.

SPECIAL PROCEDURES AND PROBLEMS

Fulguration

The Bugbee electrode, or resectoscope, may be used to destroy small lesions, 2 to 3 mm in size, by electrofulguration (Fig. 22-6). The depth of penetration through the bladder wall, with this technique, is approximately 2 mm.

This procedure is useful in patients who have been diagnosed previously with bladder cancer by appropriate biopsy, histologic evaluation, or who have small recurrences. This procedure is also for lesions near the bladder-neck, at the 12-o'clock position, that may be inaccessible to the standard resectoscope. The Bugbee electrode, with an Albarran catheterizing bridge, may reach and destroy such lesions successfully. However, fulguration destroys the cellular morphology and does not give us any information as to the degree of bladder wall invasion. We would prefer to use a cold-cup biopsy to obtain an adequate specimen for the pathologist and then fulgurate the base with the Bugbee electrode.

Lasers

Recently, Argon and YAG-neodymium lasers have been used in the management of superficial bladder tumors. Smith and

Dixon have pointed out that the Argon laser is particularly useful in lesions smaller than 1 cm.[20] The depth of penetration is about 1 mm. Conversely, the YAG-neodymium laser is capable of affecting a transmural thermal coagulation of the bladder wall, allowing treatment of larger tumors. The limited penetration of the Argon laser provides a higher margin of safety. Beisland and Seland noted that local recurrence, using a YAG-neodymium laser, was 4.8% versus 31.6% for transurethral resection of bladder tumors.[21] Presumably, electroresection of the tumors allows viable cells to become free and to implant on the urothelium. It is also possible that lymphatics may be sealed by the laser and thus prevent local spread and subsequent recurrence. The technique for laser therapy is discussed in detail in Chapter 23.

Problem Locations

Lesions at the dome of the bladder, particularly when they are near the bladder-neck, may be difficult to resect. Usually suprapubic pressure will bring the lesion into view, allowing the surgeon to resect it. However, if this cannot be done, a perineal urethrostomy can be performed. By circumventing the suspensory ligament of the penis, a better angle may be obtained through the perineal urethrostomy, thus allowing resection of lesions at the dome of the bladder and near the bladder-neck.

A perineal urethrostomy is performed over a grooved, #24 sound. The urethral mucosa is identified and secured with 0 chromic stay sutures. The resectoscope is introduced and the lesions are then removed. Following the procedure, the catheter is brought out through the perineal urethrostomy and the incision is packed open. After removal of the catheter, the perineal urethrostomy usually heals within 24 hours (Fig. 22-7).

When the lesions are on the lateral bladder wall, resection may evoke the obturator nerve reflex. This will result in adductor spasm of the leg as well as movement of the bladder. This may also result in perforation and extravasation from the bladder as the surgeon attempts to remove the lesion. In such instances, the patient may be given a general anesthetic and a neuromuscular blocking agent, such as succinylcholine, to prevent the obturator reflex. Another solution is to block the nerve with a local anesthetic as it exists through the obturator foramina, as described by Augspurger et al.[22] Occasionally, reduction of the electrical current, or stimulation of the bladder with the coagulation current and then resection when the neuromuscular junction is refractory, permits an unimpaired resection.

In a patient who is undergoing transurethral resection of his prostate for symptoms of bladder outlet obstruction, an unsuspected bladder carcinoma may be occasionally found. Laor et al. have shown that simultaneous resection of bladder tumors and the prostate has little influence on the occurrence of subsequent urothelial tumors from implantation of tumor cells in the raw prostatic fossa.[23]

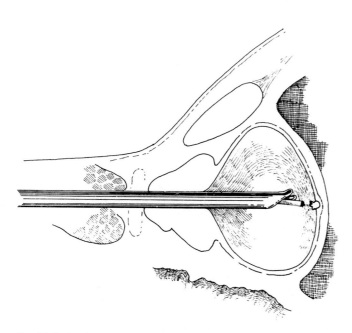

FIG. 22-6. Small 2- to 3-mm lesion destroyed by Bugbee electrode.

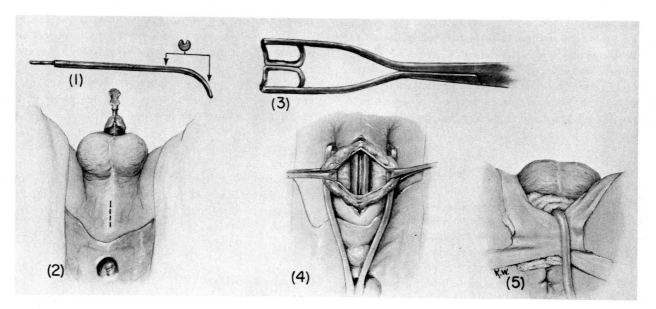

FIG. 22-7. Technique for perineal urethrostomy. (1) Grooved van Buren sound. (2) Site of perineal incision over sound. (3) Conger clamp. (4) Allis clamps on urethral edge expose steel sound. (5) Completed urethrostomy. (From Melchior, J., Valk, W. L., Foret, J. D., and Mebust, W. K.: Transurethral resection of the prostate via perineal urethrostomy: Complete analysis of 7 years of experience. J. Urol., *111:*640, 1974. Copyright 1974, the Williams and Wilkins Co., Baltimore.)

Fifteen percent of bladder carcinomas will be found to involve the ureteral orifice. These should be resected without regard to the ureteral orifice. If there is associated hydronephrosis, one may assume that this is an invasive tumor and, therefore, transurethral resection probably will not be the definitive mode of therapy. Fulguration should be kept to a minimum to help prevent stenosis of the orifice. Seventy percent of patients who have had the ureteral orifice and intramural portion of the ureter resected, will have vesicoureteral reflux postoperative.[24]

Rees et al. have noted that if the urine was sterile, there would appear to be no apparent damage to the kidney from reflux.[25] Recently, there has been some evidence that patients who develop reflux may be more prone to developing upper tract transitional cell carcinoma, as compared to those who do not have reflux.[26] Therefore, they must be followed very carefully.

Should there be extensive fulguration of the ureteral orifice, it may be advisable to insert an indwelling ureteral stent to avoid hydronephrosis from secondary edema as well as subsequent stricture formation.

INTRAVESICAL CHEMOTHERAPY

Intravesical chemotherapy to reduce recurrence and progression of superficial bladder carcinoma has been available for over 20 years. Which patients will benefit, with which drug, remains controversial. Furthermore, how frequently should intravesical chemotherapy be given and for what period of time? Part of the problem has been the difficulty in defining the natural history of superficial bladder carcinoma and the failure to use carefully controlled comparative studies.

In a series of 414 patients with stage-TA carcinoma and follow-up for a prolonged period of time, Fitzpatrick found that if the patient had no recurrence at 3-month/recystoscopy, the disease pattern followed a much more benign course.[8] Seventy-nine percent of these patients had no further recurrence. However, if there was a recurrence at 3 months, then only 10% had no further recurrence. Large tumor size and tumor multiplicity had a poor prognosis regarding recurrence and progression, in those with stage-TA lesions. He also studied age in relationship to prognosis. The incidence of recurrence, if the patient was 30 years or less, was under 8%. However, if the patient was age 30 to 40 and had a stage-TA lesion, the recurrence rate was 54%.

Patients with stage-T1 lesions usually have a higher histologic grade and are associated with a higher incidence of recurrence and progression, as compared to Stage TA. However, all T1 patients do not progress or recur. It has been our practice to withhold prophylactic intravesical chemotherapy until the first recurrence.

Of the agents available, thiotepa, Adriamycin, mitomycin-C, and BCG have been used in sufficient numbers and in controlled studies, to make some judgment as to the relative efficacy in the prevention of recurrence and progression of superficial carcinoma of the bladder.

Herr and Laudone, in reviewing intravesical chemotherapy for superficial bladder carcinoma, concluded that thiotepa appeared to be relatively ineffective. Adriamycin and mitomycin-C were moderately effective but BCG was superior in preventing or delaying recurrences.[18] The reduction in the number of patients who experienced tumor recurrence, over one year relative to TUR alone, was less than 10% for thiotepa, 20% for Adriamycin and mitomycin-C, and greater than 40%

for BCG. Furthermore, they concluded that BCG, in the high-risk patient with superficial bladder cancer, delayed the disease progression, prolonged the period of bladder preservation, and increased survival.

There are a number of doses and therapeutic regimes in the literature for each intravesical chemotherapeutic modality. The issue is "if a little is good, is a lot better"? Most regimes have an induction phase, i.e. chemotherapy weekly for 6 weeks followed by a monthly or bimonthly maintenance program. How long therapy should be given is unclear. Huland et al. have suggested that their long-term mitomycin is more beneficial than a short-term of perioperative intravesical mitomycin.[27] However, there is no controlled data to support protracted, prophylactic intravesical chemotherapy. Furthermore, there are risks of side effects from these agents, high costs, and patient inconvenience with prolonged therapy. We can only conclude that intravesical chemotherapy and BCG are effective, but further work needs to be done to clarify dosage and length of therapy.

Side Effects

Thiotepa has been shown to cause myelosuppression in 18% of patients. Chemical cystitis and urinary tract infection may occur in 2 to 40% of patients. Adriamycin has not been associated with myelosuppression although 50% have bladder irritative symptoms that may result in cessation of therapy. Mitomycin-C does not cause myelosuppression either. The most common side effect was bladder irritative symptoms, occurring in 10 to 15% of patients. Furthermore, these patients may get a chemical dermatitis if there is spillage of the urine, containing the mitomycin, on the skin during voiding. BCG usually causes an intense local inflammatory change in the bladder, resulting in dysuria, urgency, and frequency.

Serious systemic side effects are uncommon with BCG. Fever was noted in 4%, pneumonitis or hepatitis in 0.9%, arthralgia in 0.5%, ureteral obstruction in 0.3%, and bladder contracture in 0.2%. Systemic infection with BCG is rare and can be treated with antituberculous medication. The primary contraindication to BCG would appear to be patients with active tuberculosis and those who are significantly immunosuppressed.[18] Further details about immunotherapy and chemotherapy of bladder carcinoma are discussed in Chapters 45, 47, and 48.

CONCLUSION

Transurethral resection of superficial bladder carcinoma is the primary modality of treating existing lesions. Other modalities, such as lasers, continue to be evaluated. Sessile, invasive carcinoma may be occasionally treated by transurethral resection. The incidence of recurrence and progression depends on the initial stage, histologic grade, multiplicity of tumors, size of tumors, nuclear ploidy, and environmental factors. Adjuvant chemotherapy and immunotherapy has been found to be definitely useful in retarding recurrence and progression.

REFERENCES

1. SILVERBERG, E., and LUBERA, J. Cancer statistics. Ca-A. Cancer J. Clinicians, 39:3, 1989.
2. MELICOW, M. M. Histological study of vesical urothelium intervening between gross tumors in total cystectomy. J. Urol., 68:261, 1952.
3. PAGE, B. H., LEVISON, V. B., and CURWREN, M. B. The site of recurrence of non-infiltrating bladder tumors. Br. J. Urol., 50:237, 1978.
4. TORTI, F. M., LUM, B. L., and ASTON, D. Superficial bladder cancer—the primary of grade in the development of invasive disease. J. Clin. Oncol., 5:125, 1987.
5. ENGLAND, H. R., PARIS, A. M., and BLANDY, J. P. The correlation of T1 bladder tumor history with prognosis and follow-up requirements. Br. J. Urol., 53:593, 1981.
6. JORDAN, A. M., WEINGARTEN, J., and MURPHY, W. M. Transitional cell neoplasms of the urinary bladder: Can biologic potential be predicted from histologic grading? Cancer, 60:2761, 1987.
7. MALMSTROM, P-U., BUSCH, C., and NORLEN, B. J. Recurrence, progression and survival in bladder cancer: A retrospective analysis of 232 patients with >/ 5-year follow-up. Scand. J. Urol. Nephrol., 21:185, 1987.
8. FITZPATRICK, J. M. Superficial bladder cancer: Natural history, evaluation and management. AUA Update Series, 7(Lesson 11):82, 1989.
9. ENGBERG, A., SPANGBERG, A., and URNES, T. Transurethral resection of bladder tumors under local anesthesia. Urology, 22:385, 1983.
10. MacDERMOTT, J. P., et al. Cephradine prophylaxis in transurethral procedures for carcinoma of the bladder. Br. J. Urol., 62:136, 1988.
11. WOLF, H., and HOJGAARD, K. Prognostic factors in local surgical treatment of invasive bladder cancer, with special reference to the presence of urothelial dysplasia. Cancer, 51:1710, 1983.
12. NATIONAL BLADDER CANCER COLLABORATIVE GROUP. Surveillance, initial assessment, and subsequent progress of patients with superficial and subsequent bladder cancer in a prospective longitudinal study. Cancer Res., 37:2907, 1977.
13. BRACKEN, R. B., McDONALD, M. W., and JOHNSON, D. E. Cystectomy for superficial bladder cancer. Urology, 28:459, 1981.
14. SOTO, E. A., FRIEDEL, G. H., and TILTMAN, A. J. Bladder cancer seen in giant histologic sections. Cancer, 39:447, 1977.
15. BARNES, R. W., et al. Survival following transurethral resection of bladder carcinoma. Cancer Res., 37:2895, 1977.
16. WOLF, H., et al. Transurethral surgery in the treatment of invasive bladder cancer (T1 and T2). Scand. J. Urol. Nephrol. 104(Suppl.):127, 1987.
17. PROUT, G. R., JR., GRIFFIN, P. P., and DALY, J. J. The outcome of conservative treatment of carcinoma in situ of the bladder. J. Urol., 138:766, 1987.
18. HERR, H. W., and LAUDONE, V. P. Intravesical therapy for superficial bladder cancer. AUA Update Series, 8(Lesson 12):90, 1989.
19. SOLOWAY, M. S., and MASTERS, S. Urothelial susceptibility to tumor cell implantation—influence of cauterization. Cancer, 46:1158, 1980.

20. SMITH, J. A., and DIXON, J. A. Argon laser phototherapy of superficial transitional cell carcinoma of the bladder. J. Urol., *131:*655, 1984.

21. BEISLAND, H. O., and SELAND, P. A prospective study on neodymium-YAG laser irradiation versus TUR in the treatment of urinary bladder cancer. Scand. J. Urol. Nephrol., *20:*209, 1986.

22. AUGSPURGER, R., and DONOHUE, R. E. Prevention of obturator nerve stimulation during transurethral surgery. J. Urol., *123:*170, 1980.

23. LAOR, E., GRABSTALD, H., and WHITMORE, W. F. The influence of simultaneous resection of bladder tumors and prostate on the occurrence of prostatic urethral tumors. J. Urol., *126:*171, 1981.

24. FREED, S. Vesicoureteral reflux following transurethral resection of bladder tumors. J. Urol., *116:*184, 1976.

25. REES, R. M. The effect of transurethral resection of the intravesical ureter during the removal of bladder tumors. Br. J. Urol., *41:*2, 1969.

26. DE TORRES MATEOS, J. A., et al. Vesicorenal reflux and upper urinary tract transitional cell carcinoma after transurethral resection of recurrent superficial bladder carcinoma. J. Urol., *138:*49, 1987.

27. HULAND, H., et al. Long-term mitomycin-C instillation after transurethral resection of superficial bladder carcinoma: Influence on recurrence, progression and survival. J. Urol., *132:*27, 1984.

Laser Therapy for Carcinoma of the Bladder

Joseph A. Smith, Jr.

Laser technology has played an increasing role in urologic surgery. In some situations, lasers have offered no advantages over existing techniques and are used infrequently. In other settings, lasers have proved to be the treatment of choice. Although the most widespread endoscopic use of lasers in urology has been in the treatment of bladder cancer, there is no consensus regarding its value, and opinions range between profound enthusiasm and extreme skepticism. Neither of these attitudes is appropriate because laser treatment simply is an alternative to electrocautery resection. There are as yet no proved, definitive therapeutic advantages. On the other hand, treatment can often be performed with decreased patient morbidity and overall treatment expense. In addition, laser treatment offers a means for potential definitive endoscopic management of invasive bladder cancer in some patients.

INDICATIONS FOR LASER TREATMENT

There are several possible reasons why a laser may be indicated for treatment of bladder cancer. A great deal of discussion has centered around possible therapeutic advantages.

Because noncontact thermal destruction of tumors occurs, researchers have theorized that the recurrence rate due to implantation may be decreased.[1] Several series have established that laser treatment is at least as effective as electrocautery resection in eradicating grossly visible tumors.[2,3] In fact, some series show a substantial decrease in both local and overall recurrence of superficial bladder cancer in patients treated by laser compared to patients treated by electrocautery resection.[4,5] Sealing of lymphatic vessels by laser energy has been observed when a vital dye has been injected into the bladder,[1] but has not been demonstrated with more sensitive radioisotope studies.

Overall, although some data support a lower recurrence rate, there are no proved definitive therapeutic advantages for laser treatment of bladder cancer compared to electrocautery resection. Most of the rationale, then, for use of the laser centers around a consistently demonstrated decrease in patient morbidity.

The primary tissue effects of a laser when used to treat bladder cancer are due to thermal coagulation and protein denaturation. Because of this phenomenon, no bleeding occurs during laser treatment. In addition, the rapid heating of nerve endings and the relatively regular zone of thermal necrosis achieved with a laser cause less patient discomfort than a comparable electrocautery application. Laser treatment can be performed without anesthesia and usually with only modest patient discomfort. Laser fibers are flexible and can be inserted through flexible cystoscopes, further decreasing the discomfort of cystoscopy.

Obturator nerve spasm does not occur with laser energy. Tumors in diverticula can be treated without bladder perforation. Ureteral stenosis has not been observed even after treatment of tumors directly overlying the intramural ureter or ureteral orifice.

Even after a transmural coagulation, the bladder maintains its structural and architectural integrity. Thus, urinary extravasation is not a primary concern postoperatively. This, coupled with the lack of bleeding, obviates the need for Foley catheter drainage of the bladder. Thus, laser treatment of bladder cancer can easily be performed on an ambulatory outpatient basis without anesthesia. Postoperative bladder spasms and voiding discomfort usually are less severe after laser treatment than after electrocautery resection.

These putative advantages generally are irrelevant for treatment of invasive bladder cancer because minor improvements in morbidity are unimportant. However, laser treatment can extend the therapeutic margin some 5 to 7 mm beyond that obtained by electrocautery resection. Therefore, treatment of muscle-invasive bladder cancer could be performed without bladder perforation or bleeding. Difficulty in predicting the penetration depth of the laser energy, clinical understaging of invasive bladder cancer, and the inability to thermally coagulate tumors of greater size than stage $T3_b$ are limitations of laser treatment, but the procedure is especially useful in patients who are poor candidates for alternative therapy because of advanced age or poor overall health.

TUMOR STAGING

Because a laser causes thermal coagulation of tissue in a noncontact fashion, material is not retrievable for histologic examination in the usual manner. This has caused concern that understaging could occur when treating a presumed superficial lesion. In fact, several series have demonstrated that adequate tumor staging can be performed with laser therapy and that local recurrence rates compare extremely favorably (and may be superior) to those obtained with electrocautery resection.[3,4]

The most important criterion for patient selection is the visible appearance of the tumor. Lesions that have a characteristic papillary appearance and emanate from a stalk are unlikely to be anything other than low grade and low stage. On the other hand, lesions that appear more sessile or those associated with cytologic examinations positive for malignant cells should probably be treated with electrocautery resection so that deep muscle specimens can be examined. When laser treatment is performed, the malignant histology and tumor grading can be verified by taking cold cup biopsies from the tumor base. As an alternative, the laser-coagulated tissue maintains sufficient structural integrity that biopsies taken after laser treatment can be interpreted. Electrocautery resection followed by laser surgery to the base of the tumor has its proponents, but there seems little advantage to such a combined approach.

EQUIPMENT

Several parameters influence the depth of penetration of a laser, including the wavelength. Therefore, selection of an appropriate laser is essential. Fibers for endoscopic delivery of carbon dioxide laser energy have not been perfected and the wavelength (10,600 nanometers) is rapidly absorbed in a fluid medium. An argon laser has a spectral emission between 488 and 513 nanometers. Thermal coagulation and some vaporization occur, but penetration depths are limited. A KTP532 laser has a wavelength of 532 nanometers. Some vaporization occurs under water.

The wavelength that has been used most frequently for treatment of bladder tumors is 1,060 nanometers, a neodymium:YAG laser. Neodymium:YAG laser energy is readily transmitted via small flexible fibers. Light at this wavelength is poorly absorbed by water and body pigments. Thus, there is a relatively deep tissue penetration (Fig. 23-1).

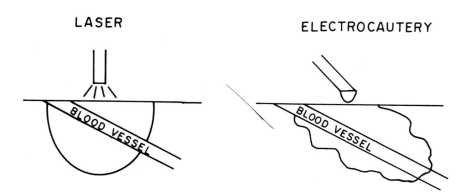

LASER   ELECTROCAUTERY

FIG. 23-1. A Nd:YAG laser produces a 3- to 5-mm zone of thermal necrosis. In contrast to electrocautery, a relatively uniform, conical area of tissue injury is observed.

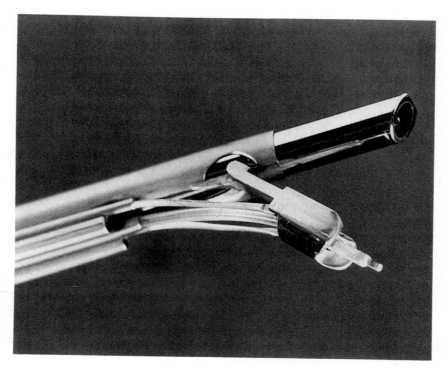

FIG. 23-2. A Nd:YAG laser fiber is flexible and can be inserted through standard rigid or flexible cystoscopes. A modified Albarran apparatus may be used to deflect the fiber tip.

Laser treatment can be performed through either a rigid cystoscope with a modified Albarran apparatus or a flexible cystoscope (Fig. 23-2). A 600-micron fiber is used with a rigid cystoscope. When flexible instruments are used, a 400-micron fiber is preferable to allow full deflection of the instrument tip.

Tips constructed of sapphire or other materials have been designed for contact use with neodymium:YAG laser fibers. Various configurations are available. These tips greatly increase the energy density and, thereby, the cutting effect of a neodymium:YAG laser. Some tissue vaporization also occurs. Because there is little forward scatter of the laser energy when contact tips are used, they have been proposed as a safer method for treatment of bladder cancer. However, treatment is slower, coagulation is less efficient, and there is less penetration of the bladder wall to eliminate small microextensions of the tumor.

TREATMENT TECHNIQUE

SUPERFICIAL BLADDER CANCER. Laser treatment may be performed in any area suitably equipped for cystoscopy in which adequate electrical power supply and water for cooling of the laser are available. The operating surgeon and other personnel in the immediate operating area (including the patient) should wear appropriate eye protection. For a neodymium:YAG laser, a special green tinted lens is necessary. Alternatively, a lens cap with an appropriate filter may be used once the fiber is inserted through the cystoscope.

When the laser is switched from the standby to the operate mode, an aiming beam becomes operative. The aiming beam usually is from a flash lamp source or a helium neon laser. Because the wavelength of a neodymium:YAG laser is invisible, the aiming beam defines the point of impact. The tip of the fiber is positioned 1 or 2 mm away from the surface of the tumor. Tumors larger than 2 cm are difficult to treat with laser energy alone. The primary limiting factor is the depth of the exophytic portion of the tumor, since 3 to 5 mm of penetration can be anticipated. As the superficial areas of the tumor are treated, the debris can be dislodged with the tip of the fiber or cystoscope to expose the deeper portions of the tumor. Debris that sticks to the tip of the fiber should be removed with a saline-soaked sponge.

A power output of 35 to 40 watts is chosen. Treatment is continued in a given area until a white color indicative of adequate thermal necrosis is observed (Fig. 23-3). Treatment is best performed as a dynamic process rather than a series of adjacent static impulses.[6] To accomplish this, it often is better to operate the laser with a continuous output rather than on a defined pulse duration. The beam should not be held in contact with a given area for more than two or three seconds. Visible changes in the tumor determine treatment adequacy.

On many patients, treatment can be performed without an anesthetic. The decision to proceed under local anesthesia depends partly upon the number and size of tumors, their location within the bladder, and the patient's anticipated pain tolerance. The laser energy itself is perceptible as a burning

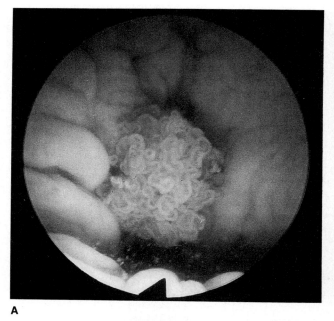

A

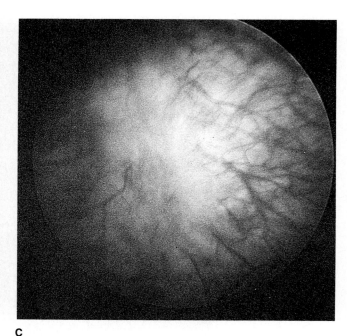

C

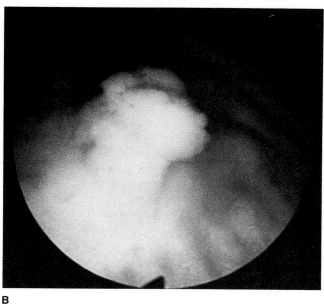

B

FIG. 23-3. *A*, Papillary transitional cell carcinoma of the bladder. *B*, After Nd:YAG laser treatment, the tumor undergoes a white discoloration characteristic of adequate thermal necrosis. *C*, After the tumor has sloughed, a pale white scar is seen without evidence of residual tumor.

sensation, but usually the amount of discomfort is slight and can be easily tolerated. Even though a transmural injury may be created, the bladder maintains its structural and architectural integrity. Therefore, a Foley catheter is not necessary postoperatively.

Tumors overlying the ureteral orifice or extending just inside the intramural ureter may be treated with laser energy. There are no reports of stenosis of the ureteral orifice or ureteral obstruction after laser treatment (Fig. 23-4). The thin wall of a bladder diverticulum raises concern for treatment of any tumors within bladder diverticula. However, small tumors within bladder diverticula have been successfully treated by neodymium:YAG laser. A coagulation necrosis without perfo-

ration of the diverticulum is observed, and a shriveling effect is often seen.

INVASIVE BLADDER CANCER. The technique that has been used for endoscopic application of laser energy in the treatment of invasive bladder cancer involves a preliminary electrocautery resection. This procedure is performed to establish the diagnosis as well as to debulk the tumor.[7] It is best to wait several days between resection and treatment in order to allow bleeding to cease and lysis of any overlying blood clots that may interfere with delivery of the laser energy.

Because the energy is being applied to an irregular resection crater, visible changes are unreliable predictors of pene-

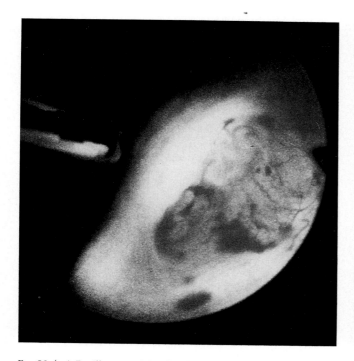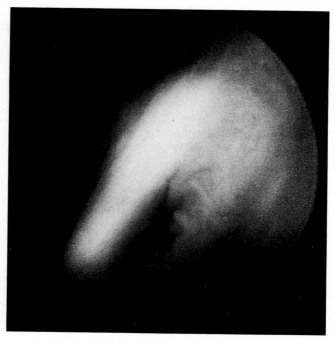

FIG. 23-4. *A*, Papillary transitional cell carcinoma extending just inside left ureteral orifice. *B*, After Nd:YAG laser treatment (35 watt × 3 seconds), the orifice has healed without residual tumor or stenosis.

tration depth. Energy should be systematically applied over the entire tumor crater as well as some of the surrounding, normal-appearing mucosa for a distance of at least 1 cm. Because transmural coagulation is the goal, a power output of 40 to 50 watts is used. Treatment is maintained in a given area for 3 to 4 seconds.

Because treatment of invasive bladder cancer often involves delivery of higher total energy than with superficial tumors, general or regional anesthesia is preferred. In addition, a simultaneous electrocautery debulking may be performed if necessary. Foley catheter drainage of the bladder is not mandatory postoperatively.

RESULTS

Beisland and Seland examined the local recurrence of superficial bladder tumors in a randomized study of electrocautery resection and laser treatment.[8] They found a significantly decreased local recurrence rate in the laser-treated patients. In most series, local tumor recurrence has been apparent in 2 to 8% of patients treated with a neodymium:YAG laser,[9] a figure that compares favorably to that for electrocautery resection.

Hofstetter has reported bowel perforation in 2 of 500 patients treated with a neodymium:YAG laser.[1] At the University of Utah, bowel perforation has not been observed in our experience with 210 patients. Nevertheless, anecdotal reports of small bowel perforation continue to emerge, and caution should be maintained, especially in treating lesions of the bladder dome.

Predictably, results for treatment of invasive bladder cancer have correlated closely with the clinical stage of the tumor. For stage T2 lesions (B1), no tumor recurrence has been observed with a minimum of 6 months follow-up in 12 of 15 patients (80%) in the University of Utah series. For stage $T3_a$ tumors, recurrence has occurred in approximately one third of patients, with less favorable results for those with stage $T3_b$ tumors.

CONCLUSION

Neodymium:YAG laser treatment of superficial bladder cancer can be performed with minimal patient morbidity. Bleeding does not occur, and the ability to perform the procedure without anesthesia or postoperative Foley catheter drainage imparts significant advantages over electrocautery resection. Concerns regarding the inability to stage laser-treated tumors adequately have largely been eliminated. The results of treatment are at least equal to those achieved by alternative methods and, perhaps, superior in some patient groups.

Only a minority of patients with invasive bladder cancer should undergo laser therapy as primary treatment. Difficulty in predicting penetration depth and inaccuracies in clinical staging are the primary limitations of treatment. Ideally, patients who are not candidates for alternative treatment (generally radical surgery) should be offered laser therapy if they have tumors that clinically are judged to be stage $T3_b$ or less. Treatment can be performed with low morbidity, and other therapeutic alternatives are not eliminated should laser therapy prove to be unsuccessful.

REFERENCES

1. HOFSTETTER, A., and FRANK, F. Laser use in urology. In: *Surgical Application of Lasers.* Edited by J. A. Dixon. Chicago, Year Book Medical Publishers, 1983, pp. 146.

2. MALLOY, T. R., and WEIN, A. J. Laser treatment of bladder carcinoma and genital condylomata. Urol. Clin. North Am., *24:*26, 1987.

3. SMITH, J. A., JR., and MIDDLETON, R. G. Bladder cancer. In: *Lasers in Urologic Surgery.* Edited by J. A. Smith, Jr. Chicago, Year Book Medical Publishers, 1985, pp. 52.

4. HOFSTETTER, A., et al. Endoscopic neodymium:YAG laser application for destroying bladder tumors. Eur. Urol., 7:278, 1981.

5. BEISLAND, H. O. Neodymium:YAG laser in the treatment of urinary bladder carcinoma and localized prostatic carcinoma. J. Oslo City Hosp., *36:*63, 1986.

6. SMITH, J. A., JR. Endoscopic applications of laser energy. Urol. Clin. North Am., *13:*405, 1986.

7. SMITH, J. A. Laser treatment of invasive bladder cancer. J. Urol., *135:*55, 1986.

8. BEISLAND, H. O., and SELAND, P. A prospective randomized study on neodymium:YAG laser irradiation versus TUR in the treatment of urinary bladder cancer. Scand. J. Urol. Nephrol., *20:*209, 1986.

9. STAEHLER, G., et al. The use of the neodymium:YAG lasers in urology: indications, technique and critical assessment. J. Urol., *134:*1155, 1985.

Cystectomy for Bladder Cancer

Donald G. Skinner

The successful management of carcinoma of the bladder depends on several factors: the grade and stage of the initial tumor, evidence of multicentricity and, in particular, the proper and timely selection of treatment from a wide range of therapeutic methods.

Once the diagnosis of a high-grade or muscle-invading tumor has been established, efforts should be made to rule out metastatic disease. Appropriate studies include chest roentgenogram, bone scan correlated with bone roentgenograms for suspicious areas, and liver function tests. Radioisotopic liver scan is performed only if liver function studies show abnormalities. If there is no evidence of metastatic disease, aggressive therapy should be planned. Other diagnostic efforts to stage the localized primary tumor, including ultrasound, computerized tomography (CT), and magnetic resonance imaging (MRI), have become a routine part of the staging workup for many urologists. However, the accuracy of CT in predicting transmural invasion or the involvement of pelvic lymph nodes is less than 75% in most studies, with both over- and understaging common. MRI has not proved to be substantially better. Therefore, we do not routinely obtain these studies before operation.

The successful management of high-grade tumors or invasive tumors of any grade usually requires aggressive therapy. Rarely a high-grade, unifocal, or grade 2 muscle-invasive tumor may be responsive to transurethral or segmental resection. In such cases, it is essential that the urologist obtain random mucosal biopsies remote from the tumor and make certain there is no atypia or evidence of carcinoma in situ. Close follow-up by cystoscopic and cytologic studies to detect recurrence is necessary. Any overt high-grade tumor associated with mucosal atypia or carcinoma in situ (even though the primary tumor may not be invasive) or any recurrence following initial conservative treatment of a unifocal high-grade tumor warrants radical cystectomy.

Radical cystectomy implies the en bloc removal of the anterior pelvic organs: the prostate, seminal vesicles, and bladder with its visceral peritoneum and perivesical fat in men, and the urethra, bladder, cervix, vaginal cuff, uterus, ovaries, and anterior pelvic peritoneum in women. A pelvic iliac lymph node dissection of varying extent is usually included, but it should be denoted together with the term radical cystectomy to clarify whether a meticulous dissection was performed. The operation is sometimes called an anterior exenteration with bilateral pelvic iliac lymph node dissection, particularly in women.

235

This is the optimal ablative surgical procedure for the treatment of invasive carcinoma of the bladder in the properly selected patient who is an appropriate surgical risk. Many urologic oncologists have used planned, preoperative radiation therapy before radical cystectomy.[1] Results indicate that doses up to 5,000 rads have no significant impact on the operation in terms of morbidity or the ability to perform the operation successfully as described. Previous radiation therapy in excess of 6,000 rads, however, is associated with increased surgical morbidity and mortality.[2] It is usually not feasible or safe to perform a pelvic node dissection in such patients because of the dense desmoplastic radiation-induced pelvic fibrosis frequently associated with accumulated doses of this magnitude.

In 1984, we reported a comparison of 100 patients receiving preoperative radiation therapy with 97 treated by operation alone, and found no significant difference in survival or pelvic recurrence rates.[3] Recently, two other centers have confirmed this finding.[4] Therefore, we no longer use preoperative radiation routinely for our cystectomy patients.

PREOPERATIVE PREPARATION

In general, patients are admitted by 9:00 A.M. the day before operation. They continue a regular or low-roughage diet through breakfast the morning of the day before the operation, thereafter taking only clear liquids by mouth until the midnight before the operation. At 9:00 A.M. the day before the operation, 120 ml of Neoloid, a palatable emulsion of castor oil, are given by mouth. Patients then receive 1 g orally of neomycin at 10:00 A.M., 11:00 A.M., 12 noon, 1:00 P.M., 4:00 P.M., 8:00 P.M., and 12 midnight, and 1 g orally of erythromycin base at 12 noon, 4:00 P.M., 8:00 P.M., and 12 midnight.[5] This intestinal preparation is of short duration and is exceedingly effective in cleansing and decompressing the small and large intestines. It also prevents dehydration associated with prolonged catharsis, renders enemas unnecessary, and maintains good nutritional support.

Patients older than 50 years of age routinely undergo prophylactic digitalization before radical cystectomy, unless there is a specific contraindication. Digoxin is given orally: 0.5 mg on admission, 0.25 mg the afternoon before the operation, and 0.125 mg that evening. No digoxin is given the morning of the operation. Evidence suggests that prophylactic preoperative digitalization may reduce the incidence of intraoperative or postoperative arrhythmias and the development of congestive heart failure in elderly patients undergoing a surgical procedure of considerable magnitude, such as cystectomy.[6,7] This dosage schedule has not resulted in toxicity in any of more than 500 patients.

Preoperative hydration with Ringer's lactate or 5% dextrose with 0.5 normal saline solution at 125 ml per hour is initiated intravenously the afternoon before the operation. One of the most important preparations for the procedure is the determination of the ileal stoma site. This decision is made jointly by the surgeon and the enterostomal therapist, while examining the patient in the supine, sitting, and standing positions. Optimal stomal placement is essential to postoperative management, patient acceptance of the procedure, and ability to care for the ileostomy effectively. In patients opting for continent urinary diversion, the position for the ileostomy location may be lower (well caudal to the belt or underwear line), and close to the pubis for concealment, since these patients do not wear an external appliance skin folds or creases are unimportant. However, if cosmetic concealment is of little concern to the patient, placement higher on the abdominal wall may facilitate intermittent catheterization.

SURGICAL TECHNIQUE

Position

The patient is placed in the hyperextended supine position (Fig. 24-1). A catheter is routinely placed in the bladder, which is then drained.

Incision

The operation commences with a midline incision. The anterior rectus sheath is incised, the rectus muscle is retracted laterally, and the posterior rectus sheath and peritoneum are entered in the superior part of the incision. As the peritoneum and posterior rectus fascia are incised inferiorly, care is taken to identify the urachal remnant, which should be circumscribed so that it can be removed en bloc with the bladder. Similarly, if the patient has had a previous segmental resection or cystotomy through a vertical incision, that incisional tract should be circumscribed full thickness, to be removed en bloc with the bladder.

When the peritoneal cavity has been opened, a careful intra-abdominal exploration is necessary to determine the extent of disease, to search for possible intrahepatic metastatic disease, and to detect concomitant unrelated disease. All intra-abdominal adhesions should be incised and freed at this time.

Dissection

A right-angle Richardson retractor is used to elevate the right abdominal wall, and the surgeon mobilizes the ascending colon and peritoneal attachments to the small intestinal mesentery (Fig. 24-2). The ascending colon and peritoneal attachments to the small intestine mesentery are triangular, with the ileocecal region the apex of this triangle, the retroperitoneal transverse portion of the duodenum the base, the medial portion of the descending left colonic mesentery the left border of the triangle, and the peritoneal attachment to the ascending colon (avascular line of Toldt) the right side of the triangle. This mobilization is an important part of setting up the surgical field to perform a cystectomy and is necessary for proper subsequent packing of the intra-abdominal contents.

The left colon and sigmoid mesentery are widely mobilized by incising the avascular line of Toldt along the left gutter. This dissection extends up to the lower pole of the left kidney, and

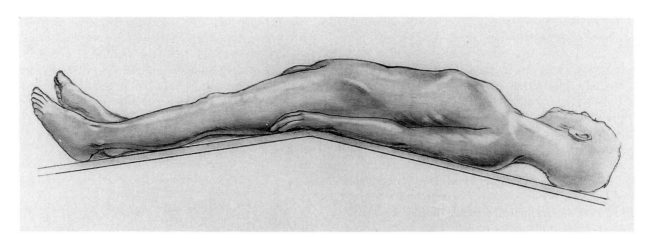

FIG. 24-1. Proper position of the patient for cystectomy. Hyperextension of the table opens up the pelvis and facilitates exposure. (From Skinner, D., and Lieskovsky, G., eds. *Diagnosis and Management of Genitourinary Cancer.* Philadelphia, W. B. Saunders Co., 1988, p. 608. Reproduced by permission of W. B. Saunders Co.)

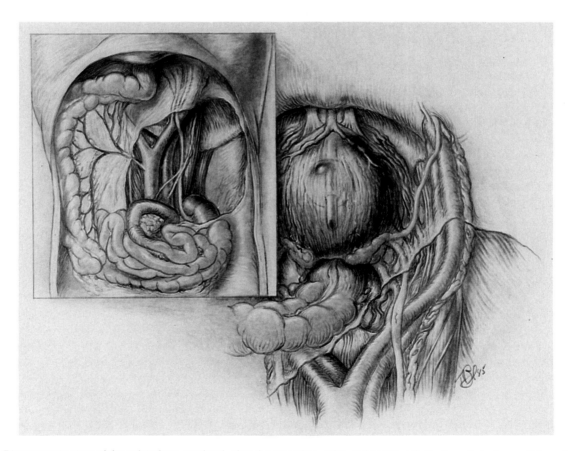

FIG. 24-2. Diagrammatic view of the pelvis from overhead, after the ascending colon and peritoneal attachments to the small bowel mesentery have been mobilized up to the level of the duodenum (inset). This mobilization is important to allow the bowel to be packed in the epigastrium and to provide exposure to the area of the aortic bifurcation for initiation of the node dissection. (From Skinner, D., and Lieskovsky, G., eds. *Diagnosis and Management of Genitourinary Cancer.* Philadelphia, W. B. Saunders Co., 1988, p. 609. Reproduced by permission of W. B. Saunders Co.)

the sigmoid mesentery is mobilized from the sacral promontory and distal aorta up to the origin of the inferior mesenteric artery. In this way, the base of the sigmoid mesentery is dissected from the sacral promontory with numerous adherent bands divided so that the left ureter can eventually be brought under the mesentery without angulation or tension.

A self-retaining retractor is positioned. We prefer to use a Finochietto retractor. The right colon and small intestine are packed in the epigastrium with three moist laparotomy pads and a moist towel rolled to the width of the abdomen. No attempt is made to pack the descending colon, which should be left as mobile as possible. There is an art to successful packing that greatly facilitates the operation. In general, the surgeon's left hand should be used to position the small intestine. Open, moist laparotomy pads can be swept along the palm of the left hand using the right hand to tuck the pad under the viscera to be packed. It is best to pack each gutter and then to pack the remaining small intestine with the third laparotomy pad. The rolled moist towel can then be positioned to finish the packing; it should lie horizontally above the level of the aortic bifurcation. Occasionally a large Deaver retractor on the rolled towel facilitates the cephalad exposure, but usually the region above the aortic bifurcation is readily visible without retraction (Fig. 24-3).

At this point both ureters are dissected in the deep pelvis to several centimeters beyond the point at which they cross the common iliac arteries. Two large right-angle hemoclips are placed on the distal mobilized ureter, 1.5 to 2.0 cm apart, and the ureter is divided just proximal to the distal hemoclip. A small portion of the proximal ureter is further mobilized cephalad and tucked out of harm's way beneath the rolled towel packing. Usually a medial vessel needs to be clipped and divided to allow adequate mobilization.

Proximal and Distal Limits

The proximal extent of the lymph node dissection is initiated 1 to 2 cm above the aortic bifurcation. All fibroareolar and lymphatic tissue is dissected from the distal aorta and vena cava extending laterally to the genitofemoral nerve, which represents the lateral limits of the dissection. Large or medium hemoclips are placed on the proximal limits of dissection to reduce lymphatic leak, but the distal fibroareolar lymphatic tissue is not clipped unless a vessel is identified, because that tissue will be removed. In women the infundibulopelvic ligament (suspensory ligament of the ovary) is ligated and divided, including the ovarian vein.

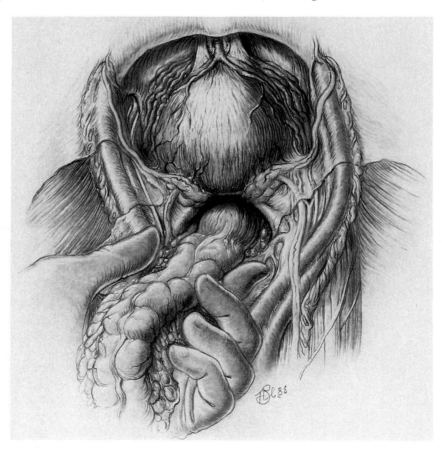

FIG. 24-3. Diagrammatic view of the pelvis after the ascending colon and small bowel have been packed in the epigastrium. Note that the sigmoid mesentery is being mobilized off the sacral promontory and distal aorta. This procedure facilitates the node dissection and allows the left ureter to pass under the sigmoid mesentery without angulation. (From Skinner, D., and Lieskovsky, G., eds. *Diagnosis and Management of Genitourinary Cancer.* Philadelphia, W. B. Saunders Co., 1988, p. 610. Reproduced by permission of W. B. Saunders Co.)

All tissue is swept from the distal aorta, vena cava, and common iliac vessels, over the sacral promontory into the deep pelvis. The common iliac arteries are mobilized, and care must be taken to secure small arterial and venous branches running on the sacral promontory. The cautery can be helpful in this area because hemoclips are often dislodged, and annoying bleeding can result if these vessels are not well controlled.

After the proximal portion of the dissection is complete, a finger is passed under the pelvic peritoneum over the external iliac artery and vein to the femoral canal. The opposite hand can be used to sweep the peritoneum from the undersurface of the transverse abdominis fascia to connect with the dissection from above. This technique elevates the peritoneum and defines the limits of lateral peritoneum to be excised. The elevated peritoneum is incised medial to the testicular vessels in men and lateral to the ovarian vein in women, with the vas deferens in men and the round ligament in women clipped and divided. These are the only structures of consequence encountered in this divided tissue.

A large right-angle rake retractor is used to elevate the lower abdominal wall. Tension on this retractor should be directed to the ceiling, not caudally, and the distal round ligament in women and spermatic cord in men should be retracted to provide maximum visualization of the region of the femoral canal.

All fibroareolar and lymphatic tissue is dissected from the distal external iliac artery and vein circumferentially. Medium hemoclips are meticulously placed on the distal tissue to prevent lymph leakage. The deep circumflex iliac vein represents the distal limits of dissection along the artery, the genitofemoral nerve represents the lateral limits, and the pectineal (Cooper's) ligament represents the medial distal limits of dissection. The lymph node of Cloquet (or Rosenmüller) represents the distal limits of lymphatic dissection medial to the external iliac vein in the femoral canal, and afferent lymphatics into this node should be clipped. The external iliac artery and vein are then circumferentially dissected. The surgeon should look for an accessory obturator vein draining into the back wall of the external iliac vein at this level. This vessel, present in approximately 40% of patients, is ligated and divided.

When the distal limits of the dissection have been defined and the dissection completed, the proximal portion of the external iliac artery and vein are skeletonized. A small muscular artery and venous branch are usually found along the proximal portion of the external iliac vessels, but other major vascular branches are not usually encountered. The fibroareolar tissue overlying the psoas can be incised medial to the genitofemoral nerve. On the left side, the genitofemoral nerve often pursues a more medial course and may be related intimately to the vessels; if so, it is excised.

Obturator Dissection

At this point the external iliac vessels are retracted medially, and a gauze sponge is used to dissect bluntly all fibroareolar and lymphatic tissue from the lateral wall of the pelvis. The tissue is pushed with one or two sponges into the obturator fossa (Fig. 24-4). The vessels are then retracted laterally and, with traction, using the left hand, the surgeon can bluntly sweep all lymphatic and fibroareolar tissue out of the obturator fossa. Great care must be exercised to identify and protect the obturator nerve and not tear the internal iliac vein. The nerve is carefully dissected free and retracted laterally so that the index finger of the left hand can be placed medial to that nerve, parallel to the endopelvic fascia. The second finger is passed along the endopelvic fascia medial to this region, which isolates the obturator vessels between the two fingers, medial to the obturator nerve. These vessels should be ligated at this time and divided, allowing the obturator group of nodes to be swept medially with the specimen. When the obturator fossa has been dissected free, the lateral pedicle is developed.

The next step is perhaps the most important in the safe performance of a radical cystectomy. With countertraction by the left hand, the left index finger is gently swept medial to the internal iliac artery in the deep pelvis, parallel to the sweep of the sacrum, extending all the way to the endopelvic fascia. This technique helps define two pedicles, one extending from the anterior pelvic organs to the internal iliac vessels, and the other extending posteriorly to the rectum. Again using the left hand with the index finger behind the lateral pedicle for countertraction, the surgeon further skeletonizes the internal iliac artery (Fig. 24-5). The first branch from the posterior portion of the internal iliac artery, the posterior superior gluteal artery, should be identified and protected if possible. A right-angle clamp can be passed carefully behind the internal iliac artery distal to the posterior superior gluteal artery. The internal iliac artery is ligated at this level. Occasionally, because of the extent of disease or anatomic variation, it is necessary to ligate the internal iliac artery proximal to its first posterior muscular branch. Some patients in whom this is done complain of buttock claudication with exercise postoperatively, but this sequela can be avoided by preserving the posterior superior gluteal artery whenever possible.

The lateral pedicle is divided between large hemoclips all the way to the endopelvic fascia or as far as technically feasible (see Fig. 24-5). Blunt dissection with the index finger allows development of the plane and protection of the rectum. Large right-angle hemoclip appliers are ideally suited for proper placement of clips. It is important to position the dual set of clips as far apart as possible so that at least 0.5 to 1.0 cm of tissue projects beyond each clip as the pedicle is divided. This positioning prevents the clips from becoming dislodged, which leads to troublesome bleeding.

Posterior Dissection

When the lateral pedicle has been divided, attention is drawn to the posterior pedicle. A large clamp can be placed on the urachal peritoneal remnant in men, and a double-hook thyroid tenaculum can be placed on the body of the uterus in women to give anterior traction for visualization of the cul-de-sac or

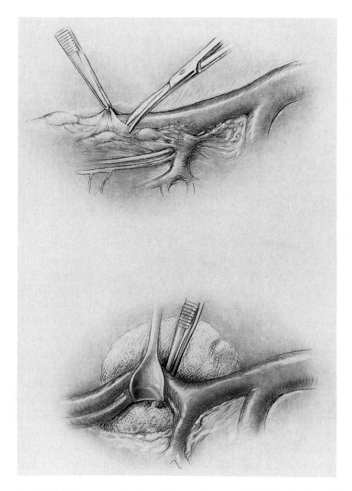

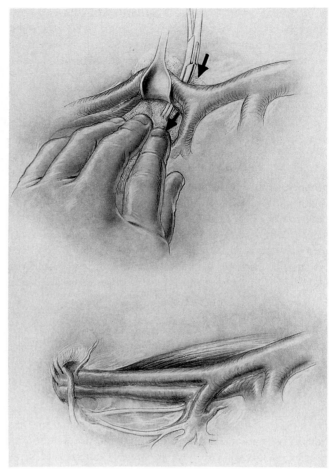

Fig. 24-4. Diagrammatic view of the technique of skeletonization of the external iliac artery and vein. A gauze sponge is used to dissect out the obturator fossa, sweeping all fibroareolar and lymphatic tissue, en bloc, toward the bladder. (From Skinner, D., and Lieskovsky, G., eds. *Diagnosis and Management of Genitourinary Cancer.* Philadelphia, W. B. Saunders Co., 1988, p. 612. Reproduced by permission of W. B. Saunders Co.)

the pouch of Douglas. The peritoneum lateral to the rectum is incised, extending the incision anteriorly into the cul-de-sac to join the incision from the opposite side. The anterior and posterior peritoneal reflections meet in the cul-de-sac to form Denonvillier's fascia, which extends caudally to the urogenital diaphragm, and constitutes an important anatomic boundary in men between the posterior surface of the prostate and seminal vesicles and the anterior surface of the rectum (Fig. 24-6). The peritoneal incision in the cul-de-sac should be made immediately on the rectal side rather than on the bladder side so that the plane between the posterior leaf of Denonvillier's fascia and the anterior rectal wall is developed (Fig. 24-7). This incision allows entry into Denonvillier's space. In this plane, the rectum can easily be swept from the bladder, seminal vesicles, and prostate in men and from the posterior vaginal wall in women. If the peritoneal incision in the cul-de-sac is made anteriorly, entry may occur between the two layers of Denonvilliers' fascia or anterior to that fascial plane, making dissec-

tion of the rectum difficult with increased risk of incidental rectal injury. Occasionally, carcinoma may obliterate this plane, or previous high-dose radiation therapy may cause severe fibrosis, making dissection of this plane difficult. In instances where patients have received previous high-cumulative-dose radiation (greater than 6,000 rads), dissection of this plane can be greatly facilitated by an initial perineal dissection.[2]

A hand should be used to finish the dissection of this plane with posterior motion to sweep the rectum from Denonvillier's fascia and to develop the posterior pedicles (Fig. 24-8). This motion thins and develops the posterior pedicle, facilitates use of hemoclips, and protects the rectum from injury during division of the posterior pedicles. When the posterior pedicles have been defined, they are clipped and divided all the way to the endopelvic fascia in men, which is also incised on the ipsilateral side of the prostate and swept from the posterior and side wall of the prostate (see Fig. 24-8).

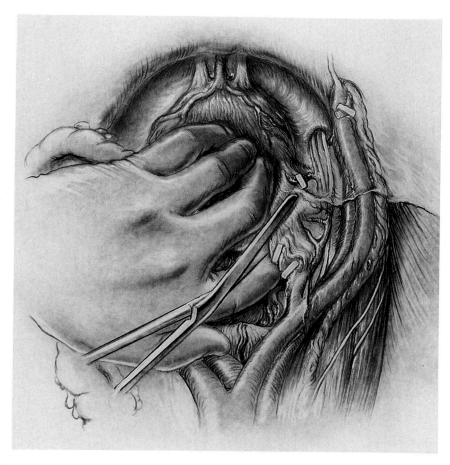

FIG. 24-5. The left hand is used to define the right lateral pedicle, extending from the bladder to the hypogastric artery. To develop this plane, the surgeon inserts the index finger just behind the hypogastric artery. This thin vascular pedicle can then be clipped and divided all the way to the endopelvic fascia. Traction with the left hand defines the pedicle, allows direct visualization, and protects the rectum from injury. (From Skinner, D., and Lieskovsky, G., eds. *Diagnosis and Management of Genitourinary Cancer.* Philadelphia, W. B. Saunders Co., 1988, p. 614. Reproduced by permission of W. B. Saunders Co.)

In women the posterior pedicles, including the cardinal ligaments, are clipped and divided for approximately 4 to 5 cm beyond the cervix. At this point the posterior vaginal wall is opened and the vagina is circumscribed anteriorly. The anterior vaginal wall is dissected from the posterior wall of the bladder down to the region of the urethra. This maneuver further defines the two distal posterior pedicles extending from the bladder to the lateral aspect of the vagina on either side. These pedicles are clipped and divided distally, freeing the bladder from its posterior attachments except for the urethra. In some patients with large, deeply penetrating posterior tumors, it may be advantageous to remove the anterior vaginal wall completely; the lateral vaginal wall is then incised down to the location of the urethral meatus.

A similar dissection is performed on the opposite side. Right-handed surgeons customarily switch to the opposite side of the table to initiate the dissection on the left side. When the lateral and posterior pedicles have been delineated, the surgeon usually returns to the ipsilateral side of the operating table to facilitate clipping and dividing the pedicles.

Anterior Dissection

When the posterior and lateral dissections have been completed, attention is drawn anteriorly for the first time. In men the puboprostatic ligaments should be identified and sharply divided close to the pubis. Next, a right-angled clamp should be passed just anterior to the membranous urethra under the dorsal venous complex. This large venous complex can then be ligated with No. 2-0 silk and sharply divided close to the apex of the prostate.[8] In patients who have undergone a previous segmental resection or open prostatectomy, this plane can be difficult to develop. In such situations, this part of the operation can be greatly facilitated by incising the periosteum of the pubis with the cautery. A periosteal elevator can be used to develop the subperiosteal plane easily down to the region of the urethra.

Once the venous complex has been divided, the membranous urethra comes into view and can be stretched several centimeters above the urogenital diaphragm. A large curved pedicle clamp is placed on the urethra just beyond the apex of

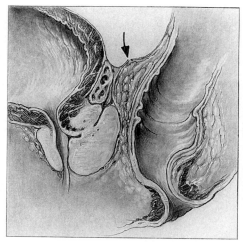

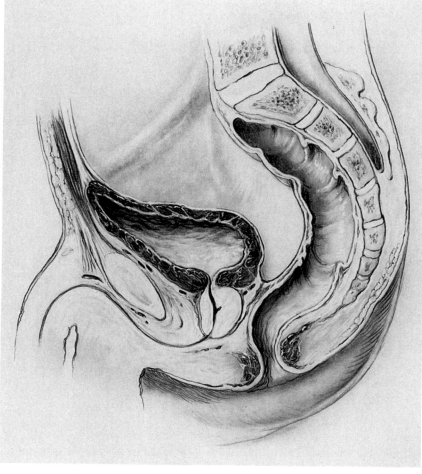

Fig. 24-6. Illustration of the formation of Denonvillier's fascia. Note that it is derived from a fusion of the anterior and posterior peritoneal reflections, and that Denonvillier's space lies behind the fascia. Therefore, to successfully enter this space to facilitate mobilization of the anterior rectal wall off Denonvillier's fascia, the incision in the cul-de-sac should be close to the peritoneal fusion at the anterior rectal wall and not close to the bladder (arrow). See inset for detail. (From Skinner, D., and Lieskovsky, G., eds. *Diagnosis and Management of Genitourinary Cancer.* Philadelphia, W. B. Saunders Co., 1988, p. 615. Reproduced by permission of W. B. Saunders Co.)

the prostate (Fig. 24-9). Care must be taken in placing this clamp to avoid rectal injury. In addition, the end of the clamp must extend beyond the urethra to avoid spilling vesical contents after the urethra is divided. The index finger of the left hand is placed beyond the clamp, and the urethra is divided with the catheter distal to the clamp. Placement of the finger prevents rectal injury during division of the urethra. The entire specimen is then removed. In selected male patients in whom lower urinary tract reconstruction is planned using an intestinal reservoir to the urethra, a series of 2-0 chromic sutures are placed circumferentially into the urethra to facilitate that anastomosis.

In women, once the urethropubic ligaments have been divided, a large curved Kocher clamp is placed on the urethra, and the anterior vaginal wall is opened distally and incised circumferentially around the urethral meatus. The vaginal cuff is closed longitudinally with interrupted 0 Dexon or chromic

sutures. Preservation of the anterior vaginal wall, when feasible, results in a functional vagina. When the anterior vaginal wall is removed because of the local extent of the primary tumor, closure results in a small, largely obliterated vagina. It is important to suspend the closed vagina on each side to the pectineal (Cooper's) ligament to prevent vaginal prolapse or development of an enterocele.

In both men and women, a figure-of-eight 0 chromic or Dexon suture is placed through the levator ani muscles anteriorly immediately adjacent to the pubis unless lower urinary tract reconstruction is planned. This effectively controls venous bleeding from the dorsal vein of the penis and the large venous plexus found in this region. Inspection of the side walls of the pelvis ensures that all bleeding is controlled, and a dry laparotomy pad is placed in the deep pelvis. In selected patients, controlled hypotensive anesthesia can effectively reduce blood loss and requirement of blood replacement.[9]

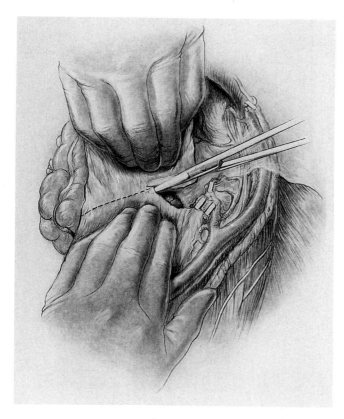

instances, the patient is placed in the hyperextended frogleg position. A two-team surgical approach is used to simultaneously dissect out the urethra within the corpora spongiosum while the cystectomy portion of the operation is being completed from above.[10] This approach allows for an en bloc removal of the entire urethra with the cystoprostatectomy specimen without prolonging the operative procedure.

In most instances, the pathologic findings of the cystectomy specimen determine who is a candidate for secondary urethrectomy. The histologic findings of carcinoma in situ or overt transitional cell carcinoma in the prostatic urethra indicate a secondary urethrectomy. In patients with multifocal disease or carcinoma in situ remote from the primary tumor, secondary urethrectomy is performed only when saline urethral washings performed 4 months after cystectomy and yearly thereafter reveal malignant cells. We prefer not to perform routine urethrectomy for two reasons: First, this proce-

FIG. 24-7. The peritoneum lateral to the rectum is incised down to the cul-de-sac, where the incision is extended anteriorly over the rectum to join the incision from the opposite side. It is important that the peritoneal incision be made precisely at its junction with the anterior rectal wall so that the plane behind Denonvillier's fascia can be developed safely. (From Skinner, D., and Lieskovsky, G., eds. *Diagnosis and Management of Genitourinary Cancer.* Philadelphia, W. B. Saunders Co., 1988, p. 616. Reproduced by permission of W. B. Saunders Co.)

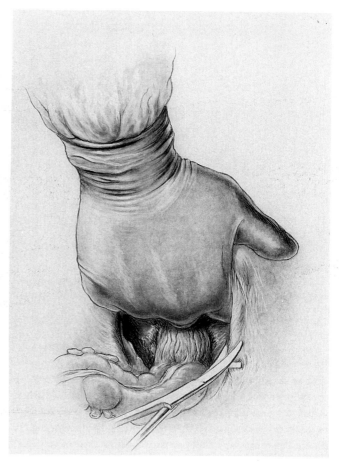

Major bleeding from the region of the dorsal vein has not been a factor in more than 500 consecutive patients, and it has not been necessary to use a Foley catheter inserted through the penis to control bleeding. In fact, that maneuver may contribute to a higher incidence of pelvic abscess. In the rare patient in whom the pelvis continues to ooze, a large Hemovac has been used and left on suction for 24 to 48 hours. In patients undergoing continent urinary diversion, a doubled one-inch Penrose drain is left in the pelvis.

A formal gastrostomy is carried out before closure of the abdomen for easier management of postoperative intestinal suction and feeding, obviating the discomfort and disadvantages of prolonged nasogastric intubation.

MANAGEMENT OF THE URETHRA

In women urethrectomy is routinely performed with cystectomy. In men, en bloc urethrectomy is done only when an overt tumor is seen in the membranous urethra or carcinoma is noted to invade the distal prostatic urethra. In these rare

FIG. 24-8. Once the peritoneum of the cul-de-sac has been incised, the anterior rectal wall can be swept off the posterior surface of Denonvilliers' fascia, thereby defining the posterior pedicle that extends from the bladder to the lateral side of the rectum on either side. (From Skinner, D., and Lieskovsky, G., eds. *Diagnosis and Management of Genitourinary Cancer.* Philadelphia, W. B. Saunders Co., 1988, p. 616. Reproduced by permission of W. B. Saunders Co.)

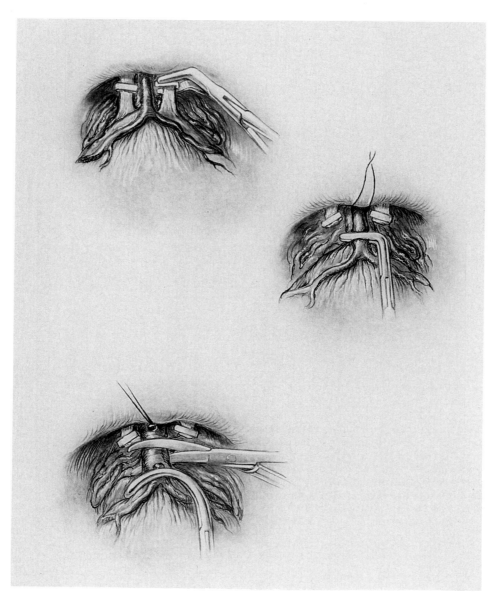

FIG. 24-9. The final step in performing a cystectomy is division of the puboprostatic ligaments (*A*) leaving the bladder attached only by the urethra. Next the dorsal vein of the penis and Santorini's venous plexus should be ligated with No. 2-0 silk and divided. This maneuver is accomplished by passing a right-angle clamp over the membranous urethra and under the venous complex once the puboprostatic ligaments have been divided (*B*). A large curved pedicle clamp can then be placed on the stretched membranous urethra, which is divided distal to the clamp (*C*). The specimen can then be removed. (From Skinner, D., and Lieskovsky, G., eds. *Diagnosis and Management of Genitourinary Cancer.* Philadelphia, W. B. Saunders Co., 1988, p. 617. Reproduced by permission of W. B. Saunders Co.)

dure is seldom necessary because a new urothelial carcinoma develops in the retained urethra in fewer than 10% of patients undergoing cystectomy. Although pelvic recurrence after cystectomy may present itself as a bloody discharge from the urethra, it is important to differentiate failure of the primary operation from failure because of development of a new urothelial carcinoma in the retained urethra. Second, most male patients whose tumor does not involve the prostatic urethra prefer continent lower urinary tract reconstruction using an ileal reservoir with bilateral ureteroileal urethrostomy.

A secondary urethrectomy with the patient positioned correctly is a simple operation with low morbidity and can be reserved for the few patients who really need it. We prefer to do a secondary urethrectomy 4 to 6 months after cystectomy. The operation can be performed at the time a penile prosthesis is inserted.

COMMENTARY

Between 1971 and 1988, 621 patients were explored with the intention of performing a single-stage radical cystectomy with en bloc pelvic iliac lymph node dissection and urinary diversion for cure of primary urothelial carcinoma of the bladder. Eighteen patients (3%) were found to have unresectable disease, usually extensive disease above the aortic bifurcation. Urinary diversion and a total cystectomy were performed in these patients unless the ureters were involved or encased by tumor. This course provided reasonable palliation in eliminating bleeding, urgency, and strangury. Because of serious medical problems, 6 patients (1%) were deemed not to be surgical candidates. 597 patients underwent the operation with the intent of cure. The postoperative mortality, defined as death from any cause before leaving the hospital or within 30 days of the operation regardless of location, was 1.7% (10/587). From 1971 to 1978, most of these patients were treated with high-dose short-course preoperative radiation therapy and single-stage radical cystectomy for the management of invasive bladder carcinoma.[11] Data from that study were analyzed for morbidity. Early postoperative complications prolonging hospitalization occurred in 46 of 165 patients (28%). It should be emphasized that 119 patients suffered no complication, and their average hospitalization was only 12.7 days.

It has been our policy since 1971 to administer sodium warfarin (Coumadin) for postoperative prophylactic anticoagulation. Coumadin (20 mg) is given through the gastrostomy tube in the recovery room, usually followed by 10 mg the following day unless the patient's prothrombin time is above 14 seconds. In such patients the dose is reduced to 5 or 2.5 mg the second day. Therefore, optimal prophylactic anticoagulation requires maintenance of a prothrombin time between 15 and 18 seconds or one and one half to two times the control, with oral doses ordered daily according to the day's prothrombin time. If the patient's prothrombin time exceeds 21 seconds, anticoagulation should be reversed with phytonadione (AquaMEPHYTON) because the complications of excessive anticoagulation exceed possible benefits. Use of this procedure has virtually eliminated pulmonary embolism in this group of high-risk patients.

Further analysis of data from patients undergoing radical cystectomy for management of invasive bladder carcinoma reveals important implications regarding node involvement relative to extent of primary disease. Table 24-1 reveals the incidence of positive nodes according to pathologic (P) stage. Although the incidence of positive nodes increased with in-

TABLE 24-1. *Incidence of Positive Nodes According to Primary Pathology in 197 Consecutive Patients Undergoing Bilateral Pelvic Iliac Lymph Node Dissection with En Bloc Radical Cystectomy for Bladder Cancer 1971–1982.*

	PO	P1S–P1	P2	P3A	P3B	P4
N−	18	67	36	14	44	18
N+	—	5	9	4	24	8
%N+	0	7%	25%	28%	55%	44%

(From Skinner, D. G. Urol. Clin. North Am., 8:353, 1981. By permission of W. B. Saunders Co.)

creasing depth of penetration of primary tumor, 7% of patients with a pathologically superficial tumor and 25% of patients with superficial muscle invasion had already had metastases to the pelvic nodes. This finding supports treatment of the pelvic nodes whenever cystectomy seems indicated for carcinoma. Five-year survival curves indicate that approximately 33% of patients with positive nodes can be cured by a pelvic node dissection.[12] Perhaps standard fractionation radiation therapy of 4,000 to 5,000 rads can sterilize pelvic nodal metastatic disease, but it is unlikely that 1,600 to 2,000 rads can control metastatic disease in these patients. Whenever cystectomy is indicated for the treatment of transitional cell carcinoma of the bladder, the high incidence of nodal metastatic disease implies there is a need to treat that area effectively. A pelvic node dissection can lead to cure in some patients with minimal metastatic disease and identifies patients at high risk for the development of disseminated disease. In these instances, the early use of systemic adjuvant chemotherapy may have a beneficial impact resulting in a delay in relapse.[13]

In summary, a single-stage radical cystectomy with bilateral pelvic iliac lymph node dissection and urinary diversion can be performed with an acceptably low surgical mortality and morbidity. Attention to preoperative preparation affects surgical mortality and morbidity. The operation remains the optimal procedure for the management of multifocal or invasive bladder cancer.

REFERENCES

1. Skinner, D. G., Tift, J. P., and Kaufman, J. J. High dose, short course preoperative radiation therapy and immediate single stage radical cystectomy with pelvic node dissection in the management of bladder cancer. J. Urol., *127*:671, 1982.
2. Crawford, E. D., and Skinner, D. G. Salvage cystectomy after irradiation failure. J. Urol., *123*:32, 1980.
3. Skinner, D. G., and Lieskovsky, G. Contemporary cystectomy with pelvic node dissection compared to preoperative radiation therapy plus cystectomy in management of invasive bladder cancer. J. Urol., *131*:1069, 1984.
4. Crawford, E. D., Das, S., and Smith, J. A., Jr. Preoperative radiation therapy in the treatment of bladder cancer. Urol. Clin. North Am., *14*:781, 1987.
5. Nichols, R. L., et al. Effect of preoperative neomycin-erythromycin intestinal preparation on the incidence of infectious complications following colon surgery. Ann. Surg. *178*:453, 1973.
6. Burman, S. O. The prophylactic use of digitalis before thoracotomy. Ann. Thorac. Surg., *14*:359, 1972.
7. Pinaud, M. L. J., Blanloeil, Y. A. G., and Souron, R. J. Preoperative prophylactic digitalization of patients with coronary artery disease—a randomized echocardiographic and hemodynamic study. Anesth. Analg. *62*:865, 1983.
8. Walsh, P. C., Lepor, H., and Eggleston, J. C. Radical prostatectomy with preservation of sexual function: Anatomical and pathological consideration. Prostate, *4*:473, 1983.
9. Ahlering, T. E., Henderson, J. B., and Skinner, D. G. Controlled

hypotensive anesthesia to reduce blood loss in radical cystectomy for bladder cancer. J. Urol., *129*:953, 1983.

10. WHITMORE, W. F., JR., and MOUNT, B. M. A technique of urethrectomy in the male. Surg. Gynecol. Obstet., *131*:303, 1970.

11. SKINNER, D. G., CRAWFORD, E. D., and KAUFMAN, J. J. Complications of radical cystectomy for carcinoma of the bladder. J. Urol., *123*:640, 1980.

12. SKINNER, D. G. Management of invasive bladder cancer: A meticulous pelvic node dissection can make a difference. J. Urol., *128*:34, 1982.

13. SKINNER, D. G., DANIELS, J. R., and LIESKOVSKY, G. Current status of adjuvant chemotherapy after radical cystectomy for deeply invasive bladder cancer. Urology, *24*:46, 1984.

CHAPTER
25

Partial
Cystectomy

Frank Mayer
E. David Crawford

The attractiveness of partial cystectomy in the management of invasive bladder carcinoma is obvious for the following reasons:

1. Normal voiding is maintained because the lower urinary tract is left intact.
2. Male erectile function is not affected because the surgical margins do not cross the neurovascular bundles inferiorly.
3. The patient's general medical condition is of less concern because the operating time is much shorter than that of a radical cystectomy with urinary diversion.

Additionally, patient acceptance of the procedure is high, as they perceive segmental resection as a much less traumatic and disfiguring operation when compared to radical cystectomy with urinary diversion. They are not faced with the need to wear an external appliance (in the case of an ileal conduit) or to frequently catheterize an abdominal stoma (in the case of a continent reservoir).

Nonetheless, there are potential disadvantages to segmental resection of invasive bladder carcinoma. Transitional cell carcinoma, the predominant histologic subtype of bladder cancer, often affects multiple areas of urothelium. During the work-up of a patient with bladder carcinoma, intraepithelial neoplasia may be missed by multiple random biopsies and, at the time of segmental resection, occult carcinoma may be left untreated. This "field effect" theory of transitional cell carcinoma is used as one argument against performing partial cystectomy for invasive cancer of the bladder.

Tumor seeding of the cystotomy incision is a well-documented phenomenon and is evidence for tumor spillage during partial cystectomy.[1,2] As will be discussed later, however, steps may be taken to lower the chance of tumor spillage and seeding. The high local recurrence rate is another argument against segmental resection of invasive bladder carcinoma. Roughly 40 to 70% of appropriately selected patients treated by partial cystectomy will develop local recurrence and possibly require a second procedure for treatment of their disease.[3–6] Thus, the aforementioned advantages must be weighed against the above-noted disadvantages prior to recommending partial cystectomy to an individual with invasive bladder cancer.

EPIDEMIOLOGIC CONSIDERATIONS

During 1989, approximately 47,000 new cases of bladder cancer will be diagnosed in the United States,[7] and 20% of these cases will have been classified as invasive at diagnosis. Of the 80% of bladder cancer cases that are found to be superficial at diagnosis, 10 to 15% will fail conservative therapy and progress to invasive disease.[8,9] Thus, roughly 10,000 cases per year of bladder carcinoma will require some form of surgical treatment. With studies showing that 2.5 to 6.0% of patients presenting with primary bladder carcinoma are suitable candidates for partial cystectomy, it is evident that this is not a frequently performed procedure.[1,10]

ETIOLOGIC CONSIDERATIONS

Although human exposure to various carcinogens has been linked epidemiologically to the development of bladder cancer, it is also suspected that individual host factors also play a part in tumor development and tumor invasion. In over 50% of all cases of bladder carcinoma, the patient gives either a history of significant exposure to industrial arylamines or a significant history of cigarette smoking.[11] Unusually high doses of sodium cyclamate and sodium saccharine induce bladder tumors in laboratory animals, but these artificial sweeteners have not been shown epidemiologically to cause bladder tumors in humans.[12] Attempts at implicating coffee drinking with the development of bladder cancer are met with difficulty because of the widespread consumption of coffee and the confounding variables of concomitant cigarette smoking and artificial sweetener use in the population of coffee drinkers. Chronic irritation of bladder mucosa by the long-term use of indwelling catheters and by chronically infected urine has been shown to increase the risk for squamous metaplasia and for the development of squamous cell carcinoma.[13] Chronic infestation of the urothelial tract by the Schistosoma ova is a well-known risk factor for the development of squamous cell carcinoma of the bladder in Egypt, where the parasite is endemic.

Although it is believed that some subgroups of the population are predisposed to the development of cancer, no genetic predisposition of the development of bladder cancer has been proven. Current research into the host factors responsible for the initiation of bladder tumors centers around the study of oncogenes and amino acid metabolism. No unified concept regarding neoplastic transformation in bladder mucosa has been formulated, but it has been postulated that environmental carcinogens may lead to the development of superficial bladder cancer, while individual host factors may be involved in the progression to early invasive cancer.[14]

SELECTION OF PATIENTS

Several authors have set forth criteria for the selection of patients to undergo segmental resection.[3,15,16] The following list represents conservative guidelines for partial cystectomy:

1. Solitary, primary lesion
2. Histologic type of transitional cell carcinoma or adenocarcinoma
3. High grade tumor: grades II, III, or IV
4. Invasive tumor: stages T_1 or T_2 (A to B_1)
5. Location of tumor on posterior wall and upper hemisphere most desirable
6. Inaccessibility to adequate transurethral resection (in stage-A disease)
7. Location of tumor in vesical diverticulum
8. Palliation of the poor-risk patient with bladder cancer or other primary tumor of pelvic origin

Contraindications to partial cystectomy include:

1. Presence of carcinoma-in-situ on random bladder biopsy
2. Involvement of bladder neck or prostatic urethra with cancer
3. Extravesical disease.

Low-grade, low-stage disease (grade I, stages 0 to A) is best treated by transurethral resection with or without intravesical chemo- or immunotherapy. Multifocal invasive carcinoma, carcinoma-in-situ refractory to intravesical therapies, and squamous cell carcinoma of the bladder, require radical cystectomy with urinary diversion because of the more aggressive nature of the disease.

Some authors include stage T_{3A} (B_2) disease in their selection criteria for partial cystectomy; however, better results can be obtained with radical cystectomy for these patients. Five-year survival rates for patients with stage T_{3A} disease treated by radical cystectomy range from 26 to 73% with a mean of 48%.[17-20] Five-year survival rates of 18 to 45%, with a mean of 37%, have been achieved with partial cystectomy under similar circumstances.[4,21,22] It must be emphasized that the above studies did not stratify patients according to histologic grade and, with the relatively small number of patients in each study with stage-T_{3A} disease, it is entirely possible that no true difference exists between either treatment modality. Nevertheless, it has long been believed that stage T_{3A}-disease behaves more closely to stage-T_{3B} disease than to stage-T_2 disease, and radical cystectomy has been considered the better therapeutic choice for patients with stage-T_{3B} disease.

PREOPERATIVE EVALUATION AND MANAGEMENT

Cystoscopy

All patients with adequate creatinine clearance should undergo intravenous pyelography to delineate upper tract anatomy, and to demonstrate any upper tract pathology, including tumor. Those patients with borderline creatinine clearance or with poor quality IVP should have retrograde pyelography performed at the time of definitive cystoscopy. At cystoscopy, urine cytology should be collected along with random bladder biopsies and a wide transurethral resection of the bladder tumor (TURBT). An extensive TURBT with fulguration of the site prior to partial cystectomy is associated with a low tumor implantation rate (1.5%).[1]

Other Staging Studies

Routine preoperative serum chemistries, urinalyses, urine cultures, and sensitivities, along with liver function tests, should be obtained. Chest roentgenogram is useful both for preoperative staging purposes and for comparison during postoperative surveillance. Computed tomography (CT) of the pelvis is reasonably helpful in demonstrating gross pelvic lymphadenopathy, while CT of the abdomen may reveal liver and other visceral metastases—especially when elevated liver enzymes raise the suspicion for metastatic disease. Routine preoperative bone scintigraphy is not recommended.[23] In patients with bone pain and elevated serum alkaline phosphatase levels, bone scan with or without site-specific plain x-ray may be diagnostic for bony metastasis.

Radiation Therapy

The patient should be treated with 1,000 to 1,600 rads of external beam radiation to a 15 cm by 15 cm portal over a 3- to 4-day period. Short-course, high-dose external beam radiation therapy has been shown by vanderWerf-Messing to greatly reduce the incidence of tumor seeding, without increasing perioperative morbidity.[24] Segmental resection should be undertaken within 2 days after completion of radiation therapy.

Antibiotics

Every attempt should be made to sterilize the urine preoperatively. If preoperative cultures show no growth of pathogenic bacteria, a first generation, parenteral cephalosporin infused 30 minutes prior to the skin incision and continued for 48 hours postoperatively should suffice for perioperative coverage. If the urine is infected preoperatively, antibiotics should be initiated 3 days prior to the planned procedure and continued for 7 days postoperatively. Oral antibiotics administered on an outpatient basis are adequate for routine urinary tract infections, although more complicated urinary tract infections may require earlier hospitalization with intravenous antibiotics prior to surgery.

The short course bowel preparation advocated by Lieskovsky and Skinner (a modification of the Nichol's bowel prep) is effective in cleansing and decompressing the bowel and carries few untoward side effects.[25] The morning before surgery, the patient takes 120 ml of Neoloid (a castor oil preparation) orally, followed by 1 gm Neomycin orally at 1000, 1100, 1200, 1300, 1600, 2000, and 2400 hours, and 1 gm Erythromycin base at 1200, 1600, 2000, and 2400 hours. In the authors' experience, this regimen is better tolerated than the polyethylene glycol (Go-Lytely) preparation, which requires that the patient drink 4 L of the solution over a short time period and often requires parenteral antiemetics or a nasogastric tube for the patient to finish ingesting the solution.

Bladder preparation

A second cystoscopy is performed immediately prior to starting the partial cystectomy. The tumor site is circumscribed by linear fulguration with the Bugby electrode at a distance of 2 cm from the margins of the tumor (Fig. 25-2). A three-way Foley catheter is placed and 30 mg of Thiotepa in 30 ml of sterile water is instilled intravesically to help reduce the likelihood of tumor implantation after cystotomy.[26,27]

SURGICAL TECHNIQUE

The patient is positioned supine with hyperextension at the lumbo-sacral spine, which affords better visualization of the deep pelvis. The patient is prepped and draped in the usual manner with the urethral catheter included in the sterile field. Just prior to performing the low midline incision, the bladder is drained of the thiotepa and distended with 250 ml of normal saline. The Foley catheter is clamped. The incision is then taken down to the peritoneum in the usual fashion. After entering the peritoneal cavity, the liver, colon, and para-aortic lymph nodes are palpated for metastases and for unrelated pathologic disorders. A Balfour retractor is placed and a bilateral pelvic lymphadenectomy is performed. Suspicious lymph nodes are sent for frozen sectioning and immediate pathologic diagnosis. That portion of the parietal peritoneum closely adherent to the dome of the bladder is left with the bladder, while the rest of the peritoneum is closed with a running suture of 3-0 chromic catgut.

The bladder is then packed away from the other pelvic organs with lap sponges, as this step contributes to a lower tumor implantation rate once the bladder is entered.[1] The initial cystotomy is carefully performed so as to not involve the tumor itself, to allow for an adequate (2 cm) margin of resection around the tumor, and to preserve at least one-half to one-third of the bladder volume after the resection (Fig. 25-1).

Babcock clamps are placed on the cut edges of the initial cystotomy, and gentle lateral traction applied. The cystotomy is extended carefully, until adequate exposure of the tumor site and the intended margin of resection is achieved. The free edges of the bladder are retracted with four Allis clamps (Fig. 25-2). A self-retaining retractor is avoided as it may cause undue trauma to the bladder mucosa or contribute to tumor disruption and spillage.

The tumor site, with the already demarcated 2 cm margin of bladder, is sharply excised (Fig. 25-3). Frozen sections are obtained from the cut edges of the bladder wall to assure that the margins are free of disease prior to closure of the bladder. In the event that the ureteral orifice is in close proximity or involved with tumor, resection of the distal ureter followed by ureteroneocystostomy with stenting is carried out.

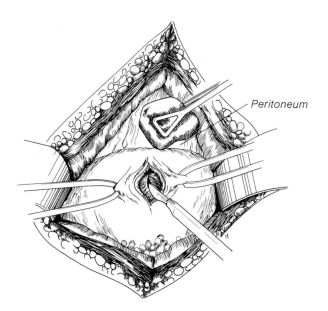

FIG. 25-1. The bladder is exposed through a midline incision. An initial cystotomy is made in a longitudinal manner and away from the tumor. The peritoneum, which already has been opened for thorough intraperitoneal exploration is closed before the bladder is incised.

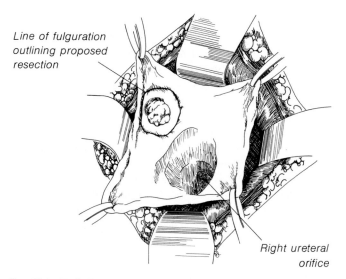

FIG. 25-2. With the cystotomy complete, the tumor is fully exposed, with the intended margin of resection marked by the line of fulguration. Exposure is aided by Allis clamps applied to cut edges of the bladder.

The bladder is then irrigated with sterile water and hemostasis is assured. The cystotomy is closed in two layers. First, full thickness sutures utilizing 0-chromic catgut are placed in an interrupted fashion. This suture line is then oversewn with a running 2-0 chromic suture incorporating the seromuscular layer (Figs. 25-4 and 25-5).

A 1/2″ Penrose drain is placed in the most dependent part of the pelvis and brought out through the skin via a separate stab wound. A three-way indwelling urethral catheter is inserted to allow for continuous bladder irrigation in the event of persistent gross hematuria postoperatively. The lap sponges

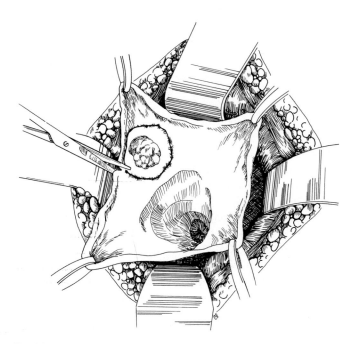

FIG. 25-3. Excision of the bladder tumor, along with a 2-cm cuff of normal tissue is carried out along the line of fulguration. Ureteral catheters may be employed if resection is near an orifice. If the tumor's location dictates, the orifice and distal ureter may be sacrificed, which requires a ureteroneocystostomy.

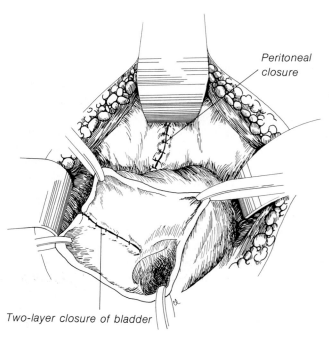

FIG. 25-4. The defect created by excision of the bladder tumor is closed in two layers. Also shown is the single-layered peritoneal closure.

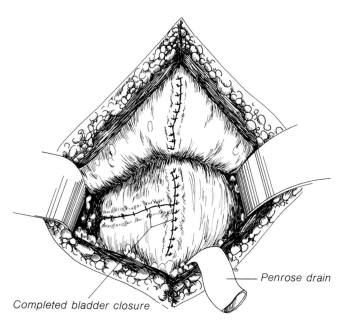

Completed bladder closure — Penrose drain

FIG. 25-5. A urethral catheter is placed prior to completing watertight closure of the bladder. Cystotomy drainage may be employed for troublesome bleeding. Penrose drains are placed, and the wound is closed with nylon retention sutures and No. 1 chromic catgut sutures on the midline fascia.

are removed and the pelvis is copiously irrigated. Hemostasis is once again assured. The rectus sheath, the deep and superficial fascia, and the skin are closed according to the surgeon's preference.

POSTOPERATIVE MANAGEMENT

Prophylaxis against deep venous thrombosis may be initiated either intraoperatively or immediately postoperatively by employing sequentially activated pneumatic antiembolism stockings on the lower extremeties. Ideally, the patient should be ambulating with assistance the night of the operation, thus obviating the need for the above stockings. Prophylactic anticoagulation with either subcutaneous heparin or oral coumadin is not without risk and is not routinely indicated in the post-operative care of the patient undergoing partial cystectomy. However, if the patient gives a history consistent with a hypercoaguable state or with past episodes of thromboembolism, then parenteral heparin or oral coumadin may be required.

Prophylactic parenteral antibiotics should be administered for only 48 hours postoperatively and in most cases is followed by oral antibiotics continued for 7 to 10 days after surgery. Continuous bladder irrigation may be used for persistent gross hematuria. The indwelling urethral catheter may be removed (along with the ureteral stent if one was placed) after 1 week. The Penrose drain is removed when the dressing sponges overlying it stay dry for one day. Urinary frequency will be encountered postoperatively; nevertheless, the patient should be reassured that the bladder will expand to accommo-

date near normal capacity and the patient's voiding pattern should eventually normalize.[28]

Postoperative adjuvant systemic chemo- or immunotherapy is not likely to be of benefit to the patient who has undergone partial cystectomy for bladder carcinoma, although no studies to date have addressed this issue. Likewise, it is unknown whether a regimen of postoperative adjuvant intravesical chemo- or immunotherapy would decrease the tumor recurrence rate. Only with randomized studies incorporating large numbers of subjects could these questions be answered. Inasmuch as only about 5% of patients presenting with invasive bladder carcinoma are suitable candidates for segmental resection, it is doubtful that any single institution would amass adequate numbers of subjects to achieve statistical significance, necessitating a multicenter cooperative study to resolve the above questions.

Patients selected to undergo partial cystectomy must be followed closely after surgery with periodic chest roentgenogram, urine cytology, cystoscopy, and necessary transurethral bladder biopsies of any suspicious recurrence. Recurrence of bladder cancer has been demonstrated in 30 to 70% of patients treated by partial cystectomy.[3–6] Thus, both the patient and the physician must be prepared for a lifelong surveillance program. Additionally, during preoperative counseling, the patient must be made aware that he or she may require further procedures (including salvage cystectomy and urinary diversion) in the future, should he or she suffer a recurrence of bladder cancer after partial cystectomy.

CONCLUSION

With improvements in surgical and anesthetic techniques and the widespread use of postoperative intensive care unit monitoring, many patients whose general medical condition would otherwise preclude extensive oncologic procedures are being successfully carried through radical surgery. Improvements in the design of implantable penile prostheses along with the advent of continent urinary diversion have effectively eliminated the important drawbacks of radical cystectomy. Further refinements in surgical techniques, including nerve-sparing cystoprostatectomy and anastomosis of continent urinary reservoirs to the membraneous urethra, offer the prospect of maintenance of normal erectile ability and micturition.[29–32] Clearly, the current trend in bladder cancer surgery is moving away from conservative therapy toward a radical extirpative surgery combined with reconstruction of the lower urinary tract with intestinal segments. Nevertheless, partial cystectomy will always play a role in the management of a select population of patients with invasive bladder cancer. At the same time, recent developments of effective chemotherapeutic and radiotherapeutic regimens have also kindled future hopes of treating invasive bladder carcinomas with probable bladder preservation. Partial cystectomy occupies a unique position between these two contrasting therapeutic trends. In a properly selected population, with meticulous adherence to surgical details, partial cystectomy can achieve both the objectives of cancer control and bladder preservation.

REFERENCES

1. Novick, A. C., and Stewart, B. H. Partial cystectomy in the treatment of primary and secondary carcinoma of the bladder. J. Urol., *116:*570, 1976.
2. Wallace, D. M., and Bloom, H. J. G. The management of deeply infiltrating (T_3) bladder carcinoma: Controlled trial of radical radiotherapy versus preoperative radiotherapy and radical cystectomy. Br. J. Urol., *48:*587, 1976.
3. Utz, D. C., and DeWeerd, J. H. The management of low-stage, low-grade carcinoma of the bladder. In *Genitourinary Cancer.* Edited by D. G. Skinner and J. B. deKernion. Philadelphia, W. B. Saunders Co., 1978, p. 263.
4. Cummings, K. B., Mason, J. T., Correa, R. J., Jr., and Gibbons, R. P. Segmental resection in the management of bladder carcinoma. J. Urol., *119:*56, 1978.
5. Merrell, R. W., Brown, H. E., and Rose, J. F. Bladder carcinoma treated by partial cystectomy: A review of 54 cases. J. Urol., *122:*471, 1979.
6. Schoborg, T. W., Sapolsky, J. L., and Lewis, C. W., Jr. Carcinoma of the bladder treated by segmental resection. J. Urol., *122:*473, 1979.
7. Silverberg, E., and Lubera, J. A. Cancer statistics, 1989, CA *39:*3, 1989.
8. Althausen, A. F., Prout, G. R., Jr., and Dal, J. J. Non-invasive papillary cancer of the bladder associated with carcinoma in situ. J. Urol., *116:*575, 1976.
9. Heney, N. M., et al. Superficial bladder carcinoma: Progression and recurrence. J. Urol., *130:*1083, 1983.
10. Utz, D. C., Hanash, K. A., and Farrow, G. M. The plight of the patient with carcinoma in situ of the bladder. J. Urol., *103:*160, 1970.
11. Cole, P. A population-based study of bladder cancer. In *Host Environment Interactions in the Etiology of Cancer in Man.* Edited by R. Doll and I. Vodopija. Lyon, IARC, 1973, p. 83.
12. Armstrong, B., and Doll, R. Bladder cancer mortality in diabetics in relation to saccharin consumption and smoking habits. Br. J. Prev. Soc. Med., *29:*73, 1975.
13. Kaufman, J. M., et al. Bladder cancer and squamous metaplasia in spinal cord injury patients. J. Urol., *118:*967, 1977.
14. Droller, M. J. Transitional cell cancer. In *Campbell's Urology.* 5th Edition. Edited by P. C. Walsh, R. F. Gittes, A. D. Perlmutter, and T. A. Stamey. Philadelphia, W. B. Saunders, 1986, p. 1353.
15. Brannan, W., et al. Partial cystectomy in the treatment of transitional cell carcinoma of the bladder. J. Urol., *119:*213, 1978.
16. Skinner, D. G., and Lieskovsky, G. Management of invasive and high-grade bladder cancer. In *Diagnosis and Management of Genitourinary Cancer.* Edited by D. G. Skinner and G. Lieskovsky. Philadelphia, W. B. Saunders Co., 1988, p. 298.
17. Long, R. T. L., et al. Carcinoma of the urinary bladder (comparison with radical, simple, and partial cystectomy and intravesical formalin). Cancer, *29:*98, 1972.
18. Whitmore, W. F., Jr., et al. Radical cystectomy with or without prior irradiation in the treatment of bladder cancer. J. Urol., *118:*184, 1977.
19. Pearse, H. D., Reed, R. R., and Hodges, C. V. Radical cystectomy for bladder cancer. J. Urol., *119:*216, 1978.
20. Montie, J. R., Straffon, R. A., and Stewart, B. H. Radical cystectomy without radiation therapy for carcinoma of the bladder. J. Urol., *131:*477, 1984.
21. Resnick, M. I., and O'Conor, V. J., Jr. Segmental resection for carcinoma of the bladder: Review of 102 patients. J. Urol., *109:*1007, 1973.
22. Utz, D. C., et al. A clinicopathologic evaluation of partial cystectomy for carcinoma of the urinary bladder. Cancer, *32:*1075, 1973.
23. Lindner, A., and DeKernion, J. B. Cost-effective analysis of precystectomy radioisotope scans. J. Urol., *128:*1181, 1982.
24. vanderWerf-Messing, B. Carcinoma of the bladder treated by suprapubic radium implants. Eur. J. Ca., *5:*277, 1969.
25. Skinner, D. G., and Lieskovsky, G.: Technique of radical cystectomy. In *Diagnosis and Management of Genitourinary Cancer.* Edited by D. G. Skinner and G. Lieskovsky. Philadelphia, W. B. Saunders Co., 1988, p. 607.
26. Burnand, K. A., et al. Single-dose thiotepa as adjuvant to cystodiathermy in treatment of transitional cell bladder carcinoma. Br. J. Urol., *48:*55, 1976.
27. Byar, D., and Blackard, C. Comparisons of placebo, pyridoxine, and topical thiotepa in preventing recurrence of stage I bladder cancer. Urology, *10:*556, 1977.
28. Baker, R., et al. Subtotal cystectomy and total bladder regeneration in treatment of bladder cancer. JAMA, *168:*1178, 1958.
29. Ghoneim, M. A., et al. Appliance-free, sphincter-controlled bladder substitute: Urethral Kock pouch. J. Urol., *138:*1150, 1987.
30. Walsh, P. C., and Mostwin, J. L. Radical prostatectomy and cystoprostatectomy with preservation of potency. Results using a new nerve-sparing technique. Br. J. Urol., *56:*694, 1984.
31. Schlegel, P. N., and Walsh, P. C.: Neuroanatomical approach to radical cystoprostatectomy with preservation of sexual functions. J. Urol., *138:*1402, 1987.
32. Kock, N. G., et al. Replacement of bladder by urethral Kock pouch: Functional results, urodynamics and radiological features. J. Urol., *141:*111, 1989.

CHAPTER
26

Salvage Cystectomy after Irradiation Failure

William Nabors
E. David Crawford

I n the United States, radical cystectomy is the standard treatment for invasive bladder cancer. Radiation therapy is offered to those who will not, or can not undergo cystectomy. An unknown percentage of those who fail will become candidates for salvage cystectomy.

British urologists have for many years advocated radiation therapy, with cystectomy reserved for those who do not respond, or for those who relapse. Jenkins et al. recently published a review of 182 patients treated in this manner. Their overall, corrected five-year survival was 40%. Fifty eight percent of the patients had persistence or recurrence of their cancer, and thus were potential candidates for salvage cystectomy.[1]

HISTORICAL PERSPECTIVES

The first attempt to remove a bladder tumor surgically was made during the 1700's by LeCat, who removed the tumor with forceps introduced through the female urethra.[2] Little progress was made in the surgical ablation of bladder tumors, however, until Thompson described the perineal-digital ap-

proach in the late 1800's.[3] This was followed by Billroth's description of the open suprapubic method.[4]

The current surgical technique of cystectomy had its beginning in 1887 when Bardenheuer described removal of the bladder and implantation of the ureters into the bowel.[5] Unfortunately, he was unable to implant the ureters, and the patient died in the early postoperative period. Cystectomy did not gain great popularity until the 1940's, with the development of satisfactory methods of diversion, better anesthesia, fluid therapy, and effective antibiotics. Though these advances sparked interest in cystectomy, the goal of long-term survival remained elusive.

Radiation therapy for bladder cancer began in 1906.[6] At that time it was felt to be an unsatisfactory method of treatment.[7] Even with the development of newer methods of radiation, the survival rates have remained dismal when radiation therapy alone is employed.

In an effort to improve local control and survival, several groups are reporting the use of concomitant radiation therapy and chemotherapy. These studies include radiation therapy and Misonidazole,[8] radiation therapy and concomitant

253

5-Fluorouracil,[9] upfront MCV followed by radiation therapy plus Cisplatin,[10] and radiation therapy plus Cisplatin.[11-14] Follow-up times are short and it remains to be seen if the higher local response rates reported will translate to higher 5-year survival rates.

SELECTION OF PATIENTS

Patients selected for salvage cystectomy are those who have biopsy-proven tumor recurrence or those who have crippling irritative bladder symptoms after definitive radiation therapy. Patients undergoing this procedure should have a thorough metastatic evaluation, including chest roentgenogram, bone scan with spot films and/or biopsy of suspicious areas, and liver profile and scan if functional tests prove abnormal. Bimanual examination under anesthesia and palpation of lymph node areas are generally unrewarding because of the radiation-produced fibrosis. CT scans have not proven universally useful, for it is not possible to distinguish between radiation induced fibrosis and tumor. The remainder of the preoperative evaluation and preparation is discussed in Chapter 24.

SURGICAL PROCEDURE

The 5-year survival rate of patients undergoing salvage cystectomy is 37 to 51.5%. Operative deaths range from 0 to 14%. Crawford and Skinner, in a review of 37 patients undergoing salvage cystectomy, revealed that the selective use of an initial perineal approach in most patients, and the use of staged cystectomy after preliminary urinary diversion in high-risk patients, resulted in decreased morbidity and mortality rates (Table 26-1).

Should a rectal laceration occur during cystectomy, a diverting colostomy should be performed at the time of repair. Primary closure alone is associated with a higher morbidity and mortality. (Table 26-2).

Certain modifications in the technique of radical cystectomy (see Chapter 24) are necessary. The classic radical cystectomy is generally not feasible because skeletonization of

TABLE 26-1. *Relationship of Staged and/or Perineal Approach to Early Complications*

	NUMBER OF PATIENTS	NUMBER OF COMPLICATIONS
Staged Procedure		
With Perineal Approach	7	—
Without Perineal Approach	6	1 (16%)
Single-Stage Procedure		
With Perineal Approach	8	2 (25%)
Without Perineal Approach	16	5 (31%)
Total	37	8 (24%)

*From Crawford, E. D., and Skinner, D. G.: Salvage cystectomy after irradiation failure. J. Urol, *123*:32, 1980. Copyright 1980, The Williams & Wilkins Co., Baltimore.

TABLE 26-2. *Results of Treatment of Rectal Laceration*

SERIES	RECTAL LACERATIONS	TREATMENT	OUTCOME
Crawford and Skinner[16]	1	Colostomy	Successful
Smith and Whitmore[17]	2	Colostomy (1) Delayed Colostomy (1)	Death Death
Swanson, et. al.[18]	2	Colostomy	Successful
Freiha and Faysal[19]	3	Primary closure (2)	Pelvic abcess (2)
		Primary closure with colostomy	Successful
Konnak and Grossman[20]	3	Primary closure	Death (1) Leak (1) requiring colostomy

the pelvic vessels and removal of the lymph nodes are generally not possible because of the fibrosis produced by higher doses of irradiation. Therefore, a total cystectomy is performed, which consists of surgical removal of the pelvic peritoneum, bladder, prostate, and seminal vesicles in males, and anterior exenteration in females. We have found that, in male patients, there is often a dense desmoplastic radiation fibrosis in the pelvis that makes it difficult to separate the prostate from the rectum. With the initial perineal approach, the rectum can be separated from the prostate under direct vision, rather than by performing the dissection deep in the pelvis through the abdominal incision.

Patients undergoing this procedure often have concomitant medical problems that increase the operative and perioperative risk (perhaps thus justifying radiation as the primary therapy). In our experience, a staged procedure, consisting of preliminary urinary diversion followed by cystectomy in 4 to 6 weeks, significantly reduces the morbidity and mortality in the high-risk patient.

Proper position of the patient is extremely important when the early perineal approach is performed. The patient is placed in the exaggerated lithotomy position, with sandbags beneath the sacrum, bringing the perineum parallel to the table (Fig. 26-1). The perineal area is prepared and draped, and a sterile towel is sutured anterior to the anal opening to isolate it from the operative field. A Lowsley retractor is passed through the urethra into the bladder. A curved skin incision is made 1.5 cm anterior to the anus and carried posterior and lateral to the medial aspect of the ischial tuberosities.

The superficial perineal fascia is then divided sharply, and with blunt dissection, the ischiorectal fossae are developed lateral and anterior to the rectal wall (Fig. 26-2). The central tendon of the perineum is isolated and sharply divided. The rectal sphincter is identified posteriorly, and a bifid retractor is placed in the wound. The rectal fascia is identified and, with a sharp and blunt dissection, a plane is established anterior to the rectal wall. The rectourethralis muscle is encountered in

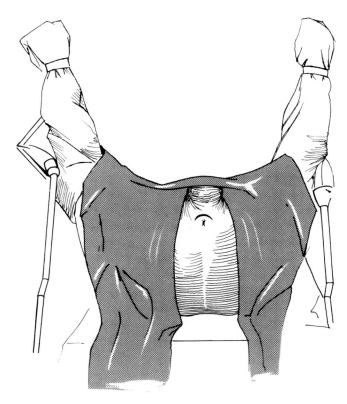

Fig. 26-1. Exaggerated lithotomy position. Lowsley retractor is passed per the urethra into the bladder. A sterile towel (not shown) is sutured anterior to the anus.

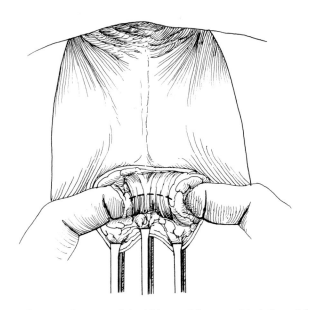

Fig. 26-2. Development of the ishiorectal fossae and isolation of the central tendon of the perineum.

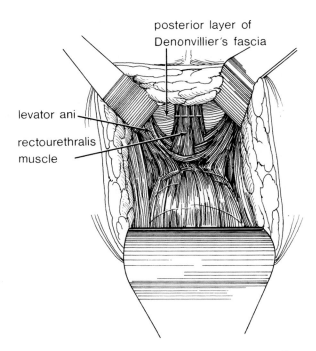

Fig. 26-3. Rectourethralis muscle is encountered in the midline and divided.

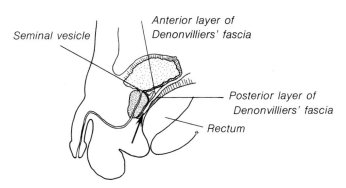

Fig. 26-4. Arrow indicates the plane of dissection. The anterior layer of Denonvillier's fascia must be incised in order to mobilize the seminal vesicles.

the midline and divided sharply (Fig. 26-3). The anterior layer of Denonvillier's fascia fuses with the prostatic capsule and must be entered sharply to continue the dissection cranially around the seminal vesicles (Fig. 26-4). The lateral aspects of the incision are developed and the procedure is completed. We do not divide the urethra at this time because this would constitute a premature commitment to cystectomy.

The rectum is inspected for any lacerations and the incision is closed in two layers. A Penrose drain is left in place for 48 hours or until most of the drainage subsides. Cystectomy is then undertaken as described in Chapter 24.

The initial perineal approach requires approximately 30 minutes of operative time. This initial investment results in time saved when the abdominal portion of the cystectomy is performed. More importantly, the risk of rectal laceration in a heavily irradiated field is reduced.

REFERENCES

1. JENKINS, B. J., et al. Reappraisal of the role of radical radiotherapy and salvage cystectomy in the treatment of invasive (T2/T3) bladder cancer. Br. J. Urol., *62*:343, 1988.

2. MURPHY, L. J. T. From the renaissance to the nineteenth century. In *The History of Urology.* Edited by L. J. T. Murphy. Springfield, Charles C. J. Thomas, 1972.

3. THOMPSON, H. *Tumours of the Bladder.* London, J & A Churchill, 1884.

4. BILLROTH, T. Extirpation eines Harnblasenmyoms nach vorausgehenden tiefen und hohen Blasenschnitt (C. Gussenbauer). Arch. Klin. Chir., *18*:411, 1875.

5. BARDENHEUER, B. *Der Extraperitonealer Explorativschnitt.* Stuttgart, Enke, 1887.

6. GRAY, A. L. The roentgen ray treatment of malignant disease of the bladder through a suprapubic incision: Report of a case. Am. J. Surg., *20*:307, 1906.

7. RICHES, E. Surgery and radiotherapy in urology: The bladder. J. Urol., *90*:339, 1963.

8. ABRATT, R. P., et al. Radical irradiation and misonidazole for T2 Grade 3 and T3 bladder cancer: 2 year follow up. Int. J. Radiat. Oncol. Biol. Phys., *10*:1719, 1984.

9. ROTMAN, M., et al. Treatment of advanced bladder carcinoma with irradiation and concomitant 5-Fluorouracil infusion. Cancer, *59*:710, 1987.

10. MARKS, L. B., et al. Invasive bladder carcinoma: Preliminary report of selective bladder conservation by transurethral surgery, upfront MCV(Methotrexate, Cisplatin, and Vinblastin) chemotherapy and pelvic irradiation plus Cisplatin. Int. J. Radiat. Oncol. Biol. Phys., *15*:877, 1988.

11. SHIPLEY, W. U., et al. Cisplatin and full dose irradiation for patients with invasive bladder carcinoma: A preliminary report of tolerance and local response. J. Urol., *132*:899, 1984.

12. JAKSE, G., and FROMMHOLD, H. Combined radiation and chemotherapy for locally advanced bladder cancer. In *Progress and Controversies in Oncological Urology.* New York, Alan R. Liss Inc., 1984, p. 365.

13. SHIPLEY, W. U., et al. Treatment of invasive bladder cancer by Cisplatin and radiation in patients unsuited for surgery. JAMA, *258*:931, 1987.

14. SAUER, R., et al. Preliminary results of treatment of invasive bladder carcinoma with radiotherapy and cisplatin. Int. J. Radiat. Oncol. Biol. Phys., *15*:871, 1988.

15. JOHNSON, D. E., LAMY, S., and BRACKEN, R. B. Salvage cystectomy after radiation failure in patients with bladder carcinoma. South. Med. J., *70*:1279, 1977.

16. CRAWFORD, E. D., and SKINNER, D. E. Salvage cystectomy after irradiation failure. J. Urol., *123*:32, 1980.

17. SMITH, J. A., JR., and WHITMORE, W. F., JR. Salvage cystectomy for bladder cancer after failure of definitive irradiation. J. Urol., *125*:643, 1981.

18. SWANSON, D. A., et al. Salvage cystectomy for bladder carcinoma. Cancer, *47*:2275, 1981.

19. FREIHA, F. S., and FAYSAL, M. H. Salvage cystectomy. Urology, *23*:496, 1983.

20. KONNAK, J. W., and GROSSMAN, H. B. Salvage cystectomy following failed definitive radiation therapy for transitional cell carcinoma of bladder. Urology, *26*:550, 1985.

21. BOCCON GIBOD, L., LELEU, C., and STEG, A. Salvage cystectomy: The case for a combined abdominoperineal approach. Eur. Urol., *10*:370, 1984.

Continent Urinary Diversion: An Overview

"It usually requires a considerable time to determine with certainty the virtues of a new method of treatment and usually still longer to ascertain the harmful effects."
ALFRED BLALOCK (1899–1964)

Sakti Das

For nearly 40 years ileal loop diversion has remained the surgical standard for diversion or substitution of the lower urinary tract. Various short- and long-term complications have led to modifications and use of other parts of the intestine as the conduit. Despite all these improvements in surgical techniques and quantum advances in the external appliances, an external conduit diversion remains a poor substitution for the lower urinary tract and an unsatisfactory alternative for the patients in regard to their body image and quality of social life. Urologists of the 1980s have responded to these concerns with a dedicated interest in the development of continent urinary diversion. Historically, the evolution of continent diversion actually represents a renascence of the original urinary diversion with ureterosigmoidostomy, which intended to avoid external appliances.

PRINCIPLES OF CONTINENT URINARY DIVERSION

Continent urinary diversion implies a diversion or substitution of the lower urinary tract upon which the patient has reason-able control of elimination. Such a diversion should ideally fulfill the following criteria:

1. The reservoir fashioned to substitute for the lower urinary tract should collect and store urine under low pressure.
2. Damage to the upper urinary tract should be prevented by avoiding high reservoir pressure and obstruction at any point in the onward egress of urine.
3. The diversion must prevent reflux into the upper urinary tract.
4. The diversion should not cause recurrent infections from stasis or reflux.
5. The diversion should not cause deleterious fluid or electrolyte and acid-base imbalances.
6. Malabsorptive nutritional disorders should be minimized.
7. Continence should be maintained so that the patients can control the emptying of the reservoir at socially acceptable and convenient intervals.

TYPES OF CONTINENT DIVERSION

In 1852 Simon attempted to divert urinary drainage in his patient by creating a communication between the ureters and the rectum.[1] The development of continent diversion since then has continued with several ingenious technical innovations during the last several decades. The major milestones in this journey toward ideal continent diversion can be classified as follows:

1. Continent urinary reservoir attached to an intact urinary sphincter mechanism: enterourethrostomy using ileal segment, ileal pouches, detubularized ileocecal and sigmoid colon.
2. Continent urinary reservoir using a surrogate sphincter mechanism:
   a. Using the anal sphincter, the choices are ureterosigmoidostomy, rectal bladder with abdominal fecal colostomy, or rectal bladder with juxta-anal fecal colostomy.
   b. Artificial sphincter devices.
3. Continent urinary reservoir with abdominal stoma for intermittent catheterization.
   a. Continence is dependent upon intussuscepted segments of ileum (Kock pouch and its variations).
   b. Continence is dependent upon the intussuscepted ileocecal valve.
   c. Continence is based upon the ileocecal valve and plicated ileum (Indiana pouch) or tapered ileum (Miami pouch).

Enterourethrostomy

The enterourethrostomy procedures work as a bladder substitution with a suitable intestinal segment for the purpose of collection and storage of urine. Emptying of this reservoir is achieved by spontaneous urethral voiding or by intermittent urethral catheterization. Because of the inherent necessity of preserving a competent outlet sphincter mechanism and the urethral conduit, it is essential to adhere to stringent selection criteria before these operations are undertaken. The short length of the female urethra and the relative weakness of the pelvic outlet musculature of women preclude these operations in female patients unless one considers additional procedures such as artificial sphincter implantation, and intussusception or plication continence mechanisms, proximal to the reservoir outlet. In addition, because most of the urethra is left behind along with the proximal sphincter mechanism, enterourethrostomy is contraindicated in the presence of urethral carcinoma, carcinoma at the bladder neck, and diffuse carcinoma in situ. Careful follow-up with urethroscopy and cytology is essential in all patients postoperatively. Camey reported that in about 15% of the patients it is difficult to bring the ileum up to the urethra because of the short ileal mesentery.[2]

Such difficulties are not encountered with ileocolonic[3] or sigmoid colonic[4] segments.

The most frustrating morbidity with enterourethrostomy is enuresis. Most of these patients are continent during the day; however at night when the perineal musculature is relaxed, they often develop enuresis. Setting an alarm to wake up and void every 2 to 3 hours, perineal exercises, and the use of alpha-adrenergic medications can help improve the situation often to a socially acceptable state.

Various techniques of detubularization and longitudinal division of circular muscles with or without add-on ileal patch have been advocated to create a low-pressure commodious reservoir with improvement in day and night continence.

Ureterosigmoidostomy

Several modifications of Simon's original concept of diverting urinary drainage into the sigmoid colon remained popular until Bricker established the ileal conduit diversion in 1950.[5] With increasing experience and follow-up, a number of serious complications of ureterosigmoidostomy have become evident. The early complications relate to obstruction or leakage of the ureterocolonic anastomosis. Among chronic complications, recurrent pyelonephritis occurs in at least 50% of the patients even after successful nonrefluxing ureteral implantation. Incidence of renal calculi and ureteral obstruction due to anastomotic scarring increases with time. Hyperchloremic hypokalemic acidosis is a unique electrolytic disturbance described by Ferris and Odel in 1950.[6] Recently, reports of adenocarcinoma developing commonly at the ureteral implantation site have been a subject of major concern, especially for younger patients.[7] Because of these prohibitive morbidities, modern urologists are less inclined to consider ureterosigmoidostomy even though many patients may find such a diversion appealing. In properly selected candidates with normal upper urinary tracts, unimpaired renal function, good anal sphincter tone, and no history of local radiation therapy, and for those who are intelligent enough to control and initiate rectal voiding, ureterosigmoidostomy may still be considered a preferred alternative of continent diversion.

Rectal Bladder with Abdominal Colostomy

To obviate the problem of recurrent infection from fecal contamination and electrolytic imbalances in ureterosigmoidostomy, the sigmoid colon can be disconnected and brought out as a colostomy. The remaining rectum with the implanted ureters works as a continent urinary reservoir. The colostomy is managed with daily colonic enemas and normally does not require elaborate external collecting appliances. Postoperative electrolyte imbalances are virtually absent even in patients with large rectal bladders. Frequent urination and nocturnal leakage can be effectively controlled with imipramine. Recurrent pyelonephritis, however, continues to be a problem in about 30% of the patients.[8]

Rectal Bladder with Juxta-anal Colostomy

In this ingenious operation a rectal bladder is constructed. Instead of performing an abdominal colostomy, the surgeon brings the transected proximal sigmoid colon down through the anal sphincter and sutures it to the perineum in the form of a neoanus for fecal elimination. The intact anal sphincter is supposed to provide continence for both urine and feces.[9] Various modifications of this surgical principle have met with sporadic success. In general, urologists have been hesitant to accept this procedure because of the technical difficulty as well as inconsistent outcome.

Artificial Sphincter for Continence of Substituted Bladder

Light and Scott have reported successful use of artificial sphincteric devices to achieve continence after substitution of bladder with the ileocolonic pouch.[10] In patients with an absent or predictably damaged sphincter mechanism, the prosthesis has been implanted as a primary procedure at the time of creation of the urinary reservoir. If, however, sphincteric weakness becomes apparent with postoperative incontinence, the artificial sphincter cuff can be placed around the bulbar urethra at a later date.

Continent Urinary Reservoir with Abdominal Stoma

The evolution of continent abdominal stoma dates back to 1899 when Watsuji described intussuscepted nipple construction for gastrostomy.[11] Urologists and enteric surgeons for many years strived for the creation of the ideal continent internal reservoir. In 1950 Gilchrist and associates successfully used the ileocecal segment as a continent urinary reservoir.[12] They subsequently reported an impressive 94% continence in 40 patients followed for 10 years. With the end of the ileum brought out as a stoma, continence was maintained by virtue of the antiperistaltic direction of the conduit flow, a competent ileocecal valve, and the small size of the stoma. Subsequent workers failed to reproduce such a high rate of continence, probably because of the high pressure generated in the intact cecum. However, the idea of a continent, catheterizable reservoir was firmly established. During the next several decades workers in different parts of the world developed various procedures of continent diversion with gratifying results.[13–17] Authors in the subsequent chapters have elaborated on the procedures now popular in the United States.

The sudden interest in continent diversion demands a cautious appraisal of the information accrued so that continued search for the ideal diversion can be pragmatic. The following clinicopathologic considerations require evaluation:

IMPACT ON RENAL FUNCTION. Although long-term results are not yet available, 2 to 5 years of follow-up have not indicated any deterioration of glomerular filtration rate or serum creatinine levels.[17,18] Any long-term effects of chronic bacteriuria, occasional reflux, and reservoir pressure on the kidneys of patients with continent urinary reservoir are yet unknown.

INFECTION. Continent reservoirs with cutaneous stoma often harbor bacterial colonies, whereas the urine in enterourethrostomy patients is sterile. Whether the antibodies of intestinal mucosa against intestinal bacteria or the antimicrobial defense mechanism of urine renders the bacteria of the reservoir urine less virulent is a matter of continued research. Upper urinary tract infections are certainly infrequent with continent urinary diversion, especially in the presence of nonrefluxing ureteral systems.

ELECTROLYTE AND ACID BASE IMBALANCES. The mechanism and effects of electrolyte and ion exchanges between urine and serum across the bowel mucosa have been subjects of academic curiosity and research since Boyd in 1931 reported chronic acidosis[19] and Ferris and Odel in 1950 observed hyperchloremic acidosis following ureterosigmoidostomy.[6] In both the ileum and colon, the fluid and electrolyte transfer occurs as an active process of absorption and secretion. Bicarbonate absorption depends upon the rates of cation and anion exchanges. Because of selective hyperabsorption of chloride more than the sodium ions, a net loss of bicarbonate ions in the lumen results in acidosis. Potassium flux in the bowel, however, is a passive process to maintain electrical neutrality when sodium is absorbed. Additional potassium loss can occur from chronic diarrhea as well as from diuresis secondary to water absorption.

Minor degrees of hyperchloremic acidosis have been observed following enterourethrostomies and in catheterizing continent reservoirs.[20] The incidence of significant electrolytic imbalance varies widely from less than 1% to 65% in different series.[18,21] The factors influencing the incidence and degree of metabolic alterations include: (1) the absorptive and secretory nature and capacity of the intestinal segment interposed in the urinary tract, (2) the interval of urinary contact with the bowel mucosa, (3) the surface area of bowel mucosa as modified by the length and configuration of the bowel segment, (4) the baseline renal function and its capacity to withstand additional electrolytic changes, and (5) the histologic and functional alterations of the mucosal villi, the extent of which depends on the time elapsed since the surgical procedure.

Deleterious electrolytic derangements have certainly been less common in patients with continent reservoir and intestinal substitution of bladder compared to those following ureterosigmoidostomy. However, periodic postoperative monitoring of electrolytes and acid base status is essential so that corrective therapy with hydration, alkalizing medications, chlorpromazine, or nicotinic acid can be instituted appropriately in the event of any metabolic alterations.

MALABSORPTION AND NUTRITIONAL CONSIDERATIONS. Impaired absorption of water, fat, electrolytes, and vitamin B_{12} can result from resection of long segments of the small intestine. Vitamin B_{12} is absorbed from the terminal ileum. Fortunately, even in continent diversions utilizing the ileocecal segments, megaloblastic anemia secondary to vitamin B_{12} deficiency is uncommon, probably because of the minimal daily requirement and relatively large storage reserve of vitamin B_{12}. Use of larger segments of ileum may cause steatorrhea due to impaired lipid digestion, bile salt deficiency, and diarrhea from hurried transit of the intestinal contents. Overall incidence of postoperative diarrhea is uncommon and, if present, usually subsides in 3 to 4 months. Vitamin B_{12} deficiency has been reported.[17] Patients should be followed for years because the body reserve may become depleted.

CARCINOGENESIS. Clinically in patients with ureterosigmoidostomy and experimentally in the laboratory it has been proved that a close apposition of urothelium and colonic mucosa in the presence of urine and feces leads to a high incidence of adenocarcinoma of colonic origin at the anastomotic suture line.[22] It is conjectured that urinary nitrates may be converted to active carcinogen nitrosamine by the fecal bacteria.[23] Colonic epithelium further alters nitrosamine into a more actively carcinogenic hydroxylated form. Because modern continent urinary diversions are excluded from fecal stream, chances of carcinogenesis may be minimized. Moreover, in experimental animals, ileal epithelium proved to be immune to carcinogenesis.[7] Continent urinary reservoirs constructed from small intestine may therefore have the least propensity toward malignant transformation. The issue of carcinogenesis under similar circumstances of urinary diversion is riddled with ignorance and conjectures. Whether chronic bacterial colonies in a continent urinary reservoir are also capable of converting carcinogens in the long run will be determined by further research and clinical vigilance.

RESERVOIR PRESSURE AND CONFIGURATION. An ideal reservoir constructed from the shortest bowel segment should store an adequate volume of urine under low pressure. Because the opened or detubularized bowel segments allow a larger capacity and low reservoir pressure, they cause less damage to the kidneys. Hinman has elegantly analyzed the principles involved in the construction of an ileal reservoir.[24] The important factors in consideration are the configuration, accommodation, viscoelasticity (compliance), and contractility. Geometric equation proves that simple longitudinal opening of a tube and folding it back on itself as a pouch virtually doubles the capacity from that of a same length of unopened tube. The reservoir or pouch thus created, because of its larger radius, also accommodates a larger volume at physiologic pressure (Laplace's law). The larger radius with greater mural tension is more compliant and has larger capacity at low pressure. Longitudinal opening of the bowel prevents synchronized circular contractions with their resultant rise of pressure. Hinman concludes that only operations involving detubularization will benefit from the consequent alterations in geometry, accommodation, compliance, and contractility that reduce harmful contractions and, at the same time, yield the largest capacity from the shortest segment of bowel.

In 1950, Eugene Bricker, the pioneer of modern urinary diversion, stated, "The concept of radical and amputative surgery could be carried to such a stage that what was left with the patient became a consideration of equal importance to that which was removed." Our continued research into these considerations of the biologic alterations and complications of urinary diversion has widened our understanding and expanded our concerns to include maintaining self-image and improving overall quality of life.

In the absence of effective systemic therapy, cystectomy remains the therapeutic choice for patients with invasive bladder cancer. Cystectomy itself, irrespective of the mode of urinary diversion, could profoundly affect mental and emotional attitudes, personal and sexual relationships, working abilities, and leisure activities. The most obviously disruptive effect on the patient's lifestyle, however, results from the external urinary diversion. Avoiding the use of an external appliance is the major concern for the patients and relates directly to their body image and social convenience. Whether a catheterizable continent reservoir or the more anatomic enterourethrostomies will be preferable remain to be seen.

There is no panacea in medicine. In selecting alternatives, we should remember that the operation that causes least alteration, provided cure is not vitiated, will afford the greatest quality of life. However, the physician must evaluate each individual's situation in relation to what is technically feasible for the surgeon and what is personally acceptable to the patient.

REFERENCES

1. SIMON, J. Ectopia vesicae (absence of the anterior walls of the bladder and pubic abdominal parietes); operation for directing the orifices of the ureters into the rectum; temporary success; subsequent death; autopsy. Lancet, 2:568, 1852.
2. CAMEY, M., and LEDUC, A. L'enterocystoplastie avec cystoprostatectomie totale pour cancer de la vessie. Ann. Urol., 13:114, 1979.
3. GIL-VERNET, J. M., JR. The ileocolonic segment in urologic surgery. J. Urol., 94:418, 1965.
4. HRADEC, E. A. Bladder substitution: indications and results in 114 operations. J. Urol., 94:406, 1965.
5. BRICKER, E. M. Bladder substitution after pelvic evisceration. Surg. Clin. North Am., 30:1511, 1950.
6. FERRIS, D. O., and ODEL, H. M. Electrolyte pattern of the blood after bilateral ureterosigmoidostomy. J.A.M.A., 142:634, 1950.
7. GITTES, R. F. Carcinogenesis in ureterosigmoidostomy. Urol. Clin. North Am., 13:201, 1986.

8. GHONEIM, M. A., SHEHAB-EL-DIN, A. B., ASHAMALLAH, A. K., and GABAL-LAH, M. A. Evolution of the rectal bladder as a method for urinary diversion. J. Urol., *126*:737, 1981.

9. TACCIUOLI, M., LAURENTI, C., and RACHELI, T. Sixteen years' experience with the Heitz Boyer-Hovelacque procedure for exstrophy of the bladder. Br. J. Urol., *49*:385, 1977.

10. LIGHT, J. K., and SCOTT, F. B. Total reconstruction of the lower urinary tract using bowel and the artificial urinary sphincter. J. Urol., *131*:953, 1984.

11. WATSUJI, H. (cited by SKINNER, D. G., BOYD, S. D., and LIESKOVSKY, G.) Clinical experience with the Kock continent ileal reservoir for urinary diversion. J. Urol., *132*:1101, 1984.

12. GILCHRIST, R. K., MERRICKS, J. W., HAMLIN, M. H., and RIEGER, I. T. Construction of a substitute bladder and urethra. Surg. Gynecol. Obstet., *90*:752, 1950.

13. KOCK, N. G., et al. Urinary diversion via a continent ileal reservoir: Clinical results in 12 patients. J. Urol., *128*:469, 1982.

14. SKINNER, D. G., BOYD, S. D., and LEISKOVSKY, G. Clinical experience with the Kock continent ileal reservoir for urinary diversion. J. Urol., *132*:1101, 1984.

15. ASHKEN, M. H. An appliance-free ileocecal urinary diversion: Preliminary communication. Br. J. Urol., *46*:631, 1974.

16. BENCHEKROUN, A. Continent cecal bladder. Br. J. Urol., *54*:505, 1982.

17. MANSSON, W. The continent cecal reservoir for urine. Scand. J. Urol. Nephrol., *85*:8, 1984.

18. KOCK, N. G., et al. The continent ileal reservoir (Kock pouch) for urinary diversion. World J. Urol., *3*:146, 1985.

19. BOYD, J. D. Chronic acidosis secondary to ureteral transplantation. Am. J. Is. Child., *42*:366, 1931.

20. McDOUGAL, W. S. Bladder reconstruction following cystectomy by uretero-ileo-colourethrostomy. J. Urol., *135*:698, 1986.

21. THUROFF, J. W., et al. The Mainz pouch (mixed augmentation ileum and cecum) for bladder augmentation and continent diversion. J. Urol., *136*:17, 1986.

22. STARLING, J. R., UEHLING, D. T., and GILCHRIST, K. W. Value of colonoscopy after ureterosigmoidostomy. Surgery, *96*:784, 1984.

23. STEWART, M., HILL, J. M., PUGH, R. C. B., and WILLIAMS, C. B. The role of N-nitrosamine in carcinogenesis at the ureterocolic anastomosis. Br. J. Urol., *53*:115, 1981.

24. HINMAN, F., JR. Selection of intestinal segments for bladder substitution: Physical and physiological characteristics. J. Urol., *139*:519, 1988.

Ileal Conduit Urinary Diversion

Jerome P. Richie

The challenge of devising a practical and effective alternative means of elimination of urine when the bladder could no longer function properly dates back to 1851, when John Simon diverted the flow of urine into the bowel.[1] The first crude attempts involved crushing clamps or placement of foreign bodies to establish a fistula between the ureter and rectum, and most patients died of peritonitis or uremia. Tizzoni and Poggi, in 1888, were the first to transplant ureters into an isolated loop of ileum interposed between the ureters and the urethra.[2]

The close proximity of the sigmoid colon and the attractive advantage of an intact sphincter mechanism made implantation of the ureters into the intact sigmoid colon a logical alternative for urinary diversion. As early as the 1880's, numerous investigators were attempting to solve the problems of uretero-intestinal anastomoses into the intact sigmoid colon. Ureterosigmoidostomy was the procedure of choice for urinary diversion from 1880 until 1950. The techniques developed for use with ureterosigmoidostomy are worthy of review, as much of our current knowledge about urinary diversion rests upon these techniques.

The problem of reflux, especially of fecally contaminated material, was recognized as a potential problem with this form of urinary diversion. Coffey, in 1911, heralded the modern era of uretero-intestinal diversion.[3] He was studying the problem of prevention of reflux in the biliary system and in ureterosigmoidostomy, and devised a flap valve or "tunneled" technique (Coffey I). With this technique, the slit end of the ureter was introduced into the bowel and attached by a transfixing suture, with the muscular coat of bowel and peritoneum sutured over the ureter in a submucosal gutter. Charles Mayo was the first to use this technique clinically and the technique became known as the Coffey-Mayo operation. Subsequent work with intubated ureteral stents led to the description of the Coffey II operation in 1927.

Numerous investigators described techniques for implantation of ureters into the colon. There was, however, general dissatisfaction because of high mortality and morbidity. All of these techniques relied upon scarring and slough of the distal end of the ureter and resulted in varying and unpredictable amounts of obstruction at the uretero-intestinal anastomosis. Nesbit, in 1949, provided a major breakthrough with the creation of a direct elliptical spatulated anastomosis with suture approximation of ureteral mucosa to bowel mucosa.[4] This technique, however, did not solve the problem of reflux.

Leadbetter and Clarke, with a farsighted accomplishment, combined the tunneled technique of Coffey and the elliptical mucosa to mucosa anastomosis of Nesbit, thereby describing the "combined" technique in 1950.[5] This technique has withstood the test of time and remains the preferred technique for ureterocolonic anastomoses for colonic conduits. An equally effective and innovative technique, the open transcolonic implantation, was provided by Goodwin and associates in 1953.[6] This technique, similar to a Leadbetter-Politano ureteral reimplant in the bladder, allows creation of a submucosal tunnel from within the lumen of the sigmoid colon.

The results of ureterosigmoidostomy were far from ideal, but other reasonable options for urinary diversion were limited. The known complications could be attributed to obstruction, reflux, and pyelonephritis. Hydronephrosis was reported in 32% of patients, pyelonephritis 57% and electrolyte abnormalities in 46% of patients, even with nonrefluxing anastomoses.[7] Ureterosigmoidostomy was a contributing factor in the demise of many of these patients. The major alternatives included colostomy with rectal bladder or rectal pouch and colostomy through the rectal sphincter. None of these procedures produced satisfactory long-term results.

The end of the ureterosigmoidostomy era was heralded by several factors. Ferris and Odel, in a classic paper, explained the method of hyperchloremic acidosis as the troubling electrolyte abnormality. They related this problem to the increased absorption of urinary contents, especially chloride, resulting from prolonged contact of urine with bowel mucosa.[8] Furthermore, the incidence of colon carcinoma has been reported in up to 11% of patients.[9] At the same time, Bricker popularized the creation of a cutaneous conduit, initially from the colon at the time of pelvic exenteration and subsequently from the distal ileum.[10] The conduit form of diversion had the advantage of shortened contact time of mucosa with urine and lessened the likelihood of hyperchloremic acidosis, a significant change from the previous systems of ureterosigmoidostomy. Surgeons, disappointed with the short- and long-term results of ureterosigmoidostomy, easily accepted this new form of diversion and it rapidly became the procedure of choice after radical cystectomy. In 1954, Bill and associates described ileal conduit procedures for children, and many people with benign bladder dysfunction such as neurogenic bladder or myelodysplasia, underwent urinary diversion for social reasons.[11] The short term follow-up was quite impressive and hyperchloremic acidosis and pyelonephritis were much less of a problem than with ureterosigmoidostomy. However, as long-term data became available, ileal conduits were discovered to be far from an ideal form of urinary diversion.

Stomal stenosis was noted in up to 25% of patients, many of whom required several revisions of the ileal conduit stoma. Pyelonephritis and calculi formation were noted in 10 and 15% of patients. Most importantly, in patients with normal pyelographic appearance of the kidney prior to diversion, 8% had shown signs of deterioration within 3½ years after diversion.[12] Follow-up studies up to 10 years post diversion confirmed this high rate of deterioration of the kidneys. Although stenosis or technical problems could be defined as the cause of deterioration in some patients, there remained a number who suffered renal damage for no apparent cause. Reflux, especially of infected urine, had to be considered a contributing factor as it had in patients with ureterosigmoidostomy.

Dissatisfaction with the ileal conduit lead to the third era of urinary diversion, the addition of anti-reflux (colonic conduits). Mogg, in 1966, popularized the colon conduit.[13] The conduit form prevented the problems of electrolyte absorption, and the antireflux tunnel, borrowed from the developments in the ureterosigmoidostomy era, diminished the problems of reflux and renal deterioration. Strong laboratory evidence supported the superiority of nonrefluxing colonic conduits over ileal conduits; pyelonephritis after 3 months of diversion in an animal preparation was reduced from 83% in ileal conduits to 13% with colon conduits.[14] Clinical experience has attested to the long-term superiority of colonic conduits.

The fourth era of urinary diversion is the continent cutaneous diversion or orthotopic bladder. Although many complex procedures had been described previously, difficulties with infection, the need for catheterization, and the complexity of the procedures in general had precluded widespread acceptance. Medical advances, especially the acceptance of the use of intermittent self catheterization, have changed the premise for construction of continent supravesical diversion procedures. Experience with continent diversions after proctocolectomy lead Kock to adapt this technique to continent ileal reservoirs for urinary diversion.[15] Vast clinical experience has been gained and recorded with the use of a long segment of ileum with nipples to prevent reflux and provide continence.[16] A variety of techniques has been described for use of a long segment of ileum or the ileocecal segment and entire right colon, with a variety of techniques to prevent reflux and provide continence. The continent cutaneous diversions and orthotopic bladder will be discussed in detail in chapters 27, 29–31.

The ideal bladder substitute has yet to be described. Conduits are currently the procedure of choice for urinary diversion, but many problems remain. The construction of the conduit requires exact and meticulous attention to detail, as complications may rapidly lead to mortality as well as increased morbidity. This section will deal with our preference for urinary diversion in patients with benign and malignant disease and will include technical preparation as well as certain "tricks of the trade."

INDICATIONS

The majority of urinary diversion procedures are performed after radical cystectomy for carcinoma of the bladder. In such patients, several factors must be taken into consideration.

1. One must be cognizant of the multifocal nature of urothelial tumors and be certain that the remaining urothelial system is free of carcinoma prior to urinary diversion. Frozen sections of the distal ureteral margins should suffice to exclude carcinoma in situ of the ureter.
2. In selection of the proper conduit, consideration must be taken of the amount of prior therapy, especially radiation therapy. Large fields and high doses of radiation

therapy, especially in a patient with prior abdominal surgery, may render the distal ileum and distal ureter dangerous because of the likelihood of improper healing. Careful observation of the bowel at the time of initial exploration and prior to excessive manipulation is essential to avoid usage of bowel that has been damaged by radiation.

3. One must consider the age of the patient and the overall prognosis. With only a 50 to 60% 5-year survival rate, the potential problems of reflux and renal deterioration, especially in the fully developed adult kidney, may not outweigh the risks inherent in creation of antireflux anastomosis. Indeed, one may utilize the freely refluxing anastomosis to obtain retrograde studies of the ureters and renal pelves for follow-up of the patient after radical cystectomy and Bricker urinary diversion.

4. In creation of a sigmoid conduit, the surgeon relies upon anastomoses between the middle and superior hemorrhoidal arteries for adequate blood supply to the distal colonic segment. Because the hypogastric artery is ligated during cystectomy, the blood supply to the distal colon may be tenuous.

For the above reasons, our conduit of choice after cystectomy is the distal ileal conduit. In patients with increased amounts of radiation therapy, a jejunal or transverse colonic conduit may be selected, preferably without an antireflux mechanism. In selected patients, continent cutaneous diversion or orthotopic bladder may be considered. These techniques are time consuming and may place the patient at increased risk if there are substantial medical problems. Patient motivation is an important factor, because many of these newer procedures can carry a higher morbidity and reoperation rate than the standard ileal conduit urinary diversion. Nonetheless, in selected patients, these alternatives are reasonable to consider.

In patients who undergo total exenteration, the colonic conduit is clearly the procedure of choice. This technique obviates an ileo-ileal anastomosis, and the distal colonic blood supply (rectosigmoid) is of no concern. We would reserve the nonrefluxing conduit predominantly for children with benign disease or for patients with neurogenic bladder who require diversion. Preservation of the remaining renal function is a significant concern for long-term survival of these patients.

PREOPERATIVE PREPARATION

Bowel preparation for the patient who will undergo ileal conduit diversion need not be as stringent as for the patient in whom a colonic segment will be utilized. Nonetheless, the routine preparation in all patients should consist of both mechanical and antibiotic measures in order to lessen potential complications of wound infection and sepsis. Although longer-term mechanical cleansing and clear liquid diet was the preparation of choice, in this day and age, with reduced hospital stays, patients are generally admitted the afternoon before surgery. In such circumstances, GoLytely can be utilized orally for effective mechanical bowel cleansing.[17] Neomycin, 1 g orally every hour for 4 doses and then every 4 hours, and Erythromycin base, 1 g orally 4 times daily, are begun one day preoperatively.[18] This regimen effectively inhibits growth of anaerobic bacteria.

The patient should be well hydrated preoperatively with 1 L of 0.9% sodium chloride given intravenously during the night before surgery. A central venous catheter may be placed and its position verified by X-ray.

Selection of the stomal site is a critical and important preoperative step. The preferred placement is midway between the umbilicus and the anterior superior iliac spine, in the right lower quadrant for a right-handed patient (Fig. 28-1A). The stoma should be just medial to the lateral border of the rectus muscle. The selected site should avoid bony protuberances, previous surgical scars, or areas of unevenness in the subcutaneous tissues. The aid of an experienced enterostomal therapist preoperatively is invaluable, both for the selection of the stomal site and for effective preoperative instruction of the patient and family. The site should be evaluated with the patient in supine, sitting, and standing positions, and if any question exists, the patient may wear an appliance filled with saline for several hours in order to verify proper positioning.

ILEAL CONDUIT

The patient is placed in the supine position with the table slightly extended, thereby widening the distance between the costal cartilage and the true pelvis. A left paramedian incision is preferred, with extension to the symphysis pubis if cystectomy is to be performed in conjunction with the ileal conduit diversion (Fig. 28-1A). Fascial layers are divided in line with the incision, and the peritoneal cavity entered. Careful attention must be paid at the time of initial exploration to the condition of the distal ileum. Radiation enteritis is manifest by pale discoloration of the bowel or numerous hyperemic vessels on the surface of the bowel serosa.

Preparation of Ureters

Posterior peritoneotomies are performed where the ureters cross the common iliac arteries, and a right-angled clamp and then moistened umbilical tape is passed underneath the ureter. Dissection should allow most of the periureteral adventitia to remain with the ureter in order to prevent ischemia. The ureters should be mobilized distally to well below the iliac vessels and then divided between chromic ligatures or large hemoclips. This will allow the proximal ureter to dilate, thereby facilitating the uretero-enteric anastomoses. If in conjunction with the cystectomy, sections of the proximal ureter should be analyzed for presence of frank carcinoma or carcinoma in situ. The ureters are mobilized craniad to the level of the lower pole of the kidney (Fig. 28-1B). Stay sutures of 4-0 chromic are placed at the cut end of the ureter to facilitate

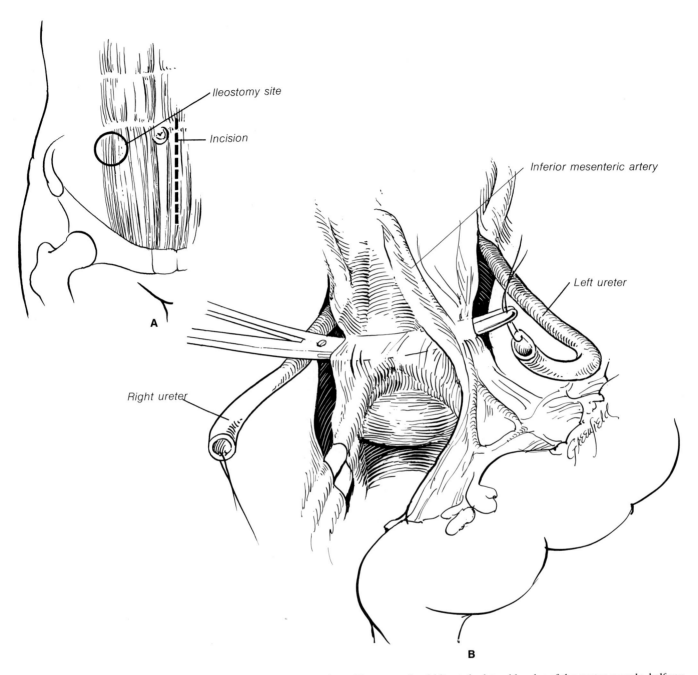

FIG. 28-1. *A,* Ideal placement for the stoma in the right lower quadrant. The stoma should lie at the lateral border of the rectus muscle, halfway between the umbilicus and the anterior superior iliac spine. A left paramedian incision is preferred. *B,* A tunnel has been created underneath the sigmoid mesentery and the left ureter is being pulled through the newly created tunnel. Stay sutures of 4.0 chromic catgut minimize manipulation of the ureteral mucosa.

mobilization and to reduce damage to the ureter by excessive use of forceps.

A tunnel must be created posterior to the colonic mesentery and anterior to the great vessels to allow the left ureter to be brought to the right side. This tunnel should allow the left ureter to swing across in a gentle arc with absolutely no tension. The effective craniad limit of the tunnel is the inferior mesenteric artery. Blunt and sharp dissection can be used to free the area and hemostasis can be obtained with small hemo-

clips. The left ureter is then drawn through the tunnel to lie in close proximity to the right ureter near the psoas muscle (Fig. 28-1*B*).

Preparation of Ileal Segment

In the absence of radiation changes, the preferred segment is the distal ileum, approximately 10 to 15 cm proximal to the ileocecal valve. The anatomy is relatively constant and permits dissection of the mesentery just medial to the ileo-colic artery, basing the selected segment on the last branch of the superior mesenteric artery prior to the bifurcation (Fig. 28-2). A segment approximately 25 cm in length should be selected, with longer segments chosen for more obese patients or those in whom the segment must be placed in an unusual position. The mesenteric incision should be much longer for the distal segment, as it will be necessary to provide length to reach the cutaneous surface. The proximal mesenteric incision should be short in order to protect the blood supply to the isolated segment (Fig. 28-2). If any question exists regarding the blood supply to the isolated segment, cross-table illumination will reveal the mesenteric arcades. A ¼ in. Penrose drain is placed at the proximal and distal ends of the proposed mesenteric incisions and the peritoneal reflection is divided. Small vessels in line with the mesenteric incisions are doubly clamped, divided, and ligated with 4-0 silk ligatures. The mesentery is

cleared from the bowel surface for a distance of 2 to 3 cm, and bowel clamps are applied. The clamps are placed in a 45° angle away from the antimesenteric surface on the intact bowel side, and straight across at a 90° angle on the conduit side (Fig. 28-2). This maneuver avoids ischemia of the antimesenteric side of the proximal and distal bowel segments to be anastomosed by entero-enterostomy.

Incision of the proximal bowel segment is performed first, and the conduit end immediately closed with a running Parker-Kerr suture of 3-0 chromic. A running layer of vertical mattress sutures is placed to close the butt end of the loop and reinforced by a second running layer of seromuscular mattress sutures, creating a double inverting seromuscular closure (Fig. 28-3A). Additional reinforcement is provided by interrupted Lembert sutures of 4-0 silk in the seromuscular portion of the bowel only (Fig. 28-3). Prompt closure of the proximal end of the loop insures an isoperistaltic segment. The distal end of

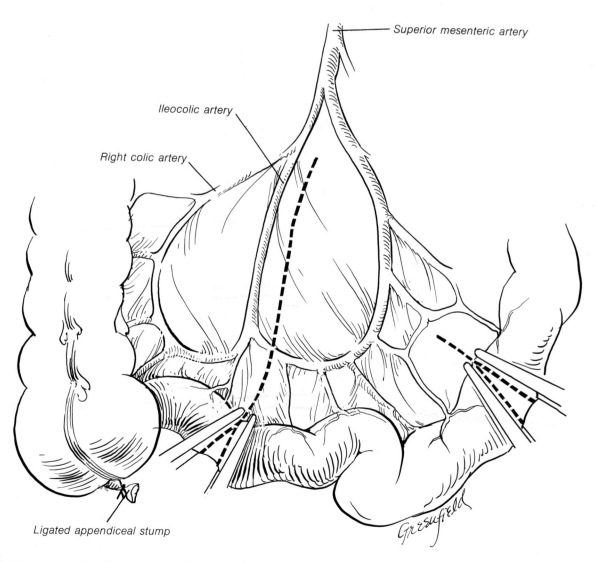

Fig. 28-2. Mesenteric incision for the creation of an isolated ileal conduit. A short proximal incision and a longer distal mesenteric incision ensure adequate mobility without compromise of blood supply. Clamps are placed at a 45° angle on the intact bowel side to prevent ischemia.

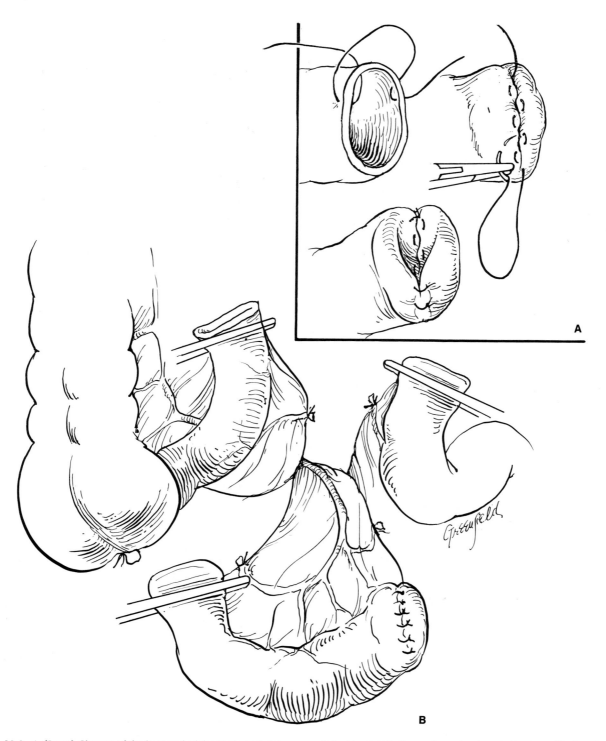

Fig. 28-3. *A*, (Inset) Closure of the butt end of the ileal conduit is accomplished by double-layered running inverted sutures (Parker-Kerr) and is reinforced by a separate layer of interrupted 4-0 silk sutures. *B*, The isolated ileal conduit is positioned caudad in preparation for entero-enterostomy.

the conduit is divided between clamps and the segment allowed to drop caudad (Fig. 28-3*B*). A standard entero-enterostomy is performed. We prefer a two-layer closure with interrupted 4-0 silk sutures for each layer (Fig. 28-4). The mesenteric window is closed with interrupted 4-0 silk sutures with care taken not to compromise the blood supply to the entero-enterostomy.

Ureteroileal Anastomosis

The bowel is packed out of the way and the closed end of the loop is placed near the psoas muscle to estimate the appropriate length for the ureters. The left ureter is then divided and spatulated on its medial border and a stay suture is placed to minimize trauma (Fig. 28-5*A*). Care must be taken to ensure

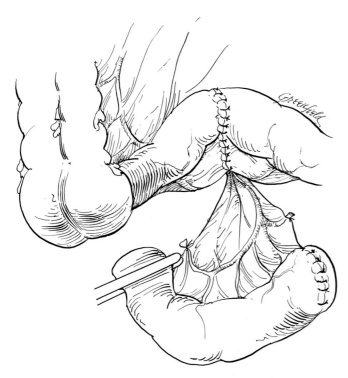

FIG. 28-4. Enteroenterostomy has been completed and the mobile isolated segment is ready to receive the ureters.

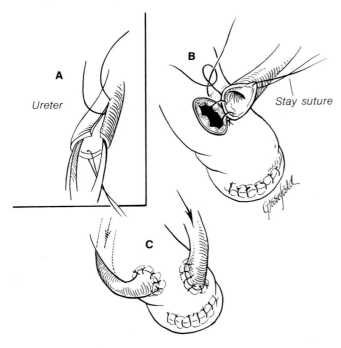

FIG. 28-5. (Inset) *A*, Elliptical spatulation of the ureter is performed and the apical suture is placed. Note the use of forceps to spread the ureter and to prevent handling of the mucosa. Note also the stay suture placed at the 12-o'clock position to aid in completion of the anastomosis. *B*, The apical suture of the ureteroileal anastomosis has been completed and additional sutures are being placed in staggered fashion. The stay suture on the 12-o'clock position of the ureter aids in manipulation of the ureter from side to side for better visualization. *C*, Both ureteral anastomoses have been completed. The right ureteroileal anastomosis is 1 cm distal to the left anastomosis, preventing ischemia between the two anastomoses.

that the ureter has not been twisted or angulated. A small ellipse of serosa and mucosa is removed sharply approximately 2 cm from the closed end of the loop. Forceps placed into the lumen of the ureter allow exact placement of sutures of 5-0 coated Vicryl (cutting needle) without trauma to the ureteral mucosa. The apical suture is placed first and approximated to the ileum by incorporating a small amount of mucosa and a larger amount of serosa, and is tied with the knots on the outside (Fig. 28-5*B*). This technique allows the ureter to extend into the enterotomy and obviates tension of the anastomosis. The stay suture is used to manipulate the ureter from side to side, allowing precise placement of alternating interrupted sutures until the anastomosis is secure. Five to 6 sutures will usually suffice and stents are not utilized routinely. The last two or three sutures are placed and tagged, and a fine right-angle ensures the patency of the ureter and the ileal opening prior to the final closure. A similar procedure is performed for the right ureter, with placement on the right side of the loop approximately 1 cm more distal from the closed end of the loop (Fig. 28-5*C*).

Once the anastomoses are completed, the closed end of the ileal conduit is sutured to the psoas muscle or sacral promontory with one or two seromuscular sutures of 4-0 silk. Great care must be taken to prevent angulation of the ureters during this step. No attempt is made to place the anastomoses into the retroperitoneal space, because radical cystectomy, performed concomitantly in many cases, makes this impossible. The small trap that is left between the sigmoid mesentery and the base of the ileal loop should be closed carefully with interrupted 4-0 silk sutures to prevent internal small bowel herniation and possible obstruction.

Stomal Preparation

The muscular layers of the abdominal wall are grasped with heavy Kocher clamps and the subcutaneous tissue is grasped with towel clips and held at the approximate level of closure prior to construction of the ileal stoma. This technique will avoid shifting or shuttering of the muscular layers during wound closure with subsequent obstruction of the ileal conduit. At the preselected site (marked by a scratch or tatoo prior to skin preparation), an ellipse of skin and subcutaneous tissue approximately the size of a quarter is excised with the orientation along Langer's line (Fig. 28-6*A*). A plug of subcutaneous fat is removed with care not to undermine the cutaneous edges of the incision, and the anterior rectus fascia is exposed at the lateral border of the rectus muscle. Army-Navy retractors or lateral perineal retractors are helpful in providing the exposure in obese patients. A cruciate incision is made in the anterior rectus fascia, creating an opening large enough to admit two fingers (Figs. 28-6*B* and 28-6*C*). The rectus muscle may be separated by blunt dissection with Kelly clamps, with care taken to avoid the inferior epigastric vessel (Fig. 28-6*D*). A cruciate incision is made in the posterior rectus fascia and peritoneum, with care taken to avoid injury to the underlying bowel (Fig. 28-6*E*). The opening should easily permit two fin-

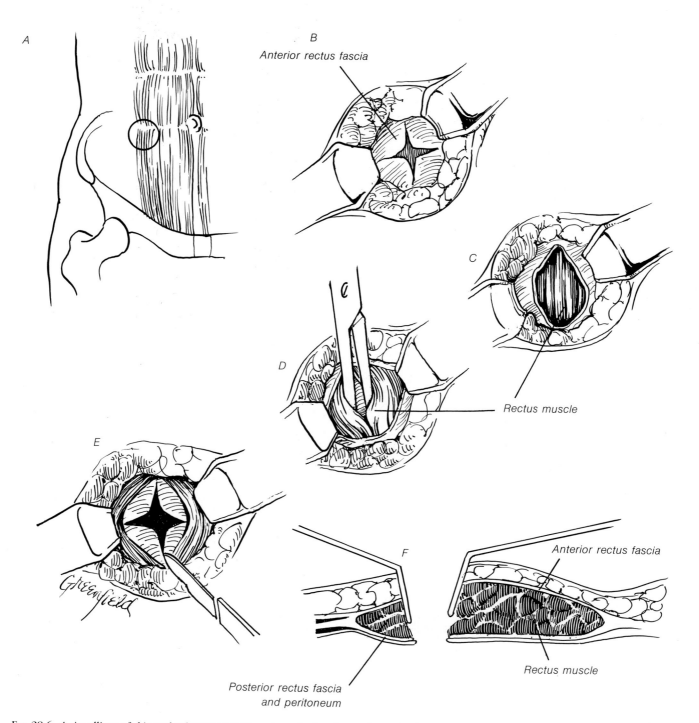

FIG. 28-6. *A*, An ellipse of skin and subcutaneous tissue is excised at the predetermined stomal site. *B* and *C*, A cruciate incision is made in the anterior rectus fascia, exposing the rectus muscle. *D*, The rectus muscle is separated in line with the incision. *E*, A cruciate incision is made in the posterior rectus fascia and peritoneum. *F*, Lateral view of the stomal creation. Note the cone-shaped appearance preventing undermining of the skin edge.

gers to pass without tension. Slight angulation from the skin surface through the various layers will create a cone-shaped opening and prevent any problem with dead space (Fig. 28-6F).

Prior to delivery of the loop through the stomal site, four quadrant sutures of 3-0 chromic catgut are placed through the anterior rectus fascia and the posterior rectus fascia and are temporarily clamped. This technique excludes the rectus mus-

cle and allows a firm anchoring of the ileal loop to both the anterior and posterior rectus fascia, thereby preventing herniation. The ileal segment is then brought through the opening and should protrude at least 3 to 4 cm above the skin level (Fig. 28-7A). If this can be accomplished without tension, the tagged anterior and posterior rectus fascia sutures are placed through the seromuscular layer of the emerging ileum and are tied (Fig. 28-7A). Additional sutures may be placed between the anterior rectus fascia and the seromuscular layer of the ileum to close any additional gaps and prevent herniation. Eversion of the stoma is created by a modified Brooke technique. It is imperative that a protruding or "bud" stoma be created rather than a flat or level stoma because of subsequent problems of application of the appliance and leakage. Quadrant sutures of 4-0 Dexon are placed through the subcuticular tissue just at the cutaneous margin, through the seromuscular layer of the ileum, approximately 1 cm above the fascial fixation, and through the full thickness of the bowel at its distal edge (Fig. 28-7B). Placement of four quadrant sutures in this fashion will allow turning of the stoma upon itself, much like the French cuff of a sleeve, and allow fixation with a good protruding stoma (Fig. 28-7C). Additional sutures may be placed between the subcuticular tissue and the mucosa of the everted stoma. Care must be taken in the area of the mesentery at 12 to 1 o'clock to prevent strangulation or compromise of the blood supply. Protrusion of the stoma at least 1 cm above the skin level allows effective diversion of efflux into the external collecting system and should prevent ileostomy dysfunction in well over 90% of all patients.[19] The completed ileal conduit is illustrated in Figure 28-8. Stents are not rou-

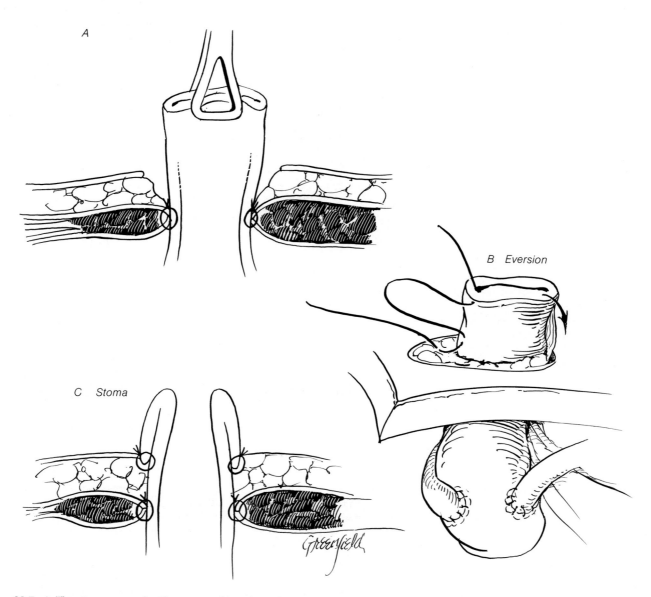

FIG. 28-7. A, The stoma, grasped with a noncrushing clamp, has been delivered to well above the skin level. Fixation sutures of 3-0 chromic incorporate anterior rectus fascia, posterior rectus fascia, and seromuscular portion of the emerging ileal loop. This effectively excludes the rectus muscle. B, Maturation of the stoma is accomplished by interrupted sutures in the subcuticular layer, emerging ileum, and full-thickness ileum. Four quadrant sutures are placed. C, Tying the four quadrant sutures results in a French cuff with a double layer of ileum, creating a bud or protruding stoma.

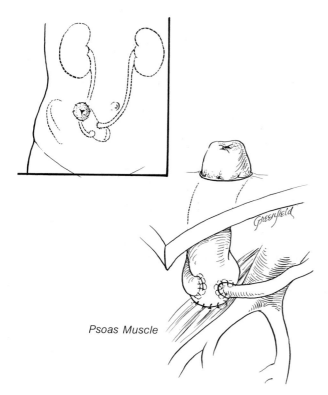

FIG. 28-8. Completed ileal loop. The ileal conduit has been anchored to the psoas muscle and the ureters lie without tension or angulation. A protruding bud stoma has been created.

Psoas Muscle

tinely used unless the patient has been irradiated or there is concern about the healing potential of the patient. Other authors, however, prefer to use stents routinely.[20]

In patients who are moderately obese or in patients with a short thick mesentery to the bowel, the ileal segment cannot be easily brought above the skin level without excessive tension on the mesentery. In these instances, a loop-end ileostomy should be fashioned according to the method of Turnbull (Fig. 28-9A–C).[21] The most mobile part of the ileal loop is thereby selected to be brought through the opening in the anterior abdominal wall and should protrude easily at least 4 to 5 cm above the skin level. The closed distal end of the loop may reside within the peritoneal cavity and lie in a subcutaneous position. The loop is fixed to the anterior rectus fascia with interrupted sutures of 3-0 chromic. Turnbull recommended placement of glass rod underneath the stoma, but fixation at the fascial level will obviate the need for the glass rod. The functional end of the ileal conduit should be placed caudad, and the loop is opened transversely ⅘ths of the way around the circumference near the junction of the defunctionalized limb and the cutaneous tissue. Thus, the loop is opened on its distal side near the level of the skin. Eversion of the mucosa and maturation to the subcuticular tissue with in-

terrupted sutures of 4-0 Dexon produce a prominent functional loop directed caudad and a recessive nonfunctioning loop directed craniad (Fig. 28-9B). The completed loop (Fig. 28-9C) has a prominent functional limb and a small defunctionalized distal limb. The clear-cut advantage of this technique is obviation of tension on the ileal loop mesentery. The stoma's advantage and ease of construction have made it my procedure of choice in obese patients. Emmott et al. have compared end versus loop stomas and feel that the loop stomas are superior because of better blood supply and less ischemia.[22]

In patients with severe pulmonary problems or neurogenic bladder, in whom prolonged ileus may be anticipated, a gastrostomy tube may be placed. Otherwise, a nasogastric tube is left for several days until active bowel sounds are present. A No. 10 closed-suction drain (Jackson-Pratt) is utilized routinely. A 16-French red rubber catheter is sewn into the loop to prevent obstruction from edema.

Postoperative Care

Nasogastric drainage is established by low intermittent suction for 3 to 4 days until bowel function is adequate as manifest by bowel sounds and passage of flatus. Adequate hydration in the postoperative period is important, and the use of volume expanders is necessary in conjunction with radical cystectomy. Instructions by an enterostomal therapist are important for the care of the ileostomy and for the fitting of the permanent appliance.

A postoperative urinary pouch is applied in the operating room. My preference is one of the vinyl pouches cut to fit the diameter of the stoma with an additional ¹⁄₁₆ in. clearance between the stoma and the opening in the face plate. Karaya washers are to be avoided because they react with the urine and produce a gelatinous mass with swelling. Attendance by an enterostomal therapist in the postoperative period will help familiarize the patients with the stoma and the proper techniques for applying the collecting device.

Permanent equipment of plastic pouches with various mounting rings, belts, and valves for emptying the urine are available and can be fitted in the postoperative period. However, shrinkage of the stoma will occur over the first several weeks and may necessitate ordering a smaller size face plate with time. The ileostomy should be recalibrated for shrinkage approximately 3 to 4 weeks postoperatively and again 6 weeks later. A maximum distance of ¹⁄₁₆ in. should exist between the stoma and face plate; otherwise, skin reaction with urine will occur.

Follow-up periodic visits with the enterostomal therapist are important at 3 months, 6 months, and 1 year postoperatively, to ensure adequate manipulation of the stomal appliance. Loop cultures and residual urine should be measured at each visit. An intravenous pyelogram should be obtained early in the postoperative period and again at 6 months to 1 year postoperatively.

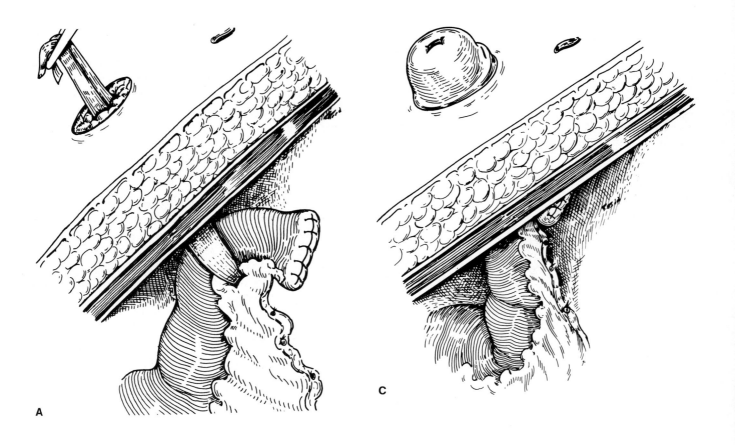

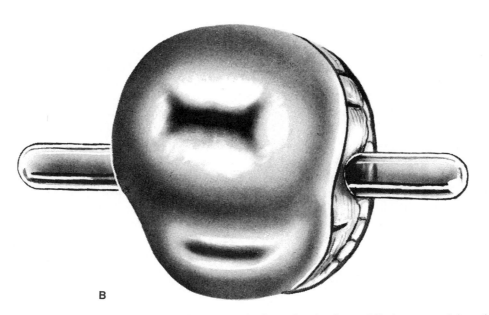

FIG. 28-9. Turnbull end-loop ileostomy. *A*, The distal end of the ileal loop has been closed and an umbilical tape passed through the mesentery in preparation for delivery of the loop into the created stomal opening. *B*, The loop has been opened four fifths of the way across the nonfunctional segment, creating a protuberant functional limb and a recessive nonfunctional limb. The glass rod is optional and may be obviated by fascial fixation sutures. *C*, Completed Turnbull stoma with the functioning loop pointed caudad and a short nonfunctioning loop craniad. This technique produces an excellent stoma without tension on the mesentery.

REFERENCES

1. Simon, J. Ectopic vesical (absence of the anterior walls of the bladder pubic abdominal parietes); operation for diverting the orifices of ureters into the rectum: temporary success: subsequent death: autopsy. Lancet, 2:568, 1852.

2. Tizzoni, G., and Poggi, A. Die wiederherstelung der Harnblase: experimentelle untersuchungen. Zbl. Shir., 15:921, 1911.

3. Coffey, R. C. Physiologic implantation of the severed ureter or common bile duct into the intestine. JAMA, 56:397, 1911.

4. Nesbit, R. M. Ureterosigmoid anastomosis by direct elliptical connection: A preliminary report. J. Urol., 61:728, 1949.

5. Leadbetter, W. F., and Clarke, B. G. Five years' experience with ureteroenterostomy by the "combined" technique. J. Urol., 73:67, 1954.

6. Goodwin, W. E., et al. Open, transcolonic uretero-intestinal anastomosis. Surg. Gynecol. Obstet., 97:1, 1953.

7. Wear, J. B., Jr., and Barquin, O. P. Ureterosigmoidostomy. Long-term results. Urology, 1:192, 1973.

8. Ferris, D. O., and Odel, H. M. Electrolyte pattern of the blood after bilateral ureterosigmoidostomy. JAMA, 142:634, 1950.

9. Zabbo, A., and Kay, R. Ureterosigmoidostomy and bladder exstrophy: A long-term followup. J. Urol., 136:396, 1986.

10. Bricker, E. M. Bladder substitution after pelvic evisceration. Surg. Clin. North Am., 30:1511, 1950.

11. Bill, A. H., Jr., et al. Urinary and fecal incontinence due to congenital abnormalities in children: Management by implantation of the ureters into an isolated ileostomy. Surg. Gynecol. Obstet., 98:565, 1954.

12. Richie, J. P. Intestinal loop urinary diversion in children. J. Urol., 111:687, 1974.

13. Mogg, R. A. The treatment of neurogenic urinary incontinence using the colonic conduit. Br. J. Urol., 37:681, 1965.

14. Richie, J. P., Skinner, D. G., and Waisman, J. The effect of reflux in the development of pyelonephritis in urinary diversion: An experimental study. J. Surg. Res., 16:256, 1974.

15. Kock, N. G., et al. Urinary diversion via a continent ileal reservoir: Clinical results in 12 patients. J. Urol., 128:469, 1982.

16. Skinner, D. G., Boyd, S. D., and Lieskovsky, G. Clinical experience with the Kock continent ileal reservoir for urinary diversion. J. Urol., 132:1101, 1984.

17. Wishnow, K. I., et al. Effective outpatient use of polyethylene glycolelectrolyte bowel preparation for radical cystectomy and ileal conduit urinary diversion. Urology, 31:7, 1988.

18. Nichols, R. L., et al. Effect of preoperative neomycinerythromycin intestinal preparation on the incidence of infectious complications following colon surgery. Ann. Surg., 178:453, 1973.

19. Artz, C. P., and Hardy, J. D. *Management of Surgical Complications*. 3rd Edition. Philadelphia, W. B. Saunders Co., 1975.

20. Regan, J. B., and Barrett, D. M. Stented versus nonstented uretero-ileal anastomoses: Is there a difference with regard to leak and stricture? J. Urol., 134:1101, 1985.

21. Weakley, F. L., and Turnbull, R. B., Jr. Special intestinal procedures. In *Operative Urology*. Edited by B. H. Stewart. Baltimore, Williams & Wilkins, 1975.

22. Emmott, D., Noble, M. J., and Mebust, W. K. A comparison of end versus loop stomas for ileal conduit urinary diversion. J. Urol., 133:588, 1985.

CHAPTER
29

Continent Cutaneous Diversion: Kock Pouch

Stuart D. Boyd

Donald G. Skinner

Gary Lieskovsky

The continent cutaneous urinary diversion is not an original concept of the 1980s. Current advances in this field owe their success to surgical pioneers such as Kock and Gilcrist, whose work in this area began over 30 years ago.[1,2] Kock's continent ileal reservoir for urinary diversion is a modification of the continent ileostomy that he developed in the 1960's for patients undergoing proctocolectomy for ulcerative colitis. The main feature of his urinary diversion is the creation of a reservoir that has extremely low internal pressures with afferent and efferent intussuscepted valves that prevent reflux and provide continence. Kock and his associates have shown how detubularized, double-folded ileal reservoirs demonstrate pressure characteristics and absorptive capacities unique among the various intestinal segments.[3–7] These reservoirs could maintain a much lower internal pressure compared to the cecal reservoirs. This low pressure was found to be critical for the long-term viability of the diversion. Another advantage of using ileum instead of colon was observed in the effect of continuous urine expo-

sure on bowel morphology and transport capacity. In the ileal reservoir, the villi become increasingly atrophic over time and the transport of water and solutes across the mucosa decreases. No such beneficial structural changes have been demonstrated in the colon.

Our own series of continent ileal reservoirs for urinary diversion now exceeds 600 patients. A number of technical modifications and adjustments to Kock's original description have been made at our institution. These are aimed at reducing the incidence of late complications and the need for reoperation.[8–10] The reservoir has also been modified for use in lower urinary tract reconstruction (bladder substitution) with primary anastomosis to the urethra in selected patients. Our experience has demonstrated that continent diversions are not too difficult to perform or maintain. In fact, continent diversions, whether to the skin or to the urethra, should be able to replace conduit diversions in most instances. In the future, patients will demand to be informed about these types of diversions and about the associated quality-of-life issues.[12]

274

SELECTION AND EVALUATION OF PATIENTS

Any patient who is a candidate for a urinary diversion is potentially suitable for a cutaneous Kock reservoir, as long as adequate bowel is available and life expectancy is reasonable. The patients should have the intelligence, maturity, and manual dexterity to care for their own diversion. The presence of prior radiation therapy does not preclude the procedure. We have performed continent diversions on a number of patients who have received up to 6500 rads of pelvic radiation. In these cases, one certainly has to be more careful in selecting the bowel segment, and patients who have had other abdominal operations prior to their radiation therapy will have an increased risk of complication. Radiated bowel will have a decreased compliance and the resulting reservoir will take longer to get up to its maximum capacity.

Over the last few years, bladder substitution procedures have become increasingly popular among the male patients (Fig. 29-1). The ability to void per urethra after cystectomy obviously can have a tremendous impact on a patient's quality of life. Bladder substitution, however, cannot be used in male patients with transitional cell carcinoma where the tumors extend into the prostatic urethra because these patients should probably undergo simultaneous or subsequent urethrectomy. Complete bladder substitution is not that effective in females because of the lack of an effective external sphincteric mechanism. Obesity does not appear to be an overriding factor in any patient. Unlike Camey, we have not had to abort any procedure for fear that a thick ileal mesentery would not allow the reservoir to reach to the skin or to the urethra.[11]

If conversion of an ileal conduit to a continent Kock pouch is being contemplated, it is important to radiographically examine the uretero-ileal anastomoses prior to surgery. If there is free reflux up the ureters on a loop-o-gram and no evidence of ureteral obstruction on intravenous urogram, the base of the old conduit with its implanted ureters may be preserved. At surgery, this portion of the conduit may be anastomosed directly to an appropriately shortened afferent limb of the Kock pouch.

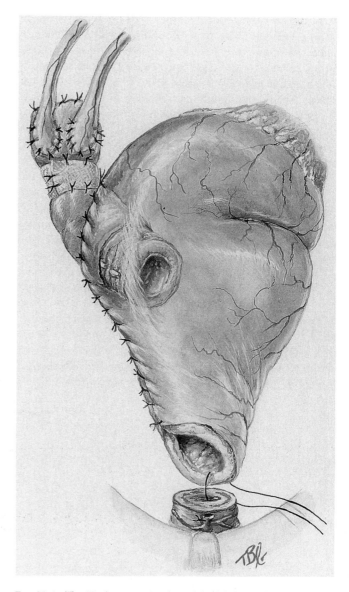

Fig. 29-1. The Kock reservoir adapted for bladder substitution with direct anastomosis to the urethra for internal urinary diversion. The procedure is not applicable in females or in males with bladder cancer, where the tumor extends into the prostatic urethra.

PREOPERATIVE PREPARATION

Patients are typically admitted to the hospital 1 day prior to surgery and placed on a clear liquid diet. A laxative such as Neoloid is administered the morning of the preoperative day and oral Neomycin and Erythromycin base given on that afternoon and evening. Good hydration is maintained by initiating intravenous fluids that night. Routine preoperative parenteral nutrition is not used unless the patient's serum albumin/total protein levels are low. The enterostomal therapist is invaluable in preparing cutaneous diversion patients prior to surgery. Detailed patient instruction by a dedicated therapist prior to and after the surgery makes the postoperative transition and the catheterization experience much smoother and easier.

The enterostomal therapist also provides necessary input in predetermining the general location of the cutaneous stoma. The stoma site can usually be low on the abdominal wall because avoidance of skin folds for ostomy bag placement is not a factor.

SURGICAL PROCEDURE

The patient is placed in a hyperextended supine position in order to widen the distance between the ribs and the pelvis. A midline abdominal incision is made, curving to the left of the umbilicus and extending to the pubis if a cystectomy is to be performed in conjunction with the diversion. When a simultaneous cystectomy is being performed, that portion of the procedure should be completed first. In patients being converted from a previous ileal conduit diversion, a similar amount of time as that needed for the cystectomy will probably be spent delineating the old conduit and mobilizing the intestine. At this time, if the preoperative radiologic evaluations of the ileal conduit reveal that the uretero-ileal anastomoses are still in good condition, the base of the old conduit, with is implanted ureters, should be delineated and saved. We have had one case where the ileal conduit was found to be greater than 80 cm in length and the entire continent diversion was created out of the old ileal conduit. The more likely scenario, however, is that just the base of the conduit will be saved for anastomosis end-to-end to an appropriately shortened afferent limb of the pouch.

In the patient without prior diversion, the ureters should be mobilized early, well below the iliac vessels, and divided between large ligaclips. This will allow the proximal ureter to dilate during the case and facilitate the ureteroileal anastomoses. A tunnel should be created beneath the mesentery of the descending colon and anterior to the great vessels to allow the left ureter to smoothly swing over to the midline. This tunnel should be just below the inferior mesenteric artery.

Selection of the Ileal Segment

The segment of ileum to be used for the diversion must first be delineated (Fig. 29-2). If there has not been a prior bowel anastomosis, and in the absence of radiation-induced changes, the distal ileal division (efferent end) should be made approximately 15 to 20 cm from the cecum. This will allow for a long mesenteric division in the avascular plane between the terminal branch of the superior mesenteric artery and the ileocolic artery. This division can be made back to the base of the mesentery and will provide the necessary length and mobility for the diversion to easily reach the skin. If there is an existing ileal conduit, the prior small bowel anastomosis should be identified and excised. The prior mesenteric division should be opened for its full extent and the efferent end of the pouch begun at this point.

Silk sutures are used to mark off the individual segments of the reservoir: 17 cm for the efferent (distal) limb, 22 cm for each of the two arms of the reservoir, and 17 cm for the afferent (proximal) limb. Approximately 5 cm of ileum proximal to the afferent end is discarded, along with a small triangular wedge of mesentery. This provides improved mobility to the pouch and to the small bowel anastomosis, and because this mesentery division will be quite short, an excellent blood sup-

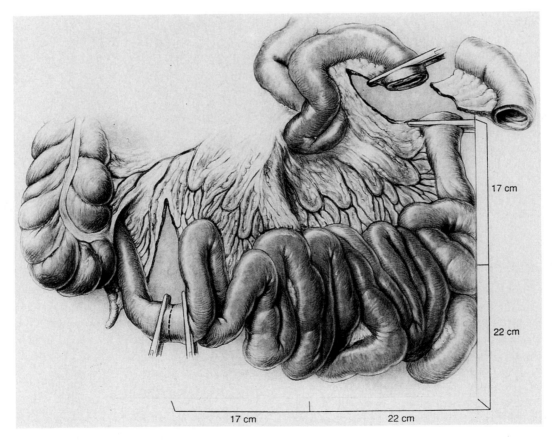

FIG. 29-2. Ileum delineated for the Kock pouch: 17 cm for the efferent limb, 22 cm for each of the two segments of the reservoir, and 17 cm for the afferent limb. A 5-cm wedge of ileum and mesentery is resected proximal to the afferent limb to provide better mobility. (From Skinner, D. G., Boyd, S. D., and Lieskovsky, G. Creation of the continent Kock ileal reservoir as an alternative to cutaneous urinary diversion. In *Genitourinary Cancer.* Edited by D. G. Skinner and G. Lieskovsky. Philadelphia, W. B. Saunders Co., 1988.)

ply to the pouch is ensured. The small bowel continuity is re-established with a standard, sutured or stapled enteroenterostomy, depending on the surgeon's preference. The mesenteric defect is closed with running #2-0 chromic sutures, with care taken not to impinge upon the mesentery to the reservoir or to compromise the blood supply to the enteroenterostomy. The end of the afferent limb is closed with a running Parker-Kerr #3-0 chromic suture, and is reinforced by a second running layer of seromuscular mattress sutures, creating a double inverting seromuscular closure. If stapling is used, we recommend that this end be oversewn with 3-0 PGA suture so that the staple line is definitely excluded from the urine.

Construction of the Reservoir

The two 22-cm ileal segments for the reservoir are directed caudally in a "U" shape (Fig. 29-3). Prior to opening the reservoir, the segments are apposed with a running 3-0 PGA suture placed in the serosa just above the mesentery on each side. The reservoir is then opened with the cautery knife by incising the ileal segments just above the apposing suture line (Fig. 29-4). This incision should be extended for 2 to 3 cm up the afferent and efferent limbs, along their antimesentery border, so that when the nipple valves are constructed, they will be well separated. This aids both in the closure of the pouch and in subsequent endoscopic evaluation of the mature pouch. The back wall of the reservoir is closed with two layer running 3-0 PGA suture (Fig. 29-5). This back wall closure extends just for the length of the reservoir segments and does not extend up into the opening in the afferent and efferent limbs.

Construction of Valves

The antireflux and continence valves are created from the afferent and efferent limbs by intussuscepting the bowel. The intussusception is made easier and more secure by first dividing the mesentery beneath the portion of the limb to be intussuscepted (Fig. 29-6). The cautery knife is used to create the mesentery opening for 8 cm along the bowel's serosal surface. The windows of Deaver in the mesentery are incised and the individual vessels picked up with forceps and cauterized. If the mesentery is not stripped away, it may serve as the leading edge for later slippage or extussusception of the valve.

An additional opening in the mesentery is made one vascular arcade distal to the 8-cm opening just created. A 2-cm strip of PGA mesh is passed through this additional opening to serve as an anchoring collar for the base of the nipple valves. Marlex mesh was originally used for this purpose, but Marlex tends to be erosive and can become a source of infection and stone formation. We have now abandoned using Marlex mesh as an anchoring collar after our initial 150 cases.

The intussusception of the nipple valves is accomplished by passing two Allis forcep clamps just over half way up the open limb to the anchoring collar, grasping the mucosa, and inverting the ileum into the pouch (Fig. 29-7). A valve at least 5 cm long will be created, still leaving a 1-cm lip of pouch at

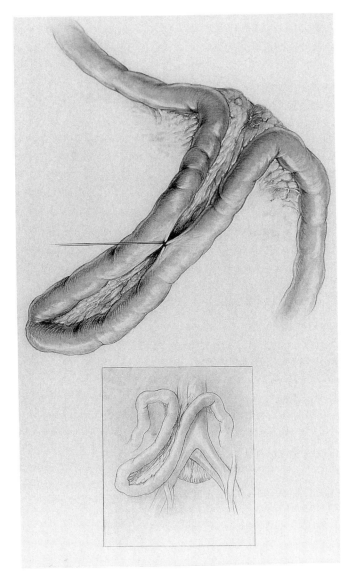

FIG. 29-3. The reservoir segments are directed caudally in a "U" shape. (From Skinner, D. G., Boyd, S. D., and Lieskovsky, G. Creation of the continent Kock ileal reservoir as an alternative to cutaneous urinary diversion. In *Genitourinary Cancer*. Edited by D. G. Skinner and G. Lieskovsky. Philadelphia, W. B. Saunders Co., 1988.)

the opening for subsequent reservoir closure. Non-crushing staples are used to secure the valves (Fig. 29-8). Until recently, we had been using a standard TA-55 stapler with 4.8 mm staples to apply three rows of parallel staples as shown. The TA-55 stapler utilizes a pin that leaves a pin hole that needs to be separately sutured closed at the base of each staple line. This pinhole has been noted to be the occasional site of a valve fistula. We have now switched to using either a special, pinless TA-55 or a custom GIA stapler that places a double row of staples without a knife and does not create a pinhole. We have also found that it is necessary to place only two double rows of staples rather than three rows. This creates a well-vascularized but still well-secured valve. The staple rows should be placed

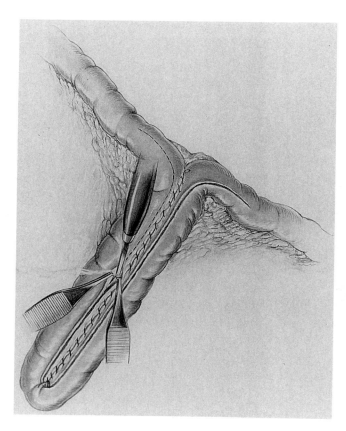

FIG. 29-4. The inner walls of the reservoir segments are apposed with running #3-0 PGA sutures and opened with the cautery knife. The incision is extended for 2 to 3 cm up the afferent and efferent limbs along their antimesenteric border. (From Skinner, D. G., Boyd, S. D., and Lieskovsky, G. Creation of the continent Kock ileal reservoir as an alternative to cutaneous urinary diversion. In *Genitourinary Cancer.* Edited by D. G. Skinner and G. Lieskovsky. Philadelphia, W. B. Saunders Co., 1988.)

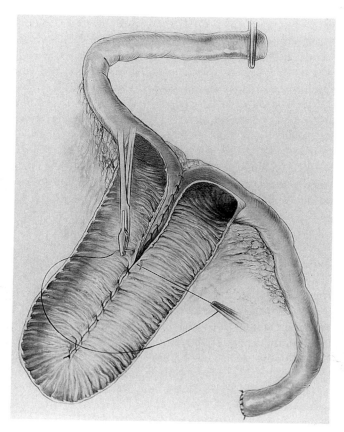

FIG. 29-5. The reservoir segments are opened and the back wall of the reservoir is closed in a watertight manner with two layers of running #3-0 PGA sutures. (From Skinner, D. G., Boyd, S. D., and Lieskovsky, G. Creation of the continent Kock ileal reservoir as an alternative to cutaneous urinary diversion. In *Genitourinary Cancer.* Edited by D. G. Skinner and G. Lieskovsky. Philadelphia, W. B. Saunders Co., 1988.)

in the anterior half of the valve, leaving the posterior side free so that another row of staples can subsequently fix the nipple to the back wall of the pouch. Do not be alarmed if the tip of the nipple valve appears dusky or congested. The overall length of the valve, once it has healed, should always be much longer than the needed functional length of 2.5 cm. The staples at the base of the valves are the most important for preventing valve slippage and these staples bury themselves well beneath the mucosa. Because the staples at the tip of the nipple valves really do not contribute to the maintenance of the valve, and because they are more likely to remain exposed and become a potential site for stone formation, the distal six staples are removed from the corresponding end of the staple cartridge prior to stapling.

The effectiveness of the nipple valves are further ensured by fixing them to the back wall of the reservoir. This can be accomplished by either of two methods (Fig. 29-9). We prefer to slip the outer arm of the stapler between the two leaves of the valve, with the other arm remaining outside the reservoir, and staple the valve to the back wall, posteriorly just next to

the mesentery. This places only two layers of tissue in the stapler, one wall of the nipple valve and the wall of the pouch, while fixing the valve in a secure fashion. A standard, full-length staple cartridge is utilized. A secondary technique is also demonstrated in Figure 29-9. This requires making a small opening in the back wall of the pouch near the tip of the valve. The outer arm of the stapler is passed through this opening from the outside and advanced up the inside of the valve. When stapled, this fixes the full thickness of the valve to the back wall just lateral to the mesentery. The small opening in the reservoir is closed with #3-0 PGA sutures. With either technique, two additional #3-0 PGA sutures are used to further secure the tip of each valve to the pouch wall (Fig. 29-10). The secure fixation of the nipple valve to the pouch wall not only helps prevent long-term valve slippage but also increases the efficiency of the antireflux and continence mechanisms as the reservoir fills and stretches.

Prior to fixation of the PGA mesh collar, it is soaked in tetracycline solution (250 mg in 10 cc normal saline), to help it incite more a fibrous reaction at the base of the valve. The

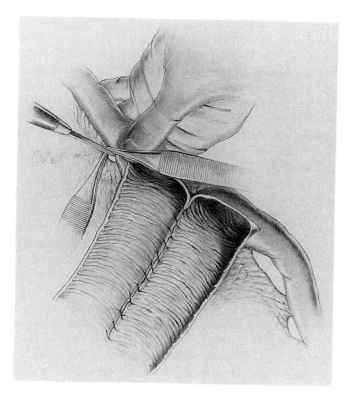

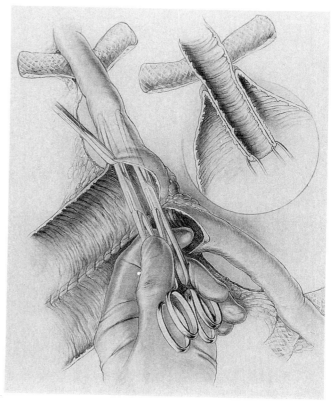

Fig. 29-6. An 8-cm mesenteric window is opened with the cautery knife beneath the portion of each limb to be intussuscepted. The window should begin 1 cm back from the opening of the limb into the reservoir. A second 1-cm window in the mesentery is made one vascular arcade beyond to accommodate each anchoring collar. (From Skinner, D. G., Boyd, S. D., and Lieskovsky, G. Creation of the continent Kock ileal reservoir as an alternative to cutaneous urinary diversion. In *Genitourinary Cancer.* Edited by D. G. Skinner and G. Lieskovsky. Philadelphia, W. B. Saunders Co., 1988.)

Fig. 29-7. One-cm anchoring collars of PGA mesh are positioned in their mesenteric openings. Two Allis forcep clamps are passed up each limb just over half way to the anchoring collar, the mucosa is grasped, and the ileum intussuscepted, creating a nipple valve at least 5 cm long. (From Skinner, D. G., Boyd, S. D., and Lieskovsky, G. Creation of the continent Kock ileal reservoir as an alternative to cutaneous urinary diversion. In *Genitourinary Cancer.* Edited by D. G. Skinner and G. Lieskovsky. Philadelphia, W. B. Saunders Co., 1988.)

mesh is anchored to the base of the valves and the ileal limb with sutures of #3-0 PGA (Fig. 29-10). One should not include the mesentery in these sutures. The collar further stabilizes the valves and also serves as an anchoring point for fixing the efferent valve and limb to the abdominal wall. A 30-French Medina catheter can be passed up the nipple valve and through the mesh site while the mesh is being sutured. This will allow the mesh to be affixed snugly without being too tight. The redundant mesh can be excised.

Reservoir Closure

The reservoir is completed by folding the ileum in the opposite direction to which it was opened and suturing it closed (Fig. 29-11). The closure is accomplished with a two layer, running #3-0 PGA suture, which is meticulously placed to ensure water tightness. The principle of opening, folding, and closing is important as it causes the motor activities of the different ileal segments of the pouch to counteract them-

selves, thus creating an extremely low pressure reservoir. This helps assure the long-term viability of the diversion.

Ureteroileal Anastomoses

The bowel is packed out of the way and the proximal closed end of the afferent limb is secured to the tissue overlying the sacral promontory with #3-0 PGA suture (Fig. 29-12). Each ureter is carefully trimmed to an appropriate length, spatulated, and anastomosed to a small opening created on each side of the afferent limb. The anastomoses are accomplished in a standard end-to-side fashion using interrupted #4-0 PGA suture.[13] Approximately eight sutures are usually required. After each anastomosis is half completed, the ureters are stented with 8-French infant feeding tubes that are perforated with extra holes and fed up through the afferent limb and valve to remain indwelling in the pouch. We remove these stents endoscopically in approximately 3 weeks. One may also elect to bring the stents out through the reservoir wall to the

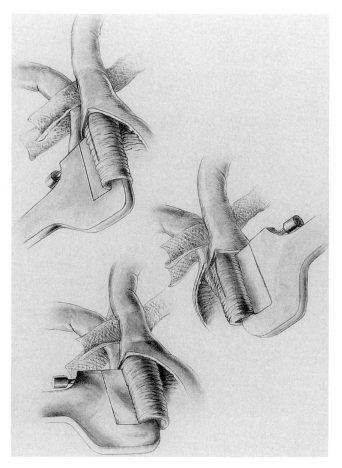

Fig. 29-8. The nipple valves are first stabilized by stapling two or three times with special pinless TA-55 or knifeless GIA staplers. Note that the distal 6 staples are preremoved from the staplers. (From Skinner, D. G., Boyd, S. D., and Lieskovsky, G. Creation of the continent Kock ileal reservoir as an alternative to cutaneous urinary diversion. In *Genitourinary Cancer.* Edited by D. G. Skinner and G. Lieskovsky. Philadelphia, W. B. Saunders Co., 1988.)

skin, or out the efferent limb through the stoma, to monitor their drainage individually in the immediate postoperative period. We have found the manipulation required to get the stents out to the skin to be time consuming and unnecessary.

Stoma Preparation and Pouch Fixation

The stoma can usually be located low on the right side of the abdomen, overlying the rectus muscle. An approximate site for the stoma can be made preoperatively by the enterostomal therapist, but the exact site should be selected after the pouch is created so that the efferent limb can reach the skin as perpendicular to the pouch as possible. This is especially important in the obese patient. Once the stoma site is determined, a 2-cm (nickel-sized) plug of skin is removed. The subcutaneous fat is opened directly beneath the stoma with the cautery knife, and the anterior rectus fascia is exposed. A 3-cm vertical incision is made through the rectus fascia, and the muscle and

peritoneum are split just widely enough to accommodate the tips of two fingers. Two horizontal mattress sutures of #1 PGA are then passed through each side of the anterior rectus fascial opening, and positioned correspondingly through each side of the efferent anchoring collar and the base of the valve (see Fig. 29-12). These sutures should be separately color coded to avoid any confusion and to maintain the alignment when the efferent limb is brought up through the stoma site. Before the sutures are tied, an additional 1-cm strip of Marlex mesh is anchored with #1 Nylon suture to the posterior rectus fascia, just cephalad and lateral to the abdominal wall opening for the stoma. This Marlex strut is brought through the window of Deaver in the mesentery adjacent to the PGA mesh (see Fig. 29-12). An Allis clamp is used to carefully bring the efferent limb up through the stomal opening, while being certain not to cross the mattress sutures. The mattress sutures are securely tied, thus fixing the base of the efferent valve to the rectus fascia. When the sutures are properly placed and tied, the efferent limb should exit the pouch without angulation. The Marlex strut is then further sutured to the posterior rectus fascia medial to the mesentery with another #1 nylon suture (see Fig. 29-12). The Marlex serves to secure the mesentery side of the limb, without risk of erosion, and prevents parastomal hernias and concomitant catheterization difficulties. The redundant efferent limb above the skin line is excised. A flush or slightly recessed stoma is completed by suturing the ileum circumferentially to the skin with interrupted #3-0 PGA. A slightly recessed stoma will usually allow the stoma site to constrict down to the size of the catheter over the first few months and give an even better cosmetic appearance to the stoma.

A 30-French Medina catheter is placed through the stoma site and positioned centrally in the pouch. Normal saline is instilled through the catheter to make certain that the pouch can be easily irrigated in the postoperative period and to check the water tightness of the suture lines. After being properly positioned, the catheter is secured at the stoma site with two #1 nylon sutures. A 1 in. Penrose drain is placed through a separate stab incision in the abdominal wall and positioned below the pouch. The abdomen is then closed.

POSTOPERATIVE CARE

The general care of these patients in the immediate postoperative period will be the same as for patients undergoing cystectomy and ileal conduit diversion. Gastric drainage, either by a nasogastric tube or gastrostomy tube, is maintained until bowel function is adequate, usually noted in 4 to 5 days. Hydration is maintained initially by intravenous fluids. Patients are encouraged to resume a normal diet as soon as possible and to begin early ambulation. The one unique care feature of the continent diversion is the need to periodically irrigate the reservoir with normal saline to make certain that it stays clear of mucous. Typically, the Medina catheter is rinsed every 4 hours with 30 to 60 cc of normal saline. By the third postoperative day, patients are instructed in self-irrigation techniques

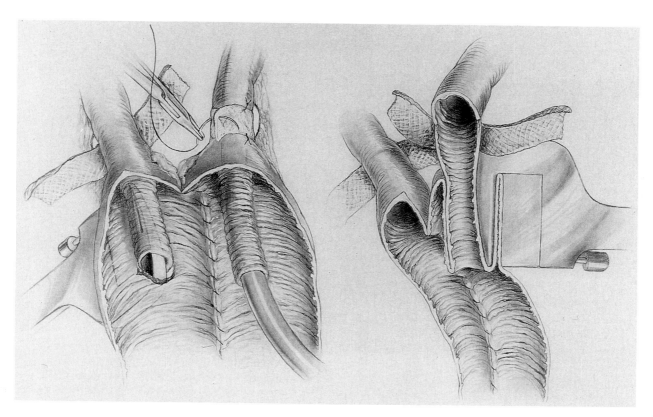

FIG. 29-9. The nipple valves are further fixed to the back wall of the reservoir utilizing either of two methods. The preferred technique is demonstrated on the right. The arm of the stapler is inserted from the outside, next to the mesentery, between the two leaves of the valve, and the stapler is fired, fixing one leaf of the valve to the back wall. A secondary method is shown on the left. A hole is made in the back wall of the reservoir opposite the tip of the valve. The arm of the stapler is passed through the hole, up the inside of the valve, and fired. The hole in the back wall is closed with #3-0 PGA. The PGA mesh anchoring collar is firmly sutured to the base of each valve and limb with a Medina catheter temporarily in place to determine the sizing. (From Skinner, D. G., Boyd, S. D., and Lieskovsky, G. Creation of the continent Kock ileal reservoir as an alternative to cutaneous urinary diversion. In *Genitourinary Cancer*. Edited by D. G. Skinner and G. Lieskovsky. Philadelphia, W. B. Saunders Co., 1988.)

so that they can do this themselves. Once patients are self reliant, they can be discharged to home health care, usually within 8 to 10 days of the operation. It is extremely important that patients keep themselves well hydrated and continue the catheter irrigation at home. Discharge medication should include an oral antibiotic.

The Medina catheter remains indwelling in the reservoir for 3 weeks. At the end of the 3 weeks, the patients are readmitted for a 1-day stay. A Kockogram (cystogram of the pouch) is performed, followed by an intravenous urogram. If the system is well healed, the catheter is removed and the patient is instructed in self-catheterization techniques. The ureteral stents are endoscopically removed at this time. Catheterization is begun at 2- or 3-hour intervals. If no difficulties are encountered during the 24-hour stay, the Penrose drain can be removed and the patient discharged. The ideal catheters for home use are 18 or 20 French Coudé tip, reusable catheters. Each patient usually maintains a supply of two or three catheters. Catheters can be kept in a plastic lined bag and easily carried in a purse for women or in a tobacco pouch for men. The catheterization interval is usually increased by

1 hour each week while at home. The goal after 4 to 6 weeks is to have patients catheterize themselves every 6 hours during the day and be able to sleep through the night. Patients should be instructed to be independent and to feel free to travel. Oral antibiotics are usually maintained until the catheterization schedule has stabilized. All patients wear a small absorbency pad over their stoma to prevent mucous spotting of their clothing. The pads are removed for swimming or bathing.

RESULTS

The overall early and late complication rates for patients undergoing cystectomy and continent diversion should not differ significantly from what we see in patients undergoing cystectomy and ileal conduit urinary diversion. The late complications unique to continent cutaneous diversions usually involve continence problems. Leakage of urine from the stoma sufficient to warrant reoperation occurred in 10 to 15% of our patients in the early part of our series. The problem was usually totally correctable at surgery by resecuring or replacing the continence valve.[14] It is hoped that the newer methods of

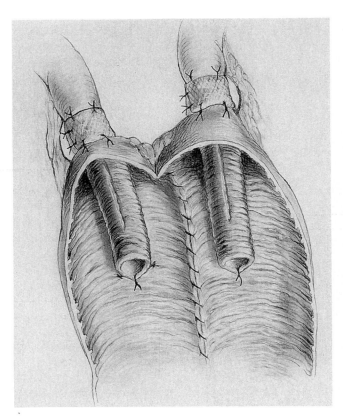

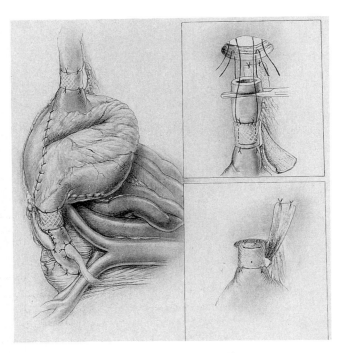

FIG. 29-10. The fixation of the valves is completed by suturing the tips of the valves to the reservoir wall with #3-0 PGA. (From Skinner, D. G., Boyd, S. D., and Lieskovsky, G. Creation of the continent Kock ileal reservoir as an alternative to cutaneous urinary diversion. In *Genitourinary Cancer*. Edited by D. G. Skinner and G. Lieskovsky. Philadelphia, W. B. Saunders Co., 1988.)

FIG. 29-12. The end of the afferent limb is fixed over the sacrum and a standard ureteroileal end-to-side anastomoses is performed. After the stoma site is selected and a 2-cm skin plug is removed, two horizontal mattress sutures of #1 PGA are fixed to the anterior rectus fascia and correspondingly on each side of the anchoring collar and the base of the efferent valve. A 1-cm strut of Marlex mesh is passed through the mesenteric opening for the anchoring collar and is sutured to the posterior fascia laterally with #1 nylon. The efferent limb is pulled up through the stoma, the mattress sutures tied, and the Marlex strut sutured medially to the posterior fascia. (From Skinner, D. G., Boyd, S. D., and Lieskovsky, G. Creation of the continent Kock ileal reservoir as an alternative to cutaneous urinary diversion. In *Genitourinary Cancer*. Edited by D. G. Skinner and G. Lieskovsky. Philadelphia, W. B. Saunders Co., 1988.)

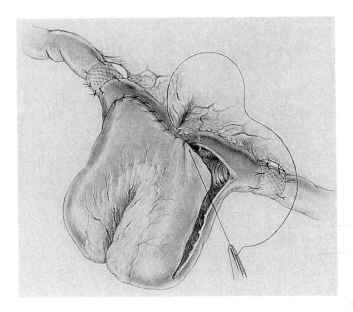

FIG. 29-11. The reservoir is completed by folding the ileum back on itself and suturing with two-layer, running #3-0 PGA. (From Skinner, D. G., Boyd, S. D., and Lieskovsky, G. Creation of the continent Kock ileal reservoir as an alternative to cutaneous urinary diversion. In *Genitourinary Cancer*. Edited by D. G. Skinner and G. Lieskovsky. Philadelphia, W. B. Saunders Co., 1988.)

nipple fixation, and the use of the Marlex strut and the pinless stapler will reduce this rate. Problems with catheterization in the cutaneous Kock diversion occur in only 1% of patients if our method of stabilization of the efferent limb is used. The antireflux mechanism of the Kock diversion has a 98% reliability, which is difficult to obtain by any other method. The incidence of ureteroileal stenosis is 3%, similar to that seen in a standard ileal conduit. Electrolyte problems are rare and so far vitamin B12 deficiency has not been noted in significant numbers though vitamin B12 replacement theoretically may be necessary after 5 to 10 years.

Patient satisfaction with the continent Kock diversion is excellent. Only 1% of our patients have requested conversion of their continent diversion to a conduit type diversion. There is no question that in the areas of self-confidence, self-image, interpersonal relations, and sexual desires, a significant difference exists between Kock pouch patients and ileal conduit patients, as continent diversion is favored. The most vocal advocates of continent diversion remain those Kock pouch patients who previously have had a noncontinent urinary diversion.

REFERENCES

1. Kock, N. G., et al. Urinary diversion via a continent ileal reservoir: Clinical results in 12 patients. J. Urol., *128*:469, 1982.

2. Gilcrist, R. K., et al. Construction of substitute bladder and urethra. Surg. Gynecol. Obstet., *90*:752, 1950.

3. Kock, N. G. Ileostomy without external appliances: A survey of 25 patients provided with intra-abdominal intestinal reservoir. Ann. Surg., *173*:545, 1971.

4. Kock, N. G., et al. Changes in renal parenchyma and the upper urinary tracts following urinary diversion via a continent ileum reservoir. An experimental study in dogs. Scand. J. Urol. Nephrol. *49*(Suppl.):11, 1978.

5. Kock, N. G., et al. Urinary diversion via a continent ileum reservoir: Clinical experience. Scand. J. Urol. Nephrol., *49*(Suppl.):23, 1978.

6. Kock, N. G. Continent ileostomy: Historical perspective. *Alternatives to Conventional Ileostomy.* Edited by R. Dozois. Chicago, Year Book Medical Publishers, 1985, pp. 133–145.

7. Berglund, B., Kock, N. G., and Myrvold, H. E. Volume capacity and pressure characteristics of the continent cecal reservoir. Surg. Gynecol. Obstet., *163*:42, 1986.

8. Skinner, D. G., Boyd, S. B., and Lieskovsky, G. Clinical experience with the Kock continent ileal reservoir for urinary diversion. J. Urol., *132*:1101, 1984.

9. Skinner, D. G., Lieskovsky, G., and Boyd, S. D. Technique of creation of a continent internal ileal reservoir (Kock pouch) for urinary diversion. Urol. Clin. North Am., *11*:741, 1984.

10. Skinner, D. G., Lieskovsky, G., and Boyd, S. D. Continuing experience with the continent ileal reservoir (Kock pouch) as an alternative to cutaneous urinary diversion: An update after 250 cases. J. Urol., *137*:1140, 1987.

11. Camey, M. Bladder replacement by ileocystoplasty following radical cystectomy. Semin. Urol., *5*:8, 1987.

12. Boyd, S. D., et al. Quality of life survey of urinary diversion patients: Comparison of ileal conduits versus continent Kock ileal reservoirs. J. Urol., *138*:1386, 1987.

13. Ritchie, J. P. Techniques of ureterointestinal anastomoses and conduit construction. In *Genitourinary Cancer Surgery.* Edited by E. D. Crawford and T. A. Borden. Philadelphia, Lea and Febiger, 1982, p. 227.

14. Lieskovsky, G., Skinner, D. G., and Boyd, S. D. Complications of the Kock pouch. Urol. Clin. North Am., *15*:195, 1988.

Continent Cutaneous Diversion Using the Ileocecal Segment

Randall G. Rowland

atient and physician awareness of the possibility of a continent urinary reservoir has created a tremendous interest and demand for continent diversions. Many different styles of reservoirs have been described in the literature. After reviewing them all, several principles come forward from the successful procedures. First, a reservoir must have a volume at least equivalent to that of a normal bladder. The reservoir must be compliant and have low pressure over the entire range of filling. In order to accomplish this high degree of compliance and low pressure, detubularization of the bowel segment(s) has been necessary. Detubularization also increases the volume of the reservoir for a given amount of bowel segment that is used. Hinman reviewed the geometry involved in this concept.[1] He demonstrated that if a cylindrical piece of bowel were split longitudinally and folded over, the reduction of the length in half and the doubling of the diameter would increase the volume of the reservoir twofold.

Because continent diversion involves the creation of a receptacle with a reservoir function, the antireflux mechanism of ureteral implantation into the reservoir is extremely important. A review of the literature reminds us that the majority of reservoirs are colonized. With this colonization, if reflux

would occur, there would be a propensity for the development of pyelonephritis.

The final major principle is that of establishing a reliable continence mechanism. Certainly, the adult patient who is accustomed to being continent and requires a urinary diversion after an extirpative procedure for a malignancy, demands a high degree of reliability in terms of the continence mechanism.

The three surgical procedures that will be reviewed in this manuscript, the Indiana continent urinary reservoir, the Duke pouch, and the Mainz pouch, all address the general principles outlined above. Each of these procedures will be reviewed. It is important for urologists to have several alternatives available to allow selection of the most appropriate procedure for a given patient.

THE INDIANA CONTINENT URINARY RESERVOIR

The Indiana continent urinary reservoir is based on an ileocecal segment reservoir initially described by Gilchrist and his associates in 1950.[2] In this procedure, the cecum and a portion of the ascending colon were left as a tubular structure and

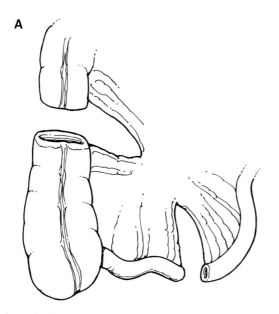
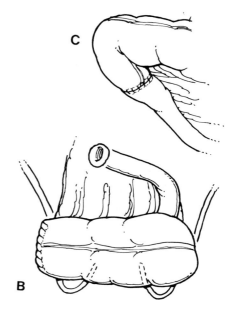

FIG. 30-1. *A*, A nondetubularized ileocecal segment was used to create the Gilchrist pouch. *B*, The ureters were tunnelled into the colon through submucosal tunnels in an antirefluxing manner. The cephalad end of the ascending colon segment was closed transversely. The efferent limb was led out as a stoma without plication or intussusception. *C*, An ileocolostomy was performed with a two-layer technique.

were used to create a reservoir. The efferent limb of the reservoir was a segment of the terminal ileum. The ileocecal valve was left unaltered. The ureters were tunnelled into the wall of the cecum in an antirefluxing fashion. Figure 30-1*A–C* illustrates the original Gilchrist procedure. In the initial experience at Indiana University, minor modifications were made on the Gilchrist procedure. The cecum and the ascending colon were left as a tubular structure; however, the efferent limb and the ureteral implantations were modified as shown later in this chapter. In the initial experience with ten patients, half of the patients were incontinent because of the development of high pressure contractions within the reservoir. All five of these patients were converted to a low pressure reservoir by detubularizing the cecal segment.

Based on this early experience, the construction of the reservoir was modified by adding an ileal patch on the pouch to detubularize the reservoir. Figure 30-2*A–C* illustrates this procedure.[3]

An additional simplification or modification of the construction of the pouch was described in 1987 by Rowland and his associates. This involved taking a longer segment of the cecum and ascending colon (25 to 30 cm in length) and dividing it over virtually its entire length along its antimesenteric border. The cephalad end was folded down to the caudal end, and the reservoir was closed transversely. The segment of bowel used and the technique for reconfiguration are shown in (Figs. 30-3 and 30-4*A–C*).[4]

An additional modification in the ileocolostomy has been made recently. Initially, an end-to-end, two-layered anastomosis had been performed with spatulation of the terminal ileum

to compensate for the size discrepancy in the two bowel segments. Recently an end-to-side stapled anastomosis was performed as shown in (Fig. 30-5*A–C*). This simplified and streamlined the technique considerably.

The continence mechanism has been created by plication of the terminal ileal segment. Initially, approximately 10 to 12 cm of terminal ileum had been preserved. Lembert sutures were used to plicate the entire efferent limb as shown in (Fig. 30-6*A–C*). After an initial experience, a second layer of running sutures was placed to reinforce the Lembert sutures and to prevent complications because of potential pulling out of the initial layer of Lembert sutures.

The ureteral implantations were performed as tunnelled anastomoses through the tenia in the manner of Leadbetter. Figure 30-7*A–D* illustrates this portion of the procedure.

The results of the initial experience of the Indiana continent urinary reservoir were reported in 1987.[4] In the first 29 patients, the overall continence rate during the daytime was 96% and 94% at night. The average volume on catheterization was in the range of 400 to 500 ml. The adult patient was able to remain dry for an average of 4¼ hours between catheterizations.

More recent, long-term follow-up on 91 patients was reported at the American Urological Association meeting in 1989.[5] In this report, the overall continence rate was 92%. Of 81 patients that had primary detubularization of the reservoir, 13.9% of the patients required reoperation based on efferent problems consisting of incontinence or stomal problems. Only 3.8% of the patients required reoperation for problems with the ureteral colonic anastomoses.

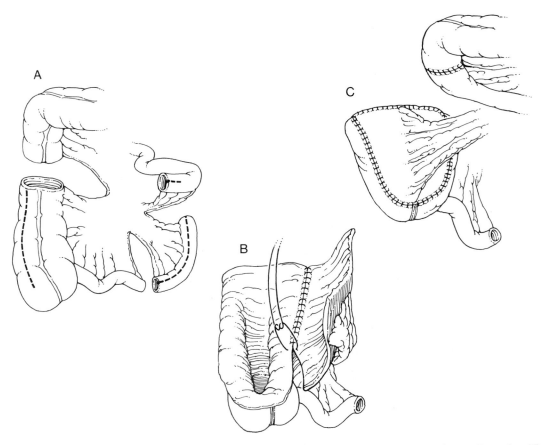

Fig. 30-2. *A*, The Indiana continent urinary reservoir is created with a detubularized segment of cecum and ascending colon. The dashed lines indicate incisions in the bowel segments. An isolated ileal segment is created to use as the patch on the pouch. *B*, The patch is anastomosed to the pouch using a two-layer technique with absorbable synthetic braided suture. The inner layer consists of a running simple suture and the outer layer consists of a running Lembert suture with every other stitch being locked. *C*, This illustration shows the globular configuration of the detubularized reservoir. An end-to-end, two-layered ileocolostomy is performed.

Because of the problems with the efferent limb and stoma, further modifications were made based on the report by Bejany and Politano.[6] Bejany and Politano's experience with a stapled tapered distal ileum was encouraging. A modification of this technique has been adopted and is illustrated in (Fig. 30-8*A–F*). This varies from the technique reported by Bejany and Politano in that Lembert sutures, rather than purse-string sutures, are used to reinforce the ileocecal valve. A recent review of 15 patients with stapled efferent limbs indicates a 100% continence rate. Only one repeat surgical procedure has been required and this was the first patient that was treated in this manner. The patient's efferent limb was 12 cm in length and, with the stapling, elongation occurred to the point that the efferent limb was difficult to catheterize because of kinking of the redundant efferent limb. After shortening the efferent limb to approximately 8 cm, the patient has had no further difficulties with catheterization. Based on this experience, all of these subsequent efferent limbs have been made approximately 8 to 10 cm in length and catheterization is no longer a problem. The stapled efferent limb also creates a small flush stoma approximately, 1 cm in diameter.

In summary, the Indiana continent urinary reservoir is currently created by taking a 25 to 30-cm segment of cecum and ascending colon as illustrated in (Fig. 30-3). If an appendectomy has not been performed prior to the procedure, it is done at some point during the procedure. The ileocolostomy is performed in a stapled manner as shown in (Fig. 30-5*A–C*). A Heinecke-Mikulicz reconfiguration is carried out as shown in (Fig. 30-4). A stapled tapering of the efferent limb is carried out as shown in (Fig. 30-8). Ureteral implantation is either by the tunnelled tenial implantation as shown in (Fig. 30-7*A–D*) or as an alternative, a LeDuc type of implantation can be carried out as shown in (Fig. 30-9*A–D*).[7] Care must be taken with this procedure so that the ureters are implanted in such a manner that they will not be affected by the folding over of the reservoir when the Heinecke-Mikulicz reconfiguration is performed.

An alternative to the Heinecke-Mikulicz reconfiguration is the placement of an ileal patch on the cecum and ascending colon, in circumstances where the patient's cecum and ascending colon are shorter than normal. If this condition is encountered, a 15 to 20 cm segment of cecum and ascending colon is used with a 15 to 18 cm patch of ileum. The technique used has been illustrated in (Fig. 30-2). Preliminary urodynamic studies of these two different methods of detubularization of the cecum and ascending colon do not

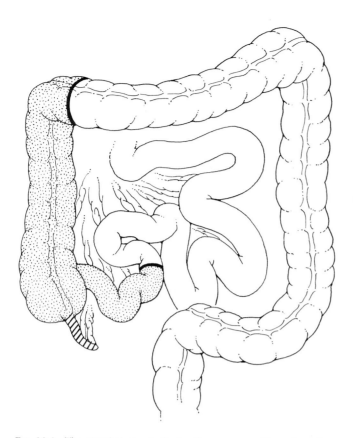

show any significant difference in the capacities or pressures of the reservoirs. The Heinecke-Mikulicz type of procedure is chosen under most circumstances because of the simpler surgical technique with less suturing involved.

The recent changes described in the creation of the Indiana continent urinary reservoir have not only increased the continence rate, but have significantly decreased the operative time required to create the reservoir. With the use of the stapled ileocolostomy and the stapled efferent limb, a reservoir requires approximately 2 to 3 hours for completion.

Long-term follow-up will be required to assess the results of this procedure. However, from preliminary evaluations, it would appear that the reoperation rate and complication rate of this procedure are equivalent to that of the gold standard, the ileal conduit.

PATIENT SELECTION AND PREOPERATIVE EVALUATION

Because creation of a continent urinary reservoir is a more complicated and time-consuming procedure, and patient adaptation to the continent reservoir takes between 1 to 2 months compared to 1 to 2 weeks for a patient with an ileal conduit, it is appropriate that the patient should have a life expectancy of at least 1 year. Patients with a shorter life ex-

FIG. 30-3. The stippled area indicates the segment of bowel used to create the Indiana continent urinary reservoir that will be reconfigured using a Heinecke-Mikulicz technique. An appendectomy is performed. Approximately 25 to 30 cm of cecum and ascending colon and 8 to 10 cm of terminal ileum are used.

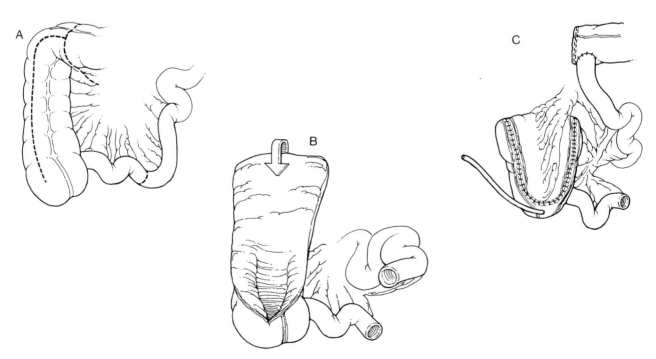

FIG. 30-4. *A*, The dashed lines indicate the incision in the antimesenteric surface of the cecum and ascending colon. Only a 1 to 2 cm cap of cecum is spared from the detubularization. *B*, The cephalad portion of the detubularized cecum is folded over for transverse closure of the reservoir. In those patients in whom the ureters will be tunnelled into the tenia, the reservoir can be closed prior to ureteral implantation. If a LeDuc type of anastomosis is to be used, the ureters must be placed prior to closure of the reservoir. *C*, The Heinecke-Mikulicz reconfiguration of the cecum and ascending colon gives a globular configuration to the reservoir. A cecostomy tube is placed in the cecum prior to closure of the reservoir. An ileocolostomy can be performed with either a hand sewn or stapled technique.

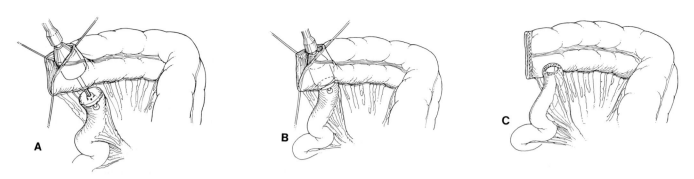

Fig. 30-5. *A*, An end-to-side stapled anastomosis is used to perform the ileocolostomy. Usually a 25 mm diameter stapling cartridge is used to create the anastomosis. The terminal ileum is fixed to the stapling device with a purse-string suture around the shaft of the stapler between the staple cartridge and the anvil. *B*, The staple cartridge is fired, anastomosing the ileum to side of the transverse colon. *C*, The end of the transverse colon is closed with a double row of intestinal staples. The mesenteric window is closed with interrupted silk sutures.

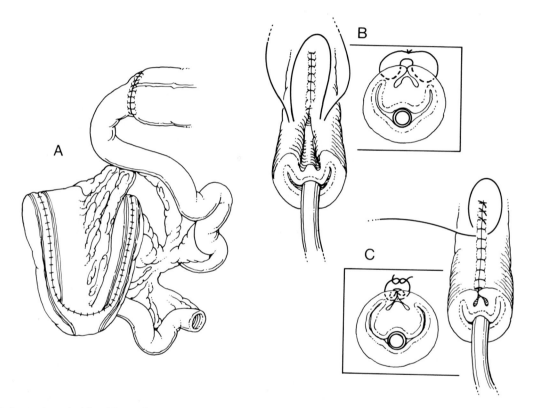

Fig. 30-6. *A*, Approximately 10 to 12 cm of terminal ileum will be used to create the efferent limb. *B*, Plication of the efferent limb is accomplished from the ileocecal valve to the portion that will become the stoma using 3-0 silk interrupted Lembert sutures. The sutures are placed approximately half way around the ileum on the antimesenteric surface. Plication is performed over a 12-French red-rubber catheter. The sutures are placed approximately 8 to 10 mm apart. Once the entire length of terminal ileum is plicated, the 12-French catheter is replaced with an 18-French catheter to be certain that the larger catheter will pass into the reservoir without difficulty. The reservoir is filled with saline. The catheter is withdrawn and pressure is placed on the reservoir to test the continence mechanism. If continence is not achieved, some additional sutures are placed particularly near the ileocecal valve, to reinforce the valve for continence. *C*, Once both the ability to catheterize the reservoir and the continence has been confirmed, a second row of running 3-0 silk sutures are placed over the Lembert sutures to reinforce the first row without further change in the size of the efferent limb.

pectancy will spend too great of a portion of their time becoming accustomed to their continent reservoir to appreciate its benefits fully. Because a continent reservoir requires more care than an ileal conduit, the patient must be highly motivated and have a strong desire to be appliance free. A strong self-image is mandatory. The patient must also have a moderate degree of manual dexterity to facilitate intermittent catheterization of the reservoir. Neurologic problems such as previ-

ous strokes, multiple sclerosis, or Parkinson's disease are contraindications to the procedure. There is no absolute upper age limitation for the procedure. The patient must be evaluated more on the other criteria listed above rather than strictly age.

Preoperatively, the patient is evaluated with an air contrast barium enema if he is 40 years in age or older, or has any history of bowel disease. The presence of multiple diverticuli

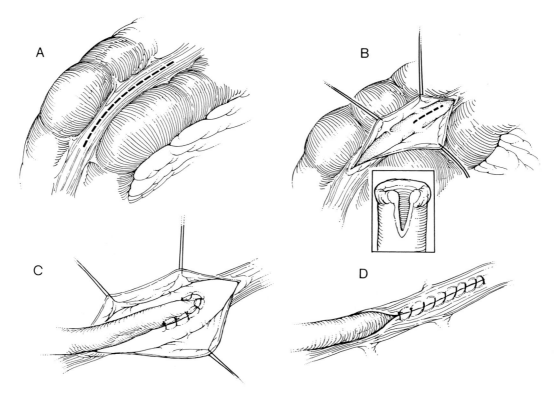

FIG. 30-7. *A*, After the appropriate location for anastomosis between ureter and the reservoir has been determined, a tenial incision is made of approximately four times the diameter of the ureter. *B*, The flaps of the tenia are dissected to make a tunnel for the ureteral implantation. A mucosal incision, approximately 1 cm long is made in the distal end of tenial tunnel. The ureter is spatulated, as shown in the insert, to create a larger anastomosis. *C*, A ureteral mucosal anastomosis is made with interrupted 5-0 monofilament absorbable sutures. *D*, The tenia is reapproximated over the ureter with a running nonabsorbable suture. The adventitia of the ureter is caught with every other suture to help assure fixation of the ureter within the tunnel. Five or 8-French ureteral stents are usually placed up the ureter and are led out through the anterior wall of the reservoir.

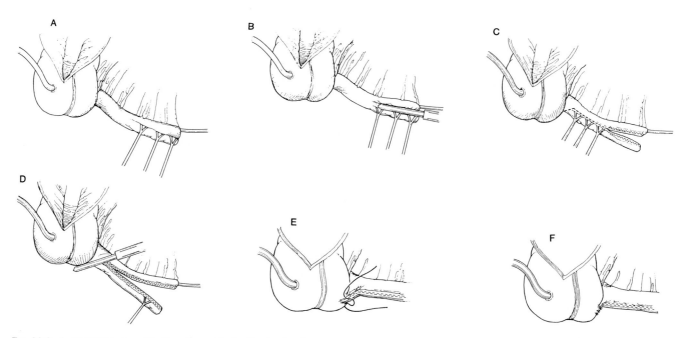

FIG. 30-8. *A*, An improvement in the efferent limb plication has been made by using gastrointestinal staples. Babcock clamps are used to grasp the antimesenteric surface of the ileum. A 12-French catheter is placed through the lumen. *B*, The gastrointestinal stapler is placed in such a manner that there is no redundant tissue left against the catheter along the mesentery. *C*, After the stapler has been activated, additional sets of staple cartridges are used to complete the resection of the redundant antimesenteric surface of the terminal ileum as shown by the dashed lines. *D*, The distal portion of the terminal ileum must be resected at an angle in order to have the staple cartridge avoid entrance into the cecum. *E*, The angulation of the last portion of the staples creates a funneled shaped portion of the very terminal distal ileum. This funnel shaped portion is converted to a straight tubular structure by the use of 4 or 5 Lembert sutures of 3-0 silk. *F*, The placement of the Lembert sutures converts the funnel shaped ileocecal junction into a straight tubular structure and reinforces the ileocecal valve.

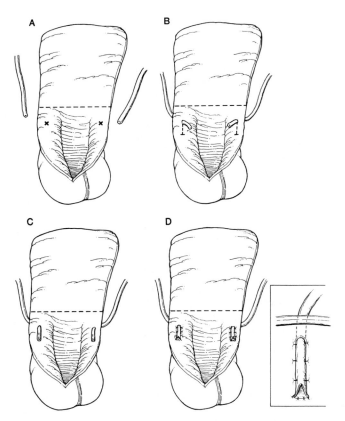

FIG. 30-9. *A*, A LeDuc type of grooved implantation of the ureter into the colon is an acceptable alternative to the tunnelled tenial anastomosis. The X's indicate the location of the hiatus of the ureter on either side. These must be located below the point at which the reservoir will be folded over for closure. The line of folding is indicated by the transverse dashed line. *B*, The ureters have been led through the wall of the reservoir. The dashed lines extending from the ureteral hiatus on each side indicates the mucosal incision to be made that will create a groove for implantation of the ureters. *C*, The ureters are laid in the grooves the length of which are three to four times the diameter of the ureters. The distal portion of the ureter is spatulated. *D*, The ureter is secured in the groove with absorbable sutures, as indicated by the insert.

in the right colon is a relative contraindication to the procedure. Certainly if any polyps are present, these must be treated and evaluated for malignancy prior to considering the use of the cecum and ascending colon for a urinary reservoir. Previous resection of colon or a significant resection of small bowel would also be a contraindication to the procedure. The patients with inflammatory bowel diseases are also excluded from consideration. Because there is some resorption of urinary products through the bowel mucosa, the patients must have nearly normal renal function in order to be eligible for this procedure (serum creatinine less than 2.0 mg/dl). Finally, as part of the preoperative evaluation, a stomal site should be selected. This is not nearly as critical as it is in the case of an ileal conduit, because an appliance is not needed. In the case of a patient who is undergoing conversion from an ileal conduit to a continent reservoir, it is often advantageous to place the stoma in the left lower quadrant, particularly if the patient has a parastomal hernia or a rather large stoma in the right

lower quadrant. This allows repair of the hernia with mesh if necessary and also allows creation of a smaller stoma in the left lower quadrant. On occasion, the previous larger stoma can be reduced in size by placing subcutaneous sutures in the stoma site and reducing the skin opening to a size compatible with the new smaller stoma, which would be approximately 1 cm in diameter.

PREOPERATIVE AND POSTOPERATIVE CARE

The patient is normally admitted to the hospital 36 to 48 hours prior to surgery. A mechanical and antibiotic bowel prep is carried out. The patient is given intravenous fluids the night before surgery to prevent dehydration. Postoperatively, a cecostomy tube is left in the reservoir along with ureteral stents. The stents are usually brought out through separate stab wounds in the anterior wall of the reservoir and are led out along side the cecostomy tube through the abdominal wall. These should be secured to the patient's skin separately so that they can be removed independently as needed.

In the immediate postoperative period, the nursing staff is asked to irrigate the reservoir through the cecostomy tube every 3 or 4 hours. This is necessary to remove the mucous from the reservoir that is secreted by the bowel segments. It is extremely important that the catheter does not become obstructed and that the reservoir does not become overdistended in the initial postoperative period. Usually, no catheter is left through the efferent limb in the postoperative period.

Stentograms are performed on the 7th postoperative day if the patient has recovered bowel function. If there is free flow of urine around the stents into the reservoir, the stents are removed.

The patient is usually discharged from the hospital with the cecostomy tube in place along with a closed drainage system such as the Jackson-Pratt drain. The patient returns at approximately 3 weeks after surgery for a 2-day admission to the hospital. At that time, the patient has an x-ray of the pouch performed by gravity filling with contrast material through the cecostomy tube. If no leak or reflux into the ureters is noted, an intravenous pyelogram is performed. The upper tracts are observed for evidence of hydronephrosis. Mild bilateral hydronephrosis is often seen in the postoperative period. This usually resolves. If the x-ray studies as outlined above are satisfactory, the patient's cecostomy tube is clamped and the patient is taught intermittent catheterization. It is important that the patient remain in the hospital during this time period so that if the patient encounters any difficulty in catheterization, assistance may be rendered to prevent overdistention of the reservoir. Once the patient has learned intermittent catheterization and is performing this successfully, the cecostomy tube and the closed drainage tube are removed. The patient is observed for an additional 24 hours and, if the patient continues to self-catheterize satisfactory, he is discharged.

Initially, the patient is asked to catheterize every 2 to 3 hours during the daytime and every 3 to 4 hours at night. If the patient remains dry, without any evidence of leakage for at

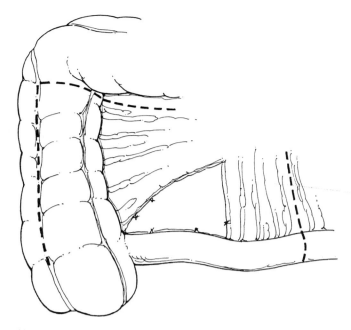

FIG. 30-10. The dashed lines indicate the incisions to be made in the bowel and mesentery for creation of a Duke pouch. A window of the mesentery of the terminal ileum has been excised for a distance of approximately 8 cm along the bowel. This allows intussusception of the ileum through the ileocecal valve.

least a 1-week period, the patient is then encouraged to gradually increase the time interval between catheterizations. It will normally take 4 to 8 weeks for the patient to achieve a capacity of 400 to 500 ml, which gives them a time interval between catheterizations of 4 to 6 hours. Approximately half of the patients sleep all night and the remainder will catheterize once during the night. The patients usually cover their stoma with a small piece of gauze or a piece of a thin feminine panty liner. The patient is asked to irrigate the reservoir 3 or 4 times per day from the time of the initial hospital discharge. Once the patient is performing intermittent catheterization, the frequency of irrigation can be decreased. Usually within 1-

2 months the patient can irrigate the reservoir once or twice a day. The frequency of irrigation is determined by the amount of mucous present in the urine. Mucous production gradually decreases with time. The patients are asked to irrigate the reservoir at least once a day long-term to make certain that they do not become obstructed with inspissated mucous.

LONG-TERM FOLLOW-UP

The patient is usually evaluated approximately 1 month after he has been started on intermittent catheterization. At that time, a BUN, creatinine, and a set of serum electrolytes are checked. Most patients will have a mild, clinically insignificant hyperchloremic acidosis. If there is no evidence of change in renal function, then the patient is asked to return for a pouchogram and an intravenous pyelogram within a 6-month period. If these examinations show no evidence of reflux or hydronephrosis, the patient is followed with pouchograms and intravenous pyelograms on an annual basis. The patient's BUN, creatinine, and electrolytes should be checked every 3 to 4 months. If any significant alteration in these values is observed, the patient must be more fully evaluated with x-ray studies and, if necessary, urodynamic studies to evaluate the function of the reservoir. Until longer-term follow-up is available, annual pouchograms and IVPs, along with chemical evaluations of the patient's renal function, are recommended.

THE DUKE POUCH

Webster and King described an ileocecal reservoir that appears to be a variant of the Mansson reservoir.[8,9] Figure 30-10 shows the preparation of the ileocecal segment. The ileocecal valve is intussuscepted to create the continence mechanism. Figure 30-11A–C shows the remainder of the construction of the pouch with fixation of the intussuscepted ileal nipple to the posterior wall of the pouch. The cecum and ascending colon are detubularized by incising the segment along the antimesenteric surface and bringing one of the cephalad corners down to the apex of the antimesenteric incision. The efferent

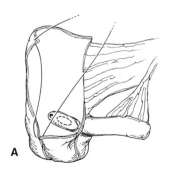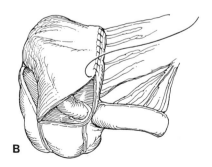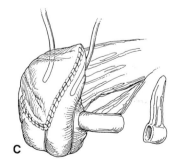

FIG. 30-11. A, The intussusception of the ileum through the ileocecal valve has been accomplished. The intussuscepted nipple is secured to the posterior reservoir wall with multiple sutures. The mucosa of the posterior wall is incised and anastomosed to the posterior wall of the nipple. The suture from the cephalad portion to the apex of the antimesenteric incision indicates the manner in which the cecum will be detubularized. B, The sutures show the continuation of the closure of the reservoir which again detubularizes the cecum and ascending colon. C, The ureters are tunnelled in through the colonic wall in an antirefluxing manner. The excess of the efferent limb is trimmed off to create a straight efferent segment to promote the ease of catheterization.

FIG. 30-12. The dashed lines indicate the incisions for creation of the Mainz pouch. Approximately 15 to 20 cm of cecum and ascending colon are used along with 30 to 40 cm of terminal ileum.

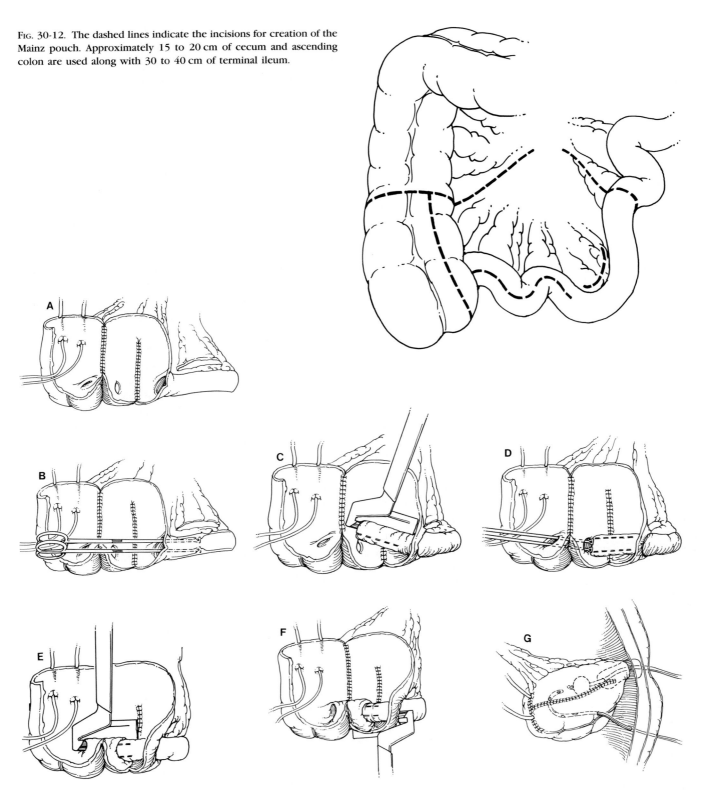

FIG. 30-13. *A*, The ureters are led through the wall of the colon in an antirefluxing manner. Stents are usually placed and led through the anterior wall of the reservoir. The ileocecal valve is maintained intact. The most distal portion of the terminal ileum is incised along the antimesenteric surface and formed into an inverted 'U' shaped configuration. This is anastomosed to the cecum to form the anterior wall of the reservoir. *B*, The more proximal portion of the terminal ileum is intussuscepted using Babcock clamps. *C*, Staple cartridges are used to fix the intussusception of the ileal segment in three or four places. *D*, The intussuscepted ileal nipple is led through the native ileocecal valve. *E*, The intussuscepted ileal segment is fixed within the ileocecal valve using an additional staple cartridge. *F*, A final staple cartridge is used to help secure the intussuscepted nipple to the anterior wall of the reservoir. *G*, The ureters are led into the reservoir through antirefluxing tunnels. A catheter is placed through the efferent limb as well as a cecostomy tube for adequate drainage in the postoperative period. The efferent limb is arranged with a short, straight course to promote the ease of catheterization.

limb is trimmed to an appropriate length to allow a straight efferent segment that will promote the ease of catheterization. The ureters are tunnelled into the colon in an antirefluxing manner. A satisfactory experience in a limited number of cases has been reported.[8] Based on the experience reported on the Kock pouch,[10] stabilization of the intussuscepted nipple that functions as the efferent limb continence mechanism has been a considerable problem. The experience in the Duke pouch has been limited, and long-term results have not yet been reported. The other principles of creation of a satisfactory continent urinary reservoir, detubularization of the reservoir segment and creation of an antirefluxing ureterocolonic anastomosis, have been satisfied by this technique.

THE MAINZ POUCH

Thuroff and his associates reported the creation of a mixed augmentation ileum 'n zecum (Mainz) reservoir.[11] Figure 30-12 indicates the bowel segments that are used. The cecum and ascending colon are used to create the posterior wall of the reservoir and a 'U' shaped patch of terminal ileum is used to create the anterior portion of the reservoir. The continence mechanism relies on intussusception of an ileal segment through the ileocecal valve. Figure 30-13A–G shows the creation of the reservoir with its intussuscepted continence mechanism. In 1988, results of 100 cases using a Mainz type of reservoir were presented.[12] Fifty-one of these cases were continent urinary reservoirs. The continence rate was 96% in this group of patients. This procedure has also undergone a great deal of evolution. The intussuscepted ileum was unsatisfactory in their experience until it was passed through the native ileocecal valve, which apparently reinforced the continence mechanism created by the intussusception. With these modifications, the Mainz pouch seems to address all three principles for a satisfactory continent urinary reservoir.

CONCLUSION

Three different continent urinary reservoirs have been presented. Each of these addresses the basic principles involved in creating a satisfactory reservoir. Long-term follow-up will help us understand which of these procedures will give satisfactory outcome based on preservation of renal function as well as continence and convenience for the patient. All of these patients will need to be watched long-term for potential metabolic alterations such as acidosis or the development of an anemia based on malabsorption of vitamin B-12 by the terminal ileum. Also, the possibility of the development of tumors within the isolated bowel segment must be considered. Certainly the experience in the literature would indicate that the incidence of tumor in isolated bowel segments is low. However, there are multiple reports in the literature of this event. Periodic visualization of the upper tracts and of the reservoir, by radiographic and endoscopic techniques, will help us discover any significant incidence of malignancies within the urinary diversion.

Finally, emphasis needs to be placed on the evaluation of the subjective factors such as patient motivation and self-image, in addition to medical factors such as renal function, bowel function, and manual dexterity, in order to help make appropriate recommendations to a patient regarding his or her form of urinary diversion.

REFERENCES

1. HINMAN, F. Selection of intestinal segments for bladder substitution: Physical and physiological characteristics. J. Urol., *139:*519, 1988.
2. GILCHRIST, R. K., et al. Construction of a substitute bladder and urethra. Surg. Gynecol. Obstet., *90:*752, 1950.
3. ROWLAND, R. G., MITCHELL, M. E., and BIHRLE, R. The cecoileal continent urinary reservoir. World J. Urol., *3:*185, 1985.
4. ROWLAND, R. G., et al. The Indiana continent urinary reservoir. J. Urol., *137:*1136, 1987.
5. SCHEIDLER, D. M., et al. Update on the Indiana continent urinary reservoir. Abstract 532, American Urological Association Meeting, Dallas, May, 1989.
6. BEJANY, D. E., and POLITANO, V. A. Stapled and nonstapled tapered distal ileum for construction of a continent colonic urinary reservoir. J. Urol., *140:*491, 1988.
7. CAMEY, M., and LEDUC, A. L'enterocystoplastie avec cystoprostatectomie totale pour cancer de la vessie. Ann. Urol., *13:*114, 1979.

8. WEBSTER, G. D., and KING, L. R. Further commentary: Cecal bladder. In *Bladder Reconstruction and Continent Urinary Diversion.* Edited by L. R. King, A. R. Stone, and G. D. Webster. Chicago, Yearbook Medical Publishers, 1987, pp. 209–223.
9. MANSSON, W. The continent cecal urinary reservoir. In *Bladder Reconstruction and Continent Urinary Diversion.* Edited by L. R. King, A. R. Stone, and G. D. Webster. Chicago, Yearbook Medical Publishers, 1987.
10. SKINNER, D. G., LIESKOVSKY, G., and BOYD, S. D. Continuing experience with the continent ileal reservoir (Kock pouch) as an alternative to cutaneous urinary diversion: An update after 250 cases. J. Urol., *137:*1140, 1987.
11. THUROFF, J. W., et al. The Mainz-pouch (mixed augmentation ileum 'n zecum) for bladder augmentation and continent urinary diversion. World J. Urol., *3:*179, 1985.
12. THUROFF, J. W., et al. 100 cases of Mainz-pouch: Continuing experience and evolution. J. Urol., *140:*283, 1988.

CHAPTER
31

Continent Diversion to the Urethra (Bladder Substitution)

Fuad S. Freiha

The ileal conduit is the most commonly used form of urinary diversion following cystectomy. It is an unattractive sequela to the treatment of localized carcinoma of the bladder. Many patients refuse and many physicians delay recommending cystectomy, a potentially curative procedure, because of the need for a urostomy. It is possible that many more patients will accept cystectomy earlier in the course of bladder cancer and improve their chances for long-term survival if the urostomy, with its social and medical drawbacks, can be eliminated and if a reservoir can be substituted for the bladder.

1988 marked the 100th anniversary of bladder substitution. In 1888, Tizzoni and Poggi excised the bladder of a dog and implanted the ureters into an isolated segment of bowel. They then anastomosed the bowel segment to the neck of the bladder, creating a receptacle for the urine.[1] Since then, a multitude of operations have been described. But, the modern day enthusiasm for bladder substitution should be credited to Maurice Camey of France. Camey performed his first enterocystoplasty in 1958, and devoted the next 30 years to modifying and perfecting this operation.[2]

In this chapter, we will describe and illustrate several of these operations and discuss their advantages and disadvantages. The suture materials, stents, catheters, and drains mentioned in the text are what the author uses and may be changed to fit the preference of the reader. Furthermore, stenting ureterointestinal anastomoses and the different types of anastomoses described are practices that the author follows, but may be modified by the reader to conform with his or her own methods.

PATIENT SELECTION

The ideal patient for bladder substitution is a relatively young male who does not need a urethrectomy as part of his treatment, and who has not had prior high-dose irradiation to the bladder. The first bladder substitution operation done at Stanford was in September, 1984. Of the 150 patients who underwent cystectomy between September, 1984 and January, 1989, only 48 (32%) were candidates for bladder substitution. Forty-four of these patients had the operation. Of the remaining four patients, two elected to have the standard ileal conduit, and in the other two, no intestinal segment could reach the membranous urethra because of a thick and obese mesentery. Patients who were not candidates for the bladder substitution either needed a urethrectomy concomitant with the cystectomy, were undergoing salvage cystectomy for failure of definitive irradiation, or were females.

SUBSTITUTION USING SMALL INTESTINE

The Camey Operation

Following a standard cystoprostatectomy with careful preservation of the membraneous urethra, a 40-cm segment of ileum is chosen so that its midportion can reach the urethra without tension. This segment, with its mesentery, is isolated, and the continuity of the bowel is re-established with an ileo-ileostomy (Fig. 31-1). A defect 1 cm in diameter is created in the wall of the antimesenteric border of the ileal segment 3 to 4 cm to the right of the midpoint to make the left limb longer. This is done because this limb has to travel over the rectosigmoid to meet the left ureter above the iliac vessels. A 20-French, 6-hole catheter, and two 8-French pediatric feeding tubes are passed per the urethra into the pelvic cavity. One feeding tube is passed through the defect created in the ileal segment, into the left limb, and is used as the left ureteral stent. The other feeding tube and the 6-hole catheter are passed through the defect into the right limb of the ileal segment. The feeding tube is used as a right ureteral stent and the 6-hole catheter is used for drainage. The 6-hole catheter is placed in the right limb so that it will lie in the direction of peristalsis rather than against it. This will help prevent its extrusion by peristaltic waves (Fig. 31-1A).

The urethro-ileal anastomosis is then performed over the feeding tubes and catheter, using six through-and-through sutures of 0 or 2-0 chromic catgut placed at 12-, 2-, 4-, 6-, 8-, and 10-o'clock, respectively (Fig. 31-1A).

The uretero-ileal anastomoses are performed outside of the pelvic cavity, lateral to the common iliac arteries. Each end of the ileal segment is opened for a distance of 4 cm to facilitate working within the lumen. The ureter is brought into the ileal lumen through the posterior wall about 2 cm from the end of the segment (Fig. 31-1B). The ureter is fixed to the wall of the ileum, where it passes through with three or four seromuscular sutures of 4-0 chromic catgut. A 3-cm incision is made in the mucosa of the ileum, starting at the site of entry of the ureter and going distally. A strip of mucosa 3 to 4 mm wide is excised or the edges of the mucosal incision are spread apart to create a trough of denuded ileal wall onto which the ureter will lie (Fig. 31-1B). The ureter is fixed onto this trough with interrupted sutures of 4-0 chromic catgut placed on both sides, between the edges of the incised mucosa and the side walls of the ureter (Fig. 31-1C). Note that this is not an implantation into a submucosal tunnel. This would be almost impossible to perform in the ileum. Excess ureter is cut splayed open and is fixed in that manner to the ileal mucosa. The feeding tubes are placed into the ureters and are advanced up to the renal pelvises. The open ends of the ileal segments are closed with a running through-and-through 3-0 chromic catgut suture and an inverting layer of interrupted 3-0 silk sutures (Fig. 31-1D). Each limb of the ileal segment is fixed to the psoas muscle, lateral to the common iliac artery, with two or three sutures of 2-0 chromic catgut.

The 6-hole catheter is taped to the penis and the ureteral stents are taped to the catheter. The ureteral stents are removed on the 7th or 8th postoperative day. The catheter is removed on the 21st postoperative day.

The average length of the procedure is 6 hours which is, in our experience, 2 hours longer than for a standard cystectomy

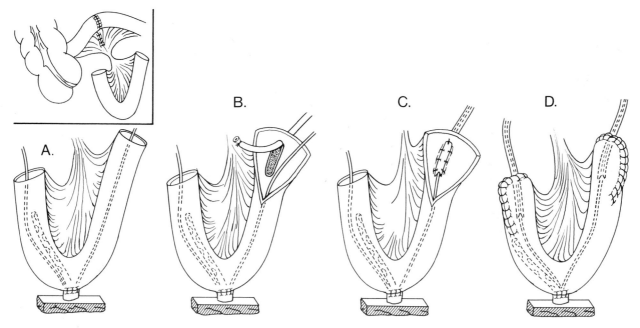

FIG. 31-1. The Camey enterocystoplasty.

and ileal conduit. It is possible to perform a nerve-sparing cystoprostatectomy prior to the Camey procedure.

RESULTS. Fifteen patients have undergone the Camey enterocystoplasty at Stanford and 14 have complete daytime continence. The average time to regain full control is 10 weeks, with a range of 6 weeks to 6 months. One patient remained incontinent and needed an artificial sphincter. Daytime voiding and frequency varies between 2 and 4 hours and bladder capacities are 400 to 800 cc. All patients have enuresis unless they are willing to wake up and void two to three times during the night. Of the eight patients who have been studied with cystograms, only one has reflux.

Urodynamic evaluation of several patients reveals high amplitude contractions that increase with increasing volume, generating intraluminal pressures of up to 100 cms of water (Fig. 31-2). Patients are usually unaware of these contractions, which do not cause incontinence.

COMPLICATIONS. The most common complication of the Camey enterocystoplasty, in our experience, is early extrusion of the catheter, which necessitates replacement under fluoroscopic guidance to avoid disruption of the urethroileal anastomosis.

One patient developed a superficial wound infection. Three patients developed urinary tract infections, two with *Staphylococcus epidermidis* and one with *Klebsiella sp.* One patient was left with minimal and stable bilateral ureteroileal anastomotic stenosis without deterioration in renal function. Electrolyte disturbances have not been encountered, even in those patients who have acquired large bladder capacities and who can last for several hours without voiding.

Despite the high incidence of enuresis, the Camey enterocystoplasty has been well accepted by all the patients and well received by the referring physicians.

The Modified Camey Procedure

To eliminate the tubular nature of the reservoir and to decrease intraluminal pressure, Camey recently described a modification to his original operation.[3] The ileal segment is opened at its antimesenteric border and is folded into a U-shaped configuration (Fig. 31-3A). The adjacent sides of the

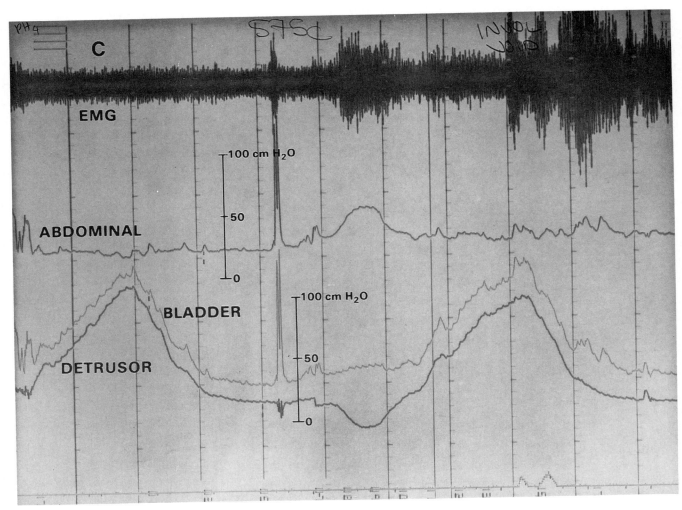

FIG. 31-2. Cystometrogram of a Camey enterocystoplasty showing high-amplitude contractions with pressures up to 100 cm H_2O with increasing volumes.

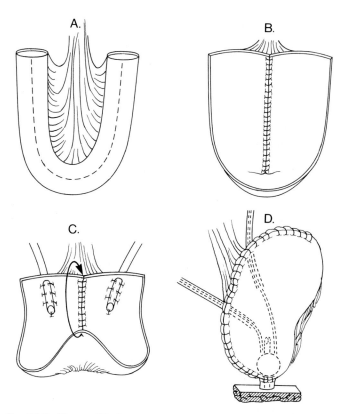

FIG. 31-3. The modified Camey enterocystoplasty with detubularization of the ileal segment.

bowel is re-established. The distal 30 cm will be used to create a pouch and the proximal 15 cm will be used to intussuscept and form a valve. The distal 30 cm are opened along the anti-mesenteric border and folded into a U-shaped configuration (Fig. 31-4A). The adjacent edges of the U are joined by running sutures of 3-0 PGA (Fig. 31-4B). The peritoneum on either side of the mesentery of the distal 10 cms of the proximal 15 cm is stripped off the mesentery to allow better adhesion when the intussusception is created (Fig. 31-4B). The proximal, intact ileal segment is then intussuscepted into the open ileum for a distance of 5 cms and is held in place by three or four rows of staples using the TA-55 automatic stapler and by several 3-0 silk seromuscular sutures placed at the outer base of the nipple (Fig. 31-4C). The opened distal segment is folded up (Fig. 31-4C) and is closed with running sutures of 3-0 PGA (Fig. 31-4D). A defect 1 cm in diameter is created in the most dependent part of the pouch. A 20-French Foley catheter and two No. 8 feeding tubes are introduced per urethra into the pelvic cavity. A long clamp is introduced through the proximal ileal segment, through the valve, and out through the created defect, to grasp the feeding tubes and bring them through the pouch and valve and out the proximal end, to stent the ureter-

U are joined together with running sutures of 3-0 polyglycolic acid (PGA), thus creating a patch of opened ileum (Fig. 31-3B). The ureters are brought into the luminal side of the opened ileum and antireflux ureteroileal anastomosis, similar to that in the Camey procedure, are performed. The ileal patch is then folded up (Fig. 31-3C) and the edges are sutured with running 3-0 PGA (Fig. 31-3D). Before completing the closure, a defect 1 cm in diameter is created in the most dependent part of the reservoir for the urethroileal anastomosis. A 20-French Foley catheter and 2 No. 8 feeding tubes are placed intraurethrally and into the reservoir. The feeding tubes are advanced into the ureters to stent the ureteroileal anastomosis, and the Foley catheter will drain the reservoir. Closure of the reservoir is then completed and the urethroileal anastomosis is performed with 2-0 or 0 chromic catgut sutures (Fig. 31-3D).

Advantages of the modified Camey procedure relate to elimination of peristaltic activity generated by tubular structures, thus decreasing intraluminal pressure. The reservoir created by the modification is easier to drain.

The Urethral Kock's Pouch (Hemi-Kock)

In 1986, Ghoneim et al. reported on a modification of the original Kock pouch. This modification eliminates one valve and anastomoses the pouch to the urethra.[4]

A 45-cm ileal segment is isolated and the continuity of the

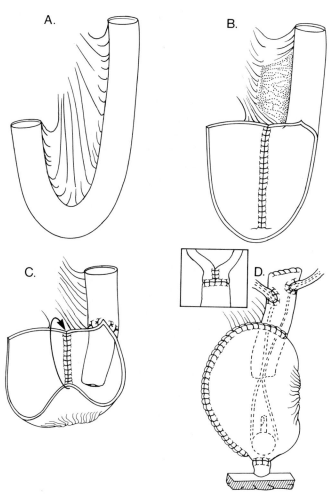

FIG. 31-4. The Hemi-Kock operation.

oileal anastomosis. The urethroileal anastomosis is accomplished over the Foley catheter using six, 2-0 or 0 chromic sutures (Fig. 31-4D). The ureters are joined to the proximal intact ileal segment either separately end-to-side or together, and the common lumen is anastomosed to the ileum, end-to-end, using 4-0 chromic catgut (Fig. 31-4D).

The advantages of the Hemi-Kock are several. The valve is an effective means of preventing reflux. The ureteroileal anastomoses are simple and are less often associated with stenosis. The length of the proximal ileal segment allows for resection of longer segments of distal ureters and, therefore, a safer margin. The main disadvantage is the use of staples, as these may lead to stone formation.

RESULTS. Twenty-eight patients at Stanford have undergone the Hemi-Kock, or a slight modification of it, and 25 are available for evaluation. All 25 patients have gained daytime control in an average time of 8 weeks and a range of 4 weeks to 4 months. Four patients can sleep through the night without enuresis but the rest are enuretic unless they wake up and void one to three times during the night. Daytime frequency of voiding ranges between 4 and 8 hours, with bladder capacities ranging from 400 to 1000 cc.

Reflux has not been encountered in any of the several patients studied with cystograms (Fig. 31-5). Urodynamic evaluation reveals lower amplitude contractions and lower intraluminal pressures (Fig. 31-6).

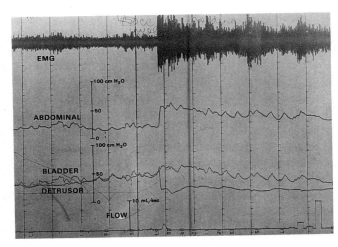

FIG. 31-6. Cystometrogram of a Hemi-Kock showing lower-amplitude contraction and lower pressures than the Camey enterocystoplasty.

Ileal Reservoir without Valve

In 1988, Studer et al. reported on the use of an ileal low-pressure reservoir without an intussusception into the pouch.[5] A 60-cm ileal segment is isolated and both ends are closed with a running suture of 3-0 PGA. The distal 40 cm are opened along the antimesenteric border (Fig. 31-7A).

The authors describe three different types of ureteroileal anastomoses, but only one will be mentioned here because it

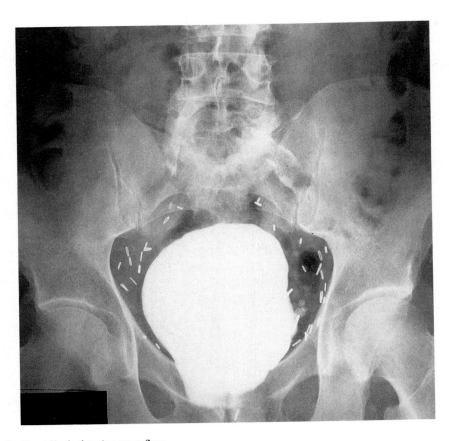

FIG. 31-5. Cystogram of a Hemi-Kock showing no reflux.

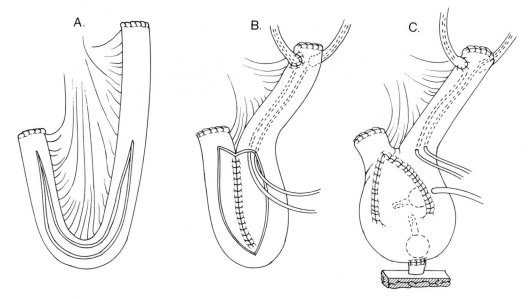

FIG. 31-7. Ileal reservoir without valve.

is the simplest and most intriguing: a stented, simple, end-to-end anastomosis of the ureters into the proximal end of the unopened 20 cm of the proximal ileal segment. It is unknown whether an antireflux mechanism between a low-pressure reservoir and the ureters in patients with sterile urine is necessary. Furthermore, the 20-cm long isoperistaltic ileal segment between the ureters and the reservoir, under slow, low-pressure filling, may have its own antireflux properties.

The opened, distal 40 cm are folded into a U-shaped configuration and the medial sides are joined together with running sutures of 3-0 PGA (Fig. 31-7B). The U is cross-folded and its lower anterior wall is closed with 3-0 PGA running sutures. A defect 1 cm in diameter is created in the most dependent part of the U and this is anastomosed to the urethra over a balloon catheter, using absorbable sutures of either 0 or 2-0 chromic or PGA. A "cystotomy" tube is inserted and the ureteral stents are brought out through separate holes (Fig. 31-7C). The rest of the pouch is closed.

The advantages of this procedure are its simplicity and the ease with which it is performed. No major complications have been encountered during a relatively short period of follow-up and only time will tell whether or not the lack of an antireflux mechanism will lead to upper tract deterioration.

Modification of the "Studer" Reservoir

For the past year, the author has been performing a modification of the procedure described by Studer et al. in order to try to increase the inherent antireflux properties of the 20-cm long isoperistaltic tubular proximal segment of the ileum.

The pouch is completed and anastomosed to the urethra before the ureteroileal anastomosis is performed. The wall of the proximal segment of the ileum is circumferentially imbricated at three or four different levels with interrupted 3-0 silk seromuscular sutures, thus creating a series of intraluminal valves (Fig. 31-8) that will gradually dampen the reflux pressure as the ureteroileal anastomosis is approached. The ureters are then joined together and the common lumen is anastomosed to the end of the ileal segment with 4-0 chromic catgut over No. 8-French feeding tubes. Figure 31-9 is a cystogram, done at 6 months, showing no reflux.

SUBSTITUTION USING THE ILEOCECAL SEGMENT

In 1965, Gil-Vernet popularized the use of the ileocecal segment for use in urologic surgery.[6] Since then, a number of different modifications have been described.

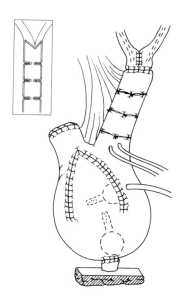

FIG. 31-8. Modification of the ileal reservoir (Freiha) to prevent reflux by circumferentially imbricating the proximal segment.

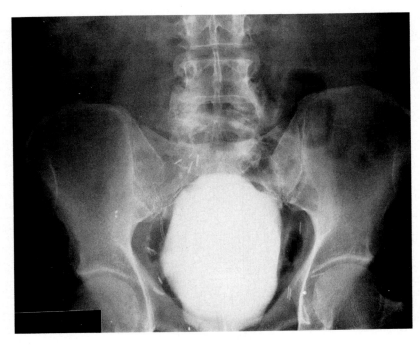

Fig. 31-9. Cystogram of a modified ileal reservoir (Freiha) showing no reflux.

The Gil-Vernet Ileocecal Bladder

A segment of terminal ileum, the ileocecal valve, cecum, and ascending colon are isolated as a unit and the continuity of the bowel is established by an ileo-ascending colostomy. An appendectomy is done. The proximal end of the ileum is closed and the ileocecal valve is reinforced by several seromuscular sutures of interrupted 3-0 silk. The open end of the ascending colon is partially closed to reduce the lumen to a diameter of 1 cm for the urethrocolic anastomosis (Fig. 31-10A). The reservoir is rotated counterclockwise 180° and the urethra is anastomosed to the reduced lumen of the ascending colon over a balloon catheter, using interrupted sutures of 2-0 or 0 chromic or PGA. The ureters are then anastomosed to the terminal ileum, end-to-side (Fig. 31-10B).

The Khafagy Modification of the Ileocecal Bladder

In 1987, Khafagy et al. updated their experience with the ileocecal bladder and reported perfect control of micturition in 82% of patients and preservation of renal configuration in 92%.[7]

Ten cm of terminal ileum and 20 cm of cecum are isolated on the ileocolic artery, and an ileo-ascending colostomy is performed. The ureters are anastomosed to the ileum. The cut end of the cecum is closed in two layers using 3-0 chromic catgut. Appendectomy is performed. The most dependent part of the cecum is anastomosed to the urethra over a balloon catheter (Fig. 31-11).

These are simple operations to perform but, because of the tubular nature of the reservoir and the mass contraction of the cecum, high pressures can be generated and lead to incontinence and eventual incompetence of the ileocecal valve and reflux.

The Mainz Pouch

The Mainz Pouch was originally designed for continent supravesical diversion. However, in 1988, Scharfe et al. reported on its use for bladder substitution.[8] The cecum and 40 cm of terminal ileum are isolated and opened along the antimesenteric border, leaving a 20-cm segment of tubular ileum proximally for the creation of the antireflux valve and for the ureteroileal anastomosis (Figs. 31-12A and 31-12B). The adjacent edges of

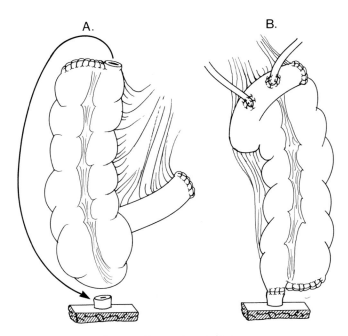

Fig. 31-10. The Gil-Vernet ileocecal cystoplasty.

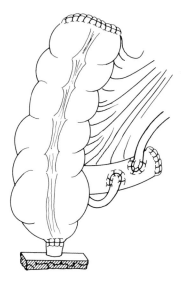

FIG. 31-11. The ileocecal bladder as described by Khafagy et al.

the open bowel are sutured together with running 3-0 PGA. The tubular ileum is intussuscepted into the common lumen and is held in place with staples and with seromuscular sutures of 3-0 silk placed circumferentially at the proximal site of intussusception (Fig. 31-12C). The pouch is folded together,

side-to-side, and is closed with running 3-0 PGA sutures. A defect 1 cm in diameter is created in the most dependent part of the cecum and is anastomosed to the urethra over a balloon catheter. Instead of joining the ureters to the cecum as originally described, the ureters are anastomosed to the ileum, either end-to-side or joined together and anastomosed end-to-end (Fig. 31-12D).

Ileocecal Reservoir without Valve

In 1988, Marshall described an ileocecal pouch with the ureters implanted into the cecum, thus eliminating the need for a valve and for intussusception.[9] Creation of the pouch is similar to that of the Mainz pouch, except that the most proximal 10 cm of ileum are eliminated. After the posterior bowel edges are approximated, a segment of the cecal wall, 6 to 8 mm in diameter, is excised in the most dependent part of the cecum. The mucosa is everted over the edges and the urethrocecal anastomosis is performed over a balloon catheter using five 2-0 PGA sutures. The left ureter is brought to the right side under the colonic mesentery and both ureters are implanted into the cecal wall separately, using a standard submucosal tunnel with a mucosa to mucosal anastomosis over 8-French feeding tubes. A "cystostomy" tube is left in place and is

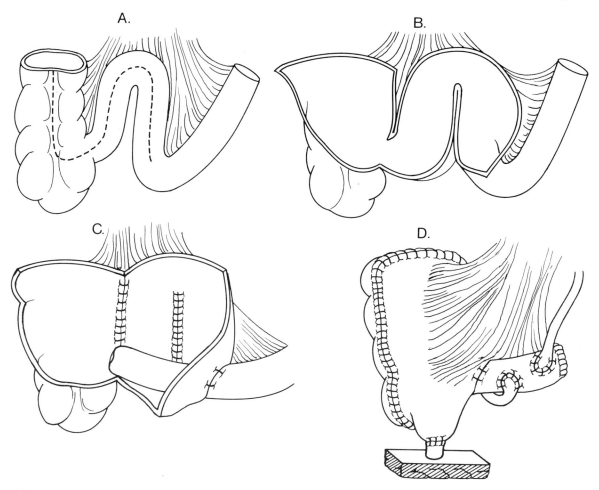

A.

B.

C.

D.

FIG. 31-12. The Mainz pouch.

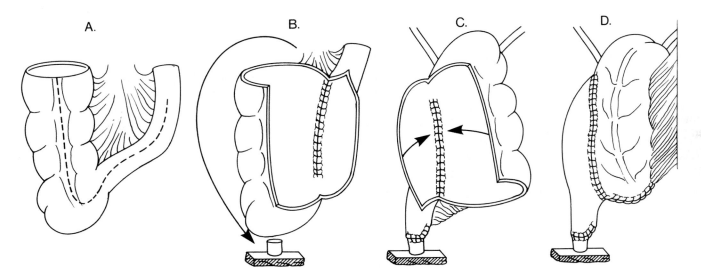

FIG. 31-13. Le Bag.

brought out through the skin along with the ureteral stents. The pouch is then closed. Marshall recommends hitching the pouch to the psoas muscle to stabilize the ureteral implantation, fixing it to the anterior abdominal wall at the site of cyctostomy, and placing a Marshall-Marchetti type suture between the anterior wall of the pouch and the undersurface of the pubic bone or the rectus muscle.

Le Bag

In 1986, Light and Englemann described the ileocolonic pouch, Le Bag, for total replacement of the bladder.[10] Both the cecum and approximately 15 cm of the terminal ileum are isolated and opened along the antimesenteric border, except for the most proximal 2 to 3 cm of the ileal segment (Fig. 31-13A). The medial edges are approximated with running 3-0 PGA sutures (Fig. 31-13B). The pouch is rotated counterclockwise 180° and the proximal ileum is anastomosed to the urethra over a balloon catheter. The ureters are implanted into the cecum using the standard antireflux submucosal tunnel with mucosa to mucosa anastomosis (Fig. 31-13C). Closure of the pouch is completed (Fig. 31-13D).

The major drawback of this procedure is the interposition of the tubular segment between the reservoir and the urethra. No matter how small this segment is, it will peristalse and generate high pressures that are transmitted to the urethra causing urgency and incontinence. This operation can be modified to eliminate this tubular segment, avoid rotation of the cecum, and anastomose the most dependent part of the cecum to the urethra.

SUBSTITUTION USING COLON

Partially Detubularized Right Colon

In 1986, Goldwasser et al. described the use of the right colon for bladder replacement.[11] The cecum, the ascending colon, and the hepatic flexure are isolated and opened along the antimesenteric tenia down to the cecum (Fig. 31-14A). The termi-

nal ileum is closed and an appendectomy is performed. The ureters are implanted into the back wall of the cecum using the standard antireflux submucosal tunnel, with mucosa to mucosa anastomosis. The most dependent part of the cecum is anastomosed to the urethra over a balloon catheter. The opened ascending colon and hepatic flexure are folded down and are closed with running 3-0 PGA sutures (Fig. 31-14B).

The Sigmoid Pouch

Whenever the small intestine or the ileocecal segment are not available for bladder substitution, it is often possible to use the sigmoid colon.

The sigmoid colon, which is usually between 20 and 30 cm long, is isolated and a colo-colostomy is performed (Fig. 31-15A). The sigmoid is opened along the antimesenteric border and the medial edges are approximated with running 3-0 PGA sutures (Fig. 31-15B). The open patch is then folded at a right

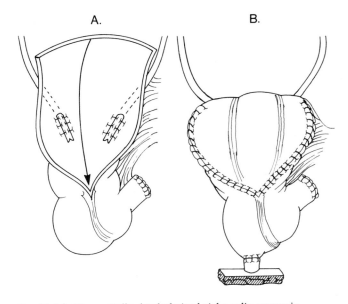

FIG. 31-14. The partially detubularized right colic reservoir.

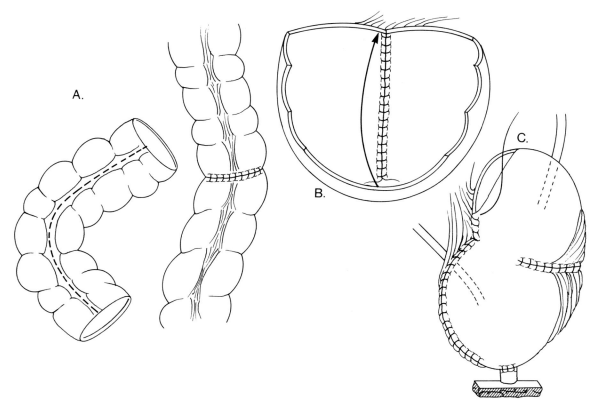

Fig. 31-15. The Sigmoid pouch.

angle to the longitudinal axis of the colon and partially closed with running 3-0 PGA sutures (Fig. 31-15*B*). The most dependent part of the pouch is anastomosed to the urethra over a balloon catheter. The ureters are then implanted into the wall of the sigmoid using the standard antireflux submucosal tunnel technique with mucosa to mucosa anastomosis. Closure of the pouch is completed (Fig. 31-15*C*). Ureteral stents may be used and can be brought in along the urethral catheter or through the bowel wall.

CONCLUSION

Coupled with the nerve-sparing technique for preservation of potency, bladder substitution has added a new dimension to the treatment of localized bladder cancer. Although the ileal conduit remains the standard, the urologist should be equipped to offer the suitable patient an alternative to the ileal conduit. We have described and illustrated 12 different reservoirs. The majority work well and serve the purpose for which they were designed. The practicing urologist needs to familiarize himself or herself with only two or three.

The author has performed more than 50 different bladder substitutions and, based on his experience, offers the following recommendations:

1. Avoid using tubular bowel.
2. Avoid interposing a tubular segment between the reservoir and the urethra.
3. If possible, avoid using terminal ileum so as not to interfere with vitamin B-12 and folate absorption, the effects of which may not become clinically detectable for years because of the rich body stores of these substances.
4. Small intestine produces less mucous than the large bowel.
5. Frequent irrigation of the catheter postoperatively to clear it of mucous is an absolute necessity in order to avoid retention, over distention, and blow-out of the reservoir.
6. Advise the patient that while daytime control is almost sure to return, enuresis is common unless he wakes up and voids two to three times during the night.

REFERENCES

1. Tizzoni, G., and Poggi, A. Die Wiederhestellung der Harnblase. Experimentalle Untersuchungen. Zentralbl. Chir., *15*:921, 1888.
2. Camey, M., and LeDuc, A. L'enterocystoplastie apres cystoprostatectomie total pour cancer de vessie. Ann. Urol. (Paris), *13*:114, 1979.
3. Camey, M. Radical cystectomy with ileocystoplasty: 30 year experience. Eur. Urol., *14*(Suppl. 1):27, 1988.
4. Ghoneim, M., et al. Cystectomy and diversion for carcinoma of the bilharzial bladder. In *Management of Advanced Cancer of Prostate and Bladder.* Edited by Smith, P. H., and Pavone-Macaluso, M. New York, Alan R. Liss, 1988, pp. 315–319.

5. STUDER, E., CASANOVA, G., and ZINGG, F. Bladder substitution with an ileal low-pressure reservoir. Eur. Urol., *14*(Suppl. 1):36, 1988.

6. GIL-VERNET, J. The ileocolic segment in urologic surgery. J. Urol., *94*:418, 1965.

7. KHAFAGY, M., et al. Radical cystectomy and ileocecal bladder reconstruction for carcinoma of the urinary bladder. A study of 130 patients. Br. J. Urol., *60*:60, 1987.

8. SCHÄRFE, T., et al. Mainz Pouch for augmentation, bladder substitution or continent urinary diversion. Eur. Urol., *14*(Suppl. 1):32, 1988.

9. MARSHALL, F. Creation of an ileocolic urinary bladder post cystectomy. J. Urol., *139*:1264, 1988.

10. LIGHT, J., and ENGLEMANN, U. Le Bag: Total replacement of the bladder using an ileocolonic pouch. J. Urol., *136*:27, 1986.

11. GOLDWASSER, B., BARRETT, D., and BENSON, R. Bladder replacement with use of detubularized right colonic segment: Preliminary report of a new technique. Mayo Clin. Proc., *61*:615, 1986.

CARCINOMA OF THE TESTIS

Testicular Cancer: An Overview

Michael Sarosdy

Testicular carcinoma is a rare form of cancer, but it has a disproportionate impact because of the age group most commonly affected, namely young men in their twenties and early thirties. In addition to this group, two other age groups comprise the trimodal frequency distribution of testis cancer, with lesser peaks seen in infants and males over 60.[1] Thus, testis cancer must be considered across the age groups in the differential diagnosis of scrotal and testicular masses.

A systematic multidisciplinary approach to patients with testis cancer over the past 20 years has led to significant improvements in the treatment of this disease. Because the majority of testicular cancers are of germ cell origin and have a high rate of metastasis, a large proportion of patients (40 to 50%) have disseminated disease at the time of diagnosis. Prior to the advent of platinum-based chemotherapy, survival of patients with metastases was poor and inversely related to the bulk of the metastatic disease. Platinum-based chemotherapy protocols have produced such dramatic results in the treatment of testicular carcinoma that current studies are aimed at maintaining the excellent results possible while reducing the toxicity of therapy. The stratification of patients according to the likelihood of response is also allowing the tailoring of

chemotherapy such that some good-risk patients may be treated adequately with only four cycles of a two-drug regimen or three cycles of a three-drug regimen.[2,3] Such progress in the treatment of a rare cancer underscores the value of cooperative group efforts in treating urologic cancer patients.

INCIDENCE

Testicular malignancies are relatively rare, with an incidence of 3.7 per 100,000 per year. In 1989, there will be approximately 5,700 new cases in the U.S., with about 350 deaths from testis cancer.[4] In addition to the trimodal frequency distribution mentioned above, certain histologic tumor types have predilections for specific age groups.[5] Infants tend to acquire teratomas and embryonal carcinomas but not seminomas or choriocarcinomas. Embryonal carcinoma and teratocarcinoma occur primarily in patients between 25 and 35, choriocarcinoma between 20 and 30, and seminoma between 35 and 60. In men over 60, the most common testicular neoplasm is lymphoma, while the most common germ cell tumor is seminoma. Seminoma is also the most common germ cell tumor overall, comprising 40% of germ cell tumors of the testis.

In addition to the age differences, several other interesting characteristics have been found concerning the incidence of this malignancy. Blacks are known to have an incidence of testis cancer about one-third that of whites, a difference that is found worldwide.[6] The incidence of malignancy is higher in cryptorchidism, a correlation that does not subside completely with orchiopexy.[7] A familial tendency has been recognized in monozygotic twins, dizygotic twins, nontwin brothers, and in fathers and their offspring.[8-11] Synchronous or metachronous bilateral tumors occur in 2 to 3% of males with testis cancer, and a history of cryptorchidism is present in nearly two-thirds of these men.[1,12]

ETIOLOGIC CONSIDERATIONS

Although the exact cause of testicular cancers remains obscure, there is growing evidence of a genetic predisposition,[13] as well as strong evidence implicating cryptorchidism, as noted above. The risk of tumor development is also higher with greater degrees of cryptorchidism, i.e. the rate for malignancy is higher in abdominal cryptorchidism than in inguinal cryptorchidism.[14] Although the true increase in risk of tumor development in cryptorchidism is not clear, it is probably on the order of 10 to 40 times the risk in a male with normally descended testes.[15,16] Seminoma occurs most commonly in cryptorchid testes that develop cancer, followed in frequency by embryonal, teratocarcinoma, and choriocarcinoma. It should be noted that it has been reported that between 5 and 10% of men with a history of cryptorchidism develop a malignancy in the contralateral, normally-descended testicle (if CIS is included).[17]

PATHOLOGIC CONSIDERATIONS

Roughly 95% of testicular malignancies are of germ cell origin and are referred to as germ cell tumors. Germ cell tumors are classically categorized according to the following histologic types: seminoma, embryonal carcinoma, teratoma, and choriocarcinoma.[18-20] They may occur in pure form (40%) or as a mixture of cell types (60%). There have been six attempts to classify these cancers meaningfully since 1941, and the system devised by Dixon and Moore in 1952 is still the one most commonly used in the United States.[19] It is a system based on prognostic groups, and includes the five categories shown in Table 32-1. Discussion of pathologic types will, therefore, follow the Dixon and Moore classification.

Seminoma

Classic seminoma accounts for about 40% of all testicular neoplasms, and presents most frequently in the fourth and fifth decades.[21] It usually forms a sharply demarcated mass on gross examination, with a whitish tan or pink appearance on its cut surface.[22] Its histologic appearance is often referred to as a monotonous uniformity, with sheets of polyhedral cells separated into compartments by fibrous septae (Fig. 32-1). A lymphocytic infiltrate is often present, and nuclei are large, round,

TABLE 32-1. *Classification and Incidence of Testicular Tumors**

	TUMOR TYPE	INCIDENCE (%)
I	Seminoma (pure)	40
II	Embryonal carcinoma ± seminoma	25
III	Teratoma ± seminoma	5–9
IV	Teratoma with embryonal carcinoma (teratocarcinoma) or choriocarcinoma, or both, ± seminoma	25
V	Choriocarcinoma ± seminoma, ± embryonal carcinoma, ± teratoma	1–3

*Adapted from Dixon, F. J., and Moore, R. A. Clinicopatholic study. Cancer, 6:427, 1953.

and centrally located. Classic seminomas are defined as those with fewer than three mitotic figures per high power field in ten high power fields. Anaplastic seminomas are those that have three or more mitotic figures per high power field in ten fields. It was formerly thought that the anaplastic forms of seminoma carried a worse prognosis than classic seminoma.[23] However, that clinical implication is no longer considered as clear-cut, as there is evidence that stage for stage, a seminoma with a high mitotic index behaves no differently than a classic seminoma.[24,25]

Spermatocytic seminoma is a rare but distinct form of seminoma. It accounts for about 7% of seminoma and is most common in the older males, with patients in one series averaging 65 years old.[26] It is an indolent tumor, with low metastatic potential. The cut surface is usually soft, with a gelatinous appearance, often with cystic degeneration. Microscopically, three cell types are present and the nesting pattern of classic seminoma is missing, as is the lymphocytic infiltrate (Fig. 32-2). The most common cell is a medium-sized cell with a round nucleus and fine granular chromatin; smaller cells are present that resemble lymphocytes but are probably degenerate; and

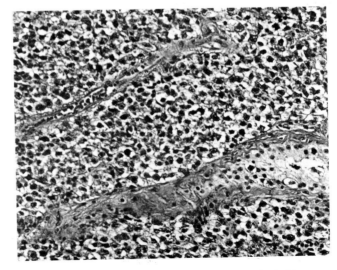

FIG. 32-1. Pure seminoma (original magnification X 450). (Courtesy of William A. Black, M.D.)

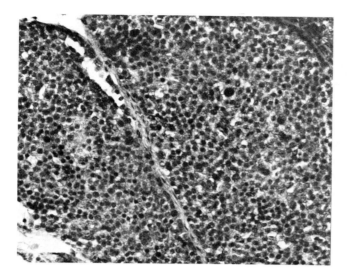

FIG. 32-2. Spermatocytic seminoma (original magnification X 400). (Courtesy of William A. Black, M.D.)

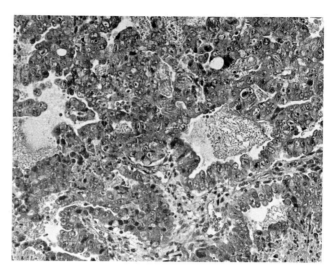

FIG. 32-3. Embryonal carcinoma (original magnification X 400). (Courtesy of William A. Black, M.D.)

giant cells with abundant eosinophilic cytoplasm and single or multiple nuclei are seen. These tumors are not associated with nonseminomatous elements.[22]

Nonseminomatous Germ Cell Tumors

Nonseminomatous germ cell tumors are thought to represent a spectrum of malignancies that arise from an undifferentiated progenitor that retains the ability to express a variety of histologic types. Embryonal carcinoma is thought to be the most primitive and clinically behaves aggressively. The other end of the spectrum is occupied by teratocarcinoma, which has a more organized appearance and behaves less aggressively. The extreme histologic type of neoplasm in this line is in fact a benign tumor by definition, mature teratoma. The histologic makeup of nonseminomatous tumors is important clinically, with the presence of embryonal carcinoma now considered to be a relative contraindication to surveillance therapy as an option for patients with nonseminomatous tumors (see treatment, below).

Embryonal Carcinoma

Embryonal carcinoma is a more aggressive tumor, and in its pure form accounts for about 20 to 25% of testicular cancers. It has a variegated or gray-red appearance on gross sectioning, often with areas of focal hemorrhage and necrosis (Fig. 32-3).[22] A variety of patterns is seen histologically, including highly anaplastic areas as well as more differentiated areas with acinar and tubular patterns. Cellular borders are usually less sharp than with seminoma, and multiple mitotic figures and multiple nucleoli are often seen.

Histologic evidence of yolk sac differentiation is often found in embryonal tumors.[27] Although the yolk sac tumor is considered to be an infantile form of embryonal cancer, also termed endodermal sinus tumor, it may be present in 40 to

45% of the adult form of embryonal cancers and probably represents focal differentiation of the embryonal component. It demonstrates a typical lacy, reticular pattern histologically and a pathognomonic "Schiller-Duval body" (Fig. 32-4). Serum levels of AFP are usually higher when yolk sac tumors are present compared to levels found in the presence of pure embryonal carcinomas.

Teratocarcinoma

Teratocarcinoma is a tumor that, according to the Dixon and Moore classification, lies between the more aggressive embryonal carcinomas and the benign adult (mature) teratoma. Grossly, the cut surface is a blend of cystic and solid areas, with the latter areas representing the poorly differentiated components. The cystic spaces demonstrate mature elements,

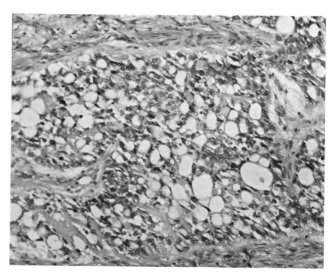

FIG. 32-4. Endodermal sinus tumor (original magnification X 400). (Courtesy of William A. Black, M.D.)

often interspersed with cartilaginous tissue. The histologic appearance is, therefore, one of an admixture of elements ranging from embryonal to mature, benign tissue types such as muscle, cartilage, and epithelium.[22]

Teratoma

Histologically benign by definition, these tumors contain no identifiable malignant elements but instead consist of two or more elements from the germinal layers. Solid and cystic areas alternate on gross sectioning as in teratocarcinomas, but no malignant elements are present microscopically. Instead, mature cartilage, smooth muscle, and epithelial-lined cysts are often seen. Despite careful study to exclude malignant elements, metastasis may occur in up to one-third of the patients with mature teratoma.

Choriocarcinoma

Choriocarcinoma is one of the most aggressive and lethal of the human cancers. Fortunately, it is relatively rare, particularly in the pure form (0.003%).[20] Grossly, there are focal hemorrhages on the cut surface. The diagnosis rests on the presence of syncytiotrophoblastic giant cells in intimate contact with cytotrophoblasts (Fig. 32-5). Syncytiotrophoblasts alone are not uncommonly found in embryonal carcinoma or teratocarcinoma, so caution must be exercised to avoid calling the latter choriocarcinoma when cytotrophoblasts are not present. Syncytiotrophoblasts are large eosinophilic giant cells with hyperchromatic nuclei. Cytotrophoblasts are sheets of cells that have abundant clear cytoplasm with single nuclei and sharp, distinct borders.

Carcinoma In-situ

Carcinoma in-situ is a characteristic abnormality of the seminiferous tubules found in association with a variety of conditions, including infertility, cryptorchidism, and adjacent to a

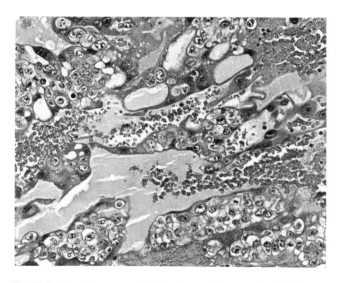

FIG. 32-5. Choriocarcinoma (original magnification X 400). (Courtesy of William A. Black, M.D.)

germ cell neoplasm in an undescended testis.[28] Waxman has described the characteristics of carcinoma in situ as abnormal germ cells with malignant morphologic characteristics, large and hyperchromatic nuclei, frequent mitotic figures, and malignant cells lining the seminiferous tubules or within the lumen of the tubules.[29] Although the exact incidence is not known, carcinoma in situ has been reported in 1% of infertile males and in up to 4% of males with a history of cryptorchidism.[28]

The clinical implications of the diagnosis of carcinoma in-situ remain unclear. However, Skakkebaek has reported the development of frank carcinoma of the testis within 5 years in 50% of infertile males followed with this diagnosis.[28] For this reason, future attention to this entity will be necessary to determine whether early therapy might be appropriate.

SERUM TUMOR MARKERS

The development and use of assays to measure the biologic activity of tumors has played a large role in the successes seen in the clinical management of patients with testicular cancer. The measurement of serum alpha-fetoprotein (AFP) and the beta subunit of human chorionic gonadotropin (HCG) do not completely predict the presence or absence of metastatic disease, but the use of these markers does provide positive guidance for making the diagnosis, clinical staging, and measuring the response to chemotherapy.[30] An understanding of the limits as well as the utility of these markers is most important in order to fully benefit from their clinical availability.

Alpha-fetoprotein is a glycoprotein with a molecular weight of about 70,000. It is produced by fetal yolk sac, the liver, and the gastrointestinal tract. It is a major protein in human fetuses, reaching a peak at about the 12th week of gestation, after which it declines. By 1 year of age, it is generally not detectable. AFP is produced in about 70% of germ cell tumors by yolk sac and embryonal carcinomas. It is not produced by seminomatous tumors. An elevation of AFP in a patient with a tumor reported histologically as a seminoma should prompt re-examination of the specimen by the pathologist for the nonseminomatous elements that must be present. AFP has a serum half-life of approximately 5.5 days.[31]

Human chorionic gonadotropin (HCG) is a glycoprotein with a molecular weight of approximately 38,000, and is normally secreted by the trophoblastic tissues of the placenta. It consists of two different polypeptide chains, an alpha and a beta. The alpha subunit is similar to the alpha subunits of luteinizing hormone, follicle-stimulating hormone, and thyroid-stimulating hormone, all produced in the pituitary gland. However, the beta subunit is different in structure from the beta subunit of the pituitary hormones, and is, therefore, antigenically distinct.[32] In germ cell tumors, it is the syncytiotrophoblastic cells that make HCG. Forty to 60% of nonseminomatous germ cell tumors produce HCG, and it may also be produced in up to 30% of patients with "pure" seminoma. The half-life of HCG is roughly 24 hours (although it is much shorter for the two subunits individually, the metabolic degradation time reflects the half-life of the entire molecule).[33]

Several additional markers may be elevated in patients with testis cancer. The most important one is probably lactic acid dehydrogenase (LDH). LDH, particularly the isoenzyme fraction LDH-1, is elevated in about 60% of patients with nonseminomatous tumors. Like AFP, it is nonspecific, but LDH does provide an additional marker with which to follow the patient whose tumor does produce it. A few of the additional nonspecific markers that may be elevated are undergoing investigation and include the pregnancy-specific protein SP-1, placental alkaline phosphatase (P1AP), fibronectin, and the "F9-like" cell-surface antigens.

AFP and HCG measurements in patients with testicular masses or cancer can be used for diagnosis, staging, monitoring of response to therapy, and prognosis. Because most seminomas and many nonseminomatous tumors do not produce either marker, only positive assays aid in the diagnosis of scrotal masses as testis cancer. Negative assays have no value and should not be considered capable of ruling out the presence of malignancy. The mainstay of diagnosis continues to be histologic examination of the mass. However, the fact that up to 90% of nonseminomatous tumors will have elevations of one or both markers at the time of diagnosis makes their use necessary as well as helpful (Table 32-2).[30]

Serum markers may be helpful in staging patients clinically after orchiectomy, but again, because of the absence of marker elevation in all tumors, negative assays are of no benefit. Patients with elevated preorchiectomy markers may be followed with serial markers after orchiectomy to see if the decay follows the curve predicted by the marker's known half-life. Failure to follow that predicted curve indicates a nontesticular source of marker production, such as from any metastatic focus. This is most helpful when radiographic studies such as abdominal CT scanning are negative. However, there is a direct correlation between pathologic stage of disease and the percentage of patients with elevated markers, ranging in one collected series from 37% in stage IIA to 84% in stage IIC (Table 32-3).[30] The high rate of false negatives should be kept in mind when considering the employment of surveillance rather than retroperitoneal lymphadenectomy to more accurately stage a patient with clinical stage-A nonseminomatous testis cancer. Again, elevated markers are helpful, but the absence of elevated markers does not rule out metastatic disease.

The most useful role of AFP and beta-HCG determinations in testis cancer is in monitoring the response to therapy for those with metastatic disease. This is true both during initial chemotherapy and after successful induction of remission. During initial chemotherapy, persistence of elevated marker levels without decay indicates a failure of the frontline choice of drugs and dictates the need to change to a different combination of drugs.[30] The same is true if the markers decay but reach a plateau without normalizing. Conversely, a rapid return to normal does not warrant shortening the number of courses. Also, radiographic evidence of residual disease after chemotherapy is still considered grounds for a "postchemo" retroperitoneal lymph node dissection (RPLND), even if the markers normalized during chemotherapy. This is the situation in 20 to 50% of patients with nonseminomatous tumors who have residual disease after chemotherapy, and RPLND is necessary in this setting because this tissue may represent teratoma, seminoma, scar, or marker-negative nonseminomatous cancer.[35,36] Finally, in patients with normalized radiographs and markers after chemotherapy, recurrent elevation of one or both markers may be the first sign of relapse. If definite and progressive, such marker elevation alone may be considered grounds for the initiation of salvage chemotherapy.

A more controversial and less well-defined use of markers in testis cancer is in prognosticating a patient's likelihood of responding to "standard" chemotherapy. In the past, tumor marker elevations alone did not seem to predict the response to chemotherapy, but appeared rather to do so only in association with bulk of disease.[36-38] Rapid half-life decline of elevated markers during chemotherapy was shown to predict more favorable outcome than for those patients whose markers declined much more slowly.[30,39] In 1983, Bosl and associates reported the results of a multivariate analysis of several different prognostic factors that did show predictive values of three factors when taken together.[40] These were the logarithm of the serum values of LDH and HCG and the total number of sites of metastasis (rather than volume). This particular formula is discussed later in this chapter, under Clinical Staging.

TABLE 32-3. *Frequency of elevated prelymphadenectomy marker levels in patients with NSGCT*

| | STAGE OF DISEASE | | | |
REFERENCE	II_A	II_B	II_C	TOTAL (%)
Scardino and Skinner[34]	6/12	12/22	5/5	23/39(59)
Lange et al.[70]	7/15	11/15	8/10	26/40(65)
Friedman et al.[71]	1/11	18/40	8/10	27/61(44)
Total (%)	14/38(37)	41/77(53)	21/25(84)	76/140(54)

From Lange, P. H., and Raghaven, D. Clinical applications of tumor markers in testicular cancer. In: *Testis Tumors*. Edited by J. P. Donohue. Baltimore, Williams & Wilkins, 1983.

TABLE 32-2. *Preorchiectomy marker levels at the University of Minnesota*[30]

DIAGNOSIS	ELEVATED AFP OR HCG LEVELS (%)
Benign intrascrotal mass (N = 43)	0(0)
Seminoma (N = 70)	16(23)
NSGCT	
Stage I (N = 32)	22(69)
Stage II-II (N = 57)	50(88)

From Lange, P. H., and Raghaven, D. Clinical applications of tumor markers in testicular cancer. In: *Testis Tumors*. Edited by J. P. Donohue. Baltimore, Williams & Wilkins, 1983.

DIAGNOSIS

Testicular cancer most commonly presents as a painless, hard mass or "swelling" noted by the patient. Some will report a dull ache or sense of fullness, and occasionally patients may report acute pain, probably related to hemorrhage into the tumor. There is often a long delay between onset of symptoms and diagnosis, with both patients and physicians responsible for that delay. A complete physical exam should be performed when testicular cancer is suspected, including a careful examination of the testicle and the left supraclavicular area. A testicular tumor is usually firm, relatively nontender, and contained within the tunica of the testis. The tunica albuginea presents a natural barrier to direct spread of the tumor, and local involvement of the epididymis or cord occurs in only 10 to 15% of cases. Masses contained within the epididymis are usually distinguishable upon close palpation. Small hydrocøeles should not make careful examination difficult, though large ones might. Although aspiration of a large hydrocøele in order to facilitate examination is not unreasonable, a trans-scrotal ultrasound study may be preferred to avoid tumor cell spillage. Transillumination is also still helpful in distinguishing small, tense hydrocøeles from tumors.

The size of a testicular tumor does not correlate with the presence or absence of metastases. Testis cancers tend to be fast-growing, with a doubling time estimated to be 10 to 30 days. 95% of patients dying from testis cancer do so within 2 years. The fast doubling time is probably responsible for the fact that 40 to 50% of patients have metastatic disease at the time of presentation and diagnosis. One-fourth of these or roughly 10% of all patients will present with symptoms of metastatic disease.[41] Those symptoms may include cough or dyspnea, abdominal fullness, nausea, vomiting, weight loss, bone pain, peripheral or central nervous system symptoms, or unilateral leg edema. Five to ten percent may have evidence of gynecomastia or other signs of estrogen excess.

The differential diagnosis includes epididymitis, epididymal or tunica albuginea cyst, hydrocele, hernia, hematoma, varicocele, and spermatocele. If a 2-week course of appropriate antibiotics does not significantly improve a case of presumptive epididymitis, surgical exploration is indicated.

Patients undergoing exploration for possible testis cancer should have a clot drawn prior to surgery. Should a tumor be found, marker assays may then be obtained to establish the patient's preorchiectomy baseline. For those with elevated preorchiectomy markers, a persistent elevation or slower-than-expected decay indicates metastatic disease, even if all radiographic staging studies are normal.

CLINICAL STAGING

Lymphatic spread is common to all germinal tumors, with choriocarcinoma spreading by vascular routes as well. The primary route of lymphatic spread is to the aortocaval nodes, with subsequent cephalad extension to the cisterna chyli, thoracic duct, and supraclavicular nodes. Retrograde spread is often seen to the lower lumbar, iliac, and pelvic nodes when massive retroperitoneal disease is present. Abdominal CT scanning with contrast is the study of choice for staging patients after the diagnosis is made. Although a plain chest x-ray will rule out bulky intrathoracic disease, a chest CT will detect smaller amounts of disease, and it is simple to obtain this at the same time as the abdominal CT scan. The intravenous urogram is of much less value today than it was in the past because a moderate amount of retroperitoneal disease may not be detected, although it would be on CT. While pedal lymphangiography does provide visualization of the retroperitoneal lymph nodes, its value over CT scanning is minimal, and such studies are more difficult to obtain. Tesoro-Tess and associates showed that CT and lymphangiography each have an individual diagnostic sensitivity of about 75% and, when used together, a cumulative sensitivity of about 90% results.[42] However, the use of both tests together increased the false-positive rate from 25 to 37%. He and most urologists feel that such a relatively small gain in diagnostic accuracy is not worthwhile in patients undergoing staging RPLND. It is important that lymphangiography and CT both be obtained in all patients being considered for surveillance (see below).

Several additional studies may be indicated in some patients, but as a rule, they are not obtained routinely. Radionucleide liver scans are necessary only if liver involvement is suggested by physical findings or elevations of liver enzymes (not including LDH). Similarly, bone and brain scans are obtained only if indicated by physical exam or elevated alkaline phosphatase, as metastases to these sites tend to occur late in the disease process.

Treatment after initial clinical screening is based on categorization of patients as early-stage disease or advanced disease. Although a more precise classification is employed to predict response to chemotherapy, a simple classification based upon the volume of gross disease detected in the above studies suffices for initial management. Although several staging systems are used for testis cancer, the one most widely used is that proposed by the Memorial Sloan-Kettering Cancer Center (modified Walter Reed scheme in parentheses):

Stage A (I)	Tumor confined to the testis
Stage B1 (IIA)	Minimal nodal spread, microscopic only and with less than 6 nodes involved, none greater than 2 cm
Stage B2 (IIB)	Grossly positive nodal disease, or more than 6 nodes positive in retroperitoneum.
Stage B3 (IIC)	Massive retroperitoneal disease, including palpable abdominal mass
Stage C (III)	Metastases above the diaphragm or involvement of solid visceral organs, brain, or bone.

Early disease stages include A, B1, and B2. Advanced disease includes stages B3 and C.

TREATMENT

Therapy is initiated by an appropriately performed orchiectomy, which should be through an inguinal incision. Scrotal surgery to make the diagnosis is an error, and occasionally results in scrotal recurrence or spread to inguinal lymph nodes. Most, but not all, blood-borne metastases occur in conjunction with lymphatic spread. The histologic diagnosis and clinical staging as outlined above dictate further therapy. An algorithm based on histology and clinical staging is shown in Figure 32-6.

Nonseminomatous Germ Cell Tumors

CLINICAL STAGE A (PATHOLOGIC STAGE A, B1, AND MOST B2's). Considerable controversy arose several years ago over the treatment of these patients, partly because of the success experienced in treating patients with more advanced disease. In the past, pathologic staging of these patients had been accomplished by retroperitoneal lymph node dissection as outlined by Donohue and others.[43,44] Because only 20 to 30% of patients had positive nodes, the surgery was negative in the majority, and roughly 10% of the negative patients eventually showed recurrence in the chest. Lack of seminal emission or ejaculatory impotence occurred in the majority of patients because of interruption of the sympathetic nerves, though improved modified node dissections and nerve-sparing dissections have been developed that preserve ejaculation in the majority of node-negative patients.[45-47] However, abdominal recurrences were seen in less than 2%, and those with chest recurrences were detected early. With appropriate followup and chemotherapy when needed, cure rates for all clinical stage-A patients, regardless of pathologic stage, approached 100%.

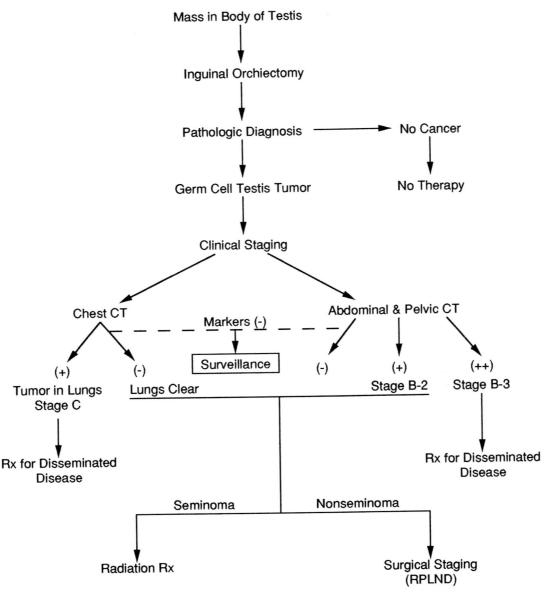

FIG. 32-6. The diagnosis, clinical staging, and assignment to treatment groups for all testis cancers. (Adapted from Rowland, R. G., and Donohue, J. P. Testicular cancer: Innovations in diagnosis and treatment. Semin. Urol., 6,3:223, 1988.)

The concept of observation or surveillance for clinical stage-A patients was introduced under the hypothesis that 70 to 80% of patients would be spared a needless lymphadenectomy, while near-100% survival would be maintained by the efficacy of chemotherapy.[48–50] To date, this has been achievable in only a highly selected group of patients and at much cost, both in terms of radiographic studies and the intensive chemotherapy required for many of those who progress.[51,52] Reasons for this include the higher degree of difficulty in detecting retroperitoneal recurrence (or progression) than pulmonary disease, as well as the fast growth rates of such tumors.[51] Thus, it has proven necessary to perform abdominal CT scanning every 2 months during the first 2 years of surveillance in all patients, in addition to bimonthly serum markers and chest x-rays. Herr and associates have identified several histologic features of the primary tumor that may place a patient at increased risk of developing retroperitoneal progression while on surveillance.[53] These include the presence of embryonal carcinoma, spermatic cord involvement, and vascular invasion in the tumor. Presently, patients having tumors with such histologic features should be excluded from surveillance and instead undergo staging retroperitoneal lymph node dissection (RPLND). Additional patients who should undergo this procedure are those judged to be poorly compliant for the rigorous followup required by surveillance therapy. For the remaining patients, strict adherence to close radiographic and marker followup is mandatory. It should also be noted that as of this writing, several centers no longer recommend surveillance therapy for the reasons outlined above.[51] It is our practice not to offer surveillance to patients, and it has been our experience that almost all patients are agreeable to RPLND when the facts are outlined to them as above. Such pathologically staged patients are then assigned to observation or chemotherapy according to the algorithm in Fig. 32-7, based on the following information.

Patients who are found to be pathologic stage A, with negative nodes at RPLND, are still at risk of recurrence in the chest, approximately 10%. As with all patients rendered clinically disease free, they should undergo close followup, with serum markers and chest x-ray monthly during the first year and bimonthly during year two. Quarterly followup is then suggested for 1 to 2 additional years.

Patients who are found to be pathologic stage B1 or B2 at RPLND have been shown to do well, whether they receive adjuvant chemotherapy postoperatively or are followed to the time of recurrence and only then treated with chemotherapy.[54] Scardino argues that because of a 13 to 37% recurrence rate in untreated B1 and B2 patients, all should have adjuvant chemotherapy utilizing less chemotherapy than an "intense" therapeutic regimen.[55] Using single-agent actinomycin D followed by one course of bleomycin and velban weekly for 5 to 10 weeks, he and Skinner reported a reduction in the relapse rate for stage-B1 and B2- patients from 33 to 14%, with a 3-year survival rate of 95%.[56] Utilizing slightly more drug, Vugrin and associates reported no relapses among 33 stage-B1 patients treated with a "mini-VAB" regimen of vinblastine, actinomycin D, and bleomycin. However, Einhorn and associates argue against adjuvant chemotherapy, despite their own success with it. In a randomized trial comparing two cycles of platinum, velban, and bleomycin (PVB) or mini-VAB immediately after RPLND, versus four cycles of PVB or VAB-VI at the first evidence of relapse, the Testicular Cancer Intergroup Study reported survival of 98 to 99% in both groups.[54] Importantly, Einhorn argues, chemotherapeutic toxicity was avoided altogether in the 51% who did not relapse after randomization to the observation arm, yet salvage was not compromised. However, those who relapsed required four courses of chemotherapy. Based on the differences in toxicity for mini-VAB versus PVB, it would therefore seem reasonable to utilize mini-VAB for adjuvant therapy and reserve more toxic platinum-based therapeutic regimens for those patients who do relapse after observation. Either course of action should salvage 99% of *compliant* patients.

STAGES B3 AND C. These patients are recognized clinically as having retroperitoneal or supradiaphragmatic disease, and should receive intense chemotherapy after orchiectomy is performed (Fig. 32-8). Although the majority of patients will do well with present treatment programs, some have such advanced disease states that even more aggressive and toxic programs are justified from the outset. Three systems were developed to classify patients into risk categories: the Samuels or MD Anderson Classification groups minimal disease and advanced disease, while the Einhorn or Indiana Staging System classifies patients as minimal, moderate, or advanced (Tables 32-4 and 32-5). Both systems and several other factors were investigated for prognostic accuracy in a Southeast Cancer Study Group trial comparing PVB alone or with doxorubicin.[57] The extent of disease as defined by the Indiana system and the number of elevated markers were found to be statistically significant predictors of response to therapy. In a prospective test of the Indiana classification system, the likelihood of a favora-

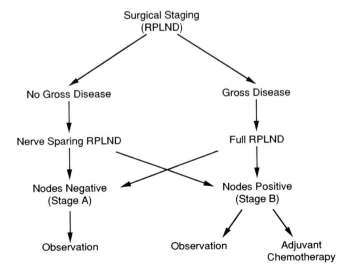

FIG. 32-7. Diagnosis, staging, and treatment of clinical stage-A testis cancer. (Adapted from Rowland, R. G., and Donohue, J. P. Testicular cancer: Innovations in diagnosis and treatment. Semin. Urol., 6,3:223, 1988.)

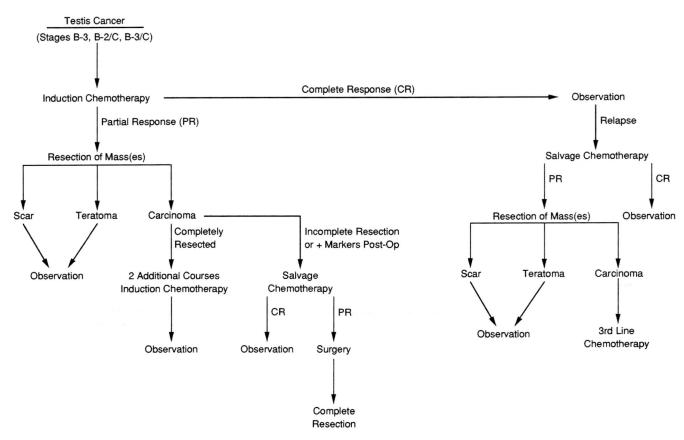

Fig. 32-8. Treatment scheme for disseminated testis cancer at Indiana University. (Adapted from Rowland, R. G., and Donohue, J. P. Testicular cancer: Innovations in diagnosis and treatment. Semin. Urol., *6,3*:223, 1988.)

ble response to therapy for minimal, moderate, or advanced disease was found to be 99%, 90%, and 58%, respectively. The third system that also has been shown to be a significant predictor of response was the TOTMET formula reported by Bosl and referred to earlier.[40] Patients who in these systems are found to have either minimal or moderate disease or "good risk" (Bosl), are treated with standard chemotherapy. The remainder are candidates for more aggressive, generally investigative protocols designed for poor-risk patients.

The standard chemotherapy today for patients with favorable prognosis is three cycles of platinum, etoposide (VP-16), and bleomycin, or the VAB-VI regimen (cyclophosphomide, velban, actinomycin-D, bleomycin, and platinum).[34,58] If all radiographic studies and markers normalize as they do in 70 to

TABLE 32-4. *M.D. Anderson Classification of Extent of Disease*

A*: Minimal pulmonary disease; no more than 5 lesions per lung field, none larger than 2 cm

B†: Pulmonary disease more advanced than A; includes hilar and mediastinal involvement

C*: Minimal abdominal ± minimal pulmonary disease (abdominal involvement <D)

D†: Advanced abdominal ± pulmonary disease; palpable abdominal mass, obstructive uropathy, lateral ureteral deviation, liver metastases

E*: Elevated marker only

F†: CNS, bone, extra-abdominal lymph node involvement

*Minimal disease
†Advanced disease

TABLE 32-5. *Indiana University Staging System*

Minimal Extent
1. Elevated markers only
2. Cervical nodes (±nonpalpable retroperitoneal nodes)
3. Unresectable nonpalpable retroperitoneal disease
4. Fewer than 5 pulmonary metastases per lung field and largest <2 cm (±nonpalpable retroperitoneal nodes)

Moderate Extent
5. Palpable abdominal mass only (no supradiaphragmatic disease)
6. Moderate pulmonary metastases; 5 to 10 per lung field and largest <3 cm, or solitary pulmonary metastasis of any size >2 cm (±nonpalpable retroperitoneal disease)

Advanced Extent
7. Advanced pulmonary metastases: primary mediastinal germ cell tumor or >10 metastases per lung field or multiple pulmonary metastases with largest >3 cm (±nonpalpable retroperitoneal disease)
8. Palpable abdominal mass plus supradiaphragmatic disease
9. Liver, bone, or CNS metastases

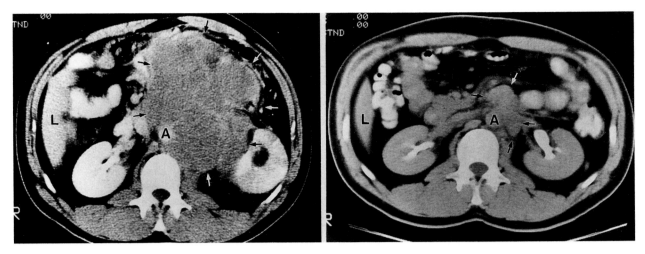

FIG. 32-9. *A*, Postorchiectomy CT scan showing massive retroperitoneal and retroperitoneal adenopathy. *B*, After four cycles of platinum, VP-16, and bleomycin, CT shows residual disease with normal markers. Histology of resected tissue showed scar and fibrous tissue only. The patient was in remission 24 months later (L: Liver, A: Aorta).

80% of cases, such patients may be followed closely without additional surgery. However, should residual disease be present after adequate chemotherapy as reflected by normalization of markers, resection of that residual tissue should be performed, whether in the lungs, the mediastinum, or in the retroperitoneum (Fig. 32-9). Such residual tissue should be resected, since 40% will have scar, 40% will have teratoma and 20% will have cancer.[59] Donohue and associates have shown that certain findings may be used to avoid postchemotherapy RPLND in selected patients who do not completely normalize their abdominal CT scan. However, verification of these findings by other centers should precede universal adoption of these guidelines.[60] These features include a 90% or greater reduction in the volume of the retroperitoneal mass using a precise mathematic formula to calculate volume, and the absence of any teratomatous elements after a meticulous histologic study of the primary tumor. In their experience, 20% of patients who would otherwise have undergone resection of residual tissue after a partial response might have been suitable for close followup and possibly could have been spared surgery.

Many patients with residual thoracic disease after adequate chemotherapy will also have residual retroperitoneal disease. Such dual-site residual disease may be approached through a thoracoabdominal incision or a median sternotomy-midline abdominal incision, or by sequential abdominal and thoracic procedures.[61,62] Those with residual pulmonary disease only may be approached through unilateral or bilateral thoracotomies, as indicated.

For those patients who undergo complete resection of residual tissue after chemotherapy, and who are found to have only benign tissue (scar or teratoma), no additional chemotherapy is required. Should carcinoma be present, additional chemotherapy is employed, usually two courses of the same regimen that they received initially.[63]

Although several recent trials have indicated that favorable, good-risk patients may do just as well with only platinum and etoposide as with the three drugs, data is not yet available on long-term relapse rates in patients so treated.[2,3] Such therapy should not yet be offered to patients except in clinical trial settings.

Occasional patients are seen who do not experience normalization of markers or significant decrease in metastatic disease with standard chemotherapy. These patients are said to have platinum-refractory disease, and should be switched early to a regimen containing ifosfamide. An alternative approach being studied in such patients is high-dose chemotherapy with autologous bone marrow transplant, utilizing such an agent as carboplatinum, an analog of cisplatinum.

By means of initial platinum-based chemotherapy and surgical resection of residual tissue followed by additional chemotherapy in those with persistent carcinoma, approximately 80% survival is obtainable in all patients with stages B3 and C disease. Those with minimal or moderate disease should have survival rates approximating 95%, with survival of 60 to 70% seen in those with extensive disease. Fortunately, the latter are a small percentage of patients with testis cancer.

Seminoma

CLINICAL STAGE-A. Because of the radiosensitivity of seminoma, clinical stage-A patients normally receive 2500 to 3500 rads to the aortocaval and ipsilateral inguinopelvic areas. Such therapy is well tolerated, and 5-year survival is 97%.[64] Those with clinical stage-B2 disease are also treated with abdominal radiotherapy, although supradiaphragmatic radiotherapy is not performed today as it once was for this stage. Survival should approach 85%.

CLINICAL STAGES B3 AND C. Such patients in the past were treated with radiotherapy to the abdomen, with additional treatment to the mediastinum and the supraclavicular area. Survival after this therapy was much poorer than for similar stages of non-seminomatous tumors, and it was found that chemotherapy could not be tolerated after such widespread radiotherapy. It has been recognized that survival is better if such patients are treated initially with the same platinum-based chemotherapy as is used in nonseminomatous tumors. Survival rates equal to those of nonseminomatous tumor patients have been reported for patients with seminomas using such therapy.[65] One difference with respect to nonseminomatous tumor patients is that most urologists do not feel that resection of residual tissue is necessary after chemotherapy for seminoma. The Indiana group recently reported relapse in only 3 of 22 patients having residual tissue after chemotherapy, supporting the approach of close followup rather than surgery in such patients.[66]

Seminoma that produces HCG carries a worse prognosis than classic seminoma and must be watched closely.[67] If HCG levels normalize after orchiectomy, the patient will likely do well with adjunctive radiotherapy to the retroperitoneum (as there is probably no tumor there).[68] Should the HCG level not normalize, there is probably a focus of nonseminomatous element present somewhere. Such patients appear to do much better with platinum-based chemotherapy, similar to those with clinical stage-B3 and C disease.

EXTRAGONADAL GERM CELL TUMORS

These tumors are rare, but that their origin is distinct from testicular primaries is clear. They may arise in the mediastinum, retroperitoneum, sacrococcygeal region, and the pineal gland. Extragonadal germ cell tumors are thought to arise from either displaced primitive germ cells or from the persistence of pluripotent cells in sequestered primitive rests. Both males and females may be affected, and patients tend to present with metastatic disease. Survival appears to be much better since the advent of platinum-based chemotherapy.[65]

PEDIATRIC TESTIS CANCERS

Testis tumors in children constitute 1 to 2% of solid childhood tumors. The peak incidence is at about 2 years of age. In contrast to adults, germ cell tumors account for only about 75% of pediatric testis tumors; the rest are a combination of relatively uncommon tumors. Yolk sac tumors account for 75% of these germ cell tumors. This tumor is similar to embryonal carcinoma, and has been termed embryonal, infantile embryonal, endodermal sinus tumor, Telium's tumor, and orchidoblastoma. Yolk sac tumors differ from adult embryonal tumors in that only 15 to 20% will metastasize. Thus, if there is no evidence on radiographic studies of disease in the chest or retroperitoneum and markers fall to normal after orchiectomy, the current recommendation is for close surveillance for the development of distant disease rather than for staging lymphadenectomy. When chemotherapy is necessary, vincristine, adriamycin, and cyclophosphamide (VAC) is the combination used.

CONCLUSION

Tremendous progress has been made in the last 20 years in the treatment of testicular cancer, with the overall 5-year survival rate increasing from 60 to 93%.[4] The early, dramatic results in curing patients with bulky metastatic disease have been replaced by the less glamorous but no-less dramatic reduction in therapeutic toxicity for the majority of patients. The necessity of continuing clinical studies remains, as investigators attempt to decrease the toxicity and the cost of therapy for those with limited disease, yet find more effective therapy for those few patients with advanced disease.

REFERENCES

1. MORSE, M. J., and WHITMORE, W. F. Neoplasms of the Testis. In *Campbell's Urology*. Edited by P. C. Walsh, R. F. Gittes, A. D. Perlmutter, and T. A. Stamey. Philadelphia, W. B. Saunders, 1986.
2. RAGHAVAN, A., et al. Deletion of bleomycin from therapy for good prognosis of advanced testicular cancer: A prospective randomized trial. In: Proc. Am. Soc. Clin. Oncol. 5:97, 1986.
3. BOSL, G. J., et al. A randomized trial of etoposide + cisplatin versus vinblastine + bleomycin + cisplatin + cyclophosphamide + dactinomycin in patients with good-prognosis germ cell tumors. J. Clin. Oncol., 6:1231, 1988.
4. SILVERBERG, E., and LUBERA, J. A. Cancer statistics. CA, 39:3, 1989.
5. KUHN, C. R., and JOHNSON, D. E. Epidemiology. In: *Testicular Tumors*. Edited by D. E. Johnson. Flushing, Medical Examination Publishing Co., 1972.
6. SHERMAN, F. P., CIAVARRA, V. A., and COHEN, M. J. Testis tumors in negroes. Urology, 2:318, 1973.
7. WHITAKER, R. H. Management of the undescended testis. Br. J. Hosp. Med., 4:25, 1970.
8. GULLEY, R. M., KOWALSKI, R., and NEUHOFF, C. F. Familial occurrence of testicular neoplasms: A case report. J. Urol., 112:620, 1974.
9. LEVEY, S., and GRABSTALD, H. Synchronous testicular tumors in identical twins. Urology, 6:754, 1975.

10. ADEEB, N. E., and GRECO, P. A. Malignant testicular tumors in non-twin brothers. Urology, 6:98, 1975.
11. SILBER, S. J., CITTAN, S., and FRIEDLANDER, G. Testicular neoplasm in father and son. J. Urol., 108:889, 1972.
12. SOHVAL, A. R. Testicular dysgenesis in relation to neoplasm of the testicle. J. Urol., 75:285, 1956.
13. DEWOLF, W. C. Somatic deletion of chromosome 6 DNA in human teratocarcinoma. J. Urol., 137:437A, 1987.
14. CAMPBELL, H. E. Incidence of malignant growth of the undescended testicle. Arch Surg., 44:353, 1942.
15. HENDERSON, B. E., et al. Risk factors for cancer of the testis in young men. Int. J. Cancer, 23:598, 1979.
16. GILBERT, J. B., and HAMILTON, J. B. Studies in malignant testis tumors: Incidence and nature of tumors in ectopic testis. Surg. Gynecol. Obstet., 71:731, 1940.
17. BERTHELSEN, J. G., et al. Screening for carcinoma in situ of the contralateral testis in patients with germinal testicular cancer. Br. Med. J., 285:1683, 1982.
18. FRIEDMAN, N. B. Pathology of testicular tumors. In: *Genito-urinary Cancer*. Edited by D. G. Skinner and J. B. DeKernion. Philadelphia, W. B. Saunders, 1978.
19. DIXON, F. J., and MOORE, R. A. Tumors of the male sex organs. In:

Atlas of Tumor Pathology. Fascicles 31b and 32. Washington, D.C., Armed Forces Institute of Pathology, 1952.

20. MOSTOFI, F. K., and PRICE, E. B., JR. Tumors of the male genial system. In: *Atlas of Tumor Pathology.* 2nd Series, Fascicle 8. Washington, D.C., Armed Forces Institute of Pathology, 1973.

21. MOSTOFI, F. K. Testicular tumors: Epidemiologic, etiologic and pathologic features. Cancer, *32:*1186, 1973.

22. NOCHOMOVITZ, L. E. The pathology of germ cell tumors of the testis. In: *Testis Tumors.* Edited by J. P. Donohue. Baltimore, Williams & Wilkins, 1983.

23. KADEMIAN, M., BOSCH, A., and CALDWELL, W. L. Anaplastic seminoma. Cancer, *40:*3082, 1977.

24. PERCARPIO, B., et al. Anaplastic seminoma. An analysis of 77 patients. Cancer, *43:*2510, 1979.

25. JOHNSON, D. E., GOMEZ, J. J., and AYALA, A. G. Anaplastic seminoma. J. Urol., *114:*80, 1975.

26. ROSAI, J., SILBER, I., and KHODADOUST, K. Spermatocytic seminoma. I: Clinicopathologic study of six cases and review of the literature. Cancer, *24:*92, 1969.

27. TALERMAN, A. The incidence of yolk sac tumor (endodermal sinus tumor) elements in germ cell tumors of the testis in adults. Cancer, *36:*211, 1975.

28. SKAKKEBAEK, N. E., BERTHELSEN, J. G., and MULLER, J. Carcinoma in-situ of the undescended testis. Urol. Clin. North Am., *9:*377, 1982.

29. WAXMAN, M. Malignant germ cell tumor in-situ in a cryptochid testis. Cancer, *38:*1452, 1976.

30. LANGE, P. H., and RAGHAVAN, D. Clinical applications of tumor markers in testicular cancer. In: *Testis Tumors.* Edited by J. P. Donohue. Baltimore, Williams & Wilkins, 1983.

31. GITLIN, D., and BOESMAN, M. Serum alpha-fetoprotein, albumin, and gamma-G-globulin in the human conceptus. J. Clin. Invest., *45:*1826, 1966.

32. VAITUKAITIS, J. L. Secretion of human chorionic gonadotropin by tumors. In: *Carcino-Embryonic Proteins,* Vol. 1. Edited by F. G. Lehmann. Amsterdam, Elsevier/North Holland Biomedical Press, 1979.

33. VAITUKAITIS, J. L. Human chorionic gonadotropin: A hormone secreted for many reasons. N. Engl. J. Med., *301:*324, 1979.

34. SCARDINO, P. T., et al. The value of serum tumor markers in the staging and prognosis of germ cell tumors of the testis. J. Urol., *118:*994, 1977.

35. LANGE, P. H., MCINTIRE, K. R., and WALDMANN, T. A. Tumor markers in testicular tumor: Current status and future prospects. In: *Testicular Tumors: Management and Treatment.* Edited by L. E. Einhorn. New York, Masson Publishing, 1980.

36. SCARDINO, P. T., and SKINNER, D. G. Germ cell tumors of the testis: Improved results in a prospective study using combined modality therapy and biochemical tumor markers. Surgery, *86:*86, 1979.

37. SCARDINO, P. T., et al. The value of serum tumor markers in the staging and prognosis of germ cell tumors of the testis. J. Urol., *118:*994, 1977.

38. FRIEDMAN, A., VUGRIN, D., and GOLBEY, R. B. Prognostic significance of serum tumor biomarkers (TM), alpha-fetoprotein (AFP), beta subunit of human chorionic gonadotropin (bHCG), and lactate dehydrogenase (LDH) in nonseminomatous germ cell tumors (NSGCT). In: Proc. Am. Soc. Clinic. Oncol., *21:*323, 1980.

39. THOMPSON, D. K., and HADDOW, J. E. Serial monitoring of serum alpha-fetoprotein and chorionic gonadotropin in males with germ cell tumors. Cancer, *43:*1820, 1979.

40. BOSL, G. J., et al. Multivariate analysis of prognostic variables in patients with metastatic testicular cancer. Cancer Res., *43:*3403, 1983.

41. BOSL, G. J., et al. Impact of delay in diagnosis on clinical stage of testicular cancer. Lancet, *2:*970, 1981.

42. TESORO-TESS, J. D., et al. Lymphangiography and computerized tomography in testicular carcinoma: How accurate in early stage disease? J. Urol., *133:*967, 1985.

43. DONOHUE, J. P. Retroperitoneal lymphadenectomy: The anterior approach including bilateral suprahilar dissection. Urol. Clin. North Am., *4:*509, 1977.

44. ROWLAND, R. G., et al. Accuracy of preoperative staging in stages A and B non-seminomatous germ cell testis tumors. J. Urol., *127:*718, 1982.

45. PIZZOCARO, G., SALVEONI, R., and ZINONI, F. Unilateral lymphadenectomy in intraoperative stage I nonseminomatous germinal testis cancer. J. Urol., *134:*485, 1985.

46. RICHIE, J. P. Modified retroperitoneal lymphadenectomy for patients with clinical stage I testicular cancer. Semin. Urol., *6:*216, 1988.

47. JEWETT, M. A. S., et al. Retroperitoneal lymphadenectomy for testis tumor with nerve sparing for ejaculation. J. Urol., *139:*1220, 1988.

48. SOGANI, P. C., et al. Orchiectomy alone in the treatment of clinical stage I nonseminomatous germ cell tumor of the testis. J. Clin. Oncol., *2:*267, 1984.

49. PECKHAM, M. J., et al. Orchiectomy alone in testicular stage I nonseminomatous germ cell tumours. Lancet, *1:*678, 1982.

50. JEWETT, M. A. S. Nonoperative approach for the management of clinical stage A nonseminomatous germ cell tumors. Semin. Urol., *2:*204, 1984.

51. PIZZOCARO, G., et al. Difficulties of a surveillance study omitting retroperitoneal lymphadenectomy in clinical stage I nonseminomatous germ cell tumors of the testis. J. Urol., *138:*1393, 1987.

52. SAGALOWSKY, A. I. Expectant management of stage A nonseminomatous testicular tumors. In: *Genitourinary Cancer.* Edited by T. L. Ratliff and W. J. Catalona. Boston, Martinus Nijhoff Publishers, 1987.

53. HERR, H. W., et al. Selection of testicular tumor patients for omission of retroperitoneal lymph node dissection. J. Urol., *135:*500, 1986.

54. WILLIAMS, S. D., et al. Early stage testis cancer: The testicular cancer intergroup study. In: *Adjuvant Therapy of Cancer V.* Edited by S. E. Salmon. Philadelphia, Grune and Stratton, 1987.

55. SCARDINO, P. T. Adjuvant chemotherapy is of value following retroperitoneal lymph node dissection for nonseminomatous testicular tumors. In: *Testis Tumors.* Edited by J. P. Donohue. Baltimore, Williams & Wilkins, 1983.

56. SKINNER, D. G., and SCARDINO, P. T. Relevance of biochemical tumor markers and lymphadenectomy in management of nonseminomatous testis tumors: Current perspective. J. Urol., *123:*378, 1980.

57. BIRCH, R., et al. Prognostic factors for favorable outcome in disseminated germ cell tumors. J. Clin. Oncol., *4:*400, 1986.

58. EINHORN, L. H., et al. A comparison of four courses of cisplatin, VP-16 and bleomycin (PVP₁₆B) in favorable prognosis disseminated germ cell tumors: A southeastern cancer study group (SECSG) protocol. In: Proc. Am. Soc. Clin. Oncol., *7:*120, 1988.

59. DONOHUE, J. P., and ROWLAND, R. G. The role of surgery in advanced testicular cancer. Cancer, *54:*2716, 1984.

60. DONOHUE, J. P., et al. Correlation of computerized tomographic changes and histological findings in 80 patients having radical retroperitoneal lymph node dissection after chemotherapy for testis cancer. J. Urol., *137:*1176, 1987.

61. TIFFANY, P., et al. Sequential excision of residual thoracic and retroperitoneal masses after chemotherapy for stage III germ cell tumors. Cancer, *57:*978, 1986.

62. MANDELBAUM, I., et al. The importance of one-stage median sternotomy and retroperitoneal node dissection in disseminated testicular cancer. Ann. Thorac. Surg., *36:*524, 1983.

63. SEITZ, D. E., et al. Chemotherapeutic approaches to the treatment of testicular cancer. Semin. Urol., *6:*238, 1988.

64. SHIPLEY, W. U. Radiation therapy for patients with testicular and extragonadal seminoma. In: *Testis Tumors.* Edited by J. P. Donohue. Baltimore, Williams & Wilkins, 1983.

65. WILLIAMS, S. D., and EINHORN, L. H. Chemotherapy of disseminated testicular cancer. In: *Testis Tumors.* Edited by J. P. Donohue. Baltimore, Williams & Wilkins, 1983.

66. SCHULTZ, S., et al. Management of post-chemotherapy residual mass in patients with advanced seminoma: Indiana University experience. In: Proc. Am. Soc. Clin. Oncol., *7:*119, 1988.

67. LANGE, P. H., et al. Serum alpha-fetoprotein and human chorionic gonadotropin in patients with seminoma. J. Urol., *124:*472, 1980.

68. MAUCH, P., WEICHSELBAUM, R., and BOTNICK, L. The significance of positive chorionic gonadotropins in apparently pure seminoma of the testis. Int. J. Radiat. Oncol. Biol. Phys., *5:*887, 1979.

69. ROWLAND, R. G., and DONOHUE, J. P. Testicular cancer: Innovations in diagnosis and treatment. Semin. Urol., *6,3:*223, 1988.

70. LANGE, P. H., McINTIRE, K. R., and WALDMANN, T. A. Tumor markers in testicular tumor: Current status and future prospects. In: *Testicular Tumors: Management and Treatment.* Edited by L. E. Einhorn. New York, Masson Publishing, 1980.

71. FRIEDMAN, A., VUGRIN, D., and GOLBEY, R. B. Prognostic significance of serum tumor biomarkers (TM), alpha-fetoprotein (AFP), beta subunit of human chorionic gonadotropin (bHCG), and lactate dehydrogenase (LDH) in nonseminomatous germ cell tumors (NSGCT). In: Proc. Am. Soc. Clin. Oncol., *21:*323, 1980.

CHAPTER
33

Radical
Inguinal
Orchiectomy

James E. Gottesman

Radical inguinal orchiectomy has been the primary diagnostic and therapeutic choice for testicular neoplasms for the last 90 years, having been formally established at the turn of the century by the work of Stinson, Chevasso, and others.[1,2] The rationale for the use of radical orchiectomy as opposed to transcrotal orchiectomy includes the early control of the venous and lymphatic portals, the removal of the surrounding paratesticular fascial layers (where tumor infiltration may be present), and a distinctly lower incidence of scrotal and inguinal recurrences.[3]

Transcrotal orchiectomy, or open testicular biopsy, has been associated with a 24% incidence of recurrence in the scrotum or spread into inguinal lymphatic channels.[4] However, surrounding scrotal or inguinal node involvement is unusual in a properly performed radical inguinal orchiectomy. A recent Testicular Cancer Intergroup study suggested that orchiectomy performed via the scrotal approach does not portend lowered survival rates, if treated with aggressive local surgical salvage and followed closely.[5] However, the potential wound contamination with tumor cells and local recurrence clearly jeopardizes patient care and cannot be recommended. Even for patients who have undergone a previous inguinal or scrotal operation with possible alteration of lymphatic drainage, the radical orchiectomy approach gives the lowest incidence of local tumor recurrence. In addition, operative and perioperative morbidity with radical orchiectomy has been found to be minimal, similar to that associated with a simple hernia repair.

INDICATIONS

Radical orchiectomy is indicated when a tumor of the testicle or paratesticular structures is suspected. To date, preoperative suspicion of the presence of testicular tumor is largely based on physical examination and clinical history. Scrotal ultrasonography may be helpful in suggesting a preoperative diagnosis, but exploration is mandatory if a testicular tumor is suspected.

Assays for testicular tumor markers, human chorionic gonadotropin (β-HCG) and alpha-fetoprotein (α-FP) have become valuable adjuncts in the treatment and followup of testicular tumors. Positive testicular tumor marker assays indicate the presence of a testicular neoplasm. However, many testicular tumors, especially pure seminomas, are not usually associated with elevation of these markers. Because of this, the decision to explore a testicle should not be based on negative results of marker assays alone. In all patients, preoperative markers should be measured as baseline for future reference.

SURGICAL PROCEDURE

The patient is placed in the supine position, and either general or conduction anesthesia is given. Preparation and draping should include the scrotum and the ipsilateral abdomen below the umbilicus (Fig. 33-1). The upper scrotum need not be shaved, unless the tumor is so large (larger than 15 cm) that the inguinal delivery is expected to be a problem.

Incision

The skin incision is made for a length of approximately 8 to 10 cm, just above and parallel to the inguinal ligament (Fig. 33-2); a transverse incision is acceptable and may be cosmetically preferable. The dissection is carried sharply through the subcutaneous fat. The two or three large veins encountered are divided and tied with 3-0 polyglactin (Vicryl) sutures or coagulated.

The external fascia (external oblique aponeurosis) is cleared from the overlying fat, and the external inguinal ring is identified (Fig. 33-3A). The external fascia is generously incised parallel to its fibers through the external ring, after it has been separated from the underlying muscles and nerve (Fig. 33-3B). Incision through the ring is important for later delivery of the testicle. Care is taken to avoid disturbing the ilioinguinal nerve, which is dissected free and isolated above or below the aponeurotic fascia with hemostats (Fig. 33-4A).

Technique

The inferior aspect of the external fascia (Poupart's or inguinal ligament) is elevated with hemostats. Working in the lateral-

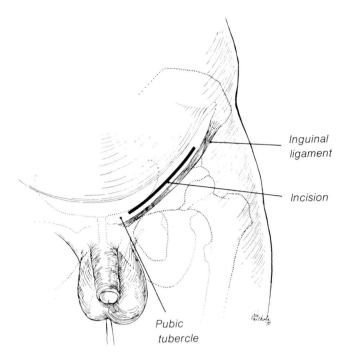

FIG. 33-2. Proposed line of incision parallel to inguinal ligament, approximately 8 cm long.

to-medial direction, the spermatic cord is reflected superiorly off the inguinal ligament with a Kitner (peanut) sponge until the pubic tubercle is clearly identified and cleared from the spermatic cord contents (Fig. 33-4A). The superior aspect of the external fascia is then similarly elevated, and the spermatic cord is reflected inferiorly until the tubercle is once again isolated (Fig. 33-4B). With this technique, all the fascial layers and lymphatics of the spermatic cord, including the cremaster muscle, will be within the Penrose drain, which is then placed around the spermatic cord at the level of the pubic tubercle (Fig. 33-5A).

The spermatic cord is elevated using the Penrose drain for traction and dissected toward the internal ring. A perforating cremasteric vessel is usually identified, divided, and tied as it enters the spermatic cord with a 3-0 Vicryl ligature. The cord is further dissected back to the internal ring. The spermatic cord is then firmly occluded, using a soft rubber-shod clamp or a Penrose drain in tourniquet fashion secured with a hemostat (Figs. 33-5B). The clamp or drain should be applied at least 1 inch from the internal ring, so that division of the spermatic cord at the level of the internal ring does not require release and replacement of the tourniquet effect.

The testicle can then be mobilized through the scrotum and inguinal canal by external upward pressure on the testicle and scrotum (Fig. 33-6). Testicular delivery may be difficult, however, with larger tumors. Inspection of the scrotal-inguinal junction reveals Scarpa's fascia often to be the cause of the difficult mobilization; incision of this fascia usually permits delivery of the testicle. For extremely large testicular tumors,

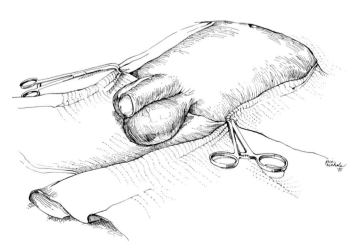

FIG. 33-1. Draping procedure for left radical orchiectomy.

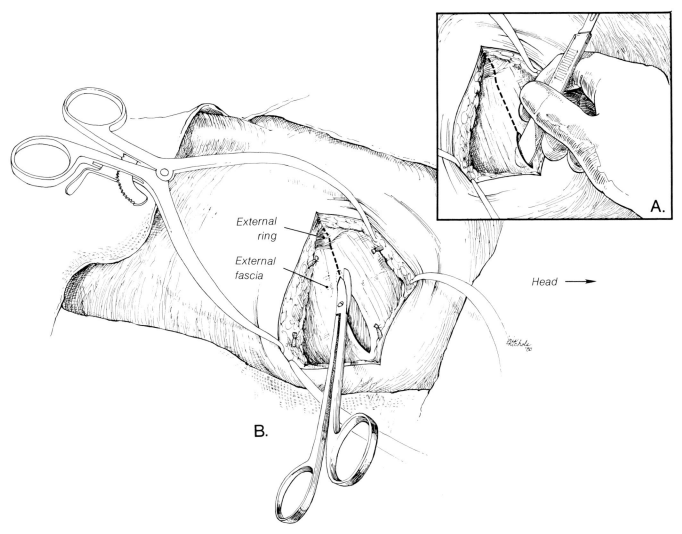

External ring

External fascia

Head →

A.

B.

FIG. 33-3. *A*, The external ring is identified and the fascia is incised. The underlying muscle and nerve are bluntly separated from the fascia. *B*, The fascia is incised along the course of its fibers through the external ring.

an extension of the incision into the upper scrotum may be necessary, but care must be taken not to enter the tunica vaginalis, and to extend the incision only as far as necessary to allow removal of the testicle.

After the testicle has been delivered through the groin incision, upward traction of the testicle is applied. The inferior aspects of the testicle and tunica vaginalis are then clamped and divided from the scrotal skin and superficial fascial investments (Fig. 33-7) and tied with 3-0 Vicryl (Figs. 33-7 and 33-8). The scrotal skin should not be included in the clamps unless the unusual circumstance of scrotal involvement is encountered. If so, a generous portion of scrotum should be removed en bloc with the tumor.

The testicle, now freed inferiorly, is isolated with towels and inspected (Fig. 33-8). If the pathologic nature of the process is in question, biopsy and frozen-section analysis can be performed without danger of contaminating the wound with tumor cells. If the process suggests testicular tumor (grossly or microscopically), the testicle is wrapped securely with

towels and sponges so as not to contaminate the wound, and the orchiectomy is completed (Fig. 33-9).

Attention is turned to the internal inguinal ring, where the anterior medial aspect of the cord is inspected for hernia. If found, the hernia sac must be dissected back to the internal ring. The sac may now be opened and a finger placed within the peritoneal cavity to palpate the regional nodes. The hernia sac is then closed with a 3-0 nonabsorbable synthetic (Nurolon) suture-ligature.

More likely, no hernia sac will be found, and the peritoneum need not be opened, because the information to be gained is usually minimal. The spermatic vessels and vas are then identified and dissected well into the internal ring (Fig. 33-9). The vessels and vas deferens are clamped separately, divided, and tied with 2-0 Nurolon ligatures. Nonabsorbable sutures are essential for this ligature because of the need to identify them if a radical retroperitoneal node dissection is later indicated. The testicle and spermatic cord are then delivered off the wound.

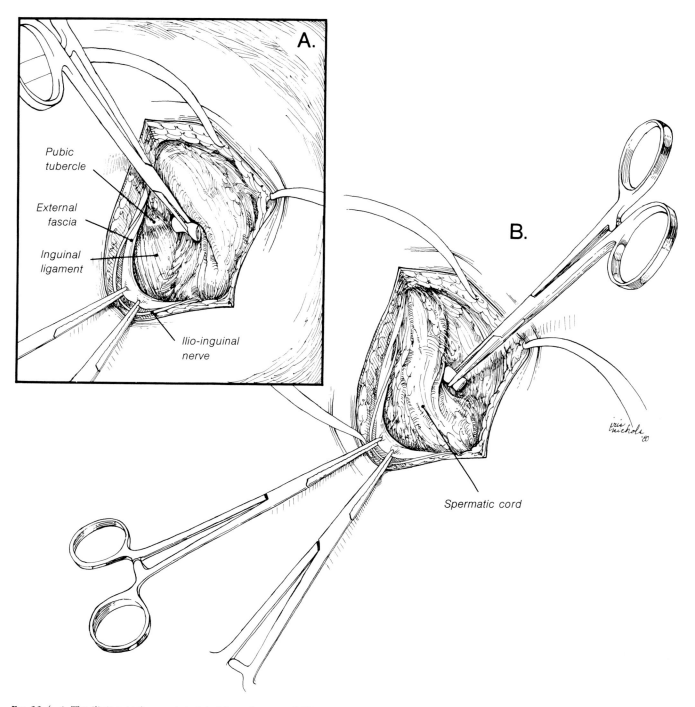

A.

Pubic
tubercle

External
fascia

Inguinal
ligament

Ilio-inguinal
nerve

B.

Spermatic cord

FIG. 33-4. *A,* The ilioinguinal nerve is isolated from the wound. The spermatic cord is reflected superiorly off the inguinal ligament, exposing the pubic tubercle. *B,* Spermatic cord is mobilized inferiorly off the external fascia, again exposing the pubic tubercle.

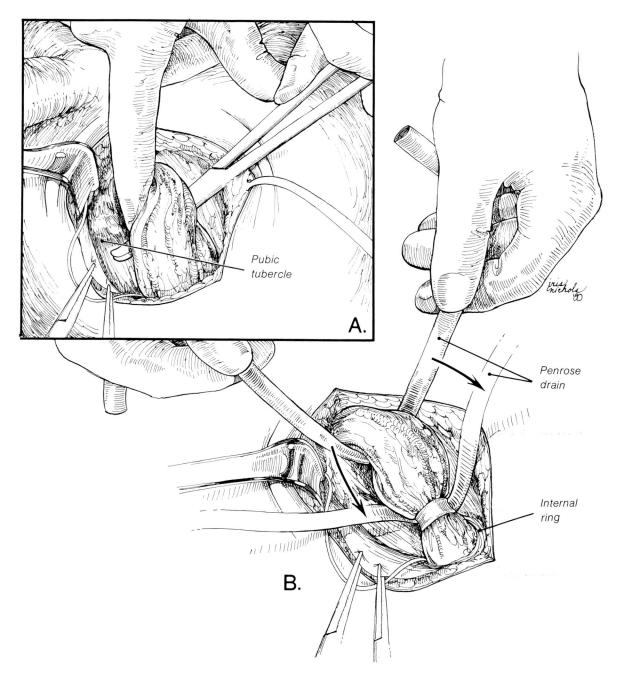

FIG. 33-5. *A*, A Penrose drain is placed around the spermatic cord at the level of the pubic tubercle. *B*, After the cremasteric vessels have been divided, the Penrose drain is doubled around the spermatic cord and clamped securely, 1 inch from the internal ring.

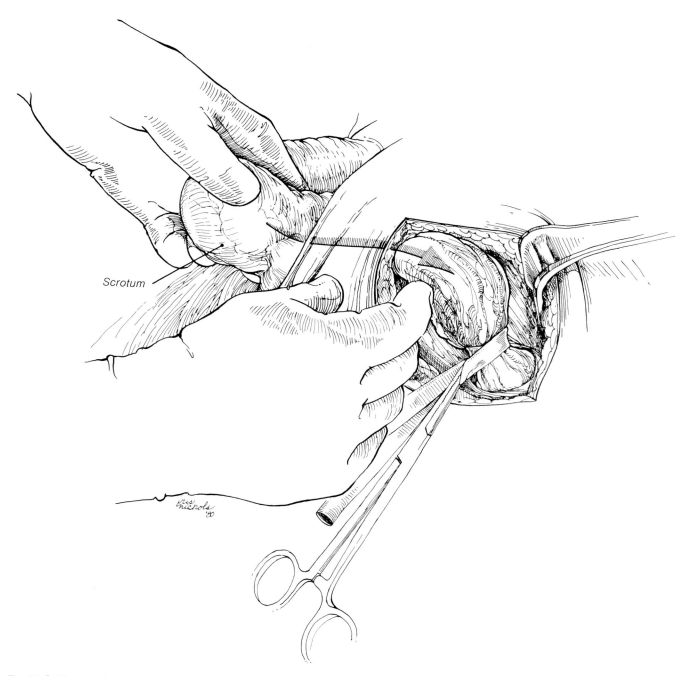

Scrotum

FIG. 33-6. The testicle is delivered into the inguinal incision by external upward pressure on the testicle.

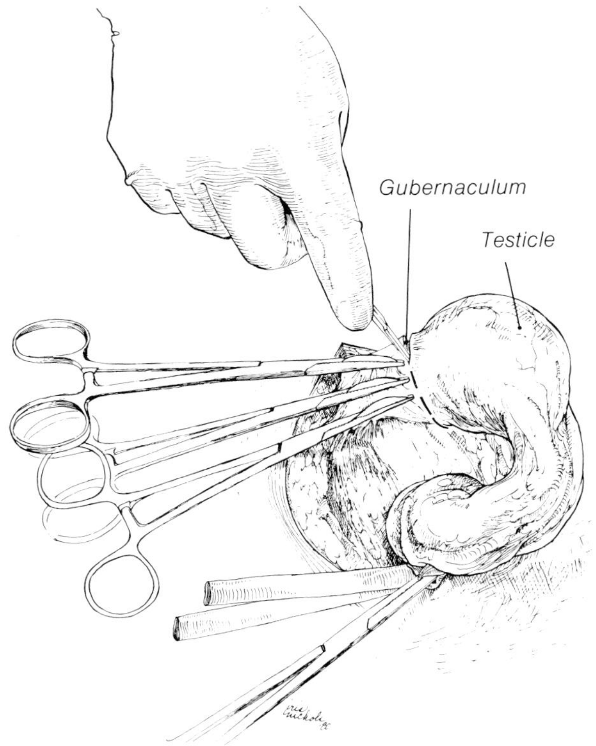

FIG. 33-7. (*Left*) The gubernaculum is divided, freeing the testicle from scrotal investments.

Gubernaculum

Testicle

FIG. 33-8. (*Bottom*) Divided ends of the gubernaculum are tied. The testicle is placed on a clean, sterile towel and isolated from the wound so that it may be inspected and, if indicated, a biopsy should be performed without contamination.

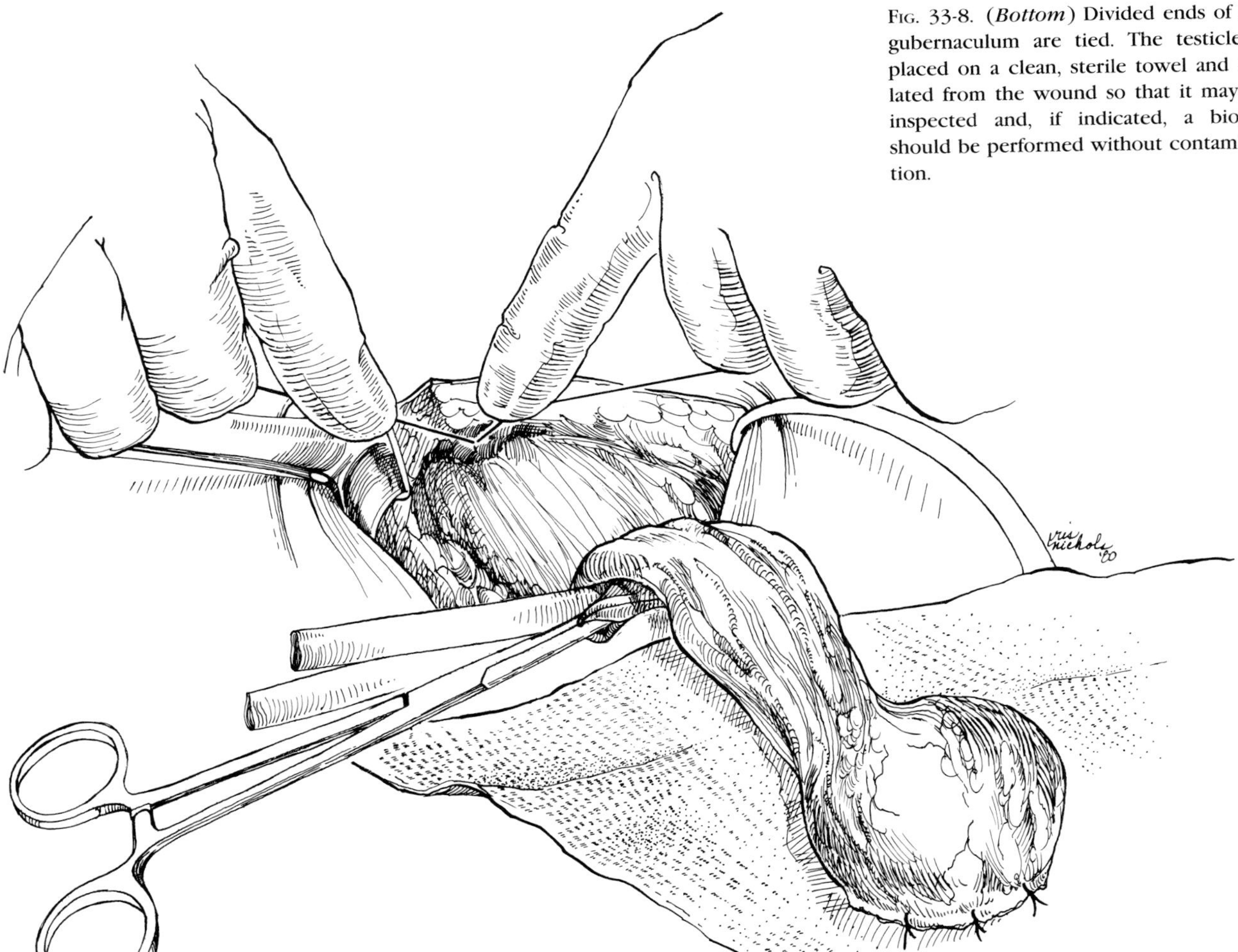

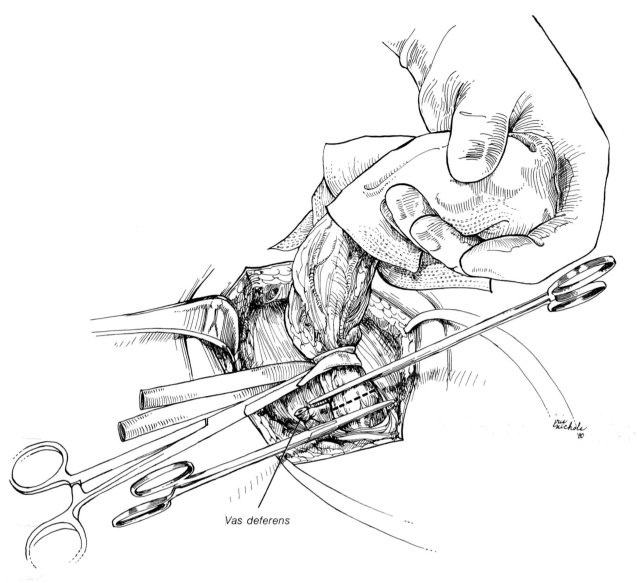

FIG. 33-9. Prior to orchiectomy, the testicle is wrapped with a towel to prevent contamination. The vas deferens and spermatic vessels are individually ligated with nonabsorbable suture.

Closure

Hemostasis is checked, and the wound is irrigated with saline. If the inguinal floor seems somewhat lax, a standard Bassini hernia repair may be done, with the conjoined tendon brought to the shelving edge of the inguinal ligament with interrupted No. 0 Vicryl or No. 0 Nurolon sutures (Fig. 33-10A). If the inguinal floor seems secure, reinforcement is not necessary. The external fascia is closed with interrupted 3-0 Vicryl sutures, and the subcutaneous tissue in heavier individuals is closed with 3-0 Vicryl (Fig. 33-10B). The skin is approximated with clips (Fig. 33-10C) or with a subcuticular running suture of 4-0 Vicryl. A sterile dressing is then applied.

NOTE ON PATHOLOGY

The pathologist should be given specific instructions regarding examination of the specimen. In addition to the testicle and tumor, the pathologist should carefully scrutinize, grossly and microscopically, the peritesticular tissues and cord structures, including the marked ends of the spermatic vessels. Although tumor type is most important; vascular, lymphatic, peritesticular, and cord involvement are important prognostic features that may dictate choice between subsequent aggressive or conservative management.

POSTOPERATIVE CARE

The patient can usually be started on a general diet and ambulation the day of the procedure. Ice packs may be placed on the scrotum to keep swelling to a minimum. Antibiotics are not used routinely. Narcotic pain medication in moderate doses is often needed for the first 24 hours. Oral analgesics with codeine may be needed for the first 4 to 5 days.

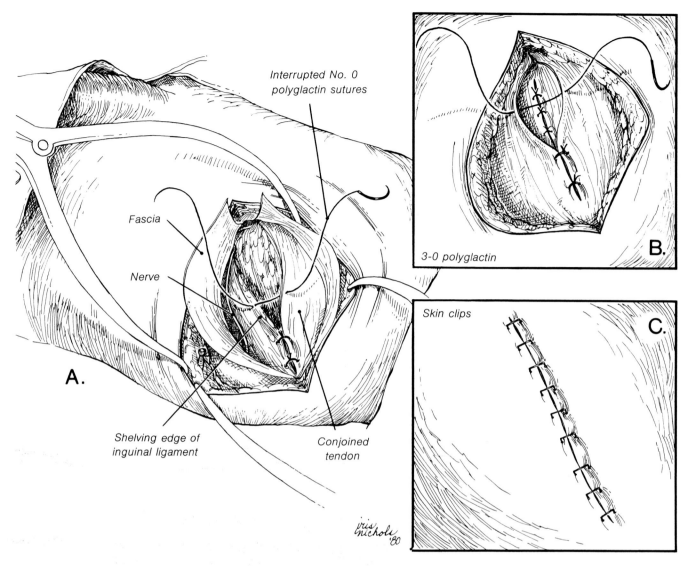

FIG. 33-10. *A*, When the inguinal floor appears lax after the orchiectomy, a formal hernia repair is performed, bringing the conjoined tendon to the inguinal ligament using interrupted No. 0 nonabsorbable synthetic (Nurolon) or No. 0 polyglactin (Vicryl) sutures. *B*, The external fascia is closed with interrupted sutures. *C*, The skin is closed with staples.

REFERENCES

1. Stinson, J. C. A new operation for malignant disease of the testicle—The necessity of a more extensive operation than castration for carcinoma, sarcoma, etc. of the testicle. Med. Rec. Dec., *52*:623, October 30, 1897.
2. Chevasso, M. Le traitement churgical des cancers du testicule. Rev. Chir., *41*:628, 1910.
3. Markland, C. Special problems in managing patients with testicular cancer. Urol. Clin. North Am., *4*:427, 1977.
4. Dean, A. L., Jr. The treatment of teratoid tumors of the testes with radium and x-ray. J. Urol., *13*:149, 1925.
5. Giguere, J. K., et al. The clinical significance of unconventional orchiectomy approaches in testicular cancer: A report from the Testicular Cancer Intergroup Study. J. Urol., *139*:1225, 1988.

Thoracoabdominal Retroperitoneal Lymphadenectomy

P. G. Wise

P. T. Scardino

During the decade of the 1970's, germ cell tumors of the testis yielded to improvements in diagnosis and therapy and in most cases can now be considered a conquered disease. Although the development of effective platinum-based chemotherapy has played the greatest role in this achievement, refinements in both the technique and timing of retroperitoneal dissection have also made an important contribution.

There are three major reasons why retroperitoneal lymphadenectomy remains a cornerstone of the management of patients with nonseminomatous germ cell tumors. First, although the operation is formidable, it can be done safely. Even the loss of ejaculation can be avoided by limiting the dissection to areas of high probability of disease occurrence in low-stage disease. Second, in conjunction with serum alpha fetoprotein and beta chain human chorionic gonadotropin, as well as chest tomograms, the procedure accurately stages the extent of the disease providing the best indication for prognosis. Third, a thorough, proper, meticulous lymphadenectomy can remove all retroperitoneal node-bearing tissue that has a significant risk of harboring metastases, thereby minimizing the risk of local retroperitoneal recurrence.

This chapter reviews the historical origins of retroperitoneal lymphadenectomy, presents the rationale for the procedure, describes the operative technique for a thoracoabdominal approach, and indicates the complications of this procedure. Finally, the merits and results of lymphadenectomy with or without adjuvant chemotherapy are briefly reviewed, and a plan of periodic postoperative evaluations is mentioned. Our focus is on patients with early-stage (A, B1, and B2), nonseminomatous tumors. Patients with advanced disease (B3 or C) are not treated initially with retroperitoneal dissection but rather with intensive combination chemotherapy.

HISTORICAL PERSPECTIVES

Systematic and accurate accumulation of information about the lymphatic drainage of the testes began with the studies of the metastatic deposits of testicular tumors in the retroperitoneum by Most, published in 1898.[1] Building on this early work, Cuneo and Marcille, in 1901, identified four to eight lymphatic channels from each testis, which drain to the periaortic lymph nodes near the renal hilum, the embryologic site of origin of the testis.[2] On the right side, one lymphatic channel drained to the external iliac nodes just below the bifurcation of the common iliac artery. This demonstrates that the lymphatic drainage of the testes is distinct from that of the scrotum, which drains to the inguinal and distal iliac nodes.

Jamieson and Dobson, in 1910, injected dye into the testes of stillborn fetuses and observed the primary site of drainage of each testis.[3] They reported that the dye from the right side drained to the interaortocaval, preaortic, and precaval nodes. Left-sided drainage was primarily to the left para-aortic and pre-aortic nodes.

In the late 1950's and 1960's, using modern radiologic techniques, it was shown that the lymphograms obtained by injecting dye into the lymphatics of the foot did not routinely opacify these lumbar nodes, but funicular injections clearly confirmed Jamieson and Dobson's original work.[4-6] Direct injection of contrast media into the lymphatics of the spermatic cord distinctly shows that there is frequent crossover (especially from the right to the left), retrograde filling of the lower lumbar nodes that occurs bilaterally, and that lymphatic drainage from both testes flows to the thoracic duct and, in most cases, to the left supraclavicular node as well.

Prior to these later studies, even before the turn of the century, surgeons began to extend the field of resection hoping to improve the poor results of orchiectomy when used as the sole treatment for testicular tumors. In 1897, Stinson reported on the use of radical inguinal orchiectomy, which became established as the proper surgical procedure for control of the primary tumor.[7] Kocher performed a transperitoneal exploration but found unresectable nodal metastatic deposits as early as 1883. The first successful transperitoneal resection of large nodal metastases was performed by Roberts in 1902. However, the patient died postoperatively.[8] Cuneo, who as previously mentioned had accurately described the anatomy of the testicular lymphatics, deserves credit for being the first to successfully resect all of the retroperitoneal node-bearing tissue in a patient with positive nodes. This patient remained alive with no evidence of disease for at least 3 years.[9]

In 1907, Howard reported his experience with 36 patients treated by orchiectomy alone for testicular tumors. Fifty percent developed massive retroperitoneal metastases, 75% developed documented recurrent disease, and only 6% of those followed survived.[10] These universally poor results stimulated surgeons to attempt to improve the surgical technique of retroperitoneal lymphadenectomy. Chevassu subsequently modified Cuneo's lateral extraperitoneal approach, and others reported limited success with improvements of this method.[11-13] Surgical extirpation of the retroperitoneal nodes became the cornerstone of therapy in 1948 when Lewis, employing the Hinman operation, reported 192 operations without a single mortality.[14] His 5-year survival rate for 28 patients with nonseminomatous tumors, treated by orchiectomy, retroperitoneal lymphadenectomy, and radiation therapy, was 46%.

The rationale and results thus established, attention was turned to refining the procedure to safely and completely remove all retroperitoneal node-bearing tissue. The limits of

the area of resection were expanded until the dissection included all nodal tissue from the suprarenal regions bilaterally, to the bifurcation of the aorta, from ureter to ureter, in addition to the ipsilateral common iliac nodes. The mapping of the nodal metastasis by Donohue and associates has allowed the reduction of the area of resection without much increase in the risk of recurrence for certain stages of the disease (Fig. 34-1).[15] The following narrative will describe the historical events and procedures that have permitted modern urologists to tailor the field of dissection to the individual patient.

Sweet initially described the thoracic approach for carcinoma of the esophagus just proximal to the gastroesophageal junction.[16] Chute, Soutter, and Kerr adapted this approach for greater exposure in removing renal tumors.[17] Cooper, Leadbetter, and Chute modified the approach to allow for wide exposure of the primary lymphatic drainage of the testes near the renal vessels.[50] Skinner and Leadbetter reported their series of 58 patients in 1971.[18] The average hospital stay was 8 to 10 days, there was only one major operative complication, there were no operative mortalities, and the survival rate was 90% if the nodes were uninvolved and 56% if the nodes were involved.

Extension of the dissection to the contralateral side was difficult using the thoracoabdominal approach described by Cooper and associates. Although their results were satisfactory, anatomic studies and clinical experience pointed to the need for a bilateral (ureter to ureter) dissection should involvement of the contralateral nodes be found at the time of surgery. With his report in 1959, Patton established the infrahilar bilateral dissection with no operative deaths and minimal complications.[19] This was soon followed by accounts of Staubitz and Whitmore and others,[20-21] confirming the efficacy of this approach.

Skinner modified and extended the thoracoabdominal incision to facilitate a complete bilateral dissection, including the ipsilateral suprahilar and contralateral hilar region. This modification is particularly suited for resection of large retroperitoneal masses, but the wide exposure lends itself to a complete resection in the case of early-stage testicular cancer, in which a completely extraperitoneal dissection can be accomplished.[22]

Donohue and associates, however, reported a retroperitoneal recurrence cephalad to the renal vessels in a patient with no involvement of the infrahilar nodes after a bilateral transabdominal dissection. Based on this experience and on the evidence for suprahilar lymphatic drainage from the testis, he developed an extended bilateral transperitoneal approach to include mobilization of the pancreas and bilateral para-aortic suprahilar resection.[23] The results have been excellent, with 93% of patients with no nodal involvement and 67% with involved nodes remaining alive and continuously free of disease after 2 years. Skinner reported a continuously disease-free survival rate of 95% with no nodal involvement, and a 71% survival rate in patients with involved nodes who did not receive chemotherapy, or who received single-agent adjuvant chemotherapy.[24] The transperitoneal infrahilar dissection

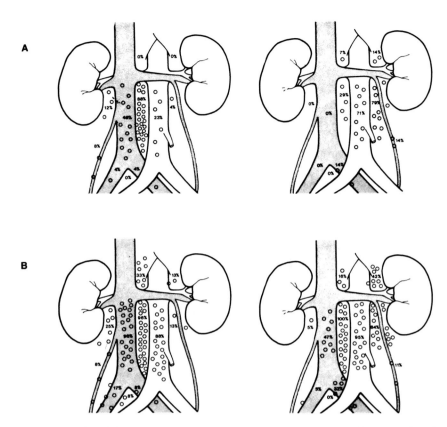

FIG. 34-1. Distribution of retroperitoneal nodal metastases in early-stage, nonseminomatous testicular cancer based on the appearance of the nodes during the operation. *A,* Grossly negative (Stage B1); *B,* Grossly positive (Stage B2). Reproduced with permission from Donohue J. P., Zachary J. M., Maynard B. R.: Distribution of nodal metastases in nonseminomatous testis cancer. J. Urol., *128:*315, 1982. © by Williams & Wilkins, 1982.

remains the most popular procedure used today, but the thoracoabdominal and transperitoneal suprahilar procedures have attracted increasing numbers of adherents, in view of the data indicating a substantial incidence of suprahilar metastases, especially in the presence of grossly involved nodes.[25]

RATIONALE FOR SURGICAL TREATMENT

Surgical resection of metastatic deposits in the retroperitoneal lymph nodes and the lungs was the most effective form of therapy before the era of platinum-based chemotherapy. Survival rates with surgical intervention alone have been excellent in patients with resectable nodal metastases. In 1979, Whitmore reviewed the long-term survival rates of patients treated with orchiectomy and lymphadenectomy and no other therapy. The rate was 63% in patients with nodal disease and 87% in those without nodal disease.[21] Therefore, testicular cancer can be considered one of the few malignant tumors in which a surgical cure can be obtained in patients with metastatic disease. Lymphadenectomy is a cornerstone of effective treatment and not simply a staging procedure in this disease.

With the advent and widespread use of effective chemotherapy, the role of lymphadenectomy needed to be redefined. Questions arose concerning whether or not a radical orchiec-

tomy should be followed by chemotherapy alone rather than retroperitoneal lymphadenectomy. The operative procedure should be retained for the following reasons: effective chemotherapy is associated with considerable morbidity and an occasional mortality (almost all series have reported mortality rates in 1 to 5% of patients treated for advanced disease[26–29]); the acute toxicity (nausea, vomiting, anorexia, weight loss, alopecia, stomatitis, fever, skin rash, and neurotoxicity) rivals, if not exceeds, that of the surgical procedure; the long-term teratogenic and oncogenic effects of the agents currently used in intensive combination chemotherapy are still not well documented; and azoospermia appears to persist for years, if not permanently.[30]

There is currently a large body of literature regarding experience with retroperitoneal lymphadenectomy from many authors in a variety of medical centers, reporting series with low morbidity and virtually no mortality (Table 34-1).[18,20,21,24,25,31,32] The only long-term sequela has been loss of ejaculation. The mechanism of this is not well understood, but probably relates to the sympathetic and hypogastric neurectomy incidental to the procedure. In an empirical effort to develop more limited operations that would remove all of the lymph nodes in low-stage disease yet still leave the contralateral sympathetic chain as well as the nerves that course over

TABLE 34-1. *Morbidity and Mortality Following Thoracoabdominal Retroperitoneal Dissection for Nonseminomatous Testicular Carcinoma.*[45]

PATHOLOGIC STAGE	NUMBER OF PATIENTS	NUMBER OF COMPLICATIONS		NUMBER OF DEATHS
		MAJOR	MINOR	
A	56	3	3	0
B1	12	0	0	0
B2	29	0	0	0
B3	12	2	0	1
C	40	7	3	1

the bifurcation of the aorta that are responsible for ejaculation, several groups have designed various operations to remove all of the lymph nodes in certain anatomic areas at high risk for metastases.[33-35] If the nerves are spared, the risk of loss of the ability to ejaculate is substantially diminished. With the anatomically limited operation we use (Figs. 2A & 2B), all the node-bearing tissue at risk of harboring metastases can be removed and ejaculation preserved in over 85% of patients.[36] Another approach is to identify and preserve the sympathetic ganglia and the fibers that course obliquely along the aorta or that traverse the lateral border of the aorta and form the hypogastric plexus. Donohue et al. and Jewett et al. have shown that in 90% of patients in whom these nerves were preserved, ejaculation was preserved as well.[37,38]

Finally, with the advent and clinical use of rectal probe electroejaculation,[39] the issue of loss of ejaculation, if a thorough retroperitoneal lymph node dissection *is* necessary, should no longer be the determining factor when deciding on a course of therapy for a testicular tumor.

An additional argument raised against retroperitoneal lymphadenectomy concerns the patient with no clinical evidence of metastases after radical orchiectomy, that is, a clinical stage-A patient. Some have suggested that a thorough staging evaluation that includes tumor markers, CT scans, and lymphograms, can reliably detect metastatic disease, so that if the results of these studies are normal, no additional therapy is necessary. The patient would have to be followed closely, and upon progression of the disease, could be treated with full-course chemotherapy with or without retroperitoneal lymphadenectomy.

There are several limitations to this apparently conservative approach. Strict criteria must be met before enrolling a patient in a surveillance protocol. The retroperitoneum is a difficult and somewhat expensive region to monitor. Meticulous staging is mandatory and should include a technically successful lymphogram. The CT scan must be interpreted by experienced personnel and repeated at frequent intervals. The serum tumor-marker levels must decline within their expected half life. Any patient who falls into the high-risk group

pathologically, which includes patients with embryonal carcinoma, tumor extending beyond the tunica albuginea (T2-4), vascular invasion, or lymphatic invasion, will have a risk of progression of approximately 45 to 50%.[40] We believe such patients are not candidates for a surveillance protocol. The patient must be reliable and available to return for frequent CT scans and serum tumor-marker assays. The physician must take responsibility for recalling those individuals who do not return for routine follow-up appointments.

Among the patients who progress and require chemotherapy, most will become infertile, and those that require retroperitoneal lymph node dissection are more likely to lose ejaculation because the margins of dissection will be wider.[41,42]

In the largest series reported to date, the progression rate was approximately 32% at 5 years, indicating that these patients are initially understaged.[43] Approximately 6% of patients whose nodes have been resected and are pathologically negative eventually will have progression of their disease outside of the retroperitoneum. Therefore, 26% of patients considered to have clinical stage A disease, harbor metastases in the retroperitoneal lymph nodes. Among the high-risk group, the percentage approximates 40 to 45%. These are the patients for whom a lymph node dissection can provide more accurate staging and prognostic information.

With several reports of a 100% survival rate for pathologic stage-A disease and 93 to 96% for stages B1 and B2 disease treated with retroperitoneal dissection with adjuvant (or rescue) chemotherapy,[23,24] it seems unwise to abandon this diagnostic and therapeutic procedure, when at least 87% of stage-A patients and 63% of stage-B patients are cured by an operation alone and may never require intensive chemotherapy.

MARGINS OF DISSECTION

Knowing the pattern of lymphatic drainage and consequent metastatic spread from left- and right-sided tumors (see Fig. 34-1) allows the surgeon to plan the margin of the retroperitoneal dissection in each stage of disease. For patients with a residual tumor mass following chemotherapy, or with large (>2 cm) positive nodes, a bilateral ureter to ureter, suprahilar-to-aortic bifurcation dissection, including the ipsilateral common iliac lymph node, should be performed.[44] For patients whose nodes appear negative at the time of surgery, the dissection is designed to remove all the nodes that are at risk of harboring metastases, yet preserve the contralateral sympathetic chain and hypogastric plexus (Figs. 34-2A and 34-2B).

Although similar results can be achieved by either a transabdominal or thoracoabdominal approach, we have preferred the latter. The major advantages of a transabdominal procedure are the ease of the incision and the access it provides to both suprahilar regions. The advantages of the thoracoabdominal incision are the wide exposure of the operative field, access to the ipsilateral lung and mediastinum for palpation and excisional biopsy of suspicious lesions, and a completely extraperitoneal dissection, which decreases the risks of ileus, pancreatitis, and subsequent adhesions.

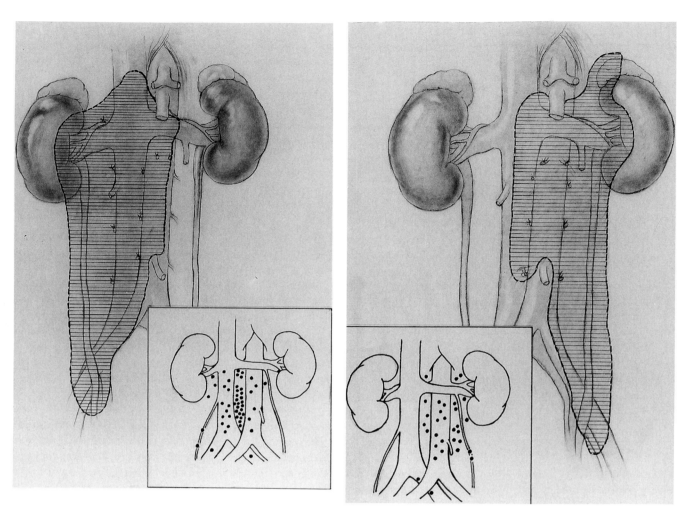

FIG. 34-2. Limits of modified nerve-sparing retroperitoneal lymph node dissection on the right side (*A*) and on the left side (*B*) for patients with grossly negative nodes. The dissection is complete within the anatomic area identified, and designed to remove all nodes likely to contain metastases (see Fig. 34-1) yet preserve the contralateral sympathetic chain and hypogastric plexus. Insets show margins of dissection overlaid on distribution of nodes in Stage B1.

PREOPERATIVE PREPARATION

As soon as the tissue diagnosis is established and the appropriate staging studies are completed, retroperitoneal dissection may proceed. Autologous blood donation (two units) is recommended if the operation will not be unduly delayed. The patient is admitted to the hospital the day before surgery for vigorous hydration. Moderate hypervolemia is induced by administering 5% dextrose in one-half normal saline at 150 ml/hr overnight. This hydration, along with mannitol given intravenously just prior to the dissection of the renal vessels, maximizes renal blood flow and minimizes the risk of arterial thrombosis or renal ischemic injury from vasospasm. For convenience, routine preoperative studies may be carried out the day of admission and should include a complete blood count, electrolyte and creatinine determinations, and a chest X-ray. An enema may be administered for evacuation of the large bowel, but this is not routine. Once the patient is anesthetized, a nasogastric tube and a Foley catheter are placed.

SURGICAL PROCEDURE

General endotracheal anesthesia can be maintained with a variety of safe agents. The anesthesiologist should be forewarned if the patient has been treated with a full course of bleomycin. Though controversial, we believe that it is prudent to avoid high percentages of inspired oxygen. Sodium nitroprusside-induced hypotension has been reported as a successful adjunctive measure to reduce blood loss. With hypotensive anesthesia, the incidence of blood transfusions decreased from 50 to 32%, the transfusion rate decreased from an average of 1.44 units per patient to 0.48, and the mean blood loss from 1341 to 920 ml. This technique was especially helpful for patients with more advanced retroperitoneal disease (Stages

B2 and B3).[45] An epidural catheter may be placed preoperatively for postoperative infusion of analgesics for pain control.

Position

The following text and illustrations describe a left thoracoabdominal incision. The key to success with any incision is proper initial positioning. After the patient has been completely anesthetized, intubated, and a nasogastric tube placed, his torso is brought flush with the left side of the operative table. The soft tissue of the flank, that area between the 12th rib and the iliac crest, lies directly over the break in the table. The hips are kept as flat as possible by triangulation of the right leg, padding all pressure points with pillows or small sections of egg-crate mattress material, and secured to the moveable parts of the table with wide tape (Fig. 34-3A).

The chest is rotated 20 to 30° to the opposite side, and supported by a thin roll of sheets under the left thorax. The left arm is secured to a padded Kraus arm support, which is attached to the right rail of the table (Fig. 34-3B). Free-standing Mayo stands or rigid wooden arm supports cannot easily accommodate necessary changes in the table during the procedure. Another roll is firmly fixed against the right abdomen, caudal to the break in the table, to secure the patient in position.

Incision

Place the incision high enough so that the renal pedicle will be in the center of the operative field. In order to do this, one need not count ribs, but simply choose the rib over which a line drawn will, when carried medially, transect a point midway between the xiphoid and the umbilicus. Before reaching this point, the incision is carried caudally in a paramedian fashion (Fig. 34-3C). With the index and long fingers exerting firm pressure on either side of the rib, the electrocautery is used to divide the muscles directly over the rib. The rib is subsequently resected subperiosteally, whether the eighth, ninth, or tenth (Fig. 34-4).

The anterior rectus sheath is divided and the incision is carried laterally toward the bed of the resected rib. The external and internal oblique muscles are divided with electrocautery. Because the abdominal muscles and diaphragm insert into the ribs or the costochondral junction, the key to developing the retroperitoneal plane is to insinuate the Mayo scissors beneath the costal margin and spread (Fig. 34-5A), then resect this segment of costal margin, allowing the peritoneum to bulge up into the wound. The transversus abdominis muscle is bluntly divided in the direction of its fibers and the rectus muscle is mobilized laterally and divided, leaving only the posterior rectus sheath covering the peritoneum (Fig. 34-5B).

Mobilization of the Peritoneum

The peritoneum is usually firmly attached to the linea alba; however, by careful use of blunt and sharp dissection, the peritoneum can be completely mobilized from the posterior rectus sheath to the midline (Fig. 34-6). With a delicate sweeping motion, palm facing upward, the surgeon separates the peritoneum from the posterior rectus sheath, incising the latter as the mobilization proceeds. With the left hand over a laparotomy pad exerting postero-inferior traction on the peritoneal envelope, and counter traction on the incised edge of the costochondral margin, the peritoneum is mobilized off the diaphragm by gently sweeping the peritoneum posteriorly with the aid of a sponge stick and scissors, for dense adhesions (Fig. 34-7). If the dissection is carried too closed to the peritoneum, it will shred; if it is too close to the diaphragm, troublesome bleeding will result from the incised muscle fibers. This dissection is continued until exposure of the white central tendon of the diaphragm is obtained. The diaphragm is incised in the direction of its fibers to avoid transecting the innervation and vascular supply.

A Finochietto or Fordor retractor is placed so that the cut costal margins will interdigitate with the openings of the blades. Towel clips can be used to secure the margins (Fig. 34-7).

The ipsilateral lung may be palpated for nodules, and any suspicious areas should be excised. The peritoneum is subsequently dissected away from Gerota's fascia. By elevating the peritoneum, an avascular plane can be identified by the fine areolar strands that extend from this structure to Gerota's fascia. This plane is developed until the left renal vein is identified. This maneuver elevates the pancreas and duodenum, allowing for identification of the junction of the renal vein with the inferior vena cava, the superior mesenteric artery, the aorta and the origins of both renal arteries and the entire retroperitoneum. Care must be taken to clip the large retroperitoneal lymphatics that often join the lacteals draining the intestinal tract at this level (Fig. 34-8A). Gerota's fascia, and the kidney within, can be quickly dissected bluntly away from the quadratus lumborum and psoas muscles to the aorta.

Superior Margin of Dissection

The superior mesenteric artery, passing anteriorly over the left renal vein, can be easily identified because it forms the upper limit of mobilization of the tissue anterior to the aorta. The lymphatics overlying the root of the superior mesenteric artery are elevated with a fine, right-angle clamp, secured with clips, and divided (Fig. 34-8). Large lacteals, running parallel with the superior mesenteric artery, can be a source of significant postoperative lymph collection if they are not appropriately ligated. Proceeding posteriorly, the tissue is dissected off the superior mesenteric artery, over the aorta, and down to the left crus of the diaphragm. Inferior traction on the kidney places tension on the band of tissue between the adrenal gland and the aorta. This tissue is clipped and divided, allowing mobilization of the upper pole of the kidney and allowing ready identification of the origin of the left renal artery. The dissection at the base of the superior mesenteric artery is also carried to the right, over the aorta and inferior vena cava, to the

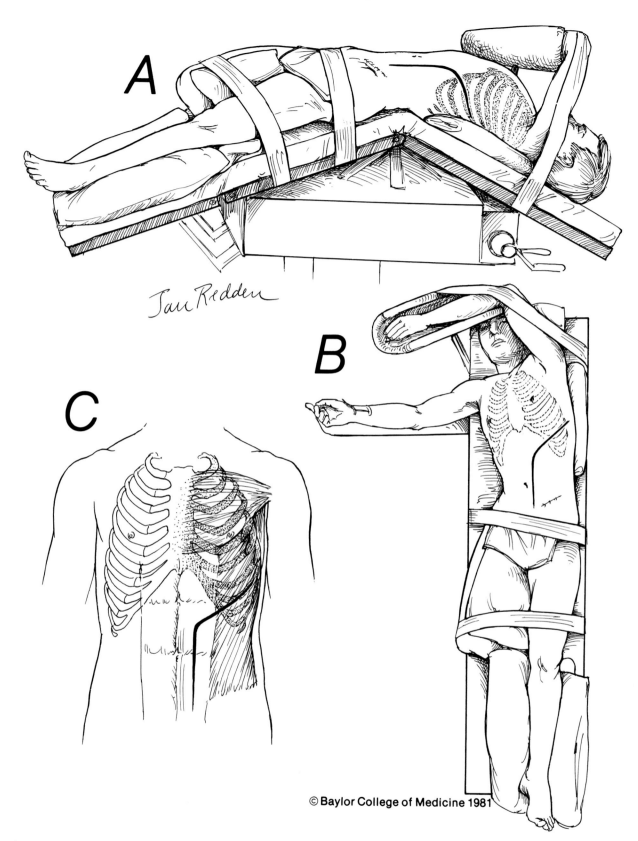

Jan Redden

© Baylor College of Medicine 1981

Fig. 34-3. Position and incision for left thoracoabdominal retroperitoneal lymphadenectomy. A, The soft tissue of the flank is placed directly over the break in the table, with the contralateral leg triangulated and the ipsilateral leg straight. The table is maximally hyperextended. B, The right arm rests on an arm board; the left arm is elevated on a well-padded Kraus support. C, The incision begins over the rib at the left posterior axillary line, is directed towards a point midway between the xiphoid and the umbilicus, and then turns over the abdomen to become a paramedian incision.

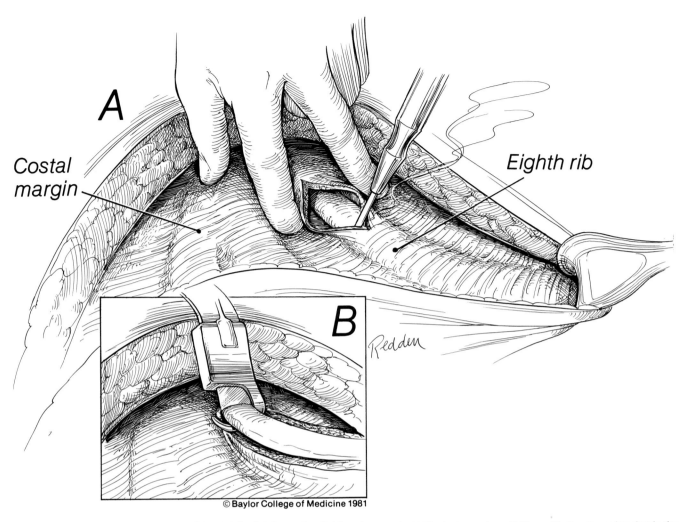

Costal margin

Eighth rib

A

B

Redden

© Baylor College of Medicine 1981

FIG. 34-4. *A*, A subperiosteal excision of the eighth rib is begun by dividing the muscles with electrocautery. *B*, The guillotine is used to divide the rib proximally and distally.

origin of the right renal vein. This completes the superior margin of dissection.

Exposure of the Great Vessels

The tissue overlying the renal vein is divided, and the adrenal and spermatic veins are ligated and divided, allowing the renal vein to be retracted anteriorly, exposing the left renal artery and the aorta. The tissue overlying the aorta is divided longitudinally down to the level of the inferior mesenteric artery (Fig. 34-9). If the lymph nodes are grossly positive, this artery is divided, allowing exposure of the interaorto-caval tissue and the vena cava to the level of the bifurcation of the aorta. The dissection of this tissue is facilitated by inserting a finger between the adventitia of the aorta and the thick envelope of fibroareolar lymphatic tissue. If the lymph nodes appear grossly negative, the right lateral margin of the dissection is the lateral border of the inferior vena cava above the inferior mesenteric artery (Fig. 34-10), and the anterior surface of the

aorta down to the inferior mesenteric artery, leaving the interaortocaval tissue below the inferior mesenteric artery undisturbed, to avoid damage to the sympathetic nerves responsible for emission and ejaculation.

To adequately remove all the tissue from around the aorta, the latter must be completely mobilized by identifying, isolating, ligating, and dividing all of the lumbar arteries from the renal vessels to the bifurcation. Because hemoclips tend to become dislodged during further dissection, 3-0 silk ties are used to ligate the lumbar arteries (see Fig. 34-10).

A bolus of mannitol is given to help protect renal function during the dissection around the renal vessels. Dissection and removal of Gerota's fascia is one technique to ensure complete and safe removal of all the lymph-bearing tissue around the renal hilum. We have found that it is equally possible to remove all of the lymph-bearing adipose tissue medial to the kidney, in the area of the renal hilum, without removing all of Gerota's fascia. On the left side, the ipsilateral adrenal is usually removed because of its intimacy with the lymph nodes in

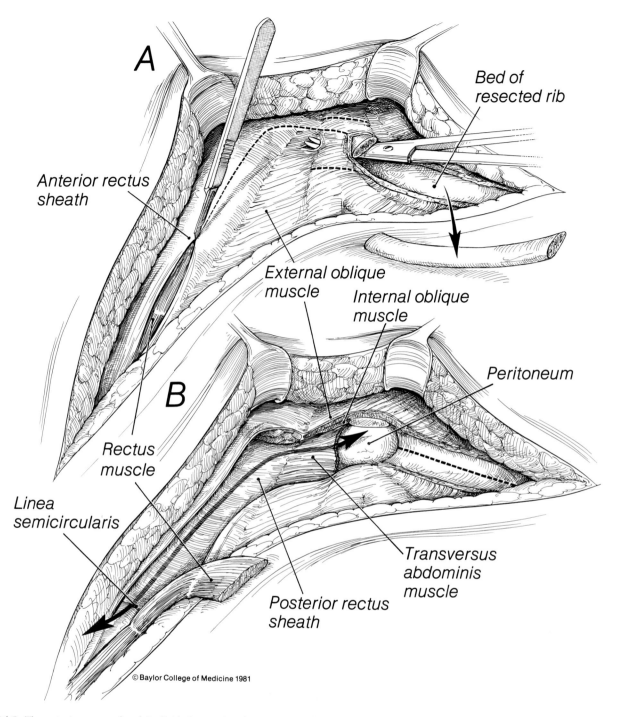

FIG. 34-5. The anterior rectus sheath is divided, exposing the rectus muscle, and the incision is carried laterally to the bed of the resected rib. The Mayo scissors are inserted immediately beneath the costal margin, and a segment of the margin is resected. *B*, The peritoneum immediately bulges through the defect in the costal margin making the extraperitoneal plane evident. The rectus muscle is divided and retracted laterally.

the left suprahilar area. For a right-sided dissection, the adrenal is not removed, to avoid the possible, though rare, incidence of iatrogenic adrenal insufficiency. With the kidney completely mobilized both anteriorly and posteriorly, the lymphatic tissue at the hilum can be dissected away from the renal artery, vein, and pelvis. With these structures in view, the tissue can be split anteriorly and swept posteriorly. The lymph nodes just below the left renal pelvis are the most frequent

sites of metastases from left-sided tumors and must be completely removed.

Dissection Between the Great Vessels

The left renal vein is retracted inferiorly, exposing both the left and right renal arteries (Fig. 34-11). The tissue surrounding these arteries is clipped, divided, and swept inferiorly. The

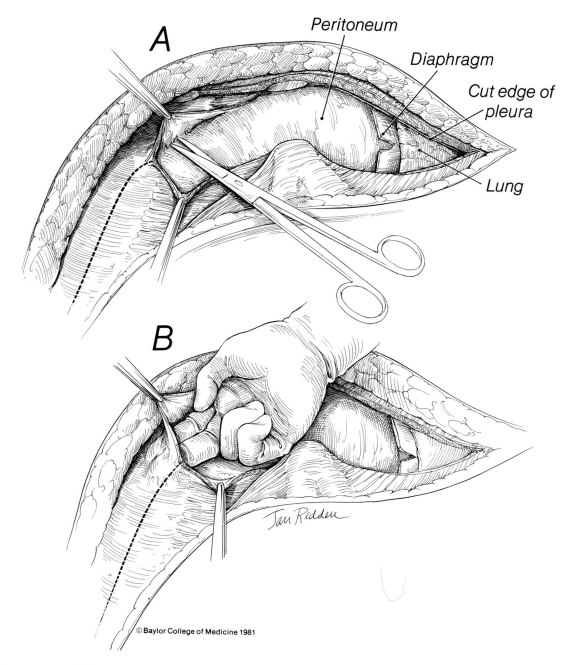

A

Peritoneum

Diaphragm

Cut edge of pleura

Lung

B

Jan Redden

© Baylor College of Medicine 1981

FIG. 34-6. The transversus abdominis is bluntly divided and the posterior rectus sheath is dissected from the peritoneum by sharp (A) and blunt (B) dissection. The periosteum of the rib is divided laterally, entering the pleural cavity and exposing the left lung.

posterior margin of dissection, the white fascial fibers of the prevertebral ligament, is clearly visualized (Fig. 34-12). The left lumbar veins are ligated and divided and the vena cava is rolled to the right, exposing the right lumbar veins. The inter-aortocaval tissue is clipped just medial to the right lumbar veins, sparing the right sympathetic chain in the groove between the psoas muscle and the vertebral column. This packet of tissue is swept inferiorly and to the left, under the completely mobilized aorta, down to the level of the inferior mesenteric artery if the nodes appear negative, or to the bifurcation of the aorta (if the nodes appear grossly positive).

The left sympathetic chain cannot be spared if all of the node-bearing tissue is to be removed (Fig. 34-13A). The ureter is bluntly dissected from the specimen and retracted laterally. The spermatic vessels are traced to the internal inguinal ring, and are removed below the ligature left at the time of radical orchiectomy. Finally, the nodes anterior and lateral to the common iliac artery are removed for approximately 3 to 4 cm distal to the bifurcation of the left iliac artery. The lateral margin of the pelvic dissection is the genitofemoral nerve.

A careful survey of the entire field of dissection is undertaken to assure adequate perfusion of the kidneys, meticulous

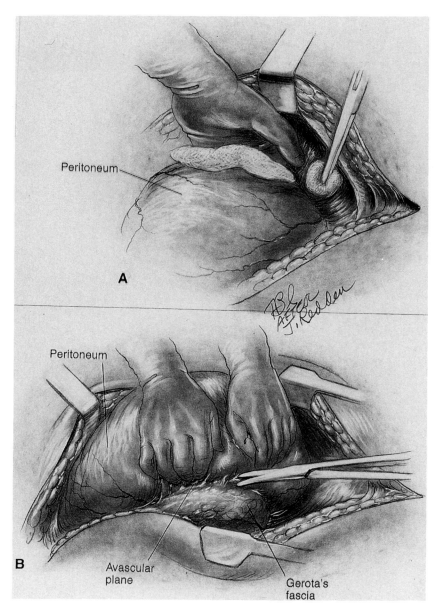

Peritoneum

A

Peritoneum

B

Avascular
plane

Gerota's
fascia

FIG. 34-7. Mobilization of the peritoneum to accomplish an extraperitoneal dissection: *A,* With retraction inferiorly on the peritoneum and superiorly on the costal margin, the diaphragm can be swept off the peritoneum with a moistened sponge stick. *B,* Once the central tendon of the diaphragm is exposed and Gerota's fascia is completely mobilized from the lumbar muscles posteriorly to the level of the aorta, the peritoneum is dissected away from Gerota's fascia anteriorly in the avascular plane.

hemostasis, and secure ligation of all lymphatics, especially at the superior and inferior margins of the dissection (Fig. 34-13).

Closure

Closure is facilitated if the break is taken out of the table. The diaphragm is closed securely in two layers with a running 2-0 polyglycolic acid (Dexon "S") or coated polygalactin (Vicryl) sutures. To prevent prolonged serous drainage from the thoracotomy tube, a watertight closure of the diaphragm is essential. The No. 28 Argyl tube is placed one interspace above or below the incision and positioned with its tip just below the apex of the lung prior to closure of the thoracic portion of the incision.

The thoracic portion of the incision is closed with No. 1 Dexon "S" or coated Vicryl all layer, figure-of-eight, interrupted sutures that are individually placed before any are tied. The three medial sutures pass through the diaphragm, completely sealing the pleura from the retroperitoneal space. The abdominal portion of the incision is closed in layers using interrupted No. 1 Dexon or Vicryl sutures. The transudate from the denuded portion of the retroperitoneum is reabsorbed in a matter of days, therefore, drains to this area are discouraged.

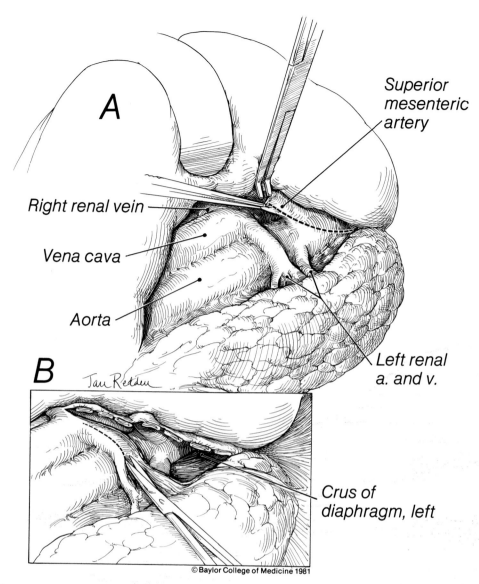

Right renal vein

Vena cava

Aorta

Superior mesenteric artery

Left renal a. and v.

Crus of diaphragm, left

© Baylor College of Medicine 1981

Fig. 34-8. *A*, Once the left renal vein is identified, it leads the surgeon to the aorta and left renal artery posteriorly, and to the superior mesenteric artery superiorly. Dissection is begun at the base of the superior mesenteric artery, where the numerous small lymphatics are clipped and divided to expose the adventitia. The dissection is continued medially along the aorta towards the left crus of the diaphragm. *B*, The superior margin of this dissection must be ligated or clipped with hemoclips to prevent lymphatic leakage. The dissection is continued to the right side over the inferior vena cava to the origin of the right renal vein.

POSTOPERATIVE CARE

Because no intraperitoneal dissection is required, the postoperative ileus resolves rapidly, and the nasogastric tube can usually be removed by the second or third postoperative day.

With the extensive dissection required, the large denuded surface of the retroperitoneum results in third-space fluid loss comparable to that seen with severe pancreatitis or a large third-degree burn. To maintain normal intravascular volume, these patients require massive infusions of albumin solution and saline. The typical patient will receive 3000 to 4000 ml of saline and 1000 to 1500 ml of 5% albumin (but no blood products) during the operation. Postoperatively, the 5% dextrose and saline infusion is continued at the rate of 150 ml/hr and 5% albumin is infused at 50 ml/hr for 18 to 24 hours and gradually tapered.

Volume status is adequately monitored by measurements of the hematocrit, vital signs, and urine output. By the third postoperative day, the urine output will increase significantly, signalling the resorption of the large third-space fluid load and parenteral fluids are, therefore, curtailed. Central venous and arterial lines are helpful adjuncts in patients with massive abdominal disease, but are not mandatory in young, generally healthy patients with minimal disease.

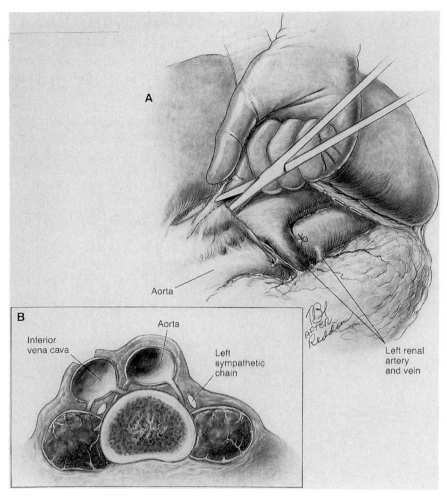

FIG. 34-9. Exposure of the great vessels. *A*, The adrenal and spermatic venous branches of the left renal vein are divided so that the vein can be retracted inferiorly and the origin of the left renal artery identified. The node-bearing tissue over the aorta is divided inferiorly to the inferior mesenteric artery. *B*, This cross-sectional view below the renal hilum illustrates the dissection.

The tube thoracostomy is connected to a closed, vented suction, at 15 to 20 cm negative water pressure. A chest film is obtained in the recovery room to assure proper placement of the tube, and full expansion of the lung. When the drainage has decreased to less than 100 ml per day, and no fluid or pneumothorax is evident on the chest x-ray, the tube is removed; usually on the second or third postoperative day. The hospital stay ranged from 5 to 49 days in one series, with a mean of 11.2 days.[46] For those patients without complications, the mean stay was 9.6 days.

COMPLICATIONS

This approach has been used in patients ranging in age from 15 to 65 years, with a surprisingly low complication rate. The most frequent intraoperative complication, though rare, has been injury to the renal vessels, which can almost always be repaired, avoiding a nephrectomy. Meticulous dissection of

the tissue around the renal hilum may result in vasospasm, which, if severe, could lead to parenchymal ischemia or arterial thrombosis. Vigorous preoperative and intraoperative volume expansion with albumin and mannitol, as previously mentioned, can be supplemented with direct irrigation of the artery with lidocaine or papaverine, to prevent or reverse the vasospasm.

Major injury to the renal vein can usually be repaired and nephrectomy is seldom necessary. Bleeding from an avulsed lumbar vessel may occur, but can be avoided by individual ligation of each pair distal to the renal vessels. Fine cardiovascular suture such as 5-0 polypropylene (Prolene), and delicate Allis forcep clamps, should be available to repair defects in the major vascular structures, which can occur if small vascular branches are avulsed during the dissection.

Major postoperative complications, including wound infection, prolonged atelectasis or pneumonia, prolonged thoracotomy tube drainage, prolonged ileus, and minor complications

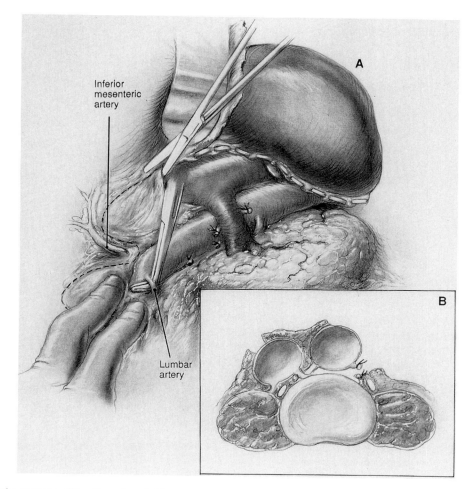

FIG. 34-10. Defining the margins of the dissection: *A*, The superior margin of dissection has been established. The tissue along the right lateral border of the vena cava is clipped and divided inferiorly to the level of the inferior mesenteric artery (IMA). Mobilization of the aorta requires ligation and division of all lumbar arteries between the renal artery and the IMA. Below the IMA only the left lumbar arteries are divided. *B*, Cross-sectional view.

have been reported in 6 to 8% of patients.[20,47] Delayed bleeding, lymphoceles, thrombophlebitis, and pulmonary emboli have been rare.

In over 900 reported cases, there has been only one operative death. This was caused by a pulmonary embolus 3 weeks after the procedure.[48]

ADJUVANT CHEMOTHERAPY AND FOLLOW-UP

There is no evidence that adjuvant chemotherapy, particularly low-dose chemotherapy, will substitute for an incompletely performed retroperitoneal lymphadenectomy in which tumor-containing lymph nodes have been left behind. For patients in whom the lymph nodes are negative after a complete retroperitoneal dissection, the recurrence rate has been reported as 6%.[23] These patients require no further therapy.

For patients with positive lymph nodes, we recommend two courses of cisplatin and etoposide. The Intergroup study, sponsored by the National Cancer Institute, showed that the relapse rate in such patients can be reduced from 47 to 3% with short-course chemotherapy (cisplatin, bleomycin, and vinblastin).[49]

Whether or not adjuvant chemotherapy should be given to these patients is a matter of judgement. The advantages include a reduced recurrence rate and low morbidity compared to intensive rescue chemotherapy regimens. Mortality is comparable whether adjuvant or rescue chemotherapy is used. The major disadvantage is the exposure of all patients to agents that only some patients need. It has not been demonstrated that the use of short-course adjuvant chemotherapy diminishes the response rate to intensive combination chemotherapy for patients who recur.

After definitive treatment for early-stage tumors, the patients must be monitored carefully and regularly. We perform a physical examination, with special attention to the supraclavicular nodes, the breasts, the abdomen, and the contralateral

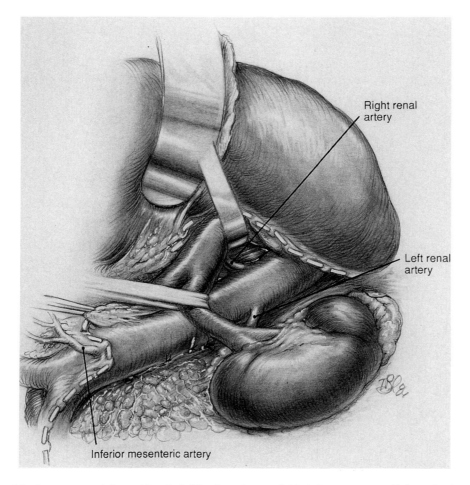

FIG. 34-11. Dissection of the interaortocaval tissue. After the left lumbar veins are divided, the vena cava and left renal vein are retracted to expose the right renal artery. Once this artery is freed, the tissue just superior to it can be mobilized as a packet, clipped, divided, and swept inferiorly along the prevertebral fascia.

testis, every 2 months for the first year, every 3 months for the second year, every 4 months for the third year, every 6 months for the fourth and fifth years, and annually thereafter. Serum determinations of beta-HCG and alpha-fetoprotein are assayed and a chest roentgenogram is obtained at each of these office visits. Other studies are performed as indicated. All patients are instructed to perform self-examination of the testis at monthly intervals up to age 50.

Acknowledgment

We are grateful for the editorial assistance of Carolyn Schum, M.A., Medical Editor, Scott Department of Urology.

REFERENCES

1. Most, I. Ueber maligne Hodengeschwulste und ihre Metastaten. Arch. Pathol. Anat. Phys. Klin. Med., *154:*138, 1898.
2. Cuneo, B., and Marcille, M. Topographie des ganglions iliopelviens. Bull. Soc. Anat. (Paris) 6s, III, 653, 1901.
3. Jamieson, J. K., and Dobson, J. F. The lymphatics of the testicle. Lancet, *1:*493, 1910.
4. Busch, F., Sayegh, E., and Cheanult, O. Some uses of lymphangiography in the management of testicular tumors. J. Urol., *93:*490, 1965.
5. Chiappa, S., et al. Combined testicular and foot lymphography in testicular carcinoma. Surg. Gynecol. Obstet., *123:*10, 1966.
6. Wahlquist, L., Hulten, L., and Rosencrantz, M. Normal lymphatic drainage of the testis studied by funicular lymphography. Acta Chir. Scand., *132:*454, 1966.
7. Stinson, J. C. A new operation for malignant disease of the testicle— The necessity of a more extensive operation than castration for carcinoma, sarcoma, etc. of the testicle. Med. Rec., *52:*623, 1897.

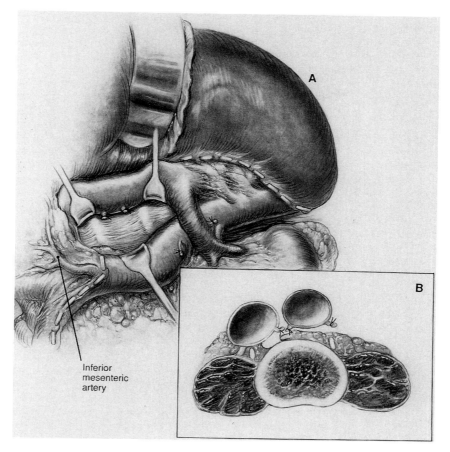

Inferior
mesenteric
artery

Fig. 34-12. *A,* The lateral margin of the dissection is established beneath the vena cava by clipping and dividing just to the left of the right lumbar veins. The interaortocaval and periaortic tissue can then be passed beneath the mobilized aorta. *B,* The tissue anterior, medial, and posterior to the vena cava is taken, but the right sympathetic chain and right lumbar veins are left intact. All of the interaortocaval tissue is removed down to the level of the inferior mesenteric artery. The aorta is lifted anteriorly, allowing the specimen to be passed beneath it as the dissection continues along the prevertebral fascia.

8. ROBERTS, J. B. Excision of the lumbar lymphatic nodes and spermatic vein in malignant disease of the testicle. Ann. Surg., *36:*539, 1902.

9. DEW, H. R. *Malignant Disease of the Testicle: Its Pathology, Diagnosis, and Treatment.* New York, Hoeber, 1926.

10. HOWARD, R. J. Malignant disease of the testis. Practitioner, *79:*794, 1907.

11. HINMAN, F. The operative treatment of tumor of the testicle. JAMA, *63:*2009, 1914.

12. HINMAN, F., JOHNSON, C. M., and CARR, J. L. The clinicopathologic classification of tumors of the testis in relation to prognosis. Trans. Am. Assoc. Genitourin. Surg., *34:*211, 1941.

13. YOUNG, H. H. Neoplasms of the urogenital tract. In *Young's Practice of Urology.* Volume 1. Edited by H. H. Young and D. M. Davis. Philadelphia, W. B. Saunders Co., 1926.

14. LEWIS, L. G. Radical orchiectomy for tumors of the testis. JAMA, *137:*828, 1948.

15. DONOHUE, J. P., ZACHARY, J. M., and MAYNARD, B. R. Distribution of nodal metastases in nonseminomatous testis cancer. J. Urol., *128:*315, 1982.

16. SWEET, R. H. Carcinoma of the esophagus and the cardiac end of the stomach. JAMA, *135:*84, 1971.

17. CHUTE, R., SOUTTER, L., and KERR, W. S. JR. Value of thoracoabdominal incision in removal of kidney tumors. N. Engl. J. Med., *241:*951, 1949.

18. SKINNER, D. G., and LEADBETTER, W. F. The surgical management of testis tumors. J. Urol., *106:*84, 1971.

19. MALLIS, N., and PATTON, J. F. Transperitoneal bilateral lymphadenectomy in testis tumors. J. Urol., *80:*501, 1971.

20. STAUBITZ, W. J., EARLY, K. S., MAGOSS, I. V., and MURPHY, G. P. Surgical management of testis tumors. J. Urol., *111:*205, 1974.

21. WHITMORE, W. F., JR. Surgical management of adult germinal testis tumors. Semin. Oncol., *6:*55, 1979.

22. SKINNER, D. G. Considerations for management of large retroperitoneal tumors: use of the modified thoracoabdominal approach. J. Urol., *117:*605, 1977.

23. DONOHUE, J. P., EINHORN, L. H., and WILLIAMS, S. D. Is adjuvant chemotherapy following retroperitoneal lymph node dissection for nonseminomatous testis cancer necessary? Urol. Clin. North Am., *7:*747, 1980.

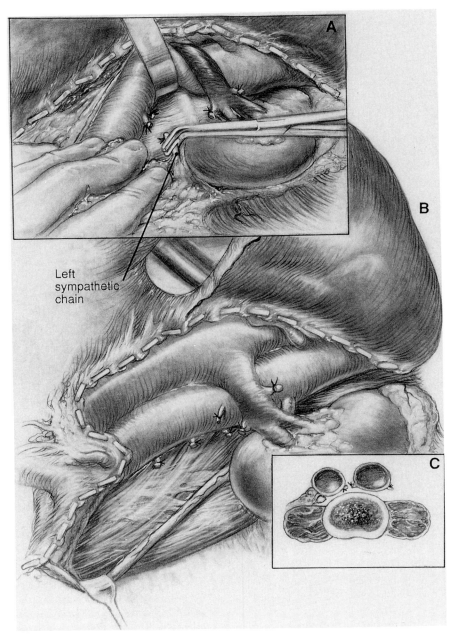

Fig. 34-13. Completion of the dissection: *A,* The small perforating vessels along the left paravertebral groove must be clipped as the specimen is removed. The left sympathetic chain cannot be spared if all of the periaortic nodes are to be removed. *B,* Overview and *C,* cross-section of the field after the specimen is removed.

24. SKINNER, D. G., and SCARDINO, P. T. Relevance of biochemical tumor markers and lymphadenectomy in management of nonseminomatous testis tumors: Current perspective. J. Urol., *123*:378, 1980.

25. DONOHUE, J. P. Surgical management of testicular cancer. In *Testicular Tumors: Management and Treatment.* Edited by L. H. Einhorn. New York, Masson Publishing USA, Inc., 1980, p. 29.

26. EINHORN, L. H., and DONOHUE, J. P. Combination chemotherapy in disseminated testicular cancer: The Indiana University experience. Semin. Oncol., *6*:87, 1979.

27. SAMSON, M. D., et al. Vinblastine, bleomycin and cisdichlorodiammine-platinum (II) in disseminated testicular cancer: Preliminary report of a Southwest Oncology Group Study. Cancer Treat. Rep., *63*:1663, 1979.

28. ANDERSON, T., et al. Chemotherapy for testicular cancer: Current status of the National Cancer Institute combined modality trial. Cancer Treat. Rep., *63*:1687, 1979.

29. SAMUELS, M. L., et al. Combination chemotherapy in germinal cell tumors. Cancer Treat. Rev., *3*:185, 1976.

30. THACHIL, J. V., JEWETT, M. A. S., and RIDER, W. D. The effects of

cancer and cancer therapy on male fertility. J. Urol., *126:*141, 1981.

31. Lewis, L. G. Radioresistant testis tumors: Results in 133 cases: five-year followup J. Urol., *69:*841, 1953.

32. Johnson, D. E., Bracken, R. B., and Blight, E. M. Prognosis for pathologic stage I nonseminomatous germ cell tumors of the testis managed by retroperitoneal lymphadenectomy. J. Urol., *116:*68, 1976.

33. Fossa, S. D., et al. Unilateral retroperitoneal lymph node dissection in patients with nonseminomatous testicular tumor in clinical stage I. Eur. Urol., *10:*17, 1984.

34. Pizzocaro, G., Salvione, R., and Sanoni, F. Unilateral lymphadenectomy in interoperative stage I nonseminomatous germinal testis cancer. J. Urol., *134:*485, 1985.

35. Weissbach, L., Boedefeld, E. A., and Oberdorster, W. Modified RLND as a means to preserve ejaculation. In *Testicular Cancer.* Edited by S. Koury et al. New York, Alan R. Liss, 1985.

36. Scardino, P. T. The extent of retroperitoneal lymph node dissection for nonseminomatous testicular cancer. Presented at the International Symposium on Therapeutic Progress in Urological Cancers, Paris, June 29–July 1, 1988.

37. Donohue, J. P. et al. Preservation of ejaculation following nerve-sparing retroperitoneal lymphadenectomy (RPLND). J. Urol., *139:*206A, 1988.

38. Jewett, M. A., et al. Retroperitoneal lymphadenectomy for testis tumor with nerve sparing for ejaculation. J. Urol., *139:*1220, 1988.

39. Shaban, S. F., Seager, S. W. J., and Lipshultz, L. I. Clinical electroejaculation. Med. Instrum., *22:*77–81, 1988.

40. Scardino, P. T., and Wise, P. G. Thoracoabdominal retroperitoneal lymphadenectomy for testicular cancer. In *Diagnosis and Management of Genitourinary Cancer,* 2nd Edition. Edited by D. G. Skinner and G. Lieskovsky. Philadelphia, W. B. Saunders Co., 1987, pp. 779–801.

41. Pizzicaro, G., Salvoni, R., and Zanomi, F. Surveillance or lymph node dissection in clinical stage I nonseminomatous germinal testis cancer. Br. J. Urol., *57:*759, 1985.

42. Sogani, P. C., et al. Orchiectomy alone in the treatment of clinical stage I nonseminomatous germ cell tumor of the testis. J. Clin. Oncol., *2:*267, 1984.

43. Freedman, L. S., et al. Histopathology in the prediction of relapse of patients with stage I testicular teratoma treated by orchiectomy alone. Lancet, *2:*294, 1987.

44. Wise, P. G., and Scardino, P. T. Thoracoabdominal retroperitoneal lymphadenectomy for non-seminomatous testicular cancer. Urol. Clin. North Am., *10:*371, 1983.

45. Stirt, J. A., Korn, E. L., and Reynolds, R. C. Sodium nitroprusside-induced hypotension in thoraco-abdominal radical retroperitoneal lymph node dissection. Br. J. Anaesth., *52:*1045, 1980.

46. Skinner, D. G., Melamud, A., and Lieskovsky, G. Complications of thoracoabdominal retroperitoneal lymph node dissection. J. Urol., *127:*1107, 1982.

47. Einhorn, L. H., and Williams, S. D. The management of disseminated testicular cancer. In *Testicular Tumors: Management and Treatment.* Edited by L. H. Einhorn. New York, Masson Publishing USA, Inc., 1980, p. 117.

48. Scardino, P. T. Thoracoabdominal retroperitoneal lymphadenectomy for testicular cancer. In *Genitourinary Cancer Surgery.* Edited by E. D. Crawford and T. A. Borden. Philadelphia, Lea & Febiger, 1982, pp 271–289.

49. Williams, S. D., et al. Immediate adjuvant chemotherapy versus observation with treatment at relapse in pathological stage II testicular cancer. N. Engl. J. Med., *317:*1433, 1987.

50. Cooper, J. F., Leadbetter, W. F., and Chute, R. The thoraco-abdominal approach for retroperitoneal gland dissection: Its application to testis tumors. Surg. Gynecol. Obstet., *90:*486, 1950.

Anterior Transabdominal Approach for Radical Retroperitoneal Lymphadenectomy: Anatomy and Nerve-Sparing Technique

Paul H. Lange
Michael K. Brawer

RETROPERITONEAL NEUROANATOMY

To understand the relationship between the retroperitoneal lymphadenectomy (RPL) and the preservation of ejaculation, one must first understand the relevant neuroanatomy (Fig. 35-1).[1] Emission is mediated by sympathetic fibers from the T12 to L3 thoracolumbar spinal cord. These nerve fibers travel within the lumbar sympathetic trunk and leave the trunk at all spinal levels within the midretroperitoneum as peripheral nerve rami (usually called lumbar splanchnic nerves). They contain both preganglionic and postganglionic fibers. The lumbar splanchnic

nerves converge toward the midline over the lower abdominal aorta forming the superior hypogastric plexus, which is variably located anterior to the lower aorta below the inferior mesenteric artery and/or below the aortic bifurcation. The sympathetic fibers leave the hypogastric plexus and travel within the pelvic nerves to innervate the vas deferens, seminal vesicles, prostate, and bladder neck. The aforementioned neuroanatomy controls emission, which is different from ejaculation. Emission implies the delivery of semen into the proximal urethra whereas ejaculation involves the propulsion of semen from the posterior urethra. Ejaculation is mediated by combined autonomic and somatic innervation originating at the

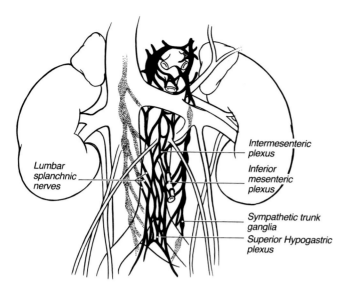

FIG. 35-1. Neuroanatomy of the sympathetic fibers controlling ejaculation.

Labels in figure:
Lumbar splanchnic nerves
Intermesenteric plexus
Inferior mesenteric plexus
Sympathetic trunk ganglia
Superior Hypogastric plexus

sacral and lumbar spinal cord levels. Sympathetic fibers tighten the bladder neck region, while pudendal somatic innervation from S2 to S4 causes relaxation of the external urethral sphincter and rhythmic contraction of the bulbocavernosus and ischiocavernosus muscles. Afferent impulses for emission and ejaculation are mediated by stimulation of the pudendal nerves by touch or vibration. In this chapter, ejaculation will be used to describe both emission and ejaculation. However, the reader should realize that in most cases, the threat to fertility that occurs with RPL results from damage to the neuropathways controlling emission.

To avoid damage to emission, one must understand the detailed neuroanatomy of the lumbar sympathetic trunk and splanchnic nerves. These nerves leave the sympathetic chain at variable levels within the midretroperitoneum. Some of the nerves leave to join a series of plexus anterior to the aorta between the superior and inferior mesenteric arteries. These nerves are usually within the field of dissection and sacrificed. Additional lumbar splanchnic nerves leave the lumbar sympathetic trunk and join the nerve plexus at or below the inferior mesenteric artery or anterior and posterior to the aortic bifurcation and proximal common iliac vessels to join the superior hypogastric plexus. These obliquely directed lumbar splanchnic nerves are the ones that can be preserved during RPL within the field of dissection.

The lumbar sympathetic trunk is located in a groove between the psoas muscle and vertebral column. It lies beneath the inferior vena cava on the right side and below the lateral edge of the aorta on the left side. There is considerable variation in the number and location of ganglia among individuals and there may be asymetry within the same man. The lumbar sympathetic trunk is usually well out of "harm's way" but is still susceptible to injury, especially when gaining hemostasis of the lumbar arteries and veins. These vessels course posterior and medial to the trunk but may pass anterior or posterior

to it. At the renal hilum, the relationship between the lumbar vessels and the sympathetic trunk can be used to identify the latter. At the renal hilum, two large lumbar veins exit the vena cava and course posteriorly and just medial to the sympathetic trunk and usually to the second lumbar ganglia. The right lumbar vein enters the inferior vena cava immediately caudal to the junction with the renal veins. The left lumbar vein usually joins the inferior border of the left renal vein near its junction with the spermatic vein. As will be discussed, the lumbar splanchnic nerves can be initially identified by locating them as they converge onto the lower aorta or by first finding the sympathetic trunk at the level of the renal hilum or below and tracing the nerves inferiorly, or a combination of both maneuvers. It is best to ligate and divide the lumbar veins early at the level of the inferior vena cava and left renal vein and then carefully follow their course posteriorly until the sympathetic trunk is located. The trunk can also be located by palpation because it is a hard cord-like structure similar in consistency to the vas deferens. Once identified, the trunk and many of the lumbar splanchnic nerves can be dissected from the lymphatic tissue. During this stage, it is imperative that the lumbar arteries and veins not be injured as they enter the back because in the process of achieving hemostasis, the sympathetic trunk may be injured.

RPL and Fertility

Opinions about the effect of lymphadenectomy on fertility have changed dramatically over the last 6 years. Previously, there was unanimous agreement in the literature that most of the patients who underwent RPL were rendered infertile because the procedure, of necessity, damaged the sympathetic nerve fibers involved in ejaculation. This perceived morbidity was the major impedence behind initiation of expectant therapy trials for patients with clinical stage-I disease. With the recent modification of lymphadenectomy techniques, a high percentage of men who undergo the operation for clinical stage-I disease can expect preservation of ejaculation.[1]

The two major factors in the preservation of ejaculation following lymphadenectomy are (1) adherence to certain surgical boundaries of dissection, thus avoiding potential injury to the nerves, and (2) meticulous dissection of the lumbar splanchnic nerves within the field of lymphadenectomy. The identification and dissection of nerves will be discussed in detail subsequently. The rationale for the surgical boundaries, their description, and their indications is discussed here.

Over the years, it has become evident that limiting the lymphadenectomy to a unilateral dissection will leave neuropathways significantly intact to preserve ejaculation in up to 75 to 90% without compromising cure in patient with no visible disease at surgery. Our boundaries for the modified unilateral lymphadenectomy are illustrated in (Fig. 35-2). Several comments about these boundaries are important:

1. Experts' opinions vary slightly in the exact limits of dissection, but the basic principles emanate from (1) previ-

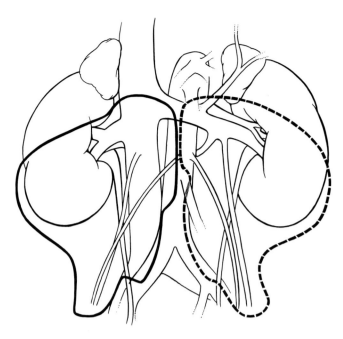

Fig. 35-2. Anatomic boundaries or right- and left-sided retroperitoneal lymph node dissection.

ous careful mapping studies that identified the location of metastasis for each clinical stage, and (2) the anatomy of the lymphatic drainage of the testes. The right testicular lymphatics drain to the midline and to the left side as it ascends, whereas the left testis drains to the region of the left renal vein and stays to the left of the aorta, unless blocked by cancer.

2. The neuroanatomy of ejaculation reveals that the most important areas to preserve are the final common pathways of the lumbar splanchnic nerves as they join the superior hypogastric plexus. Therefore, on the side contralateral to the neoplasm, the nerves at or below the inferior mesenteric artery are the most important.

3. Because the neuroanatomy is variable between individuals, preservation of ejaculation is not absolute after a unilateral dissection. Therefore, in patients who can have a unilateral dissection (vide infra), preserving as many of the ipsilateral lumbar sacral nerves as possible increases the chances of preservation of ejaculation. In patients requiring a more extensive dissection, preserving the nerves within the dissection field is essential if preservation of ejaculation is to have any chance of success. Thus, regardless of whether dissection is unilateral or bilateral, preservation of the appropriate lumbar splanchnic nerves within the dissection field is desirable if technically possible and compatible with optimal cancer control.

The indications for dissection boundary areas are as follows:

1. A unilateral dissection is appropriate for cure if the patient is clinical stage-A before surgery and no disease is found during surgery (see Fig. 35-2).
2. If low volume (microscopic only) disease is found at surgery and is located sufficiently superior to the inferior mesenteric artery, a bilateral dissection can be limited to the area above the inferior mesenteric artery. In these circumstances, contralateral dissection can probably be avoided below the inferior mesenteric artery and aortic bifurcation. Although the low recurrence rates seem to justify these modified bilateral dissection boundaries, some experts contend that all patients with even microscopic disease should have a complete bilateral dissection.
3. In patients with visible disease or microscopic disease near the contralateral inferior mesenteric artery, a complete bilateral dissection should be performed. Even in these circumstances, preservation of the appropriate nerves within the dissection field can be accomplished in some cases and ejaculation has been preserved.[2] Currently, it is controversial whether cancer control is acceptable in these situations and for now the surgeon should exercise his best judgement.

EVALUATION OF THE PATIENT

Once the diagnosis of nonseminomatous germ cell testicular tumor is established, metastatic evaluation should include serial serum AFP and hCG levels, a CT scan of the abdomen, a chest x-ray, and probably a full-lung tomography of the chest. A bipedal lymphangiogram is not advised. A CT of the abdomen must include good opacification of the small bowel, especially the 3rd and 4th part of the duodenum because these bowel segments are sometimes confused with bulky metastasis. In thin patients without much retroperitoneal fat, CT may need to be supplemented by ultrasonography.

Retroperitoneal lymphadenectomy should be advised only for the patient who has no evidence of disease or only positive markers (stage A or B1) or for patients with demonstrable metastasis located in the retroperitoneum that are smaller than 5 cm in total diameter.[3,4] Those patients with evidence of bulky retroperitoneal disease or distant metastasis should initially receive chemotherapy with cytoreductive retroperitoneal lymphadenectomy reserved for those patients who experience partial remission but have persistent abdominal masses.[5-7]

PREOPERATIVE PREPARATION

Candidates for retroperitoneal lymphadenectomy should be fully appraised of the procedure and its complications, including the potential for loss of ejaculation. Alternative therapies, especially the surveillance approach, should be discussed. If fertility is an issue, the fertility status of the man should be determined either by history or by semen analysis and, where appropriate, sperm banking should be encouraged. Preoperative medical assessment should ensure good renal, pulmonary, and cardiac reserve especially in those patients who have had previous chemotherapy. Good hydration and a full mechanical bowel prep should be administered.

SURGICAL PROCEDURE

Incision

A transabdominal retroperitoneal lymphadenectomy usually entails a midline incision from xiphoid to pubis. It is important to extend the incision completely to, and even around, the xiphoid because the extra length taken here significantly improves access to the superior mesenteric artery. This incision can be further extended into the chest through a sternotomy, a left costal incision, or rarely, a right costal incision. A classic thoracoabdominal incision can be used instead of a midline incision. However, this is more cumbersome to perform and close although it does allow performance of an extraperitoneal dissection, therefore diminishing postoperative ileus and the risk of small bowel adhesions. This approach is also sometimes advantageous in the obese or muscular patient. Retraction is best handled with two Balfour retractors or one of the large self-retaining ring retractors.

Exposure

For both right and left testis tumors, if a unilateral dissection is planned, it is usually best to divide the mesenteric attachments in order to mobilize the entire small bowel and right colon (Fig. 35-3). After the abdomen is explored by palpation, an incision is made in the right colonic gutter just medial to the line of Toldt and this is carried up to the hepatic flexure which is taken down (Fig. 35-4). The incision is then extended along the duodenum to the foramen of Winslow and a Kocher maneuver is performed. The incision is continued around the cecum and obliquely cephalad along the route of the mesentery through the ligament of Treitz. By sharp and blunt dissection, the small bowel and right colon mesentery are retracted upward. At the left margin of the posterior peritoneal incision, the inferior mesenteric vein is encountered and may be divided for additional exposure without any significant postoperative consequences. In this way, the anterior surface of Gerota's fascia can be separated from the under surface of the bowel, pancreatic head and body, duodenum, and cecum. After placing the bowels on the chest in a plastic bag, a laparotomy pad is placed on the superior mesenteric artery and pancreas, and elevated with a Harrington retractor to better expose the upper retroperitoneum. It is important to release this retraction from time to time, especially in bulky patients, in order to ensure good bowel circulation and to prevent postoperative pancreatitis. After these maneuvers, exposure for right-sided tumors is complete and the actual dissection can begin (Fig. 35-5). For left-sided tumors, mobilization of the left

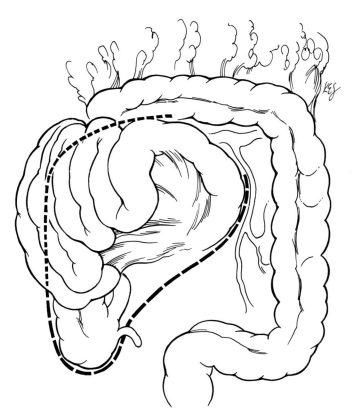

FIG. 35-3. Line of incision in posterior peritoneum to mobilize the right colon and small intestine. The incision extends from the foramen of Winslow, down the right colon, and around the root of the small bowel to the ligament of Treitz.

colon medially must be done in addition to or, rarely, instead of the right colon and small bowel mobilization (vide infra). An appendectomy is usually not performed.

Dissection

The time-honored method for removing the lymphatic tissue from around the inferior vena cava aorta and its major branches is the so-called "split and roll" technique of Donohue (Fig. 35-6). Basically the nodal package is split anteriorly over the inferior vena cava, aorta, and renal vessels, and rotated off the vessels until the lumbar arteries and veins are encountered. These can be sacrificed or preserved. The vessels are then retracted upward using vascular loops and the tissue behind and between is removed. Although methods of nerve sparing have modified the detection approach somewhat, the split and role technique is still the basic approach for RPL.

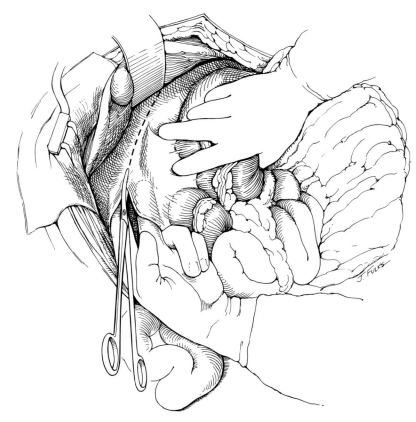

Fig. 35-4. The hepatic flexure may be taken down to gain additional exposure.

Right-sided RPL

For right-sided, nerve-sparing unilateral lymphadenectomies, dissection is usually begun at the junction of the left renal vein and vena cava (Fig. 35-7). The adventitia of the left renal vein is split just cephalad to its superior border (to aid suprahilar dissection if appropriate) and the tissue is pulled inferiorly. It is usually best to expose the left renal vein into the left renal hilum, and ligate and divide the left adrenal vein even if the dissection is to be unilateral (Fig. 35-8). The adventitial tissue in front of the inferior vena cava is also split from just above the right renal hilum all the way to its bifurcation, because no lumbar splanchnic nerves are in this area. Dissection is continued around the vessels so that vascular loops can be placed around the right renal vein and serially in several places on the inferior vena cava beginning superiorly just below the renal veins. In placing these loops, care must be taken not to injure the lumbar veins on the right side of the vena cava because

they serve as a landmark for identifying the right lumbar sympathetic trunk. During the dissection of the vena cava, the right testicular vein is usually encountered. This must be ligated and divided carefully usually with suture ligatures because bleeding there can be troublesome. Finally, the aorta is exposed. Tissues overlying the aorta are split anteriorly, beginning at the left renal vein or (usually easier) by beginning at the superior mesenteric artery and continuing underneath the left renal vein (Fig. 35-9). After encircling the aorta with vascular loops just below the renal arteries, the tissue is rolled to the right, exposing the origin of the right renal artery, which is then encircled. The superior aortocaval lymphatic package is "squared out" by dividing it superiorly at the level of the right renal artery (usually with clips) and this package is pulled down (Fig. 35-10).

The aortic adventitial split is carried out only about 5 cm below the renal vein usually to the testicular arteries, and both arteries are usually sacrificed without adverse affects to the

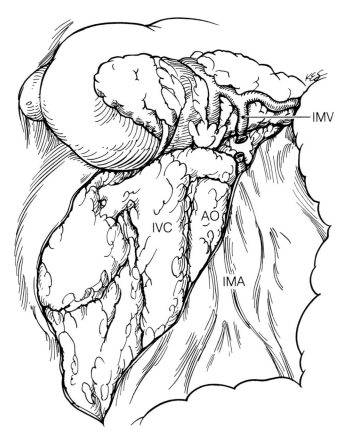

FIG. 35-5. Appearance of retroperitoneum after Kocher maneuver and full mobilization of the small intestine and the ascending colon. The inferior mesenteric vein has been ligated and divided for further exposure.

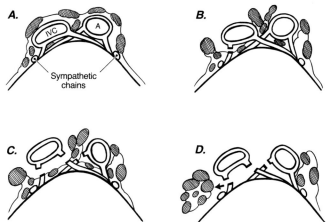

FIG. 35-6. An axial view of the split and roll technique of Donohue with preservation of the lymph node package lateral to the aorta.

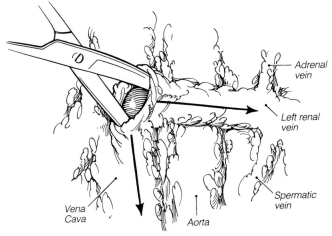

FIG. 35-7. The retroperitoneal dissection is begun by incising the tissue over the left renal vein and its junction with the inferior vena cava.

contralateral testis, provided the blood supply to the vas deferens is not injured. This split should not be carried more inferiorly at this time because important right-sided lumbar splanchnic nerves may begin to extend over the aorta beyond this point.

The next important step is to visualize the appropriate lumbar splanchnic nerves. This can be done by finding those nerves that lie within the nodal tissue surrounding the right side of the aorta at the level of the inferior mesenteric artery and below (Fig. 35-11), by finding the lumbar sympathetic trunk and tracing the nerves inferiorly, or by using both maneuvers.

Finding the lumbar sympathetic trunk deserves special comment. With the vena cava pulled up with vascular loops, the flaps of nodal tissue are dissected off its surface, thus exposing the lumbar veins. An appropriate lumbar vein is carefully dissected dorsally to the junction between the psoas muscle and the vertebral column, at which point the lumbar sympathetic chain is easily found visually or by palpation because it has a solid cord-like feel. The first or second lumbar vein that enters the vena cava below the renal veins is often a good landmark to follow to the sympathetic trunk. The lumbar veins can be preserved or ligated as appropriate but care must

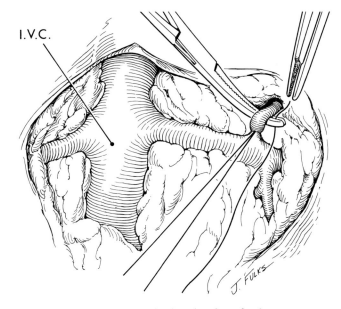

FIG. 35-8. Exposure of the left adrenal and renal veins.

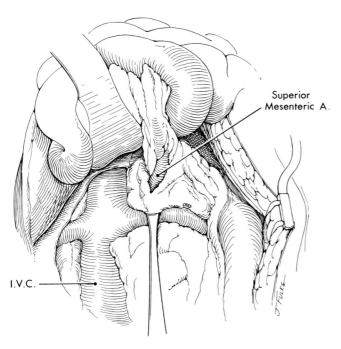

Fig. 35-9. Demonstration of tissue to be removed from between the great vessels and at the level of the superior mesenteric artery.

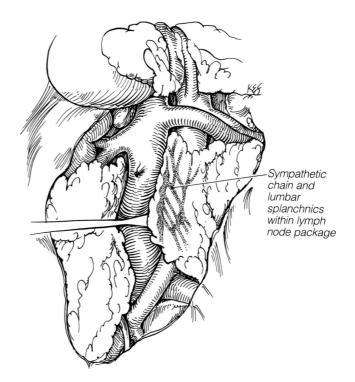

Fig. 35-11. The upper lymph node dissection has been completed and the vena cava skeletonized. The lower lymph node package between the great vessels containing the lumbar sympathetic fibers remains intact.

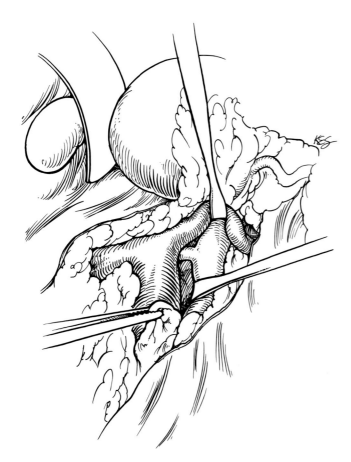

Fig. 35-10. Completion of the upper right-sided lymph node dissection between the great vessels.

be taken that they do not tear as they cross the sympathetic chain because damage to the trunk can occur in attempts at controlling bleeding (Fig. 35-12). Once the sympathetic trunk and/or lumbar splanchnic nerves are found, they can be dissected from the lymphatic tissue over and under it throughout its course from the sympathetic trunk to its destination into a plexus on the lower aorta or bifurcation (Fig. 35-13). During this dissection, the nerves often split into several branches. Not all branches can be spared, especially those that interdigitate with the periaortic nerve plexus above the inferior mesenteric artery. Usually, 2 to 3 main branches can be preserved without compromising the right-sided aortic node dissection.

It is often best to complete the dissection lateral to the vena cava either before or just after the lumbar splanchnic nerves are dissected free, saving the lower interaortocaval dissection for last. The superior aspect of the right lateral lymph node package is squared off at the right renal artery and vein. Usually the lower half of Gerota's fascia is also taken because this facilitates dissection in the right renal hilum. Next, the ureter is separated from the nodal package to just beyond the common iliac vessels. Finally, dissection is continued over the lower vena cava and right common iliac vessels to the right common iliac bifurcation or midway to the right external iliac vessels. On the common iliac vessels, it is important to take

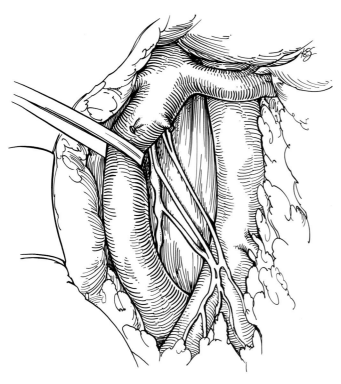

FIG. 35-12. Completion of node dissection between the great vessels for a right-sided tumor with preservation of the sympathetic chain and lower lumbar sympathetic nerves.

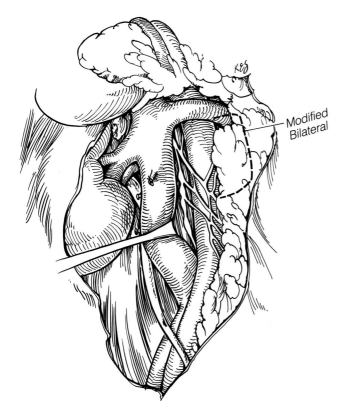

FIG. 35-13. Completion of the right-sided node dissection with preservation of the right sympathetic chain and lumbar splanchnic nerves. Boundaries for a modified bilateral node dissection are indicated.

only the tissue anterior to the vessels because the sympathetic chain and some lumbar splanchnic nerves can course under these vessels. Unless mandated by lymph node metastasis found intraoperatively, the area between the aortic bifurcation and the internal iliac and obturator areas should not be dissected. The right lateral dissection should now be connected only by the spermatic vessel pedicle that courses toward the internal inguinal ring.

Removing the inguinal part of the spermatic vessels can be troublesome. By sharp and blunt dissection, the spermatic vessels and a strip of peritoneum are isolated to the internal ring. The vas is ligated and divided as it turns into the pelvis. Using a large retractor, an assistant elevates the lower abdominal wall exposing the internal ring. At the internal ring, the induration and suture from the previous orchiectomy can be palpated but initially is not seen until further exposed by sharp dissection. Grasping the distal strip of cord with a right angle clamp is helpful in this dissection. Eventually the distal cord, together with the suture, comes free. If the suture is not visible in the specimen, it must be found usually by further intra-abdominal dissection of the internal ring or rarely by reopening the inguinal incision. These maneuvers are especially important if there is no firsthand knowledge of the orchiectomy procedure.

The final and most crucial area of dissection is removal of the interaortocaval package. If no metastases are found, the left boundary is the midaorta inferiorly to the inferior mesenteric artery at which point dissection curves to the right, leaving the aorta obliquely so that it courses over only half of the right common iliac artery (see Fig. 35-2). This deviation is necessary because throughout this and subsequent dissection, the lymph node package must be freed from the two to three identified right lumbar splanchnic nerves. As these nerves reach the aortic bifurcation, they tend to branch into plexes that cannot be dissected from the lymph node package and are therefore best avoided. Finally the package is freed from the posterior and inferior attachments between the great vessels. This dissection is tedious because the lumbosacral nerves and sympathetic trunk must be avoided and troublesome lumbar arteries and veins must be ligated or avoided. Here one should remember that the dissection proceeds superior to the vessels and dissections deep between the aorta, vena cava, and left common iliac vein are usually not necessary. With completion of this dissection, the final lymph node package for a unilateral right-sided nerve-sparing lymphadenectomy is removed (see Fig. 35-13).

If high-positioned microscopic lymph node metastasis are found, the surgeon may elect to proceed to a bilateral dissection, in which case the left colon should be reflected (vide infra) (Fig. 35-14). Alternatively, especially if microscopic lymph node metastasis is found in the upper retroperitoneum, the surgeon may legitimately decide to perform a modified bilateral dissection; that is, remove the tissue package lateral to the aorta to the level of the inferior mesenteric artery. The boundaries of this package are the left renal vessels, the left spermatic vein and ureter, the aorta, and the inferior mesenteric artery (Fig. 35-13). This dissection can be performed

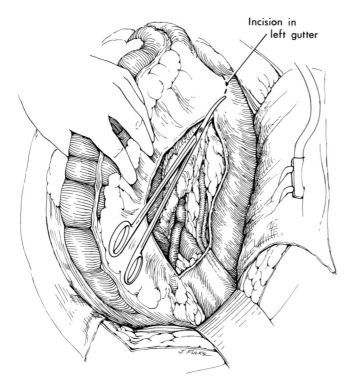

FIG. 35-14. The left colonic gutter is opened to expose the retroperitoneum. The upper lymph node package for a left-sided lymph node dissection is developed with the colon reflected medially.

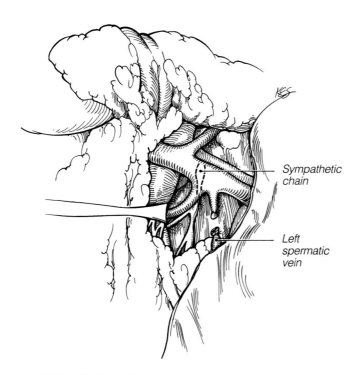

FIG. 35-15. The large lumbar vein draining into the left renal vein crosses the sympathetic chain and serves as a landmark for its identification.

medial to the colonic mesentery. Details of this dissection are presented in the discussion of a left-sided lymphadenectomy.

Left-sided RPL

To preserve the left lumbar splanchnic nerves, the left colon must be reflected medially, incising the left gutter lateral to the descending colon (see Fig. 35-14). The left dissection can be done completely lateral to the colon but usually the splenic flexure must be taken down to do so. Most surgeons prefer to first mobilize the right colon and small intestine as previously described, and then reflect the left colon medially up to but not including the splenic flexure. In this way, the upper left lymphadenectomy is performed either with the colon positioned medially or laterally, depending on the circumstances.

The upper left unilateral dissection is begun by isolating the left renal vein and ligating the left adrenal vein as previously described. In addition, the left spermatic vein is ligated at its junction with the left renal vein. Next, the aorta is exposed above and/or below the renal vein, the origin of the left renal artery is isolated, and vascular loops are placed around the aorta and renal artery. During this process, a first lumbar artery inferior to the renal artery and the first lumbar vein that usually enters the left renal vein or the left spermatic vein at their junction must be identified as they will aid in finding the left sympathetic trunk (Fig. 35-15). This trunk may be visualized at this time and, if difficulty is encountered, should be avoided until a later part of the dissection. Finally, the left lymphatic package is reflected laterally off the aorta to midway between the renal artery and inferior mesenteric artery at which point maneuvers to identify the left lumbar splanchnic nerves are begun. The left splanchnic nerves are best seen with the colon reflected medially. Although slightly more difficult to identify and dissect than those on the right, these nerves may be first identified as they join the inferior mesenteric artery nerve plexus or by finding the left sympathetic trunk and tracing it superiorly or inferiorly. Only the left half of the aorta is dissected to the inferior mesenteric artery, and only the lateral part of the aorta is dissected more caudally. Next, the superior and lateral part of the lymph node package should be developed. On the left side it is important to clear out the left renal hilum completely. This may require some suprahilar dissection (vide infra) and removal of half or even all of the Gerota's fascia. This is because the left testicular lymphatic drainage site is higher than the right (i.e., at the left renal vein). If microscopic nodes are found, removal of all of Gerota's fascia and even the left adrenal gland may be prudent. Next, the ureter is dissected from the package to below the pelvic rim and the lateral border of the package is developed to the internal inguinal ring. Finally the lymphatic package is separated from the lumbar splanchnic nerves and sympathetic trunk and dissection then extended inferiorly over the lateral lower aorta and anterior and lateral aspect of the left common iliac vessels to their bifurcation or to the mid portion of the left external iliac vessels. The cord is dissected from the inguinal ring as previously described and the left lymphatic package is removed (Fig. 35-16).

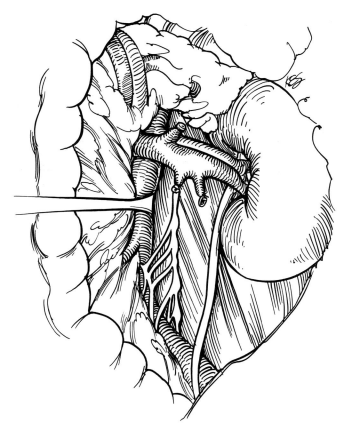

aorta so that important fibers are not sacrificed. Dissection in the lower aorta and at the aortic bifurcation should be minimal. Dissection must proceed both medial and lateral to the colon.

2. The suprahilar dissection is tedious, especially at the portion lateral to the aorta. The inferior vena cava, aorta, and renal arteries should be fully dissected and encircled with vascular loops. The inferior aspect of the superior mesenteric artery should be exposed, excising the tough neural tissue overlying it and the adjacent aorta. Dissection along the aorta reveals the right and left diaphramatic cura, which can be incised occasionally revealing nodes in the retrocural space. The package is developed by cleaning off the right and left cura, the medial border of the suprarenal vena cava, across and along the dorsum of the renal arteries, and laterally along the border of the adrenal gland. It is important to note that most of the important nodal tissue is below the surface of the cura and posterior to the aorta. Occasionally it is best to take down the splenic flexure, reflect the colon medially, and approach the left side of the dissection by removing the adrenal gland and Gerota's fascia (Fig. 35-17).

FIG. 35-16. Completed left-sided dissection with preservation of left sympathetic chain and lumbar splanchnic nerves. The colon is reflected medially.

Bilateral and Suprahilar Lymphadenectomy

Bilateral and suprahilar dissections should be performed when significant microscopic or visible metastatic disease is found intraoperatively. The boundaries for a bilateral dissection are a composite of the right and left unilateral dissections, except at the inferior contralateral extent, where the boundary ends at the mid common iliac area and, of course, the contralateral spermatic cord is not taken. The advisability of nerve-sparing attempts in these situations is unproven although several centers have shown that it is technically feasible (even for cytoreductive surgery) often with preservation of ejaculation, and they are currently testing the therapeutic outcome of these maneuvers. Suffice it to say that considerable discretion by the surgeon is required and, if disease is suspected near the boundaries or significantly within the nerve-sparing areas, the nerve-sparing procedure should then be abandoned. This is especially true if teratomatous elements are present in the patient's tumor, because adjuvant chemotherapy is less likely to succeed in ensuring cure.

The salient aspects of the bilateral and suprahilar dissection can be summarized:

1. The inferior mesenteric artery usually must be sacrificed but should be ligated significantly distal to the

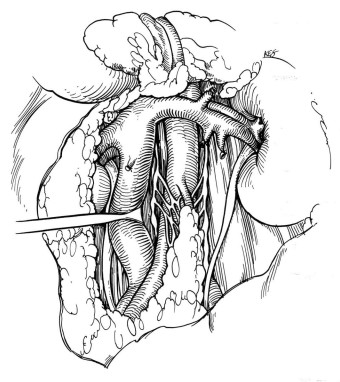

FIG. 35-17. Completion of bilateral retroperitoneal lymphadenectomy with preservation of both sympathetic chains and lower lumbar splanchnic nerves. Lymphatic tissue and the accompanying nerves are spared on the aorta below the inferior mesenteric artery and below the aortic bifurcation.

Closure

After hemostasis and the vascular integrity of the kidneys have been assured, the posterior peritoneum is reperitonealized if possible. This is done by joining the root of the small bowel mesentery to the base of the mesentery of the descending colon using a running chromic suture. The wound is usually closed with interrupted sutures. A nasogastric tube or gastrostomy tube is left in place for 5 to 7 days.

Postoperative Care

Most patients have a smooth postoperative course. Prolonged ileus often necessitates continued nasogastric suction and intravenous alimentation until intestinal motility returns. Elevated levels of serum amylase are occasionally encountered and also require delay in oral feeding. Postoperative anticoagulation should be avoided. Parenteral alimentation is sometimes necessary, particularly in patients who have previously received chemotherapy.

REFERENCES

1. LANGE, P. H., CHANG, W. Y., and FRALEY, E. E. Fertility issues in the therapy of nonseminomatous testicular tumors. Controversies in urologic oncology. Urol. Clin. North Am. *14*:731, 1987.
2. JEWETT, M. A. S., et al. Retroperitoneal lymphadenectomy for testis tumor with nerve sparing for ejaculation. J. Urol., *139*:1220, 1988.
3. LANGE, P. H., and FRALEY, E. E. Controversies in the management of low volume stage II nonseminomatous germ cell testicular cancer. Semin. Oncol., *15*:324, 1988.
4. LANGE, P. H., LIGHTNER, D. J., and FRALEY, E. E. Surveillance vs early lymphadenectomy for patients with stage I nonseminomatous germ cell testicular tumors. Ad. Urol., *2*:41, 1989.
5. WILLIAMS, S. D., et al. Treatment of disseminated germ cell tumors with cisplatin, bleomycin and either vinblastine or etoposide. N. Engl. J. Med., *316*:1435, 1987.
6. WILLIAMS, S. D., et al. Immediate adjuvant chemotherapy vs observation with treatment at relapse in pathological stage II testicular cancer. N. Engl. J. Med., *317*:1433, 1987.
7. EINHORN, L. H., et al. Cancer of the testes. In *Cancer: Principles and Practice of Oncology.* Edited by T. T. DeVita, Jr., S. Helman, and S. A. Rosenberg. Philadelphia, J. B. Lippincott Co., 1985, p. 979.

SECTION
VIII

CARCINOMA OF THE PENIS AND URETHRA

Penile and Urethral Carcinoma: An Overview

Julian Wan

H. Barton Grossman

P enile cancer is uncommon in North America and Europe and accounts for less than 1% of all cancers in men in the United States.[1-3] In other countries, most notably Latin America, Africa, and Asia, carcinoma of the penis is more common and can represent as much as 15% of all male cancers.[4-7] Squamous cell carcinoma is the most common histology of primary penile cancer. Poor genital hygiene and phimosis may play a role in the etiology of penile cancer. Cancer of the penis is almost unknown in people who practice circumcision early in infancy.[2,6,7] Penile cancers usually originate as a lesion on the surface of the penis or prepuce and may present as one of a spectrum of precancerous dermatologic lesions that either coexist with squamous cell carcinoma or precede their development.

PRECANCEROUS LESIONS

Leukoplakia

Leukoplakia appears as one or more whitish plaques or scaly patches, usually around or involving the meatus. It is seen with chronic irritation or inflammation and is often associated with diabetes mellitus. Leukoplakia is often found adjacent to or contiguous with a cancer. It is unclear whether leukoplakia is truly precancerous or is simply associated with penile carcinoma. If limited to the foreskin, circumcision is the recommended treatment. In other areas, excisional biopsy with close follow-up is recommended.[8,9]

Erythroplasia of Queyrat

Erythroplasia of Queyrat is a variant of carcinoma in situ that is characterized by a red, velvety, well-marginated lesion usually found on the glans or foreskin. It can be solitary or multiple, appearing as round or oval papules. Pain and pruritus are rare. Erosion and ulceration usually signify the development of invasive carcinoma. When these precancerous lesions are limited to the glans, topical 5-fluorouracil may be used as the initial treatment.[8] If topical treatment is unsuccessful, surgical excision is recommended. Laser therapy is an effective treatment alternative.[10] Overall, one in five cases of erythroplasia will progress to invasive cancer; one in ten will present with evidence of squamous cell carcinoma and of these, one in fifty will have lymph node metastases at the time of diagnosis. Therefore, a careful evaluation for metastases is recommended and close follow-up is essential.

Bowen's Disease

Bowen's Disease is a rare intraepithelial carcinoma of the penis. Histologically it resembles erythroplasia of Queyrat, but can also involve the epithelium of the hair follicles. It appears as a solitary dull red plaque that is rarely painful. Distant visceral cancer is found in 25% of the patients with Bowen's disease.[9] Approximately half of the cases will progress to invasive squamous cell carcinoma of the penis.[8] The recommended treatment is wide excision with a 5-mm margin and removal of the underlying subcutaneous fat to ensure complete removal of the cancer. Mohs' micrographic surgical technique has been used successfully for this lesion.[11]

Balanitis Xerotica Obliterans

Balanitis xerotica obliterans is a localized variant of lichen sclerosis et atrophicus, which is frequently limited to the glans and prepuce. It is usually benign but has rarely been associated with the subsequent development of squamous cell carcinoma.[8] The involved area is thin, scaly, and dry. Ulceration and fissure formation may cause pruritus and pain. The onset is insidious. With meatal involvement, the lesion can extend to the fossa navicularis. The initial treatment is with topical steroid cream followed by local excision if unsuccessful. Lesions on the foreskin require circumcision. When meatal involvement leads to significant stenosis, meatotomy is recommended.[2,3,8]

Buschke-Loewenstein Tumor

The Buschke-Loewenstein tumor or giant condyloma acuminatum has a gross and microscopic appearance similar to benign condylomata, but is locally invasive. The papova virus associated with ordinary condyloma acuminatum has not been demonstrated in Buschke-Loewenstein tumors. Complete surgical excision is the recommended treatment.[8] Topical agents and radiation therapy have been ineffective.[9,12] Partial or complete penectomy is often required if there is extensive involvement of the penile shaft.[13]

ETIOLOGIC CONSIDERATIONS

As noted earlier, penile cancer is rare in North America and Europe but common elsewhere in the world. No known causative agent has been isolated, although there is a strong link with poor genital hygiene and phimosis. Squamous cell carcinoma of the penis is extremely rare in populations who practice circumcision. It is nearly unheard of in Jews who circumcise during infancy, and it occurs infrequently in Muslims, who circumcise between the ages of 4 and 9.[6,14] The most common coexisting abnormality with squamous cell carcinoma of the penis is phimosis, which is found in up to 75% of the patients.[1,2,15,16] Although phimosis is statistically more common among patients with penile cancer than it is among the general population, it is unlikely that this is the direct cause of the

disease.[17] It is hypothesized that the resulting closed preputial cavity promotes the development of penile cancer by an unidentified carcinogen.[6,7] Smegma, the debris of desquamated epithelial cells on the inner surface of the prepuce, has been implicated as the putative carcinogenic agent. However, experimental evidence documenting the carcinogenic role of smegma in penile cancer is unclear. Some investigators have demonstrated the induction of invasive carcinomas when smegma was introduced into the vaginas of mice,[18] but others have not documented this effect.[19] No convincing association has been found between penile cancer and other factors such as age, race, occupation, or venereal disease exposure.[2,3,20] A possible etiologic role of viruses has been considered. The development of cervical carcinoma in women has been linked to the presence of the human papillomavirus.[21] This observation and the finding that bleomycin, an anti-viral agent, is an active agent for the treatment of squamous cell carcinoma of the penis, led to the hypothesis that there may be a viral association.[22] Although genital herpes virus (HSV-II) has been recovered from penile cancer specimens, no causative relationship has yet been made, and it was observed that herpes virus could often be recovered from male genitourinary specimens taken at random.[22] It should be noted, however, that some studies have suggested a threefold increase in the incidence of cervical carcinoma in sexual partners of men with penile cancer.[2,23]

PATHOLOGIC CONSIDERATIONS

Squamous Cell Carcinoma

Squamous cell carcinoma of the penis constitutes the vast majority of cases of penile cancer. If untreated, the natural history of this disease is characterized by progressive tumor growth with destruction of the glans, prepuce, and eventually the penile shaft. Buck's fascia acts as the initial barrier to invasion and limits the development of early hematogenous metastasis. The earliest path of dissemination is through the lymphatic route. The regional lymph nodes of the penis are the superficial and deep inguinal lymph nodes. The lymphatics of the prepuce and penile skin drain into the superficial inguinal nodes, which in turn connect with the deep inguinal lymph nodes. The lymphatics of the glans, urethra, and corpus spongiosum may drain to either the superficial or deep inguinal lymph nodes. It is important to remember that the lymphatic drainage crosses the midline permitting the development of contralateral metastasis.[1] Detectable distant metastases are uncommon and usually occur late in the course of the disease. If left untreated, death usually occurs within 2 years.[2,24]

Basal Cell Carcinoma

Basal cell carcinoma of the penis is rare and usually presents as a well-defined lesion with clear borders and a depressed center. These neoplasms are slow to metastasize and can usually be treated adequately by local excision with wide margins.[25]

Melanoma

Melanoma of the penis is a rare neoplasm with a poor prognosis.[26] The glans is the most common site for penile melanoma, with two-thirds of the lesions occurring in this location. Metastases to regional lymph nodes are found in approximately 40% of the patients at the time of diagnosis. Hematogenous metastases to the liver, lung, brain, and elsewhere also occur. Wide local excision is essential. Only small distal lesions should be considered for partial penectomy. Other tumors should be treated by total penectomy. Lymph node dissection is advisable because of the high incidence of lymphatic metastasis.[3,26]

Other Tumors

Kaposi's sarcoma, once limited to elderly men, is now seen in greater numbers with the advent of AIDS.[27] Biopsy is mandatory before beginning any definitive treatment because only 50% of mesenchymal tumors of the penis will be malignant.[9] Wide local excision without lymph node dissection is the recommended initial treatment for malignant mesenchymal tumors.[2]

Secondary tumors of the penis most commonly arise from adjacent pelvic organs. The leading site of origin is the bladder (31%), followed in frequency by the prostate (28%), and the recto-sigmoid (15%). Metastases from the kidney, testis, and lung also occur. Common presenting symptoms are priapism and local swelling from metastatic involvement of one or both of the corpora cavernosa. Therapy in these aggressive lesions is palliative with surgical excision or radiation.[28]

DIAGNOSIS AND STAGING

Diagnosis

Penile cancer is most commonly diagnosed during the sixth and seventh decades of life. However, neoplasms in children and teens have been reported.[1,9,16,17,29] A penile mass, lump, or nodule is found in approximately 50% of the cases, and a non-healing penile sore or ulcer is seen in 35%.[1,3] Phimosis may hide the lesion and create a long period of delay. The glans is the most common site (approximately 45%) with the foreskin being involved in 20%.[3] Tumors limited to the foreskin and glans are infrequently (5 to 11%) associated with nodal metastases.[24] Larger tumors are more likely to have nodal metastases.[16] The average interval between initial discovery of the penile lesion by the patient and presentation to a physician is 10 months.[1,3–5] All penile lesions of questionable etiology and behavior should be biopsied. A high index of suspicion is needed in the workup of any unusual inflammatory lesion because penile carcinoma can coexist with other benign lesions.

Staging and Prognosis

No universal system to stage penile cancer exists. Two systems are commonly used. The older and more widely used is that of Jackson.[30]

JACKSON STAGING SYSTEM FOR PENILE CANCER

Stage I	Tumor limited to glans and prepuce
Stage II	Invasion into penile shaft or corpora
Stage III	Proven operable regional (inguinal) lymph node metastasis
Stage IV	Tumor invading adjacent structures, inoperable regional lymph node metastasis or distant metastasis

The other major staging system is that devised by the American Joint Committee on Cancer.[31]

AMERICAN JOINT COMMITTEE STAGING SYSTEM FOR PENILE CANCER

TO	No primary tumor
Tis	Carcinoma-in-situ
Ta	Noninvasive verrucous carcinoma
T1	Tumor invades subepithelial connective tissue
T2	Tumor invades corpus spongiosum or cavernosum
T3	Tumor invades urethra or prostate
T4	Tumor invades other adjacent structures
NO	No nodal involvement
N1	Metastasis in a single, superficial inguinal node
N2	Metastases in multiple superficial inguinal nodes
N3	Metastasis in deep inguinal or pelvic lymph node(s)
MO	No distant metastasis
M1	Distant metastasis

Based on the clinical staging of Jackson, about 55% of patients will present with stage-I disease, 15% with stage-II, 25% with stage-III, and 5% with stage-IV.[3,4,14,30] Increasing clinical stage is associated with a worsening prognosis. The 5-year survival rate for stage-I is 66 to 90%, stage-II 50 to 64%, stage-III 20 to 24%, and stage-IV 0 to 5%.[3,24] Because associated inflammatory and infectious processes are common, the clinical assessment of lymph nodes is subject to error. It has been found that 30 to 60% of patients will present with clinically palpable nodes.[2,5,9] However, when lymphadenectomy is performed in these patients who present with enlarged regional nodes, only about 50% will have proven metastases.[2,3,32] Patients whose regional lymph nodes are clinically benign and who have a lymphadenectomy will have an 18% incidence of occult nodal metastases.[3]

Because of the significant error in clinical staging, additional diagnostic methods have been employed. Pedal lymphangiography in combination with fine-needle aspiration cytology of retroperitoneal pelvic and abdominal lymph nodes has been reported to be accurate in 83% of cases.[33] Pelvic metastasis is a poor prognostic sign.[34] Percutaneous fine-needle aspiration biopsy of the inguinal and iliac nodes may prove to be an efficient, relatively noninvasive means of ascertaining nodal involvement.[35–37]

The accurate assessment of the status of the regional lymph nodes is important because of its impact on therapy. Lymphadenectomy performed on patients with proven regional metastases will result in a 5-year survival rate of 50 to 88%.[2,24,38] In comparison, patients with inguinal metastases who do not undergo lymphadenectomy rarely survive 2 years and almost never survive 5 years.[2,24]

TREATMENT

Penile Tumor

The treatment of the primary penile tumor is usually surgical. Small tumors limited to the foreskin can be treated with circumcision, although there is a high recurrence rate of up to 50%.[38] Tumors involving the glans or distal shaft are usually excised by partial penectomy with a 2-cm, tumor-free margin. To preserve as much normal tissue as possible, several alternative methods of therapy have been employed with good success. Small, superficial lesions on the glans can be treated with laser therapy.[10] Larger lesions can be excised with a minimum of normal tissue by using Mohs' micrographic surgical technique.[11] When the tumor involves the proximal shaft or base of the penis, a total penectomy with creation of a perineal urethrostomy is recommended. Rarely, the whole penis and scrotum will have to be removed en bloc to gain local control.[39]

Radiation therapy as an alternative to surgical therapy is appealing because an intact penis is maintained. A 5-year survival rate of about 60% has been reported with 17% of patients with clinically negative inguinal lymph nodes progressing to regional metastases.[3] Radiation therapy will fail to control local disease in about 30% of cases, necessitating salvage by partial or complete penectomy. The delay created does not appear to compromise survival.[29] Urethral strictures are common after radiation therapy (40%).[40] Occasionally, severe radiation complications may require secondary penile amputation.[30] Radiation therapy appears best suited for those patients who refuse surgery and have small, superficial tumors and for those who have inoperable metastases.[2,29] Radiation therapy for clinically positive inguinal nodes has a high local failure rate. Furthermore, prophylactic radiation therapy to clinically benign nodes does not prevent the development of subsequent nodal metastases.[3,16]

Systemic chemotherapy has usually been employed in the management of advanced disease. Bleomycin, methotrexate, and cisplatin demonstrate modest activity as single agents. The role of chemotherapy in combination with surgery or radiation therapy has not yet been established.[41,42]

Management of Regional Lymph Nodes

The treatment of choice for regional lymphatic metastasis is ilioinguinal lymphadenectomy. When regional metastasis is evident, there is little doubt as to the course of action. However, controversy remains regarding the role of prophylactic lymphadenectomy in the face of clinically negative lymph nodes. Because there is a 20% incidence of occult microscopic nodal metastases, some investigators recommend bilateral ilioinguinal lymph node dissection with all penile cancers.[32,38,40] Prophylactic lymphadenectomy may result in an improvement in survival in patients with clinically negative

nodes. However, ilioinguinal lymphadenectomy is associated with considerable morbidity including phlebitis, pulmonary embolism, wound infection, flap necrosis, and lymphedema.[43] In addition, the theoretical advantage gained from early excision will benefit only 20% of the patients with clinically negative nodes. In an effort to identify the patients with subclinical nodal metastases, sentinel node biopsy has been proposed by Cabanas.[44] This procedure is based on the hypothesis that the initial site of lymphatic spread is an area in association with the superficial epigastric vein. Cabanas showed that when the sentinel lymph node biopsy was negative, inguinal node metastases were absent. In patients with positive sentinel lymph node biopsy, 80% had no other spread and 20% had additional regional spread. These findings have been confirmed,[45] but there are also reports of deep inguinal and iliac metastases with prior negative bilateral sentinel lymph node biopsy.[29,46] The role of sentinel lymph node biopsy remains controversial. When lymph node dissection is performed on unilateral palpable nodes, the risk of contralateral positive nodes is 20 to 25%.[9] Because of this finding, when unilateral positive nodes are found at the time of presentation, a bilateral inguinal dissection should be performed. However, the risk of bilateral disease appears to be less in those patients with clinically negative nodes who have been followed and subsequently develop unilateral disease. In these patients, only a unilateral dissection is recommended.[2,15,32]

URETHRAL CARCINOMA

Urethral carcinoma is uncommon and is notable for being the only urologic cancer that is more frequent in women than men.[47] Standardization of therapy has been difficult to achieve because the small number of cases makes prospective studies virtually impossible. Most data have been collected at large referral centers over decades during which philosophies and techniques have changed, further complicating the analysis of data.[48–57]

Anatomy

The male urethra is approximately 21 cm in length and is divided into five sections: fossa navicularis, penile (pendulous), bulbous, membranous, and prostatic. The mucosa of the urethra changes as it courses from the fossa navicularis to the prostate (Fig. 36-1). The fossa navicularis and the meatus are lined with stratified squamous epithelium. The penile or pendulous urethra has stratified or pseudostratified columnar epithelium. This continues through the bulbomembranous urethra where it changes into transitional epithelium in the prostate. A simple functional classification divides the male urethra into two divisions, an anterior division composed of the fossa navicularis and penile urethra, and a posterior division composed of the bulbous, membranous, and prostatic urethra. The lymphatic drainage of the anterior urethra parallels that of the glans and corpus spongiosum and drains into the deep inguinal lymph nodes. The posterior urethra drains

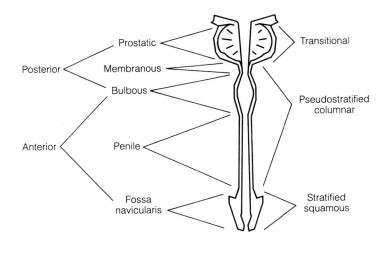

Prostatic — Transitional

Posterior — Membranous

Bulbous — Pseudostratified columnar

Anterior — Penile

Fossa navicularis — Stratified squamous

J Wan 1989

FIG. 36-1. Male urethral anatomy: Histology and organization.

into the external iliac, the obturator, and the internal iliac lymph nodes.[51,58]

The female urethra is about one-fifth the length of the male urethra. The distal two-thirds is lined with stratified squamous epithelium and the proximal third is lined with transitional epithelium.[49] Like the male urethra, the female urethra has an anterior portion comprising the distal one-third of the urethra and a posterior portion comprising the remaining proximal two-thirds (Fig. 36-2). The distal third drains into the inguinal nodes and the proximal two-thirds drain into the pelvic lymph nodes.[51,58]

Incidence

Primary urethral carcinoma represents less than 1% of all male cancers.[51] Among women, it represents less than 0.02% of all genitourinary cancers.[48] The peak incidence in men occurs between 50 and 70 years of age, while among women it tends to occur between 45 and 65 years of age.[48,50,53,59] Urethral cancers are unique among genitourinary cancers as they are far more common in women than in men.[51]

Pathologic Considerations

Male urethral cancer usually occurs in the posterior portion. Most of the cases (59%) are found in the bulbomembranous urethra, 33% occur in the penile urethra, and 7% are found in the prostate urethra.[60] In women, about 50% occur in the distal urethra.[51,57,61] As the epithelium of the urethra changes, the type of cancer encountered will also vary. In men, 70 to 80% of the cases are squamous cell carcinoma, 20% are transitional cell carcinoma, and 5% are adenocarcinoma.[52,54,60] In women, approximately 70% are squamous cell carcinoma,

15% are transitional cell carcinoma, and 15% are adenocarcinoma. There are also occasional sarcomas, melanomas, and other neoplasms.[26,52,54,57,61]

Etiologic Considerations

There is no known cause for urethral cancer. Male urethral cancer has been associated with infections and strictures. A history of urethral strictures will be found in 25 to 75% of men with urethral cancer.[47,53,56] Strictures are observed to occur most frequently at the bulbomembranous urethra, the site of most urethral cancers. These findings suggest a possible role for chronic irritation as an initiating or predisposing factor. However, others have argued that the label of stricture disease may actually represent misdiagnosis of an early unrecognized cancer.[52] Approximately one-third to one-half of patients will also have a history of venereal disease.[53,56] However, any direct causative link with urethral cancer is doubtful because venereal disease is much more prevalent than urethral cancer. Furthermore, a strong etiologic role for venereal disease would likely result in a male rather than a female preponderance.[52,54] Similar factors such as chronic irritation from micturition, coitus, pregnancy, or recurrent infection, have been implicated in the development of female urethral cancer, but again no direct causality has been proven.[52]

Signs and Symptoms

Male urethral cancer most often presents as urinary obstruction (50%). A periurethral mass or abscess is found in 30 to 40% of men. Urinary fistulas, hematuria, and urethral discharge are seen in 20 to 22% of the patients.[53,56,60] Women with urethral cancer most frequently present with bleeding

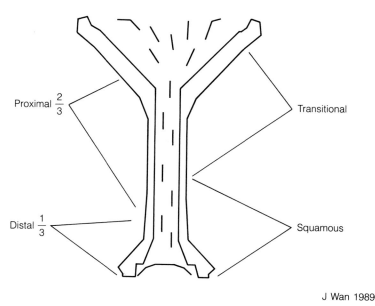

Proximal $\frac{2}{3}$

Distal $\frac{1}{3}$

Transitional

Squamous

J Wan 1989

Fɪɢ. 36-2. Female urethral anatomy: Histology and organization.

and dysuria (40 to 50%).[48,55,61] The clinical course prior to diagnosis is usually insidious and the symptoms can be mistaken for an infection. The average delay from the onset of symptoms to the time of diagnosis is 5 to 6 months.[52–54]

DIAGNOSIS AND STAGING

Diagnosis

As with penile cancer, the diagnosis of urethral cancer requires a high index of suspicion. The symptoms of urethral cancer mimic those of much more frequent and benign disorders such as strictures, urethritis, prostatitis, and cystitis. Among men, the more distal lesions tend to present earlier because they are more likely to become symptomatic at an earlier stage. A much longer delay in presentation is seen with more proximal lesions. In men, a palpable periurethral mass is commonly found, but only the most distal lesions are easily visible. Distal urethral tumors in women are usually visible as growths protruding from or attached to the urethral meatus.[47,52] Careful palpation of the inguinal lymph nodes is especially important in staging the patient. Unlike penile carcinoma, there is rarely the extensive inflammation or infection that confuses the significance of regional adenopathy. A clinical finding of palpable lymph nodes usually signifies regional spread of disease. Cystourethroscopy with adequate biopsies and careful bimanual examination are required to make a definitive diagnosis and stage the disease. There may be an inflammatory response in the tissue surrounding the cancer that can cause a shallow biopsy to give a misleading benign diagnosis. Regional lymph nodes can be assessed by computed tomography and lymphangiography. Distant metastases are present in one-third of the patients at the time of death.[52,62]

Staging

There is no universally accepted staging system for urethral cancer. Commonly employed staging systems for male and female urethral cancer are presented below.

STAGING SYSTEM FOR MALE URETHRAL CANCER[56]

Stage O	Confined to mucosa, carcinoma in situ
Stage A	Into but not beyond lamina propria
Stage B	Into but not beyond corpus spongiosum or prostate
Stage C	Beyond corpus spongiosum or prostatic capsule
Stage D1	Inguinal or pelvic lymph node metastasis
Stage D2	Distant metastasis

STAGING SYSTEM FOR FEMALE URETHRAL CANCER[58]

Stage O	Confined to mucosa, carcinoma in situ
Stage A	Into but not beyond lamina propria
Stage B	Into urethral muscle
Stage C	Invasion of adjacent organs
Stage D	Metastasis

Among both men and women, no correlation between histologic type and survival has been found. Prognosis depends largely on the clinical stage at presentation.[48,56]

Treatment

A variety of therapeutic modalities has been implemented in the management of urethral cancer. However, the rarity of the disease has made prospective studies virtually impossible. In general, the distal lesions are more easily treated and have the best prognosis.

MALE URETHRAL CANCER

Carcinoma of the male distal urethra is treated with partial penectomy with a 2-cm, tumor-free margin. Should there not be a sufficient penile stump to allow an adequate stream, total penectomy and perineal urethrostomy should be performed. In the absence of positive lymph nodes, this will result in a 5-year survival of approximately 50%.[52,53,56,58] Superficial and localized lesions may be treated with local or transurethral resection.[63] However, this carries an increased risk of local recurrence.[53] Failure to gain local control is a poor prognostic sign. Urethrectomy without penectomy is also not recommended because of the potential hazard of failure to control an otherwise localized disease.[47] Tumors in the posterior urethra, especially those in the bulbomembranous urethra, require en bloc cystoprostatectomy. This extensive surgical excision as therapy for posterior urethral lesions was described by Marshall in 1957.[64] To achieve adequate margins, it may be necessary to remove parts of the pubic rami.[65] Despite the institution of radical surgical resection, the experience with posterior urethral cancer in males has been disappointing. Kaplan and associates in 1967 found the 5-year survival rate with aggressive surgical intervention to be only 20%, and Ray and associates in 1977 reported a similar overall 5-year survival rate of 21%.[53,56] The results with radiation therapy for posterior urethral tumors are even more dismal, with none of 36 patients surviving 5-years.[53] Anterior urethral tumors treated with radiation as primary therapy have a 5-year survival of 18 to 25%.[52,53] The use of preoperative radiation has been advocated by some investigators, but the role of combination therapy has yet to be defined.[52,54]

FEMALE URETHRAL CANCER

Superficial lesions in the anterior urethra can be treated with local excision or transurethral resection.[52,54] For more advanced lesions, partial urethrectomy is recommended if adequate margins can be achieved. Survival rates of up to 90% are attainable.[52] Radiation therapy, alone or in combination with surgery, can be employed as an alternative method of treatment. Weghaupt and associates reported a 71%, 5-year survival rate in patients with anterior lesions treated with a combination of brachy and teletherapy.[57] Prempree and associates reported a 100% 5-year, disease-free survival in treating distal urethral cancer with interstitial radium implants.[66] Bracken and associates, reporting the results of treatment of both anterior and posterior urethral tumors, found combined therapy with radiation and surgery to be superior to either modality alone in preventing the development of recurrences. The combined treatment group had a 22% recurrence rate versus 46% for the radiation group and 64% for the surgery group.[48] Tumors in the posterior urethra or tumors affecting the entire urethra have a more dismal prognosis. These tumors usually present at a high stage and 50% will have pelvic lymph node metastases.[52] If no gross involvement of the pelvic nodes exists, the recommended therapy is anterior exenteration. The survival rate at 5 years for posterior tumors is 11 to 21%.[49,55,61] Radiation alone has had poor results. Peterson and associates found only a 13% 5-year survival rate in patients treated with radiation alone.[55] Desai and associates noted similar dismal results with a 5-year survival rate of 17% in patients with posterior urethral cancer.[49] However, Weghaupt and associates reported a favorable 5-year survival rate of 50% using a combination of intracavitary and external beam radiation.[57] An integrated approach using preoperative external beam radiation has been recommended, but its role has not yet been defined.[52,54]

Chemotherapy

There is little clinical data on which to base a recommendation regarding the role of systemic chemotherapy in the treatment of urethral cancer. Agents such as methotrexate, cisplatin, adriamycin, and vinblastine are being evaluated.[47,52]

Management of Lymph Nodes

Ilioinguinal lymphadenectomy should be performed on all patients with groin masses because there is a high correlation between palpable nodes and regional lymphatic metastases. Patients with benign inguinal areas should be evaluated by computed tomography and/or lymphangiography with biopsy of any suspicious lymph nodes.[54] The role of sentinel lymph node biopsy in patients with clinically negative nodes is undefined. In patients with clinically negative nodes, careful followup is needed. The subsequent development of palpable nodes requires lymphadenectomy.[47,52]

Prognosis

The prognosis is grim even when there is no evidence of clinical metastasis. The 5-year survival for men with benign nodes and distal tumors is 50%. However, the survival for bulbomembranous disease is only about 5%. The 5-year survival of prostatic urethral cancer is 23%, which may be because of the inclusion of superficial transitional cell carcinomas. The overall 5-year, disease-free survival of male urethral cancer for stages A, B, C, and D is 100%, 80%, 17%, and 20% respectively. Women with distal tumors have a 5-year survival rate of 50%. The 5-year survival of women with tumors in the proximal or entire urethra is only 13%.[47]

TRANSITIONAL CELL CARCINOMA OF THE PROSTATIC URETHRA

The majority of transitional cell carcinomas found in the prostatic urethra are associated with a prior or coexisting bladder tumor and are treated by transurethral resection, with or without intravesical chemotherapy, or cystoprostatourethrectomy.

Patients undergoing radical cystectomy for transitional cell carcinoma of the bladder have a 4 to 14% risk of subsequently developing urethral recurrence.[52] Urethral washings for cytologic examination are a sensitive method for following the urethra after radical cystectomy.[67]

Primary transitional cell carcinomas arising from the prostatic ducts are rare. They are usually high-grade lesions that present like other urethral cancers with obstructive symptoms

and bleeding. The prostate, on rectal examination, is frequently hard, making the examiner suspicious of prostate adenocarcinoma. One-quarter of the patients will indeed have a coexisting prostatic adenocarcinoma.[68] Hormonal therapy is ineffective. Transurethral resection is also inadequate, and aggressive treatment is recommended including radical cystectomy with urethrectomy and urinary diversion. Few patients survive 5 years.[68]

REFERENCES

1. BUDDINGTON, W. T., KICKHAM, C. J. E., and SMITH, W. E. An assessment of malignant disease of the penis. J. Urol., 89:442, 1963.
2. SCHELLHAMMER, P. F., and GRABSTALD, H. Tumors of the penis. In Campbell's Urology. Edited by P. C. Walsh, R. F. Gittes, A. D. Perlmutter, and T. A. Stamey. Philadelphia, W. B. Saunders, 1986, pp. 1583–1606.
3. SUFRIN, G., and HUBER, R. Benign and malignant lesions of the penis. In Adult and Pediatric Urology. Edited by J. Y. Gillenwater, J. T. Grayhack, S. S. Howards, and J. W. Duckett. Chicago, Year Book Medical Publishers, 1987, pp. 1448–1483.
4. RAJU, G. C., NARAYNSINGH, V., and VENU, P. S. Carcinoma of the penis in the West Indies: A Trinidad study. Trop. Geogr. Med., 37:334, 1985.
5. RIVEROS, M., and LEBRON, R. F. Geographic pathology of cancer of the penis. Cancer, 16:798, 1963.
6. SHABAD, A. L. Some aspects of etiology and prevention of penile cancer. J. Urol., 92:696, 1964.
7. SHABAD, A. L. The experimental production of the penis tumours. Neoplasma, 12:635, 1965.
8. MIKHAIL, G. R. Cancers, precancers, and pseudocancers on the male genitalia. J. Dermatol. Surg. Oncol., 6:1027, 1980.
9. PERSKY, L., and DEKERNION, J. Carcinoma of the penis. CA, 36:258, 1986.
10. BOON, T. A. Sapphire probe laser surgery for localized carcinoma of the penis. Eur. J. Surg. Oncol., 14:193, 1988.
11. BROWN, M. D., ZACHARY, C. B., and GREKIN, R. C. Penile tumors: Their management by Moh's micrographic surgery. J. Dermatol. Surg. Oncol., 13:1163, 1987.
12. KRAUS, F. T., and PEREZ-MESA, C. Verrucous carcinoma. Cancer, 19:26, 1966.
13. GERSH, I. Giant condylomata acuminata (carcinoma-like condylomata or Buschke-Loewenstein tumors) of the penis. J. Urol., 69:164, 1953.
14. DAGHER, R., SELZER, M. L., and LAPIDES, J. Carcinoma of the penis and anti-circumcision crusade. J. Urol., 110:79, 1973.
15. EKSTROM, T., and EDSMYR, F. Cancer of the penis: A clinical study of 229 cases. Acta. Chir. Scand., 115:25, 1958.
16. FRALEY, E. E., et al. Cancer of the penis: Prognosis and treatment plans. Cancer, 55:1618, 1985.
17. HELLBERG, D., et al. Penile cancer: Is there an epidemiological role for smoking and sexual behavior? Br. Med. J., 295:1306, 1987.
18. PRATT-THOMAS, H. R., et al. The carcinogenic effect of human smegma: An experimental study. Cancer, 9:671–680, 1956.
19. FISHMAN, M., FRIEDMAN, H. F., and STEWART, H. L. Local effect of repeated application of 3,4-benzpyrene and of human smegma to the vagina and cervix of mice. J. Natl. Cancer Inst., 2:361, 1942.
20. JOHNSON, D. E., FUERST, D. E., and AYALA, A. G. Carcinoma of the penis: Experience with 153 cases. Urology, 1:404, 1973.
21. ZDERIC, S. A., et al. The diagnosis and management of genital infections with the human papillomavirus. AUA Update. Volume 7, Lesson 34, 1988.
22. THOMAS, J. A. Penile carcinoma and viruses. J. Urol., 128:307–308, 1982.
23. GRAHAM, S., et al. Genital cancer in wives of penile cancer patients. Cancer, 44:1870, 1979.
24. MUKAMEL, E., and DEKERNION, J. B. Early versus delayed lymph-node dissection versus no lymph-node dissection in carcinoma of the penis. Urol. Clin. North Am., 14:707, 1987.
25. FEGEN, J. P., BEEBE, D., and PERSKY, L. Basal cell carcinoma of the penis. J. Urol., 104:864, 1970.
26. BEGUN, F. P., et al. Malignant melanoma of the penis and male urethra. J. Urol., 132:123, 1984.
27. CATANESE, A. J., TESSLER, A. N., and MORALES, P. AIDS and the urologist: Part 1. AUA Update. Volume 8, Lesson 1, 1989.
28. ABESHOUSE, B. S., and ABESHOUSE, G. A. Metastatic tumors of the penis: A review of the literature and a report of two cases. J. Urol., 86:99, 1961.
29. FOSSA, S. D., et al. Cancer of the penis: Experience at the Norwegian radium hospital 1974. Eur. Urol., 13:372, 1987.
30. JACKSON, S. M. The treatment of carcinoma of the penis. Br. J. Surg., 53:33, 1966.
31. BEAHRS, O. H., HENSON, D. E., HUTTER, R. V. P., and MYERS, M. H. Manual for Staging of Cancer. 3rd Edition. Philadelphia, J. B. Lippincott Co., 1988.
32. CATALONA, W. J. Role of lymphadenectomy in carcinoma of the penis. Urol. Clin. North Am., 7:785, 1980.
33. WAJSMAN, Z., GAMARRA, M., and PARK, J. J. Transabdominal fine needle aspiration of retroperitoneal lymph nodes in staging of genitourinary tract cancer (correlation with lymphography and lymph node dissection findings). J. Urol., 128:1238, 1982.
34. SRINIVAS, V., et al. Penile cancer: Relation of extent of nodal metastasis to survival. J. Urol., 137:880, 1987.
35. PISCIOLI, F., SCAPPINI, P., and LUCIANI, L. Aspiration cytology in the staging of urologic cancer. Cancer, 56:1173, 1985.
36. PISCIOLI, F., POLLA, E., and PUSIL, T. Aspiration cytology of cutaneous metastatic melanoma and epidermoid carcinoma of the penis. Am. J. Dermatopathol., 8:472, 1986.
37. SCAPPINI, P., et al. Penile cancer: Aspiration biopsy cytology for staging. Cancer, 58:1526, 1986.
38. McDOUGAL, W. S., et al. Treatment of carcinoma of the penis: The case for primary lymphadenectomy. J. Urol., 136:38, 1986.
39. YOUNG, H. H. A radical operation for the cure of cancer of the penis. J. Urol., 26:285, 1931.
40. GRABSTALD, H., and KELLEY, C. D. Radiation therapy of penile cancer: Six to ten year follow-up. Urology, 15:575, 1980.

41. AHMED, T., SKLAROFF, R., and YAGODA, A. Sequential trials of methotrexate, cisplatin, bleomycin for penile cancer. J. Urol., *132:*465, 1984.

42. MEYERS, F. J. Penile cancer chemotherapy. Recent Results. Cancer Res., *85:*143, 1983.

43. JOHNSON, D. E., and LO, R. K. Complications of groin dissection in penile cancer. Urology, 24:312, 1984.

44. CABANAS, R. M. An approach for the treatment of penile carcinoma. Cancer, *39:*456, 1977.

45. FOWLER, J. E., JR. Sentinel lymph node biopsy for staging penile cancer. Urology, 23:352, 1984.

46. PERINETTI, E., CRANE, D. B., and CATALONA, W. J. Unreliability of sentinel lymph node biopsy for staging penile carcinoma. J. Urol., *124:*734, 1980.

47. SAROSDY, M. F. Urethral Carcinoma. AUA Update. Volume 6, Lesson 13, 1987.

48. BRACKEN, R. B., et al. Primary carcinoma of the female urethra. J. Urol., *116:*188, 1976.

49. DESAI, S., LIBERTINO, J. A., and ZINMAN, L. Primary carcinoma of the female urethra. J. Urol., *110:*693, 1973.

50. GRABSTALD, H., et al. Cancer of the female urethra. JAMA, *197:*835, 1966.

51. GRABSTALD, H. Tumors of the urethra in men and women. Cancer, *32:*1236, 1973.

52. HOPKINS, S. C., and GRABSTALD, H. Benign and malignant tumors of the male and female urethra. In *Campbell's Urology.* Edited by P. C. Walsh, R. F. Gittes, A. D. Perlmutter, and T. A. Stamey. Philadelphia, W. B. Saunders, 1986, pp. 1441–1462.

53. KAPLAN, G. W., BULKLEY, G. J., and GRAYHACK, J. T. Carcinoma in the male urethra. J. Urol., *98:*365, 1967.

54. PALMER, T. E., and McCULLOUGH, D. L. Urethral carcinoma. In *Adult and Pediatric Urology.* Edited by J. Y. Gillenwater, J. T. Grayhack, S. S. Howards. and J. W. Duckett. Chicago, Year Book Medical Publishers, 1987, pp. 1315–1327.

55. PETERSON, D. T., et al. The peril of primary carcinoma of the urethra in women. J. Urol., *110:*72, 1973.

56. RAY, B., CANTO, A. R., and WHITMORE, W. F., JR. Experience with primary carcinoma of the male urethra. J. Urol., *117:*591, 1977.

57. WEGHAUPT, K., GERSTNER, G. J., and KUCERA, H. Radiation therapy for primary carcinoma of the female urethra: A survey over 25 years. Gynecol. Oncol., *17:*58, 1984.

58. LEVINE, R. L. Urethral cancer. Cancer, *45:*1965, 1980.

59. BOULDAN, J. P., and FARAH, R. N. Primary urethral neoplasms: Review of 30 cases. J. Urol., *125:*198, 1981.

60. SRINIVAS, V., and KHAN, S. A. Male urethral cancer: A review. Int. Urol. Nephrol., *20:*61, 1988.

61. SRINIVAS, V., and KHAN, S. A. Female urethral cancer: An overview. Int. Urol. Nephrol., *19:*423, 1987.

62. MAYER, R., FOWLER, J. E., JR., and CLAYTON, M. Localized urethral cancer in women. Cancer, *60:*1548, 1987.

63. KONNAK, J. W. Conservative management of low grade neoplasms of the male urethra: A preliminary report. J. Urol., *123:*175, 1980.

64. MARSHALL, V. F. Radical excision of locally extensive carcinoma of the deep male urethra. J. Urol., *78:*252, 1957.

65. SHUTTLEWORTH, K. E. D., and LLOYD-DAVIES, R. W. Radical resection for tumours involving the posterior urethra. Br. J. Urol., *41:*739, 1969.

66. PREMPREE, T., AMORNMARN, R., and PATANAPHAN, V. Radiation therapy in primary carcinoma of the female urethra. Cancer, *54:*729, 1984.

67. WOLINSKA, W. H., et al. Urethral cytology following cystectomy for bladder carcinoma. Am. J. Surg. Pathol., *1:*225, 1977.

68. GREENE, L. F., et al. Primary transitional cell carcinoma of the prostate. J. Urol., *110:*235, 1973.

Carcinoma of the Penis: Management of the Primary

Si medicamenta vincuntur, hic quoque scalpello quicquid corruptum est, sic ut aliquid etiam integri trahat, praecidi debet. (If medicaments fail, in this case whatever is corrupted should be cut away with a scalpel, so far that some sound tissue is also removed.)— Celsus[1]

Sakti Das
E. David Crawford

Excision of a presumed cancerous lesion of the penis with a margin of healthy tissue as recommended by Celsus is probably one of the earliest definitive therapies of carcinoma chronicled in the history of medicine. Nearly two millenia later however, various aspects of treatment of penile carcinoma still remain controversial. With the advent of our understanding of the regional anatomy, mode of spread, and lymphatic drainage, the surgical approaches to cancer of the penis continues to evolve. Therapeutic philosophies are still clouded by issues such as personal convictions and small numbers of patients in individual series'. Larger, collective reports spanning over long periods often include complex amalgamation of different therapies, inadequate data regarding pathologic grade and stage, and inherent ambiguity in the clinical staging of penile carcinoma.

HISTORICAL PERSPECTIVES

The famous anatomist Morgagni in 1761 mentioned the procedure of partial amputation of the penis performed by Valsalva.[2] The first detailed description of curative surgery for carcinoma of the penis has been credited to Thiersch in 1875.[3] In 1886, MacCormac advocated total amputation of the penis and bilateral inguinal lymphadenectomy.[4] Curtis,[5] in 1898, essentially reaffirmed this approach and in 1907, Young[6] recommended en bloc bilateral lymphadenectomy along with removal of the primary carcinoma of the penis. The excellent anatomic study of Daseler and associates in 1948 detailed the lymphatic anatomy of the inguinofemoral region and established the surgical feasibility and technique of radical excision of ileo-inguinal lymph nodes.[7] Baronofsky further modified this dissection with transposition of the sartorius muscle to cover the denuded femoral vessels.[8]

The significant postoperative morbidity following ileo-inguinal lymphadenectomy soon became an issue of major concern. In 1977, Cabanas claimed that the sentinel lymph nodes located at the epigastrico-saphenous junction were the first echelon of lymphatic metastases from penile carcinoma.[9] If, on biopsy, these nodes appear uninvolved, then a formal lymphadenectomy could be avoided. Several investigators subsequently objected to such approach as unreliable with reports of patients developing incurable inguinal metastases following negative sentinel node biopsy.[10,11] Further modifications with limited lymph node dissection have been proposed recently,[12] but available clinical data is inadequate for any valid conclusion.

PATHOLOGIC CONSIDERATIONS

Carcinoma-in-situ

Carcinoma-in-situ of the penis include three histologically identical entities with distinctive clinical features and natural history. They are erythroplasia of Queyrat (EQ), Bowen's disease, and Bowenoid papulosis. EQ and Bowen's disease occur as erythematous plaques on glans penis and prepuce in males around 50 years of age. Bowen's disease is characterized by higher incidence of associated internal malignancies.[13] Bowenoid papulosis appear as multiple papules on the penile shaft in younger patients aged between 20 and 40 years with no evidence of invasion of the dermis.[14] About 20 to 50% of the patients with EQ and Bowen's disease can develop invasive carcinoma.[15]

Squamous Cell Carcinoma

Macroscopically, carcinoma of the penis initially appears as a small nodule, an indolent ulcer, or a papillary verrucous lesion on the glans penis or prepuce. Advanced lesions are often large, fungating with rolled edges and central ulceration, and show induration from deep invasion of the corpora.

Histologically, penile carcinomas are essentially typical examples of squamous cell carcinomas that are well to moderately differentiated. Well-organized papillary structures with hyperkeratosis and acanthosis are interspersed with areas of infiltration of the dermis or invasion of the corium. The majority of the cells are orderly in appearance like those in a condyloma (Fig. 37-1). Disorganized foci with cells of various size, shape, pleomorphic neuclii, loss of polarity, and abnormal mitosis characterize the malignant histologic picture.

Carcinoma of the penis commonly metastasize via the lymphatics into the regional ileo-inguinal lymph nodes. Despite the rich vascularity and multiple venous system of the penis, hematogenous spread is rare. Distant metastases occur in about 10% of patients with advanced carcinoma of the penis.

THE PRIMARY TUMOR

Biopsy

Initial biopsy is mandatory for histologic confirmation of the carcinoma. Assessment of the grade, infiltration or invasion of the adjacent deep or lateral tissues aids in treatment planning. We usually remove a 1-cm, elliptical wedge centered on the margin of the growth, thereby ensuring adequate removal of neighboring normal tissue to check for infiltration (Fig. 37-2). The wound is approximated with a single suture of 3-0 chromic catgut for hemostasis. Biopsy can be done as a separate procedure or one can proceed with planned excisional surgery after immediate frozen section confirmation of the diagnosis.

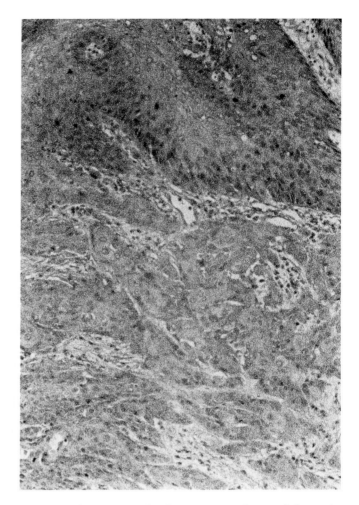

FIG. 37-1. Photomicrograph of squamous carcinoma of the penis. H & E × 400.

Non-surgical Therapeutic Alternatives

Carcinoma-in-situ lesions are often amenable to topical therapy with 5-fluorouracil cream.[16] Radiation therapy should be employed for larger lesions refractory to topical chemotherapy. Successful use of CO_2 laser and liquid nitrogen cryosurgery in sporadic cases have been reported.[17,18] Persistent disease in post-treatment biopsy calls for surgical excision. Because of the deeper involvement of the dermal appendages in Bowen's disease, earlier surgical intervention often becomes necessary.

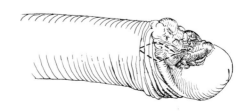

FIG. 37-2. Wedge biopsy.

Radiation therapy for squamous cell carcinoma of the penis, despite its obvious cosmetic and psychologic advantage in preserving the phallic anatomy and function, has remained controversial. The results and reports are confusing because of the lack of uniformity in modes of delivery of radiotherapy, prolonged time to regression, and histologic persistence of tumor following therapy. We offer definitive radiotherapy as a choice to the select group of young patients with tumors less than 3 cm in diameter that are clinically noninvasive and have no palpable inguinal adenopathy. Complications including telangiectasia, edema, pain, urethral stricture, scarring, and penile deformity do occur with the therapeutic radiation dosage. Patients failing radiotherapy with recurrence or persistence of tumor are treated by salvage amputation of the penis.[19,20]

We do not recommend systemic chemotherapy as definitive treatment for the primary carcinoma of the penis. Despite the initial enthusiastic report of Ichikawa with Bleomycin,[21] the experience in this country of similar therapy has been limited with less than encouraging results. The collective review of the world literature by Blum revealed only 10% complete response out of 67 patients treated with Bleomycin therapy.[22]

Other reports of successful nonamputative treatment include cryosurgery for verrucous carcinoma[23] and Neodymium-YAG laser therapy[24] for localized squamous carcinoma of the penis. Further clinical trials are necessary to substantiate the usefulness of these therapies over excisional surgery.

SURGICAL TREATMENT OF THE PRIMARY TUMOR

Our therapeutic goal is the complete excision of the primary tumor with adequate margins free of tumor. Noninvasive carcinoma limited to the prepuce can be treated by a wide circumcision with a 2-cm margin of clearance. Several reports of high recurrence rate underscore the need for careful followup of patients treated with circumcision alone.[25,26] Selected cases of superficial carcinoma on the penile shaft can be treated by wide excision followed by reconstruction with split thickness skin graft or scrotal skin. Multiple deep and lateral biopsies are examined to ensure complete excision. Alternatively, selected lesions can be excised with a minimum amount of normal tissue employing Moh's micrographic surgical technique.[27]

Carcinoma involving the glans penis and the distal shaft are better managed by partial amputation of the penis excising 1.5 to 2 cm normal tissue proximal to the tumor margin. This should leave a 2.5- to 3-cm stump of penis to allow directable micturition in an upright posture. If the penile stump appears marginally short at surgery, phallic length can be augmented by dividing the suspensory ligament of the penis and mobilizing lateral skin flaps to the prepubic area. In cases of large invasive tumors that are proximal, a total amputation of the penis is indicated to ensure an adequate tumor-free margin. The urethral stump brought out as a perineal urethrostomy allows more convenient micturition in a sitting position.

Partial Amputation of the Penis

Preoperative culture studies are done of the lesion and urine. Accordingly, appropriate parenteral antibiotics are started preoperatively and continued for 24 hours. A cleansing enema on the evening before surgery reduces the possibility of postoperative fecal soiling of the dressing and wound.

After a thorough povidone-iodine scrub, the tumor-containing distal penis is covered and isolated by a sterile glove finger or condom. A rubber tourniquet is applied to the root of the penis. The skin incision is started dorsally over half the circumference of the penis at about 1.5 cm proximal to the margins of the tumor. Two ends of the incision are carried proximally along the shaft for about 1 cm and then continued ventrally to complete the circumference (Fig. 37-3A). The subcutaneous superficial veins are electrocoagulated. Underneath the dorsal Buck's fascia, the deep dorsal vein and dorsal arteries are ligated with 3-0 chromic catgut and divided. The corpora cavernosal bodies are sharply amputated 2 cm proximal to the tumor. The central cavernosal arteries are clamped and ligated. The urethra is dissected free from the corpus spongiosum and divided in such a manner that about 1 cm stump projects beyond the transected corpora (Fig. 37-3B). The corporal ends are closed with horizontal mattress sutures of 2-0 chromic catgut incorporating the Buck's fascia, tunica albuginea, and the intercavernous septum. The tourniquet is released and hemostasis is checked. The urethral end is

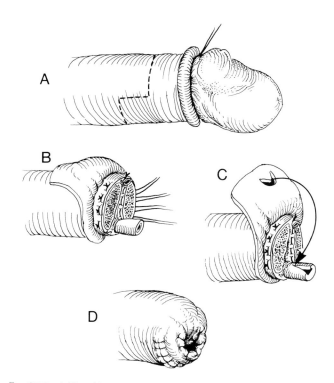

Fig. 37-3. *A*, The skin incision is outlined. *B*, The corporal bodies are transected and closed with horizontal mattress sutures. The urethral stump is dissected to project 1 cm beyond the divided corpora. *C*, A crescentic buttonhole in the dorsal skin flap is made for anastomosis of the spatulated urethra. *D*, The completed urethrocutaneous anastomosis and the skin flaps are reapproximated.

spatulated dorsally and pulled out through a 1 cm crescentic buttonhole in the dorsal skin flap (Fig. 37-3C). The proximal flap of the buttonhole is sutured to the urethral spatulation. Urethrocutaneous anastomosis is completed with interrupted 4-0 chromic catgut sutures. Skin flaps are approximated ventrally with interrupted 3-0 chromic catgut sutures (Fig. 37-3D). An 18-French Foley catheter is left indwelling.

Total Amputation of the Penis

Total amputation is indicated for proximal lesions with invasion. A vertical elliptical incision around the root of the penis is extended into the upper half of the median scrotal raphe (Fig. 37-4A). The skin, subcutaneous tissue, and dartos layer are divided. Dorsally, at the root of the penis, the deep dorsal vein and dorsal arteries are identified beneath the Buck's fascia and divided between 3-0 silk ligatures. In front of the sym-

physes pubes, the fundiform and the suspensory ligament of the penis are divided with electrocautery, allowing proximal displacement of the corporal bodies (Fig. 37-4B).

Ventrally, the urethra is dissected from the corpora and transected just distal to the bulbar area (Fig. 37-4C,D). Further dissection is aided by traction on the proximal urethral end. The corpora cavernosa are dissected up to the ischiopubic rami, suture ligated with 2-0 polyglycolic acid suture, and transected (Fig. 37-4E,F). It is not necessary to completely dissect the corpora off the bone unless an extensive infiltrating carcinoma appears too proximal. The urethra is dissected up to the area of the urogenital diaphragm to ensure its eventual unangulated straight course to the perineal urethrostomy site. At the midperineum a 1-cm ellipse of skin and subcutaneous tissue are removed (Fig. 37-5A). The urethra is tunnelled to this opening, spatulated, and anastomosed to the skin with interrupted 4-0 chromic catgut sutures (Fig. 37-5B). The pri-

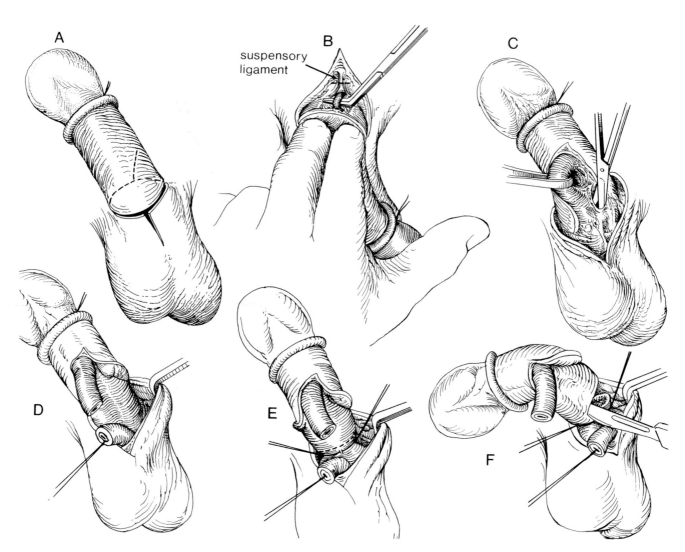

FIG. 37-4. *A,* The skin incision is outlined. *B,* The fundiform and suspensory ligament of the penis are divided. The deep dorsal vein is divided between ligatures. *C,* The urethra is dissected off the corpora. *D,* The urethra is transected. *E,* The ligature of the corpora cavernosa is sutured. *F,* The corpora cavernosa are transected.

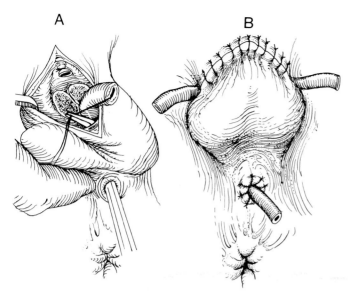

FIG. 37-5. *A,* Site of perineal urethrostomy. *B,* Urethrocutaneous anastomosis and transverse closure of skin incision.

mary incision is closed transversely to allow elevation of scrotum away from the perineal urethrostomy (Fig. 37-6). A small Penrose drain is brought out through the lateral ends of the incision. A urethral catheter is left indwelling.

For carcinoma infiltrating the corpora dorsally without any urethral involvement, Bissada has proposed a urethra-sparing total amputation.[28] The pendulous urethra is dissected completely off the corpora. Amputation of the corpora is carried out in the usual manner and the dissected urethra is buried in the scrotum with its end brought out as scrotal urethrostomy. Subsequent phallic reconstruction using scrotal flap is simplified by preservation of the urethra.

Postoperative Management

The Penrose drain is removed after 24 hours. The urethral catheter is removed on the fifth postoperative day. At subsequent visits, the urethral neomeatus should be sounded with metal bougies to check and prevent stenosis. If inguinal adenopathy is evident, oral antibiotics are continued for 6 weeks. Management of regional lymph nodes are discussed in Chapter 38.

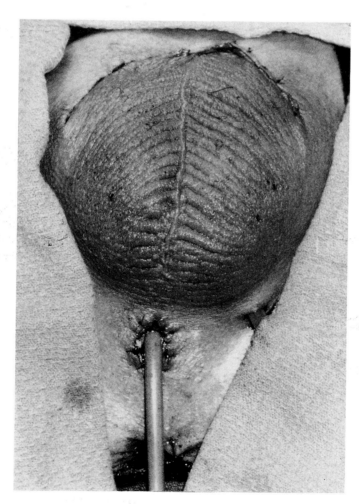

FIG. 37-6. Perineal urethrostomy following the total amputation of the penis.

REFERENCES

1. CELSUS, C. Celsus de Medicina, Translated by W. G. Spencer. Loeb Classical Library Service. Cambridge, Harvard University Press. Volume 2. 1935, p. 276.
2. MORGAGNI, G. B. *The Seats and Causes of Disease.* Book IV, Letter L, Article 50, 1761.
3. LEWIS, L. G. Young's radical operation for the cure of cancer of the penis. A report of 34 cases. J. Urol., *26*:295, 1931.
4. MacCORMAC, W. Five cases of amputation of the penis for epithelioma. Br. Med. J., *1*:343, 1886.
5. CURTIS, B. F. *American Textbook of Diseases of The Skin.* Philadelphia, W. B. Saunders, 1898, p. 76.
6. YOUNG, H. H. A radical operation for the cure of cancer of the penis. J. Urol., *26*:285, 1931.
7. DASELER, E. H., ANSON, B. J., and REIMANN, A. F. Radical excision of the inguinal and iliac lymph glands. Surg. Gynecol. Obstet., *87*:679, 1948.
8. BARONOFSKY, I. A. Technique of inguinal node dissection. Surgery, *33*:886, 1953.
9. CABANAS, R. M. An approach for the treatment of penile carcinoma. Cancer, *39*:456, 1977.
10. PERINETTI, E., CRANE, D. B., and CATALONA, W. J. Unreliability of sentinel lymph node biopsy for staging penile carcinoma. J. Urol., *124*:734, 1980.
11. deKERNION, J. B. Ilioinguinal lymphadenectomy in Genitourinary cancer surgery. Edited by E. D. Crawford and T. Borden. Philadelphia, Lea and Febiger, 1982, p. 318.
12. CATALONA, W. J. Modified inguinal lymphadenectomy for carcinoma of penis with preservation of saphenous veins: Technique and preliminary results. J. Urol., *140*:306, 1988.
13. GRAHAM, J. H., and HELWIG, E. B. Erythroplasia of Queyrat. Cancer, *32*:1396, 1973.
14. KOPF, A. W., and BART, R. S. Tumor Conference II: Multiple Bowenoid papules of the penis: A new entity? J. Dermatol. Surg. Oncol., *3*:265, 1977.
15. MIKHAIL, G. R. Cancers, precancers and pseudocancers on the male genitalia. J. Dermatol. Surg. Oncol., *6*:1027, 1980.
16. TOLIA, B. M., CASTRO, V. L., MOUDED, I. M., and NEWMAN, H. R. Bowen's disease of the shaft of the penis: Successful treatment with 5-fluorouracil. Urology, *7*:617, 1976.
17. ROSENBERG, S. K., and FULLER, T. A. Carbon dioxide rapid superpulsed laser treatment of erythroplasia of Queyrat. Urology, *16*:181, 1980.
18. SONNEX, T. S., RALFS, I. G., MARIA, P. D., and DAWBER, R. P. R. Treatment of erythroplasia of Queyrat with liquid nitrogen cryosurgery. Br. J. Urol., *106*:581, 1982.
19. GRABSTALD, H., and KELLEY, C. D. Radiation therapy of penile cancer. Urology, *15*:575, 1980.
20. KREIG, R. M., and LUK, K. H. Carcinoma of the penis. Review of cases treated by surgery and radiation therapy 1960–1977. Urology, *18*:149, 1981.
21. ICHIKAWA, T., NAKANO, I., and HIROKAWA, I. Bleomycin treatment of the tumors of penis and scrotum. J. Urol., *102*:699, 1969.
22. BLUM, R. H., CARTER, S. K., and AGRE, K. A clinical review of bleomycin-a new antineoplastic agent. Cancer, *31*:903, 1973.
23. HUGHES, P. S. H. Cryosurgery of verrucous carcinoma of the penis. Cutis, *24*:43, 1979.
24. ROTHENBERGER, K., et al. The neodymium-YAG laser in the treatment of penis carcinoma. In: Proc. 4th Cong. Int. Soc. Laser Surg., Tokyo, 1981.
25. GURSEL, E. O., et al. Penile cancer. Urology, *1*:569, 1973.
26. NARAYANA, A. S., et al. Carcinoma of the penis: Analysis of 219 cases. Cancer, *49*:2185, 1982.
27. BROWN, M. D., ZACHARY, C. B., and GREKIN, R. C. Penile tumors: Their management by Moh's micrographic surgery. J. Dermatol. Surg. Oncol., *13*:1163, 1987.
28. BISSADA, N. K. Post circumcision carcinoma of the penis: II. Surgical management. J. Surg. Oncol., *37*:80, 1988.

CHAPTER
38

Carcinoma of the Penis: Management of the Regional Lymphatic Drainage

Sakti Das
E. David Crawford

During the 19th century, the evolution of medical knowledge regarding lymphatic anatomy and lymphatic permeation by neoplasms advanced the surgical rationale of removal of the draining lymphatics as an integral part of the management of malignant neoplasms. For penile carcinoma, the pioneering report of MacCormack in 1886 established the concept of regional lymphadenectomy.[1] This was further championed by Curtis (1898)[2] and Young (1907).[3] Daseler in 1948 detailed the lymphatic distribution of the groin,[4] which is still considered the anatomic template for surgical dissection in ileoinguinal lymphadenectomy.

Carcinoma of the penis is among the few malignancies where removal of both the primary and draining lymphatics is of proven therapeutic value. The formidable morbidity associated with this extensive dissection, however, raises the question of critical selection of patients where the benefit of the procedure may justify the possible risks. Patients with clinically evident nodal metastasis, without documented distant metastasis, present a clear indication for ileoinguinal lymphadenectomy. Similar indication can be extended to those with a high probability of lymph node involvement. In the presence of positive lymph node metastases, 80% of the patients succumbed to their disease within 3 years when treated only with excision of the primary tumor.[5] In contrast, 50 to 66% 5-year survivals have been achieved by lymphadenectomy in stage-III patients.[6] Therefore, the therapeutic role of ileoinguinal node dissection in most patients with positive inguinal nodes is unquestionable.

The rationale for prophylactic lymphadenectomy in patients without demonstrable lymph node metastases remains controversial. Unfortunately, clinical evaluation of inguinal adenopathy is grossly inadequate because, in nearly half the instances, the palpable inguinal nodes in penile cancer patients are secondary to infection rather than metastatic involvement. Conversely, in clinically negative groins, 20% will harbor microscopic metastasis. If only stage-II patients were analyzed, the percentage of clinically nonpalpable metastases could be as high as 66%.[6] To obviate this high risk of false-negative clinical assessment, Cabanas proposed the sentinel lymph node biopsy.[7] He observed through lymphangiograms that the first echelon of metastatic drainage from penile carcinomas was the sentinel node located near the junction of the superficial epigastric and the greater saphenous vein. If on biopsy this sentinel node appears uninvolved, formal lymphadenectomy may not be necessary. Several authors have subsequently refuted Cabanas' proposal with reports of later development of inguinal metastases in patients with negative bilateral sentinel node biopsies.[8,9]

Luciani and associates have reported on cytologic examinations of fine-needle aspirates from nodes opacified by pedal lymphangiography.[10] The lymph nodes remain radiologically detectable for up to 9 months following the lymphangiography, allowing serial repeat aspiration cytologies.

In the absence of histologic documentation of inguinal node metastases, our decision for lymphadenectomy is based on the stage of the carcinoma of the penis. Stage-I or noninvasive tumors do not usually metastasize to lymph nodes, and are solely treated by wide excision or partial amputation with a 2-cm margin of clearance from the tumor. Stage-II tumors, with corporal invasion, have a high incidence of 40 to 66% lymph node metastases. Prophylactic ileoinguinal lymphadenectomy is expected to yield up to an 88% 5-year survival in these patients.[6] Stage-III patients with evident inguinal lymph node metastases require lymphadenectomy.

In summary, we recommend ileoinguinal lymphadenectomy under the following circumstances:

1. When inguinal lymphadenopathy persists after 6 weeks of adequate antimicrobial therapy following amputation or wide excision of the primary penile carcinoma.
2. When inguinal node metastases are histologically confirmed by biopsy or cytologic examination of fine-needle aspirates.
3. When inguinal adenopathy subsequently develops in a patient with a history of penile carcinoma.
4. In patients with stage-II or invasive carcinoma either clinically evident or proven by imaging studies (cavernosography[11] or magnetic resonance imaging).
5. When there are extensive lesions located proximally near the root of the penis.

ANATOMICAL CONSIDERATIONS FOR ILEOINGUINAL LYMPHADENECTOMY

The surgery of ileoinguinal lymph node dissection is fraught with morbid complications that are often directly related to the technique of surgical dissection. A proper conception of the lymphatic distribution, the vascular supply, and the extent or limits of necessary dissection, are imperative for a therapeutic lymphadenectomy with minimal morbidity.

Lymphatic Drainage of the Penis

Penile lymphatics are essentially divided into two sets. Those draining the prepuce and penile skin converge and coalesce into larger lymphatic trunks in the dorsum of the penis. These channels course toward the root of the penis, then pass laterally to terminate into the superficial inguinal nodes on both

sides. A more extensive network of lymphatics draining the glans penis course along the corona to the dorsum and merge to form larger vessels that follow the dorsal vein of the penis to the symphyseal area to ultimately drain into the superficial and deep inguinal nodes. Corporal lymphatics essentially follow the same pathway as that of the glans penis. Further efferent drainage of inguinal lymphatics occurs through lymph channels located in the femoral canal into external iliac and pelvic nodes.

Regional Anatomy

The superficial fascia of the lower abdomen and thigh is composed of two layers; the superficial fatty layer (Camper's fascia) and the deeper fibroelastic layer (Scarpa's fascia). The deep fascia enveloping the muscles of the thigh and gluteal region is called the fascia lata. It is attached superiorly to the posterior surface of the iliac crest, sacrum, sacrotuberous ligaments, ischium, pubic arch, symphysis pubes, pubic crest, and inguinal ligament. Distally, it is attached at the knee to the condyles of the femur and tibia and to the head of the fibula. Fascia lata is thinnest on the medial side and thickest on the lateral aspect of the thigh.

The superficial fatty layer of the superficial fascia of the abdomen continues uninterrupted into the lower extremity. The deeper fibroelastic layer, however, fuses with the fascia lata about 2 cm below the inguinal ligament.

The skin and subcutaneous tissue of the groin are supplied by the superficial external pudendal, superficial circumflex iliac, and superficial epigastric arteries. These vessels course in the superficial fatty layer of the superficial fascia and run parallel to the inguinal ligament. Because of this transverse or horizontal disposition of the blood vessels in the superficial fascia of the groin, a transverse incision is more likely to preserve adequate blood supply to the margins of the incision.

The femoral triangle is an anatomic area on the anterior thigh. It is bounded superiorly by the inguinal ligament as its base, laterally by the sartorius, and medially by the adductor longus. The adductor canal at the confluence of sartorius and adductor longus forms its apex. Its floor is formed by the fascia covering the iliopsoas and pectineus muscles. Its roof is formed by the fascia lata. The deep group of inguinal lymph nodes are located in the femoral triangle in the vicinity of the femoral vessels.

The greater saphenous vein, originating from the foot, ascends to the anteromedial aspect of the thigh. Coursing all along in the superficial fascia of the lower extremity, it ultimately passes through the fossa ovalis, an opening in the fascia lata 3 to 4 cm below the medial aspect of the inguinal ligament. The greater saphenous vein pierces the loose cribriform fascia covering the fossa ovalis and terminates into the femoral vein. At this site, the femoral vein and artery are encased in the femoral sheath, a funnel-like projection of the transversalis fascia (anteriorly) and the iliacus fascia (posteriorly). These blend to the adventitia of the femoral vessels at about a 4-cm distance from the inguinal ligament. The femoral sheath contains three distinct compartments, the most medial being the femoral canal, which contains the lymphatics and the lymph nodes. The middle compartment is occupied by the femoral vein, and the lateral compartment contains the femoral artery. The femoral nerve courses lateral to the femoral artery in a plane deep to the iliacus fascia (Fig. 38-1).

Inguino-femoral Lymph Node Distribution

The lymph nodes in this area are divided into both superficial and deep groups. The superficial inguinal nodes, along with the greater saphenous vein and its tributaries, are located within the membranous layer of the superficial fascia (Scarpa's fascia) of the femoral triangle, sandwiched between the superficial fatty layer (Camper's fascia) and the fascia lata. Daseler categorized the superficial inguinal nodes into different zones. Four quadrant zones were outlined by horizontal and vertical lines drawn at the saphenofemoral junction. Daseler's fifth quadrant was the saphenofemoral junction (Fig. 38-2). Quadrant: 1 lymph nodes are located around the superficial circumflex iliac vein. Quadrant 2, located in the superior medial area, contains lymph nodes around the superficial epigastric and superficial external pudendal vein. Of particular importance in Daseler's dissection was the fact that lymph nodes were often detected 1 cm above the inguinal ligament. Quadrant 3 is inferomedial in position and contains nodes around the greater saphenous vein. The inferolateral quadrant 4 contains lymph nodes clustered around the lateral accessory saphenous vein and termination of the superficial circumflex iliac vein. Each quadrant may contain several lymph nodes or may be completely void of them. The superficial nodes send their efferents to the glands of deeper location situated along the femoral vessels (deep inguinal nodes) and then into the retroperitoneal iliac chain in the pelvis.

The deep inguinal nodes are situated beneath the fascia lata in the femoral triangle. They form a small chain of nodes in the adipose tissue surrounding the femoral vessels within the femoral sheath. Distally, they may extend into the adductor canal

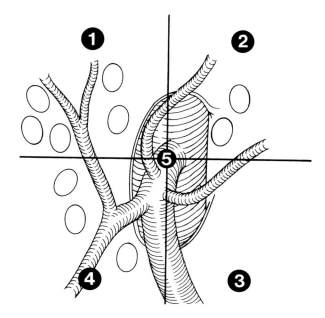

FIG. 38-2. Zonal division of superficial inguinal nodes according to Daseler.

and proximally, they continue underneath the inguinal ligament to merge with the external iliac chain. The most consistent member of the deep inguinal group is the node of Cloquet or Rosenmuller, located in the femoral canal medial to the femoral vein.

ILEOINGUINAL LYMPHADENECTOMY

Oral antibiotic therapy during the 6-week period following treatment of the primary lesion of the penis helps in reducing infectious inflammation of the inguinal lymph nodes. A low residual diet on the day before surgery and a cleansing enema on the night before surgery minimizes the risk of bowel movements and wound contamination in the immediate postoperative period. Parenteral broad-spectrum antibiotics are started just prior to surgery. Intermittent compressive stockings are applied to the lower extremities.

Although a variety of incisions and approaches have been proposed by individual advocates, we prefer to start with a midline suprapubic incision for bilateral pelvic lymphadenectomy, followed by curvilinear groin incisions for inguinal dissection (Fig. 38-3A). In patients with clinically or histologically positive inguinal adenopathy, or with invasive and extensive primary lesions, we recommend bilateral groin dissection. However, when an initially negative groin develops adenopathy during follow-up, unilateral dissection only of the involved side is recommended. The patient is positioned supine with a roll under the sacrum. The ipsilateral thigh is abducted, externally rotated, and flexed at the knee (Fig. 38-3B). A urethral catheter is left indwelling. The entire abdomen and thighs are prepared and draped.

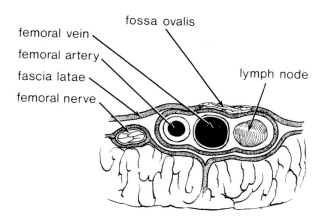

FIG. 38-1. Femoral sheath.

fossa ovalis

femoral vein

femoral artery

fascia latae

femoral nerve

lymph node

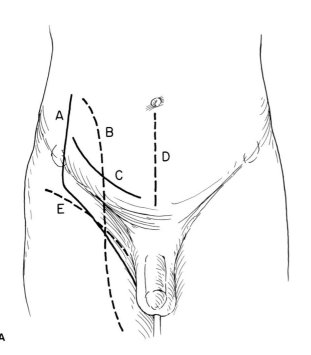

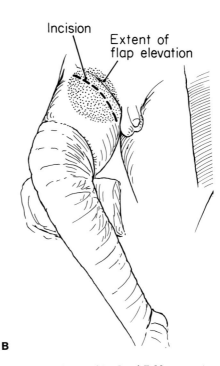

Incision

Extent of flap elevation

A

B

FIG. 38-3. *A,* Incisions employed for ileoinguinal lymphadenectomy. The skin-bridge technique is depicted in *C* and *E.* My current recommendation is a suprapubic midline incision coupled with a curvilinear thigh incision (*D* and *E*) *B,* Patient position for right ilioinguinal lymphadenectomy. The leg is abducted at the thigh, flexed at the knee, and externally rotated. An indwelling urethral catheter is inserted and the scrotum draped out of the operative field.

PELVIC LYMPHADENECTOMY

A midline incision is made from the umbilicus to the symphyses pubes. Extraperitoneal pelvic lymphadenectomy (see Chapter 16) is carried out on the ipsilateral or more involved side, taking down node-bearing adipose connective tissue around the distal common iliac artery, external iliac vessels, internal iliac artery, and the obturator fossa. If gross nodal metastases are evident and proven on frozen section analysis, then an inguinal lymphadenectomy is not warranted. If the nodes are negative, contralateral pelvic lymph node dissection is carried out with frozen section examination. In contrast to pelvic lymphadenectomy for prostatic carcinoma, the lymph node dissection is carried beyond the circumflex iliac vessels further distally, down to and behind the inguinal ligament, with special attention to dissecting nodal tissue from the femoral canal (Fig. 38-4). The dissected pelvic lymph nodal mass is removed separately at the level of the inguinal ligament. We believe that any attempt at en bloc removal of pelvic and inguinal nodes, without actual division of the inguinal ligament, is an exercise in futility. The wound is closed in layers without a drain.

INGUINAL LYMPHADENECTOMY

A curvilinear incision is made in the upper thigh, starting below the anterior superior iliac spine, running 5 to 10 cm distal and parallel to the inguinal ligament, and ending medi-

ally up to the prominent adductor longus tendon. The goal of the dissection is to clear the superficial and deep inguinal lymph nodes located in the femoral triangle.

Meticulous attention is devoted to developing viable skin flaps. The skin flaps should include the superficial fatty layer of the subcutaneous adipose tissue leaving only a thin layer of membranous Scarpa's fascia containing the superficial lymph

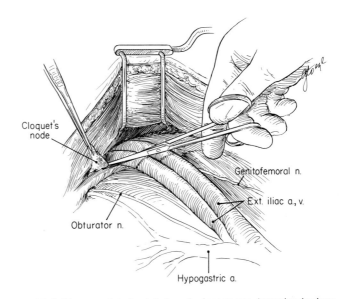

Cloquet's node

Genitofemoral n.

Ext. iliac a., v.

Obturator n.

Hypogastric a.

FIG. 38-4. The completed pelvic lymphadenectomy. Attention is given to the meticulous removal of the contents of the femoral canal.

nodes. Initially, skin edges are carefully handled with skin hooks, then grasped manually to finally be lifted up with Deaver retractors. We prefer to develop the skin flaps up to the margins of the femoral triangle, except proximally, as this flap is carried up to about 2 cm above the inguinal ligament (Fig. 38-5).

Starting superiorly, the fibrofatty tissue of the Scarpa's fascia is sharply divided down to the external oblique aponeurosis and then dissected towards the inguinal ligament (Fig. 38-5). Subcutaneous vessels are carefully electrocoagulated or divided between fine catgut ligatures throughout the dissection to ensure hemostasis and to minimize lymph leakage. Medially, the node-bearing tissues are stripped from the adductor longus muscle and dissection is continued to clear the femoral canal. The femoral vein and artery enclosed in femoral sheath, lies immediately lateral. The fascial sheath overlying the vessels is stripped to expose the vein and the artery (Fig. 38-6). Lateral to the femoral artery, the femoral nerve is noted shining underneath the fascia covering the iliacus muscle. We do not dissect the nerve and its branches because no significant nodal tissue exist in this area. Dissecting laterally, the origin of the sartorius muscle from the anterior superior iliac spine is exposed. With medial traction on the dissected superior block of tissues, the fibrofatty tissue and fascia covering the sartorius muscle are sharply divided downward to define the lateral boundary of the femoral triangle (Fig. 38-7). With downward traction on the dissected tissues, stripping of the femoral vessels is resumed. All fibrofatty and nodal tissues are

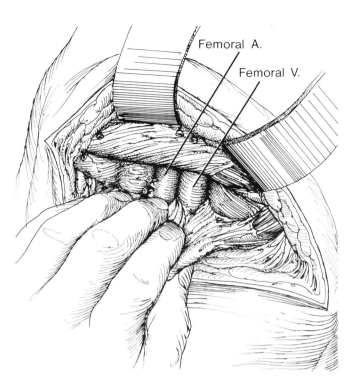

FIG. 38-6. En bloc dissection is continued in the femoral sheath clearing the tissues anterior to the femoral vessels.

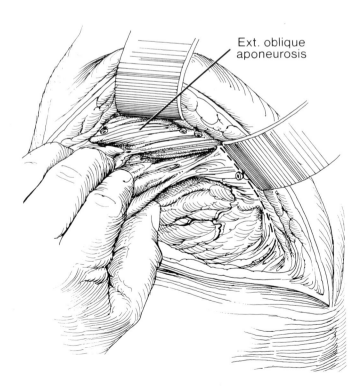

FIG. 38-5. Proximal skin flap is developed. Fibrofatty superficial fascia is dissected down to external oblique aponeurosis.

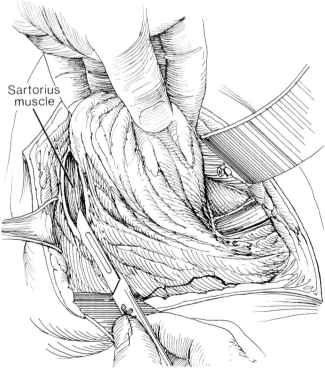

FIG. 38-7. Outer limit of dissection at the lateral margin of the femoral triangle.

meticulously dissected off the anterolateral aspect of the femoral artery and vein. Lifting the vessels and clearing the posterior aspect is not necessary as there are usually no draining lymph nodes behind the vessels. The profunda femoris branch arises from the posterior aspect of the femoral artery at about 3 cm distal to the inguinal ligament. This important arterial branch should be identified and carefully preserved. As the femoral vein is dissected, the termination of the greater saphenous vein is noticed passing through the fossa ovalis. The greater saphenous vein is ligated and divided at its junction with the femoral vein (Fig. 38-8). The edges of the fossa ovalis are divided medially, where it continues as fascia lata covering the adductor longus. All the tissues and fascia lata covering the medial margin of adductor longus are sharply divided downwards until they join the lateral dissection along the medial margin of the sartorius muscle. At the distal limit of the inferior dissection, the greater saphenous vein is encountered again and divided between ligatures (Fig. 38-9). We have proposed that preservation of the greater saphenous vein with meticulous skeletonization may be therapeutically effective with added benefit of reduced chance of postoperative edema of the lower extremities. There are no controlled study available in support or against this conjecture. Centrally, the stripping of the anterior aspect of the femoral vessels is continued up to the apex of the femoral triangle, removing the deep inguinal glands en block with the rest of the specimen.

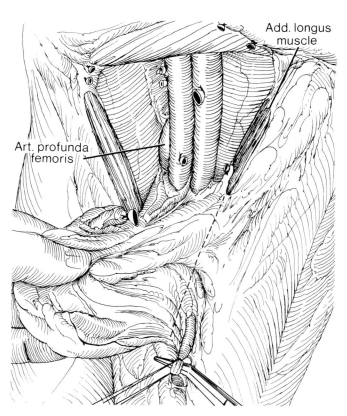

FIG. 38-9. Distal limit of dissection at the apex of the femoral triangle. The greater saphenous vein is again ligated and divided.

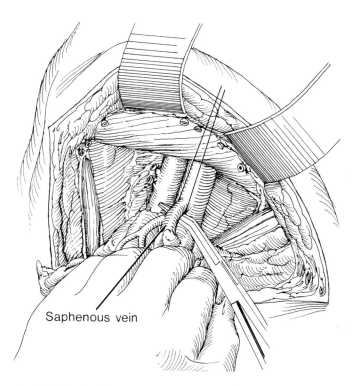

FIG. 38-8. Further dissection in the floor of the femoral triangle. Ligation and division of the greater saphenous vein.

WOUND CLOSURE

The wound is irrigated with saline and any visible bleeding or lymphatic oozing is controlled. The inguinal ligament is sutured to the Cooper's ligament with interrupted 2-0 silk sutures to close the empty femoral canal medial to the femoral vein. The sartorius muscle is dissected off its origin from the anterior superior iliac spine. It is partially mobilized medially to cover the femoral vessels and is secured to the inguinal ligament with interrupted 2-0 silk horizontal mattress sutures (Fig. 38-10). The subcutaneous tissue of the lower flap is anchored to the underlying muscles with interrupted 4-0 polyglycolic acid sutures. This eliminates the dead spaces and prevents fluid collections in the wound (Fig. 38-10). A 7 mm Jackson-Pratt suction drain is inserted through the distal flap (Fig. 38-11). Several millimeters of excess skin are removed from the edges of the skin flaps. The use of intravenous fluorescin and Wood's lamp helps delineate viable skin edges.[12] The skin edges are reapproximated with interrupted 4-0 Prolene sutures. So that the vascularity of the skin flaps may not be compromised, sterile dressings are applied and secured loosely to avoid pressure.

POSTOPERATIVE CARE AND COMPLICATIONS

The patient is maintained on bedrest for 7 days. The lower extremities are kept in intermittent compressive stockings and

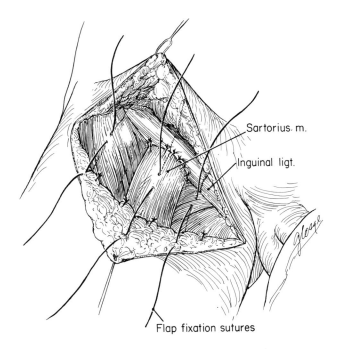

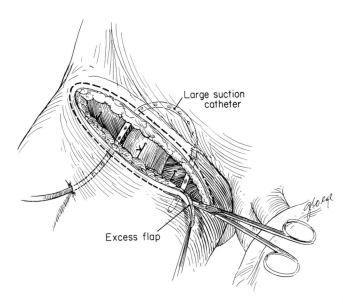

Fig. 38-11. The excess skin is excised. A large suction catheter is inserted distal to the lower flap and is coiled under the upper and lower flaps.

FIG. 38-10. The sartorius muscle is sharply detached from its origin at the iliac spine and displaced medially. Care must be taken to preserve blood supply to the muscle, which enters posteriorly near its midportion. Silk fixation sutures are employed to secure sartorius to the inguinal ligament.

elevated during bedrest. The urethral catheter is removed after 48 hours. The suction drain is removed when the 24-hour drainage output becomes less than 30 cc's. This usually occurs 5 to 7 days postoperatively when the patient starts ambulating. Anticoagulation with mini-dose Heparin levels adjusted according to the partial thromboplastin times is continued during the bedrest period to prevent thrombophlebitis.[13] Necrosis of the skin flaps can occur if the skin flaps are traumatized or dissected too thin and thereby devascularized. Meticulous intraoperative care should be exercised during the development of the skin flaps to prevent such complications. Wound infection is an uncommon complication unless the surgery was performed on an ulcerated or infected groin. Infection can precipitate necrosis of the compromised skin flaps. Established wound necrosis is treated by debridement and split thickness skin grafting. Postoperative lymphedema of the lower extremity has been reported in up to 40% of patients. Edema may be transient or permanent, affecting the distal leg or the whole lower extremity. Treatment includes support stockings, elevation, and the judicious use of diuretics.

REFERENCES

1. MacCormack, W. Five cases of amputation of the penis for epithelioma. Br. Med. J., *1*:343, 1886.
2. Curtis, B. F. *American Textbook of Diseases of the Skin.* Philadelphia, W.B. Saunders, 1898, p. 76.
3. Young, H. H. A radical operation for the cure of cancer of the penis. J. Urol., *26*:285, 1931.
4. Daseler, E. H., Anson, B. J., and Reimann, A. F. Radical excision of the inguinal and iliac lymph glands. Surg. Gynecol. Obstet., *87*:679, 1948.
5. Staubitz, W. J., Lent, M. H., and Oberkircher, O. J. Carcinoma of the penis. Cancer, *8*:371, 1955.
6. Scott McDougal, W., Kirchner, F. K. Jr., Edwards, R. H., and Killion, L. T. Treatment of carcinoma of the penis: The case for primary lymphadenectomy. J. Urol., *136*:38, 1986.
7. Cabanas, R. M. An approach for the treatment of penile carcinoma. Cancer, *39*:456, 1977.
8. Perinetti, E., Crane, D. B., and Catalona, W. J. Unreliability of sentinel lymph node biopsy for staging penile carcinoma. J. Urol., *124*:734, 1980.
9. deKernion, J. B. *Ilioinguinal Lymphadenectomy in Genitourinary Cancer Surgery,* Edited by E. D. Crawford and T. A. Borden. Philadelphia, Lea & Febiger, 1982, p. 318.
10. Luciani, L., Piscioli, F., Scappini, P., and Pusiol, T. Value and role of percutaneous regional node aspiration cytology in the management of penile carcinoma. Eur. Urol., *10*:294, 1984.
11. Crawford, E. D., and Dawkins, C. A. Cancer of the penis. In *Diagnosis and Management of Genitourinary Cancer,* Edited by D. G. Skinner and G. Lieskovsky. Philadelphia, W. B. Saunders, 1988, p. 554.
12. Smith, J. A., Jr., and Middleton, R. G. The use of fluorescin in radial inguinal lymphadenectomy. J. Urol., *122*:754, 1979.
13. Leyvraz, P. F., et al. Adjusted versus fixed-dose subcutaneous heparin in the treatment of deep vein thrombosis after total hip replacement. N. Engl. J. Med., *309*:954, 1983.

Surgical Management of Urethral Carcinoma*

Peter R. Carroll

Urethral carcinoma is rare. Although Thiaudierre published the first report in 1834, little more than 1,500 cases have been reported in the English-language literature since then. It generally arises during the sixth and seventh decades of life, is the only genitourinary cancer that is more common in women than men (0.02% of cancers in women), and occurs more commonly in whites than blacks. Because of the substantial anatomic differences between the male and female urethra, management in each sex must be considered separately.

Most reports of these rare cancers, even from large referral institutions, include both relatively small numbers and substantial variation among individual tumors because of differences in tissue structure, grade, site, and anatomic extent. Thus no consensus has been reached on the optimal management. Presently, treatment decisions must be based on the biologic characteristics of the tumor (i.e., stage, grade, and site), the morbidity of each mode of treatment, and its ability to eradicate or control the malignancy.

MALE URETHRAL CARCINOMA

Anatomy

The male urethra is approximately 21 cm long and can be divided into three regional segments: prostatic, membranous, and penile.[1] (Fig. 39-1) The prostatic urethra, approximately 3-cm long, is surrounded by prostatic tissue and contains the ejaculatory and prostatic ducts. The membranous urethra, the thickest and shortest segment (averaging between 2 and 2.5 cm), is surrounded by smooth and skeletal muscle, the latter constituting the external urinary sphincter. The penile urethra, the longest segment, is contained within the corpus spongiosum and extends from the pelvic floor musculature to the external urinary meatus (approximately 15 cm). The proximal portion, the bulbar urethra, is expanded in a fusiform fashion and is covered by the bulbospongiosus muscle. As the pendulous urethra approaches the meatus, it widens once again to form the fossa navicularis. The posterior urethra comprises of the prostatic and membranous portions and the anterior urethra the penile segment (bulbar and pendulous). However, most authors will describe lesions in the bulbar urethra as being posterior lesions because of their similar prognosis to tumors of the membranous urethra.

The epithelial lining of the urethra varies: transitional in the prostatic urethra; pseudostratified or stratified columnar in the membranous, bulbar, and penile segments; and stratified squa-

*Supported by a Clinical Oncology Career Development Award from the American Cancer Society.

mous epithelium at the urinary meatus (see Fig. 39-1). Paired bulbourethral glands, Cowper's glands, lie within the deep perineal compartment of the urogenital diaphragm surrounding the membranous urethra. The paired ducts of these glands run distally into the corpus spongiosum and open into the bulbar urethra. Numerous submucosal glands, the glands of Littré, can be found along the anterior urethra.

The urethra is surrounded by structures with a rich blood supply. The internal pudendal artery, a branch of the hypogastric artery, gives rise to two arteries that supply the anterior urethra: the bulbar and urethral arteries. The former supplies the bulbar urethra and bulbospongiosum; the latter supplies the corpus spongiosum. The glans penis is supplied by the deep dorsal artery, which lies below Buck's fascia between the dorsal veins and nerves.

A thorough knowledge of regional anatomy and the lymphatic drainage of the urethra is essential to tumor staging and treatment planning. Generally, lesions of the anterior urethra drain into the inguinal lymph nodes and lesions of the posterior urethra into the pelvic lymph nodes. The lymphatics of the glans penis and the penile urethra drain into the deep subinguinal lymph node group underneath the fascia lata and medial to the femoral vein. There are generally only one to three lymph nodes in this group,[2] which then drain into the external iliac lymph node chain.

If a urethral carcinoma invades the corpus cavernosum or penile or scrotal skin, more extensive inguinal nodal metastases may occur. These structures drain into the superficial inguinal lymph nodes, which are contained (along with the saphenous vein) within the superficial fascia of the thigh in an area bounded by the inguinal ligament, the sartorius muscle, and the adductor longus muscle. The number of lymph nodes in this group varies considerably, and they can be divided into five groups according to their relationship with the junction of

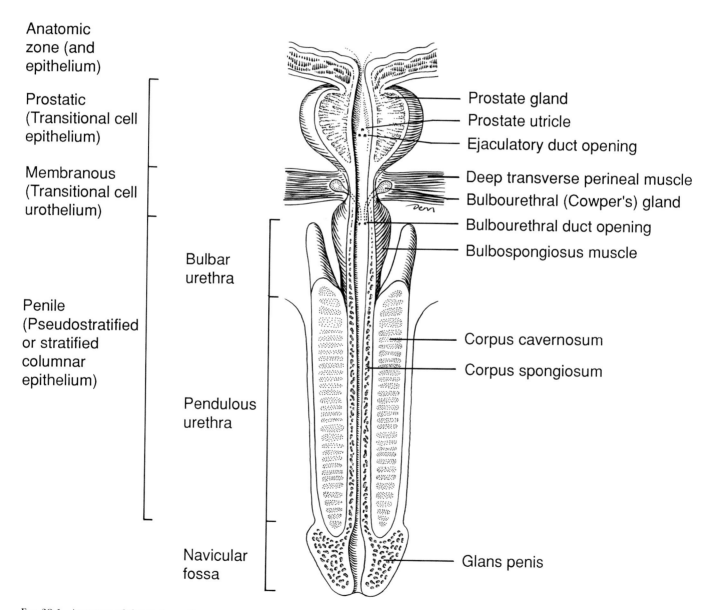

Anatomic zone (and epithelium)

Prostatic (Transitional cell epithelium)

Membranous (Transitional cell urothelium)

Penile (Pseudostratified or stratified columnar epithelium)

Bulbar urethra

Pendulous urethra

Navicular fossa

Prostate gland
Prostate utricle
Ejaculatory duct opening
Deep transverse perineal muscle
Bulbourethral (Cowper's) gland
Bulbourethral duct opening
Bulbospongiosus muscle

Corpus cavernosum
Corpus spongiosum

Glans penis

FIG. 39-1. Anatomy of the male urethra.

the saphenous and femoral veins.[3] Generally, lymphatic channels from the penis and scrotum drain into the central and medial segments.

The bulbar, membranous, and prostatic urethral segments drain into three lymphatic channels,[4] one channel travels with the dorsal vein underneath the suspensory ligament to drain into the external iliac lymph node chain (generally 8 to 10 lymph nodes are found in this region); another channel travels along the course of the internal pudendal artery to empty into the obdurator lymph node group (4 to 8 lymph nodes); a third channel empties into the presacral lymph nodes. The lymphatic drainage may vary considerably in individual cases depending on the extent of the tumor and whether it obstructs the primary lymphatic drainage system.

The perineum is bounded by the pubic symphysis anteriorly, the ischial tuberosities laterally and the coccyx posteriorly (Fig. 39-2). The urogenital diaphragm lies anterior to a line drawn between the ischial tuberosities, and the anal triangle lies posterior to this line. The posterior urethra is most often approached surgically through the urogenital diaphragm. Deep to the skin and subcutaneous fat is the membranous continuation of the superficial fascia of the anterior abdominal wall, the Colles' fascia. Beneath this fascial layer is the superficial space of the perineum in which are three paired muscles: bulbospongiosus, ischiocavernosus, and transversus perinei superficialis. The bulbospongiosus muscle lies in the midline covering the bulb of the penis; laterally, the ischiocavernosus muscle extends from the ischium to the pubic arch covering the crura of the penis; at the base of the superficial space, the paired transverse perinei superficialis muscles extend from the ischium laterally to the perineal body centrally. The deep perineal space is covered by a perineal membrane. Within this space lie striated muscular components of the external urinary sphincter, the transversus perinei profundus muscles, and Cowper's glands. Deep to this region lies a deep fascial layer covering the obdurator internus muscles.

Blood to this region is supplied by branches of the internal pudendal artery. An inferior branch, the inferior hemorrhoidal,

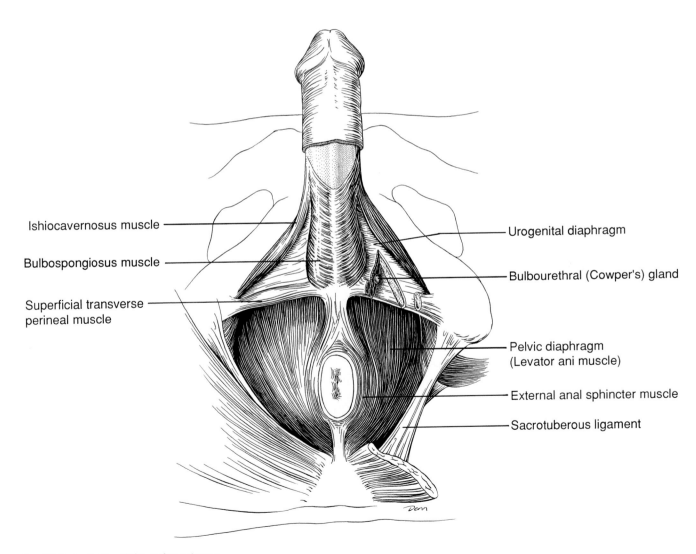

Ishiocavernosus muscle

Bulbospongiosus muscle

Superficial transverse perineal muscle

Urogenital diaphragm

Bulbourethral (Cowper's) gland

Pelvic diaphragm (Levator ani muscle)

External anal sphincter muscle

Sacrotuberous ligament

FIG. 39-2. Anatomy of the male perineum.

supplies the anal triangle. Anterior branches supply the urogenital diaphragm. One branch enters the superficial space to supply the superficial perineal musculature and then extends forward as the posterior scrotal artery. Deep branches enter the deep compartment running along the perineal membrane to supply the sphincter muscles of this layer. As mentioned previously, the internal pudendal artery supplies the bulbar and urethral branches.

Histopathology and Pathophysiology

Because the epithelial lining varies along the course of the urethra, histologic findings also will vary. The most common histologic type is squamous carcinoma (77%).[5–13] Most are moderate and high-grade tumors.[6,8,11] Primary transitional cell carcinoma accounts for 16%. Of carcinomas originating in the bulbar, membranous, and prostatic urethras, 85% are squamous cell carcinoma; of all primary carcinomas of the prostatic urethra, 90% are transitional cell. The latter should be differentiated from the more common finding of regional extension of bladder transitional cell carcinoma. Urethral adenocarcinoma is rare (6%) and must be differentiated from extension of a primary adenocarcinoma of the prostate. The exact origin of this histologic type is the subject of some speculation, but it may arise in the periurethral glands of Cowper or Littré or from areas of metaplasia.[14,15] Rarely, it will resemble clear cell adenocarcinoma of the female genital tract (characterized by cells with abundant clear cytoplasm and pleomorphism). These carcinomas must be differentiated from benign, nephrogenic adenomas. Melanoma is a rare tumor of the male urethra.[16] The most common site of origin is the meatus or fossa navicularis. Other, usually metastatic, tumor types have been reported. The most common metastatic tumors are from the prostatic, colon, and bladder carcinomas.[17,18]

Approximately 35% of male urethral carcinomas occur in the anterior urethra (meatus, fossa navicularis, and pendulous) and 65% in the posterior urethra (bulbar, membranous, and prostatic). Urethral carcinoma must be differentiated from benign urethral lesions including urethral cysts, polyps, and condylomata acuminata.

Metastases to regional lymph nodes occur in approximately 14 to 30% of patients, but have been reported in up to 50%.[6,13,19] Distant metastases are rare at the time of presentation (10 to 14%).[11,13] The most common sites include the liver, lung, and skeleton.

Risk factors for urethral carcinoma are not as yet definitive. A high association (27 to 88%) exists with a history of urethral stricture disease or infection. These may promote metaplasia of the urethral epithelium and the subsequent progression to squamous cell malignancy. Alternatively, stricture disease may have been a misdiagnosis in a patient with urethral carcinoma and obstructive voiding symptoms. The relatively high association with a history of venereal disease raises the possibility that a sexually transmitted agent might be responsible for tumor development. Interestingly, Grussendorf-Conen and colleagues demonstrated the presence of human papillomavirus (HPV-6) DNA within the nuclei of a primary squamous cell carcinoma of the male urethra.[20] Such viral DNA can be commonly found in condylomata acuminata, but has not been thought to be associated with a high rate of carcinogenesis.

Analysis of tumor DNA content by flow cytometry has been used to predict prognosis and progression rates for a variety of urologic tumors, including urethral carcinoma. Those found to have a normal DNA content (diploid) tend to be of lower stage, and progress less frequently (18%) than those with an abnormal, higher DNA content (aneuploid) (93%). Patients with diploid tumors have a higher 5-year survival rate than patients with aneuploid tumors (85 vs. 20%). Squamous cell carcinomas of the bulbomembranous urethra are more likely to exhibit aneuploidy than tumors of the penile urethra (69 and 29%, respectively).[21] Measurement of DNA content by flow cytometry may add prognostic information not gained by examining individual tumor grade or stage alone.

Diagnosis and Staging

Signs and symptoms of urethral carcinoma can vary widely. More common symptoms include bleeding (34%), obstructive voiding (40%), and dysuria or frequency (28%). The more common signs in men include a palpable mass (40%); the less common, an abscess or fistula of the perineum or genitalia.

A careful evaluation is required to confirm the diagnosis and to assess the anatomic extent. Precise staging will allow selective and appropriate management. Patients with low-stage lesions may be spared extensive surgery, radiation, or chemotherapy with their attendant morbidity, whereas patients with more extensive tumors can be offered early aggressive management. Unfortunately, a staging system based on a tumor, node, metastasis (TNM) classification scheme has not been developed for urethral carcinomas as it has been for other genitourinary malignancies. Presently, most clinicians use those staging systems developed by Ray and associates or Levine (Table 39-1).

Staging begins with a careful physical examination noting the presence of a urethral mass (size, site, and any fixation), fistula formation, infection, and regional or distant lymphadenopathy. Biopsy, preferably under anesthesia, is the single most important method of diagnosis and local tumor staging. Tumor size, extent, and location should be carefully estimated. If possible, the bladder and most proximal urethral segments should be examined to note the proximal extent of the tumor and the presence of bladder involvement.

Retrograde urethrography has been the primary imaging technique for local disease (Fig. 39-3). This is now well complemented by magnetic resonance imaging (MRI) (Fig. 39-4), which allows for multiplanar imaging and excellent soft tissue contrast. Regional extension may be better estimated with this technique than with the conventional methods of urethrography or computerized tomography (CT). Although cavernosography has been used to assess the extent of primary or

TABLE 39-1. *Staging of Male Urethral Carcinoma*

RAY (MEMORIAL) STAGING SYSTEM

Stage 0	Confined to the mucosa only (in situ)
Stage A	Into but not beyond the lamina propria
Stage B	Into but not beyond the substance of the corpus spongiosum or into but not beyond the prostate
Stage C	Direct extension into tissue beyond the corpus spongiosum (corpora cavernosa, muscle fat, fascia, skin, direct skeletal involvement) or beyond the prostatic capsule
Stage D1	Regional metastases including inguinal and pelvic lymph nodes (with any primary tumor)
Stage D2	Distant metastases (with any primary tumor)

LEVINE STAGING SYSTEM

Stage 0	In situ (limited to mucosa)
Stage A	Submucosal (not beyond submucosa)
Stage B	Into but not beyond the substance of the corpus spongiosum (corpora cavernosa, muscle, fat, fascia, skin, direct skeletal involvement) or beyond the prostatic capsule
Stage C	Direct extension into tissue beyond the corpus spongiosum (corpora cavernosa, muscle, fat, fascia, skin, direct skeletal involvement) or beyond the prostatic capsule
Stage D	Metastasis 1. Inguinal lymph nodes 2. Pelvic lymph nodes below the bifurcation of the aorta 3. Lymph nodes above the bifurcation of the aorta 4. Distant

metastatic penile carcinomas, its use in urethral carcinoma has been limited.[22] Similar information may be gained noninvasively with MRI.

Inguinal lymph node metastases may be assessed with physical examination, CT, or MRI (Fig. 39-5). Pelvic lymphadenopathy is best assessed radiographically with CT or MRI. Chest radiography and bone scan will complete staging in most patients.

Treatment of Localized Disease: Alternatives to Surgery.

Selected low-grade and -stage urethral malignancies may be managed with local resection. Squamous cell tumors suitable for such an approach would be low-grade squamous papillomas of the meatus or fossa navicularis.[23] These may be excised with standard transurethral resection techniques or the CO_2 or neodynium/YAG laser. Patients managed in such a fashion require careful surveillance and often adjunctive treatment with topical chemotherapy is warranted. This approach has been successful in patients with low-grade, superficial transitional cell carcinomas of the urethra, usually associated with a history of bladder carcinoma.[5,24]

Invasive, higher grade lesions of the urethra require more aggressive treatment to cure the malignancy and prevent local progression. Radiation has had variable success.[5,7,8,10,25] Long-term survival is uncommon (approximately 15%), and local recurrence arises in the majority who receive irradiation alone. Radiation seems most effective for small-volume lesions of the anterior urethra that are minimally to moderately invasive. The delivery of interstitial radiation with modern techniques may allow for more accurate treatment with limited morbidity.[26] Radiation may be an important palliative in treating patients with unresectable local tumor or symptomatic metastatic disease.

Chemotherapy has been used in only a small number of patients with localized urethral carcinoma. Pure transitional cell carcinoma of the prostatic and membranous urethra has been treated with cisplatin-based combination chemotherapy: methotrexate, vinblastine, doxorubicin, and cisplatin.[27] A complete clinical response was seen in 3 of 5 patients. The combination of irradiation and chemotherapy has had relatively good success in squamous cell tumors of the anus and esophagus and should be investigated further for the management of urethral carcinoma.[28]

Surgery seems to be more effective than radiation for invasive tumors. In patients with anterior urethral carcinoma, local recurrence has been documented in approximately 8% and 5-year survival in approximately 55%. Carcinoma of the posterior urethra frequently presents at an advanced stage and therefore carries a poorer prognosis: 5-year survival is approximately 24% [5,7–11,13,29,30] and local recurrence is more common (approximately 20%).

The surgical approach to invasive urethral carcinoma varies with the site, size, and volume of the tumor. Anterior carcinoma often can be excised preserving an adequate margin of resection with less extensive surgery than that required for posterior tumors.

Anterior Urethral Carcinoma

Preoperative preparation should include prophylactic antibiotic therapy in patients with no evidence of infection. A broad-spectrum antibiotic administered perioperatively is usually adequate. With evidence of infection, a broad-spectrum antibiotic combination should initially be followed by specific treatment once culture results are available. Surgery should be delayed until the inflammatory process has resolved or stabilized. Usually a limited bowel-cleansing program is instituted the day before surgery.

Patients undergoing distal or segmental urethrectomy alone may be placed in the standard lithotomy position. Those patients requiring excision of the more proximal urethral segments with construction of a perineal urethrostomy or complete urethrectomy after previous cystectomy should be placed in the extreme or exaggerated lithotomy position (Fig.

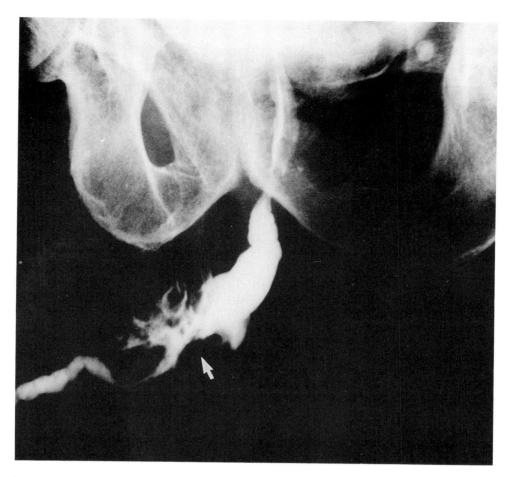

Fig. 39-3. An extensive bulbar urethral carcinoma demonstrated by retrograde urethrography (arrow).

39-6) with the legs in stirrups rotated in a cephalad direction. A rolled towel can be placed underneath the sacrum to ensure that the perineum is almost parallel with the floor. All pressure points should be padded carefully.

Rarely, noninvasive lesions may be managed by segmental urethrectomy followed by end-to-end reanastomosis of the proximal and distal urethral segments (which should be examined intraoperatively with frozen sections to ensure complete excision of the carcinoma). A distal urethrectomy alone, with preservation of the corpora cavernosa, is indicated in only those rare patients with superficial or minimally invasive lesions of the anterior urethra. An inverted U, or curvilinear, incision is made extending just medial to and between the ischial tuberosities (Figs. 39-7 and 39-9). For more distal exposure, a midline incision can be added at the apex. The subcutaneous tissue is divided and the bulbocavernosus muscle is incised in the midline. Dissection proceeds along the urethra distally toward the meatus, with gradual mobilization resulting in inversion of the penis. At the glans, the penis is inverted back to its normal anatomic position. An incision is made around the entire meatus. The meatus and fossa navicularis are separated from the surrounding spongy tissue of the glans, thereby completing dissection of the penile and distal bulbar

segments of the urethra. The meatal incision is closed with 3-0 or 4-0 chromic sutures. Glanular drainage usually is not necessary. The most proximal part of the urethral dissection is then completed. The midbulbar urethra should be mobilized proximally, preserving its extensive blood supply. A small ellipse of skin is excised in the midline at the base of the original incision, and a tunnel is created in the subcutaneous tissue by blunt dissection. The urethra is spatulated and anastomosed to the skin with interrupted 3-0 absorbable suture material. A small Penrose or Jackson-Pratt drain is left along the area of dissection and is brought out in a separate lateral skin incision. The subcutaneous layers are brought together with interrupted 2-0 or 3-0 absorbable suture material. The original skin incision is closed similarly, and the drain is left in place approximately 48 hours or until drainage becomes minimal.

Frankly invasive lesions of the anterior urethra require either partial or total penectomy. Very distal lesions can be managed with partial penectomy, a procedure similar to that for management of primary penile carcinoma (see Chap. 37). For more proximal lesions of the anterior urethra, partial penectomy may not allow for sufficient reconstruction of the penile urethra to direct the urinary stream or ensure a tumor-free margin. These should be managed with total penectomy and

FIG. 39-4. MRI of an extensive bulbomembranous urethral carcinoma. *A,* T1-weighted transaxial view showing invasion of ischium (I). *B,* Sagittal view showing dilated prostatic urethra (PU), large urethral carcinoma (arrow), and corpus cavernosum (CC).

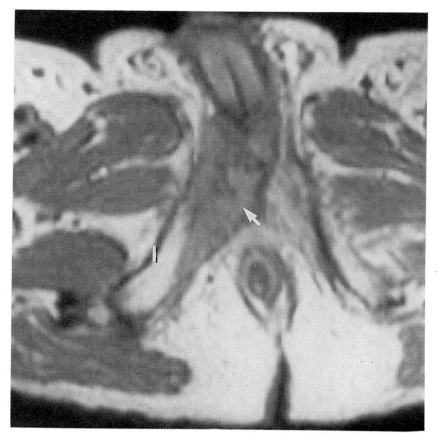

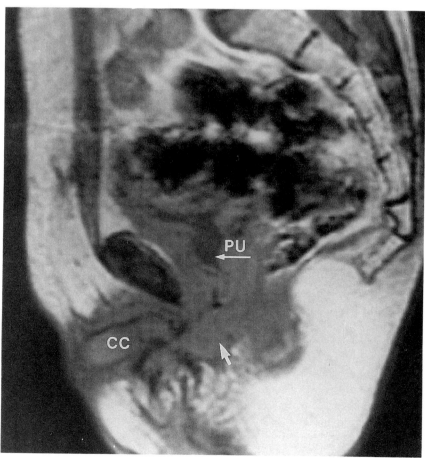

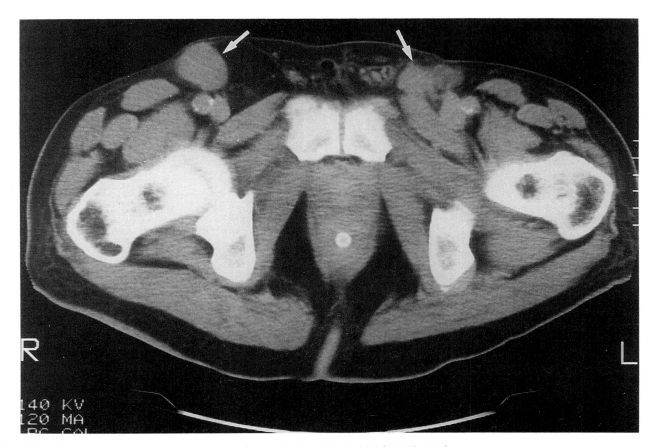

FIG. 39-5. CT showing bilateral inguinal metastases (arrows) just anterior to the femoral vessels.

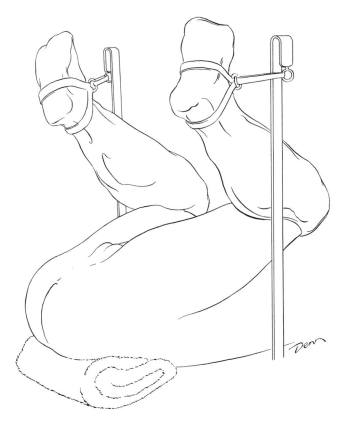

FIG. 39-6. Extreme or exaggerated lithotomy position.

FIG. 39-7. Penectomy, urethrectomy, and creation of a perineal ure-throstomy. *A,* Incision around base of penis. *B,* Perineal incision made allowing proximal dissection and easy exposure of the entire bulbar urethra and crura. Urethra incised and dissected free proximally. The corpora cavernosae have been incised and closed underneath the pubis. *C,* Perineal urethrostomy completed.

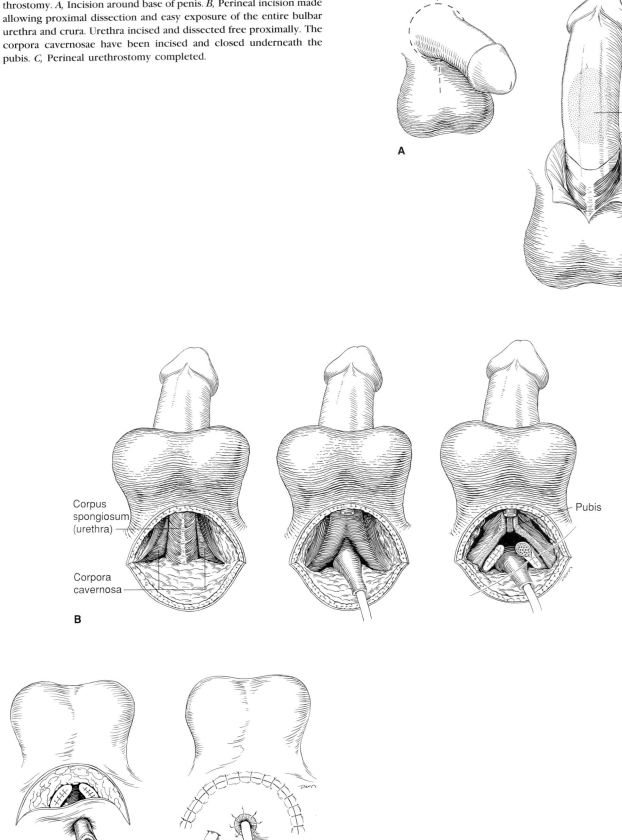

creation of a perineal urethrostomy (see Fig. 39-7). The patient should be placed in the extreme lithotomy position. An elliptical incision is made around the base of the penis and dissection should proceed proximally along the corporal bodies with care to preserve a clear margin of resection. The dorsal vessels are divided at the level of the pubic symphysis after the suspensory ligament has been divided. Dissection should proceed proximally along the corpus spongiosum until a tumor-free margin of approximately 2 cm has been achieved. For more proximal dissection, a separate perineal incision may be necessary. The spongiosum is then dissected free from the corpora cavernosa proximally. The corpus spongiosum and urethra are then divided sharply and a sample of the proximal margin is sent for frozen section review. The corpora cavernosa are divided sharply underneath the pubic symphysis and closed with interrupted 2-0 absorbable suture material. The proximal urethral segment is brought to the skin as a perineal urethrostomy.

Posterior Urethral Carcinoma

Carcinoma of the posterior urethra rarely lends itself to urethrectomy alone; resection of contiguous structures is usually required.[31] Because of the advanced nature of these lesions, preoperative radiation or combined radiation and chemotherapy should be considered in the large number in which surgical resection alone may not allow complete local tumor excision.[10,28]

Because cystectomy and urinary diversion are required for complete excision of most advanced posterior urethral carcinomas, complete bowel preparation should be performed preoperatively.[32,33] To avoid preoperative dehydration, intravenous hydration should be continued beginning the day before surgery.

Some surgeons have recommended staged procedures in which urinary diversion is performed first, followed in two weeks by cystectomy, prostatectomy, urethrectomy, and resection of contiguous structures.[10,34] However, all but the more debilitated patients should undergo a one-stage approach. Patients requiring cystectomy in combination with urethrectomy should be placed in the low lithotomy position to permit simultaneous abdominal/pelvic and perineal exposure. A midline or paramedian incision extending form the pubic symphysis to midway between the umbilicus and xiphoid is made. An initial laparotomy with bilateral pelvic lymphadenectomy is performed first to exclude visceral metastases or extensive metastases to the pelvic or retroperitoneal lymph nodes. The bladder and prostate should be mobilized as for excision of invasive bladder carcinoma. Dissection should proceed to that point where the bladder is completely mobilized along its lateral and posterior margins. The puboprostatic ligaments need not be incised because the pubic symphysis will be completely or partially removed later.

After completion of the pelvic lymphadenectomy and preliminary mobilization of the bladder, the perineal dissection should begin. Extensive carcinomas often require en bloc resection of the penis and all or a portion of the scrotum (Fig. 39-9).[35] An elliptical incision is made around the base of the penis and through or around the scrotum (depending on the extent of the tumor). The incision is deepened superiorly, allowing ligation of the dorsal vasculature, incision of the suspensory ligament of the penis, and exposure of the pubic symphysis. The lateral dissection should extend to the fascial covering of the adductor musculature bilaterally. Orchiectomy is often necessary in patients who require complete scrotal excision. The inferior incision should be deepened by incising the muscles of the superficial perineal space—bulbospongiosus, ischiocavernosus, and transverse perinei superficialis—to allow mobilization of the bulbomembranous urethra and visualization of the deep perineal fascia. Those striated muscles attached to the pubic symphysis and medial aspect of the inferior pubic ramus (adductor longus, gracilis, adductor brevis, obdurator internus, levator ani, and portions of the adductor magnus) are transected at their insertions with a periosteal elevator and the electrocautery. All or a portion of the pubic symphysis and inferior pubic rami are then resected with a Gigli saw (Fig. 39-8). A curved Kocher clamp is passed from the perineum just lateral to the inferior pubic ramus through the obdurator foramen into the pelvis. The tip of the clamp should be directed medially to prevent damage to the obdurator nerve or vessels. One end of a Gigli saw is grasped and brought to the perineum. The Kocher clamp is then passed medial to the inferior pubic ramus and ischium into the pelvis and the second end of the Gigli saw grasped and brought to the perineum. A similar procedure is performed on the opposite side. A Gigli saw is then passed around the pubic symphysis. A Kocher clamp is passed through the obdurator foramen more anteriorly on either side of the pubic symphysis. Each end of a Gigli saw is grasped and brought to the perineum. Laterally and upwardly beveled osteotomies are made through both inferior pubic rami and the inferior aspect of the pubic symphysis, respectively. Usually only the inferior rim of the pubic symphysis rather than the entire pubis need be resected to ensure an adequate margin of resection. This completes the dissection, because the bladder and prostate had been mobilized previously. Urinary diversion or, in selected patients, construction of a continent urinary reservoir is then performed.

The perineal wound, which is often large, should be drained and closed with scrotal skin, if available. Large defects may be closed with gracilis myocutaneous flaps. An omental flap may also be used to fill the pelvis and separate the intestine from the perineal wound.

In selected cases in which the carcinoma is confined to the most proximal portions of the urethra, the corpora cavernosa may be spared and the penis preserved. The abdominal and pelvic portions of the procedure should proceed as described. The perineal dissection would begin with an inverted U incision between and just medial to the ischial tuberosities. The posterior and lateral dissection would be similar to that described; however, anteriorly the corpora cavernosa can be incised at the crura, preserving the overlying skin and dorsal vasculature. The pubic symphysis need not be resected. Seg-

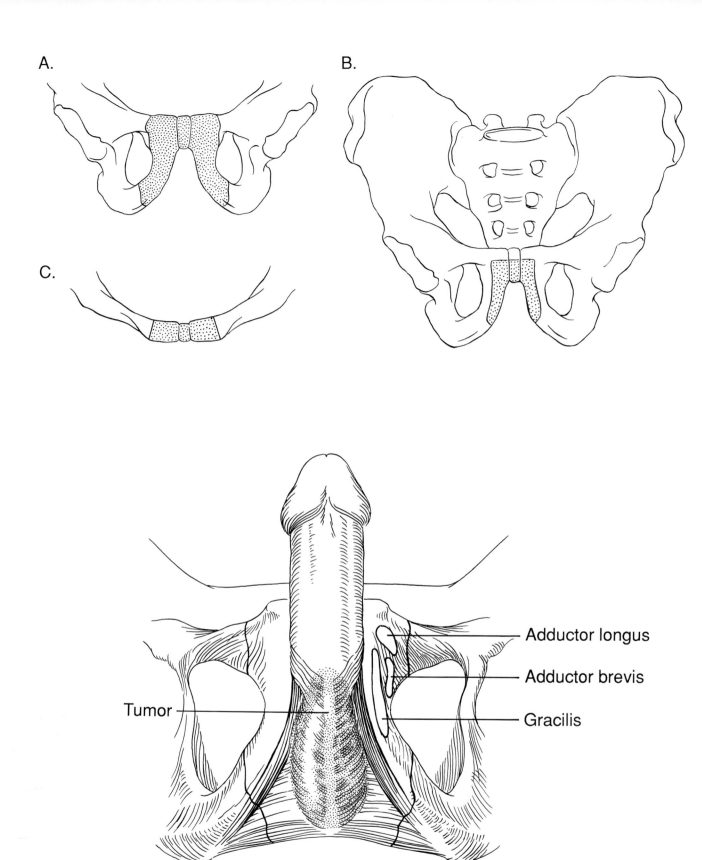

A.

B.

C.

Adductor longus

Adductor brevis

Gracilis

Tumor

FIG. 39-8. Excision of high-stage urethral carcinoma. Shaded areas represent portions of pelvis excised for higher (*A*) or lower volume (*B*) urethral carcinomas. *C*, Cephalad view of pelvis showing beveling of pubic bone incision to allow pubic symphysis to be lifted out. *D*, En bloc excision of posterior urethral carcinoma. Structures to be excised outlined.

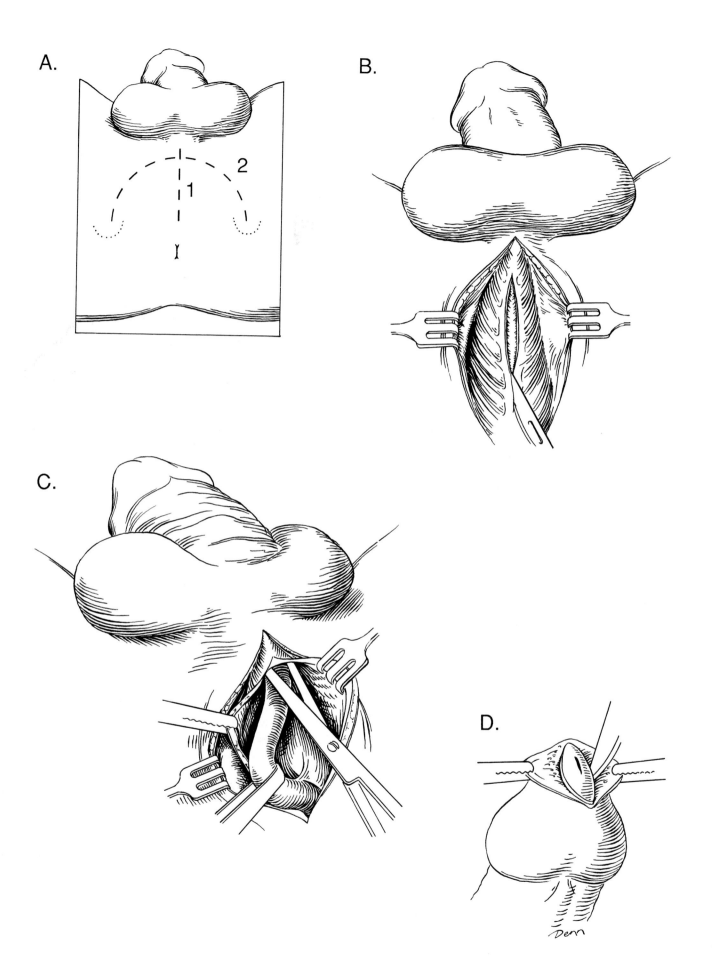

A.

B.

C.

D.

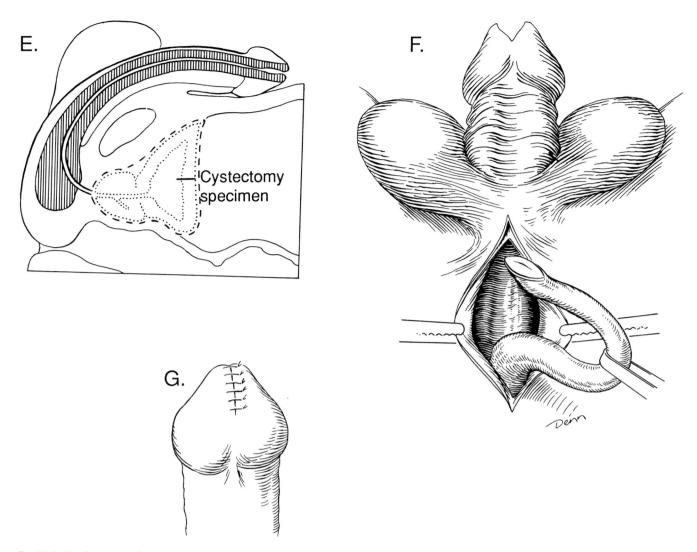

FIG. 39-9. Urethrectomy after previous cystectomy. *A,* Choice of incisions: midline, vertical incision (*1*), or inverted U incision (*2*). *B,* Exposure of bulbar urethra. *C,* Dissection along bulbar urethra proceeds anteriorly toward meatus. *D,* Excision of meatus and fossa navicularis. *E,* Sagital view of urethra showing its relationship with pelvic floor; previously excised cystectomy specimen outlined. *F,* Excision of distal urethra. *G,* Closure of glans penis.

mental resection of the urethra and corpus spongiosum with primary urethral realignment or use of a skin substitute has also been performed in rare cases.[13,36]

Regional Disease

Approximately 14 to 30% of patients will have inguinal lymph node metastases at the time of presentation.[6,11,13] Although inguinal lymph node metastases are more common with invasive carcinomas of the anterior urethra, they may be present in up to 28% of patients with invasive bulbomembranous tumors.[11] A higher rate of distant relapse is to be anticipated, but ileoinguinal lymphadenectomy may be curative for small-volume disease and may be palliative in limited high-stage disease. Extended survival has been reported.[11]

The indications for ileoinguinal lymphadenectomy are not as well defined for urethral as for penile carcinoma. However, it seems advisable in those patients with suspected (palpable) or confirmed (biopsied) inguinal lymph node metastases who have no evidence of more distant disease. Patients with no evidence of disease may be followed carefully with periodic physical examination of the inguinal lymph nodes. Should lymphadenopathy develop, more extensive disease must be excluded by bone scan, chest x-ray and CT or MRI of the pelvis and abdomen before ileoinguinal lymphadenectomy is performed (see Chap. 38).

Treatment of Metastatic Disease

Relatively few patients present with distant metastases. Cisplatin-based chemotherapy (i. e., MVAC, CISCA, and CMV) is effective in metastatic transitional cell carcinoma,[37,38] but has not been used extensively for squamous cell carcinoma of the urethra because of its rarity and low rate of metastasis.[39] The experience is broader in squamous cell carcinoma of the penis, which resembles that of the urethra. Bleomycin, methotrexate, and cisplatin have all been reported to be active single agents.[40] Various drug combinations, delivered intravenously or intra-arterially, had some efficacy in unresectable or metastatic squamous urethral carcinoma.[41] Patients with progressive local or metastatic disease who are not candidates for treatment or who have relapsed after various forms of treatment should be offered aggressive palliative care including pain medication and focal radiotherapy for isolated, painful metastases.[42]

Transitional Cell Carcinoma of the Urethra after Cystectomy

Transitional cell carcinoma of the bladder is often a multifocal urothelial disease that may involve the renal pelvis, ureter, or urethra. Approximately 4 to 10% of patients who undergo cystectomy alone will develop recurrences in the retained urethral segment,[43–48] most often proximally and rarely in the meatus.[49] All such patients should undergo careful surveillance to detect low-volume, low-stage disease amenable to urethrectomy.[50,51] Collection of urethral wash specimens for cytology and perhaps flow cytometry should be performed routinely along with careful physical examination.

Patients who require urethrectomy should be positioned in the extreme lithotomy position (Fig. 39-6). An inverted curvilinear or midline incision is made between the ischial tuberosities, which are easily palpable (Fig. 39-9). Dissection proceeds through the superficial fascial and subcutaneous layers of the perineum. The bulbocavernosus muscle is incised in the midline. Dissection proceeds along the urethra distally toward the meatus. As the dissection proceeds to the glans, the urethra is gradually mobilized resulting in inversion of the penis. At this point the penis is inverted back to its normal anatomic position and the meatus and fossa navicularis are dissected free from the surrounding spongy tissue of the glans. The meatal incision is closed with 3-0 or 4-0 chromic sutures. Attention is then directed at completing the most proximal part of the urethral dissection. The proximal bulbar urethra is further mobilized to the level of the membranous urethra. Because this is often retained after cystectomy, dissection must proceed into the deep perineal compartment of the genitourinary diaphragm. Careful and meticulous dissection along the urethra will allow complete excision without damage to any intestinal segments that may have fallen into the pelvic space above the genitourinary diaphragm after cystectomy. A drain is often left along the area of the dissection, brought through a separate incision, and removed when output becomes minimal. The subcutaneous tissue layers are closed with interrupted 2-0 or 3-0 absorbable suture material. The skin is closed in a similar fashion. A light gauze dressing is applied, reinforced with fluff gauze, and kept in place with a scrotal support.

FEMALE URETHRAL CARCINOMA

Anatomy

The female urethra is approximately 4- to 6-cm long, running from the bladder neck to the external urethral meatus, which lies just anterior to the vaginal hiatus and approximately 2 cm inferior to the glans clitoris.[1] (Fig. 39-10). The urethra is rich in collagen and elastic fibers and is therefore occluded, except during voiding. The mucous membrane is composed of transitional cell epithelium along the proximal third of the urethra and stratified squamous epithelium along the distal two thirds. Submucosal glands, lined by pseudostratified and stratified columnar epithelium, can be found opening along the entire length. The female urethra has a muscular wall composed of an inner longitudinal muscle coat continuous with the inner layer of the detrusor muscle and an outer semicircular coat continuous with the outer wall of the detrusor muscle. Somewhat arbitrarily, the female urethra can be divided into anterior and posterior segments, the former representing the distal-most third and the latter representing the proximal two thirds.

The boundaries and anatomy of the female perineum are similar to those in the male, with the major exception being that the vaginal canal separates the components of the urogenital triangle in the midline (Fig. 39-11). In addition to the transverse perinei superficialis and ischiocavernosus, the muscles of the superficial space include the sphincter vaginae, which are paired striated muscles surrounding the vagina.

The lymphatics of the distal urethra drain into the superficial and deep inguinal lymph nodes, those of the proximal urethra drain preferentially into the pelvic lymph nodes (external and internal iliac, obturator, and presacral).

Histopathology and Pathophysiology

In women, as in men, the majority of urethral cancers are squamous cell carcinomas (approximately 70%).[52–58] Transitional cell carcinomas account for approximately 15% and must be differentiated from primary bladder carcinoma. Adenocarcinomas are identified in approximately 10 to 13% of women with urethral tumors and appear to be of two histologic types: clear cell and columnar/mucinous.[59] The former must be differentiated from clear-cell tumors of the female genital tract and are characterized by cells with abundant clear cytoplasm and cellular pleomorphism.[60] The latter resembles colonic or endocervical adenocarcinoma most commonly showing tubular glands with focal papillary areas. The cells are generally columnar with regular nuclei and little pleomorphism. Adenocarcinomas are thought to arise from neoplastic differentiation of transitional cell epithelium of the urethra or glandular epithelium of the paraurethral glands. These tumors present at a higher stage and carry a worse prognosis than squamous carcinomas. In one rather large series, extension to local structures or regional lymph nodes was identified in 82% of patients, and 64% were dead of their disease within 2 years of diagnosis.[59] Melanomas account for a small number of ure-

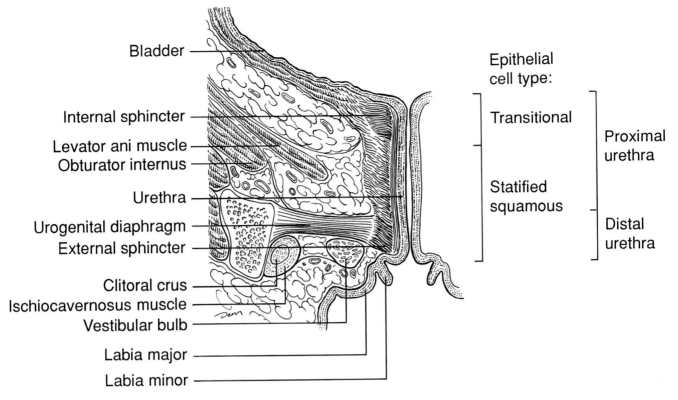

Fig. 39-10. Anatomy of the female urethra.

Bladder

Internal sphincter

Levator ani muscle
Obturator internus

Urethra

Urogenital diaphragm
External sphincter

Clitoral crus
Ischiocavernosus muscle
Vestibular bulb

Labia major

Labia minor

Epithelial
cell type:

Transitional

Statified
squamous

Proximal
urethra

Distal
urethra

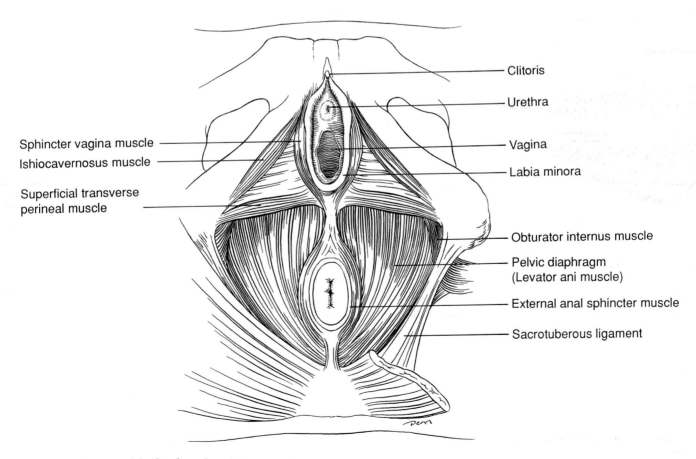

Fig. 39-11. Anatomy of the female perineum.

Sphincter vagina muscle
Ischiocavernosus muscle

Superficial transverse
perineal muscle

Clitoris

Urethra

Vagina

Labia minora

Obturator internus muscle

Pelvic diaphragm
(Levator ani muscle)

External anal sphincter muscle

Sacrotuberous ligament

thral carcinomas, and most commonly occur along the anterior urethra.[61] They also have a poor prognosis because of a higher rate of regional and metastatic disease.

Approximately 45% of urethral tumors in women are located along the anterior urethra alone, 7% in the posterior urethra alone, and 48% located along the entire urethra on clinical examination.[53,54,56] Seventy-five percent are moderately well-differentiated or poorly differentiated neoplasms (grade 2 or 3).[54,56] Urethral carcinoma must be differentiated from benign abnormalities including urethral caruncle, cyst, condylomata acuminata, urethral prolapse, and periurethral abscess.

Risk factors are not well documented. A history of significant infection or trauma is not as common in women as in men. Urethral caruncles have been found in a small percentage of women with urethral cancers. Several tumors arising within urethral diverticulae have been reported,[62] the majority being adenocarcinomas.

Approximately 28% of women with urethral carcinoma will present with metastases to inguinal lymph nodes. These are more common with high-stage lesions. Distant metastases are rare (10 to 15%).[56] As in men, the most common sites of metastases include the liver, lungs, skeleton, and brain.

Diagnosis and Staging

The most common presenting symptoms and signs of urethral carcinoma in women include bleeding (60 to 75%) obstructive voiding or incontinence (27 to 52%), irritative voiding symptoms (21 to 65%), pain (25 to 40%) and a palpable mass (6 to 40%).[54–56] A careful physical examination should be performed, noting the presence of a mass on inspecion or on bimanual palpation. Its size, color, and extent should be assessed, as well as the presence of any inguinal or supraclavicular adenopathy. A more accurate examination can be performed under anesthesia at which time the mass may be excised or biopsied. Cystoscopy should be performed, if possible, noting the proximal extent of the lesion as well as the presence of bladder involvement. The vaginal vault and cervix should be carefully examined to assess regional extension to these areas and exclude the possibility that the urethral tumor represents local infiltration by a primary tumor of the genital tract.

As in the male, extension to local structures and regional lymph nodes may be assessed with lymphangiography, CT, or MRI (Fig. 39-12). The presence of any pulmonary or bony metastasis may be assessed initially by chest x-ray and nuclear bone scan, respectively. Urethral carcinoma in women is most often staged clinically according to the schemes developed by Grabstald[56] and colleagues and Prempree[63] (Table 39-2).

Treatment of Localized Disease: Alternatives to Surgery

In women, the experience with radiation therapy is much more extensive than in men.[12,54,56,63–70] The best results have

TABLE 39-2. *Staging of Female Urethral Carcinoma*

GRABSTALD (MEMORIAL) STAGING SYSTEM

Stage 0 (Tis)	In situ (limited to mucosa)
Stage A (T1)	Submucosal (not beyond submucosa)
Stage B (T2)	Muscular (infiltrating periurethral muscle)
Stage C (T3–4)	Periurethral
C1	Infiltrating muscular wall of the vagina
C2	Infiltrating muscular wall of the vagina with invasion of vaginal mucosa
C3	Infiltration of other adjacent structures, such as bladder, labia, and clitoris
Stage D (N+/M+)	Metastasis
D1	Inguinal lymph nodes
D2	Pelvic lymph nodes below the bifurcation of the aorta
D3	Lymph nodes above the bifurcation of the aorta
D4	Distant

PREMPREE MODIFICATION STAGING SYSTEM

Stage I	Disease limited to the distal half of the urethra
Stage II	Disease involving the entire urethra, with extension to the periurethral tissues but not involving the vulva or bladder neck.
Stage III	
a	Disease involving the urethra and vulva
b	Disease invading the vaginal mucosa
c	Disease involving the urethra and bladder neck
Stage IV	
a	Disease invading parametrium or paracolpium
b	Metastases
1	Inguinal lymph nodes
2	Pelvic nodes
3	Para-aortic
4	Distant

been seen in low-stage, anterior lesions where local control and long-term survival rates are favorable. Such lesions are amenable to an integrated approach whereby patients receive 4,000 to 4,500 cGy by external beam radiotherapy delivered initially from anteroposterior parallel-opposed fields. This is followed after 3 to 4 weeks with interstitial radiotherapy to bring the total dose to 6,500 to 7,000 cGy. The dose can be distributed homogeneously with a urethral template attached to a vaginal cylinder. Needle placement and radioactive seed distribution are tailored to the site and size of the individual tumor.

Radiotherapy alone with either external beam radiotherapy or a combination of external beam and interstitial radiotherapy has not been as effective for posterior or higher-stage urethral carcinomas. Local recurrence is common and survival limited. Most series report complication rates of approxi-

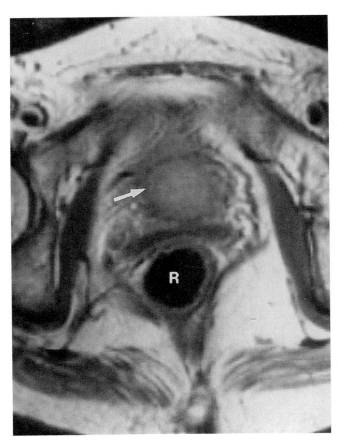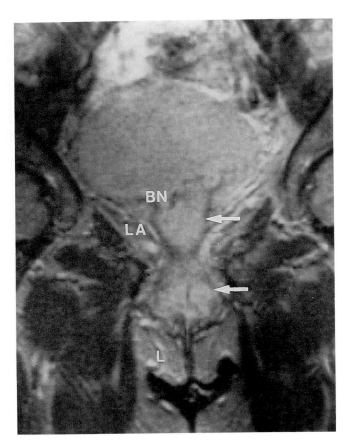

Fig. 39-12. MRI of female urethral melanoma (arrows). *A,* T1-weighted transaxial view of tumor anterior to rectum (R). *B,* Coronal view showing hour-glass appearance of tumor (arrows). Tumor involves entire urethra above and below genitourinary diaphragm. Bladder neck (BN), levator ani (LA), and labia (L).

mately 15 to 25% (range 0 to 42%) (Table 39-3). Complications include urinary incontinence, urethral stricture, local tissue necrosis or ulceration, fistula or abscess formation, and osteomyelitis.

Owing to the high likelihood of local persistence and recurrence after radiotherapy, some investigators are exploring the efficacy of concomitant radiotherapy and chemotherapy.[28,70] Such an approach has merit, as certain chemotherapeutic agents act as radiosensitizers.

Surgery has been used in all stages of disease, although more often for advanced disease because of the high failure rate of radiation alone. However, the local recurrence rate is often high and survival limited, even with aggressive surgical management (Table 39-4). Patients treated with radiation therapy followed by anterior exenteration may have fewer local recurrences than those patients treated with either surgery or radiation therapy alone.[58,72] The preoperative use of chemotherapy in addition to radiation may permit better downstaging and more complete surgical excision.

Surgical Techniques

Certain low-volume and low-stage carcinomas (i.e., stages O, A, B, or I) of the anterior urethra may be completely excised with an adequate margin and preservation of urinary conti-

nence. The distal one half of the urethra may be excised without risking postoperative continence. Patients should be placed in the standard lithotomy position. The labia minora should be sutured laterally with silk sutures and a weighted speculum placed in the vagina to allow clear visualization of the periurethral area (Fig. 39-13). A 16 or 18 Fr urethral catheter is inserted to facilitate the dissection. A circumferential incision is made around the urethra inferior to the clitoris. The incision should extend widely around the tumor. The anterior urethra is freed from surrounding tissue by careful, sharp dissection. Once a clear margin has been achieved, the urethra may be transected. Frozen sections should be taken on both the proximal and distal margins of resection to ensure complete tumor excision. Bleeding points should be grasped with fine forceps and cauterized. The urethral meatus should be reconstructed with interrupted 3-0 chromic suture material. Postoperatively, pain and discomfort are usually limited and the patient is often ready for discharge on the first postoperative day. The catheter is left in place for 5 to 7 days.

Higher stage tumors (i.e. B, C, or II, III) require more aggressive surgery, and preoperative radiation with or without chemotherapy should be considered in all but the lowest volume disease (generally external beam radiation to approximately 4,500 cGy). The concurrent administration of chemotherapeutic agents with synergistic antitumor activity (i.e.,

TABLE 39-3. *Radiotherapy for Female Urethral Carcinoma*

AUTHOR	PATIENTS	LOCAL RECURRENCE	SURVIVAL (2–5 YEAR)	COMPLICATIONS
Pointon and Poole-Wilson[12]	92	NS	46%	0%
Desai et al.[54]	14	NS	39%	NS
Grabstald et al.[56]	29	69%	24%	NS
Monaco et al.[57]	8	NS	75%	NS
Bracken et al.[58]	50	46%	32%	42%
Prempree et al.[63]	14	36%	71%	21%
Antoniades[64]	20	25%	50%	30%
Mayer et al.[65]	5	100%	40%	NS
Weghaupt et al.[66]	62	NS	65%	NS
Klein et al.[69]	3	0	66%	0

*NS = not stated.

mitomycin, 5-fluorouracil, and cisplatin) should be considered in locally aggressive lesions. Most high-stage urethral tumors will require complete anterior exenteration. Rarely, a patient may be managed by urethrectomy alone with preservation of the bladder, but they will require a suprapubic catheter or construction of a continent stoma.

Preoperative preparation is similar to that in men: complete bowel preparation, intravenous hydration, and antibiotic prophylaxis previously. The patient should be placed in the low lithotomy position, which allows for both abdominal and perineal exposure. A midline incision is made from over the pubic symphysis to midway between the umbilicus and xiphoid. The abdomen and retroperitoneum are inspected for the presence of metastatic disease. A bilateral pelvic lymphadenectomy is then completed. The bladder and uterus (and usually the ovaries) are mobilized and excised (see Chap. 24). However, the dissection is not completed at this point. The vagina is opened just distal to the cervix and the incision is extended down either side approximately two-thirds of its length. Blood vessels in this posterior pedicle are clamped and ligated sequentially. The entire lateral and anterior segments of the vagina should remain attached to the specimen to pre-

TABLE 39-4. *Surgery Alone for Female Urethral Carcinoma*

AUTHOR	PATIENTS	LOCAL RECURRENCE	SURVIVAL* (2–5 YEARS)
Grabstald et al.[56]	26	54%	39%
Bracken et al.[58]	11	64%	45%
Mayer et al.[65]	10	60%	30%
Moinuddin et al.[71]	5	40%	40%
Monaco et al.[57]	5	0%	100%

*Disease-free survival for patients followed more than 24 months.

serve a tumor-free margin of resection. On occasion, the entire vagina is resected. At this point, attention is directed to the perineal dissection.

A semicircular incision is made beginning at the level of the previous incisions in the posterior vaginal wall. This should extend laterally to include both labia minora (Fig. 39-14). The clitoris should be included within the anterior limits of the incision for removal of large tumors that extend anteriorly. The incision is deepened anteriorly to expose the periosteum of the pubic symphysis and laterally through the muscular elements of the urogenital triangle until the periosteum of the inferior pubic ramus is reached. The insertions of the adductor muscles along the inferior pubic ramus may be incised with the periosteal elevator and electrocautery. The distal third of the vagina may be incised on either side to join with the vaginal incisions made during the pelvic part of the dissection.

The pubic arch resection is completed next in a fashion similar to that for men. Laterally and upwardly beveled osteotomies are made through both inferior pubic rami and the inferior aspect of the pubic symphysis, respectively. Usually only the inferior rim of the pubic symphysis rather than the entire pubic symphysis need be resected to ensure an adequate margin of resection. The entire specimen is then removed and hemostasis achieved. An omental flap or polyglycolic acid mesh is placed within the pelvis to separate the intestines from the perineal incision and prevent a future enterocele or fistula. The vaginal remnant, if present, is brought anteriorly and sutured to the vulvae with running or interrupted 2-0 or 3-0 absorbable suture material. The perineal wound can be closed primarily or with myocutaneous gracilis flaps if a large defect is present. In selected patients, bilateral myocutaneous gracilis flaps can be used to create a functional vagina. Closed pelvic and perineal drainage systems are placed and routine abdominal closure is completed.

Postoperative complications are similar to those described for radical cystectomy. In addition, osteitis pubis and adductor

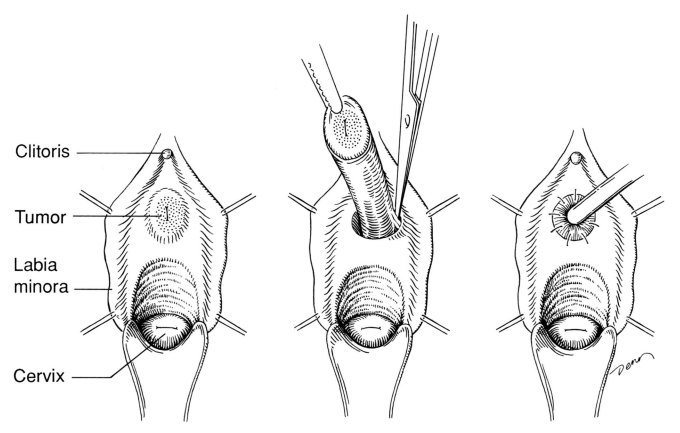

Clitoris

Tumor

Labia
minora

Cervix

FIG. 39-13. Anterior urethrectomy for female urethral carcinoma.

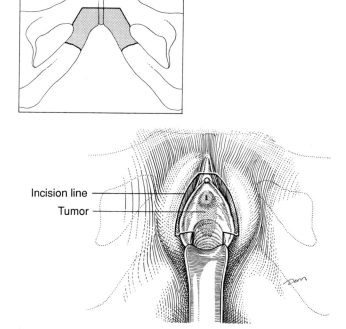

Incision line

Tumor

FIG. 39-14. Excision of high-stage urethral carcinoma in women. Skin incision outlined. Exact limits of the skin incision depend on the size and extent of the tumor. Clitoris should be excised when the urethral carcinoma is large or extends anteriorly. Area of pubic arch to be excised is shaded (in box). The entire pubic symphysis can be excised when the tumor is large to ensure an adequate margin of resection.

muscle spasms have been reported in a few patients. Rarely, a patient will develop sacroiliac instability secondary to complete pubic arch excision.

Regional and Metastatic Disease

Approximately 28% of women with urethral carcinoma will present with metastases to inguinal lymph nodes (Table 39-5). Management is similar to that described for men. Ileoinguinal lymphadenectomy should be performed for biopsy-proven inguinal metastases or palpably enlarged inguinal lymph nodes. In patients with unresectable inguinal metastases or distant metastases, systemic chemotherapy should be considered.

CONCLUSION

Urethral carcinomas are rare human malignancies. Low-volume and low-stage tumors can be treated with a variety of surgical or radiotherapeutic techniques designed to preserve genitourinary function. Unfortunately, high-volume and high-stage carcinomas frequently present with advanced local and regional disease not amenable to either excision or radiation alone. An integrated management approach should be considered. The use of neoadjuvant chemotherapy should be investigated in an attempt to increase downstaging and the likelihood of complete tumor excision.

TABLE 39-5. *Lymph Node Involvement in Female Urethral Carcinoma*

| AUTHOR | INGUINAL LYMPH NODES | | PELVIC LYMPH NODES |
	CLINICALLY POSITIVE	HISTOLOGICALLY POSITIVE	
Grabstald et al.[56]	25/79 (32%)	22/24 (92%)	13/26 (50%)
Weghaupt et al.[66]	19/62 (14%)	7/7 (100%)	
Pointon and Poole-Wilson[12]	46/132 (35%)		
Desai et al.[54]	6/16 (33%)	2/6 (33%)	
Monaco et al.[57]	5/23 (22%)	2/5 (40%)	

REFERENCES

1. TANAGO, E. A. Anatomy of the lower urinary tract. In: *Campbell's Urology.* 5th Ed. Edited by P. C. Walsh, R. Gittes, A. D. Perlmutter, and T. A. Stamey. Philadelphia, W. B. Saunders, Co., 1986.

2. JOHNSON, D. E., and AMES, F. C. Surgical anatomy and lymphatic drainage of the ilioinguinal region. In: *Groin Dissection.* Edited by D. E. Johnson and F. C. Ames. Chicago, Year Book Medical Publishers, 1985.

3. DASELAR, E. H., ANSON, B. J., and REIMANN, A. F. Radical excision of the inguinal and iliac lymph glands: A study based on 450 anatomical dissections and upon supportive clinical observations. Surg. Gynecol. Obstet., 87:679, 1948.

4. HAND, J. R. Surgery of the penis and urethra. In: *Urology.* 3rd Ed. Edited by M. F. Campbell and J. H. Harrison. Philadelphia, W. B. Saunders, Co., 1970.

5. MULLIN, E. M., ANDERSON, E. E., and PAULSON, D. F. Carcinoma of the male urethra. J. Urol., *112*:610, 1974.

6. ANDERSON, K. A., and McANINCH, J. W. Primary squamous cell carcinoma of the anterior male urethra. Urology, *23*:134, 1984.

7. GUINN, G. A., and AYALA, A. G. Male urethral cancer: Report of 15 cases including a primary melanoma. J. Urol., *91*:107, 1970.

8. MANDLER, J. I., and POOL, T. L. Primary carcinoma of the male urethra. J. Urol., *96*:67, 1966.

9. KING, L. R. Carcinoma of the urethra in male patients. J. Urol., *91*:555, 1964.

10. BRACKEN, R. B., HENRY, R., and ORDONEZ, N. Primary carcinoma of the male urethra. South. Med. J., *73*:1003, 1980.

11. RAY, B., CANTO, A. R., and WHITMORE, W. F. Experience with primary carcinoma of the male urethra. J. Urol., *117*:591, 1977.

12. POINTON, R. C. S., and POOLE-WILSON, D. S. Primary carcinoma of the urethra. Br. J. Urol., *40*:682, 1968.

13. KAPLAN, G. W., BULKLEY, G. J., and GRAYHACK, J. T. Carcinoma of the male urethra. J. Urol., *98*:365, 1967.

14. SACKS, S. A. et al. Urethral adenocarcinoma (Possibly originating in the glands of Littré). J. Urol., *113*:50, 1975.

15. BOURQUE, J. et al. Primary carcinoma of Cowper's gland. J. Urol., *103*:758, 1970.

16. POW-SANG, J. M., KLIMBERG, I. W., HACKET, R. L., and WAJSMAN, Z. Primary malignant melanoma of the male urethra. J. Urol., *139*:1304, 1988.

17. IVERSON, A. P., BLACKARD, C. E., and SCHULBERG, V. A. Carcinoma of the prostate with urethral metastases. J. Urol., *108*:901, 1972.

18. SELIKOWITZ, S. M., and OLSSON, C. A. Metastatic urethral obstruction. Arch. Surg., *107*:906, 1973.

19. RICHES, E. W., and CULLEN, T. H. Carcinoma of the urethra. Br. J. Urol., *2*:209, 1951.

20. GRUSSENDORF-CONEN, E. -I., DUETZ, F. J., and de VILLIERS, E. M. Detection of human papillomavirus-6 in primary carcinoma of the urethra in men. Cancer, *60*:1832, 1987.

21. WINKLER, H. Z., and LIEBVER, M. M. Primary squamous cell carcinoma of the male urethra nuclear deoxyribonucleic acid ploidy studied by flow cytometry. J. Urol., *139*:298, 1988.

22. ESCRIBANO, G. et al. Cavernosography in diagnosis of metastatic tumors of the penis: 5 new cases and a review of the literature. J. Urol., *138*:1174, 1987.

23. KONNAK, J. W. Conservative management of low grade neoplasms of the male urethra: A preliminary report. J. Urol., *123*:175, 1980.

24. HILLYARD, R. W., LADAGA, L., and SCHELLHAMMER, P. F. Superficial transitional cell carcinoma of the bladder associated with mucosal involvement of the prostatic urethra: Results of treatment with intravesical bacillus calmette guerin. J. Urol., *139*:290, 1988.

25. RAGHAVAIAH, N. V. Radiotherapy in the treatment of carcinoma of the male urethra. Cancer, *41*:1313, 1978.

26. TICHO, B. H., PEREZ-TAMAYO, C., and KONNAK, J. W. Primary carcinoma of the distal male urethra: A case treated with lymphadenectomy and interstitial radiation therapy. J. Urol., *129*:1302, 1988.

27. SCHER, H. I. et al. Neoadjuvant M-VAC (methotrexate, vinblastine, doxorubicin and cisplatin) for extravesical urinary tract tumors. J. Urol., *139*:475, 1988.

28. JOHNSON, D. W., KESSLER, J. F., FERRIGNI, R. G., and ANDERSON, J. D. Low dose combined chemotherapy/radiation therapy in the management of locally advanced urethral squamous cell carcinoma. J. Urol., *141*:615, 1989.

29. MARSHALL, V. F. Radical excision of locally extensive carcinoma of the deep male urethra. J. Urol., *78*:252, 1957.

30. HOTCHKISS, R. S., and AMELAR, R. D. Primary carcinoma of the male urethra. J. Urol., *72*:1181, 1954.

31. SHUTTLEWORTH, K. E. D., and LLOYD-DAVIES, R. W. Radical resection for tumours involving the posterior urethra. Br. J. Urol., *41*:739, 1969.

32. CONDON, R. E. et al. The efficacy of oral and systemic antibiotic prophylaxis in colorectal surgery. Arch. Surg., *188*:496, 1983.

33. NICHOLS, R. L. et al. Efficacy of preoperative antimicrobial preparation of the bowel. Ann. Surg., *176*:227, 1972.

34. JOHNSON, D. E., and LO, R. K. Tumors of the penis, urethra and scrotum. In: *Genitourinary Cancer Management.* Edited by J. B.

DeKernion and D. Paulson. Philadelphia, Lea & Febiger, p. 219, 1987.

35. KLEIN, F. A. et al. Inferior pubic rami resection with en bloc radical excision for invasive proximal urethral carcinoma. Cancer, *51*:1238, 1983.

36. JEWETT, H. J., and OSTERLING, J. E. A simple substitute for a missing segment of the proximal anterior urethra. J. Urol., *138*:1241, 1987.

37. STERNBERG, C. N. et al. M-VAC (methotrexate, vinblastine, doxorubicin and cisplatin) for advanced transitional cell carcinoma of urothelium. J. Urol., *138*:461, 1988.

38. HARKER, W. G. et al. Cisplatin, methotrexate, and vinblastine (CMV): An effective chemotherapy regimen for metastatic transitional cell carcinoma: A Northern California Oncology Group study. J. Clin. Oncol., *3*:1463, 1985.

39. KASIMIS, B. S. Primary carcinomas of the male and female urethra. In: *Chemotherapy and Urological Malignancy.* Edited by A. S. D. Spiers. New York, Springer-Verlag, p. 106, 1982.

40. AHMED, T., SKLAROFF, R., and YAGODA, A. Sequential trials of methotrexate, cisplatin, and bleomycin for penile cancer. J. Urol., *132*:465, 1984.

41. DEXEUS, F. H., LOGOTHETIS, C. J., and SIPAHI, H. Chemotherapy for advanced squamous carcinoma of the male external genital tract and urethra. In: *Systemic Therapy for Genitourinary Cancers.* Edited by D. E. Johnson, C. J. Logothetis, and A. C. Von Eschenbach. Chicago, Year Book Medical Publishers, 1989, p. 255.

42. HANKS, C. W., ed. Pain in cancer. Cancer Surveys, 7:1, 1988.

43. POOLE-WILSON, D. S., and BARNARD, R. J. Total cystectomy for bladder tumors. Br. J. Urol., *43*:16, 1978.

44. FAYSAL, M. H. Urethrectomy in men with transitional cell carcinoma of the bladder. Urology, *16*:23, 1980.

45. ZABBO, A., and MONTIE, J. E. Management of the urethra in men undergoing radical cystectomy for bladder cancer. J. Urol., *131*:267, 1984.

46. BEAHRS, J. R., FLEMING, T. R., and ZINCKE, H. Risk of local urethral recurrence after radical cystectomy for bladder cancer. J. Urol., *131*:264, 1984.

47. RAZ, S., McLORIE, G., JOHNSON, S., and SKINNER, D. G. Management of the urethra in patients undergoing radical cystectomy for bladder carcinoma. J. Urol., *120*:298, 1978.

48. SCHELLHAMMER, P. F., and WHITMORE, W. F. Transitional cell carcinoma of the urethra in men having cystectomy for bladder cancer. J. Urol., *115*:56, 1976.

49. SCHELLHAMMER, P. F., WHITMORE, W. F. Urethral meatal carcinoma following cystourethrectomy for bladder carcinoma. J. Urol., *115*:61, 1976.

50. WOLINSKA, W. H., MELAMED, M., SCHELLHAMMER, P. F., and WHITMORE, W. F. Urethral cytology following cystectomy for bladder carcinoma. Am. J. Surg. Pathol., *1*:225, 1973.

51. HERMANSEN, D. K. et al. Detection of carcinoma in the post-cystectomy urethral remnant by flow cytometric analysis. J. Urol., *138*:304, 1988.

52. JOHNSON, D. E., and O'CONNELL, J. R. Primary carcinoma of female urethra. Urology, *21*:42, 1983.

53. TURNER, A., and HENDRY, W. F. Primary carcinoma of the female urethra. Br. J. Urol., *52*:549, 1980.

54. DESAI, S., LIBERTINO, J. A., and ZINMAN, L. Primary carcinoma of the female urethra. J. Urol., *110*:693, 1973.

55. SRINIVAS, V., and ALI KHAN, S. Female urethral cancer—An overview. Int. J. Urol. Nephrol., *19*:423, 1987.

56. GRABSTALD, H., HILARIS, B., HENSCHKE, U., and WHITMORE, W. F. Cancer of the female urethra. JAMA, *197*:835, 1966.

57. MONACO, A. P., MURPHY, G. B., and DOWLING, W. Primary cancer of the female urethra. Cancer, *11*:1215, 1958.

58. BRACKEN, R. B., et al. Primary carcinoma of the female urethra. J. Urol., *116*:188, 1976.

59. MEIS, J. M., AYALA, A. G., and JOHNSON, D. E. Adenocarcinoma of the urethra in women: A clinocopathologic study. Cancer, *60*:1038, 1987.

60. YOUNG, R. H., and SCULLY, R. E. Clear cell adenocarcinoma of the bladder and urethra. Am. J. Surg. Pathol., *9*:816, 1985.

61. KATZ, J. I., and GRABSTALD, H. Primary malignant melanoma of the female urethra. J. Urol., *116*:454, 1976.

62. GONZALEZ, M. O., HARRISON, M. L., and BOILEAU, M. A. Carcinoma in diverticulum of female urethra. Urology, *26*:328, 1985.

63. PREMPREE, T., AMORNMARN, R., and PATANAPHAN, V. Radiation therapy in primary carcinoma of the female urethra. Cancer, *54*:729, 1984.

64. ANTONIADES, J. Radiation therapy in carcinoma of the female urethra. Cancer, *24*:70, 1969.

65. MAYER, R., FOWLER, J. E., and CLAYTON, M. Localized urethral carcinoma in women. Cancer, *60*:1548–1551, 1987.

66. WEGHAUPT, K., GERSTNER, G. J., and KUCERA, H. Radiation therapy for primary carcinoma of the female urethra: A survey over 25 years. Gynecol. Oncol. *17*:58, 1984.

67. TAGGART, C. G., CASTRO, J. R., RUTLEDGE, F. N. Carcinoma of the female urethra. Am. J. Roentgenol., *114*:145, 1972.

68. DELCLOS, L., WHARTON, J. J. T., and RUTLEDGE, F. N. Tumors of the vagina and female urethra. In: *Textbook of Radiotherapy,* Edited by G. Fletcher. Philadelphia, Lea & Febiger, 1980, p. 812.

69. KLEIN, F. A., MOINUDDIN, M., and KERSH, R. Carcinoma of the female urethra: Combined iridium Ir 192 interstitial and external beam radiotherapy. South. Med. J., *80*:1129, 1987.

70. NORI, D. et al. Metronidazole as a radiosensitizer and high-dose radiation in advanced vulvovaginal malignancies, a pilot study. Gynecol. Oncol., *16*:117, 1983.

71. MOINUDDIN, M., KLEIN, F. A., and HAZRA, T. A. Primary female urethral carcinoma. Cancer, *62*:54–57, 1988.

72. SKINNER, E. C., and SKINNER, D. G. Management of carcinoma of the female urethra. In: *Genitourinary Cancer,* Edited by D. G. Skinner, and G. Lieskovsky. Philadelphia, W. B. Saunders, Co., 1988, p. 490.

SECTION
IX

PEDIATRIC TUMORS

Pediatric Tumors: An Overview

"Pediatric cancer seen in perspective, then, puts us almost at the end of a long tunnel, looking back in one direction towards the blackness of 'no hope' and 'no cure.' Looking forward, we see a wide and open road with well-spaced way-stops en route to our final destination. Some of these way-stops surely are the development of ever more refined and precisely targeted methods of treatment, so that the increasing numbers of successfully treated children of today do not become the chronically ill adults of tomorrow. The end of the road will be reached via prophylactic and preventive measures, when cancer, as a threat to the life and limb of children, will have been eliminated forever.

Indeed, cure is not enough."[1]

G. J. D'ANGIO

Michael T. Macfarlane
Richard M. Ehrlich

The introductory quotation, written in 1975 by Dr. Giulio D'Angio, Chairman of the National Wilms' Tumor Study (NWTS), succinctly and eloquently pinpoints the current thrust in modern pediatric oncology. He further stresses that " . . . while the emphasis properly is on improving survival rates, there is a parallel effort to refine treatment, reducing it to the minimum necessary to achieve cure."[1] It could not be better expressed. The NWTS continues to be the quintessential example of accomplishment derived from cooperative endeavors between surgeons, pediatricians, oncologists, and radiation therapists.

PATHOLOGIC ENTITIES

There is a wide spectrum of tumors that afflict children and the majority of these fall into the care of the pediatric urologist. We will focus only on the malignant tumors of common occurrence; however, the more common benign tumors of children that involve the genitourinary tract such as hydronephrosis from ureteropelvic junction obstruction or reflux, and multicystic kidneys, must not be forgotten when making a diagnosis. Of the many malignant tumors that arise in the genitourinary tract of children, only *nephroblastomas* (Wilms' tumor), *neuroblastomas,* and *rhabdomyosarcomas* occur commonly. Less common malignancies include renal adenocarcinomas, transitional cell carcinomas, and testicular neoplasms. In addition, a few tumors previously considered variants of Wilms' tumor are now more generally classified as separate entities. These include *clear cell sarcoma of the kidney* (bone metastasizing renal tumor of childhood), *rhabdoid tumor of the kidney,* and *multilocular cysts of the kidney* (cystic nephroma). Clear cell sarcoma of the kidney and rhabdoid tumor were originally classified as unfavorable histologic variants of Wilms' tumor, whereas multilocular cysts of the kidney were classified as more favorable histologic variants of Wilms' tumor.

Another distinctive tumor of the infantile kidney is the *congenital mesoblastic nephroma.* This tumor tends to resemble a leiomyoma both grossly and histologically; however, it has a tendency to infiltrate locally. It is generally regarded as having a less malignant potential, at least when removed with wide surgical margins within the first 3 months of life.

DIAGNOSTIC IMAGING

Advances in imaging techniques have greatly changed the approach to diagnosis and staging of the child with a suspected malignancy. Initial evaluation with chest and plain abdominal radiographs, in conjunction with abdominal ultrasound, is now preferred. The chest films may demonstrate metastatic disease but not exclude it. Curvilinear calcifications on the plain abdominal film suggest Wilms' tumor and speckled calcifications suggest neuroblastoma. Abdominal ultrasound is non-invasive and is the simplest, method of establishing a diagnosis of a solid tumor. In addition, it provides high-quality images of the kidneys, liver, inferior vena cava (IVC), and aorta. The intravenous urogram (IVU) has substantially been replaced by the combination of ultrasound and CT. Additionally, one can obtain a plain abdominal radiograph at the conclusion of a contrast-enhanced CT scan to provide a more traditional anatomic view of the renal collecting system and the ureters.

A contrast-enhanced abdominal CT scan is the most effective staging modality to date. CT can more accurately assess local invasion or involvement of lymph nodes and IVC. In addition, chest CT is the definitive examination for the detection of pulmonary metastases.

Magnetic resonance imaging (MRI) is becoming more popular as a staging modality.

A nuclear isotope bone scan (^{99m}Tc MDP) has replaced the skeletal survey for assessing bony involvement. Nuclear scans utilizing radiolabled iodine substances such as ^{123}I MIBG or the monoclonal antibody UJ13A have been shown to be effective in identifying tissue of neuroectodermal origin such as in neuroblastomas or pheochromocytomas.[2]

WILMS' TUMOR

Despite the fact that the exceptional efficacy of chemotherapy and radiation therapy may compensate for a poorly executed nephrectomy for Wilms' tumor, the surgeon dealing with these tumors must be thoroughly familiar with the latest information regarding diagnosis and treatment. This implies a constant perusal of pertinent urologic and surgical literature and an in-depth familiarity with the guidelines of the NWTS.

Surgical treatment of Wilms' tumor is not a casual undertaking. As pointed out by Leape and associates, the surgeon assumes a critical responsibility both for accurate assessment of tumor spread and for expert, gentle extirpation.[3] Anything less may lead to upstaging and more extensive chemotherapy and radiation therapy, with their attendant morbidity and mortality. Familiarity with the complications of chemotherapy and radiation therapy is essential for the urologist to make intelligent decisions in the ongoing management of complex and enigmatic situations. These complications are further discussed in Chapter 51.

Diagnostic Considerations

It should be emphasized that it is the surgeon's responsibility to ensure a thorough preoperative evaluation, to avoid both preoperative misdiagnoses and intraoperative error. The recorded frequency of incorrect preoperative diagnoses in NWTS-1 was 5% (30 of 606 patients).[4] It is important to note that 14 of the 30 misdiagnoses represented benign lesions. In

our review of 19 of these 30 cases, we concluded that when pyelography is used alone, there will be a group of patients with retroperitoneal lesions who cannot be diagnosed with certainty.[5] These facts underscore the hazards inherent in the use of preoperative chemotherapy and irradiation in the absence of a histologic diagnosis of Wilms' tumor. Improved imaging techniques, such as CT and MRI, should improve the accuracy of preoperative diagnoses. However, NWTS-3 data demonstrate that diagnostic errors continue even when pathologic material is available.[6] Twenty-five percent of tumors entered in NWTS-3 with unfavorable histology had initially been classified as favorable histology by the contributing pathologists. Likewise, 4% of cases entered with favorable histology had been classified as unfavorable before review. An incorrect diagnosis can lead to significant under- or over-treatment when dealing with tumors as different as congenital mesoblastic nephroma or the more aggressive rhabdoid tumor or clear cell sarcoma.

Some salient points regarding preoperative evaluation deserve special emphasis. Nonvisualization of a Wilms' tumor on an intravenous pyelogram, although not conferring a worse prognosis, may be secondary to invasion of the vascular or collecting system, total parenchymal replacement, or extrinsic obstruction of the ureteropelvic junction.[7] In this setting, further preoperative investigative measures are mandatory to obviate intraoperative surprises and to plan the appropriate surgical approach. All children who have nonvisualized tumors or gross hematuria, as well as all postoperative patients with gross hematuria, should undergo cystoscopic examination. Retrograde pyelograms should also be obtained to rule out bladder and ureteral metastases.[8-11] Nephroureterectomy is the procedure of choice if ureteral implants are present. Invasion of the collecting system may also be suspected when results of urine cytologic studies are positive.[12]

An ultrasonogram is helpful, not only in differentiating between the cystic or solid nature of a renal mass, but also in detecting tumor extension into the renal vein or vena cava.[13-16] With the addition of CT and MRI, venous extension can usually be confirmed. A venacavogram can generally be avoided. Accurate assessment of venous involvement preoperatively will allow the surgeon to plan the appropriate incision and to avoid embolization during manipulation of the tumor. Despite improved imaging techniques, including ultrasound, CT, and MRI, IVC extension was missed preoperatively in one-third of NWTS-3 patients.[17]

The CT scan has become the mainstay for staging Wilms' tumors. It provides the best delineation of the lesion and determines whether invasion of contiguous structures is present. Identification of degeneration or liquefaction of the tumor is valuable information for the surgeon who wishes to obviate potential tumor rupture. MRI is becoming increasingly useful with these tumors. Its future role is yet to be defined.

Surgical Technique: Prevention of Complications

A properly planned and executed incision is one of the main factors in obviating complications of surgical treatment of

Wilms' tumor. Despite emphasis on the necessity for a generous transperitoneal incision in cases of Wilms' tumor, inadequate flank procedures continue to be performed. The flank approach is contraindicated because it results in improper staging, the abdomen and contralateral kidney cannot be explored, lymph nodes can neither be assessed nor removed, and the likelihood of tumor spill is increased.[3,18] This caveat cannot be overemphasized.

Variations of the transperitoneal approach are many, with thoracic extension suggested in unusually large upper-pole masses.[19] A formal thoracoabdominal incision in the torque position, or a supine subcostal modification of the thoracoabdominal incision, will provide superb exposure.[20–22] The thoracoabdominal approach may be helpful in the excision of an ipsilateral, solitary pulmonary metastasis.[23]

The National Wilms' Tumor Study-3 (NWTS-3) found extrarenal renal vein involvement in 11% of their patients and thrombus in the inferior vena cava (IVC) in 3%. Removal of caval or atrial thrombus resulted in complications in 43% of NWTS-3 patients.[24] Despite this, mortality was not adversely affected by vascular involvement in NWTS-3. Accurate preoperative assessment of venous extension allows proper planning of the surgical approach.

The use of preoperative chemotherapy was argued in a recent review and is presently the approach of the International Society of Pediatric Oncology (SIOP).[25] The counter argument is made by Guilio J. D'Angio, who states that tumor stage is an expression of the tumors' inherent aggressive potential. Therefore, preoperative chemotherapy downstaging produces a false negative, obscuring the need for intensive therapy.[26] Early surgical therapy is advocated by NWTS. Comparison of NWTS and SIOP data fails to demonstrate any difference in the aggregate results between these different approaches.

New Horizons in Wilms' Tumor

The DNA content of Wilms' tumor cells as measured by flow cytometry has been found to be highly accurate in identifying anaplastic tumors.[27] Hyperdiploid DNA content 1.7 to 3.2 times normal corresponds well with anaplasia. This type of technology may prove to be useful in predicting clinical prognosis. In addition, recent data concerning N-myc oncogene expression in Wilms' tumor suggests an important role for molecular genetics in our future understanding of the pathogenesis of this neoplasm.[28]

RHABDOMYOSARCOMA

Rhabdomyosarcoma (RMS) accounts for about 50% of all soft-tissue sarcomas in children, and approximately 21% will arise from the genitourinary tract (paratesticular, bladder, prostate, vagina, and uterus). As we have seen with Wilms' tumor and the NWTS group, the dramatically improved success in the treatment of children with RMS is a direct result of a multimodal team approach and the Intergroup Rhabdomyosarcoma Study (IRS). IRS-3, which was begun in 1984, continues to

define the most efficacious treatment for these devastating tumors.

Prognostic pretreatment staging has continued to be a problem with rhabdomyosarcoma. The IRS Clinical Grouping classification is the most widely used staging scheme for RMS, but is based on the type of surgery performed. However, recent modifications of the TNM system, first advocated by the International Union Against Cancer, has demonstrated prognostic validity in a study at Stanford.[29,30]

Nonsurgical therapies now comprise the initial treatment in most instances of genitourinary RMS. However, surgery, when feasible, is still required for optimal results. More than half of childhood RMS is unresectable when first diagnosed. Current chemotherapeutic regimens employ combinations of vincristine, actinomycin-D cyclophosphamide, doxorubicin, VP-16, cisplatin, and imidazolecarboxamide (DTIC). Utilization of chemotherapy with or without radiation has made extirpation of previously unresectable tumors possible without mutilating exenterative procedures. Emphasis on the quality of life without compromised survival continues to be the hallmark of therapy. Familiarity with the IRS protocol and its multimodal therapeutic branches is essential for a knowledge of the many chemotherapeutic possibilities available. Optimal treatment demands the multidisciplinary approach.

NEUROBLASTOMA

The results of treatment of neuroblastoma continue to be disappointing. Despite the better imaging modalities of ultrasound and CT, early diagnosis is a major problem. Two-thirds of all children have metastatic disease at the time of diagnosis. Radiation and chemotherapy have failed to improve the prognosis of these unfortunate children with disseminated disease.

Most primary neuroblastomas arise within the abdomen, particularly in the adrenal gland. As such, they are an important diagnostic concern for urologists, even though we will have a limited role in their therapy. Utilization of ultrasound, CT, and MRI have improved preoperative diagnosis and staging; however, histologic confirmation of the diagnosis is still necessary.

Measurement of urine catecholamines and vanillylmandelic acid can be helpful both diagnostically and prognostically. Most patients will have elevated levels despite the lack of clinical manifestations such as hypertension.[31] A ratio of vanillylmandelic acid to homovanillic acid greater than 1.5 has been associated with a better prognosis. Serum neuron-specific enolase has also shown some promise as a tumor marker for neuroblastoma. Elevated levels have been associated with poor survival.[32]

The most important prognostic factors in neuroblastomas are tumor stage, patient age at the time of diagnosis, and the primary tumor location. High stage-IV tumors continue to demonstrate dismal prognosis, whereas 90% of children with stage-I or stage-II disease (a minority of patients) can expect cure. Early diagnosis prior to 1 year of age and tumors arising in the chest or neck have also been associated with better survival.

Complete surgical resection is still the most successful form of therapy. However, this is an option in few cases because of metastases or unresectability at the time of diagnosis. Adrenal neuroblastomas will usually require a radical nephrectomy. Excision of tumor that has invaded adjacent organs is advisable although preservation of vital structures may preclude it. Postoperative radiotherapy may help control local disease under these circumstances.

Chemotherapy, utilizing cyclophosphamide, dimethyltriazenoimidazolecarboxamide (DTIC), vincristine, and doxorubicin, should be given to patients with metastatic or unre-

sectable disease. If the response is good, resection of residual tumor is an option. Despite the high rate of complete and partial responses utilizing these agents, ultimate survival does not appear to have been significantly affected. An approach to patients who have failed induction chemotherapy is to deliver supralethal chemotherapy and radiation followed by allogeneic or autologous bone marrow reconstitution.[33,34] This aggressive approach entails serious morbidity and mortality. Because the bone marrow is often already involved with tumor, methods of separating the neuroblastoma cells from the normal marrow cells utilizing monoclonal antibodies is being tried.[35] If successful, this would allow autologous marrow reconstitution in these patients.

REFERENCES

1. D'ANGIO, G. J. Pediatric cancer in perspective: Cure is not enough. Cancer, 35(Suppl.):866, 1975.

2. GORDON, I., and GOLDMAN, A. A critical approach to imaging in neuroblastoma. In Pediatric Hem/Oncology Reviews. Edited by C. Pochedly. New York, Praeger, 1985, pp. 81–103.

3. LEAPE, L. L., BRESLOW, N. E., and BISHOP, H. C. The surgical treatment of Wilms' tumor: Results of the National Wilms' Tumor Study. Ann. Surg., 187:356, 1987.

4. D'ANGIO, G. J., et al. The treatment of Wilms' tumor: Results of the National Wilms' Tumor Study. Cancer, 38:633, 1976.

5. EHRLICH, R. M., et al. Wilms' tumor, misdiagnosed preoperatively: A review of 19 National Wilms' Tumor Study I cases. J. Urol., 122:791, 1979.

6. BECKWITH, J. B. Advances in pathology. Wilms' tumor update: Current issues in management. Dial. Ped. Urol., 11:2, 1988.

7. CANTY, T. G., NAGARAJ, H. S., and SHEARER, L. S. Nonvisualization of the intravenous pyelogram—A poor prognostic sign in Wilms' tumor? J. Pediatr. Surg., 14:828, 1979.

8. TAYKURT, A. Wilms' tumor at lower end of the ureter extending to the bladder: Case report. J. Urol., 107:142, 1972.

9. PAGANO, F., and PENNELLI, N. Ureteral and vesical metastases in nephroblastoma. Br. J. Urol., 46:409, 1974.

10. STEVENS, P., and ECKSTEIN, B. Ureteral metastasis from Wilms' tumor. J. Urol., 115:467, 1976.

11. WICKLUND, R. A., and TANK, E. S. Polypoid renal pelvic lesions in children. J. Urol., 123:943, 1980.

12. HELSON, L., and HAJDU, S. I. The cytology of urine of pediatric cancer patients. J. Urol., 108:660, 1972.

13. HUNIG, R., and KINSER, J. Ultrasonic diagnoses of Wilms' tumors. Am. J. Roentgenol., 117:119, 1973.

14. SLOVIS, T. L., and PERLMUTTER, A. D. Recent advances in pediatric urologic ultrasound. J. Urol., 123:613, 1980.

15. WALZER, A., WEINER, S. N., and KOENIGSBERG, M. The ultrasound appearance of tumor extension into the left renal vein and inferior vena cava. J. Urol., 123:945, 1980.

16. GORDON, I. Imaging in pediatric genitourinary malignancy. In Pediatric Tumors of the Genitourinary Tract. Edited by B. H. Broecker and F. A. Klein. New York, Alan R. Liss, 1988, pp. 3–7.

17. RITCHEY, M. L., and KELALIS, P. P. Intravascular and intracardiac thrombi. In Wilms' tumor update: Current issues in management. Dial. Ped. Urol., 11:2, 1988.

18. GOSFELD, J. L., BALLANTINE, T. V. N., and BAEHNER, R. L. Experience with "second-look" operations in pediatric solid tumors. J. Pediatr. Surg., 13:279, 1978.

19. SIGEL, A., and CHLEPAS, S. Nephroblastoma. In Surgical Pediatric Urology. Edited by H. B. Eckstein, R. Hohenfellner, and D. I. Williams. Philadelphia, W. B. Saunders Co., 1977, p. 200.

20. SKINNER, D. G. Thoracoabdominal approach to retroperitoneal surgery. In Modern Techniques in Surgery: Urologic Surgery. Edited by R. M. Ehrlich. New York, Futura Publishing Co., 1980.

21. COLE, A. T., FRIED, F. A., and BISSADA, N. K. The supine subcostal modification of the thoracoabdominal incision. J. Urol., 112:168, 1974.

22. COLE, A. T., and FRIED, F. A. Experience with the thoraco-abdominal incision for nephroblastoma in children less than 3 years old. J. Urol., 114:114, 1975.

23. EHRLICH, R. M., and GOODWIN, W. E. The surgical treatment of nephroblastoma (Wilms' tumor). Cancer, 32:1146, 1973.

24. RITCHEY, M. L., and KELALIS, P. P. Intravascular and intracardiac thrombi. In Wilms' tumor update: Current issues in management. Dial. Ped. Urol., 11:2, 1988.

25. VOUTE, P. A., DELEMARRE, J. F. M., and deKRAKER, J. Preoperative therapy. In Wilms' tumor update: Current issues in management. Dial. Ped. Urol., 11:2, 1988.

26. D'ANGIO, G. J. Counterpoint: Preoperative therapy. In Wilms' tumor update: Current issues in management. Dial. Ped. Urol., 11:2, 1988.

27. DOUGLASS, E. C. Prognostic importance of DNA content and chromosomal rearrangements. In Wilms' tumor update: Current issues in management. Dial. Ped. Urol., 11:2, 1988.

28. RICH, M., and NISEN, P. Molecular genetics. In Wilms' tumor update: Current issues in management. Dial. Ped. Urol., 11:2, 1988.

29. DONALDSON, S. S., and BELLI, J. A. A rational clinical staging system for childhood rhabdomyosarcoma. J. Clin. Oncol., 2:135, 1984.

30. PEDRICK, T. J., DONALDSON, S. S., and COX, R. S. Rhabdomyosarcoma: The Stanford experience using a TNM staging system. J. Clin. Oncol., 4:370, 1986.

31. GRAHAM-POLE, J., et al. Tumor and urine catecholamines (CATs) in neurogenic tumors: Correlations with other prognostic factors and survival. Cancer, 51:834, 1983.

32. Zeltzer, P. M., et al. Serum neuron-specific enolase in children with neuroblastoma: Relationship to stage and disease course. Cancer, 57:1230, 1986.
33. August, C. S., et al. Treatment of advanced neuroblastoma with supralethal chemotherapy, radiation, and allogeneic or autologous marrow reconstitution. J. Clin. Oncol., 2:609, 1984.
34. August, C. S., et al. Eight years' experience in neuroblastoma patients transplanted after relapse. Proceedings of the American Association for Cancer Research, 27:203, 1986.
35. Saarinen, U. M., et al. Eradication of neuroblastoma cells in vitro by monoclonal antibody and human complement: Method for purging autologous bone marrow. Cancer Res., 45:5969, 1985.

Neuroblastoma

Alfred A. de Lorimier
Michael R. Harrison
N. Scott Adzick

Neuroblastoma is the most common malignant solid tumor in children and accounts for 7% of all childhood malignancies and 15% of malignancy deaths.[1] In the abdomen, it is second in frequency only to Wilms' tumor. Neuroblastoma originates from cells arising in the neural crest portion of the neuroectoderm.[2] These neuroblasts were destined to form the sympathetic and chromaffin portions of the nervous system. Therefore, neuroblastoma most often arises in any position along the sympathetic chain from the neck to the pelvis. Rarely, it may originate intracranially from the sphenopalatine, ciliary, or otic ganglia. Neuroblastoma may have a primary origin within the spinal canal, but spinal cord compression most often results from a dumbbell tumor that arises from the sympathetic chain and grows through the intervertebral foramen into the spinal canal. This tumor rarely develops in the extremities from major neural structures such as the sciatic nerve or the brachial plexus.[3]

Neuroblastoma arising within the olfactory nerves occurs in older age groups, demonstrates an indolent biologic behavior, and does not excrete products of catecholamine metabolism, as do those that have other sites of origin. Therefore, olfactory neuroblastoma is usually called an esthesioneuroblastoma.[4]

Some embryonic neuroblasts migrate to regions adjacent to the sympathetic ganglia and condense into clusters of paraganglia. These cells contain enzymes that convert norepinephrine to epinephrine. In histologic sections, epinephrine stains brown with chrome salts, which designates these cells as part of the chromaffin system. Chromaffin cells are typical of the adrenal medulla and may be found in clusters along the abdominal aorta, particularly at the level of the inferior mesenteric artery where they are known as the organ of Zuckerkandl.

PROGNOSTIC CONSIDERATIONS

The biologic behavior of neuroblastoma, and thus the outcome of the disease, is highly variable and correlates with the age of the patient, the site of primary origin, the stage of the disease, sex, resectability, histologic appearance, and biochemical maturity of the tumor.[5-18] Tumor markers such as serum ferritin and neuronspecific enolase and chromosome analyses for the presence of N-myc oncogene amplification, identification of aneuploidy, and the proportion of cells in the mitotic phase using flow cytometry also seem to be important prognostic indicators.

To calculate survival rates, the interval of time after which most patients will succumb to the disease should be defined. Collins introduced a concept of tumor doubling time, that is, the length of time in which a given tumor will double in size. He proposed that pediatric tumors such as neuroblastoma are congenital in origin; thus, assuming a constant rate of tumor cell division, a period of risk for the recurrence of tumor would be the patient's age at diagnosis plus 9 months (the length of gestation).[14]

Because neuroblastoma is a rapidly growing tumor, some authors have suggested that a period of 14 months is equivalent to a 5-year survival period in adult tumors.[15] A review of children who were followed by the California Tumor Registry allows a comparison of the survival rates for the interval as defined by Collins, the 14-month interval, and the 2-year interval, as related to age of the patient (Fig. 41-1).[6] Eight percent of the patients died after 14 months and 5% after 2 years; 2 of 212 patients died after the period of risk as defined by Collins. Because Collins' interval is too long for a practical definition of long-term survival, most authors use the 2-year period to define cure rate.

Age

Neuroblastoma occurs from the newborn period to adulthood. The mean age at diagnosis is 3 years. There is no difference in survival in patients between 2 and 4 years of age, 5 and 9 years of age, and in those older than 10 years.[6,11,12] The frequency and survival rates according to age group from data prior to 1976 are shown in Table 41-1.[12] With better pre- and postoperative care, the current survival in infants is 96%.[13] Age is an important variable in prognosis, and comparison of various series must be corrected for variation in the age distribution of reported cases.

Spontaneous Regression and Maturation

Of all reported cases of spontaneous "cure" of malignant tumor, neuroblastoma is the tumor most frequently involved. Infants with Stage IV-S neuroblastoma are typical examples of this phenomenon.[19,20] In the era prior to chemotherapy, there were 20 documented patients with extensive hepatic and subcutaneous metastases who received no treatment because early death was expected.[21] Upon later follow-up, they were found to have no evidence of residual disease. This phenomenon is confined to infants, for regression occurred in 72% of those under 6 months of age, in 24% of those were between 6 months and 1-year-old, with the oldest patient being younger than 18 months old. The tumors involuted and were replaced by varying amounts of scar tissue.

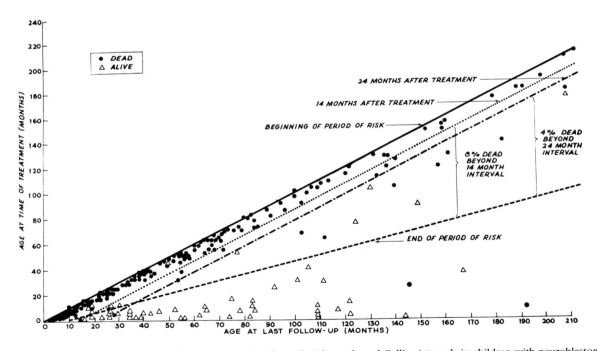

FIG. 41-1. Correlation of age at diagnosis and survival rates for 14-month, 24-month, and Collins intervals in children with neuroblastoma. Dots show deaths; triangles are survivors at the last follow-up. Note that most deaths (96%) occur within 24 months. Most survivors are children less than 2 years old. (DeLorimier, A. A., Bragg, K. V., and Linden, G. Neuroblastoma in childhood. Am. J. Dis. Child., *118*:444, 1969. Copyright 1969, American Medical Association.)

TABLE 41-1. *Incidence and Survival Rates by Age for Neuroblastoma[12]*

AGE	INCIDENCE (%)	SURVIVAL RATE (%)
0–11 months	28	55
12–23 months	19	24
over 2–4 years	53	8

TABLE 41-2. *Incidence and Survival Rates for Neuroblastoma by Location of Tumor[16]*

LOCATION	INCIDENCE IN NEONATES (%)	INCIDENCE IN ALL AGE GROUPS (%)
Neck	5.2	3.0
Mediastinum	33.0	15.8
Adrenal	36.7	55.0
Extra Adrenal	18.3	19.9
Pelvis	5.2	4.8
Unknown	1.6	1.5

Spontaneous regression of neuroblastoma actually may be more common than is clinically recognized. Beckwith and Perrin have noted cells in the adrenal glands similar to neuroblastoma in fetuses and newborns dying of unrelated causes.[22] They found an incidence of adrenal "neuroblastoma in situ" occurring once in every 250 newborns, while only 1 in 10,000 live-born infants will eventually develop clinically evident neuroblastoma. The "neuroblastoma in situ" is not found after the age of 3 months.

The 40-fold decrease in the occurrence of neuroblastoma, confined to young infants, would seem to be further evidence of spontaneous regression. However, the cells suggestive of neuroblastoma in situ may be embryonal neuroblasts, and not neoplastic cells, which eventually mature to adrenal medulla.[23]

Maturation of neuroblastoma to ganglioneuroma is also described as a mechanism of spontaneous cure. This process of maturation is frequently described, but it is rare.[24] Although there may be an actual development of neuroblastoma cells into ganglioneuroma, it is likely that the neuroblastoma elements of a ganglioneuroblastoma regress, leaving only the ganglion cells. It is unclear if ganglioneuromas themselves develop from this mechanism of maturation. Ganglioneuromas are rare in infancy and are most commonly encountered in adults.[24] Ganglioneuroma occurs four times as frequently in the mediastinum than in any other location, while a retroperitoneal origin for neuroblastoma is twice as common as it is for ganglioneuroma. It is possible that this difference in distribution for ganglioneuroma is related to the better prognosis for extra-abdominal neuroblastoma, and that it is because of spontaneous regression (perhaps maturation) in the mediastinum.

The unique biologic behavior of neuroblastoma in the young age groups has prompted intense interest in the immune mechanism of tumor control. Cells of the lymphoid series are known to be important in cell-mediated immunity. A retrospective review of the histology of neuroblastoma has shown that extensive infiltration of tumor by lymphocytes is seen in patients with longer survival.[24] However, these particular tumors also had greater degrees of differentiation than those with poor outcomes.

There has been no correlation between absolute peripheral blood lymphocyte counts and survival in neuroblastoma patients.[16] Lymphocytes from some neuroblastoma patients have been shown to have cytotoxic effects against their own tumors and against neuroblastomas from other patients in cell cultures.[27,28] In addition, the lymphocytes from some mothers and siblings of children with neuroblastoma have also shown cytotoxic effects on tissue cultured with neuroblastoma cells. However, there has been no correlation between the lymphocyte reactivity against tumor cells and the subsequent prognosis.

More recent studies have demonstrated the existence of enhancing and blocking antibodies that greatly modify the tumoricidal effect of lymphocytes.[28] In spite of the strong suggestion of an immune system, there has been no breakthrough in utilizing immunity to control neuroblastoma.

Site of Origin

The incidence of primary site of origin, with comparison between infants and all ages and the survival rate for all ages, is shown in Table 41-2.[16] This general distribution seems to be consistent in various geographic areas of the world. However, some centers have reported a disproportionately large number of intra-abdominal or mediastinal tumors, which will alter the overall prognosis of these series. The site of primary origin is an important variable in the prognosis.

Stage of Disease

Staging of neuroblastoma is important because the prognosis and intensity of treatment will vary depending upon the extent of disease. However, because of the vagaries in the natural history of neuroblastoma, there is no universal agreement of a staging system. There are currently two systems of staging that are used most often in the United States: the Children's Cancer Study Group (CCSG) staging system, and the St. Jude Children's Research Hospital/Pediatric Oncology Group (POG) staging system.[13,18] The CCSG and POG systems are defined as follows:

CHILDREN'S CANCER STUDY GROUP (CCSG)

Stage 1	Tumor confined to the organ or structure of origin.
Stage 2A	Unilateral tumor extending in continuity beyond the organ or structure of origin but not crossing the midline, which is incompletely excised. Ipsilateral and contralateral lymph nodes are microscopically negative. Intraspinous extension of tumor is stage 2.
Stage 2B	Unilateral tumor that is incompletely or completely excised and regional ipsilateral nodes are positive.
Stage 3	Tumors infiltrating in continuity beyond the midline. Tumor that overlaps the midline and does not infiltrate around midline structures is considered stage 2. A unilateral tumor with contralateral or bilateral nodes is stage 3.
Stage 4	Remote disease involving bone, parenchymatous organs, soft tissues, distant lymph node groups, or bone marrow.
Stage 4-S	Infants who would otherwise be stage 1 or 2 but who have remote disease confined to one or more of the following sites: liver, skin, or bone marrow (without evidence of bone osteolysis).

PEDIATRIC ONCOLOGY GROUP (POG)[18]

Stage A	Complete gross excision of primary tumor, with margins histologically negative or positive. Intracavitary lymph nodes not intimately adhered to, and removed with resected tumor, are histologically free of tumor. If primary is in abdomen (including pelvis), liver is histologically free of tumor.
Stage B	Incomplete gross resection of primary. The lymph nodes and liver are histologically free of tumor, as in stage A.
Stage C	Complete or incomplete gross resection of primary. The intracavitary nodes are histologically positive for tumor. The liver is histologically free of tumor.
Stage D	Disseminated disease beyond intracavitary nodes (i.e., bone marrow, liver, skin, or lymph nodes beyond the cavity containing the primary tumor).

Note that in the POG staging system, the presence of lymph node metastases is considered a variable that adversely affects prognosis. In 1988, the International Criteria for Diagnosis writing committee modified the CCSG Staging described here to gain prospective information on the importance of regional metastatic nodes.[29] Ninane et al. reviewed 33 children with CCSG stage-II tumors, and found that, of 20 children who had no lymph node metastases, 4 died of toxicity to treatment, and the remaining 16 were long-term survivors.[30] Thirteen of the 33 children had positive lymph nodes and 7 survived. It was concluded that patients with stage-II tumors and no metastatic nodes require only surgical resection, while the presence of lymph node metastases was associated with significant mortality and warranted more aggressive treatment. Hayes et al., of St. Jude Children's Research Hospital described 58 children with CCSG stage-II tumors, and 24 of 25 without lymph node metastases survived and 24 of 33 with metastatic lymph nodes survived.[31] In this group with metastatic nodes, all 5 infants survived, but 7 of 12 children older than 1 year died. In the same St. Jude's series of 36 stage-III tumors, in which all were associated with lymph node metastases, 6 of 13 children younger than 1 year old and 19 of 23 older children died. Because of their findings, the POG isolated metastatic lymph nodes as an important prognostic variable that they refer to as stage C when there is no disseminated disease.[18]

By contrast, Evans et al. reviewed 251 cases of localized and regional neuroblastoma (CCSG stage I, II and III) and noted that the survival rate was the same for 15 patients with negative nodes as it was for 93 patients with positive nodes.[13] There was no difference in survival if the nodes were attached to the primary tumor or separate from it. However, with stage-III tumors in which nodes were separated from the primary tumor, the survival was only 30%. The St. Jude Hospital/POG combined staging system does not recognize the decidedly adverse effect of neuroblastoma extending across the midline, where survival with unilateral tumors is 80% and survival with tumors extending across the midline is 50%. The POG system is not as discriminating between stages as is the CCSG system (Table 41-3).[13] Finally, the POG classification does not recognize the special group of infants with widespread tumor (stage IV-S), in which the prognosis is excellent. For these reasons, we prefer the CCSG staging system, and it is used for this discussion.

TABLE 41-3. *A Comparison of the Influence of Staging upon 5-Year Survival in the CCSG and POG Staging Systems Suggests that the CCSG Criteria are more discriminating.[13]*

	CCSG	POG
Stage I	approx. 100%	Stage A 87%
Stage II	78%	Stage B 74%
Stage III	43%	Stage C 67%

A stage-I tumor is defined as one confined to the site of origin, without local extension or regional lymph node involvement, that has been completely excised. Unlike other tumor systems, such as those arising in the kidney, stage-I neuroblastomas are not contained within an organ surrounded by normal parenchyma. Stage-I tumors may or may not have a well-defined capsule, but they have no evidence of neoplastic cells at the margin of resection. About 23% of all neuroblastoma patients have stage-I disease.

Stage-II neuroblastoma has local extension to adjacent organs or local lymph node metastasis confined to the same side of the midline as the primary tumor. In stage IIA, the tumor has been incompletely excised. Ipsilateral and contralateral nodes should be excised and proven to be negative for metastatic tumor. Intraspinal or dumbbell tumors without lymph node metastases are also classified as stage IIA and have an excellent prognosis unless the extraspinal extent of the tumor infiltrates across the midline. Intraspinal extension of abdominal or thoracic primary sites occurs in 6% to 14% of cases. Stage IIB consists of similar tumor that has been completely or incompletely excised, but ipsilateral nodes contain metastases and contralateral nodes do not. About 13% of neuroblastomas are classified as stage-II disease.

Stage-III neuroblastoma is defined as tumor infiltrating across the midline of the body. A unilateral tumor that overlaps the midline is stage II. A unilateral tumor with contralateral metastatic nodes is stage III. Stage-III tumors are almost exclusively intra-abdominal in origin, with occasional mediastinal and rarely, cervical primary tumors. Approximately 9% of neuroblastomas are stage III at diagnosis.

The staging of neuroblastoma arising from pelvic primary origin needs to be clarified because the prognosis of the midline pelvic tumors is better than that of other stage III retroperitoneal primary sites. Pelvic tumors might be staged accordingly; those completely excised are stage 1, residual gross or microscopic tumor in the area of resection or regional lymph nodes on one side only are stage II, and a pelvic tumor invading both sides of the pelvis or bilateral lymph node metastases are stage III.

Stage-IV disease consists of either lymphatic or hematogenous metastasis far beyond the area of the primary tumor. Most often, stage-IV tumors are characterized by osteolytic bone metastases. Favorite sites for bone disease are the base of the skull and calvarium, metaphyses of the long bones, vertebral bodies, and pelvis. Cervical, mediastinal, and retroperitoneal metastases may become so extensive that confluence of the nodes will produce prominent tumor masses. Rarely, metastases may appear in the liver, lungs, and brain. Approximately 40 to 60% of neuroblastomas are stage IV.

A special form of stage-IV metastatic tumor has been designated stage-IV-S. This occurs in infants and has an excellent prognosis.[19,20] At birth, or within several months subsequently, some infants develop extensive neuroblastoma throughout the liver and/or in subcutaneous fat throughout the body. These infants may also have neuroblastoma cells in the bone marrow aspirate, but there is no evidence of osteolytic metastases. If osteolytic bone lesions are found on skeletal roentgenographic survey, however, the biologic behavior of the tumor indicates a poor prognosis and the extent of the tumor is considered stage-4 and not stage-IV-S. In addition, the presence of tumor markers such as N-myc amplification, indicating a poor prognosis, identifies a stage-IV rather than a IV-S patient (see below). In some rare congenital cases, neuroblastoma has been noted in the lung, spleen, and kidney, and in other sites of metastasis not found in older children. In stage IV-S, the primary tumor is usually small, commonly arising in one or both adrenal glands. The metastatic tumors in these infants may grow rapidly and dramatically, to the extent that there may be almost as much tumor as normal tissue. The mechanical effects of this tumor bulk can be devastating, producing pulmonary distress associated with enormous enlargement of the liver. There may be severe anemia from hemorrhage in the multiple masses or replacement of the bone marrow. However, most of these infants will develop a spontaneous regression of all tumor masses after a phase of alarming growth during the first 6 to 9 months of life. From a review of 137 infants with stage-IV-S disease that was filed with the Armed Forces Institute of Pathology, Stephanson et al. identified two risk groups.[20] The high-risk group were those infants younger than 6 months old who lacked the skin metastases with liver involvement alone (29 cases), or those with liver plus bone marrow metastases (9 cases). Only 32% survived. The low-risk group was comprised of 7 to 12 month old children with any combination of metastases, or those younger than 6 months of age who had skin metastases. The survival in the low-risk group was 86%. It has been speculated that all of these tumor masses have multiple primary sites of origin or are not metastases at all.[20] Recent studies have shown that the IV-S tumors are composed of cells that are predominantly aneuploid, strongly suggesting neoplasia. However, the overall cure rate is greater than 70%; death occurs either from aggressive treatment or from physiologic impairment by the tumor masses. The incidence and overall survival rates taken from data prior to 1970 and after 1970 for the five CCSG stages of neuroblastoma are shown in Table 41-4.[6,8,11,13] The improved

TABLE 41-4. *Incidence and Survival Rates for Neuroblastoma by Stage of Tumor*[6,8,11,13]

STAGE	INCIDENCE (%)	SURVIVAL RATE (%) BEFORE 1970	SURVIVAL RATE (%) AFTER 1970
I	23	59	100
II	13	47	78
III	9	19	43
IV	44	5	15
IV-S	11	70	
TOTAL	100	29	

survival rate is probably related to better overall care of the children, rather than as a result of more effective chemotherapy.

Gender

Males are affected slightly more frequently than females, with a ratio of about 1.25 : 1. Of four series' correlating gender and survival, two suggested and one clearly indicated a better survival rate in females (30%) than in males (18%).[6,10,11] Wilson and Draper reported that the females in their series were younger and had a greater proportion of favorable sites of origin, stage, and histologic grades of tumor.[11] More recent studies fail to identify a difference in prognosis based on gender.[13]

Resectability

Clearly, the more localized the tumor, the more likely that it is resectable. Stella and associates noted that of 12 children whose tumors were completely removed, 11 (92%) survived. Nineteen of 34 patients (58%) survived when complete surgical excision was accompanied by radiation therapy given pre- or postoperatively.[10] In contrast, only 12 of 93 patients (13%) survived who had radiation or chemotherapy, but only partial resection or biopsy as the surgical treatment.[10]

In the Children's Cancer Study Group classification, the presence of residual primary tumor following operation does not change the stage of disease. However, the degree of residual primary tumor should be noted, as it is also a determinant of prognosis. Residual disease has been graded as follows:[13]

> GRADE 1—Microscopic residual tumor occurs when the surgeon does not believe there was a clean resection, or whenever there was a biopsy or previous rupture of the tumor or metastatic nodes were present.
> GRADE 2—When less than 5% of the original primary tumor remains.
> GRADE 3—When there is 5 to 25% residual tumor.
> GRADE 4—When there is more than 25% residual tumor or only a biopsy has been performed.

More than 90% of the patients with stage-I, complete excision survive, and only 44% of those with grade-4 residual tumor survive. Patients who have grade-1 or grade-2 residual tumor have an intermediate survival of 60 to 75%, which is nearly equal to those with microscopic residual disease.[13]

In one CCSG protocol, in which children with stage-III tumors received cyclophosphamide, vincristine, and DTIC plus radiation to the tumor bed, those with complete resection at original diagnosis or at a "second look" operation had a significantly better survival than those with biopsy only or those with incomplete resection of the tumor with grade-1 or grade-2 residual tumor.

Histologic Differences

Undifferentiated neuroblastoma is characterized by small, round cells containing dark-staining nuclei with little cytoplasm, closely packed together, with abundant vascular channels. With cellular elements lacking any differentiation, it may be impossible to distinguish neuroblastoma from some forms of retinoblastoma, Ewing's sarcoma, rhabdomyosarcoma, extranodal lymphoma, small cell osteosarcoma, or primitive neuroectodermal tumor (PNET).[33] These cases have been traditionally referred to as "small round-cell tumors." The differentiation of these various tumors requires electron microscopy, immunocytochemistry, and occasionally, more special techniques such as in situ hybridization with DNA or RNA probes, or cytogenetics.[33]

Shimada et al. have developed a histologic grading system based on Schwannian (stroma) and neuronal differentiation, prevalence of mitoses, and age, all of which have prognostic significance.[34] This system seems to be reproducible by various pathologists. The scheme is shown in Figure 41-2. The first dividing criterion that correlates with good prognosis is the predominance of deeply eosinophilic, Schwannian spindle-cell stroma surrounding the neoplastic cells. The stroma-rich component of Schwannian spindle cells should not be confused with neuropil, which is acellular and contains pale-staining and finely fibrillar or granular areas in the tumor. Stroma-rich tumors usually surround isolated, "well-differentiated" neuroblastoma cells, or there may be clusters of neuroblastoma cells

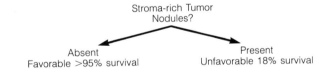

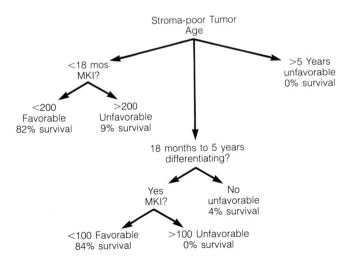

Fig. 41-2. Shimada classification of neuroblastomas.

of microscopic size intermixed with the stroma. The stroma-rich tumors comprise 20% of the total cases reviewed. However, if there are one or more macroscopic nodules or discrete masses of neuroblastoma cells within the stroma-rich tumor, the prognosis is adversely affected (Fig. 41-2).

Of the stroma-poor tumors, the age of the patient is an important determinant. Three age groups are considered: younger than 18 months, 18 months to 5 years, and older than 5 years. Within these age groups, a prognostic factor is the mitotic activity of the tumor. The number of cells in mitosis can be quantitated. It is often difficult to distinguish mitotic figures from karyorrhexis, therefore, the incidence of the two are combined for the total count. This count per 5000 cells is obtained from randomly selected, high-power microscopic fields and is called the mitosis-karyorrhexis index or MKI. In the age group younger than 18 months, an MKI above or below 200 determines prognosis.

Between 18 months and 5 years of age, an MKI below 100 defines a good prognosis, while an MKI above 100 is associated with a poor prognosis. In this age group, an additional variable is the degree of differentiation of the nuclei and cytoplasm of the neuroblasts toward a ganglioneuroma pattern. The tumor is considered to be "differentiating" when at least 5% of the cells have an enlarged vesicular nucleus and an eosinophilic cytoplasm with a distinct cell border and cell processes. If there is no differentiation of cells occurring, the prognosis is poor. In those stroma-poor tumors showing differentiation, an MKI below 100 defines a good prognosis, while an MKI above 100 has a poor prognosis. It should be noted that all of the stroma-poor specimens from children older than 5 years are associated with a poor prognosis regardless of the MKI or degree of differentiation of the tumor cells.

Shimada's classification was developed from patients who had not been treated at the time of biopsy or excision, and included all stages of disease. Subsequently, Chatton et al. reviewed pathology specimens obtained from patients with CCSG stage-III and stage-IV disease.[35] All of the stage-III tumors were reviewed prior to treatment, while many of the stage-IV tumor tissues were obtained at various times in the course of chemotherapy or radiation treatment. This study correlated well with Shimada's original results. In the stage-IV patients, the analysis of tumor tissue was just as predictive when the tissue was from the primary site or from a metastatic lesion, and it was predictive for tumor tissues obtained after various forms of treatment. In Chatton's review, calcification within a tumor was also identified as a favorable histologic finding. The survival was more than 2.75 times greater in patients who had tumors with calcification.

Chromosome Analysis

Tissue culture of neuroblastoma allows characterization of the chromosome composition and gene abnormalities. In neuroblastoma, variable lengths of deletion in the short arm of chromosome #1 (1p-) have been found beyond band 32.[37] It is speculated that the loss of DNA in this location represents a loss of suppressor or regulator genes that allows the development of neuroblastoma. The 1p- is rarely noted in stage-I, II, or IV-S tumors, but it is found in most of the stage-III and stage-IV tumors.[37] Poor prognosis is also related to the presence of diploid or hypotetraploid tumor cells, and 1p- is found in all of the tumors with these chromosomal anomalies.[37] There does not seem to be a relationship between N-myc amplification and 1p-, even though N-myc is considered to be one of the best identifiers of poor prognosis (see below). The presence of 1p- abnormalities may be a more important predictor of prognosis than other abnormal DNA/RNA variables, such as N-myc, described so far.[37]

Other abnormalities noted in 20% of cases include additional chromosomal material in the long arm of chromosome 1 and 17.[37,38] Loss of a sex chromosome is present in 30% of cases.[37,38] In addition, many neuroblastomas show varying lengths of homogeneously staining regions (HSR) within the short or long arms of various chromosomes. DNA is also present in the cytoplasm of some neuroblast cells, which are extrachromosomal paired chromatin bodies without centromeres, called double minutes (DM).[39] The finding of DM and HSR has the same connotation as amplified N-myc, predicting a poor prognosis (see below).

The N-myc Oncogene

One of the most important predictors of prognosis is analysis of the N-myc oncogene composition in the DNA of neuroblastoma cells. This proto-oncogene is normally found in the short arm of chromosome 2 (2p 23–24) as a single copy in all mammalian cells. Many neuroblastomas demonstrate amplification of the N-myc oncogene where multiple copies are present. Seeger et al. have been able to correlate prognosis with the number of N-myc copies in the tumor.[40] Those with one copy of N-myc have an overall survival rate of 65% in all stages of disease. The survival drops to 25% when 1 to 3 N-myc copies are present. There are essentially no survivors when more than 10 copies are found (see Table 41-5).[40]

TABLE 41-5. *The Relationship of Stage, Frequency of N-myc Amplification and Survival*

STAGE	(%) AMPLIFIED	SURVIVAL
I	none	100%
II	10%	85%
III	40%	50%
IV	40%	10%
IV-S	6%	95%
Ganglioneuromas	0	100%

Apparently, the presence or absence of N-myc amplification and the number of copies seem to be specific for each tumor. There is no evidence that a neuroblastoma can progress from a low number of copies to a many-fold increase, when there has been progression of disease.

Amplification of N-myc occurs in 30% of untreated patients with advanced-stage neuroblastoma. It is predictive of progressive dissemination of tumor, when originally localized. However, another 30% of patients who have progressive tumor show no amplification of N-myc. It is postulated that in these cases, the development and progression of neuroblastoma is caused by overexpression of a single copy of the N-myc oncogene in the absence of amplification, or that there are other oncogenes that may be responsible for the particularly malignant course of many neuroblastomas.[41]

DNA Analysis

Flow cytometry provides a method for measuring the DNA content of tumor cells. These studies can be performed on fresh tissue or by processing paraffin blocks. The tumor cells are treated with a fluorescent dye that binds to DNA, and the amount of fluorescence produced from each cell passed through a fluorescent-activated cell sorter is registered to quantitate the total DNA and the mitotic phase of each cell.[42-44] Normal cells and some neuroblastoma tumor cells are characterized by the normal number of 48 diploid chromosomes. Many malignant cells are hyperdiploid; that is, replication of DNA occurs by mitosis, in the absence of cellular division, which results in more than 48 chromosomes per cell (aneuploidy). In most adult tumors, excessive DNA content has been associated with a poor prognosis. However, in neuroblastoma, aneuploidy is associated with a favorable prognosis. In an analysis of 51 neuroblastomas, Hayashi et al. noted near diploid (42 to 47 chromosomes) in 11 cases, 10 of whom had stage-III and IV disease.[37] There were three cases with hypotetraploid (80 to 83 chromosomes) that had stage-IV tumors. Hyperdiploidy (50 to 56 chromosomes) were found in four tumors and near triploidy (60 to 77 chromosomes) were present in 33 tumors. With the exception of five stage-III tumors, hyperdiploid and near triploid tumors were from stage-I, II, and IV-S patients. As many as 100 chromosomes have been found in neuroblastoma cells.[37,47] Gansler et al. reported that euploid cells were present in 36% of survivors and 79% of non-survivors.[43]

Flow cytometry is also used to detect the proportion of cells in the various phases of the cellular growth cycle, and hence the rate of mitosis.[45] When there is a high proportion of cells in the DNA synthetic or S phase, G_2, and mitotic M phases, (related to the total in the quiescent G_0G_1 phases of the cell cycle) the prognosis is poor. Survivors had a mean of 21 to 22% of cells in the S, G_2, M phase, while 34% of the non-survivors had a greater number of cells in the mitotic phases.[43] The proportion of cells in the S, G_2, M phase can be

substituted for the MKI in the Shimada, as a better predictor of poor prognosis histology.[43,45]

Tumor Cell Markers for Neuroblastoma

Neuroblastoma produces five different metabolic products that can be measured in the plasma or urine. These markers are useful in establishing the diagnosis; some have prognostic significance, and some can be used to follow response to treatment and to detect recurrence of tumor. The markers that are particularly effective are serum ferritins, serum neuron-specific enolase, plasma and urine products of catecholamine metabolism, cystathionine, and gangliosides.

Neuroblastomas (as well as some hepatomas) secrete ferritins that can be measured in the serum.[46] Ferritins are normally iron-storage compounds found within the reticuloendothelial cells throughout the body, and normal serum levels range from 7 to 150 micrograms per L. Ferritins have an adverse effect on host immune mechanisms such as blocking rosette formation by T-lymphocytes with sheep cell erythrocytes, by blocking the lymphocyte response to mitogens, as well as depressing some granulocyte functions.[46] Elevated serum ferritin levels are found in about 40 to 65% of patients with stage-III or stage-IV neuroblastoma, while serum ferritins are not elevated in stage-I, stage-II, and stage-IV-S tumors. The level of serum ferritin does not seem to be related to the tumor burden, because the serum ferritin is elevated in stage-IV patients, but not in stage-IV-S patients where the tumor cells themselves contain comparable amounts of ferritin.[46] There is a correlation between the level of serum ferritin and ultimate survival in neuroblastoma. Hann et al. found that survival of children with stage-III tumors was 76% when the ferritin was negative and only 23% when the ferritin was positive.[46] In stage-IV disease, the survival was 27% with a negative serum ferritin and only 3% when the ferritin was positive. The serum ferritin level is an independent predictor of survival, unrelated to the age of the patient. The level of serum ferritin might also be used as a marker to identify tumor response to treatment.

Neuron-specific enolase (NSE) is secreted by some neuroblastomas and APUDomas.[47] The serum levels are highest and elevated most commonly with stage-III and IV disease, but they are not elevated in stage-IV-S tumors. Serum NSE may be elevated when catecholamine excretion is normal. Infants younger than 1 year of age with stage-IV disease, and children younger than 2 years of age with stage-III tumors and elevated NSE levels have a poor prognosis.[47] Neuron-specific enolase is not specific for neuroblastoma, for it may be elevated in medulloblastoma, PNET's, retinoblastoma, Wilms' tumor, Ewing's sarcoma, pancreatic carcinoma, and dysgerminoma. NSE seems to be a reliable tumor marker for following the clinical course of the disease.[47]

As might be expected of cells destined to become ganglia, neuroblastomas secrete neurotransmitters. In sympathetic ganglia, tyrosine is converted to dihydroxyphenylalanine

(DOPA), which is then metabolized to norepinephrine and, in the adrenal medulla, to epinephrine (Fig. 41-3). There are many metabolites in the degradation of DOPA, norepinephrine, and epinephrine. It is possible to measure each of these metabolites in the plasma and urine (Table 41-6).[48–50] The more malignant tumors lack the enzymes for the formation of DOPA, Dopamine, or norepinephrine. About 10% of neuroblastomas do not excrete catechols, but may produce acetyl choline, and these tumors have a particularly malignant course.[50]

The more malignant neuroblastomas are deficient in dopamine hydroxylase and do not produce norepinephrine. Therefore, they excrete the degradation products of dopamine, particularly homovanillic acid (HVA), and little of the catecholamines of norepinephrine such as vanilyllmandelicacid (VMA). In contrast, a more enzymatically differentiated neuroblastoma will produce norepinephrine, and this will be reflected in a significant excretion of VMA. Therefore, the prognosis can be predicted by the ratio of VMA to HMA; a ratio greater than one has a favorable prognosis while the predomi-

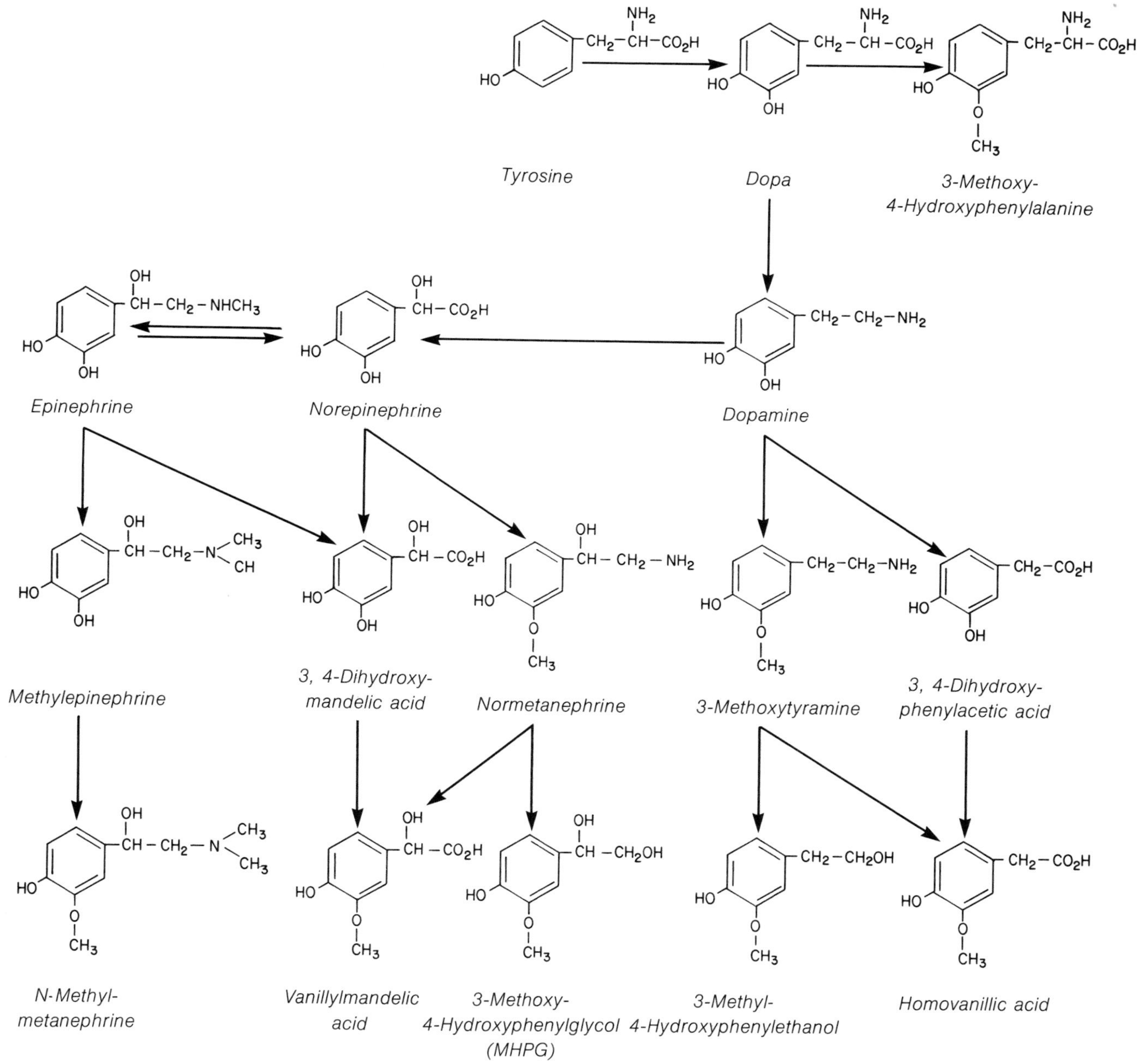

FIG. 41-3. Pathways for metabolism of dopamine, norepinephrine, and epinephrine. Children with neuroblastoma who excrete more homovanillic acid (HVA) than vanillylmandelic acid (VMA) have poorer prognoses. Presumably, this is because biologically primitive (hence more malignant) tumor lacks dopamine-B-hydroxylase to convert dopamine to norepinephrine.

TABLE 41-6. *Variations in Levels of VMA and HVA According to Age*

AGE	VMA CONCENTRATION (μ/mg CREATININE)	HVA CONCENTRATION (μ/mg CREATININE)
0–6 months	1.4–82.7	14.0–36.8
7–11 months	0.1–21.6	2.0–42.0
1–2 years	0.7–14.5	1.1–34.1
2–5 years	1.4–12.4	3.9–33.8
5–10 years	0.7–10.2	3.0–25.8
10–15 years	0.8– 8.5	1.8–22.2
over 15 years	0.8– 8.5	0.2– 3.1

nance of HVA predicts a poor prognosis.[51] Normal levels for VMA and HVA excretion in the urine are related to urinary creatinine, and are shown in Table 41-6. Unlike pheochromocytoma, neuroblastoma does not have an erratic secretory rate of catecholamine byproducts, and levels in an 8-, 12-, or 24-hour urine specimens are adequate.

A spot test of the urinary catecholamines VMA, HVA, and VLA (vanillacetic acid) in 6-month-old infants has been used as a mass screening effort for early detection of neuroblastoma in Japan.[52] The occurrence of neuroblastoma was found in 1:15,500 to 1:18,749 cases screened. In the US, we already mass screen infants for hypothyroidism, phenylketonemia, and galactosemia, and the incidence of neuroblastoma exceeds these diseases. Of the screened infants, 96% were asymptomatic and 72% had no evidence of a mass. Through the mass screening they have found that there was a higher incidence of favorable stage-I and stage-II tumors than previously published, while the distribution of the primary site of origin was the same. Screening is an appealing idea, although it might be more important when applied to an age group older than 1 to 1.5 years. The cure rate in infants is high anyway, and early detection in the older age group might discover earlier-stage disease.

The urine should also be tested for the presence of cystathionine.[52] Cystathionine is an intermediate metabolite of methionine metabolism; it is normally found in the brain, with smaller amounts present in the liver, kidney, and muscle. Cystathionine is not present in the urine of normal individuals, but it has been found in children with neuroblastoma who have had no VMA excretion. There is no correlation between the presence of cystathionine and the clinical course of the tumor, except that all patients in whom the tumor was completely controlled had no further excretion of cystathionine. However, some children stopped excreting cystathionine during active spread of the tumor.

Ganglioside G_{D2} is present in small quantities on the surface of cell walls of many normal cells, such as neurons, renal glomerulus, testicular and ovarian stroma, myometrium, and lymphoid follicles of the spleen.[54] More than 95% of neuro-

blastomas have high concentrations of G_{D2} on the cell surface and elevated serum levels.[54] It is not yet known whether there is a relationship between the serum G_{D2} and prognosis, but it is likely that it can be used to follow the clinical course of the disease. Monoclonal antibodies to G_{D2} are available and, when conjugated with radioisotopes, they may be used to locate the extent of tumor and for therapy.

Lactic dehydrogenase (LDH) and plasma carcinoembryonic antigen (CEA) may be elevated in most children with neuroblastoma.[53] LDH and CEA are elevated in many kinds of tumors (lung, breast, colon, and liver), and serial plasma determinations might be helpful in following the course of disease.

DIAGNOSIS

Symptoms and Physical Findings

In more than half of children with neuroblastoma, the initial manifestation of tumor is the presence of a mass.[15,56] The mass may be asymptomatic, but it is often associated with symptoms secondary to compression of surrounding structures, particularly the lungs, whether from a mediastinal or an intra-abdominal primary site. The mass is usually firm, irregular, and bosselated. Any grossly irregular mass extending across the midline of the abdomen is likely to be a neuroblastoma.

Frequently, the child will have recently had a normal physical examination, only to have the abrupt appearance of the mass. The tumor is often tender, and this seems to be associated with hemorrhage into the mass, which may account for the recent enlargement. High thoracic lesions may encroach upon the airway. Tumors arising from the stellate ganglion will produce Horner's syndrome, and if the tumor arises in utero, it will be associated with a lack of pigmentation of the ipsilateral iris (heterochromia).[57] Some masses extend into the intervertebral foramen, producing cord compression manifested by bladder and bowel atony, pain in the lower extremities, or anesthesia and paralysis.[58] Tumors arising in the pelvis may obstruct the bladder and rectum, and they can extend through the sciatic notch to become evident as masses in the buttocks. Edema and cyanosis of the lower extremities may occur from venous and lymphatic compression.

In approximately one-third of patients, the initial presenting symptoms result from metastases rather than from the primary tumor.[15,56] This usually occurs in older children who develop non-specific symptoms of listlessness, anorexia, weight loss, fever, vague aches and joint pains, a limp, or an unwillingness to move about. The symptoms may be confused with rheumatic fever. The base of the skull is a frequent site for metastases, producing proptosis of one or both eyes, with periorbital ecchymoses. Lymph node metastases are frequent, particularly in the cervical and supraclavicular nodes. Obvious irregularities of the skull or metaphyses of the long bones are caused by osteolytic metastases.

In infants, subcutaneous metastases will have a bluish discoloration, prompting the term "blueberry muffin baby."[59,60] Spontaneous blanching of the skin overlying the tumor nodules has been described, presumably because of local vasoconstriction from norepinephrine produced and secreted by the tumors.[61]

Hypertension occurs in 10 to 50% of children in various reported series'.[15,56] Increased catecholamine excretion by these tumors may also produce flushing and sweating. The blood pressure elevation is usually not hemodynamically significant, although there are instances in which hypertensive cardiomyopathy, similar to that occurring in patients with pheochromocytoma, requires the use of preoperative beta-adrenergic blockers to prevent perioperative hemodynamic complications. In these instances, the prognosis for cure of the tumor is excellent. Oftentimes, hypertension is not caused by catecholamines, but by compression of one or both kidneys or their blood supply.

Associated Syndromes

APUD AND VIP-PRODUCING TUMORS. In addition to producing products of norepinephrine metabolism, some neuroblastomas manufacture polypeptides similar to other APUD (amine precursor uptake, decarboxylase) tumors. APUD cells are derived from the neural crest, giving rise to the enterochromaffin cells of the gastrointestinal tract and tracheobronchial tree.[62] Neoplasms originating from APUD cells include carcinoid tumors, ACTH-producing bronchogenic carcinoma, islet cell tumors of the pancreas (insulinoma, glucagonoma, gastrinoma, and somatostatinoma), medullary carcinoma of the thyroid (which produces calcitonin), and others.

In common with some APUD tumors, neuroblastoma can secrete vasoactive intestinal peptide (VIP).[63] A syndrome of watery diarrhea, abdominal distention, hypokalemia, and acidosis has been reported in children with ganglioneuroma or ganglioneuroblastoma arising in the neck, mediastinum, and abdomen.[64] About 7% of children with neuroblastoma will have persistent watery diarrhea. This syndrome is associated with high levels of VIP in the plasma and tumor. Unlike the more common VIP-producing tumors of pancreatic or bronchial origin, increased catecholamine excretion was found in all VIP-producing ganglioneuroblastomas. VIP is a vasodilator, which may counteract some of the vasopressor effects of catecholamines. However, profound postoperative hypotension can occur following removal of the tumor, presumably because VIP has a longer hemodynamic effect than the catecholamines. Therefore, beta-adrenergic blockage with phenoxybenzamine and inhibition of the synthesis of tyrosine-containing octapeptides with metyrosine have been advocated to avoid postoperative hypovolemia and vasodilator shock.[64]

MYOCLONUS-OPSOCLONUS SYNDROME. Another syndrome occurring in approximately 2% of cases of neuroblastoma is the combination of myoclonus and opsoclonus.[65–67] These children have involuntary, uncoordinated, irregular, flickering muscular movements involving the limbs, trunk, head, and eyes that mimic cerebellar ataxia and nystagmus. The neurologic abnormality may resolve before treatment, but it usually persists for many months following resection of the tumor.

More than one-half of the children with myoclonus and opsoclonus will develop mental retardation.

Usually the neurologic abnormality is the first manifestation, preceding the discovery of the tumor by several weeks to more than a year. The neuroblastoma may be difficult to find when the cerebellar dysfunction is recognized. The tumor was located in the mediastinum in 53% of reported cases, and cervical, retroperitoneal, and pelvic primary tumor have also been reported. Seventy-one percent were favorable stage-I, II, and IV-S cases, with a survival rate of close to 100%.[66] However, even patients with stage-III and IV disease had a 71% survival rate.[66] The better prognosis in children with the myoclonus-opsoclonus syndrome is not related to a predominance in the favorable age group, because only 7% were younger than 2 years old.

The cause for the neurologic disability is unknown, but three mechanisms have been proposed: (1) neurotropic virus infecting neural crest cells and cerebellum, producing tumor transformation and encephalopathy, (2) neuroblastoma releasing a neurotoxin, and (3) antibody formation to neuroblastoma antigen producing cross reactions with cerebellar cells. The last theory is popular. The better prognosis in these patients, even with advanced-stage disease, is thought to be related to antibody control of the tumor. No cerebellar lesions have been proven at autopsy, and the immune mechanism has not been established.

OTHER ASSOCIATED DISEASES. Neuroblastoma has been associated with the clinical picture of myasthenia gravis and Cushing's syndrome, which responded promptly after excision of the tumor.[68,69] Ganglioneuroma and neuroblastoma have also been described in patients with neurofibromatosis.[70] The development of malignant pheochromocytoma and subsequent renal cell carcinoma has been reported following treatment of neuroblastoma.[71] The familial occurrence of neuroblastoma has also been described.[72]

Imaging Studies

The diagnostic evaluation requires clarification of the position of the primary tumor in relation to the surrounding normal structures and an indication of the presence of any metastases. Neuroblastoma metastasizes to local and distal lymph nodes, metaphyses of long bones, basal and parietal areas of the skull and, in infants, to the liver. Pulmonary metastases are rare. Radiologic studies include chest roentgenogram, intravenous pyelogram, CT or MRI scans of the chest, abdomen, and pelvis, and a skeletal survey (Fig. 41-4). CT and MR scans of the thoracic, abdominal, and pelvic masses provide clear definition of the tumor. More than 70% of neuroblastomas contain calcifications that can be readily detected on CT scans, thereby providing a further indication of the type of tumor. The disadvantage of the CT scan is the requirement of oral and intravenous contrast, and the radiation exposure. CT images are usually in an axial plane only. The distinct advantage of the CT scan is to demonstrate calcification within a tumor and document small

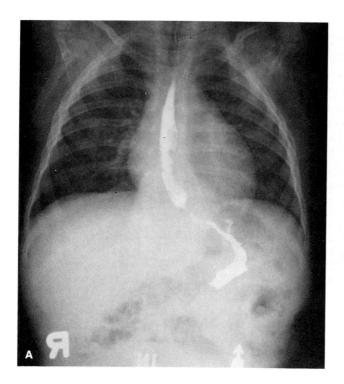

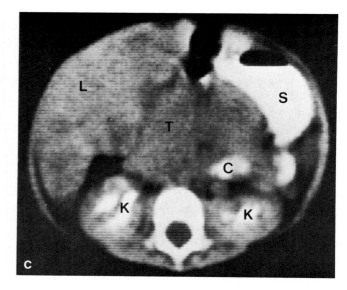

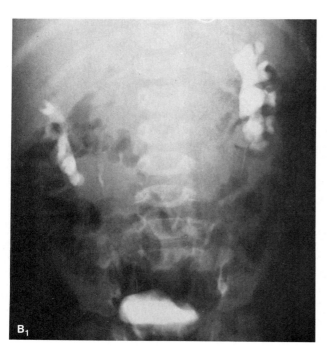

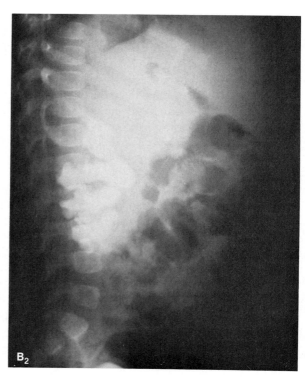

FIG. 41-4. Radiologic studies showing the appearance of neuroblastoma. *A*, Esophagram shows displacement of esophagus by an adrenal neuroblastoma extending into the posterior mediastinum through the aortic hiatus. *B*, Anterior-posterior (1) and lateral abdominal (2) radiographs of an intravenous pyelogram showing both kidneys displaced laterally by a large neuroblastoma arising from the celiac and superior mesenteric autonomic nerve plexuses. *C*, Computerized axial tomogram at the level of the second lumbar vertebra showing large celiac neuroblastoma (T) containing calcification (C). The tumor is anterior to both kidneys (K) containing contrast medium. The liver (L) is visualized, and the stomach (S) and small bowel are outlined by ingested contrast medium.

pulmonary metastases, which cannot be seen on plain chest films. However, because lung metastases are rare, a preferable study might be the MR scan.

Magnetic resonance imaging (MR) has become a valuable method for outlining tumors with respect to surrounding normal structures that can be readily accomplished in the coronal, sagittal and axial planes.[74,75] The technique is especially effective in identifying infiltration of tumor extra-durally within the spinal canal. The disadvantage of the MRI technique is the need for heavy sedation and the difficulty monitoring completely immobilized small children during the study.

An abdominal or neck mass can also be delineated by sonograms. The sonogram may be the preferred initial study, as it is noninvasive and eliminates radiation exposure. It can usually determine the relationship of the mass to surrounding structures, and it can determine whether the mass is cystic or solid.

Isotope scans of the soft tissues and bones using radionuclides such as technicium, gallium, or MIBG are essential for determining the extent of tumor (Fig. 41-5). For visualization of the primary tumor and metastases, the gallium (^{67}Ga) scan has been advocated as a prognostic indicator.[77] Most neuroblastomas do not take up gallium, but those that do seem to have a poor outcome.

Metaiodobenzylguanidine (MIBG) is a guanethidine derivative resembling norepinephrine that can be labelled with iodine 123 or 131.[78] For imaging purposes, the I 123 isotope is preferred because of the short half-life reducing radiation burden, better imaging, and the ability to use larger doses.[79] When given intravenously, it is bound to norepinephrine binding sites and then stored in neuro-secretory granules of the adrenal medulla, pheochromocytoma, and other neural crest tumors. However, uptake in the salivary glands, heart, liver and excretion in the bladder and the colon may obscure tumor.[80] MIBG scan is the preferred scanning technique because it identifies metastatic neuroblastoma in soft tissue sites of spread, as well as in bone; and it has a greater sensitivity and

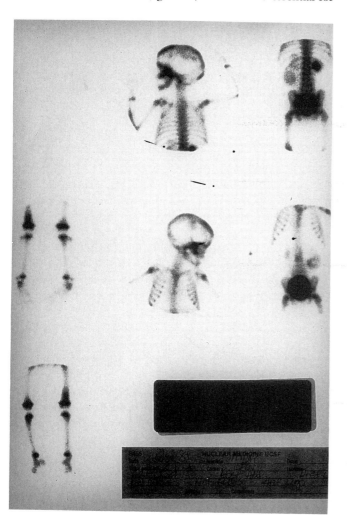
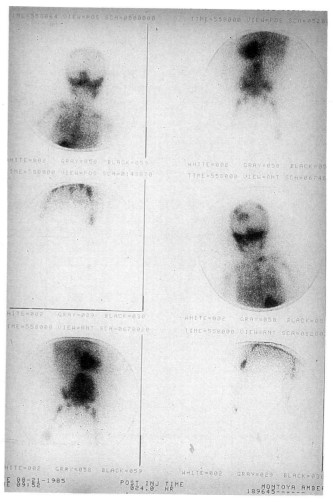

FIG. 41-5. *Left,* Technicium bone scan with uptake into tumor involving the calvarium, base of skull, left mandible, head of the scapulae and humerus bilaterally, the right ulna, thoraco-lumbar spine, retroperitoneal tumor on the left, both proximal femurs, right mid- and distal femurs, and both proximal and distal femurs. Note the concentrated technicium appearing in the right kidney and in the full bladder, which could obscure other tumor masses. *Right,* 131 I MIBG scan showing background uptake in the salivary glands, heart, and liver. There is uptake in the metastases of the calvarium and base of the skull, left clavicle and thoraco-lumbar spine, pelvis, and head of the femurs. A large, left retroperitoneal tumor is also seen. Excretion into a distended bladder obscures the lower lumbosacral spine and pelvis.

specificity than other scanning materials. However, it is slightly less sensitive than bone marrow aspiration and biopsy for detecting bone marrow metastases.[77] MIBG can localize metastases in neuroblastoma that does not produce catecholamines.

Hematologic Studies

The blood count may show anemia either from bleeding into the tumor or from bone marrow replacement by metastases. "Cogwheel" erythrocytes have been described in patients with neuroblastoma.[67] All patients with neuroblastoma should have a bone marrow aspiration and biopsy performed to help in identifying any metastatic spread.

Additional blood tests should include platelet count, prothrombin time, and partial thromboplastin time.[81] If a coagulation defect is detected, a deficit in specific clotting factors may have to be studied. Neuroblastomas are frequently highly vascular, and hemorrhage into the tumors can deplete coagulation factors. In addition, disseminated intravascular coagulopathy may occur. Blood samples for fibrinogen and fibrin-split products should be determined if coagulopathy seems to be present.

To summarize, the diagnostic evaluation of children with neuroblastoma should include the following:

1. Blood count, platelet count, prothrombin time, and partial thromboplastin time.
2. Serum BUN, creatinine, albumin, SGOT, LDH, alkaline phosphatase, neuron-specific enolase, ferritin, and glucoside G_{D2}.
3. Urine-routine analysis, 24-hour collection for VMA, HVA, dopamine, and cystathionine.
4. Bone marrow aspiration and biopsy from each iliac crest.
5. Bone scan—MIBG.
6. Skeletal survey.
7. MR or CT scan or ultrasound of the primary tumor.
8. MR scan or CT myelogram for paraspinous tumors with possible intraspinous extension.

The resected specimen should be processed for:

1. Routine histology—formalin fixed; Shimada classification.
2. Frozen section and touch preparation for immunocytochemistry.
3. Electron microscopy.
4. N-myc and immunocytology.
   a. Several tumor pieces $0.3 \times 1.0 \times 1.0$ cm should be immersed in isopentane and immediately placed in dry ice and stored at below $-20°C$ for N-myc and immunohistology analysis. This specimen should contain areas of the tumor most likely to be viable and frozen immediately after removal.

b. The bone marrow aspirate can be processed by differential sedimentation to concentrate any neuroblastoma cell present. Monoclonal antibodies for neuroblastoma can be used to identify one tumor cell in 10^5 normal marrow cells.

TREATMENT

Four modalities of treatment are used to attempt cure of neuroblastoma: surgical resection, chemotherapy, radiation therapy, including radioiodinated MIBG, and intensive chemotherapy with total-body irradiation.

The initial treatment of neuroblastoma depends on the stage of the tumor and the effect the tumor is having on adjacent structures. Stage-I and stage-II neuroblastomas are treated primarily, and possibly exclusively, by surgical resection. Stage-IV tumors, and most stage-III neuroblastomas are managed by chemotherapy initially, followed by surgical excision of remaining bulk disease and continued aggressive chemotherapy thereafter. Radiotherapy is utilized for unresectable bulk disease, to prevent possible pathologic fracture and to relieve bone pain. Total-body irradiation is also used in concert with very toxic courses of chemotherapy, which then eradicates the bone marrow and necessitates either autologous or allogenic bone marrow transplant.

Surgical Treatment

Surgical management may consist of biopsy only, partial removal, subtotal resection or debulking (i.e., removal of more than 75% of gross primary tumor), or total excision of all obvious tumor, including adjacent involved structures and lymph nodes.

Approximately 55% of children with neuroblastoma first present with localized tumors. Complete surgical resection of these tumors is of the highest priority. With the exception of infants with stage IV-S disease, and the unusual older child with limited stage-IV metastases, the most cures in neuroblastomas occur in those patients in whom the primary tumor is resected.[10,18]

The prognosis is clearly related to the extent of surgical excision. Figure 41-6 is a life table analysis of survival and extent of surgical excision showing a 94% survival when complete excision is accomplished. For those in whom excision with microscopic residual disease is present, the survival is 81%. The presence of gross residual, after debulking the tumor (grade-2 or 3 residual disease) results in a survival of 79%, while those with biopsy only have a 55% survival.[13] A poor-risk patient should have a course of radiation or chemotherapy or both, followed by a later attempt at surgical resection.

ANESTHESIA AND INTUBATION. General anesthesia and an endotracheal tube are mandatory in every case in which a neuroblastoma is to be resected. A large-bore cannula should be placed into the superior vena cava or right atrium. This is readily accomplished following general anesthesia with a percutane-

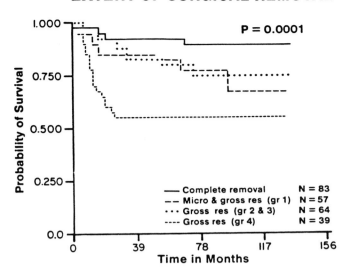

EXTENT OF SURGICAL REMOVAL

P = 0.0001

Probability of Survival

1.000
0.750
0.500
0.250
0.0

—— Complete removal   N = 83
– – Micro & gross res (gr 1) N = 57
··· Gross res (gr 2 & 3)   N = 64
---- Gross res (gr 4)   N = 39

0   39   78   117   156
Time in Months

Fig. 41-6. Life-table analysis of survival correlated with the extent of removal of local and regional neuroblastoma. (From Evans, A. E., et al. A comparison of four staging systems for localized and regional neuroblastoma: A report from the Children's Cancer Study Group. J. Clin. Oncol., in press, 1990.

ous needle puncture of the deep jugular or subclavian vein. Another peripheral extremity vein should be cannulated to provide an additional route for the administration of medications, fluids, or blood. The central venous cannula can be connected to a transducer to monitor the pressure. Central venous pressures above 10 cm of water suggest vascular volume overload or myocardial failure. However, a normal central venous pressure may be recorded in the presence of severe hypovolemia, because venous constriction occurs to preserve venous return to the heart.

Most anesthetic agents, administered in concentrations that provide muscular relaxation, depress vasomotor tone and myocardial contractility. Therefore, the plane of anesthesia may have to be maintained at a light level, with muscle relaxants used to facilitate surgical exposure. This technique will mask the magnitude of hypovolemia. Thus, the absolute level of central venous pressure must be correlated with the adequacy of perfusion, manifested by the rate of skin capillary refill following compression, by the briskness of bleeding from a fresh wound, and by the volume of urine output. Radial or pedal artery cannulation should be established for sampling of the arterial blood for blood gas and pH measurements. The presence of metabolic acidosis indicates inadequate tissue perfusion, most likely because of hypovolemia. It is helpful to place a Foley catheter in the bladder to measure the rate of urine formation. A urine flow of between 1 and 2 ml/kg/hr is desirable.

CONTROL OF BLOOD LOSS AND FLUID REPLACEMENT. Some large neuroblastomas are vascular and friable, and attempted removal produces extensive blood loss. If immediate surgical resection is indicated, rather than radiation and chemotherapy followed by a second-look procedure, the technique of deliberate hemodilution, hypothermia, and hypotension should be considered.[82] In this technique, the patient's blood is withdrawn into a citrate-phosphate-dextrose anticoagulant container, and replaced with a volume of Ringer's lactate solution and/or hetastarch three times the volume removed. Blood is withdrawn until the hematocrit value is between 15 and 20%. Because this technique greatly diminishes the oxygen-carrying capacity of the blood, it is necessary to reduce the metabolic rate of the tissues. Although anesthesia accomplishes this to some extent, deliberate induction of hypothermia to a core temperature of 32°C reduces the metabolic rate to 50% of normal.

The status of arterial and central venous blood pH, PCO_2, and PO_2 must be monitored closely. Tissue perfusion is maintained by compensatory increased heart rate and cardiac output, lower blood viscosity, and by a lowered peripheral vascular resistance. Inadequate tissue perfusion is detected by the appearance of metabolic acidosis, and requires more fluid volume. The mean blood pressure is lowered to 40 mm Hg by increasing the depth of anesthesia. The operative procedure can thus be accomplished with greatly reduced bleeding. The blood loss is replaced with equal or greater volumes of Ringer's lactate solution or hetastarch. Blood is not infused unless the mixed venous oxygen saturation falls below 50%, or metabolic acidosis persists in spite of volume replacement, or the hematocrit falls below 15%.

Upon completion of the operation, the blood that was withdrawn is warmed and replaced. To avoid the subsequent hypervolemia and cardiac failure, diuresis is induced by giving furosemide (Lasix) at 1 mg/kg intravenously. The patient is rewarmed by the heating mattress, the warmth of the operating room, heated nebulization of anesthetic gases, and irrigation of the abdomen or chest with Ringer's lactate warmed to 38°C. When the core temperature rises to 34 to 36°C, the child may be awakened. However, endotracheal ventilatory support is maintained for approximately 4 hours, until two-thirds of the infused Ringer's/hetastarch has been voided and the child has demonstrated adequate spontaneous ventilation. This technique of deliberate hemodilution, hypotension, and hypothermia allows for easier surgical removal of vascular tumors, but it also requires a team of anesthesiologists to intensively monitor metabolic responses and prolonged postoperative care.

During the course of the operative procedure, significant third-space fluid losses occur from the wound and the serosal surfaces. The composition of this fluid is essentially that of plasma, except for a much lower protein content. This fluid is not only sequestered at the operative site; capillary integrity seems to be impaired throughout the body for approximately 48 hours postoperatively. Therefore, the fluid replacement should be with Ringer's lactate or acetate solution. Dextrose (5% solution) added to the Ringer's solution is preferred, but because hyperglycemia and osmotic diuresis from glycosuria may occur with large-volume infusions, the urine and blood sugar content should be monitored. Hyperglycemia can be managed by Ringer's solution without dextrose. A large operative dissection may warrant a rate of volume infusion between 8 and 15 ml/kg/hr during the procedure.

When hemodilution and hypothermia are not utilized, the volume of blood loss must be closely measured. Dry sponges should be used so they can be weighed to identify the volume of blood loss, although this technique tends to underestimate the actual blood loss because of evaporation. The cannister used to collect blood suctioned from the wound should be calibrated to measure the volume, and it should be close to the patient to minimize dead space in the tubing. If the patient was not initially anemic, transfusion is not necessary until the blood loss exceeds 10% of the blood volume. Blood volume can be calculated as 80 ml/kg of body weight. A difficult surgical resection can result in losses equivalent to two or three times the patient's blood volume. Because transfused blood is usually refrigerated, it should be rewarmed before administration by being passed through coils of tubing placed in a water bath maintained at a temperature of at least 37°C.

CONTROL OF TEMPERATURE. When the hemodilution-hypothermia technique is not being used, normal body temperature should be preserved during the operation; this requires measurement of the core temperature with an esophageal or rectal thermometer probe. Although the metabolic rate is depressed with hypothermia under general anesthesia, upon termination of the procedure, shivering occurs, accompanied by a significant catecholamine excretion that results in an abrupt increase in the metabolic rate. Under these circumstances, the depressed, hypothermic child may be incapable of adapting to this metabolic demand, and cardiovascular and respiratory failure may occur. The child should be placed on a water mattress where the circulating fluid can be either cooled or warmed to help regulate the desired core temperature. The operating room temperature is initially maintained at about 30°C until the sterile preparation and draping is completed. The use of adherent plastic drapes is valuable to minimize heat loss. One of the most effective methods for preventing hypothermia is to use a heated humidifier to convey the anesthetic gases in the tubing connected to the endotracheal tube. This avoids large evaporative heat losses from the lung. If normal body temperature is maintained, the postoperative care will be much less intense, and there will be little risk of cardiac arrhythmia, respiratory depression, and metabolic acidosis.

Surgical Approach

The approach used in the operative procedure itself will depend on the extent to which the tumor has involved surrounding structures. Neuroblastoma does not arise within an organ that provides a clear demarcation from adjacent normal structures. Each site of origin—in the neck, mediastinum, abdomen, and pelvis—provides unique problems for the surgeon.

NECK TUMORS. In the neck, complete surgical resection is feasible for a well-circumscribed tumor of one of the cervical ganglia. However, these tumors commonly extend into the thoracic inlet and involve major vessels and nerves, such as the phrenic, vagus, and recurrent laryngeal nerves and the brachial plexus. A combined neck-and-chest incision may be required. Despite extensive exposure, microscopic residual tumor frequently remains in the vicinity of the major neurovascular structures. The potential for neurologic complications is significant, resulting in such abnormalities as Horner's syndrome, vocal cord or diaphragmatic paralysis, muscle weakness, and focal numbness of the arms and hands.

MEDIASTINAL TUMORS. In the mediastinum, complete surgical resection is probably more common than in any other site of origin. The tumor is usually densely adherent to the vertebral body and ribs, with a varying extension along the intervertebral foramen. Excision of these tumors frequently includes the affected intercostal nerves and a portion of the intercostal muscle. Block excision of the ribs or adjacent vertebral body is not indicated because a plane of resection can be accomplished subperiosteally. Rib resections may produce debilitating scoliosis in later years. Frequently, the tumor extends beyond the margin of transection in the intervertebral foramen. An MR scan or a CT myelogram may be indicated to assess the extent of intraspinous involvement.

RETROPERITONEAL TUMORS. Intra-abdominal neuroblastoma presents one of the greatest surgical challenges. A well-circumscribed, readily resectable primary tumor may be present in those children in whom the mass is discovered as a result of other symptoms, such as the myoclonus-opsoclonus syndrome. However, children who present with an abdominal mass as the dominant symptom usually have retroperitoneal tumors that are large and difficult to resect. Three types of retroperitoneal masses may be encountered: (1) adrenal, (2) celiac, and (3) non-celiac, extra-adrenal primary tumors.

ADRENAL AND EXTRA-ADRENAL TUMORS. Adrenal and extra-adrenal tumors may be well circumscribed, or they may intimately involve the adjacent kidney, aorta, or vena cava and may extend through the crura of the diaphragm into the chest. Upper abdominal tumors should be approached through an incision that can be lengthened into the chest to gain access to a mediastinal extension of tumor. In spite of the bulk of growth, most adrenal and extra-adrenal neuroblastomas can be resected of all gross tumor. The excision may require removal of the adrenal gland and adjacent kidney. Tumors arising from the lower lumbar area usually have a well-developed plane along the adventitia of the aorta and vena cava.

CELIAC TUMORS. Neuroblastomas arising from the area of the celiac and superior mesenteric autonomic nerve plexuses are the most difficult to manage. These masses extend across the midline to encircle the aorta and vena cava and the renal, superior mesenteric, and celiac vessels. Commonly, they spread into the hilus of the liver and invade the pancreas and the bowel mesentery. It is easy to underestimate the normal size of the major vessels coursing through these tumors; the vessels may be accidentally ligated, producing infarction of the bowel, liver, or kidneys.

Careful judgement is necessary before undertaking an aggressive resection. Although a kidney may be removed to allow complete excision of tumor, major vessels supplying the bowel, opposite kidney, liver, and spinal cord must not be compromised. If complete resection is not possible, the decision for biopsy or a debulking procedure must be made. Theoretically, removal of as much neoplasm as possible decreases the tumor burden for radiation and chemotherapy, and enhances the ability of the patient's own immune system to effectively eradicate residual disease. It is often better to remove sufficient tumor for histology, tumor markers, and chromosome analysis, and rely on subsequent chemoradiation therapy to reduce the tumor. "Second- and third-look" operative resection can be effective.

Unlike many other tumors, wide en bloc resection may not be possible with neuroblastoma, but dissection into the mass does not produce widespread dissemination of tumor with inevitable local recurrence. However, neuroblastoma is highly vascular; a fragmented excision and a morselling or scooping out of the tumor can produce extensive blood loss. If resection seems to be hazardous during this initial exploration, a generous biopsy should be obtained and the procedure should be terminated. The patient would then undergo intensive chemotherapy and radiotherapy so that a re-exploration in 4 to 5 months might result in a better operative resection.

PELVIC TUMORS. Pelvic neuroblastoma tends to be circumscribed and is resectable by way of a lower transabdominal approach. It is often difficult to recognize whether the poor functioning of the bladder is caused by obstruction and compression, or if the nervi erigentes are involved with tumor. In males, the presence of absence of sleep erections of the penis may help determine the integrity of the sacral autonomic nerve control. In either instance, a deep-lying tumor that has invaded the pelvic walls, or has extended to the level of the levator musculature, might preferably be treated initially by chemotherapy and possibly irradiation, to diminish the size of the tumor. A second-look procedure could result in a smaller risk of autonomic nerve injury. The prognosis for pelvic primary tumors is excellent, and it is important to preserve autonomic nerve function.

STAGE IV-S DISEASE. Resection of the primary tumor in infants with stage-IV-S disease has been advocated to accelerate involution of multiple metastases.[51] There is no evidence that this approach is effective because spontaneous regression occurs almost uniformly. However, following apparent complete regression of all gross disease, CT scans should be obtained to detect residual primary tumor. If a tumor mass persists, resection may be justified, as some of these tumors later recur and metastasize, with a fatal outcome. Because infants with stage-IV-S disease seem to develop spontaneous regression and disappearance of all metastatic tumor, there is question as to whether radiation and chemotherapy are justified in their management. The only mortality occurring in stage-IV-S tumors is because of the massive involvement of the liver producing mechanical encroachment on the lungs, intra-abdomi-

nal vessels, and the kidneys. Almost invariably, this is seen in infants within the first 6 weeks of life, when explosive growth of tumor within the liver develops. Of interest, those infants younger than 6 weeks of age, who have liver involvement without skin metastases, have only a 32% survival, but if there are associated skin metastases, 88% survive. When explosive liver enlargement occurs, chemotherapy is indicated. Cyclophosphamide and vincristine have not been uniformly effective. Therefore, newer agents such as cisplatinum, VP16 and VM26 might be considered. In desperation, a tense abdominal wall, with a greatly increased intra-abdominal pressure, has been treated by making a large abdominal wall hernia. The hernia can then be repaired after the huge liver has regressed in size.

Intraspinous Extension of Neuroblastoma

Intraspinal extension of a cervical, thoracic, abdominal, or pelvic primary tumor usually produces a neurologic deficit. Flaccid paralysis, paresis, sensory deficits, and impaired bladder and anal sphincter function require an MRI scan to outline the intra- and extraspinal extent of the tumor. Resolution of any neurologic deficit takes precedence over attempted control of the extraspinal tumor component. A laminectomy has been indicated in the past for emergency decompression when recent deterioration of nerve function developed. However, chemotherapy may be preferable to laminectomy. The combination of a laminectomy and postoperative radiotherapy has resulted in severe kyphoscoliosis, often requiring orthopedic correction. The tumor often extends three or more vertebral levels cephalad and caudad to the extension through the intervertebral foramen, and laminectomy at these multiple levels is extremely deforming. Furthermore, return of neurologic function occurs only in 40 to 65% of reported cases with laminectomy. More recently, chemotherapy has become the primary mode of treatment.[83] There seems to be prompt response to the tumor with a much greater incidence of return of good neurologic function. Long-term survival and complete control of these tumors is excellent. The amount of persistent neurologic deficit varies, depending on the severity of the original spinal cord compression.

Bad Prognosis—Stage II, III and IV Disease

Patients who present with obvious, extensive metastatic disease (stage IV) are usually seriously ill, with severe bone pain, ecchymosis, anemia from bleeding and/or replacement of bone marrow by tumor, and emaciation. These patients are not candidates for surgical intervention. It would be tempting to establish the diagnosis by removing a portion of a large primary tumor. However, confirmation of neuroblastoma can be achieved by the typical findings on imaging studies, by the presence of tumor markers in the blood and urine, and by bone marrow aspirate showing neuroblastoma cells by routine histology, monoclonal antibodies, and by N-myc amplification in the DNA. These patients will initially require intensive chemotherapy, with surgical resection of a gross residual disease deferred until maximum regression of the tumor has been achieved, which is usually before 16 weeks into therapy.

Those patients who are not so critically ill, and who do not have bone marrow involvement on bone aspiration or biopsy, require tissue diagnosis by either removal of metastatic nodes or by biopsy/excision of the primary tumor. A well-circumscribed primary tumor might be readily resected, but more often there is extensive involvement of normal structures, and therefore, only a wedge biopsy is indicated. Immediate primary resection does not improve survival, and delayed primary resection after initial chemotherapy may improve survival. The advantage of initial surgical resection is to obtain tissue that can be studied for all the prognostic indicators. More than 70% of neuroblastomas will have apparent complete or partial response to currently available chemotherapy agents. However, most often, residual tumor is present and resectable. Further, in contrast to the usually friable, very bloody tumors encountered with initial primary resection, most of the tumors, following chemotherapy, become "matured" toward ganglioneuroma and are solid, firm, rubbery, and relatively avascular. If total excision is not feasible because of involvement of large visceral blood vessels or organs, a debulking procedure is indicated. The use of an ultrasonic dissector has been helpful in removal of tumor around major blood vessels, avoiding injury to the vessels. Occasionally, a complete resection requires removal of kidney or a segment of bowel, which is justified if the remaining kidney is normal or the length of bowel resection will not produce malabsorption.

In some institutions, intraoperative focal irradiation can be given at the time of surgical resection or several days later. Following resection, the area of tumor involvement and residual disease is frequently outlined with metallic clips so that a subsequent plain abdominal x-ray will identify the involved field for external radiotherapy. These clips should be composed of tantalum, which will not produce artifactual scatter when follow-up CT scans are performed. After surgical resection or radiotherapy, aggressive chemotherapy will be required for long-term control of the tumor.

Chemotherapy

During the last two decades, there has been an increasingly aggressive use of chemotherapy to improve survival. Although both patients with stage-I tumors and most infants are long-term survivors, there are a large number of older children with more advanced stage tumors who do not survive. With the current identification of prognostic factors, the population of patients who should have the most aggressive treatment can be identified. Any patient, in any stage, who has an elevated serum ferritin, an elevated neuron-specific enolase in infants younger than 1 year old, unfavorable histology, cytogenetic studies showing diploidy or hypotetraploidy, abnormal chromosome 1, homogeneously staining regions (HSR), double minutes (DM), and particularly an amplification of N-myc, has a poor prognosis and aggressive chemotherapy is indicated.

In the 1960's and 1970's, the CCSG and POG studied single and combination chemotherapy agents causing regression of neuroblastoma. Complete or partial response rates for single agents were: peptichemio (PTC) 92%, cyclophosphamide (CPM) 59%, cisplatin (CCDP) 46%, Adriamycin (ADR) 41%, epipodophyllotoxins (VP-16, V-26) 30%, vincristine (VCR) 24%, and dacarbazine (DTIC) 14% (Table 41-7).[18] It became clear that most neuroblastomas were resistant to single agents. In those patients with disseminated disease, where there was a there was a good response, almost all developed recurrence of tumor, presumably by clones of cells that developed drug-resistance. Therefore, multi-drug therapy evolved.

Combinations of agents were tried in patients with stage-IV tumors, using varying doses and sequences of the above drugs. The combination of CPM, VCR, and DTIC resulted in survival rates of 10 to 15%. Until 1978, the best results were a 20% overall survival, where 50% of infants, 5% of children between the ages of 1 and 6 years old, and 44% of children older than 6 years of age had complete long-term regression of tumor.[84] Subsequently, Green et al. recognized the importance of aggressive induction to achieve complete responses in the early course of treatment.[85] By using CPM (which kills tumor cells in all phases of the growth cycle) daily for 7 days, they induced increased mitotic activity in the tumor. At the end of the 7-day period they then used adriamycin, which is most effective during mitosis. This regimen resulted in a 52% rate of complete remission with 15 of 35 long-term survivors. Those without complete response then received combinations of VCR and ADR, VM-26, VM-26 and ADR, VCR and DTIC, CDDP or CDDP, and VM-26, and the complete response rate was improved to 70%. Shafford et al. used pulses of CPM, VCR, CDDP, and VM-26 over a 3-day period repeated every 3 weeks and achieved a complete regression in 78% of patients. The addition of ADR did not improve the response rate.[85] However, the eventual survival was 20%, similar to many previous trials.

Newer protocols are studying as many as six drugs in combination, including CPM, VCR, DTIC, CDDP, and the podophylins. In some trials, the doses are being intensified, and continuous infusions are being used to achieve antitumor efficacy and minimize normal cell toxicity. With the initiation of therapy, the drug doses are intensified to achieve rapid reduction of tumor. This is referred to as the *induction* phase of therapy. Usually, this involves four courses of a combination of agents within 3 to 4 months. The patient is reassessed at that time using all of the imaging studies and bone marrow aspiration to identify local and metastatic disease. The second phase of treatment is referred to as a *consolidation* phase. At this time, aggressive resection of residual bulk disease and radiation therapy of residual tumor may be used. When a good response has been achieved, a third phase of therapy is begun, referred to as a *maintenance* phase, in which a combination of chemotherapy agents are used less intensively than they are in the induction phase. In all the previous trials where aggressive induction and consolidation therapy produced a complete or partial response, relapse developed frequently within

TABLE 41-7. *Chemotherapeutic Agents Available for Treatment of Neuroblastoma*

AGENT	INTRAVENOUS DOSE (MG/M^2)	TOXIC EFFECTS
Cyclophosphamide (CPM)	300–750	Nausea, vomiting, alopecia, bone marrow depression, immunosuppression, hemorrhagic cystitis, and azotemia.
Melphalan (L-PAM)	140	Nausea, vomiting, diarrhea, mucosal ulcers, hemorrhagic cystitis, alopecia, liver enzyme abnormalities, and increased ADH secretion.
Vincristine (VCR)	1.5	Local tissue necrosis, neurotoxicity, and alopecia.
Dacarbazine (DTIC)	250	Nausea, vomiting, and bone marrow depression.
Teniposide (VM-26)	15	Nausea, vomiting, alopecia, bone marrow depression, and allergic reactions.
Etoposide (VP-16)	100	Nausea, vomiting, alopecia, allergic reactions, hypotension, and pancytopenia.
Adriamycin (ADM)	35	Local tissue necrosis, nausea, vomiting, bone marrow depression, and myocardiopathy with total dose above 500 mg/m^2.
Cisplatin (CDDP)	60	Anorexia, nausea, severe vomiting, renal toxicity, hearing loss, pancytopenia, hypocalcemia, and hypomagnesemia.
Peptichemio (PTC)	1–1.5 mg/kg/day	Leukopenia, thrombocytopenia, alopecia, and phlebosclerosis.

24 weeks of treatment. Therefore, current protocols are aimed at ablation of all tumor within the 24 to 26 week interval, and there has been some deemphasis on the maintenance phase of tumor suppression. When induction has been effective, second-look or delayed primary exploration of the primary tumor is advocated in the consolidation portion of the regimen. Even when imaging studies showed no residual tumor, surgical exploration usually reveals resectable remaining tumor.

Intensive Chemotherapy and Total Body Irradiation (TBI)

The unsatisfactory results of the multiple chemotherapy regimens in the poor-prognosis patient has prompted innovative approaches to treatment. Recognizing that a 70+% complete or partial response of primary and metastatic neuroblastoma can be achieved with combination chemotherapy, and with the realization that recurrence (i.e., tumor resistance) evolves within 24 weeks, massive chemo-radiation therapy is being tried. Melphalan and total-body radiation are being added to the consolidation phase following multi-agent induction.[87] Because neuroblastoma is prone to metastasize to bone marrow, all metastatic sites are included in the radiation field. The TBI amounts to a total of 1,000 cGy. It is fractionated to 333 cGy over 3 days to minimize toxicity to the eyes and lungs, and it is known that neuroblastoma cells are less capable of repairing DNA injury than are normal tissues following sublethal radiotherapy.

As expected, massive chemo-radiation treatment produces lethal and irreversible destruction of the bone marrow. Therefore, bone marrow transplantation becomes essential. Both autologous and allogeneic transplantation are being used. The advantage of autologous marrow transplantation is the ab-

sence of morbidity from graft versus host reactions and its treatment. The bone marrow is harvested from the patient at about the 12th week of therapy. Prior to this, the bone marrow aspirate is analyzed for the presence of metastatic neuroblastoma and to ensure that the myeloid cells have recovered to at least 15×10^6 normal marrow cells.

Obviously, there is a significant risk of transplanting neuroblastoma cells back to the patient. The bone marrow is harvested at 12 weeks following the onset of chemotherapy. It is known that 75% to 85% of bone marrow samples from stage-IV patients, where no obvious neuroblastoma is seen by routine histologic methods, will contain malignant cells by immunocytologic techniques. Methods have been developed to identify as few as one neuroblastoma cell per 10^6 marrow cells, and techniques have been developed to purge the harvested bone marrow of neuroblastoma cells for transplantation.[87] The technique employs a combination of differential sedimentation, filtration, and tagging of the neuroblastoma cells with a number of monoclonal antibodies. The neuroblastoma monoclonal antibodies can be coated on magnetized beads, and when the antibody-bead-neuroblastoma cell conjugate is placed in a magnetic field, the neoplasm is removed, while the marrow stem cells are preserved. After purging the marrow, it is cryopreserved until it is required following the chemotherapy and total body radiation, at about 22 weeks into the treatment program.

Allogeneic bone marrow transplant is possible when there is an HLA-MHC-matched sibling as a donor. However, only about 25% of patients are likely to have an available matched donor. Because the neuroblastoma recipient is immunocompromised by the intensive chemo-irradiation, transfusion with even HLA-matched marrow can result in a graft versus host reaction because of a "minor" HLA mismatch. There may be a significant advantage of allogeneic marrow transplantation, because the transplanted T-cell population may be cytotoxic to residual neuroblastoma. A similar immunologic approach might be a future direction for treatment of metastatic neuroblastoma.

Other Treatment Modalities

When MIBG was found to localize in chromaffin tumors, it was natural to consider its use in the treatment of unresectable neuroblastoma, similar to the treatment of metastatic thyroid carcinoma with I 131.[88] The patient takes iodine to minimize uptake of 131 I-MIBG in the thyroid gland, and he must be isolated with precautions to protect both hospital personnel and family from contamination from the isotope. 131 I MIBG is injected intravenously over 4 to 6 hours. The drug is excreted in the urine, but the patient can be discharged from the hospital after 5 days. The radiation dose to be given is difficult to estimate because the amount of radiation received in organs such as the bone marrow cannot be measured. Although there is selective uptake in thyroid and salivary glands, heart and liver, no notable toxicity to these organs has occurred. The limiting factor has been thrombocytopenia, particularly when the patient has had intensive chemotherapy or a previous bone marrow transplant. The results have been disappointing. Although one-half of the patients may develop reduction in tumor size or stable disease, recurrence has occurred almost uniformly. It is possible that a significant problem with these results is that all of the patients have had multiple trials of other therapy, and the I 131 MIBG treatment faced a particularly resistant disease.

There is great interest in using radio-iodinated monoclonal antibodies to achieve control of metastatic disease. However, as with MIBG, uptake in normal tissues and problems providing the appropriate dose have limited the usefulness of these techniques.

Other possible methods to control systemic neuroblastoma might include chemotherapy agents tagged to neuroblastoma cell receptor sites, or perhaps a means of destroying the amplification of the N-myc oncogene, which seems to facilitate deregulation and uncontrolled proliferation of neuroblastoma cells.

CONCLUSION

The aggressiveness of therapy is based on the prognostic factors of stage, age, histology, and tumor markers. The following outline might be a guide for treatment options.

Not every variable is indicated in this scheme. For example, deletion of the short arm of chromosome 1 may outweigh all other factors such as stage or N-myc in requiring aggressive treatment. Further experience will determine if there is a discordance between the importance of serum ferritin and histology in stage-II and III tumors, or between an elevated serum gangleoside and diploidy, which will alter the approach to treatment. Only by pooling these cases in multi-institutional protocols will there be advances made in the diagnostic evaluation and treatment of this highly variable and complex tumor.

STAGE	AGE	HISTOLOGY	NSE	FERRITIN	N-MYC	TREATMENT
I	ALL	ALL	ALL	ALL	ALL	EXCISION AND OBSERVATION
II	<1	FAVORABLE	<100 UG/ML	<142 UG/ML	<3 COPIES	EXCISION AND OBSERVATION
II	<1	ALL	>100 UG/ML	>143 UG/ML	>3 COPIES	EXCISION AND CHEMOTHERAPY
II	>1	ALL	ALL	ALL	>3 COPIES	EXCISION AND CHEMOTHERAPY OR, WITH BULKY DISEASE CHEMOTHERAPY, EXCISION, AND LOCAL RT CHEMOTHERAPY
II	>1	ALL	ALL	ALL	>3 COPIES	EXCISION AND CHEMOTHERAPY
III	ALL	FAVORABLE	ALL	<142 UG/ML	<3 COPIES	EXCISION OR DEBULKING LOCAL RADIATION (RT)
III	>1	UNFAVORABLE	ALL	>142 UG/ML	>3 COPIES	CHEMOTHERAPY AND EXCISION OR DEBULKING, LOCAL RADIATION (RT) CHEMOTHERAPY
IV	<1	ALL	<100 UG/ML	ALL	<3 COPIES	EXCISION, CHEMOTHERAPY, AND AGGRESSIVE CHEMOTHERAPY
IV	>1	ALL	ALL	ALL	ALL	AGGRESSIVE CHEMOTHERAPY, EXCISION, LOCAL RT, AND AGGRESSIVE CHEMOTHERAPY TBI.
IVS	ALL	ALL	<100 UG/ML	>142 UG/ML	<3 COPIES	OBSERVATION RADIATION TO LIVER, AND VENTRAL HERNIA.
IVS	ALL	ALL	>100 UG/ML	>142 UG/ML	>3 COPIES	PROBABLY IV- NOT IVS.

REFERENCES

1. BILL, A. H., JR., HARTMANN, J. R., and BECKWITH, J. B. The unique biology of childhood tumors. Pac. Med. Surg., 75:281, 1967.

2. BLANDE, R. P. The neurocrestopathies; a unifying concept of disease arising in neural crest maldevelopment. Hum. Pathol., 5:409, 1974.

3. NEWBITT, K. A., and VIDONE, R. A. Primitive neuroectodermal tumor (neuroblastoma) arising in sciatic nerve of a child. Cancer, 37:1562, 1976.

4. KADISH, S., GOODMAN, M., and WANG, C. C. Olfactory neuroblastoma. A clinical analysis of 17 cases. Cancer, 37:1571, 1976.

5. BRESLOW, N., and MCCANN, B. Statistical estimation of prognosis for children with neuroblastoma. Cancer Res., 31:2098, 1971.

6. DE LORIMIER, A. A., BRAGG, K. U., and LINDEN, G. Neuroblastoma in childhood. Am. J. Dis. Child., 117:441, 1969.

7. GROSS, R. E., FARBER, S., and MARTIN, L. W. Neuroblastoma sympatheticum. A study and report of 217 cases. Pediatrics, 23:1179, 1959.

8. KOOP, C. E., and JOHNSON, D. G. Neuroblastoma: An assessment of therapy in reference to staging. J. Pediatr. Surg., 6:595, 1971.

9. PRIEBE, C. J., and CLATWORTHY, H. W., JR. Neuroblastoma. Evaluation of the treatment of 90 children. Arch. Surg., 95:538, 1967.

10. STELLA, J. G., SCHWEISGUTH, O., and SCHLIENGER, M. Neuroblastoma. A study of 144 cases treated in the Institute Gustave-Roussy over a period of 7 years. Am. J. Roentgenol., 108:324, 1970.

11. WILSON, L. M. K., and DRAPER, G. J. Neuroblastoma, its natural history and prognosis: A study of 487 cases. Br. Med. J., 3:301, 1974.

12. JAFEE, N. Neuroblastoma: Review of the literature and an examination of factors contributing to its enigmatic character. Cancer Treat. Rev., 3:61, 1976.

13. EVANS, A. E., et al. A comparison of four staging systems for localized and regional neuroblastoma: A report from the Children's Cancer Study Group. J. Clin. Oncol., 1990, in press.

14. COLLINS, V. P., LOEFFLER, R. K., and TIVEY, H. Observations on growth rates of human tumors. Am. J. Roentgenol., 76:988, 1956.

15. KOOP, C. E., and HERNANDEZ, R. Neuroblastoma: Experience with 100 cases in children. Surgery, 50:726, 1964.

16. POCHEDLY, C. (ed) *Neuroblastoma: Clinical and Biological Manifestations.* New York, Elsevier Biomedical, 1982, pp. 1–61.

17. GROSFELD, J. L., and BACHNER, R. L. Neuroblastoma: An analysis of 160 cases. World J. Surg., 4:29, 1980.

18. HAYES, F. A., and SMITH, E. I. *Neuroblastoma in Principles and Practice of Pediatric Oncology.* Edited by P. A. Pizzo and D. G. Poplack. Philadelphia, J. B. Lippincott, Co. 1989, pp. 607–622.

19. EVANS, A. E., BAUM, E., and CHARD, R. Do infants with stage IV-S neuroblastoma need treatment? Arch. Dis. Child., 56:271, 1981.

20. STEPHANSON, S. R., COOK, B. A., MEASE, A. D., and RUYMAMN, F. B. The prognostic significance of age and pattern of metastases in Stage IV-S neuroblastoma. Cancer, 58:372, 1986.

21. EVERSON, T. C., and COLE, W. H. *Spontaneous Regression of Cancer.* Philadelphia, W. B. Saunders, 1966.

22. BECKWITH, J. B., and PERRIN, E. V. In situ neuroblastoma: A contribution to the natural history of neural crest tumors. Am. J. Pathol., 43:1089, 1963.

23. TURKEL, S. B., and ITABASHI, H. H. The natural history of neuroblastic cells in the fetal adrenal gland. Am. J. Pathol., 76:225, 1974.

24. DYKE, P. C., and MULKEY, D. A. Maturation of ganglioneuroblastoma to ganglioneuroma. Cancer, 20:1343, 1967.

25. MARTIN, R. F., and BECKWITH, J. B. Lymphoid infiltrates in neuroblastomas: Their occurrence and prognostic significance. J. Pediatr. Surg., 3:161, 1968.

26. EVANS, A. E., et al. Factors influencing survival of children with non-metastatic neuroblastoma. Cancer, 38:661, 1976.

27. HELLSTROM, K. E., and HELLSTROM, I. Immunologic defenses against cancer. Hosp. Pract., 5:45, 1970.

28. HELLSTROM, K. E., and HELLSTROM, I. Lymphocyte-mediated cytotoxicity and blocking serum activity to tumor antigens. Adv. Immunol., 18:209, 1974.

29. BRODEUR, G. M., et al. International criteria for diagnosis, staging and response to treatment in patients with neuroblastoma. In *Advances in Neuroblastoma Research 2.* New York, A. R. Liss, 1988, pp. 509–524.

30. NINANE, J., et al. Stage II neuroblastoma. Adverse prognostic significance of lymph node involvement. Arch. Dis. Child., 57:438, 1982.

31. HAYES, F. A., GREEN, A., HUSTER, O., and KURNAR, M. Surgicopathological staging of neuroblastoma: Prognostic significance of regional lymph node metastases. J. Pediatr., 102:59, 1983.

32. HAASE, G. M., et al. Improvement in survival after excision of primary tumor in Stage IV neuroblastoma. J. Pediatr. Surg., 24:194, 1989.

33. TRICHE, T. J., and CAVAZZANA, A. O. Pathology in pediatric oncology. In *Principles and Practice of Pediatric Oncology.* Edited by P. A. Pizzo and D. G. Poplack. Philadelphia, J. B. Lippincott, Co. 1989, pp. 93–125.

34. SHIMADA, H., et al. Histopathologic prognostic factors in neuroblastic tumors: Definition of subtypes of ganglioneuroblastoma and an age-linked classification of neuroblastomas. J. Natl. Cancer Inst., 73:405, 1984.

35. CHATTEN, J., et al. Prognostic value of histopathology in advanced neuroblastoma: A report from the Children's Cancer Study Group. Hum. Pathol., 19:1187, 1988.

36. ROMANSKY, S. G., CROCKER, D. W., SHAW, K. N. F. Ultrastructural studies on neuroblastoma. Evaluation of cytodifferentiation and correlation of morphology and biochemical and survival data. Cancer, 42:2392, 1978.

37. HAYASHI, Y., et al. Cytogenetic findings and prognosis in neuroblastoma with emphasis on marker chromosome 1. Cancer, 63:126, 1989.

38. GILBERT, F., et al. Human neuroblastomas and abnormalities of chromosomes 1 and 17. Cancer Res., 44:5444, 1984.

39. BRODEUR, G. M., and SEEGER, R. C. Gene amplification in human neuroblastoma: Basic mechanisms and clinical implications. Cancer Genet. Cytogenet., 19:101, 1986.

40. SEEGER, R. C., et al. Association of multiple copies of the N-myc oncogene with rapid progression of neuroblastoma. N. Engl. J. Med., 313:1111, 1985.

41. SEEGER, R. C., et al. Expression of N-myc by neuroblastoma with one or multiple copies of the oncogene. In *Advances in Neuroblastoma Research 2.* Edited by A. E. Evans et al. New York, Alan R. Liss, 1988, pp. 41–49, 57–59.

42. KANEKO, Y., et al. Different karyotypic patterns in early and advanced stage neuroblastomas. Cancer Res., 47:311, 1987.

43. GANSLER, T., et al. Flow cytometric DNA analysis of neuroblastoma. Cancer, 58:2453, 1986.

44. LOOK, T. A., et al. Cellular DNA as a predictor of response to chemotherapy in infants with unresectable neuroblastoma. N. Engl. J. Med., 311:231, 1984.

45. OPPEDAL, B. R., STORM-MATHISEN, I., LIE, S. O., BRANDTZAEG, P. Prognostic factors in neuroblastoma: Clinical, histopathologic, and immunohistochemical features and DNA ploidy in relation to prognosis. Cancer, 62:772, 1988.

46. HANN, H. W. L., et al. Prognostic importance of serum ferritin in patients with stage III and IV neuroblastoma: The Children's Can-

cer Study Group experience. Cancer Res., *45*:2843, 1985.

47. ZELTZER, P. M., MARANGOS, P. J., EVANS, A. E., and SCHNEIDER, S. L. Serum neuron-specific enolase in children with neuroblastoma: Relationship to stage and disease course. Cancer, *57*:1230, 1986.

48. TSUCHIDA, Y., et al. Serial determination of serum neuron-specific enolase in patients with neuroblastoma and other pediatric tumors. J. Pediatr. Surg., *22*:419, 1987.

49. GITLOW, W. E., DZIEDZIC, L. B., and DZIEDZIC, S. W. Catecholamine metabolism in neuroblastoma. In *Neuroblastoma.* Edited by C. Pochedly. Acton, Publishing Sciences Group, 1976.

50. YOKOMORI, K., TSUCHIDA, Y., and SAITO, S. Tyrosine hydroxylase and choline acetyltransferase activity in human neuroblastoma. Cancer, *52*:263, 1983.

51. ALVARADO, C. S., et al. Plasma dopa and catecholamines in the diagnosis and follow-up of children with neuroblastoma. Am. J. Pediatr. Hematol. Oncol., *7*:221, 1985.

52. SAWADA, T., et al. Mass screening for neuroblastoma in infancy. In *Advances in Neuroblastoma Research.* New York, A. R. Liss, 1988, pp. 525–534.

53. GEISER, C. F., and EFRON, M. L. Cystathioninuria in patients with neuroblastoma or ganglioneuroblastoma. Its correlation to vanillylmandelic acid excretion and its value in diagnosis and therapy. Cancer, *22*:856, 1968.

54. CHEUNG, N. K., and MIRALDI, F. D. Iodine 131 labelled G$_{D2}$ monoclonal antibody in the diagnosis and therapy of human neuroblastoma. In *Advances in Neuroblastoma Research 2.* New York, A. R. Liss, 1988, pp. 595–604.

55. FRENS, D. B., BRAY, P. F., WU, J. T., and LAHEY, M. E. The carcinoembryonic antigen assay: Prognostic value in neural crest tumors. J. Pediatr., *88*:591, 1976.

56. FERNBACH, D. J., WILLIAMS, T. E., and DONALDSON, M. H. Neuroblastoma. In *Clinical Pediatric Oncology.* Edited by W. W. Sutow, T. J. Vietti, and D. J. Fernbach. 2nd Edition. St. Louis, C. V. Mosby, 1977.

57. JAFFE, N., et al. Heterochromia and Horner Syndrome associated with cervical and mediastinal neuroblastoma. J. Pediatr., *87*:75, 1975.

58. KING, D., et al. Dumbbell neuroblastomas in children. Arch. Surg., *110*:888, 1975.

59. SHOWN, T. E., and DURFEE, M. F. Blueberry muffin baby: Neonatal neuroblastoma with subcutaneous metastases. J. Urol., *104*:193, 1970.

60. SCHNEIDER, K. M., BECKER, J. M., and KRASNA, I. H. Neonatal neuroblastoma. Pediatrics, *36*:359, 1965.

61. HAWTHORNE, H. C., JR., NELSON, J. S., WITZLEBEN, C. L., and GIANGIACOMO, J. Blanching subcutaneous nodules in neonatal neuroblastoma. J. Pediatr., *77*:297, 1970.

62. WELBOURN, R. B. Current status of the apudomas. Ann. Surg., *185*:1, 1977.

63. TRUMP, D. L., LIVINGSTON, J. N., and BAYLIN, S. B. Watery diarrhea syndrome in an adult with ganglioneuromapheochromocytoma. Cancer, *40*:1526, 1977.

64. KAPLAN, S. J., et al. Vasoactive intestinal peptide secreting tumors of childhood. Am. J. Dis. Child., *134*:21, 1980.

65. ALTMAN, A. J., and BAEHNER, R. L. Favorable prognosis for survival in children with coincident opso-myoclonus and neuroblastoma. Cancer, *37*:846, 1976.

66. BERG, B. O., ABLIN, A. R., WANG, W., and SKOGLUND, R. Encephalopathy associated with occult neuroblastoma. J. Neurosurg., *41*:567, 1974.

67. WILLIAMS, T. H., HOUSE, R. F., JR., BURGERT, E. O., JR., and LYNN, H. B. Unusual manifestations of neuroblastoma: Chronic diarrhea, polymyoclonia-opsoclonus, and erythrocyte abnormalities. Cancer, *29*:475, 1972.

68. ROBINSON, M. H., and HOWARD, R. N. Neuroblastoma, presenting as myasthenia gravis in a child aged 3 years. Pediatrics, *43*:111, 1969.

69. KAGUT, M. D., and DONNELL, G. N. Cushing's syndrome in association with renal ganglioneuroblastoma. Pediatrics, *28*:566, 1961.

70. BOLANDE, R. P., and TOWLER, W. F. A possible relationship of neuroblastoma to von Recklinghausen's disease. Cancer, *26*:162, 1970.

71. FAIRCHILD, R. S., KYNER, J. L., HERMRECK, A., and SCHIMKE, R. M. Neuroblastoma, pheochromocytoma, and renal cell carcinoma. JAMA, *24*:220, 1979.

72. WONG, K., HANENSON, I. B., and LAMPKIN, B. C. Familial neuroblastoma. Clin. Nucl. Med., *5*:450, 1980.

73. MULLER, J. L., GAMSU, G., WEBB, W. R. Pulmonary nodules; Detection using magnetic resonance and computed tomography. Radiology, *153*:687, 1985.

74. BOECHAT, M. I., and KANGARLOO, H. MR Imaging of the abdomen in children. AJR, *152*:1245, 1989.

75. DIETRICH, R. B., KANGARLOO, H., LENARSKY, C., and FEIF, S. A. Neuroblastoma: The role of MR imaging. AJR, *148*:937, 1987.

76. COHEN, M. D., et al. Efficacy of magnetic resonance imaging in 139 children with tumors. Arch. Surg., *121*:522, 1986.

77. BIDANI, N., et al. Gallium scan as a prognostic indicator in neuroblastoma. Clin. Nucl. Med., *5*:450, 1980.

78. MC EWAN, A. J., et al. Radioiodobenzylguanidine for the scintigraphic location and therapy of adrenergic tumors. Semin. Nucl. Med., *15*:132, 1985.

79. SHAPIRO, B., and GROSS, M. D. Radiochemistry, biochemistry, and kinetics of ^{131}I-metaiodobenzylguanidine (MIBG) and ^{123}I-MIBG. Med. Pediatr. Oncol., *15*:170, 1988.

80. LUMBROSO, J. D., et al. Metaiodobenzylguanidine (mIBG) scans in neuroblastoma: Sensitivity and specificity: A review of 115 scans. In *Advances in Neuroblastoma Research 2.* New York, A. R. Liss, 1988, pp. 689–705.

81. MCMILLAN, C. W., GAUDRY, C. L., JR., and HOLEMANS, R. Coagulation defects and metastatic neuroblastoma. J. Pediatr., *72*:347, 1968.

82. ADZICK, N. S., et al. Major childhood tumor resection using normovolemic hemodilution anesthesia and hetastarch. J. Pediatr. Surg., *20*:372, 1985.

83. HAYES, F. A., et al. Chemotherapy as an alternative to laminectomy and radiation in the management of epidural tumor. J. Pediatr. *104*:221, 1984.

84. FINKELSTEIN, J. Z., et al. Multiagent chemotherapy for children with metastatic neuroblastoma: a report from the Children's Cancer Study Group. Med. Ped. Oncol. *6*:179, 1979.

85. GREEN, A. A., GREEN, M. D., HAYES, A., and HUSTU, H. O. Sequential cyclophosphamide and doxorubicin for induction of complete remission in children with disseminated neuroblastoma. Cancer, *48*:2310, 1981.

86. SHAFFORD, E. A., ROGERS, D. W., and PRITCHARD, J. Advanced neuroblastoma: Improved response rate using a multiagent regimen (OPEC) including sequential cisplatin and VM-26. J. Clin. Oncol., *2*:742, 1984.

87. SEEGER, R. C., et al. Bone marrow transplantation for poor prognosis neuroblastoma. In Advances in Neuroblastoma Research 2. New York, A. R. Liss, 1988, pp. 203–213.

88. HARTMANN, O., et al. The therapeutic use of I^{131} meta-iodobenzylguanidine (MIBG) in neuroblastoma: a phase II study in 12 patients. In Advances In Neuroblastoma Research 2. New York, A. R. Liss, 1988, pp. 655–667.

Testicular Tumors in Children

Julian Wan
David A. Bloom

Prepubertal testicular tumors (PPTTs) are rare. The Pathological Society of London in 1885 noted that only 18 such cases had been reported in children under the age of 10.[1] At another meeting of the same society in 1886, a dermoid cyst of the testis was reported in a 4-year-old with the comment that only 10 such cases had been recorded in 200 years.[2] In the century following these early descriptions of PPTTs, much has been learned about their histology and behavior. Yet, in spite of the various modern treatment options for benign and malignant tumors, orchiectomy is still the basic treatment.

It is estimated that 5,600 new cases of testicular cancer occur yearly in the United States, but few of these occur in prepubertal boys.[3] At Walter Reed Army Medical Center, from 1950 to 1985, only 12 out of approximately 1,100 testicular malignant tumors occurred in prepubertal boys. The types and distribution of these tumors differ from those of adult male tumors. Among prepubertal boys, 75% of testicular tumors are germ cell testicular tumors (GCTT) and 25% are non-germ cell testicular tumors (NGCTT), whereas in adults the ratio between GCTT and NGCTT is closer to 95% and 5%, respectively.[4]

Children with PPTTs tend to be at the younger end of the prepubertal age range, and newborn cases have been reported.[5] PPTTs have been associated with concomitant congenital anomalies such as bladder diverticuli, pericaval ureter, inguinal hernia, cryptorchidism, ureteral duplications, neurofibromatosis, and Down's syndrome.[6–8]

The Section on Urology of the American Academy of Pediatrics has classified PPTTs into 8 groups:

1. GCTT: yolk sac tumors, teratoma, and others
2. Gonadal stromal and interstitial cell tumors: e.g., Sertoli, Leydig
3. Gonadoblastoma
4. Tumors of supporting structures: e.g., sarcomas, fibromas
5. Leukemias, lymphomas
6. Tumor-like lesions
7. Secondary tumors
8. Paratesticular tumors

Rhabdomyosarcomas, although extratesticular, are usually discussed among PPTTs because of their similar presentation and management. To simplify our discussion, the prepubertal testicular tumors will be organized into four broad categories: GCTT, NGCTT, rhabdomyosarcoma, and miscellaneous lesions.

TYPES OF PREPUBERTAL TESTIS TUMORS

Germ Cell Testicular Tumors (GCTT)

YOLK SAC TUMOR. The yolk sac tumor (YST) is the most common PPTT, accounting for 70% of these lesions.[9] It was first distinguished from the adult form of embryonal cell carcinoma in 1951 by Magner and Bryant.[10] The term YST is derived from the work of Telium who found a similarity between it and the endodermal sinus of the rat yolk sac.[11] Others found further similarities with primitive fetal structures and proposed the terms archenteronoma and orchioblastoma.[12,13] From these beginnings, the yolk sac tumor has developed a large number of synonyms (Table 42-1).

Regardless of nomenclature, YST is a germ cell testicular tumor and not a tumor of yolk sac origin. It is curious that pure YST is rare in adults, although its elements are found in over 40% of adult mixed tumors.[14] This finding suggests that YST is not a unique pediatric testicular tumor but a tumor with patterns of differentiation dependent on age.[15] Manivel et al. proposed that different pathogenetic mechanisms are at work.[16] They note that intratubular germ cell neoplasia occurs in most adult germ cell testicular tumors. These clumps of cells, within the lumens of the seminiferous tubules, are a form of carcinoma in situ. They are found in over 85% of adult seminoma patients and in nearly 100% of adult nonseminoma germ cell testicular tumor patients. Yet, even when searched for, none were found in children with YST.[16] It has been proposed that pediatric YSTs are mono- or oligoclonal neoplasms derived from the transformation of a single or a few germ cells. These cells proliferate, and by the time the tumor is detected, the cells have already progressed to the invasive stage. This phenomenon may explain why the behavior of adult YSTs with its high frequency of mixed tumor types is different.[16]

TABLE 42-1. *Synonyms for Yolk Sac Tumor*

Adenocarcinoma with clear cells
Adenosarcoma of rete testis
Archenteronoma
Distinctive adenocarcinoma of infant testis
Endodermal sinus tumor
Extraembryonic mesoblastoma
Infantile embryonal carcinoma
Juvenile testicular embryonal carcinoma
Mesoblastoma ovaril
Mesoblastoma vitellinum
Orchidoblastoma
Schiller's tumor
Telium's tumor
Vitelline tumor

The presentation of YSTs is much like that of other prepubertal testicular tumors: a painless testicular mass is usually found incidentally. The mean age of diagnosis is 3 years, with a range from 6 weeks to 15 years. Some authors have reported a favorable prognosis for boys under two years of age, whereas others had contrary findings.[9,17,18] Overall, about 30% of boys with YST die from the disease, usually within the first two years of diagnosis.[19]

The staging system for YSTs is the same as that used for other PPTTs and adult testicular tumors. Stage I lesions are limited to the testis, stage II lesions involve the regional nodes, and stage III tumors have progressed supradiaphragmatically with distant metastases.

Yolk sac tumors spread lymphatically to the regional nodes and hematogenously to the lungs. Although there is still debate as to which route is the most prevalent, the important point is that both pathways exist and are used. Grossly the cut surface is a homogeneous grayish pink that may exhibit a mucoid or lipid texture. Histologically the tumor is characterized by small epithelial cells with a primitive appearance that varies from flat to cuboidal or even low columnar. Acinar, tubular, and papillary structures can be formed.[14] Vascular invasion and angiogenesis are additional features. Immunohistochemical staining demonstrates alpha-fetoprotein (AFP) in intracytoplasmic vacuoles as well as in extracellular hyaline globules.[20] Alpha-fetoprotein is an albumin precursor that is normally synthesized in utero by the yolk sac. Later in life it is produced by the liver and the gut. Synthesis halts at the time of birth with peak levels present at 12 to 13 weeks.[21] Postpartum elevations are usually due to abnormal synthesis caused by a hepatoma, YST, gastrointestinal tumor, or non-neoplastic hepatopathies.[22] The half-life of AFP is 3.5 to 5 days, although it can be as long as 7.7 days in low-birth-weight babies.[23] High AFP levels, while important, do not correlate with tumor volume. They do signal the persistence or recurrence of tumor after orchiectomy. False negative AFP levels have been noted in spite of retroperitoneal nodal metastases.[24] A normal AFP level, therefore, does not preclude metastases.[25]

A few decades ago, the treatment of YST consisted of orchiectomy alone. Radiation, node dissection, and chemotherapy have subsequently been applied with good results. Any discussion of treatment modalities is qualified by the fact that few centers have a large experience with YST and much of our understanding of treatments comes from the analysis of pooled data. There is debate concerning the value of the new modalities of management of a child with localized YST, and strong arguments are offered for orchiectomy and surveillance as the primary management of stage I YSTs.[26] There is reported only a 6 to 11% chance of retroperitoneal metastases in younger boys, with the lungs being most likely the site of any disseminated disease.[27,28] This observation has prompted some to treat stage I tumors solely with orchiectomy and observation. Flamant et al. treated 24 boys with stage I disease solely with orchiectomy.[29] About 20% subsequently did relapse and were salvaged with chemotherapy. The point here is that 80% were treated successfully without risking the morbidity of chemotherapy or retroperitoneal lymph node dissection. Others, however, have found that mortality appears to be much less in boys who have undergone some form of combined therapy with chemotherapy, node dissection, or radiation.[30]

Retroperitoneal lymph node dissection plays a major diagnostic and therapeutic role in the management of adult nonseminomatous GCTT. Considerable debate, however, exists regarding the role of retroperitoneal lymph node dissection in the management of YST. Unilateral retroperitoneal lymph node dissection is unequalled for diagnosis of retroperitoneal lymph nodes with minimal morbidity. For left-sided lesions, the primary target nodes are the left para-aortic nodes, whereas for right-sided lesions they are the interaortocaval nodes. The main cause of hesitation in recommending retroperitoneal lymph node dissection is possible ejaculatory failure. Standard bilateral node dissection impairs seminal emission in 75% of prepubertal patients.[31] Ephedrine stimulation may restore ejaculation and fertility in some affected patients.[32] A unilateral retroperitoneal lymph node dissection sparing the sympathetic ganglia, especially in the L3 to L5 region, probably decreases the risks of postoperative ejaculatory failure. Opponents of retroperitoneal lymph node dissection argue that absolute pathologic certainty is not required as it is possible to follow patients with serum AFP levels. Those whose levels persist or recur after orchiectomy can be rescued with chemotherapy. Further it is argued that the lymphatic route of spread has not been shown to be more significant than the hematogenous route. Until it can be shown what specific factors (e.g., age greater than 2, interval between orchiectomy and nodal metastases, presence of embryonal elements) would favor retroperitoneal lymph node dissection, its use will remain controversial.

The role of radiation therapy is limited. Although some have had good results with a combination of orchiectomy and prophylactic radiation to the retroperitoneal nodes, others have reserved radiation for those patients with positive nodes.[33] Yolk sac tumor in the retroperitoneum seems to be sensitive to radiation doses of about 3,500 rads. Because the risk of radiation injury to the spinal cord, bowel, bone marrow, testes, and kidneys in young children is significant, most centers reserve radiation for patients with localized tumor targets that are resistant to chemotherapy.

Chemotherapy is effective against YST. An unresolved question is when to treat. Some researchers favor adjuvant chemotherapy in all patients.[34,35] Others wait for radiographic evidence of disease or serum AFP elevation.[24] As with radiation therapy, the use of chemotherapeutic agents has significant risks, including hemorrhagic cystitis and testicular damage.[36,37] Nevertheless, if any residual or systemic disease is present, chemotherapy should be initiated. The specific agents and the duration of therapy should reflect the current attitudes of the pediatric oncologist on the treatment team.

Surveillance of patients not treated with retroperitoneal lymph node dissection or chemotherapy is crucial. Physical examination, serum AFP levels and chest roentgenograms should be performed regularly. A flexible schedule with progressively increasing intervals between examinations is applied so long as a disease free state is maintained. Studies can be performed 1, 3, and 6 months post orchiectomy and every 6 months thereafter for 2 to 3 years. Further lifetime follow up is then pursued on a yearly basis. Computed tomography (CT) scan of the abdomen and pelvis is recommended every 6 months during the first year following orchiectomy. Patients who have undergone radiation or chemotherapy should be followed for life because of delayed radiation effects and the chance of late secondary tumors.

The current trend of management is away from routine retroperitoenal lymph node dissection for stage I disease. The reliability of serum AFP levels is high, but not absolute. Orchiectomy with surveillance with or without adjuvant chemotherapy is satisfactory. Relapses do occur and prognosis is improved by early discovery. If any form of adjuvant therapy is rational for stage I disease, it would appear to be chemotherapy.

The team approach to the management of YST and other testicular tumors cannot be overemphasized. All treatment modalities should be represented. Procrustean protocols should be avoided. Every attempt should be made to tailor therapy to the individual patient, rather than to tailor the patient to an algorithm.

Extragonadal YST. Yolk sac tumors that manifest themselves in extragonadal locations probably arise from totipotential germ cells that migrated aberrantly. They tend to cluster along midline locations and may constitute a malignant component of a teratoma or cyst. Huntington noted that any element in a teratoma can become malignant, and such transformation is more likely to occur in embryoid than in adult tissue components.[38] Among presacral and sacrococcygeal teratomas, 21% are malignant, with the most common malignant pattern being YST.[9] O'Sullivan reported 24 patients with extragonadal primary tumors of which 17 were female.[39] The age of occurrence ranged from one day to 5 years with a mean of 21 months.[39] The most likely site was the sacrococcygeal spine, followed by the vagina, liver, nasopharynx, mediastinum, bladder, and brain. There was a 50% metastasis rate and a local recurrence rate of 20%. Despite this aggressive behavior, cures are possible with chemotherapy and primary excision. As with gonadal YST, AFP is a useful tumor marker.[15]

TERATOMA. Testicular teratoma accounts for 10 to 15% of PPTTs and is benign, unlike the potentially malignant testicular teratoma of postpubertal males. The mean age of diagnosis is 18 to 20 months. Teratomas consist histologically of multiple cysts of varying size, although one third have a solitary cyst. Like their postpubertal counterparts, various structures and tissues are found, such as cartilage, bone, muscle, nervous tissue, epidermoid tissue, ciliated epithelium, and intestinal epithelium. The diagnosis of teratoma depends on the discovery of recognizable fetal or adult tissues from all three germ cell layers. Fraley used these precise criteria to demonstrate that prepubertal testicular teratoma was benign.[40] Orchiectomy alone provides satisfactory treatment.[26,41]

ADULT TUMORS. Seminoma is the most common single cell type of GCTT in postpubertal males, but among prepubertal boys it is extremely rare. Only about 12 cases of prepubertal seminoma have been reported.[42,43] From these limited reports it appears that treatment is similar to that used with adult seminomas: operation followed by radiation with retroperitoneal lymph node dissection as needed. Embryonal carcinomas occur primarily in older boys, and their treatment, like that of seminomas, is similar to that of adult embryonal carcinomas. Although Magner and Bryant demonstrated that YST was an entity distinct from embryonal carcinoma, elements of embryonal carcinoma are found in otherwise distinctive YSTs.[10]

Non-Germ Cell Testicular Tumors (NGCTT)

The so-called interstitial cell tumors are rare in adults, but are somewhat more common in children, representing the most common prepubertal NGCTT. There are two main subgroups: Leydig cell tumors and Sertoli cell tumors. They are also known as androblastoma, arrhenoblastoma, interstitial cell tumors, granulosa stromal tumors, and gonadal stromal tumors. They may or may not be hormonally active, and are found in all age groups. The youngest reported case was in a 30-week-old 1,000-gram fetus.[44]

LEYDIG CELL TUMOR. The Leydig cell tumor (LCT) represents about 7% of all prepubertal testicular tumors and has a bimodal distribution.[45] It tends to occur between the ages of 6 and 12 in children and between the third and the seventh decade in adults. Symptoms may precede diagnosis by several years.[46] In some patients no discernible mass is noted, and random biopsies do not reveal the tumor.[47]

The tumors may first manifest themselves with precocious puberty, gynecomastia, or both.[48] Feminizing forms are more likely in postpubertal patients. Of the 38 feminizing LCTs reported by Gabrilove, 5 occurred in prepubertal boys and the rest were in patients aged 19 to 68.[47] Patients with androgen-producing LCTs usually present with evidence of precocious puberty. Early development of the penis, beard, and muscles and accelerated linear growth may occur. Unusual aggressive behavior is also seen and can sometimes be the main clinical feature.[48] Any boy with precocious puberty and a swollen testicle should be suspected of having a LCT.

Laboratory studies include elevated plasma and urinary 17-ketosteroids, which are not suppressed by the administration of exogenous corticosteroids. This observation allows differentiation from congenital adrenal hyperplasia. Leydig cell tumors are usually small brown yellowish tumors. They are pleomorphic and have many mitotic figures.

Despite these ominous findings, their behavior is usually benign. Prepubertal LCTs are unlikely to metastasize, and the designation of malignancy depends on the finding of metastases. Only about 10% of LCTs are malignant.[49] Some features suggestive of malignancy include: diameter of the primary tumor greater than 5 cm, presence of infiltrating margins, lymphatic or vascular invasion, necrosis, and more than 3 mitotic figures per high-power field.[49] Orchiectomy is usually curative, although there is one report of a case successfully managed by enucleation.[50] Retroperitoneal lymph node dissection should be considered for malignant LCT.[49] Removal of the tumor, however, may not cause regression of gynecomastia or precocious puberty. Close follow-up is needed because metastases have been found as late as 9 years after orchiectomy.[51]

SERTOLI CELL TUMOR. Sertoli cell tumors (SCT) are among the rarest of testicular tumors in children or adults. They are painless testicular masses sometimes associated with feminization. Gynecomastia is a rare finding with benign SCT, occurring in only 10 to 26% of the cases, whereas it is found in 60% of those with malignant SCT. Among prepubertal boys, the behavior of SCT is usually benign. As with the LCT, malignancy is defined by its behavior. Metastases are more common in adults, occurring in 30% of these patients.[4] Histologically, the tumor is composed of uniform eosinophilic cells with rare mitotic figures. A pathognomonic feature of SCT is the Charcot-Böttcher crystalloid.[52]

GRANULOSA CELL TUMOR. Whereas gonadal stromal tumors of the testes are mainly Leydig cell tumors or Sertoli cell tumors, the stroma also has the potential to give rise to ovarian stromal tumors such as theca and granulosa cell tumors. Male and females can have tumors containing all these cell types in either pure forms or in combinations.[53] Granulosa cell tumors comprise 15% of all gonadal stromal tumors and usually are present in patients younger than 6 months old. About 10% of granulosa cell tumors initially or ultimately show evidence of metastasis.[54] The sites of metastases are the retroperitoneal lymph nodes, liver, or lungs and almost all metastases develop within 5 months.[54] Treatment consists of orchiectomy with node dissection.

GONADOBLASTOMA. Gonadoblastomas are rare hormone-secreting tumors derived from mixtures of germ cells and interstitial cells. Nearly all patients have an underlying gonadal abnormality. These tumors do not metastasize, but may be associated with a malignant tumor within the same gonad or in the contralateral gonad. Histologically, they appear as discrete aggregates of intermixed germ cells and smaller epithelial cells that resemble immature Sertoli and granulosa cells. Two thirds of the tumors, usually in postpubertal patients, contain Leydig or lutein-type cells. In one third of the patients, the tumors occur bilaterally.

These tumors are also called dysgenetic gonadomas and gonadocytomas. They are most common in phenotypic females who may or may not be virilized, but who are likely to be found, on karyotyping, to have a Y chromosome. Fewer than 18% of the tumors in Scully's original review occurred in phenotypic males.[55] The males are usually male pseudohermaphrodites; some have mixed gonadal dysgenesis. The involved gonad is often easily identified, but may also be a streak gonad or testis. When the tumor is hormonally active, the effect is generally androgenic. In some cases the germ cells are no longer intermixed with the epithelial cells and invade the stroma. Scully refers to these tumors as germinomas and suggests that this is a malignant progression, with behavior like that of any other testicular tumor.

The recommended treatment is orchiectomy, with further treatment dictated by the concomitant malignant germ cell testicular tumor. As a general rule, a streak or dysgenetic gonad should be removed before it becomes a gonadoblastoma.[56]

LEUKEMIA AND LYMPHOMA. The testicle is the first site of extramedullary relapse in 8 to 36% of boys with leukemia.[57,58] These recurrences usually present as a painless swelling. Some do not present with a discernible change in size, but when examined carefully an irregular contour and induration are noted.[59] The leukemic infiltration involves the interstitial spaces, but may also enter the seminiferous tubules. Relapses can occur during complete marrow remission, and some protocols advise testicular biopsy prior to discontinuing therapy and then repeated biopsies during surveillance. Ultrasound scanning of the testis may be useful in screening for infiltration and in detecting subclinical nonpalpable disease, but has not replaced biopsy.[60] Standard open biopsy is performed bilaterally. Aspiration biopsy is also useful and may be positive when wedge biopsy is negative. The usual treatment of testicular relapse is local irradiation with 1,000 to 2,000 rads and the resumption of chemotherapy.[61] Others advocate chemotherapy alone without gonadal irradiation.[62]

Although it is usually a disease of older men, lymphoma may occasionally occur in prepubertal testes. Burkitt's lymphoma, a common pediatric tumor in Africa, comprised 50% of testicular tumors in one report.[63] Lymphoma is otherwise rarely mentioned in any other series on pediatric gonadal tumors. When it does occur, it incurs a poor prognosis, because the disease is invariably widely metastatic at that point. Hayes reported 4 children with testicular lymphoma and all but one succumbed within 5 months of diagnosis.[64]

Rhabdomyosarcoma

Childhood rhabdomyosarcoma is as prevalent as Wilms' tumor or neuroblastoma.[42] Only 15% of pediatric rhabdomyosarcomas involve the urogenital tract, usually occurring in prostate, bladder, and vagina. Tumors in the paratesticular site are uncommon, occurring in only 7% of all rhabdomyosarcoma patients.[65] Despite this small figure, rhabdomyosarcoma is the most common spermatic cord tumor and is more often found in children than in adults.[66] Two thirds of these patients are under 15 years old and the best prognoses have been in patients under 5 years of age.[67] The most common location has been spermatic cord (34%), followed by paratesticular region (31%), testis (15%), tunics (8%), epididymis (8%), and scrotum (4%).[66] A bimodal age distribution has been found with peaks at 4 and 16 years of age. In children younger than 10, the left side is 2.5 times more likely to be involved.

The presenting symptoms of paratesticular rhabdomyosarcoma (PTR) are painless scrotal or inguinal masses. Their growth and position may make the site of origin difficult to determine. These lesions are nodular with a rubbery texture. There are four histologic types: pleomorphic, alveolar, embryonal, and botryoid. The last three are the juvenile forms. Mostofi notes that cross-striations may help in diagnosis, but their presence is not required.[19] No useful tumor marker exists for PTR, and the diagnosis is made by examining the inguinal orchiectomy specimen. Scrotal exploration for the tumor leaves significant chance for local recurrence. The Intergroup Rhabdomyosarcoma Study Group staging system is widely recognized:

Group 1   Localized and resectable tumors.
Group 2   Grossly resected tumors with local residual disease or regional nodal tumors.
Group 3   Localized tumors not treatable by initial resection.
Group 4   Metastatic at diagnosis.

PTRs have nodal involvement in 40% of cases.[65] In contrast, patients with extremity rhabdomyosarcoma have a lymph node involvement rate of only 17% at presentation, and patients with the tumor at other genitourinary sites have a nodal invasion rate of only 5%.[68] A greater predilection for lymphatic dissemination by the paratesticular form seems probable. Because there is no useful serum marker, retroperitoneal lymph node dissection is an important diagnostic and therapeutic tool, after initial orchiectomy and distal cord resection. It also affords the opportunity to remove any residual primary tumor in the spermatic cord. We generally favor retroperitoneal lymph node dissection as part of the management of most group 1 and 2 tumors. Some centers prefer to delay retroperitoneal lymph node dissection unless lymphangiograms are positive.[69] Johnson proposed a limited conservative bilateral retroperitoneal lymph node dissection if the lymphangiogram is negative, while limiting the dissection to a left modified retroperitoneal lymph node dissection for isolated left-sided disease, and a complete bilateral dissection for right-sided disease.[68]

Chemotherapy usually involves cyclic treatment with vincristine, actinomycin, and cyclophosphamide and is usually given to group 1 and 2 patients after or instead of lymphadenectomy.[65] Children with more extensive disease are best treated initially with chemotherapy to lessen the effects of the disease with subsequent tumor resection or irradiation. Survival seems to improve with increased knowledge and experience. Johnson reported nearly a 60% median 6-year disease-free survival.[68]

Miscellaneous Lesions

The differential diagnosis of the prepubertal scrotal mass is extensive. The more common alternatives to the aforementioned testicular tumors include hernia, hydrocele, varicocele, epididymo-orchitis, and testicular torsion.[70] Other conditions that are far less common and less well known are described briefly. Most of these lesions are benign, and proper identification may permit preservation of the involved testicle. The following brief catalog and Table 42-2 list esoteric gonadal and intrascrotal lesions of childhood that may be, or may masquerade as, testicular tumors.

EPIDERMOID CYSTS. These cysts are monolayer expressions of teratomas. They are composed of keratohyaline material without skin appendages. Of 5,845 testicular tumors in the Testicular Tumor Registry, Price found 69 (1.2%) epidermoid cysts. Four diagnostic criteria are used:

1. The lesion is intratesticular.
2. The lumen contains keratinized debris.
3. The cyst is fibrous tissue with an inner lining of squamous epithelium.
4. There are no teratomatous or adnexal structures (hair or oil glands) with the testicular parenchyma.[71]

Most epidermoid cysts are found on routine or self-examination. When the lesion has been present for a long time and tumor markers are not elevated, some authors suggest frozen section and enucleation with preservation of the testis.[72-74] In postpubertal males, epidermoid cysts with parenchymal scarring or teratomatous elements are best treated as if they were teratomas.[75]

DERMOID CYSTS. These rare keratinous cysts contain skin appendages such as oil glands and hair follicles. Elements of a second germ cell layer, such as bone or cartilage, may also be present. Some have suggested that the dermoid cyst is a bilayer manifestation of teratomas whereas the epidermoid cyst is a monolayer expression.[76] Dermoid cysts have been described in patients as young as 6 months of age, in association with calculus, and have been intrascrotal yet extratesticular.[77-79]

CYSTS OF THE TUNICA ALBUGINEA. Cysts of the tunica albuginea have been described in about a dozen reports since Frater's description in 1929, and in most instances a testicular neoplasm was suspected preoperatively.[80] These lesions may be retention cysts or capsule formation after resolution of hemorrhages due to trauma, and treatment is simply excision of the cyst.[81]

CYSTIC DYSPLASIA OF THE TESTIS. This rare cystic scrotal mass is also known as ectasia of the rete testis. Multiple anastomosing irregular cysts characterize the lesion. It predominantly occurs in the mediastinum testis and spreads haphazardly, compressing the normal testicular parenchyma under the tunica albuginea. It is thought to result from failure of the precursors of the rete testes and the efferent ductules (gonadal blastema and mesonephric duct, respectively) to meet during development. Fisher reported a case in a 10-year-old with a 9-month history of progressive left scrotal swelling.[82] Three extensive cases were also described by Nistal.[83]

TABLE 42-2. *Miscellaneous Intrascrotal Lesions*

NAME	BEHAVIOR	TREATMENT	COMMENTS
Epidermoid cysts	benign	simple excision	can be confused with teratomas
Dermoid cysts	benign	simple excision	only 2 germ cell layers
Tunic cysts	benign	simple excision	? due to trauma ? retention cysts
Cystic dysplasia of testis	benign	simple excision	failure of mesonephric duct and gonadal blastema to meet ?
Papillary cystadenoma of epididymis	benign	simple excision	only benign epithelial tumor of epididymis; associated with von Hippel-Lindau disease
Meconium peritonitis	benign	none needed	preoperative KUB will show calcifications
Lymphangioma	benign	simple excision	usually involves axilla and neck; watch for lymphangitis
Hemangiomas	benign	simple excision	excise to prevent hematomas; observation in simple cases
Aberrant epididymal tissue	benign	simple excision	embryonic remnants
Pseudolymphoma	benign	none needed	hard to diagnose; treat underlying process
Adrenal rest	benign	none needed	enlarges in patients with congenital adrenal hyperplasia and mimics testicular tumors
Neurofibromatosis	malignant potential	simple excision	look for neural crest tumors
Neuroblastoma	malignant	orchiectomy	look for primary tumor in adrenals and retroperitoneum

PRIMARY EPIDIDYMAL NEOPLASMS. Epididymal neoplasms are uncommon in children. In adults and children, the most frequent epididymal neoplasm, benign or malignant, is the adenomatoid tumor or mesothelioma. It comprises about 60% of all primary epididymal neoplasms.[84] Primary tumors are rare with sarcomas being twice as common as carcinomas.[84] The papillary cystadenoma, the only known benign epithelial tumor of the epididymis, is linked to von Hippel-Lindau disease. This autosomal dominant heritable disorder is characterized by angiomatosis of the retina, cerebellum, and other organs. It is strongly associated with renal cell carcinoma, pheochromocytoma, and ependymoma. Two thirds of patients with bilateral papillary cystadenomas have von Hippel-Lindau disease. One fifth of those with unilateral lesions are also afflicted. It is therefore necessary to observe patients with papillary cystadenoma for signs of von Hippel-Lindau disease.[84,85]

MECONIUM PERITONITIS. Meconium peritonitis may cause scrotal calcification. Because testicular masses are often evaluated without abdominal roentgenograms, this diagnosis may be missed. Meconium peritonitis results from in utero perforation of the gastrointestinal tract. The meconium spills into the peritoneum and provokes a sterile inflammatory reaction resulting in calcification and fibrosis. It is often associated with atresia of the bowel, volvulus, or peritoneal bands. It can be asymptomatic and only discovered incidentally. Infants may present with hydroceles at birth; the hydroceles contain serous fluid and meconium. After birth, the meconium calcifies and hardens into a scrotal mass. The finding of abdominal and scrotal calcification may make an operation unnecessary.[86]

CYSTIC LYMPHANGIOMA. A benign tumor due to malformation of the lymphatic system, cystic lymphangioma usually occurs in the upper torso in children. It is also referred to as cystic hygroma, hygroma, or lymphangioma. The rest of the lymph system is otherwise normal. Scrotal lymphangioma has been described in several children.[87,88]

GENITAL HEMANGIOMAS. These tumors are rare. They may be painful and can extend to the perineum, abdominal wall, or thigh. To avoid risk of spontaneous or traumatic hemorrhage, surgical excision has been recommended.[89] Fewer than 40 cases have been reported of hemangiomas of the scrotum and penis. Senoh reported a scrotal hematoma in a 6-year-old child secondary to blunt trauma.[90] This was resected and identified as a cavernous hemangioma. Gotoh et al. in 1983 reported a case that suggested that prolonged temperature elevation from a large scrotal hemangioma can lead to testicular degeneration.[91] Our own experience suggests that for stable cutaneous lesions, watchful waiting and conservative therapy with topical steroids, such as 1% hydrocortisone, yield good results, with spontaneous regression.

EPIDIDYMAL ANOMALIES. Epididymal anomalies are usually associated with cryptorchidism. About 33 to 66% of patients with undescended testicles have epididymal anomalies.[92] An increase is also seen in patients with cystic fibrosis or von Hippel-Lindau syndrome, and in those whose mothers took diethylstilbestrol during pregnancy. Epididymal cysts may present as enlarging and symptomatic scrotal masses. As epididymal function, including secretions, increases with puberty and hormonal stimulation, these cysts usually become evident around puberty.[92]

TESTICULAR PSEUDOLYMPHOMA. Testicular pseudolymphoma is a reactive process than can be confused with lymphomas. Algaba reported the first case in a child.[93] A 3-year-old without prior illness was seen for a right painless testicle mass. Pseudolymphomas have also been reported in the gastrointestinal tract, especially the stomach, and in the spleen, lung, larynx, and breast. The criteria for diagnosis include: delimitation of lesion, although infiltration of adjacent structure is possible; mixed cellular infiltration with mature lymphocytes and plasma cells; and follicular distribution.[93]

ECTOPIC ADRENAL RESTS. Although harmless, ectopic adrenal rests can be confused with malignant tumors. When exposed to high levels of ACTH, aberrant adrenal tissue becomes markedly enlarged and hormonally active. Franco-Saenz performed biopsies of bilateral testicular tumors in patients with congenital adrenal hyperplasia. He found that the tumors developed from pluripotential testicular cells that, under ACTH stimulation and LH suppression, differentiated into ACTH-dependent cells that are similar to LCTs but function like adrenal cells.[94,95]

GENITOURINARY NEUROFIBROMATOSIS. This condition has been reported in only about 50 patients. Pelvic neurofibromatosis can produce urinary tract obstruction and can cause genital edema. Neurofibroma of the pelvis is thought to originate from the pelvic autonomic plexus. It can also involve the perineum, spermatic cord, and seminal vesicles. Direct involvement by neurofibromatosis can produce penile, scrotal, and labial enlargement.[96]

METASTATIC NEUROBLASTOMA. Metastatic neuroblastoma to the testis was found in only 3.8% of neuroblastoma patients in one series.[97] All had infradiaphragmatic primary tumors, and 82% had bone or bone marrow involvement. Yamashina reported the case of a 1-month-old boy born with a firm left intrascrotal mass.[98] Exploration through a scrotal incision revealed paratesticular neuroblastoma adherent to the scrotal wall.

EVALUATION OF SCROTAL MASSES IN CHILDREN

The differential diagnosis of intrascrotal masses in children must begin with consideration of torsion. When this condition is suspected, the next step is immediate exploration. A scrotal mass in a neonate is usually the curious variant of extravaginal torsion of the spermatic cord. The likely causes of intrascrotal enlargement in children are hydrocele and hernia. Trauma may produce a hematocele or may exacerbate a hernia or hydrocele. Varicoceles are often misconstrued as testicular tumors.

Careful history-taking and thorough physical examination generally suffice to define these entities. Physical examination of a child with intrascrotal enlargement is incomplete without determination of stage of sexual development and presence of gynecomastia.[99] Usually the testicle can be palpated through a hydrocele or hernia, but when this is not possible, ultrasonography can readily prove the testis to be normal. Management can then remain focused on the hydrocele or hernia. When gonadal enlargement, deformity, or induration indicate possible malignancy, there is little reason to defer further investigation with ultrasonography or surgical exploration. Before exploration, the usual tumor markers, alpha-fetoprotein and beta human chorionic gonadotropin (AFP and b-HCG), must be drawn.

Inguinal exploration offers the best approach to most intrascrotal disorders in children. When testicular tumor is among the differential diagnoses, the inguinal route is clearly preferred. The cord can be mobilized and the intrascrotal contents delivered en bloc. If testicular tumor is obvious, the entire gonad and spermatic cord below the internal inguinal ring are resected and the operative field is irrigated with sterile distilled water. If the diagnosis of tumor is not obvious, the gonad is isolated with sterile towels, much as described by Chevassu in 1910.[100] The tunica vaginalis is opened and any hydrocele fluid can be saved for cytologic study. When direct testicular exploration or biopsy is necessary, the spermatic vessels are cross-clamped and the use of iced saline slush prolongs safe testicular ischemia time as one waits for a frozen section analysis.[101] In any circumstance in which a gonad is explored, it should be palpated for induration and measured, and the morphology of testis and epididymis must be described. Appendages should be identified and removed if the testis is retained. Paratesticular tissues are inspected carefully and, if abnormal, a biopsy is performed. Extragonadal lesions are usually benign, and should be removed without jeopardy to the testis.

SUMMARY

Scrotal masses in children are occasionally caused by testicular tumors. Three quarters of these tumors are of germ cell origin. The most common is the yolk sac tumor. The primary treatment is a radical orchiectomy. Further treatment for disseminated disease should be tailored to accommodate the particular needs and limitations of the patient. Treatment should be guided by a team of physicians with representatives of pediatrics, oncology, and radiation therapy.

All solid scrotal masses should be considered malignant until proven otherwise. Control of the vascular and lymphatic channels prior to any intrascrotal manipulation is necessary and is best achieved through an inguinal approach. Once exposed, a mass can be safely examined, and a biopsy performed if necessary. Should the lesion prove benign, then excision may be possible with preservation of the testicle. Even if the lesion is malignant, cure is likely, but lifelong surveillance is necessary.

REFERENCES

1. Pathological Society of London. Meeting Minutes: Congenital sarcoma of testis. Lancet, *1*:662, 1885.
2. Pathological Society of London. Meeting Minutes: Dermoid cyst of testis. Lancet, *2*:774, 1886.
3. Silverberg, E., and Lubera, J. A. Cancer Statistics, 1988. Ca, *38*:5, 1988.
4. Brosman, S. A. Male genital tract. In: *Clinical Pediatric Urology.* 2nd Ed. Edited by P. P. Kelalis, L. R. King, and A. B. Belman. Philadelphia, W. B. Saunders Co., 1985.
5. Doyle, G. B. Embryonal carcinoma of testis in infant. Br. J. Urol., *27*:287, 1955.
6. Groot-Loonen, J. J., Voute, P. A., and deKraker, J. Testicular tumor concomitant with von Recklinghausen's disease. Med. Pediatr. Oncol., *16*:116, 1988.
7. Li, F. P., and Fraumeni, J. F., Jr. Testicular cancers in children: Epidemiologic characteristics. Natl. Cancer Inst. Bull., *48*:1575, 1972.
8. Sakashita, S. et al. Congenital anomalies in children with testicular germ cell tumor. J. Urol., *124*:889, 1980.
9. Green, D. M. The diagnosis and treatment of yolk sac tumors in infants and children. Cancer Treat. Rev., *10*:265, 1983.
10. Magner, D., and Bryant, A. J. S. Adenocarcinoma of testis occurring in infants: Report of 2 cases. Arch. Pathol., *52*:82, 1951.
11. Telium, G. Endodermal sinus tumors of the ovary and testis. Comparative morphogenesis of the so-called mesonephroma ovarii (Schiller) and extraembryonic (yolk-sac allantoic) structures of the rat's palcenta. Cancer, *12*:1092, 1959.
12. Mackinnon, A. E., and Cohen, S. J. Archenteronoma (yolk sac tumors). J. Pediatr. Surg., *13*:21, 1978.
13. Teoh, T. B., Steward, J. K., and Willis, R. A. The distinctive adenocarcinoma of the infant's testis: An account of 15 cases. J. Pathol. Bacteriol., *80*:147, 1960.
14. Mostofi, F. K., Davis, C. J., and Sesterhenn, I. A. The pathologist's view of testicular germ cell tumor management. AUA Update, *7*:18, 1988.
15. Talerman, A., Haije, W. G., and Baggerman, L. Serum alpha-fetoprotein (AFP) in patients with germ cells tumors of the gonads and extragonadal sites: Correlation between endodermal sinus (yolk sac) tumor and raised serum AFP. Cancer, *46*:380, 1980.
16. Manivel, J. C., Simonton, S., Wold, L. E., and Dehner, L. P. Absence of intratubular germ cell neoplasia in testicular yolk sac tumors in children. Arch. Pathol. Lab. Med., *112*:641, 1988.
17. Pierce, G. B., Bullock, W. K., and Huntington, R. W., Jr. Yolk sac tumors of the testis. Cancer, *25*:644, 1970.
18. Young, P. G., Mount, B. M., Foote, F. W., Jr., and Whitmore, W. F., Jr. Embryonal adenocarcinoma in the prepubertal testis. A clinicopathologic study of 18 cases. Cancer, *26*:1065, 1970.

19. MOSTOFI, F. K., and PRICE, E. B., Jr. Tumors of the male genital system. Atlas of Tumor Pathology, Second series, Fascicle 8. Washington, DC, Armed Forces Institute of Pathology, 1973.

20. SHIRAI, T., et al. Immunofluorescent demonstration of alpha-fetoprotein and other plasma proteins in yolk sac tumor. Cancer, 38:1661, 1976.

21. NARAYANA, A. S., LOENING, S., WEIMAR, G., and CULP, D. A. Serum markers in testicular tumors. J. Urol., 121:51, 1979.

22. GITLIN, D., PERRICELLI, A., and GITLIN, G. M. Synthesis of alpha-fetoprotein by liver, yolk sac, and gastrointestinal tract of the human conceptus. Cancer Res., 32:979, 1972.

23. MIZEJEWSKI, G. J., BELLISARIO, R., and CARTER, T. P. Birth weight and alpha-fetoprotein in the newborn (letter). Pediatrics, 73:736, 1984.

24. HOMSY, Y., ARROJO-VILA, F., KHORIATY, N., and DEMERS, J. Yolk sac tumor of the testicle: Is retroperitoneal lymph node dissection necessary? J. Urol., 132:532, 1984.

25. KRAMER, S. A., et al. Yolk sac carcinoma: An immunohistochemical and clinicopathologic review. J. Urol., 131:315, 1984.

26. MARSHALL, S., LYON, R. P., and SCOTT, M. P. A conservative approach to testicular tumors in children: 12 cases and their management. J. Urol., 129:350, 1983.

27. CARROLL, W. L., et al. Conservative management of testicular endodermal sinus tumors in childhood. J. Urol., 133:1011, 1985.

28. GRIFFIN, G. C., et al. Yolk sac carcinoma of the testis in children. J. Urol., 137:954, 1987.

29. FLAMANT, F., et al. Optimal treatment of clinical stage I yolk sac tumor of the testis in children. J. Pediatr. Surg., 21:108, 1986.

30. NELSON, R. P. Malignant testicular tumors in children. Urology, 10:290, 1977.

31. CROMIE, W. J., RANEY, R. B., Jr., and DUCKETT, J. W. Paratesticular rhabdomyosarcoma in children. J. Urol., 122:80, 1979.

32. LYNCH, J. H., and MAXTED, W. C. Use of ephedrine in postlymphadenectomy ejaculatory failure: A case report. J. Urol., 129:379, 1983.

33. MATSUMOTO, K., NAKAUCHI, K., and FUJITA, K. Radiation therapy for the embryonal carcinoma of testis in childhood. J. Urol., 104:778, 1970.

34. DRAGO, J. R., NELSON, R. P., and PALMER, J. M. Childhood embryonal carcinoma of testes. Urology, 12:499, 1978.

35. QUINTANA, J., et al. Infantile embryonal carcinoma of testis. J. Urol., 128:785, 1982.

36. MOSLI, H. A., CARPENTER, B., and SCHILLINGER, J. F. Teratoma of the testis in a pubertal child. J. Urol., 133:105, 1985.

37. RABINOVITCH, H. H. Simple innocuous treatment of massive cyclophosphamide hemorrhagic cystitis. Urology, 13:610, 1979.

38. HUNTINGTON, R. W., Jr., and BULLOCK, W. K. Yolk sac tumors of extragonadal origin. Cancer, 25:1368, 1970.

39. O'SULLIVAN, P., et al. Extragonadal endodermal sinus tumors in children: A review of 24 cases. Pediatr. Radiol., 13:249, 1983.

40. FRALEY, E. E., and KETCHAM, A. S. Teratoma of testis in an infant. J. Urol., 100:659, 1968.

41. ABELL, M. R., and HOLTZ, F. Testicular neoplasms in infants and children. I. Tumors of germ cell origin. Cancer, 16:965, 1963.

42. GIEBINK, G. S., and RUYMANN, F. B. Testicular tumors in childhood. Review and report of three cases. Am. J. Dis. Child., 127:433, 1974.

43. HOUSER, R., IZANT, R. J., Jr., and PERSKY, L. Testicular tumors in children. Am. J. Surg., 110:876, 1965.

44. CRUMP, W. D. Juvenile granulosa cell (sex cord-stroma) tumor of fetal testis. J. Urol., 129:1057, 1983.

45. KAPLAN, G. W., et al. Gonadal stromal tumors: A report of the prepubertal testicular tumor registry. J. Urol., 136:300, 1986.

46. COOK, C. D., GROSS, R. E., LANDING, B. H., and ZYGMUNTOWICZ, A. S. Interstitial cell tumor of the testis. Study of a 5-year-old boy with pseudoprecocious puberty. J. Clin. Endocrinol., 12:725, 1952.

47. GABRILOVE J. L., NICOLIS G. L., MITTY H. A., and SOHVAL, A. R. Feminizing interstitial cell tumor of the testis: Personal observations and review of the literature. Cancer, 35:1185, 1975.

48. JUNGCK, E. C., et al. Sexual precocity due to interstitial cell tumor of the testis: Report of 2 cases. J. Clin. Endocrinol., 17:291, 1957.

49. KIM, I., YOUNG, R. H., and SCULLY, R. E. Leydig cell tumors of the testis; a clinicopathological analysis of 40 cases and review of the literature. Am. J. Surg. Pathol., 9:177, 1985.

50. YUVAL, E., EIDELMAN, A., BEER, S. I., and VURE, E. Local excision of a virilizing Leydig-cell tumour of the testis. Br. J. Urol., 46:237, 1974.

51. SILVERBERG, S. G., THOMPSON, J. W., HIGASHI, G., and BASIN, A. M. Malignant interstitial cell tumor of the testis: Case report and review. J. Urol., 96:356, 1966.

52. WAXMAN, M., DAMJANOV, I., KHAPRA, A., and LANDAU, S. J. Large cell calcifying Sertoli tumor of the testis: Light microscopic and ultrastructural study. Cancer, 54:1574, 1984.

53. LAWRENCE, W. D., YOUNG, R. H., and SCULLY, R. E. Juvenile granulosa cell tumor of the infantile testis. Am. J. Surg. Pathol., 9:87, 1985.

54. UEHLING, D. T., SMITH, J. E., LOGAN, R., and GHOLOM-REZA, H. Newborn granulosa cell tumor of the testis. J. Urol., 138:385, 1987.

55. SCULLY, R. E. Gonadoblastoma. A review of 74 cases. Cancer, 25:1340, 1970.

56. BEHESHTI, M., et al. Neoplastic potential in patients with disorders of sexual differentiation. Urology 29:404, 1987.

57. ROSENKRANTZ, J. G., et al. Leukemic infiltration of the testis during long-term remission. J. Pediatr. Surg., 13:753, 1978.

58. STOFFEL, T. J., NESBIT, M. E., and LEVITT, S. H. Extramedullary involvement of the testes in childhood leukemia. Cancer, 35:1203, 1975.

59. SHEPARD, B. R., HENSLE, T. W., and MARBOE, C. C. Testicular biopsy and occult tumor in acute lymphocytic leukemia. Urology, 22:36, 1983.

60. PHILLIPS, G., KUMARI-SUBAIYA, S., and SAWITSHKI, A. Ultrasonic evaluation of the scrotum in lymphoproliferative disease. J. Ultrasound Med., 6:169, 1987.

61. SAIONTZ, H. I., et al. Testicular relapse in childhood leukemia. Mayo Clin. Proc., 53:212, 1978.

62. KIM, T. H., et al. Pretreatment testicular biopsy in childhood acute lymphocytic leukemia. Lancet, 2:657, 1981.

63. JUNAID, T. A. Testicular cancer in children and adolescents in Ibadan, Nigeria. Urology, 18:510, 1981.

64. HAYES, M. M., SACKS, M. I., and KING, H. S. Testicular lymphoma, a retrospective review of 17 cases. S. Afr. Med. J., 64:1014, 1983.

65. RANEY, R. B., Jr., et al. Paratesticular rhabdomyosarcoma in childhood. Cancer, 42:729, 1978.

66. OLNEY, L. E., et al. Intrascrotal rhabdomyosarcoma. Urology, 14:113, 1979.

67. LITTMANN, R., TESSLER, A. N., and VALENSI, Q. Paratesticular rhabdomyosarcoma: A case presentation and review of the literature. J. Urol., 108:290, 1972.

68. JOHNSON, D. E., McHUGH, T. A., and JAFFE, N. Paratesticular rhabdomyosarcoma in childhood. J. Urol., 128:1275, 1982.

69. OLIVE, D., et al. Para-aortic lymphadenectomy is not necessary in the treatment of localized paratesticular rhabdomyosarcoma. Cancer, 54:1283, 1984.

70. BAKER, W. C., BISHAI, M. B., and WHITE, R. W. D. Misleading testicular masses. Urology, *31*:111, 1988.

71. PRICE, E. B., Jr. Epidermoid cysts of the testis: A clinical and pathologic analysis of 69 cases from the testicular tumor registry. J. Urol., *102*:708, 1969.

72. BUCKSPAN, M. B., SKELDON, S. C., KLOTZ, P. G., and PRITZKER, K. P. H. Epidermoid cysts of the testicle. J. Urol., *134*:960, 1985.

73. COTTER, M., LAMPERT, I. A., and SALM, R. Epidermoid cysts of testis. Clin. Oncol., *10*:149, 1984.

74. MALEK, R. S., ROSEN, J. S., and FARROW, G. M. Epidermoid cyst of the testis: a critical analysis. Br. J. Urol., *58*:55, 1986.

75. BATES, R. J., PERRONE, T. L., and ALTHAUSEN, A. Simple epidermoid cysts of testis. Urology, *17*:560, 1981.

76. GILBAUGH, J. H., Jr., KELALIS, P. P., and DOCKERTY, M. B. Epidermoid cysts of the testis. J. Urol., *97*:876, 1967.

77. BLOOM, D. A., DIPIETRO, M. A., GIKAS, P. W., and McGUIRE, E. J. Extratesticular dermoid cyst and fibrous dysplasia of the epididymis. J. Urol., *137*:996, 1987.

78. FORD, J., Jr., and SINGH, S. Paratesticular dermoid cyst in 6-month-old infant. J. Urol., *139*:89, 1988.

79. GUPTA, S. K., GUPTA, S., and KHANNA, S. Dermoid cyst of scrotal raphe containing calculi. Br. J. Urol., *46*:348, 1974.

80. FRATER, K. Cysts of the tunica albuginea (cysts of the testis). J. Urol., *21*:135, 1929.

81. WARNER, K. E., NOYES, D. T., and ROSS, J. S. Cysts of the tunica albuginea testis: A report of 3 cases with a review of the literature. J. Urol., *132*:131, 1984.

82. FISHER, J. E., et al. Ectasia of the rete testis with ipsilateral renal agenesis. J. Urol., *128*:1040, 1982.

83. NISTAL, M., REGADERA, J., and PANIAGUA, R. Cystic dysplasia of the testis. Arch. Pathol. Lab. Med., *108*:579, 1984.

84. LONGO, V. J., and McDONALD, J. R. Primary neoplasms of the epididymis. J.A.M.A., *147*:937, 1951.

85. WERNERT, N., GOEBBELS, R., and PREDIGER, L. Papillary cystadenoma of the epididymis. Case report and review of the literature. Pathol. Res. Pract., *181*:260, 1986.

86. FRIEDMAN, A. P., HALLER, J. A., and GOODMAN, J. D. Sonography of scrotal masses in healed meconium peritonitis. Urol. Radiol., *5*:43, 1983.

87. MacMILLAN, R. W., MacDONALD, B. R., and ALPERN, H. D. Scrotal lymphangioma. Urology, *23*:79, 1984.

88. MERKA, S. T., BHATT, K. S., and WOOD, F. W. Cystic lymphangioma of the scrotum: A case report. J. Urol., *131*:1179, 1984.

89. KAUFMAN, D. G., et al. Benign scrotal tumors masquerading as expanding varicoceles. Urology, *29*:612, 1987.

90. SENOH H, et al. Cavernous hemangioma of scrotum and penile shaft. Urol. Int., *41*:309, 1986.

91. GOTOH, M., TSAI, S., and SUGIYAMA, T. Giant scrotal hemangioma with azoospermia. Urology, *22*:637, 1983.

92. WOLLIN, M., et al. Aberrant epididymal tissue: A significant clinical entity. J. Urol., *138*:1247, 1987.

93. ALGABA, F., SANTAULARIA, J. M., GARAT, J. M., and CUBELLS, J. Testicular pseudolymphoma. Eur. Urol., *12*:362, 1986.

94. FRANCO-SAENZ, R., et al. Cortisol production by testicular tumors in a patient with congenital adrenal hyperplasia (21-hydroxylase deficiency). J. Clin. Endocrinol. Metab., *53*:85, 1981.

95. RUTGERS, J. L., YOUNG, R. H., and SCULLY, R. E. The testicular "tumor" of the adrenogenital syndrome. A report of 6 cases and review of the literature on testicular masses in patients with adrenocortical disorders. Am. J. Surg. Pathol., *12*:503, 1988.

96. OGAWA, A., and WATANABE, K. Genitourinary neurofibromatosis in a child presenting with an enlarged penis and scrotum. J. Urol., *135*:755, 1986.

97. KUSHNER, B. H., VOGEL, R., and HAJDU, S. I. Metastatic neuroblastoma and testicular involvement. Cancer, *56*:1730, 1985.

98. YAMASHINA, M., KAYAN, H., and KATAYAMA, I. Congenital neuroblastoma presenting as a paratesticular tumor. J. Urol., *139*:796, 1988.

99. MARSHALL, W. A., and TANER, J. M. Variation in the pattern of pubertal change in boys. Arch. Dis. Child., *45*:13, 1970.

100. CHEVASSU, M. Le traitment chirurgical des cancers du testicule. Rev. Chir., *41*:620, 1910.

101. GOLDSTEIN, M., and WATERHOUSE, K. When to use the Chevassu maneuver during exploration of intrascrotal masses. J. Urol., *130*:1199, 1983.

Wilms' Tumor: Current Perspectives

Sakti Das
Arjan D. Amar

"So long as any child dies of this neoplasm or has its life impaired significantly by our therapeutic procedures, we have not achieved our ultimate goals."

J. BRUCE BECKWITH[31]

T he original description of Wilms' tumor has been credited to Rance[1] in 1814 and Wilms[2] in 1899, although the first known specimen featuring a bilateral tumor in a young child was prepared and displayed in the Royal College of Surgeons in London by the immortal John Hunter during the latter half of the 18th century.

Wilms' tumor (nephroblastoma) is an embryonal carcinoma of the kidney, representing the most common malignant neoplasm of the urinary system in children.[3] It is fifth in frequency among the childhood solid tumors. The annual incidence of Wilms' tumor in the United States is 7.8 per million children younger than age fifteen. It has no sexual, racial, or geographic predilection.

The spectacular improvement in the prognosis of Wilms' tumor is a testimony to the progress of the multimodal therapeutic approach in pediatric oncology that originated with Wilms' tumor. From a dismal 10 to 15% 2-year survival at the turn of the century,[4,5] to an approximately 90% 2-year survival at present, the signal achievements of modern combination therapy owe much to the ongoing intergroup cooperative studies conducted by the National Wilms' Tumor Study

(NWTS) in the USA,[6–8] the Medical Research Council in the UK,[9] and the International Society of Pediatric Oncology.[10,11]

PATHOLOGIC CONSIDERATIONS

These tumors are often large and encapsulated with a compressed shell of uninvolved renal tissue. The cut surface is soft and bulging with frequent areas of necrosis, focal hemorrhage, and variegated cystic spaces. Multiple small tumors may indicate nodular renal blastema, nephroblastomatosis complexes that are associated with Wilms' tumor in 44% cases.[12,13] Renal venous permeation, perinephric invasion, and lymph node metastases may be grossly evident. Wilms' tumor sometimes presents as polypoid masses in the renal pelvis or the ureter.

Microscopically, there is a protean admixture of blastemal, epithelial, and stromal cells. Blastemal cells are rounded or ovoid, with scanty cytoplasms arranged in a nodular or trabecular pattern. Intervening stromal elements frequently appear as skeletal muscles and rarely as cartilagenous, osteoid, fat, elastic, or lymphoid tissues. The epithelial components present as tubular and glomeruloid elements in various phases of nephrogenic differentiation.

Histopathologic reviews of the specimens in the initial NWTS identified four unfavorable characteristics that portend ominous prognosis. These are focal anaplasia, diffuse anaplasia, clear cell sarcoma, and rhabdoid sarcoma.[14] The NWTS-4 has eliminated rhabdoid sarcoma as a distinct tumor that can occur also at extrarenal sites. Clear cell sarcoma is still under scrutiny by NWTS-4.[15]

CLINICAL PRESENTATION AND DIAGNOSIS

The majority of Wilms' tumors present before age 7 years, with the mean age at diagnosis being 3½ years. Hereditary and bilateral cases occur earlier, at a mean of 2½ years of age.[16] Most commonly, the presenting symptom is an abdominal mass or an enlarging abdomen. The child is thriving and well, with occasional pyrexia, malaise, and anorexia. About one-third of the children complain of varying degrees of pain. Hypertension is found in 60% of patients. Gross hematuria is rare, but microhematuria is detected in about half of the patients. A smooth, firm, nontender mass is palpable unilaterally. In contrast to neuroblastoma, Wilms' tumor usually does not cross the midline.

Diagnostic imaging studies start with the standard excretory urography that reveals characteristic caliceal deformity and displacement by intrarenal mass. Peripheral curvilinear calcification secondary to hemorrhage is seen in 5 to 10% of the patients. The contralateral kidney is also evaluated for possible bilateral Wilms' tumor or associated pathologies. Nonvisualization of the affected kidney may be secondary to obstruction by ureteral or renal pelvic tumor, gross parenchymal replacement by the tumor, or renal venous and inferior vena caval permeation by tumor thrombus. We routinely carry out abdominal ultrasonography which, aside from showing the characteristic echogenecity of the tumor, helps determine the patency of the renal vein and the inferior vena cava. Inferior vena cavography is done when the ultrasonography reveals invasion or equivocal patency of the vena cava. The contralateral kidney, liver, and retroperitoneal lymph nodes are also evaluated by abdominal ultrasonography.

Computed tomography is extremely useful for better delineation of small tumors, evaluation of the contralateral kidney, retroperitoneal lymph nodes, vena caval, and contiguous spread. The utility and true potential of magnetic resonance imaging in the evaluation of Wilms' tumor is yet to be determined.

Arteriography is not necessary in the routine evaluation of Wilms' tumor except when the lesion is small and when diagnosis remains uncertain with other studies. In bilateral tumors, and in horse-shoe kidneys, angiographic knowledge of the arterial architecture is helpful before embarking on renal-sparing tumor excision.

Cystoscopy and retrograde study of the upper urinary tracts are indicated in the presence of hematuria or nonvisualization of the kidney on excretory urography. Presence of ureteral or pelvic tumors necessitate an en bloc nephroureterectomy.

GENETIC CONSIDERATIONS AND ASSOCIATED ANOMALIES

Pathogenesis of Wilms' tumor is based upon a variety of ill-defined heterogeneous elements. Possible chromosomal factors account for the heritable and nonheritable forms. Knudson and Strong suggested a two-stage mutation with the first occurring at prezygotic level and the second mutation resulting in the tumor formation of the target tissue.[17] Heritable tumors often occur at an earlier age and are more likely to be multicentric and bilateral.

Congenital anomalies most commonly associated with Wilms' tumor are aniridia, hemihypertrophy, and genitourinary malformations.[18]

Hemihypertrophy is found in 3% of the patients with Wilms' tumor.[19,20] Hamartomatous lesions like hemangioma, pigmented naevi, and neurofibromatosis also occur more frequently than in the general population.[21] About 33% of the patients with sporadic aniridia develop Wilms' tumor.[22] Earlier age incidence and bilateral Wilms' tumors are observed more often in patients with sporadic aniridia. About one-third of the patients with sporadic aniridia and Wilms' tumor have a common chromosomal anomaly in the form of 11p interstitial deletion suggesting the hypothesis of heritable mutation.[23] However, the fact that all patients with a similar chromosomal defect do not develop Wilms' tumor remains unexplained.

Recent chromosomal and biochemical studies also implicate elevated levels of insulin-like growth factor (IGF) in Wilms' tumor tissue.[24,25] The gene for IGF-II is located in the vicinity of chromosome 11p13. As a known embryonal mutagen, IGF-II may have a significant, although yet unravelled, etiologic role in the genesis of Wilms' tumor.

STAGING OF WILMS' TUMOR

The clinicopathologic staging system devised by the NWTS group is based on the combination of intraoperative findings and histopathologic examination. The stage of the disease implies the extent of the gross and microscopic tumor. Each tumor should be further designated as favorable or unfavorable histology, based on its histologic features.

STAGE I. The tumor is limited by an intact renal capsule and is completely removed without rupture or spillage. There is no residual tumor beyond the margin of excision.

STAGE II. The tumor extends beyond the capsule or there is vascular permeation outside the kidney, or it has been biopsied with local spillage. But, the tumor is completely excised with no residual tumor at the margins of excision.

STAGE III. There is residual tumor confined to the abdomen. There may be metastatic retroperitoneal lymph nodes, or diffused peritoneal spillage by a rupture or peritoneal implants, or an unresectable tumor.

STAGE IV. Tumor with hematogenous metastases.

STAGE V. Bilateral Wilms' tumor.

SURGICAL INTERVENTION

The role of surgery in the management of Wilms' tumor is the extirpation of the neoplasm as far as possible and accurate staging for further therapeutic considerations. At the same time, surgical conservatism aimed at preserving nephrons is prudent because of the available effective anticancer therapy. The child is placed supine with the back hyperextended and the affected side slightly elevated on soft rolls. A transverse transperitoneal incision is made from the tip of the twelfth rib to across the opposite rectus abdominis muscle in the epigastrium. The liver, retroperitoneal and hilar lymph nodes, and vena cava are carefully assessed by inspection and palpation. The contralateral kidney is approached by medial mobilization of the colon. The Gerota's fascia is opened widely and the kidney is thoroughly exposed so that both surfaces of the entire kidney can be examined and biopsied as necessary.

The affected kidney with the tumor is then approached by reflection of the colon. The renal artery and vein should be sequentially ligated prior to mobilization of the kidney. Radical nephrectomy is then performed. Renal mobilization should be careful and gentle to prevent rupture of the tumor. Rupture and spillage of tumor advances the stage of tumor and necessitates abdominal irradiation. We usually preserve the adrenal gland when the upper pole of the kidney is uninvolved with tumor. Regional lymphadenectomy is carried out removing the lymph nodal tissue around the ipsilateral great vessel and the renal hilar region using the technique described in Chapter 4. Any other suspicious retroperitoneal lymph nodal mass is also removed. The tumor may extend to the mesocolon, diaphragm, psoas muscle, or adjacent viscera. En bloc removal of these contiguous areas of spread with the tumor allows primary extirpation of the lesion. However, overzealous resection of the involved viscera, because of its attendant morbidity, is not recommended. Chemotherapy and radiation therapy shrinks the tumor appreciably and residual tumors can be removed more easily at subsequent exploration. All the areas of residual disease are marked with metal hemaclips to aid radiotherapy field planning. Involvement of major renal vein and vena cava are dealt with in the same manner as described in Chapter 8.

The majority of children with Wilms' tumor can now be cured with appropriate modern anticancer therapy. Ultimate prognosis depends on the stage, histopathology, and the type of multimodal therapy instituted. Because of the continued improved survival of over 80% of patients surviving at 4 years from diagnosis, NWTS is currently investigating protocols to see whether reduced therapy can be sufficient to control the disease. Chemotherapy and radiotherapy protocol against Wilms' tumor are detailed in Chapter 51.

BILATERAL WILMS' TUMOR

The reported frequency of synchronous bilateral Wilms' tumor is 4.4%. The review by Blute and associates of the 145 patients with bilateral disease entered in the NWTS registry, focuses on several important issues and recommendations.[26] It is disconcerting that despite advancement in our diagnostic acumen in about one-third of the patients the bilateral lesion was ascertained by intraoperative exploration and not diagnosed preoperatively.[27] Therefore, in every Wilms' tumor patient it is mandatory to thoroughly explore the contralateral kidney before approaching the obviously affected site.

Interesting pathologic features are the multicentricity of the tumors and the association of nephroblastomatosis in the majority of cases. Despite the large volume of disease present, 67% of the patients had only stage-I disease and unfavorable histology was evident in only 10%. The overall 3-year survival of these patients was 76%.[26] Improved prognostic factors include lower stage of disease, favorable histology, and negative lymph nodal status. Metachronous bilateral tumors are rare and probably represent a second primary involvement rather than a metastatic involvement. The prognosis is poor, with about 39% surviving 2 to 4 years following diagnosis of the second tumor.[28]

The therapeutic objective in bilateral Wilms' tumor is to maximally preserve the functional renal tissue through sequential excisions, as necessary, following effective chemotherapy and radiation therapy. Both kidneys should be widely exposed and multiple representative biopsies of the tumor and lymph nodes should be obtained to determine the stage and histology. Complete excision is to be attempted only if at least two-thirds of renal tissue can be preserved. Chemotherapy is administered postoperatively. Repeat exploration is done within 6 months and partial nephrectomy is carried out if all tumors can be excised. Otherwise, repeat biopsy and further chemotherapy is continued and radiation therapy is considered. A third-look exploration is done within 6 months from the last surgery. Surgical options at this time include bilateral partial nephrectomy, unilateral nephrectomy with contralateral partial nephrectomy or biopsy, bilateral biopsies only, and bilateral nephrectomy with eventual transplantation. Patients with unfavorable histology in one or both sides have an ominous prognosis. Following initial biopsy, triple drug chemotherapy with Actinomycin D, Vincristine, and Doxorubicin is continued for 15 months and combined with radiation to one or both flanks. More aggressive excision is carried out at second-look exploration with nephrectomy or bilateral nephrectomy considered in patients whose tumors are not irradicated by the adjuvant measures.

CONCLUSION

The saga of Wilms' tumor continues to be punctuated by jubilant cries of triumph, moanful pangs of defeat, and perennial gleams of hope. The National Wilms' Tumor Study is endeavoring to reduce the morbidity of therapy by further minimizing chemotherapy and radiation therapy in the favorable histology groups. Conversely, patients with unfavorable histology are being treated vigorously in an effort to salvage their poor prognosis. Prognostic parameters such as flow cytometric analysis of nuclear DNA ploidy are being evaluated to select patients who would benefit from a more curtailed regimen or who may need more aggressive therapy.[29] The advanced imaging systems should enable us to make specific and correct preoperative diagnosis and staging. Development of Wilms' tumor markers and other immunologic techniques that would aid in earlier diagnosis and monitoring of treatment efficacy are on the horizon.[30] In the field of surgery, more conservative renal-sparing surgery should be feasible in unilateral disease, especially in combination with effective adjuvant therapies. The sinister prognosis of lymphatic spread remains a concern and whether extensive lymphadenectomy will encompass the metastatic disease or better stage them for further therapy is being evaluated. The treatment of Wilms' tumor has proven to be a legend of success of human ingenuity and cooperative efforts, and with perseverance and scientific vigil, the prognostic future of the children afflicted with Wilms' tumor will continue to improve.

REFERENCES

1. RANCE, T. F. Case of fungus hematodes of the kidneys. Med. Phys., *32:*19, 1814.

2. WILMS, M. Die Mischgeschwuelste der Niere. Leipzig: A. Georgi, 1899.

3. YOUNG, J. L., JR., and MILLER, R. W. Incidence of malignant tumors in U.S. children. Pediatr., *86:*254, 1975.

4. WHITE, W. C. Wilms' mixed tumor of the kidney. Ann. Surg., *9:*139, 1936.

5. PRIESTLEY, J. F., and SCHULTE, T. L. The treatment of Wilms' tumor. J. Urol., *47:*7, 1942.

6. D'ANGIO, G. J., et al. The treatment of Wilms' tumor: Results of the Third National Wilms' Tumor Study. Cancer, *38:*633, 1976.

7. D'ANGIO, G. J., et al. The treatment of Wilms' tumor: Results of the second National Wilms' Tumor Study. Cancer, *47:*2302, 1981.

8. D'ANGIO, G. J., et al. Results of the National Wilms' Tumor Study. Proc. Am. Assoc. Cancer Res., *25:*183, 1984.

9. Medical Research Council's Working Party on Embryonal Tumours in Childhood. Management of nephroblastoma in childhood: Clinical study of two forms of maintenance chemotherapy. Arch. Dis. Child., *53:*112, 1978.

10. LEMERLE, J., et al. Preoperative versus postoperative radiotherapy, single versus multiple courses of Actinomycin D in the treatment of Wilms' tumor. Preliminary results of a controlled clinical trial conducted by the International Society of Pediatric Oncology (SIOP). Cancer, *38:*647, 1976.

11. LEMERLE, J., et al. Effectiveness of preoperative chemotherapy in Wilms' tumor: Results of an International Society of Pediatric Oncology (SIOP) clinical trial. J. Clin. Oncol., *1:*604, 1983.

12. BOVE, K. E., and McADAMS, A. J. The nephroblastomatosis complex and relationship to Wilms' tumor: A clinico-pathologic treatise. Perspect. Pediatr. Pathol., *3:*185, 1976.

13. MACHIN, G. A. Persistent renal blastema (nephroblastomatosis) as a frequent precursor of Wilms' tumor: A pathological and clinical review. Part 3: Clinical aspects of nephroblastomatosis. Am. J. Pediatr. Hematol. Oncol., *2:*353, 1980.

14. BECKWITH, J. B., and PALMER, N. F. Histopathology and prognosis of Wilms' tumor: Results from the first National Wilms' Tumor Study. Cancer, *41:*1937, 1978.

15. National Wilms' Tumor Study-4. Therapeutic Trial Protocol, July 7, 1986.

16. BRESLOW, N. E., and BECKWITH, J. B. Epidemiological features of Wilms' tumor: Results of the National Wilms' Tumor Study. J. Natl. Cancer Inst., *68:*429, 1982.

17. KNUDSON, A. G., JR., and STRONG, L. C. Mutation and cancer: A model for Wilms' tumor of the kidney. J. Natl. Cancer Inst., *48:*313, 1972.

18. KRAMER, S. A., and KELALIS, P. P. Wilms' tumor 1984. AUA Update Series, Volume III, Lesson 18, 1984.

19. MAURER, H. S., et al. The role of genetic factors in the etiology of Wilms' tumor: Two pairs of monozygous twins with congenital abnormalities (aniridia; hemihypertrophy) and discordance for Wilms' tumor. Cancer, *43:*205, 1979.

20. JANIK, S. S., and SEELER, R. A. Delayed onset of hemihypertrophy in Wilms' tumor. J. Pediatr. Surg., *11:*581, 1976.

21. MEADOWS, A. T., and JARRETT, P. Pigmented nevi, Wilms' tumor and second malignant neoplasms. J. Pediatr., *93:*889, 1978.

22. BRODEUR, G. M. Genetic and cytogenetic aspects of Wilms' tumor. In: *Wilms' Tumor: Clinical and Biological Manifestations.* Edited by C. Pochedly and E. S. Baum. New York, Elsevier Science Publishing Co., 1984, pp. 125–145.

23. RICCARDI, V. M., et al. The aniridia-Wilms' tumor association: The critical role of chromosome band 11p13. Cancer Genet. Cytogenet., *2:*131, 1980.

24. REEVE, A. E., et al. Expression of insulin-like growth factor II transcripts in Wilms' tumor. Nature, *317:*258, 1985.

25. SCOTT, J., et al. Insulin-like growth factor II gene expression in Wilms' tumor and embryonic tissues. Nature, *317:*260, 1985.

26. BLUTE, M. L., et al. Bilateral Wilms' tumor. J. Urol., *138:*968, 1987.

27. MESROBIAN, H. J. Wilms' tumor: Past, present, future. J. Urol., *140:*231, 1988.

28. JONES, B., et al. Metachronous bilateral Wilms' tumor. National Wilms' Tumor Study. Amer. J. Clin. Oncol., *5:*545, 1982.

29. RAINWATER, L. M., et al. Wilms tumors: Relationship of nuclear deoxyribonucleic acid ploidy to patient survival. J. Urol., *138:*974, 1987.

30. MOSS, T. J., and SEEGER, R. C. Immunology of Wilms' tumor: Its possible use in diagnosis and treatment. In: *Wilms' Tumor: Clinical and Biological Manifestations.* Edited by C. Pochedly and E. S. Baum. New York, Elsevier Science Publishing Co., 1984, pp. 83.

31. BECKWITH, J. B. Wilms' tumor and other renal tumors of childhood: An update. J. Urol., *136:*320, 1986.

CHAPTER
44

Management of Genitourinary Rhabdomyosarcoma in Children

Edmond T. Gonzales, Jr.

Rhabdomyosarcoma is the third most common solid malignant tumor in childhood (seen only slightly less often than Wilms' tumor and neuroblastoma) and is the most common soft-tissue sarcoma. This tumor ranks seventh as a cause of death from cancer in childhood.[1] Although these neoplasms can occur almost anywhere, nearly 20% arise within the true pelvis, primarily from the bladder, prostate, or vagina. In some instances, the tumor can only be classified as arising from an unspecified pelvic or retroperitoneal site. In advanced cases, it may not be possible to define an exact site of origin, because these tumors tend to be locally aggressive and to readily invade adjacent viscera. A smaller percentage of these tumors occur in the spermatic cord, usually in the immediate paratesticular area. Rhabdomyosarcomas occur at any age, although there are peaks in young childhood (2 to 6 years) and adolescence. Paratesticular lesions occur relatively more often in the older age groups.

HISTOLOGIC CHARACTERISTICS AND GROWTH PATTERNS

Rhabdomyosarcomas are thought to arise from embryonic mesenchyme and, when they occur in the genitourinary region, their propensity for developing in the prostate, trigone, vagina, and immediate paratesticular areas suggests that they originate from cells of the urogenital sinus or mesenchymal tissue of the mesonephros.[2,3] Three histologic patterns of rhabdomyosarcoma are classically recognized: (1) embryonal, a pattern seen most commonly in young children; (2) alveolar, described most often in the adolescent and generally in tumors presenting in the extremity; and (3) pleomorphic rhabdomyosarcoma, typical in adults.

The embryonal form of rhabdomyosarcoma is typical of the histologic findings from tumors arising in the pelvic region. Embryonal rhabdomyosarcoma is characterized by a primitive mesenchyme with differentiation of some of the cellular elements to the embryonal rhabdomyoblast. The rhabdomyoblast assumes several different histologic characteristics but, if sufficiently differentiated, may form cross striations (a finding seen in about one-third of cases). A significant component of mixoid cells is also commonly present.[4] Sarcoma botryoides is a term used to describe the large, bulky intraluminal polypoid masses typical of rhabdomyosarcoma of the bladder and vagina. Once thought to represent a separate category, these neoplasms also show a histologically typical embryonal pattern.

More recently, attempts have been made to classify rhabdomyosarcomas based on other cytologic characteristics. Palmer and Foulkes[5] reviewed the pathologic material from the Intergroup Rhabdomyosarcoma Study and proposed that these tumors could be classified as monomorphous, anaplastic, and mixed. In the monomorphous variety, the cells are uniform in size with constant nuclear characteristics throughout the tumor. This particular variety of rhabdomyosarcoma has an unfavorable prognosis. In the anaplastic variety, there are many bizarre and enlarged mitotic figures that also indicate an unfavorable prognosis. Both of these varieties represent only about 5% of the total population of tumors studied. The mixed variety represents nearly 80% of all tumors in the IRS study group and bodes a more favorable prognosis. Similarly, Tsokos and Triche[6] described a solid variant of rhabdomyosarcoma. Once again, this histologic description was associated with a less favorable prognosis.

Hawkins and Camacho-Valasquez studied 47 rhabdomyosarcomas from all sites and classified the tumors as either anaplastic or well differentiated.[7] Distinction was not made between embryonal, alveolar, or pleomorphic varieties. This simpler histologic classification correlated well with ultimate survival—patients with the anaplastic tumors did much worse than those whose tumors were well differentiated.

Growth patterns of rhabdomyosarcoma are somewhat predictable. Lesions of the bladder and vagina tend to spread beneath the mucosa and are seen initially as clusters of intraluminal masses. Distant metastases are infrequent at the time of presentation. Tumors arising within the prostate or from nonvisceral undetermined pelvic sites tend to spread directly along fascial planes and to disseminate earlier by both hematogenous and lymphatic routes.[8] Although the tumors often appear encapsulated, infiltration of malignant cells extends to and beyond the margin of the pseudocapsule. Raney and associates[9] studied the sites of origin for these tumors and correlated the sites with ultimate prognosis. This study demonstrated that tumors of the bladder, the prostate, and vagina had a better prognosis than tumors arising from a nonvisceral pelvic wall location. They suggested in this study that this may simply be because the lesions that are easily seen (vaginal introitus tumors), or the lesions that are likely to cause urinary obstruction (bladder and prostate), are diagnosed earlier in the course of the disease than are the deeper pelvic lesions.

Most children initially present with symptoms secondary to local growth: a palpable suprapubic mass, a visible tumor at the vaginal introitus, or obstruction to urinary outflow.

Paratesticular neoplasms are recognized as solid, nontender scrotal masses. Because of local invasion, the testis may be indistinguishable from the mass. Retroperitoneal lymphatic spread can be expected to be present in one-third of patients at the time of presentation.

TREATMENT: GENERAL CONSIDERATIONS

The treatment of rhabdomyosarcoma remains one of the more controversial topics in pediatric oncology. Until fairly recently, radical wide surgical excision was the only effective form of management for these tumors. As late as 1972, early radical extirpation was recommended for management of pelvic rhabdomyosarcoma.[3] Limited or less aggressive surgical procedures were universally associated with local recurrences.

Chemotherapy

Prior to 1966, the use of chemotherapy in this disease was limited to individual agents used in the treatment of metastases.[10–13] Responses were reported in up to 83% of cases, but these were usually of short duration. In 1966, James and associates first reported improved objective responses in one-third of patients treated with a combination of actinomycin D and vincristine.[14] In 1969, Grosfeld and colleagues also combined these agents, but used them in repeated courses, with prolonged survival in 12 of 18 patients.[15]

Shortly thereafter, several groups reported the use of a combined multidisciplinary approach to embryonal rhabdomyosarcoma and introduced the concept of "reasonable" surgical treatment for this neoplasm: wide excision of the primary tumor, but without gross sacrifice of form or function.[16–22] At the same time, Heyn reported on a prospective, controlled, randomized study of 28 patients whose tumors had been completely resected or who had only microscopic residual tumors; 86% of the patients were free of disease after 2 years when treated on a multidisciplinary protocol of surgery, radiotherapy, and combination chemotherapy (actinomycin D and vincristine)—a dramatic improvement in survival for this disease.[23] A follow-up report of the original 28 children who achieved a complete response demonstrated that 24 (85.7%) remained disease free for at least 3 years.[24]

Chemotherapeutic regimens have varied, and one should refer to the references given at the end of this chapter for dosage, schedules, and length of treatment. Most protocols have included both vincristine and actinomycin D[20] or these two agents in addition to cyclophosphamide and adriamycin.[25–27] Exelby has suggested an aggressive, seven-agent chemotherapeutic regimen that includes actinomycin D, cyclophosphamide, bleomycin, vincristine, adriamycin, methotrexate, and BCNU (carmustine).[28]

Radiotherapy

Concurrent with the development of effective chemotherapy was the observation of the benefit of radiotherapy for local control of these tumors, which extended the concept of a truly multidisciplinary approach to these lesions.[29] Dritschilo and associates have recently reported that local control of the primary tumor from a variety of sites was achieved in 96% of patients who received radiotherapy, although the majority also received chemotherapy.[30] Radiotherapy has become primary therapy for the local lesion of rhabdomyosarcoma of the orbit, head, and neck.[25] Dosage at a level of 5000 to 6000 rads is generally recommended.

INTERGROUP RHABDOMYOSARCOMA STUDY

The Intergroup Rhabdomyosarcoma Study (IRS) was organized in 1972 to evaluate various combinations of surgery, chemotherapy, and radiotherapy. In 1977 they published a most encouraging report.[26] In this study, all patients underwent excision of the primary tumor (or biopsy if the neoplasm was unresectable or involved a vital structure) and were grouped according to the following classification:

Stage I   Localized disease, completely resected

Stage II   Localized disease, microscopic residual tumor

     IIA.   Grossly resected tumor, microscopic residual tumor, no nodal involvement

     IIB.   Regional nodal disease, completely resected, no microscopic residual tumor

     IIC.   Regional nodal disease, grossly resected, but with evidence of microscopic residual tumor

Stage III   Incomplete resection or biopsy with gross residual regional disease

Stage IV   Distant metastases present at time of diagnosis

Children with stage-I disease received a combination of vincristine, actinomycin D, and cyclophosphamide (VAC), and were randomized for radiation therapy. Control was achieved in 92% of patients. The addition of radiotherapy did not improve this response.

Patients in all other stages of disease were given both chemotherapy and radiotherapy, although chemotherapeutic protocols varied. Clinical response rates of 85% for stage-II patients and approximately 50% for stages-III and -IV patients were achieved. Of particular interest is the observation that, in stage-II patients, VAC was not more effective than vincristine and actinomycin D alone.

Unfortunately, more recent reports have not shown improved response with an intensified chemotherapeutic program for the initially more advanced disease.[25,27] In addition, the possibility and incidence of late recurrence remains unknown, and children who remain disease free for as long as 7 years have returned with locally recurrent rhabdomyosarcoma.[3,28]

RHABDOMYOSARCOMA OF THE PELVIS

The treatment of rhabdomyosarcoma of the pelvis is generally considered to be a single entity, although significant differences exist between tumors in this general location depending on the site of origin. In addition, preliminary data gathered by the IRS suggests that genitourinary tumors may have more favorable prognoses than primary tumors in the extremities or in the region of the head and neck.[27]

Because of the high incidence of local recurrence after limited surgical excision, survival was rare before current concepts of therapy were established.[31] With the introduction of more radical surgical procedures (anterior or total exenteration), improved survival was obtained with bladder and vaginal tumors,[3,28,32,33] but remained dismal for primary prostatic tumors.[34] Not until the introduction of planned multidisciplinary therapy has significant improvement in survival been realized for all forms of pelvic rhabdomyosarcoma.

With improving survival and the appreciation of the effectiveness of combined, cyclic, long-term chemotherapy, as well as the recognition of the serious and morbid effects of radical surgical procedures or radiotherapy for treatment of pelvic tumors in children, surgeons and medical oncologists began to re-evaluate the primary thrust of management of these lesions. In 1975, Rivard suggested intensive chemotherapy as a primary method of management of pelvic rhabdomyosarcoma, and demonstrated reduction in primary tumor bulk with this approach, allowing more limited surgical intervention than originally planned in nine patients.[35] Belman and Baum also described a similar, although smaller, series in support of this concept.[36] The original series of Rivard was updated by Ortega.[37] Thirteen patients were included in this series. Five children had died, although three of these had metastatic disease at the time of presentation and would not have been candidates for radical surgical treatment. Only one child failed to respond to chemotherapy and required an early radical surgical procedure. Eight patients were alive without evident disease at the time of the report, although all but one also had an operation or radiation therapy as well. However, it was the authors' opinion then that less surgical intervention was required after chemotherapy than would originally have been necessary without it; and for the group as a whole, only two urinary diversions were necessary.

Other authors have observed the benefits of initial chemotherapy in the reduction of both tumor bulk and the extent of surgery, as well as in improving the quality of life for these children.[8,38] The IRS has recognized this special consideration for primary pelvic tumors and has established a subgroup within the protocol to evaluate chemotherapy as the primary and only therapy in initially resectable pelvic tumors.

Since the development of the Intergroup Rhabdomyosarcoma Study, several investigators have assessed their results in an effort to better define the appropriate relationship between chemotherapy, surgery, and radiotherapy in order to maximize survival. In 1982, Hays and associates reported the initial data from IRS-1 in 64 children with primary bladder or prostatic tumors.[39] Most of the patients underwent some initial surgical procedure followed by chemotherapy and radiotherapy, depending on the clinical group as outlined by the IRS. Fifty-three children presented without clinical evidence of metastases. Thirty-seven of these had initial surgery followed by chemotherapy or radiotherapy, and 16 were begun on a primary chemotherapy and radiotherapy program. The number of children in each treatment group and their incidence of recurrence is listed below:

INITIAL TREATMENT PROGRAM	NUMBER OF PATIENTS	RECURRENCE
Primary Bladder Tumor		
Exenteration	11	2
Partial Cystectomy	12	5
Chemo/Rad Rx	5	3
Prostatic Tumors		
Exenteration	14	0
Chemo/Rad Rx	11	2

In this initial report from the IRS, those children managed initially by aggressive surgery fared best. The authors concluded that pelvic exenteration, when combined with local radiotherapy and appropriate chemotherapy, results in a high rate of survival and contrasts sharply with the dismal survival statistics before multidisciplinary management. They expressed concern, however, that this report had not decreased the mutilative aspect of surgery of pelvic rhabdomyosarcoma and proposed a trial of more intensive primary nonsurgical efforts with frequent biopsies. Surgical excision would be reserved for incomplete responses or recurrence.

Hays et al. subsequently reported on 29 children with bladder or prostatic primaries treated initially with chemotherapy alone in an effort to preserve pelvic organ function ("Pulse VAC" at first; addition of adriamycin when response was inadequate).[40] Radiotherapy and limited surgery were included when clinical response was incomplete or in cases of recurrence. In this series, 38% of the total group of children maintained satisfactory bladder function, although only 2 of the 29 achieved this on chemotherapy only. The mortality rate was 27%. This mortality figure contrasts with a mortality of 5% in IRS-1 in children treated by exenteration (most often anterior exenteration only).

Scholtmeyer et al. reviewed 16 children (10 boys and 6 girls) with genitourinary rhabdomyosarcoma and reported a 60% overall survival.[41] However, in each case, surgical management was necessary to achieve a disease-free state. Fleming and associates presented a most encouraging report from the St. Jude Children's Research Hospital.[42] Twenty-two children were seen with genitourinary rhabdomyosarcomas (10 vaginal and 12 bladder or prostate) in the pelvis. One patient with a vaginal primary refused surgery and subsequently died despite chemotherapy and radiotherapy. The other 9 children with vaginal lesions had preoperative chemotherapy (and subsequent radiotherapy if tumor response was felt to be inadequate) followed by surgical excision in all. Eight of these children are free of disease: 7 after hysterovaginectomy only and 1 after anterior exenteration; 1 had active residual disease after surgery. Twelve children had bladder or prostate lesions. In 11 cases, preoperative chemotherapy and radiotherapy was used.

Five of these children have functioning bladders without evidence of disease. Six have active disease or are dead.

Ghavimi and associates reported on their experience with 27 patients at Memorial Sloan Kettering Cancer Center.[43] A combination of surgeries, chemotherapy, and radiotherapy were used. Eighteen patients were alive and well at the time of the report, and nine of these had a functional bladder. Primary chemotherapy failed to achieve satisfactory control of these tumors in the majority (only 2 of 27). They demonstrated that extirpative surgery followed by chemotherapy in their program gave the best overall results.

Broecker and colleagues reported the results of management for pelvic rhabdomyosarcoma from the Great Ormond Street Hospital in London.[44] From a population of 20 children, there was a survival rate of 55% and bladder salvage in half of these. Once again, their conclusion was that complete surgical resection of the tumor combined with chemotherapy and radiotherapy offers the highest chance of cure.

Green summarized the results of the three Intergroup Rhabdomyosarcoma Studies in 1987.[45] The conclusions were:

1. Aggressive, combination chemotherapy is indicated as initial therapy.
2. Patients must be followed carefully at this stage because of a high incidence of progressive disease development despite chemotherapy. Complete response to chemotherapy only is unusual.
3. After a partial response (at 6 weeks post initial therapy), consideration is given to either surgical management or radiotherapy, depending on the extent of residual disease. If total excision is possible (especially if this can be accomplished with organ salvage, i.e., partial cystectomy), surgery would be chosen rather than radiotherapy.
4. Radiotherapy may not be necessary if margins after resection are completely clear of tumor.
5. Chemotherapy must be continued postoperatively.

Other factors that correlate with survival rates are site of origin of the tumor and histologic differentiation. Raney and associates compared survival of children with bladder and prostate tumors (n = 8) with those who had a pelvic tumor arising separate from the bladder (n = 8).[9] In those patients with a bladder or prostate lesion, the tumors were smaller at presentation, showed more histologic differentiation, and demonstrated fewer distant metastases. At the time of their report, 6 of the 8 patients having either a bladder or prostate tumor were alive and thought to be free of disease; only 3 of 8 patients with primary pelvic tumors were alive and only one was apparently tumor free. The authors felt that although there were many factors that might have influenced survival, the most important seemed to be that bladder or prostate tumors caused urinary symptoms early and were picked up sooner than pure pelvic lesions.

Hawkins and Camacho-Velasquez correlated the degree of cellular anaplasia with survival in 47 cases of rhabdomyosarcoma from numerous sites.[7] Fourteen cases were felt to be anaplastic and 12 of these died. Only 10 of those 33 patients with well-differentiated tumors died.

Ragab and colleagues assessed the significance of age in the prognosis for rhabdomyosarcoma 78 [5%] of 1561 patients in the IRS as of May, 1983 were younger than 1 year of age.[46] Except for a slightly greater incidence of undifferentiated histology in the infant group (18% versus 7%), the other demographic factors did not differ significantly between the two groups. There was a somewhat higher rate of bladder/prostate/vagina primary site in the infants as compared to older children (24% versus 10%). Infants also developed more toxicity to treatment. However, overall survival was no different for the two groups. As compared to Wilms' tumor and neuroblastoma, where younger patients have a more favorable prognosis, age does not affect the prognosis of those with rhabdomyosarcoma.

It is clear after analyzing these many reports that survival is best with a combination of aggressive multimodel therapy; that chemotherapy alone is only rarely successful in completely controlling the majority of tumors, although some partial response can be expected in most; that local excision may be possible with organ preservation and that this is best assessed after a short course of intensive chemotherapy; and that radiotherapy is effective and essential if residual tumor is left behind.

The principles of management I prefer, as outlined here, are based on the observations discussed above and parallel the protocol and recommendations of the IRS. It must be emphasized, however, that controversy exists, especially regarding the timing of the surgical procedure and radiotherapy, and that the surgeon must carefully and thoughtfully consider each patient individually in regard to the location and size of the tumor and the consequences of radical surgical intervention, radiotherapy, or extensive chemotherapy.

The initial surgical treatment for suspected pelvic rhabdomyosarcoma should be limited: transurethral resection for biopsy of vesical or prostatic lesions, and direct biopsy for intraluminal vaginal lesions. It should be stressed that these polypoid neoplasms (sarcoma botryoides) often have considerable edematous mucosa overlying the submucosal tumor, and deep, "fleshy" biopsies must be obtained.

A few cases of rhabdomyosarcoma are not accessible for endoscopic biopsy and are best biopsied via an open surgical approach. At this time, dissection should be limited, and only as much tumor should be excised as can be safely removed without sacrifice of any vital organ, e.g., the bladder, genital system, or rectum. Rarely, a lesion in this area may not involve any viscera, and the biopsy may result in total removal of all grossly identifiable tumor.

After diagnosis is confirmed, chemotherapy is instituted. Protocols vary, as noted previously, but should initially include at least vincristine and actinomycin D. I prefer a more intensive program, as outlined by Ortega,[37] or that described by the IRS as "pulse-VAC." The chemotherapy is administered in short, intensive doses every 28 days and includes the following:

1. Vincristine, 2 mg/m^2 intravenously on Days 0 and 4 (maximum single dose, 2 mg)
2. Actinomycin D, 0.015 mg/kg/day intravenously for 5 days beginning on Day 0 (maximum single dose, 0.5 mg)
3. Cyclophosphamide, 10 mg/kg/day intravenously for 3 days starting on Day 0.

Re-evaluation is carried out at the end of 6 to 8 weeks (after two courses of "pulse-VAC"), with a second examination under anesthesia and endoscopic biopsy. If apparently complete or significant partial remission has occurred, continued chemotherapy alone is in order for another two courses of chemotherapy, with re-evaluation performed again upon completion. If results of this examination and biopsy continue to be negative, chemotherapy alone is again in order. The present data do not suggest that the addition of radiotherapy will improve survival.

If the biopsy is positive or if progressive disease is identified, surgical treatment or radiotherapy should be included in the therapeutic program. Radiotherapy is attractive because it does not sacrifice any vital structure, but the early and late sequelae of radiotherapy are significant. I prefer limited surgical excision before radiotherapy. However, if on exploration total exenteration appears necessary, the surgeon might consider radiotherapy in the hope that further reduction in size might allow for a more limited surgical procedure later. It is also important to emphasize here that the best survival results are in those children who have surgical removal of the tumor, even if removal requires anterior (rarely total) exenteration. In our experience, as in that of most other investigators, regression is only partial with primary chemotherapy and additional therapy will be indicated.

Most bladder lesions and all prostatic lesions will require total cystectomy and prostatectomy. A simultaneous pelvic lymphadenectomy should be accomplished to complete the staging of the tumor. The choice of urinary diversion depends on the experience and philosophy of the surgeon. Current continent diversions offer the possibility of avoiding appliances and improving body image for these children.[47] In females, pretreatment might reduce the bulk of the tumor such that simultaneous hysterectomy and vaginectomy will not be necessary. Although most vesical neoplasms arise at the level of the bladder neck and trigone, 25% of these tumors presented to the IRS appeared to arise from and to be confined to the dome of the bladder, making partial cystectomy theoretically possible after pretreatment. If the margins of the dissection show tumor or if the nodes are involved with disease, then radiotherapy can be added as the third therapeutic method.

Uterine and vaginal tumors have responded well to pretreatment chemotherapy, and a survival rate of 75% can be anticipated with chemotherapy only or with limited surgical treatment (partial vaginectomy or hysterovaginectomy), but without radiotherapy.[38,48]

Tumors arising within the confines of the bony pelvis, but without any obvious relationship to the pelvic organs and without an intraluminal component that is accessible to endoscopic observation and biopsy, constitute a particularly difficult subgroup of pelvic rhabdomyosarcoma. They are not included in the IRS study as lesions suitable for treatment with primary chemotherapy, yet they tend to infiltrate widely and are rarely suitable for primary surgical extirpation when first seen. After initial celiotomy, with removal of as much tumor as is safe, but without exenteration, primary intensive chemotherapy should be instituted.

As opposed to the bladder and vaginal lesions, I believe radiotherapy should be included as part of the initial therapy because local recurrences in my experience have been common after chemotherapy only and are generally not then amenable to surgical extirpation. After completion of the initial phase of therapy, a "second-look" celiotomy should be considered for repeated biopsy and excision of any apparent residual tumor.

In summary, the management of pelvic rhabdomyosarcoma is complex and involves the judicious use of surgical procedures, chemotherapy, and radiotherapy. It can no longer be said that primary radical surgical intervention is the preferred approach and that initial chemotherapy is reserved only for unresectable or metastatic lesions. Clinical trials are currently evaluating these concepts, but each case must still be carefully considered individually.

PARATESTICULAR RHABDOMYOSARCOMA

Paratesticular rhabdomyosarcoma is somewhat less common than pelvic lesions, and tends to occur in an older age group. In the series of genitourinary rhabdomyosarcoma reported by Exelby, 40% of the tumors were paratesticular.[28] These lesions are usually seen as firm, nontender, rapidly growing scrotal masses that may be indistinguishable from the testis.

As for any malignant scrotal mass, the initial surgical approach should be inguinal. If the tumor is accidentally approached scrotally, a hemiscrotectomy should be done. Unless the tumor is small and completely excised locally, radiotherapy should be administered to the ipsilateral hemiscrotum and to the inguinal area because, as with all rhabdomyosarcomas, the local recurrence rate is high. If local radiation is to be employed, the surgeon should consider transplantation of the contralateral testis into the thigh.

Paratesticular rhabdomyosarcoma metastasizes widely but does so primarily to the regional lymphatics.[49] Approximately one-third of patients in the original IRS had metastases to the retroperitoneal nodes at the time of presentation. Because of this, I believe all patients without evidence of hematogenous metastases at the time of presentation should still undergo a retroperitoneal lymphadenectomy. Cromie had previously suggested a complete, bilateral dissection from the level of the renal hila to the bifurcation of the aorta and then along the ipsilateral iliac vessels,[50] although others suggested that an adequate node sampling is all that is necessary. The risk of future infertility that might be averted with a more limited dissection appeared justified, in his view, by the improved staging and possible potential therapeutic benefit of a complete dissection.

More recent data, including information from IRS-2, suggests that such an aggressive approach may not be necessary. Raney and associates recently reviewed the cases of 95 boys with paratesticular rhabdomyosarcoma seen in the IRS.[51] Seventy-seven of these children were in groups I or II, and they achieved a survival rate of over 90% at three years. Twenty-eight percent of these children had positive retroperitoneal nodes, but the authors found no difference in the incidence of positive nodes or overall survival whether unilateral or bilateral retroperitoneal lymphadenectomy was performed. Therefore, it seems that a more limited node sampling, significantly reducing the risk of seminal emission failure, is appropriate.

If the retroperitoneal nodes are not involved with disease, radiotherapy can be withheld. When they are involved, radiotherapy should be directed to the retroperitoneal and mediastinal areas.

Olive et al. have suggested that retroperitoneal lymphadenectomy may not be indicated in group-I patients staged by intravenous urography and bipedal lymphangiography.[52] In a series of 18 patients (only 16 had lymphangiography), all maintained on chemotherapy, 17 have remained free of disease, most for over 2 years. At this time, though, it remains unclear just how effective chemotherapy alone is in sterilizing metastatic retroperitoneal nodes. In 6 patients in IRS-1 who relapsed in the para-aortic nodes, all died.[53] At this time, it is recommended that at least a unilateral retroperitoneal node excision be performed on all clinical group-I patients.

Chemotherapy should be continued whether the nodes are involved or not. The chemotherapeutic protocol can be modified according to the extent of recognized residual disease. In the absence of hematogenous metastases or bulky lymphatic disease, a less toxic program using vincristine and actinomycin D alone might be employed. With more extensive bulky disease, an intensive program as described for pelvic lesions would be appropriate. Through a selective, multidisciplinary program, survival can now be anticipated in greater than 90% of these neoplasms.

SEQUELAE OF THERAPY

Although the primary goal of cancer therapy in children is disease-free survival, some publications have drawn attention to the delayed sequelae of successful treatment for the primary lesion.[54-56] The effects of radical surgical extirpation are obvious and lifelong. For radical pelvic procedures, these effects include abdominal stomas, sterility, and impotence in males.

Cutaneous urinary diversion in children, especially the ileal conduit, has also been associated with a high long-term complication rate, including atrophic pyelonephritis, calculous disease, delayed loop strictures, ureterointestinal anastomotic strictures, and stomal stenosis.[57] More contemporary forms of urinary diversion, including antireflux ureterointestinal anastomoses and continent abdominal stomas, offer an improved quality of life and, possibly, a better outlook for renal preservation. These techniques are technically complex, have a high incidence of immediate postoperative complications, and remain unproven over several decades of follow-ups.[47]

The long-term effects of chemotherapy are not yet fully known. The tendency for cyclophosphamide to produce hemorrhagic cystitis is well documented, but its effects on germ cells are less clear. Adriamycin may cause cardiomyopathy and cardiac failure.

The most serious sequelae arise from the use of radiother-apy. Abnormalities in bone growth, scoliosis, chest wall deformities, and soft tissue fibrosis have all been reported. The skeletal abnormalities may be particularly disabling.[58] Radiation is a known oncogen, and increasing numbers of secondary tumors are being reported. Li and associates have calculated that the risk of a second tumor following radiotherapy for a childhood neoplasm is 17%, with the peak incidence occurring 15 to 19 years after initial therapy.[59]

REFERENCES

1. MILLER, R. W. Fifty-two forms of childhood cancer: United States mortality experience, 1960–1966. J. Pediatr., 75:685, 1969.
2. BATSAKIS, J. G. Urogenital rhabdomyosarcoma: Histogenesis and classification. J. Urol., 90:180, 1963.
3. TANK, E. S., et al. Treatment of urogenital tract rhabdomyosarcoma in infants and children. J. Urol., 107:324, 1972.
4. STOUT, A. P., and LATTES, R. Tumor of the soft tissues. In: Atlas of Tumor Pathology. Fascicle 1. Washington, D.C., Armed Forces Institute of Pathology, 1967.
5. PALMER, N., and FOULKES, M. Histopathology and prognosis in the second Intergroup Rhabdomyosarcoma Study. Proc. Am. Soc. Clin. Oncol., 2:229, 1983.
6. TSOKOS, M., and TRICHE, T. J. Primitive, "solid variant" rhabdomyosarcoma. Lab. Invest., 54:65A, 1986.
7. HAWKINS, H. K., and CAMACHO-VELASQUEZ, J. V. Rhabdomyosarcoma in children: Correlation of form and prognosis in one institution's experience. Am. J. Surg. Pathol., 11:531, 1987.
8. BARTHOLOMEW, T. H., GONZALES, E. T., STARLING, K. A., and HARBERG, F. J. Changing concepts in management of pelvic rhabdomyosarcoma in children. Urology, 13:613, 1979.
9. RANEY, B., et al. Primary site as a prognostic variable for children with pelvic soft tissue sarcomas. J. Urol., 136:874, 1986.
10. STEINBERG, J., et al. Clinical trials with cyclophosphamide in children with soft tissue sarcoma. Cancer Chemother. Rep., 28:39, 1963.
11. SUTOW, W. W. Chemotherapy in childhood cancer (except leukemia). Cancer, 18:1585, 1965.
12. SUTOW, W. W., et al. Vincristine sulfate therapy in children with metastatic soft tissue sarcoma. Pediatrics, 38:465, 1966.
13. TAN, C. T. C., GOLBEY, R. B., and YAP, C. L. Clinical experience with actinomycin-D. Ann. N.Y. Acad. Sci., 89:426, 1960.
14. JAMES, D. H., et al. Childhood malignant tumors—concurrent chemotherapy with Dactinomycin and vincristine sulfate. JAMA, 197:1043, 1966.
15. GROSFELD, J. L., CLATWORTHY, H. W., and NEWTON, W. A. Combined therapy in childhood rhabdomyosarcoma. J. Pediatr. Surg., 4:637, 1969.
16. PRATT, C. B., et al. Coordinated treatment of childhood rhabdomyosarcoma with surgery, radiotherapy and combination chemotherapy. Cancer Res., 32:606, 1972.
17. KILMAN, J. W., et al. Reasonable surgery for rhabdomyosarcoma: A study of 67 cases. Am. Surg., 178:346, 1973.
18. GHAVIMI, F., et al. Combination therapy of urogenital embryonal rhabdomyosarcoma in children. Cancer, 32:1178, 1973.
19. JAFFE, N., et al. Rhabdomyosarcoma in children—improved outlook with a multidisciplinary approach. Am. J. Surg., 125:482, 1973.
20. HEYN, R. M., et al. The role of combined chemotherapy in the treatment of rhabdomyosarcoma in children. Cancer, 34:2128, 1974.
21. EXELBY, P. R. Management of embryonal rhabdomyosarcoma in children. Surg. Clin. North Am., 54:849, 1974.
22. GHAVIMI, F., et al. Multidisciplinary treatment of embryonal rhabdomyosarcoma in children. Cancer, 35:677, 1975.
23. HEYN, R. M. The role of combined chemotherapy in the treatment of rhabdomyosarcoma in children. Cancer, 34:2128, 1974.
24. HEYN, R. M., HOLLAND, R., and JOO, P. Treatment of rhabdomyosarcoma in children with surgery, radiotherapy, and chemotherapy. Med. Pediatr. Oncol., 3:21, 1977.
25. DONALDSON, S. S., et al. Rhabdomyosarcoma of the head and neck in children. Cancer, 31:26, 1973.
26. MAURER, H. M., et al. The Intergroup Rhabdomyosarcoma Study: A preliminary report. Cancer, 40:2015, 1977.
27. RANEY, B. B., GEHAN, E. A., and MAURER, H. M. Evaluation of intensified chemotherapy in children with advanced rhabdomyosarcoma (Clinical Groups III and IV). Cancer Clin. Trials, 2:19, 1979.
28. EXELBY, P. R., GHAVIMI, F., and JEREB, B. Genitourinary rhabdomyosarcoma in children. J. Pediatr. Surg., 13:746, 1978.
29. CASSADY, J. R., et al. Radiation therapy for rhabdomyosarcoma. Radiology, 91:116, 1968.
30. DRITSCHILO, A., et al. The role of radiation therapy in the treatment of soft tissue sarcoma of childhood. Cancer, 42:1192, 1978.
31. GHAZALI, S. Embryonic rhabdomyosarcoma of the urogenital tract. Br. J. Surg., 60:124, 1973.
32. JARMAN, W. D., and KENEALY, J. C. Polypoid rhabdomyosarcoma of the bladder in children. Trans. Am. Assoc. Genitourin. Surg., 61:80, 1969.
33. WILLIAMS, D. I., and SCHISTAD, G. Lower urinary tract tumors in children. Br. J. Urol., 36:51, 1964.
34. MACKENZIE, A. R., WHITMORE, W. F., and MELAMED, M. Myosarcomas of the bladder and prostate. Cancer, 22:833, 1968.
35. RIVARD, G. E., et al. Intensive chemotherapy as primary treatment for rhabdomyosarcoma of the pelvis. Cancer, 36:1593, 1975.
36. BELMAN, A. B., and BAUM, E. S. Current trends in treatment of childhood rhabdomyosarcoma of lower genitourinary tract. Urology, 8:31, 1976.
37. ORTEGA, J. A. A therapeutic approach to childhood pelvic rhabdomyosarcoma without pelvic exenteration. J. Pediatrics, 94:205, 1979.
38. HAYS, D. M. Pelvic rhabdomyosarcomas in childhood. Cancer, 45:1810, 1980.
39. HAYS, D. M., et al. Bladder and prostatic tumors in the Intergroup Rhabdomyosarcoma Study (IRS-1). Cancer, 50:1472, 1982.

40. HAYS, D. M., et al. Primary chemotherapy in the treatment of children with bladder-prostate tumors in the Intergroup Rhabdomyosarcoma Study (IRS-II). J. Pediatr. Surg., *17*:812, 1982.

41. SCHOLTMEYER, R. J., TROMP, C. G., and HOZEBROEK, F. W. J. Embryonal rhabdomyosarcoma of the urogenital tract in childhood. Eur. Urol., *9*:69, 1983.

42. FLEMING, I. D., et al. The role of surgical resection when combined with chemotherapy and radiation in the management of pelvic rhabdomyosarcoma. Ann. Surg., *199*:509, 1984.

43. GHAVIMI, R., et al. Treatment of genitourinary rhabdomyosarcoma in children. J. Urol., *132*:313, 1984.

44. BROECKER, B. H., et al. Pelvic rhabdomyosarcoma in children. Brit. J. Urol., *61*:427, 1988.

45. GREEN, D. M. The treatment of advanced or recurrent malignant genitourinary tumors in children. Cancer, *60*:602, 1987.

46. RAGAB, A. H., et al. Infants younger than 1 year of age with rhabdomyosarcoma. Cancer, *58*:2606, 1986.

47. DECTER, R. M., and GONZALES, E. T. Bladder augmentation in the pediatric age group. Journal d' Urologie, *94*:91, 1988.

48. KUMAR, A. P. M., et al. Combined therapy to prevent complete pelvic exenteration for rhabdomyosarcoma of the vagina or uterus. Cancer, *37*:118, 1976.

49. OLNEY, L. E., et al. Intrascrotal rhabdomyosarcoma. Urology, *14*:113, 1979.

50. CROMIE, W. J., RANEY, R. B., and DUCKETT, J. W. Paratesticular rhabdomyosarcoma in children. J. Urol., *122*:80, 1979.

51. RANEY, R. B., et al. Paratesticular sarcoma in childhood and adolescence. Cancer, *60*:2337, 1987.

52. OLIVE, D., et al. Paraaortic lymphadenectomy is not necessary in the treatment of localized paratesticular rhabdomyosarcoma. Cancer, *54*:1283, 1984.

53. RANEY, E. B., et al. Prognosis of children with soft tissue sarcoma who relapse after achieving a complete response: A report from the Intergroup Rhabdomyosarcoma Study 1. Cancer, *52*:44, 1983.

54. JAFFE, N. Nononcogenic sequelae of cancer chemotherapy. Radiology, *114*:167, 1975.

55. JAFFE, N. Late side effects of treatment: Skeletal, genetic, central nervous system, and organic. Pediatr. Clin. North Am., *23*:233, 1977.

56. SCHEIN, P. S., and WINOKUR, S. H. Immunosuppressive and cytotoxic chemotherapy: Long-term complications. Ann. Intern. Med., *82*:84, 1975.

57. SHAPERO, S. R., LEBOWITZ, R., and COLODNY, A. H. Fate of ninety children with ileal conduit urinary diversion a decade later: Analysis of complications, pyelography, renal functions, and bacteriology. Urology, *114*:289, 1975.

58. JAFFE, N., et al. Childhood urologic cancer therapy-related sequelae and their impact on management. Cancer, *45*:1815, 1980.

59. LI, F. P., CASSADY, J. R., and JAFFE, N. Risk of second tumors in survivors of childhood cancer. Cancer, *35*:1230, 1975.

SECTION X

CHEMOTHERAPY

Chemotherapy, Hormonal Therapy, and Immunotherapy for Genitourinary Cancer: An Overview

F. Andrew Dorr

It is estimated that in 1989 there will be 1,010,000 newly diagnosed cancers in the United States. Cancers of the prostate, bladder, testis, and kidney will account for 178,900 of these cases. Of the 502,000 cancer deaths for 1989, nearly 10% will be attributable to genitourinary neoplasms.[1] The role of systemic therapy in the management of these diseases has expanded in recent years with new effective therapies for bladder, prostate, and kidney cancer, as well as improved therapy for testis cancer. As effective therapies are identified for advanced stages of these diseases, efforts to extend their indications in the surgical adjuvant setting have become the subject of ongoing clinical research activities.

In this chapter, an overview of the chemotherapy, hormonal therapy, and immunotherapy of each of these tumor types will be presented.

BLADDER CANCER

Background

The incidence of bladder cancer increases with age and is most commonly diagnosed in patients in their sixth and sev-

enth decades of life. It accounts for 7% of new cases diagnosed each year in men and for 3% of new cases in women. The male to female ratio of newly diagnosed bladder cancer is approximately 3:1. In 1989, 10,200 deaths will be attributable to bladder cancer.[1]

Bladder cancer is more prevalent in urban communities, suggesting a relationship with industrial carcinogens such as dyes and organic chemicals. There also appears to be a consistent etiologic link between cigarette smoking and bladder cancer. Smokers are at twice the risk of developing bladder cancer as are nonsmokers. It has been estimated that nearly half of all bladder cancer diagnosed may be related to cigarette smoking. Exposure to chemicals in the dye industry has long been correlated with bladder cancer. Specifically, exposure to aromatic amines, a class of compounds used to manufacture dyes, has been identified as a bladder carcinogen. Two aromatic amines, benzidine and 2-napthylamine, are thought to be the most potent bladder carcinogens encountered in the work place. A compound created as a byproduct in the manufacture of dyes, 4-aminobiphenyl, is another bladder carcinogen. This compound is also found in cigarette smoke. Occupations that appear to increase the risk of bladder cancer, presumably because of exposure to cancer-causing agents, include work in rubber, leather, textile and chemical industries, as well as hairdressers, machinists, metal workers, painters, printers, and truck drivers.[2]

Histology

Transitional cell carcinoma accounts for approximately 90% of the cases of bladder cancer in the United States, with squamous cell and adenocarcinoma accounting for 8% and 2%, respectively. Squamous cell cancer is the predominant histology in other areas of the world, particularly in regions where the parasitic infection, schistosomiasis, is endemic.[3]

Although 75 to 85% of patients present with superficial disease, 10 to 15% present with locally advanced tumors, and 5% have metastatic disease at presentation. For patients with superficial disease, local therapy alone is appropriate. Intravesical instillation of cytotoxic agents or BCG appears to ablate early tumors and to delay or prevent recurrent disease.[4] However, tumor recurrence with progression of grade and stage still occurs, adding to the population of patients who might benefit from systemic therapy. Patients with locally advanced and metastatic disease, however, often present without history of prior superficial bladder cancer. Despite aggressive local therapy with partial or radical cystectomy and/or radiotherapy, 40 to 80% of these patients die of disseminated disease within 3 years of diagnosis.[5-7] Regional therapy alone is not satisfactory, thus stimulating the search for effective systemic therapy.

Single-Agent Chemotherapy

The two single agents with the best documented activity in transitional cell bladder cancer are cisplatin and methotrexate (Table 45-1). Since Yagoda et al. reported a 35% partial response rate to single-agent cisplatin in 1976,[8] there have been numerous trials demonstrating its effectiveness, with response rates ranging from 15 to 65%, although it infrequently produces complete remissions.[9-23] This range in response rates is probably because of variable patient-related features such as performance status, type of prior treatment, and volume and location of disease. Moreover, bladder cancer patients often have poorly measurable disease, making accurate response assessment difficult. Despite these factors, as well as the variety of doses and schedules used, cisplatin has consistently demonstrated antitumor activity. The best reported response rates are in patients with locally advanced disease without metastases.[9-10] Responses to cisplatin usually occur within the first 6 weeks of treatment, with a median duration of response of 5 to 7 months. The large majority (more than 95%) of responses are incomplete. Although the optimal dose and schedule have not been prospectively evaluated, it appears that there is a dose response effect for cisplatin.

Methotrexate as a single agent has also been given in a wide range of doses and on varying schedules. The overall response rate reported is 30% with a range of 11 to 52%. The complete response rate with methotrexate is, like cisplatin, less than 5%. Responses usually occur within the first 4 weeks of treatment but are usually maintained for only 3 to 4 months. One study from the Royal Marsden Hospital suggested a dose response relationship. In 25 patients treated with methotrexate at 50 mg intravenously every 2 weeks, three patients experienced partial responses (12%). In contrast, among 23 patients treated with 100 mg intravenously every 2 weeks, there were 13% complete and 39% partial responses. Other small studies of low-dose compared to higher-dose methotrexate have not demonstrated a superior response rate for the higher doses evaluated.[24-28]

A third effective drug in transitional cell cancer of the urothelium is doxorubicin. Although an early study reported a response rate of 55%, subsequent studies have generally demonstrated a lower rate of antitumor efficacy with an overall response rate of 18%. Responses are also brief with doxorubicin as a single agent and complete responses have been reported only for the primary tumor, not in sites of metastases.[29-38]

Although vinblastine sulfate has been incorporated into effective multiple drug regimens, its single-agent activity has been evaluated in only one clinical trial. Vinblastine was administered at 0.10 to 0.15 mg/kg intravenously each week to

TABLE 45-1. *Active Single Agents for Urothelial Tract Cancer*

AGENT	EVALUABLE PATIENTS	NUMBER OF RESPONDERS	AVERAGED RATE (%)	RESPONSE (RANGE)	CONFIDENCE INTERVAL (95%)
Cisplatin	436	149	35	(15–65)	30–38
Methotrexate	232	70	30	(11–52)	24–36
Doxorubicin	239	43	18	(10–50)	13–23
Vinblastine	28	5	18	(—)	6–37
5-Fluorouracil	71	14	20	(15–30)	11–31
Cyclophosphamide	65	19	29	(7–52)	19–42

28 patients, the majority of whom had previously been treated with cytotoxic chemotherapy. Five (18%) partial responses were noted.[39] In a subsequent study, the same investigators combined vinblastine at 3 to 4 mg/m^2 and methotrexate at 30 to 40 mg/m^2 weekly. Eighteen of 38 patients (49%) who had received no prior chemotherapy achieved an objective response.[40]

Two additional agents that may be modestly effective in bladder cancer patients are 5-fluorouracil (5-FU) and cyclophosphamide. The overall response rate for three studies of 5-FU is 20%.[33,36,41] The activity of cyclophosphamide as a single agent is less clear. The average response rate from the several small trials was 29%, with a range of 7 to 52%.[42–44] Yagoda reported the largest experience with this drug, finding a 7% response rate in 26 patients.[44]

Combination Chemotherapy

Combinations of the active cytotoxic agents can produce response rates in as many as 50 to 70% of patients with metastatic bladder cancer. The response rates for five reported trials of cisplatin plus methotrexate range from 27 to 68% with an average of 46%.[14,15,45–47] Of particular note is the frequency of complete responses in 6 to 23% of patients. Although these response rates seem better than those reported with the single-agent studies of cisplatin and methotrexate, the only randomized trial of cisplatin alone versus the combination failed to demonstrate a significant advantage for combination therapy. In the trial from the Australian Bladder Cancer Study Group, cisplatin was given at 80 mg/m^2, with or without methotrexate, at a dose of 50 mg/m^2 on days 2 and 4 of each 4-week cycle. A 45% response rate was observed in the 49 patients treated with both drugs and a 33% response rate in 51 patients treated with cisplatin alone.[15] Although these differences are not statistically significant, a larger study might have identified meaningful differences.

The complete response rate with cisplatin plus methotrexate has provided encouragement for developing this regimen further. In vitro data has suggested a synergistic antitumor effect between vinca alkaloids and methotrexate. On this basis, as well as the promising clinical results noted above, two cisplatin-based regimens have evolved that appear to provide the most promising results of the combinations that have been evaluated. The combination of cisplatin, methotrexate, and vinblastine (CMV) was first studied by Harker et al., finding a 56% response rate in 50 patients with metastatic disease, with half of those responses being complete (Table 45-2).[48–50] The MVAC regimen (methotrexate, vinblastine, adriamycin, and cisplatin) from Memorial Sloan-Kettering Cancer Center (MSKCC) produced a 69% response rate with 36% complete responders (Table 45-3). In this study, the survival probability for patients with a complete response is estimated to be 55% at three years.[51] This represents a substantial increment compared to other reports of single-agent or combination chemotherapy in metastatic bladder cancer. Complete responses

with these combinations have been observed in visceral, soft tissue, and bony sites of metastases.[51–55]

The encouraging results of clinical trials employing either CMV or MVAC in preliminary studies in patients with metastatic disease have stimulated phase-II trials of neoadjuvant chemotherapy in patients with localized bladder cancer. In several small studies using CMV preoperatively and/or postoperatively, more than 50% of patients have responded. De Vries et al. treated 36 patients with four cycles of preoperative CMV followed by another two cycles postoperatively as consolidation therapy. Eleven of the 12 complete responders were alive and disease-free at 15 to 46 months.[56] Droz et al. treated 28 patients with two and four courses of preoperative and postoperative therapy. Twenty-one patients are alive and disease-free.[57] Although it seems that this regimen is effective in downstaging locally advanced bladder cancer, its effect on overall and disease-free survival needs to be investigated further. Most of the studies using preoperative MVAC employ two to four cycles of the combination.[58–63] Clinical complete tumor regressions were noted in all studies with pathologic confirmation frequently noted in those patients undergoing cystectomy (Table 45-4). The largest single experience is that of 41 patients with T2-T4 bladder cancers treated preoperatively with MVAC at MSKCC. There were 10 clinical complete responses and 16 clinical partial responses. Of 30 patients who underwent surgical evaluation, 33% and 17% achieved pathologic complete and partial responses, respectively.[61] These results demonstrate the efficacy of this regimen in downstaging locally advanced disease, as was seen with CMV. They also point out the difficulties in the management of these patients. Radiographic studies and physical examination are inadequate for accurately staging the primary disease and the response to therapy. Patients are encountered who are thought to have no response or, at best, a partial response to chemotherapy, who are then evaluated pathologically and found to have only fibrosis without evidence of disease. Understaging, however, is a more common problem than overstaging, with residual disease often present in patients thought to be in complete response by even the most rigorous clinical evaluation.

Combination Chemotherapy and Radiation Therapy

The conventional management of locally invasive bladder cancer has been radical cystectomy with or without preoperative radiation therapy. For patients who refuse surgery or who are unacceptable surgical candidates, radical or definitive radiotherapy has proven to be reasonably effective at controlling the local disease. As effective chemotherapy has evolved for the treatment of metastatic disease, there has been extensive clinical interest in the use of chemotherapy in combination with radiotherapy, whether as an adjuvant to radiotherapy or as a radiation sensitizer. It is hoped that these combinations will enhance local control of primary disease and eradicate subclinical metastases.

Cisplatin has been used with full-dose radiation therapy with results suggesting an improvement over the historical

TABLE 45-2. *Urothelial Tract Cancer CMV Regimen*

DOSE/SCHEDULE (mg/m^2)	REFERENCE	EVALUABLE PATIENTS	NUMBER OF RESPONSES (CR/PR)*	AVERAGE RESPONSE RATE	CONFIDENCE INTERVAL (95%)
DDP 45 d2,3 MTX 40 dl VLB 4 d3	48	19	14(6/8)	74	49–91%
DDP 100 d2 MTX 30 dl, 8 VLB 4 dl, 8	49	17	10(8/2)	59	33–82%
DDP 100 d2 MTX 30 dl, 8 VLB 4 dl, 8	50	50	28(14/14)	56	41–70%
		86	52(28/24)	60	49–71%

*Complete response rate: 33 ± 10%

results of radiation alone. Where reported, pathologic complete response rates in similarly staged patients treated with precystectomy radiation (40 Gy to 50 Gy) have ranged between 12 and 39%. In three trials, the concurrent administration of at least 40 Gy pelvic radiation and 70 to 100 mg/m^2 of cisplatin has produced complete clinical response in 70 to 77% of patients.[64–66] As noted, however, it is difficult to compare clinical and pathologic response rates among studies.

Other investigators have combined concurrent 5-fluorouracil and radiation therapy with apparent benefit.[67–68] Rotman et al. treated 19 patients with inoperable bladder cancer with this combination and reported a 62% 5-year survival. Russell et al. reported 13 complete responses in 14 patients treated with a similar regimen at a median follow-up of 7 months.[68] Operative confirmation of these response rates was generally not available, so it is likely that the pathologic complete response rate is lower; but this combined approach clearly deserves further investigation. Randomized clinical trials that will compare radiation alone to radiation plus chemotherapy, with or without surgery, should be initiated to further define the role of chemotherapy in combination with radiation in invasive bladder cancer.

Important, randomized clinical trials in bladder cancer that are ongoing in the United States can be divided into those for locally advanced disease and those for metastatic disease. Perhaps one of the most important studies is a comparison of cisplatin alone with the MVAC regimen developed at MSKCC. This study will hopefully confirm the nonrandomized data suggesting that greater antitumor effect can be achieved with combination chemotherapy, particularly by inducing complete responses. For locally advanced bladder cancer, a national high-priority study is being coordinated by the Southwest Oncology Group. In that study, patients are randomized either to immediate cystectomy or to three courses of MVAC followed by cystectomy. This study should give important information on downstaging relative to a concurrently randomized control population, as well as relative to the clinical stage at diagnosis. In addition, it will define the impact of combina-

TABLE 45-3. *Urothelial Tract Cancer MVAC Regimen*

REFERENCE	EVALUABLE PATIENTS	NUMBER OF RESPONSES (CR/PR)*	AVERAGE RESPONSE RATE (%)	CONFIDENCE INTERVAL (95%)
Sternberg et al. (1988)[51]	83	57(31/26)	69	59–79%
Soloway (1988)[52]	19	10(6/4)	53	30–75%
Chong et al. (1987)[53]	10	4(1/3)	40	12–74%
Connor, Rappaport, and Sawczuk (1987)[54]	7	6(3/3)	86	42–99%
Sheehan, Sagalowsky, Balaban, and Cox (1987)[55]	5	3(0/3)	60	15–95%
	124	80(41/39)	62	

*Complete response rate: 33 ± 9%

TABLE 45-4. *Neoadjuvant MVAC for Locally Advanced Bladder Cancer*

REFERENCE	EVALUABLE	CLINICAL CR	CLINICAL PR	TOTAL RESPONSE RATE (%)
Vogelzang et al.[58]	11	5	2	64
Lee et al.[59]	10	4	0	90
Zincke, Sen, Hahn, and Keating[60]	16	8	3	69
Scher et al.[61]	41	10	16	63
Simon et al.[62]	36	15	10	69
Bukowski, Monatie, Lee, and Ganapathi[63]	10	2	2	40
	124	44	33	62%

tion chemotherapy as prescribed in this study on long-term, disease-free, and overall survival. This study is of critical importance for understanding the optimal management of the patient with locally advanced transitional cell cancer of the urothelium.

TESTICULAR CANCER

Background

Germ cell cancer of testicular origin has been termed a model disease in the systemic treatment of advanced cancer. Patients with poor-risk metastatic disease have cure rates of less than 50% while those with good-risk disease have cure rates in excess of 80%. Although surgery and/or radiotherapy provide the primary treatment modality for early-stage disease, state-of-the-art treatment for advanced testicular cancer centers around cisplatin-based combination chemotherapy. The chemotherapeutic approach to patients with advanced seminoma and nonseminoma are similar and will be discussed together, although most seminoma patients can be considered to have good-risk disease.

Testicular cancer accounts for approximately 1% of all malignancies in men. Most of these cases occur between age 15 and 35, with estimated 1989 incidence figures of 5700 new cases and 350 deaths.[1] Trends in the 5-year survival rates for this disease in white males have shown a consistent increase between 1974 and 1976 (79%) and 1979 and 1984 (91%), while the rate for blacks in a similar population-based study did not show an improvement of similar magnitude (77% between 1974 and 1976 and 82% between 1979 and 1984). Although an overall increase in incidence has been observed over the last 30 years, the mortality rate has declined by approximately 60% since 1970,[69] partly because of improved detection and diagnostic procedures, but largely because of the development of highly effective combination chemotherapy for patients with advanced disease and improved radiotherapy for patients with disease limited to the abdomen and pelvis.

The etiology of germ cell cancer of the testis is unclear. The only known risk factors are abnormal testicular development and nondescent of the testis during fetal development. It may be that a defect within the germinal epithelium may be responsible for both maldescent and tumor formation.[70] Other hypothesized etiologic factors include environmental exposure to carcinogens and viral causes. Recently, a particular chromosomal abnormality has been identified (isochrome of the short arm of chromosome 12) in 13 of 14 tumor specimens taken from 12 patients with germ cell tumors. In addition, seven of seven germ cell tumor cell lines contained this isochrome. This abnormality may thus represent an early genetic event in the development of germ cell tumors and warrants further study.[71]

Combination Chemotherapy for Advanced Germ Cell Cancer

The evolution of combination chemotherapy for germ cell cancer has taken into consideration the potential for synergy among drugs and the pharmacokinetic interaction of these drugs, as well as their overlapping toxic effects. Vinblastine and bleomycin were shown to produce complete remission rates of 10 to 20% when used as single agents. In combination, however, the complete response rate was 40 to 50%. With the discovery of cisplatin and its extraordinary clinical efficacy in disseminated germ cell cancer, several regimens incorporating combinations of cisplatin, vinblastine, and bleomycin have been developed that produce remarkable cure rates. Indeed, the chance of cure for patients with relatively good-risk disease is so great that the most clinically relevant questions for these patients focus on toxicity reduction. Even with the most aggressive regimens identified so far, however, patients with poor-risk disease have only a modest opportunity for long-term cure. Concepts being evaluated in clinical trials for this group therefore are akin to those for most solid tumors. The value of dose intensity, the role of high-dose chemotherapy with autologous bone marrow transplantation, and the substitution of potentially more effective agents in the active regimens are all being studied in current clinical trials.

Germ Cell Tumor Prognostic Factors

Several groups have developed guidelines for assessing prognosis of patients with germ cell tumor.[72,73] These classification schemes all include the site and extent of metastases in estimating prognosis. In some classification systems, the absolute value or logarithm of tumor markers (AFP, HCG, and LDH) and the number of elevated tumor markers have been incorporated into mathematical models for predicting outcome. Perhaps the simplest staging system for clinical use is that developed at Indiana University (Table 45-6). Elevation of tumor markers is not incorporated as they were not found to better define those with minimal or moderate disease. Although in their experience, marker elevation subdivided the group with advanced disease into different subgroups, these subgroups all had relatively poor prognoses (from 45 to 73% free of disease at 2 years compared to 96% for those with minimal or moderate disease). In developing the Indiana Staging System, several parameters were not found to be predictive. These include histologic type, site of primary tumor (testicular versus extragonadal), age and performance status, and presence or absence of prior radiotherapy.[72]

In the model developed by MSKCC, the logarithm of the LDH and HCG adds to the information provided by the number of sites of metastases.[73] The mathematical model is somewhat more difficult to use in the clinical setting although it may provide more precise information about the prognosis of a given patient than other staging systems. For the present, however, these staging systems are most useful for assigning risk for clinical trials with different goals. Those with excellent prognoses should be studied in trials where reduction of toxicity is the primary objective, while those with a poorer prognosis should be evaluated in trials for which new approaches are being compared to a standard regimen.

VAB Regimen

Several different combination chemotherapy regimens have been developed that are of apparently comparable efficacy (Table 45-5). VAB refers to the combination of vinblastine,

TABLE 45-6. *Germ Cell Tumor Indiana Classification of Extent of Disease*

MINIMAL

- Elevated HCG and/or Alphafetoprotein Only
- Cervical Nodes (Nonpalpable, Abdominal Disease)
- Unresectable, but Nonpalpable, Retroperitoneal Disease
- Minimal Pulmonary Disease (Fewer than Five Per Lung Field and the Largest Smaller than 2 cm ($\pm$Nonpalpable Abdominal Disease)

MODERATE

- Palpable Abdominal Mass As Only Anatomical Disease
- Moderate Pulmonary Metastases (Five to Ten Pulmonary Metastases Per Lung Field and the Largest Smaller than 50% of the Intrathoracic Diameter or a Solitary Pulmonary Metastasis Smaller than 2 cm

ADVANCED

- Advanced Pulmonary Metastases (Exceeds Criteria for Minimal or Moderate Disease)
- Palpable Abdominal Mass Plus Pulmonary Metastases
- Hepatic, Osseous or CNS Metastases

actinomycin D, and bleomycin, which was developed at MSKCC in the early 1970's. Among 71 patients treated with this regimen in their initial experience, 14% experienced complete remissions.[74] Cisplatin was then added to the VAB combination (termed VAB-II), with a 50% complete response rate in 50 patients studied, although only 12 enjoyed long-term disease-free survival.[75] Subsequent modifications of the VAB regimen, including the addition of cyclophosphamide and the modification of doses and schedule, have produced substantially better results. There has been extensive experience with the VAB-6 regimen (Table 45-7) in patients with primary testicular germ cell tumors and in patients with extragonadal primary tumors. In the initial report of this regimen, 142 evaluable patients with primary testicular tumors were treated, with 98 (69%) experiencing complete response to chemotherapy. An additional 14 patients (10%) were converted to complete response with resection of residual masses. Ten of 19 patients (53%) with extragonadal primaries had a complete response to chemotherapy while 4 (21%) required sur-

TABLE 45-5. *Chemotherapy of Germ Cell Tumors*

REGIMEN	N	ELIGIBILITY	CR (+SURGERY)(%)	DISEASE FREE (%)
PVB	147	ALL	84	80
	121	ALL	74	80
VAB-6	82	"GOOD RISK"	96	88
	161	ALL	78	73
BEP	123	ALL	83	84
EP	82	"GOOD RISK"	93	88

TABLE 45-7. *VAB-6 Dose and Schedule*

DRUG	DOSE AND SCHEDULE	
Vinblastine	4 mg/m²	Day 1
Cyclophosphamide	600 mg/m²	Day 1
Actinomycin D	1.0 mg/m²	Day 1
Bleomycin	30 U IVP	Day 1, then
	20 U/m²	Days 1–3 by Continuous Infusion
Cisplatin	120 mg/m² IV	Day 4 with Mannitol
Repeat Every 4 Weeks × 3 But with No Bleomycin in Third Course		

gery following chemotherapy to achieve complete response. Overall, 12% of these patients relapsed, with relapse more likely in patients with extragonadal primaries (21%) than in those with testicular primaries (11%). Long-term, disease-free survival reported with this regimen was 71%.[76]

As mentioned above, recent clinical trial efforts in patients with good-risk testicular cancer have been designed to explore toxicity reduction without compromising the excellent long-term outcome. Investigators at MSKCC have recently published a randomized clinical trial in this group that compared VAB-6 with the two-drug combination of cisplatin and VP-16 (EP). The complete response to chemotherapy ± surgery (79 of 82 with VAB-6 and 76 of 82 with EP) and long-term, disease-free survival for these two regimens were identical, but patients receiving EP experienced significantly less neutropenia, emesis, mucositis, and pulmonary toxicity.[77]

In an effort to further reduce toxicity for this group of patients, the MSKCC is conducting a clinical trial in which EP is being compared to VP-16 + carboplatin. No results were available from this study at the time of this writing.

PVB Regimen

Concurrent with the development of the VAB regimens, investigators at Indiana University began studying cisplatin, vinblastine, and bleomycin (PVB). The therapeutic outcome with that original regimen is well known. Subsequent trials have demonstrated that a lower dose of vinblastine could be used, thereby reducing toxicity without decreasing efficacy, that doxorubicin does not add to the PVB regimen, that maintenance vinblastine for 2 years is unnecessary, and that VP-16 could be substituted for vinblastine without compromising survival, while reducing neuromuscular toxicity. This substitution might even improve survival. The current standard regimen recommended by Indiana University is the combination of bleomycin, etoposide (VP-16), and cisplatin (BEP) shown in Table 45-8.[78]

For patients with good-risk disease, Indiana University and the Eastern Cooperative Oncology Group (ECOG) are currently (1989) comparing the results of their BEP regimen with the two-drug regimen EP, noted above. For patients with poor-risk germ cell cancer, the BEP regimen is being compared with the same three drugs but with cisplatin given at twice the dose (40 mg/m²/day for 5 days). This trial, when completed, will provide important information about the dose response curve for cisplatin in germ cell tumors. Another study, underway in ECOG, is comparing the BEP regimen with VP-16 plus ifosfamide and cisplatin. Ifosfamide's impressive activity in patients with refractory disease suggests that it may enhance the potential for cure in those with newly diagnosed advanced disease with poor-risk features.

Salvage Chemotherapy

The development of salvage regimens for patients with germ cell tumors has produced several new leads for improving standard therapy. Both VP-16 and ifosfamide were found to produce occasional, long-term remissions in patients either relapsing after cisplatin-based chemotherapy or refractory to cisplatin. VP-16 given alone to relapsing patients was found to induce responses, but only when given with cisplatin was it found to produce an apparent cure rate of 23% in refractory patients. Ifosfamide produced a 23% response rate in 30 relapsed patients, but only one complete response was seen. However, when ifosfamide was combined with cisplatin and either vinblastine or VP-16, 12 of 56 patients had complete responses to chemotherapy and an additional 8 patients were rendered free of disease following surgery. Responses were sustained with 7 patients continuously disease free for over 2 years at the time of the report.[79] Given these data, ifosfamide has recently been approved by the FDA for germ cell cancer in second-relapse patients. The combinations used in this trial, with the choice of vinblastine or VP-16 depending on prior drug exposure, represent an effective standard approach for patients with relapsed disease.

Another treatment strategy developed by investigators at Indiana University is high-dose chemotherapy with VP-16 and

TABLE 45-8. *BEP/PVB Dose and Schedule*

DRUG	DOSE AND SCHEDULE	
Cisplatin	20 mg/m²/day IV	Days 1–5
Bleomycin and	30 U IV	Weekly
Vinblastine (PVB) or	0.15 mg/kg IV	Days 1 and 2
VP-16 (BEP)	100 mg/m² IV	Days 1–5
Both PVB and BEP Are Given Every 3 Weeks × 4		

carboplatin, a cisplatin analog with good antitumor activity in germ cell tumors, followed by autologous bone marrow transplantation. In that study, patients received a fixed total dose of VP-16 of 1200 mg/m^2, while the dose of carboplatin ranged from 900 mg/m^2 to 2000 mg/^{2}. There were 8 complete remissions with 4 being sustained in excess of 1 year. There were also 6 partial responses but 7 toxic deaths.[80] The toxic deaths were secondary to opportunistic infections and were at the highest dose levels studied. The recommended doses for further study are VP-16 at 1200 mg/m^2 and carboplatin at 1200 mg/m^2. This regimen may offer an opportunity for cure for patients with refractory disease. It may be appropriate to move this approach earlier in the disease course so that drug resistance can more likely be overcome. Alternatively, the preparative chemotherapy regimen might be altered by adding ifosfamide or another alkylating agent such as cyclophosphamide at high dose prior to autologous bone marrow reinfusion.

Other salvage approaches for germ cell tumors are essentially restricted to the development of new drugs against this tumor. Given the small numbers of these patients, drug development must be fairly targeted to those drugs that appear to be active in the setting of cisplatin resistance.

Through the careful conduct of clinical trials, the understanding of chemotherapy of germ cell tumors of gonadal and extragonadal origin has improved dramatically since the early 1970's. Patients can now be considered for treatment strategies based on the characteristics of their tumor extent and tumor markers. That 75 to 80% of patients are cured by standard cisplatin-based regimens is encouraging. Aggressive and careful administration of these regimens is required to achieve these results. There remains a need for better treatment strategies both for those with poor-risk disease and for those who relapse or progress on standard regimens.

PROSTATE CANCER

Prostate cancer is the most common cancer diagnosis in men and the third most common cause of cancer death. In men over 55, it is the leading cause of cancer death. It is estimated that 1 out of 11 men in the US will develop prostate cancer in his lifetime. In 1989, 103,000 new cases of prostate cancer are expected to occur, with about 30% of those afflicted expected to die within 5 years of diagnosis.[1]

Relatively little is known about the etiology of prostate cancer. Various aspects of sexual activity, endocrine factors, occupational exposures, and diet have been suspected of playing a role. Men who have never married have lower rates of prostate cancer, as do Jewish men, whereas rates are 50% higher among blacks than whites.[69]

The disease occurs predominantly in older males with a median age at presentation of 70 years, with more than 80% of cases occurring in men older than 60. The most common histology arising in the prostate is adenocarcinoma, accounting for 95% of tumors in this organ. Sarcoma and squamous cell histologies account for most of the remaining diagnoses. Adenocarcinomas usually originate from peripheral acinar glands although primary tumors may occur anywhere in the prostate. The disease may be multifocal within the gland. Prostate cancer is more common in the apex than in any other part of the gland. Normal growth and development of the human prostate gland requires a balanced interaction between epithelial and stromal cells as well as stimulation by androgens. The androgen dependence of prostate cancer for growth maintenance was first demonstrated in 1941. The importance of androgens for the development of prostate cancer is poorly understood but their role is critical because those castrated prior to puberty do not develop this disease.

Most patients with prostate cancer have locally advanced or disseminated disease at the time of presentation. Approximately 80% of new cases present with disease beyond the confines of the prostate gland and 40 to 50% have distant metastases. The metastatic pattern is dominated in the majority of patients by bone involvement.

For nearly 50 years, the standard treatment for patients with advanced carcinoma of the prostate has been hormone manipulation (orchiectomy or administration of estrogen). Seventy to 80% of patients show an initial response or stabilization to endocrine therapy, but the median duration of response in most studies is 1 year. The morbidity of both orchiectomy (impotence and psychologic impact of surgical castration) and estrogen therapy (impotence and cardiovascular side effects) and their unsatisfactory antitumor efficacy, have stimulated the search for more effective therapies.

Primary Hormone Therapy

Analogues of gonadotropin-releasing hormone (Gn-RH) have been introduced in the past decade with the hope of improving the efficacy and limiting the toxicity relative to standard therapies. Gn-RH analogues are synthesized by substitution of amino acids at the sixth and tenth positions of the parent decapeptide. These agonists have been found to have up to 100 times the potency of the parent compound. They function by inhibiting pituitary release of normal gonadotropin-releasing hormone, resulting in castrate levels of gonadal hormones. The most widely applied Gn-RH analogues include buserelin, goserelin, leuprolide, and decapeptyl. Only leuprolide is currently commercially available in the United States.[81]

During the 1980's, numerous clinical trials investigated the use of Gn-RH analogues in prostate cancer. Several studies were important in establishing the role of Gn-RH analogues as a means of suppressing testosterone and dihydrotestosterone to castrate levels (Table 45-9).[82–102] The clinical efficacy of these drugs appears to be equivalent to that of estrogens or surgical castration. Only one study directly comparing a Gn-RH analog with DES has been successfully completed and published. In that study from the Leuprolide Study Group, leuprolide at 1 mg per day was compared with DES at 3 mg per day in 186 evaluable, previously untreated patients with meta-

TABLE 45-9. *Gonadotropin-Releasing Hormone Analogues Results in Untreated Prostate Cancer Patients*

GN-RH ANALOG	DOSE RANGE	NUMBER EVALUATED	CR + PR (%)
Buserelin[82–91]	150 μg-2400 μg/day sq or intranasal	343	46
Goserelin[92–98]	.9 mg–3.6 mg SQ/month 50–500 μg SQ/day	346	52
Leuprolide[81,99]	1 mg SQ/day	145	37
Decapeptyl[100–102]	500 μg SQ/day 3.75 mg SQ/month	142	39

static prostate cancer. Using National Prostate Cancer Project response criteria, overall response rates, including stable disease, were essentially the same for both treatments. The complete plus partial response rate was slightly higher for the DES group (46%) than for the leuprolide group (38%), although this difference was not statistically different. Toxicities however, were substantially different, with patients receiving DES experiencing more frequent painful gynecomastia, nausea and vomiting, peripheral edema, and thromboembolism than did those patients on leuprolide. Time-to-treatment failure and median survival were virtually identical for the two treatments.[99]

One European study has compared zoladex with surgical castration in 359 patients.[103] A preliminary analysis of the study has identified no difference between the two as measured by response rates and time to progression, but additional follow-up is necessary before final conclusions can be reached. A smaller British study compared decapeptyl with surgical castration in 104 patients, with no differences identified in clinical outcome between the two treatments.[100]

Thus, it appears that medical castration with Gn-RH analogues produces comparable clinical results when compared with heretofore standard therapies. There is no evidence that increasing the dose beyond that necessary to achieve castrate testosterone levels produces additional benefit. Institution of therapy with these compounds is accompanied by a transient increase in testosterone and dihydrotestosterone levels, which is frequently accompanied by an increase in clinical or biochemical disease activity. This disease flare usually lasts less than 1 week but should be taken into consideration when planning the treatment strategy for patients with metastases to critical sites such as the vertebral spine, where stimulation of tumor growth may produce spinal cord compression.

Antiandrogens

Antiandrogens are a group of compounds that peripherally inhibit the action of testosterone by interfering with receptor binding or nuclear translocation. They generally fall into two classes: steroidal (eg, cyproterone acetate) and nonsteroidal

(eg., flutamide). Although progestational agents have an antiandrogenic effect, they appear to be less effective than standard therapies in the treatment of patients with prostate cancer.[104,105] Cyproterone acetate is a more potent antiandrogen than progestins. The European Organization for Research and Treatment of Cancer (EORTC) has compared cyproterone acetate with DES and medroxyprogesterone acetate in 175 patients with locally advanced or metastatic prostate cancer. Cyproterone acetate produced a 40% response rate and DES produced a 45% response rate. Only 26% of MPA-treated patients responded. Time to progression and survival, however, favored those treated with DES when compared to either CPA or to MPA. Thus it would appear that DES, although more toxic than CPA, offers the patient a better opportunity for long-term disease remission.[106]

Nonsteroidal antiandrogens such as flutamide have mostly been studied either as second-line therapy or in combination with orchiectomy or a Gn-RH analogue. The value of these compounds as single-agent therapy for previously untreated patients requires further study. Antiandrogens are well tolerated, with gastrointestinal toxicity manifested by diarrhea as the most commonly described side effect of flutamide. One advantage of these compounds is their potency-sparing potential, which occurs more frequently than with conventional endocrine therapies. As endocrine therapies are considered for earlier stages of prostate cancer, these potency-sparing agents may play increasingly important roles.

Combination Hormonal Therapy

The concept of combining an antiandrogen with a Gn-RH analogue or orchiectomy is based on the hypotheses that prostate cancer primarily depends on androgens and that tumor progression following conventional endocrine manipulations may result from inadequate suppression of androgens of adrenal origin. The opposing view is that prostate cancer is composed of both androgen-dependent and androgen-independent cells, with progression of disease following frontline therapy a result of uncontrolled growth of the androgen independent subpopulation. Labrie and associates reported impressive results with the combination of castration and flutamide in a nonrandomized study.[107] More recently, the combination of leuprolide and flutamide versus leuprolide plus placebo has been evaluated. Although response rates were comparable between the two treatment groups, both time to progression and survival were significantly longer for patients receiving combined therapy compared to those initially receiving single-agent leuprolide.[108] Similar studies using different Gn-RH analogues and/or different antiandrogens are underway in Canada and in Europe, with definitive results not yet reported at the time of this writing.

Secondary Hormonal Therapy

The treatment of advanced prostate cancer following progression on initial hormonal intervention is a major problem in the practice of oncology. These patients have a poor prognosis with a median survival in most studies of less than 1 year. In addition, the quality of life of these patients is generally poor because many have a poor performance status secondary to painful bony metastases that can be difficult to control. In contrast to the relative success of hormonal manipulations in patients with newly diagnosed disease, objective evidence of tumor regression in patients treated with secondary hormone therapy is rare and short-lived. The reported response rates to several agents used as second-line therapy are summarized in Table 45-10.[109-118] The different response rates reported may be attributable to differences in how response is defined and not to real differences in efficacy. The appeal of second-line hormonal therapy is the relative lack of toxicity compared to cytotoxic agents as well as the occasional responses that are seen. Nevertheless, an acceptable standard therapy following progression with front-line hormonal therapy remains to be identified.

Chemotherapy of Prostate Cancer

Over the last 15 years, multiple single-agent and combination cytotoxic agent trials were performed by various groups (Table 45-11).[119] Although symptom relief in up to 30% of patients with advanced disease may occur, that benefit is generally of limited duration. Studies conducted by the National Prostate Cancer Project compared the single-agent activity of cyclophosphamide, 5-FU, dacarbazine, nitrosoureas, methotrexate, and cisplatin with supportive therapy, defined as continued hormonal therapy with palliative radiotherapy where indicated. In the comparison of cyclophosphamide versus 5-FU versus standard therapy, 41% and 36% of those given cytotoxic therapy had not progressed compared to 19% of those managed with standard therapy. There was no difference in survival among the treatments.[120] Nevertheless, these results provided the rationale for subsequent studies that did not employ a "control" arm. There was no difference in survival. Although this study was not blinded and the endpoint was somewhat arbitrary, subsequent randomized studies have infrequently used a no-treatment control arm that has made their interpretation more difficult. One randomized study compared doxorubicin with 5-fluorouracil, in which survival was superior for those receiving doxorubicin after adjustment for prognostic factors.[121] There has not been a subsequent confirmatory trial that demonstrates a survival difference for patients treated with doxorubicin compared to those treated with palliative care or with another cytotoxic therapy. Given doxorubicin's low level of activity as measured by tumor regression, these results must be viewed with caution.

Many combinations of cytotoxic agents have been evaluated in patients with hormone refractory prostate cancer. None of these have identified a combination that was superior to the single agent to which it was being compared. Because single-agent therapy has yet to be demonstrated to be superior to supportive care alone, new approaches to the treatment of prostate cancer are needed. The use of cytotoxics earlier in the course of the disease, including concurrently with or before hormonal therapy, has yet to identify any effective combinations.[122]

Another approach has been to administer chemotherapy following androgen priming. Androgen priming may induce malignant cells into active cell cycling, thus making them more sensitive to cell-cycle-specific cytotoxic agents. Although earlier trials in androgen priming were associated with

TABLE 45-11. *Chemotherapy of Prostate Cancer Single Agent Results*

DRUG	N	CR + PR (%)
Doxorubicin	99	13
Cyclophosphamide	134	5
Cisplatin	209	12
5-Fluorouracil	148	10
Hydroxyurea	82	3
Methotrexate	58	5

Modified from Eisenberger, M. A. et al. J. Clin. Oncol., *3*:827, 1985. A re-evaluation of non-hormonal cytotoxic chemotherapy in the treatment of prostatic carcinoma.

TABLE 45-10. *Secondary Hormonal Therapy Metastatic Prostate Cancer*

DRUG	DOSE AND SCHEDULE	NUMBER EVALUATED	OBJECTIVE RESPONSE RATE (%)
Ketoconazole[109-112]	200–400 mg tid	58	19
Aminoglutethimide[113,114]	125–250 mg qid	84	11
Flutamide[115,116]	250 mg tid	97	1
Megestrol Acetate[117]	160 mg qid	37	3
Tamoxifen[118]	10–30 mg qid	17	0

substantial morbidity, more recent studies were designed to achieve a more controlled stimulatory effect.[123] Manni et al. reported a randomized trial in which 61 patients with advanced disease were treated with aminoglutethimide, cortisone acetate, and cytotoxic agents with or without fluoxymesterone (halotestin). The response rate was not significantly different between the experimental group (42%) and the control group (35%). Median duration of response was also comparable. In spite of the cautious tumor priming in the group receiving fluoxymesterone, toxicity was greater in that group and they experienced a shorter survival (10 months) than the control group (15 months).[124]

Endocrine therapy remains the only clearly effective therapy for patients with advanced prostate cancer. Sixty to 80% of newly diagnosed patients respond with tumor regression or disease stabilization, suggesting that the majority of these patients have tumors that require androgens for continued growth. Once that requirement is lost, patients relapse, usually within 1 to 3 years. Withdrawing exposure to androgens as completely as possible appears to offer the patient the best chance for a prolonged time to progression. The palliative use of secondary endocrine manipulations or cytotoxic drugs after relapse has produced limited benefit. Secondary hormonal therapy is generally ineffective in producing objective evidence of tumor regression. No chemotherapeutic agent or combination of agents has been identified that clearly produces a clinically significant benefit. The assessment of clinical benefit in patients with newly diagnosed or hormone refractory prostate cancer remains one of the challenges for future clinical trials. New technologies for evaluating and quantifying bony metastases would greatly simplify assessment of clinical efficacy of investigational therapies. In addition, sophisticated, quality-of-life measures may help identify therapies that will produce clinically significant benefits that are not detectable by objective measures.

RENAL CELL CANCER

Background

Renal cell cancer accounts for 75% of all kidney cancers and is the almost exclusive tumor histology in adults. It arises from epithelium of the distal portion of the proximal renal tubule. Three different histologic subtypes are recognized including clear cell, granular cell, and spindle or sarcomatoid variant. It seems clear that tumors of the sarcomatoid type have a worse prognosis.

In the United States, the estimated number of new cancers of the kidney and renal pelvis for 1989 is 23,100, with 10,000 deaths expected. Renal cell cancer accounts for approximately 3% of all adult malignancies and occurs twice as often in men as in women. A rise in incidence of approximately 0.8% per year has been noted in the past 14 years, with a comparable rise in mortality. Risk factors for renal cell cancer include cigarette smoking, obesity, analgesic abuse (phenacetin), and, possibly, environmental exposure to petroleum products.[125–127]

Patients with renal cell cancer frequently present with metastatic disease at the time of diagnosis, either to distant sites or within regional lymph nodes. Hormonal therapy, chemotherapy, and biologic response modifiers have been studied extensively with only the latter approach consistently showing antitumor activity.

Hormonal Therapy

Hormonal modulation of renal cell cancers was demonstrated in animal models of the tumor and provided the rationale for the study of various hormonal interventions. Progestational agents have been most extensively studied with medroxyprogesterone acetate the most common progesterone used. In a review by Hrushesky and Murphy, a 17% response rate was noted in 228 patients treated between 1967 and 1971. However, among 415 patients treated between 1971 and 1976, only a 2% response rate was seen. The difference was thought to be attributable to more objective definitions of response. In addition to progestational agents, androgens and antiestrogens have been fairly extensively studied. Objective response rates summarized from several reports have been found to be less than 10%. Combinations of different endocrine therapies have been no more successful than the experience with single-agent studies. The occasional clinical use of these drugs in patients with metastatic renal cell cancer can likely be correlated with their relative lack of toxicity and the absence of effective alternative therapies. The relatively recent development of effective biologic therapies, albeit more toxic, has made the use of endocrine therapies difficult to justify, at least as initial therapy.[128–129]

Chemotherapy

Cytotoxic therapy plays an integral role in the treatment of many solid tumors such as bladder and germ cell tumors, but as with prostate cancer, this therapeutic modality has demonstrated little or no activity against advanced renal cell cancer. Although many patients may have nonprogressive disease for a prolonged period on chemotherapy, this should not be considered evidence of benefit from that therapy because renal cell cancer can be a slow growing tumor and can be metastatic to locations in which tumor growth may be difficult to document such as bone or retroperitoneum.

Many investigational and commercially available cytotoxics have been studied in renal cell cancer. The results of these studies have been the subject of several review articles.[128,129] For the most part, cytotoxic therapy has been almost uniformly ineffective. Vinblastine, whether given as a bolus or by continuous infusion, is considered the most active agent in the treatment of renal cell cancer. As a bolus it produces tumor reduction in 7 to 31% of patients when given on a weekly schedule. The higher response rate was found to correlate with higher dose. Of 39 patients receiving 0.2 to 0.3 mg/kg/week, 31% responded, while 15% of 96 patients receiving less than 0.2 mg/kg/week responded. More recent efforts have been made to study the drug as continuous infusion, to take advantage of potentially superior pharmacokinetics. In one study of 35 optimal patients (minimal prior therapy and good performance status) only 9% were found to respond. Others have found responses to continuous infusion vinblastine to range from 0 to 16%. The composite results from these several trials thus describes an 8% response rate among 99 patients treated with continuous infusion vinblastine.[130] One recent approach to improving the efficacy of cytotoxics in renal cell cancer has been to administer fluorodeoxyuridine (FUdR) on a variable infusion schedule. On this schedule, substantially higher doses of FUdR are tolerated and of 61 patients treated on this "circadian" infusion schedule, there have been 6 complete responses and 12 partial responses in one reported study.[131] Efforts to reproduce this experience by other investigators are underway. FUdR on other schedules has not been useful in renal cell cancer.

Another report suggested that the combination of the benzopyrone, coumarin, and cimetidine, induced tumor response in 33% of 41 patients treated.[132] The mechanism of action of this combination is unknown although, if it is effective, it may work through biologic response modification rather than by being directly cytotoxic. Others have subsequently studied this combination at the same dose and schedule and in a seemingly optimal patient population, and have found no activity in 40 patients treated.[133,134] Because essentially no toxicity is seen with this combination, dose escalation studies of coumarin have been ongoing in order to identify a maximally tolerated dose and an optimal biologic dose. It remains to be convincingly demonstrated whether coumarin with or without cimetidine has significant efficacy in the treatment of renal cell cancer.

Biologic Response Modifier Therapy

Renal cell cancer is probably the tumor most commonly associated with spontaneous regression of metastases, particularly following removal or angioinfarction of the primary tumor. Although this occurs extremely rarely, it has been postulated that immune mechanisms are responsible for the apparent spontaneous remissions. Some investigators have found that patients with metastatic renal cell cancer have impaired cellular immunity in vivo. This observation led to the rationale for the evaluation of various biologic response modifiers in the treatment of renal cell cancer. These studies have included nonspecific immunomodulators, active specific immunotherapy with autologous tumor extracts, cytokines such as interferons and interleukin-2, monoclonal antibodies, and adoptive immunotherapy with lymphokine activated killer cells. The experience with nonspecific immune stimulators such as BCG is limited but has not shown significant promise thus far. Similarly, research with monoclonal antibodies is extremely active but mostly preclinical.

Interferons

Extensive experience with the interferons has been reported, particularly with various alpha-interferon preparations. Quesada reviewed the activity of recombinant alpha interferons in renal cell cancer. In 257 patients treated with several different

TABLE 45-12. *Interferons in Advanced Renal Cell Cancer*[136]

INTERFERON TYPE	N	CR + PR (%)
Leukocyte IFN	157	32 (20%)
Lymphoblastoid IFN	184	34 (17%)
Recombinant IFN-α2	330	48 (15%)
Recombinant IFN-γ	70	2 (3%)
Recombinant IFN-β	15	2 (13%)

high-dose regimens of alpha interferon, an overall response rate of 17% (range 7 to 29%) was seen from five different trials. In two trials of low-dose alpha interferon, there were no responses in 15 patients in one study of 2 million units/m²/day and a 10% response rate in 46 patients given the same dose but only three times per week.[135] Although these studies suggest a dose-response relationship for alpha interferon, there have not been direct comparisons of different doses. Variables such as scheduling of drug administration, patient selection, and subtype of interferon studied could contribute to the differences seen among these studies. Other interferon preparations have been less extensively studied but preliminary results with beta and gamma interferon suggest a lower level of activity than the alpha interferons (Table 45-12).[136]

Cytokines

Since the 1985 report by Rosenberg et al. of significant activity with the combination of interleukin-2 and lymphokine activated killer (LAK) cells in several solid tumors, there has been intense interest in this combination.[137] Interleukin-2 is a T-cell derived lymphokine that plays a central role in immune regulation. Its primary action is to stimulate mitogenesis of T cells with IL-2 receptors. Lymphoid cells that are incubated with IL-2 develop the capacity to lyse fresh tumor cells. These "lymphokine-activated killer cells" are the effector cells in the concept of adoptive immunotherapy. In the experience with adoptive immunotherapy from the National Cancer Institute, 36 patients with renal cell cancer have been treated with 4 complete responses and 8 partial responses, for an overall response rate of 33%. In their initial experience with IL-2 alone, only 1 of 21 treated patients responded.[138] A recent update of their data finds that the response rate for this combination remains at 35%, while their results with IL-2 alone have improved with 21% of 52 patients so treated having a complete or partial response.[136] Several other schedules of IL-2 with and without LAK cells have been studied, with response rates ranging from 7 to 26% (Table 45-13).[139–143] Whether ex vivo expansion of LAK cells is required to achieve the antitumor effect that has been observed is unclear. One European study found that 17% of 18 patients treated with IL-2 alone responded, while 26% of 19 patients treated with IL-2 plus LAK cells responded.[139] The National Cancer Institute is conduct-

TABLE 45-13. *Results with IL-2 + LAK Cells in Advanced Renal Cell Cancer*

STUDY	TREATMENT	N	CR + PR (%)
Philip et al.[139]	IL-2 Alone	18	3 (17%)
	IL-2 + LAK	19	6 (26%)
Weiss et al.[140]	IL-2(C.I.) + LAK	27	7 (26%)
	IL-2(Bolus) + LAK	31	6 (19%)
Marshall et al.[141]	IL-2(Low Dose) + LAK	10	1 (10%)
Bukowski et al.[142]	IL-2 Alone (Bolus)	43	3 (7%)
Fisher et al.[143]	IL-2 + LAK	32	5 (16%)
Rosenberg, Spiess, Laferniere[144]	IL-2 + LAK	72	25 (35%)
	IL-2 Alone	52	11 (21%)

ing a randomized study of IL-2 + LAK versus IL-2 alone. Final results of that study were not yet reported at the time of this writing. Therapy with IL-2 + LAK is toxic when given at the high doses employed in most of these studies, with most patients requiring intensive monitoring. IL-2 causes most of the toxicity, which includes generalized malaise, fever, nausea, vomiting, diarrhea, hepatic dysfunction characterized by hyperbilirubinemia, moderate myelosuppression, capillary leak syndrome with interstitial pulmonary edema, decrease in systemic vascular resistance, hypotension, and subsequent renal dysfunction. Efforts to improve the results of IL-2 in the treatment of renal cell cancer include modification of the scheduling in which continuous infusion is used in combination with bolus IL-2, in order to enhance the pharmacokinetic profile of the drug. PEG-IL-2 is polyethylene glycol modified IL-2 that has a longer half-life and, therefore, may also improve the pharmacokinetic profile of IL-2. Trials are ongoing with this IL-2 preparation.

In addition to IL-2 modifications, clinical trials with lymphocytes harvested from resected tumor specimens and then expanded in vitro with IL-2 are underway. These tumor infiltrating lymphocytes (TIL's) have been shown to be more potent than LAK cells in inducing regression of established metastases in animal tumor models.[144] There are not yet results from clinical trials in humans to assess whether this approach will be more effective than that seen with LAK cells.

Since 1984, systemic therapy for the treatment of renal cell cancer has begun to change the view of this disease as a resistant one. At present it is clear that the use of endocrine therapy for the treatment of renal cell cancer is highly unlikely to be of any benefit. Cytotoxic therapy may offer a modestly better chance for antitumor response than progestin therapy;

however, the recent reports of tumor response to FUdR and coumarin requires further investigation before any concrete claims of efficacy can be made.

The most promising modality for research is through biologic response modification. Alpha interferons have consistently produced tumor reduction in 15 to 20% of patients. Given their probable mechanism of action, patients with lesser tumor bulk are more likely to have responsive disease. This forms the rationale for an ongoing study in which alpha interferon is being compared to observation in the adjuvant setting. Currently, the most exciting laboratory and clinical work centers on the biologic effects of interleukin-2. Apparent synergy of IL-2 with interferon and of cytotoxics with interferon is beginning to be explored in clinical trials. Identification of tumor specific and tumor associated antigens may add yet another modality as the understanding and technology of monoclonal antibody therapy grows.

CONCLUSION

There is ample reason for optimism in the treatment of tumors of the genitourinary tract. The past decade has seen tremendous growth in our understanding of the multifaceted nature of the problems presented by these tumors. Improved definitions of prognosis for patients with germ cell cancer has allowed a more tailored approach to recommended therapy. Bladder cancer can now be considered a chemotherapy sensitive disease. We are still learning how and when to best employ these cytotoxic agents. Prostate cancer remains a refractory disease although improved endocrine therapies have become available in the past several years. As we better understand the mechanisms of control of growth of prostate cancer, drugs that interfere with these growth factors may offer a major new modality for this previously refractory disease. Finally, renal cell cancer has been shown to be responsive to therapies that modulate the host's immune response to tumor. Refinements in our understanding of the mechanisms by which immune modulation effects tumor lysis should lead to even more effective therapies.

Further clinical and laboratory studies will likely soon lead to greater advances in the treatment of these tumors. Although there have not yet been major changes in the survival of patients with prostate, kidney, and bladder cancers, significant steps have already been made toward that goal.

ACKNOWLEDGEMENT

The author wishes to thank Dr. Leo Lacerna and Ms. Linda Ferragut of the Emmes Corporation for their assistance in the preparation of this chapter.

REFERENCES

1. SILVERBERG, E., and LUBERA, J. A. Cancer statistics, 1989. CA, *39*:1, 1989.

2. MATANOSKI, G. M., and ELLIOTT, F. A. Bladder cancer epidemiology. Epidemiol. Rev., *3*:203, 1981.

3. TORTI, F. M., and LUM, B. L. The biology and treatment of superficial bladder cancer. J. Clin. Oncol., 2:505, 1984.

4. TORTI, F. M., and LUM, B. L. Superficial bladder cancer: Risk of recurrence and potential role for interferon therapy. Cancer, 59:613, 1987.

5. WHITMORE, W. F., JR. Management of bladder cancer. Curr. Probl. Cancer, 4:3, 1979.

6. ZINCKE, H., PATTERSON, D. F., UTZ, D. C., and BENSON, R. C., JR. Pelvic lymphadenectomy and radical cystectomy for transitional cell carcinoma of the bladder with pelvic nodal disease. Br. J. Urol., 47:156, 1985.

7. SKINNER, D. G. Current perspectives in the management of high-grade invasive bladder cancer. Cancer, 45:1866, 1980.

8. YAGODA, A. et al. Cis-dichlorodiamineplatinum (II) in advanced bladder cancer. Cancer Treat. Rep., 60:917, 1976.

9. FAGG, S. L. et al. Cis-diamminedichloroplatinum (DDP) as initial therapy of invasive bladder cancer. Br. J. Urol., 56:296, 1984.

10. PEARSON, B. S., and RAGHAVAN, D. First-line intravenous cisplatin for deeply invasive bladder cancer: Update on 70 cases. Br. J. Urol., 57:690, 1985.

11. SOLOWAY, M. S. et al. A comparison of cisplatin and the combination of cisplatin and cyclophosphamide in advanced urothelial cancer. Cancer, 52:767, 1983.

12. SOLOWAY, M. S. Cis-diamminedichloroplatinum II in advanced urothelial cancer. J. Urol., 120:716, 1978.

13. TRONER, M. Phase III comparison of cisplatin alone versus cisplatin, doxorubicin and cyclophosphamide in the treatment of bladder (urothelial) cancer: A Southeastern Cancer Study Group Trial. J. Urol., 137:660, 1987.

14. HUBEN, R. P., DRAGONE, N., and TOMASELLO, E. Chemotherapy of metastatic bladder cancer. RPMI Experience. J. Urol., 135:278a, 1986.

15. HILLCOAT, B. L., and RAGHAVEN, D. A randomized comparison of cisplatinum (C) versus cisplatinum and methotrexate (C + M) in advanced bladder cancer. Proc. Am. Soc. Clin. Oncol., 5:426a, 1986.

16. KHANNDEKAR, J. D. et al. Comparative activity and toxicity of cis-diamminedichloro-platinum (DDP) and a combination of doxorubicin, cyclophosphamide, and DDP in disseminated transitional cell carcinomas of the urinary tract. J. Clin. Oncol., 3:539, 1985.

17. DE LENA, M. et al. Cis-diamminedichloroplatinum activity in bidimensionally measurable metastatic lesions of bladder carcinoma. Tumori, 70:85, 1984.

18. HAREWOOD, I. M. et al. Treatment of advanced bladder cancer using cis-platinum. Aust. N.Z.J. Surg., 53:333, 1983.

19. The London and Oxford Co-operative Urological Cancer Group, Chemotherapy Sub-Committee. A phase II study of cis-platinum in patients with recurrent bladder carcinoma. Br. J. Urol., 53:444, 1981.

20. PETERS, P. C., and O'NEILL, M. R. Cis-diamminedichloroplatinum as a therapeutic agent in metastatic transitional cell carcinoma. J. Urol., 123:375, 1979.

21. HERR, H. W. Cis-diamminedichloride platinum II in the treatment of advanced bladder cancer. J. Urol., 123:853, 1979.

22. YAGODA, A. Phase II trials with cis-dichlorodiammine-platinum (II) in the treatment of urotherial cancer. Cancer Treat. Reps., 63:1565, 1979.

23. MERRIN, C. Treatment of advanced bladder cancer with cis-diamminedichloroplatinum (II). A pilot study. J. Urol., 119:493, 1977.

24. OLIVER, R. T. D. et al. Methotrexate in the treatment of metastatic and recurrent primary transitional cell carcinoma. J. Urol., 131:483, 1983.

25. OLIVER, R. T. D. Methotrexate as salvage or adjunctive therapy for primary invasive carcinoma of the bladder. Cancer Treat. Rep., 65:179, 1981.

26. NATALE, R. B. et al. Methotrexate: An active drug in bladder cancer. Cancer, 47:1246, 1981.

27. TURNER, A. G. Methotrexate in advanced bladder cancer. Cancer Treat. Rep., 65:183, 1981.

28. HALL, R. R. et al. Metho-trexate treatment for advanced bladder cancer. Br. J. Cancer, 35:40, 1977.

29. MIDDLEMAN, E., LUCE, J., and FREI, E., III. Clinical trials with Adriamycin. Cancer, 28:844, 1971.

30. O'BRYAN, R. M. et al. Phase II evaluation of Adriamycin in human neoplasia. Cancer, 32:1, 1973.

31. O'BRYAN, R. M. et al. Dose response evaluation of Adriamycin in human neoplasia. Cancer, 39:1940, 1977.

32. SCHULMAN, C. C., WESPES, E., DELCOUR, C., and STRUYVEN, J. Intra-arterial chemotherapy of infiltrative bladder carcinoma. Eur. Urol., 11:220, 1985.

33. KNIGHT, E. W., PAGAND, M., HAHN, R. G., and HORTON, J. Comparison of 5-FU and doxorubicin in the treatment of carcinoma of the bladder. Cancer Treat. Rep., 67:514, 1983.

34. GAGLIANO, R. et al. Adriamycin versus Adriamycin plus cis-diamminedichloroplatinum (DDP) in advanced transitional cell bladder carcinoma. Am. J. Clin. Oncol., 6:215, 1983.

35. YAGODA, A. et al. Adriamycin in advanced urinary tract cancer. Cancer, 39:279, 1977.

36. FOSSA, S. D., and GUDMUNDSEN, T. E. Single-drug chemotherapy with 5-FU and Adriamycin in metastatic bladder carcinoma. Br. J. Urol., 53:320, 1981.

37. PAVONE-MACALUSO, M., and EORTC GENITO-URINARY TRACT CO-OPERATIVE GROUP A. Single-drug chemotherapy of bladder cancer with Adriamycin, VM-26 or bleomycin. Eur. Urol., 2:138, 1976.

38. MERRIN, C. et al. Chemotherapy of bladder carcinoma with cyclophosphamide and Adriamycin. J. Urol., 114:884, 1975.

39. BLUMENREICH, M. S., YAGODA, A., NATALE, R. B., and WATSON, R. C. Phase II trial of vinblastine sulfate for metastatic urothelial tract tumors. Cancer, 50:435, 1982.

40. AHMED, T. et al. Vinblastine and methotrexate for advanced bladder cancer. J. Urol., 133:602, 1984.

41. SMALLEY, R. V., BARTOLUCCI, G., HEMSTREET, G., and HESTER, M. A phase II evaluation of a 3-drug combination of cyclophosphamide, doxorubicin and 5-fluorouracil in patients with advanced bladder carcinoma or stage D prostate carcinoma. J. Urol., 125:191, 1980.

42. DEKERNION, J. B. The chemotherapy of advanced bladder carcinoma. Cancer Res., 37:2771, 1977.

43. FOX, M. The effect of cyclophosphamide on some urinary tract tumours. Br. J. Urol., 37:399, 1965.

44. YAGODA, A. Chemotherapy of urothelial tract tumors. Cancer, 60:574, 1987.

45. STOTER, G. et al. Combination chemotherapy with cisplatin and methotrexate in advanced transitional cell cancer of the bladder. J. Urol., 137:663, 1986.

46. CARMICHAEL, J. et al. Cisplatin and methotrexate in the treatment of transitional cell carcinoma of the urinary tract. J. Urol., 57:299, 1985.

47. OLIVER, R. T. D., KWOK, H. K., HIGHMAN, W. J., and WAXMAN, J.

Methotrexate cisplatin and carboplatin as single agents and in combination for metastatic bladder cancer. Br. J. Urol., *58*:31, 1986.

48. WALTHER, P. J., and WALKER, R. A. Treatment of advanced bladder carcinoma with once-monthly methotrexate, vinblastine, and cisplatin. J. Urol., *137*:215a, 1987.

49. ROSENBERG, S. J., and WILLIAMS, R. D. Cis-platinum, methotrexate, and vinblastine combination chemotherapy (CMV) for advanced carcinoma of the bladder and upper urinary tract. J. Urol., *137*:216a, 1987.

50. HARKER, W. G. et al. Cisplatin, methotrexate, and vinblastine (CMV): An effective chemotherapy regimen for metastatic transitional cell carcinoma of the urinary tract. A Northern California Oncology Group Study. J. Clin. Oncol., *3*:1463, 1985.

51. STERNBERG, C. N. et al. M-VAC (methotrexate, Adriamycin and cisplatin) for advanced transitional cell carcinoma of the urothelium. Proc. Am. Soc. Clin. Oncol., *3*:156a, 1984.

52. SOLOWAY, M. S. Incorporation of M-VAC combination chemotherapy in the treatment of patients with invasive and metastatic bladder cancer. Eur. Urol., *14*:42, 1988.

53. CHONG, C. et al. M-VAC as salvage chemotherapy in transitional cell carcinoma (TCC) of the urothelium previously treated with cisplatin combination chemotherapy [Abstract]. Proc. Am. Assoc. Cancer Res., *28*:810, 1987.

54. CONNOR, J., RAPPAPORT, F., and SAWCZUK, I. S. Results with the use of MVAC in therapeutic and abjunctive settings [Abstract]. J. Urol., *4*:662, 1987.

55. SHEEHAN, R., SAGALOWSKY, A. I., BALABAN, E., and COX, J. Initial experience with M-VAC for metastatic transitional cell carcinoma (TCC) [Abstract]. J. Urol., *4*:664, 1987.

56. DE VRIES, C. R., FREIHA, F. S., TORTI, F. Combination CMV chemotherapy plus surgery for advanced urothelial carcinoma [Abstract]. Proc. Am. Soc. Clin. Oncol., *7*:418a, 1988.

57. DROZ, J. P. et al. Pilot phase II trial of pre and post-operative cisplatin, methotrexate and vinblastine in infiltrating bladder cancer: Preliminary results. 2nd Internat. Congr. Neoadjuvant Chemother., Feb. 19–21, 1988, p. 20.

58. VOGELZANG, N. J. et al. Neoadjuvant chemotherapy for locally invasive transitional cell carcinoma of the bladder (TCCB) [Abstract]. Proc. Am. Assoc. Cancer Res., *28*:809a, 1987.

59. LEE, M. L. et al. Neoadjuvant M-VAC with intra-arterial (I.A.) cisplatin (CDDP) in locally advanced transitional cell carcinoma of the bladder. Phase I/II trial. Proc. Am. Assoc. Cancer Res., *28*:757a, 1987.

60. ZINCKE, H., SEN, S., HAHN, R. G., and KEATING, J. P. Neoadjuvant chemotherapy for locally advanced transitional cell carcinoma of the bladder: Do local findings suggest a potential for salvage of the bladder? Mayo Clin. Proc., *63*:16, 1988.

61. SCHER, H. et al. Neoadjuvant M-VAC (methotrexate, vinblastine, Adriamycin and cisplatin): Effect on the primary bladder lesion. J. Urol., *139*:470, 1988.

62. SIMON, S. D. et al. Treatment of locally invasive transitional cell carcinoma of the bladder (TCCB) with chemotherapy followed by partial cystectomy or surveillance [Abstract]. Proc. Am. Soc. Clin. Oncol., *7*:957a, 1988.

63. BUKOWSKI, R. M., MONATIE, J. E., LEE, M., GANAPATHI, R. Neoadjuvant M-VAC with intra-arterial cis-platin in locally advanced transitional cell carcinoma of the bladder [Abstract]. Proc. Am. Soc. Clin. Oncol., *6*:424a, 1987.

64. JASKE, G., FROMMHOD, H., and NEDDEN, D. Z. Combined radiation and chemotherapy for locally advanced transitional cell carcinoma of the urinary bladder. Cancer, *55*:1659, 1985.

65. COPPIN, C., and BROWN, E. The GU Tumor Group. Concurrent cisplatin with radiation for locally advanced bladder cancer: A pilot study suggesting improved survival [Abstract]. Proc. Am. Soc. Clin. Oncol., *5*:382a, 1986.

66. SHIPLEY, W. U. et al. Treatment of invasive bladder cancer by cisplatin and radiation in patients unsuited for surgery. JAMA, *258*:931, 1987.

67. ROTMAN, M. et al. Treatment of advanced bladder carcinoma with irradiation and concomitant 5-Fluorouracil infusion. Cancer, *59*:710, 1987.

68. RUSSEL, K. J. et al. Transitional cell carcinoma of the urinary bladder: Histologic clearance with combined 5-Fu chemotherapy and radiation therapy. Radiology, *167*:845, 1988.

69. Annual Cancer Statistics Review including Cancer Trends: 1950–1985, NCI, NIH, DHHS, 1988.

70. EINHORN, L. H. et al. Cancer of the testes. In *Cancer Principles and Practice of Oncology.* Edited by V. T. DeVita, S. Hellman, and S. A. Rosenberg. Philadelphia, J. B. Lippincott Co., 1989, pp. 1071–1098.

71. BOSL, G. J. et al. A specific karyotypic abnormality in germ cell tumors. Proc. Am. Soc. Clin. Oncol., *8*:131, 1989.

72. BIRCH, R. et al. Prognostic factors for favorable outcome in disseminated germ cell tumors. J. Clin. Oncol., *4*:400, 1986.

73. BOSL, G. J. et al. Multivariate analysis of prognostic variables in patients with metastatic testicular cancer. Cancer Res., *43*:3403, 1983.

74. WITTES, R. E. et al. Chemotherapy of germ cell tumors of the testis. Cancer, *37*:637, 1976.

75. CHENG, E. et al. Germ cell tumor: VAB II in metastatic testicular cancer. Cancer, *42*:2162, 1978.

76. BOSL, G. J. et al. VAB-6: An effective chemotherapy regimen for patients with germ cell tumors. J. Clin. Oncol., *4*:1493, 1986.

77. BOSL, G. J. et al. A randomized trial of etoposide + cisplatin versus VAB-6 in patients with good prognosis germ cell tumors. J. Clin. Oncol., *6*:1231, 1988.

78. EINHORN, L. H. Chemotherapy of disseminated germ cell tumors. Cancer, *60*:570, 1987.

79. LOEHRER, P. J. et al. Salvage therapy in recurrent germ cell cancer: Ifosfamide and cisplatin plus either vinblastine or etoposide. Ann. Intern. Med., *109*:540, 1988.

80. NICHOLS, C. R. et al. Dose-intensive chemotherapy in refractory germ cell cancer—A phase I/II trial of high-dose carboplatin and etoposide with autologous bone marrow transplantation. J. Clin. Oncol., *7*:932, 1989.

81. EISENBERGER, M. A., O'DWYER, P. J., and FRIEDMAN, M. A. Gonadotropin hormone-releasing hormone analogues: A new therapeutic approach for prostatic carcinoma. J. Clin. Oncol., *4*:414, 1986.

82. TOLIS, G. et al. Growth inhibition in patients with prostatic cancer treated with luteinizing hormone releasing hormone agonists. Proc. Natl. Acad. Sci. U.S.A., *79*:1658, 1982.

83. BORGMANN, V. et al. Treatment of advanced prostatic cancer with LH-RH analogues. Lancet, *1*:1097, 1982.

84. ALLEN, J. M. et al. Advanced carcinoma of the prostate: Treatment with a gonadotropin releasing hormone agonist. Br. Med. J., *286*:1607, 1983.

85. KOUTSILIERIS, M. et al. Objective response and disease outcome in 59 patients with stage D2 prostatic cancer treated with buserelin or orchiectomy. Urology, *27*:221, 1986.

86. DEBRUYNE, F. M. J. Results of a Dutch trial with the LH-RH agonist buserelin in patients with metastatic prostatic cancer and results of EORTC studies in prostatic cancer. Am. J. Clin. Oncol., *11*:S33, 1988.

87. WAXMAN, J. H. et al. The first clinical use of depot buserelin for advanced prostatic carcinoma. Cancer Chemother. Pharmacol., 18:174, 1986.

88. SOLOWAY, M. S. Efficacy of buserelin in advanced prostate cancer and comparison with historical controls. Am. J. Clin. Oncol., 11:S29, 1988.

89. SCHROEDER, F. H. Metastatic cancer of the prostate managed with buserelin versus buserelin plus cyproterone acetate. J. Urol., 137:912, 1987.

90. PRESANT, C. A. et al. Buserelin treatment of advanced prostatic carcinoma. Cancer, 59:1713, 1987.

91. FALKSON, G., and VOROBIOF, D. A. Intranasal buserelin in the treatment of advanced prostatic cancer: A phase II trial. J. Clin. Oncol., 5:1419, 1987.

92. AHMED, S. R. et al. A new hormonal therapy for prostatic cancer: Long-term clinical and hormonal responses. Br. J. Urol., 58:534, 1986.

93. DEBRUYNE, F. M. J. et al. Long-term therapy with a depot luteinizing hormone-releasing hormone analogue (zoladex) in patients with advanced prostatic carcinoma. J. Urol., 140:775, 1988.

94. AHMANN, F. R. et al. A sustained release, monthly luteinizing hormone-releasing hormone analogue for the treatment of advanced prostate cancer. J. Clin. Oncol., 5:912, 1987.

95. EMTAGE, L. A. et al. Phase II study of zoladex depot in advanced prostatic cancer with special reference to criteria of response and survival. Br. J. Urol., 60:436, 1987.

96. BEACOCK, C. J. et al. The treatment of metastatic prostatic cancer with the slow release LH-RH analogue zoladex (ICI 118630). Br. J. Urol., 59:436, 1987.

97. HOLDAWAY, L. M. et al. Treatment of metastatic prostate carcinoma with the depot LH-RH analogue zoladex. Prostate, 12:119, 1988.

98. VAN CANGH, P. H., and OPSOMER, R. J. Treatment of advanced carcinoma of the prostate with a depot luteinizing hormone-releasing hormone analogue (ICI-118630). J. Urol., 137:61, 1987.

99. GARNICK, M. B. Leuprolide versus diethylstilbestrol for previously untreated stage D2 prostate cancer. Urology, 27:21, 1986.

100. PARMAR, H. et al. Orchiectomy versus long-acting D-Trp-6-LHRH in advanced prostatic cancer. Br. J. Urol., 59:248, 1987.

101. BOCCARDO, F. et al. Long-term results with a long-acting formulation of D-TRP-6-LHRH in patients with prostate cancer. An Italian prostatic cancer project (P.O.N.C.A.P.) study. Prostate, 11:243, 1987.

102. MATHE, G. et al. Phase II trial with D-TRP-6-LHRH in prostatic carcinoma: Comparison with other hormonal agents. Prostate, 9:327, 1986.

103. KAISARY, A. V. et al. A comparison between surgical orchidectomy and LH-RH analogue in the treatment of advanced prostatic carcinoma—a multi-centre clinical study. In Management of Advanced Cancer of Prostate and Bladder. Edited by P. H. Smith and M. Pavone-Macaluso. New York, Alan R. Liss, Inc., 1988, pp. 89–100.

104. VENNER, P. M. et al. Megestrol acetate plus minidose DES in the treatment of carcinoma of the prostate. Semin. Oncol., 15:62, 1988.

105. JOHNSON, D. E. et al. Medical castration using megestrol acetate and minidose estrogen. Urology, 31:371, 1988.

106. PAVONE-MACALUSO, M. et al. Comparison of diethylstilbestrol, cyproterone acetate and medroxy-progesterone in the treatment of advanced prostatic cancer: Final analysis of a randomized phase III trial of the EORTC urological group. J. Urol., 136:624, 1986.

107. LABRIE, F. et al. Combination therapy with flutamide and castration (LHRH agonist or orchiectomy) in previously untreated patients with clinical stage D2 prostate cancer: Today's therapy of choice. J. Steroid Biochem., 30:107, 1988.

108. CRAWFORD, E. D. et al. A controlled trial of Leuprolide with and without flutamide in prostatic carcinoma. N. Engl. J. Med., 321:419, 1989.

109. TRACHTENBERG, J., and PONT, A. Ketoconazole in the treatment of metastatic prostatic cancer. Lancet, 2:433, 1984.

110. WILLIAMS, G. et al. Objective responses to ketoconazole therapy in patients with relapsed progressive prostatic carcinoma. Br. J. Urol., 58:45, 1986.

111. TAPAZOGLOU, E. et al. High-dose ketoconazole therapy in patients with metastatic prostate cancer. Am. J. Clin. Oncol., 9:369, 1986.

112. JOHNSON, D. E. et al. Ketoconazole therapy for hormonally refractive metastatic prostate cancer. Urology, 31:132, 1988.

113. HARNETT, P. R. et al. Aminoglutethimide in advanced prostatic carcinoma. Br. J. Urol., 59:323, 1987.

114. SAMOJLIK, E. et al. Medical adrenalectomy for advanced prostatic cancer: Clinical and hormonal effects. Am. J. Clin. Oncol., 11:579, 1988.

115. LABRIE, F. et al. Benefits of combination therapy with flutamide in patients relapsing after castration. Br. J. Urol., 61:341, 1988.

116. DE KERNION, J. B., MURPHY, G. P., and PRIORE, R. Comparison of flutamide and emcyt in hormone-refractory metastatic prostatic cancer. Urology, 31:312, 1988.

117. CROMBIE, C. et al. Phase II study of megestrol acetate in metastatic carcinoma of the prostate. Br. J. Urol., 59:443, 1987.

118. HORTON, J., ROSENBAUM, C., and CUMMINGS, F. J. Tamoxifen in advanced prostate cancer: An ECOG pilot study. Prostate, 12:173, 1988.

119. EISENBERGER, M. A. et al. A reevaluation of nonhormonal cytotoxic chemotherapy in the treatment of prostatic carcinoma. J. Clin. Oncol., 3:827, 1985.

120. SCOTT, W. W. et al. Chemotherapy of advanced prostatic carcinoma with cyclophosphamide or 5-fluorouracil: Results of the first national randomized study. J. Urol., 114:909, 1975.

121. DEWYS, W. D. et al. A comparative clinical trial of Adriamycin and 5-fluorouracil in advanced prostatic cancer: Prognostic factors and response. Prostate, 4:1, 1983.

122. SEIFTER, E. J. et al. A trial of chemotherapy followed by hormonal therapy for previously untreated metastatic carcinoma of the prostate. J. Clin. Oncol., 4:1365, 1986.

123. SUAREZ, A. J. et al. Androgen priming and cytotoxic chemotherapy in advanced prostatic cancer. Cancer Chemother. Pharmacol., 8:261, 1982.

124. MANNI, A. et al. Androgen priming and response to chemotherapy in advanced prostatic cancer. J. Urol., 136:1242, 1986.

125. YU, M. C. et al. Cigarette smoking, obesity, diuretic use and coffee consumption as risk factors for renal cell carcinoma. J. Natl. Cancer Inst., 77:351, 1986.

126. LORNOY, W. et al. Renal cell carcinoma, a new complication of analgesic nephropathy. Lancet, 1:1271, 1986.

127. McLAUGHLIN, J. K. et al. Petroleum-related employment and renal cell cancer. J. Occup. Med., 27:672, 1985.

128. HRUSHESKY, W. J., and MURPHY, G. P. Current status of the therapy of advanced renal carcinoma. J. Surg. Oncol., 9:277, 1977.

129. HARRIS, D. T. Hormonal therapy and chemotherapy of renal cell carcinoma. Semin. Oncol., 10:422, 1983.

130. YAGODA, A., and BANDER, N. Failure of cytotoxic chemotherapy, 1983–1988, and the emerging role of monoclonal antibodies for renal cancer. Urol. Int., in press.

131. Hrushesky, W. J. M., et al. Circadian modified FUdR infusion controls progressive metastatic renal cell cancer (RCC). Proc. Am. Soc. Clin. Oncol., 8:134, 1989.

132. Marshall, M. E. et al. Treatment of metastatic renal cancer with coumarin (1,2-benzopyrone) and cimetidine: A pilot study. J. Clin. Oncol., 5:862, 1987.

133. Venook, A. P., Davenport, Y., and Tseng, A. Activity of coumarin and cimetidine in metastatic renal cell carcinoma [Letter]. J. Clin. Oncol., 7:402, 1989.

134. Herrman, R. et al. Coumarin and cimetidine in the treatment of metastatic renal cell carcinoma. Proc. Am. Soc. Clin. Oncol., 7:131, 1988.

135. Quesada, J. R. Biologic response modifiers in the therapy of metastatic renal cell carcinoma. Semin. Oncol., 15:396, 1988.

136. Linehan, W. M., Shipley, W. U., and Longo, D. L. Cancer of the kidney and ureter. In *Cancer Principles and Practice of Oncology.* Edited by V. T. DeVita, S. Hellman, and S. A. Rosenberg. Philadelphia, J. B. Lippincott Co. 1989, pp. 993–998.

137. Rosenberg, S. A. et al. Observations on the systemic administration of autologous lymphokine-activated killer cells and recombinant IL-2 to patients with metastatic cancer. N. Engl. J. Med., 313:1485, 1985.

138. Rosenberg, S. A. et al. A progress report on the treatment of 157 patients with advanced cancer using LAK cells and IL-2 or high-dose IL-2 alone. N. Engl. J. Med., 316:889, 1987.

139. Philip, T. et al. Recombinant human interleukin-2 with or without LAK cells in metastatic renal cell carcinoma: The European experience. Proc. Am. Soc. Clin. Oncol., 8:130, 1989.

140. Weiss, G. R. et al. A randomized phase II trial of continuous infusion (CI) IL-2 or bolus injection (BI) IL-2 plus LAK cells for advanced renal cell cancer. Proc. Am. Soc. Clin. Oncol., 8:131, 1989.

141. Marshall, M. E. et al. Treatment of metastatic renal cell carcinoma with "low dose" IL-2 and LAK cells. Proc. Am. Soc. Clin. Oncol., 8:135, 1989.

142. Bukowski, R. M. et al. Phase II evaluation of recombinant IL-2 in metastatic renal cell carcinoma. Proc. Am. Soc. Clin. Oncol., 8:143, 1989.

143. Fisher, R. I. et al. Metastatic renal cancer treated with IL-2 and LAK cells. Ann. Intern. Med., 108:518, 1988.

144. Rosenberg, S. A., Spiess, P., and Laferniere, R. A new approach to the adoptive immunotherapy with tumor infiltrating lymphocytes. Science, 233:1318, 1986.

Therapy of Metastatic Renal Cell Carcinoma

J. Philip Kuebler

S ymptomatic metastatic disease leads to clinical presentation in up to one third of patients with renal cell cancer. Mortality in these patients is 74% at 1 year and 96% by 3 years.[1] However, the clinical course of metastatic renal cell cancer is quite variable. Occasional patients have prolonged periods between diagnosis and development of metastases. Some may survive for 5 to 10 years with stable metastatic tumor deposits. The unpredictable course of renal cell cancer makes evaluation of treatment programs difficult. This problem is further complicated by the occurrence of spontaneous regression of metastatic disease reported in some patients. The incidence of this phenomenon is low, approximately 0.4 to 0.8%, and cannot explain the variable course of the disease.[2]

NEPHRECTOMY

There is no evidence that nephrectomy in the presence of metastatic disease increases the incidence of spontaneous regression. A retrospective review of 93 patients with metastatic renal cancer treated at MD Anderson Hospital failed to reveal a survival advantage for the 43 patients who underwent nephrectomy.[3] Middleton observed no regression of pulmonary metastases in similarly treated patients, and none survived more than 2 years.[4] Various adjuvant therapies, including radiotherapy, hormonal therapy, and chemotherapy after palliative nephrectomy, also failed to induce regression or alter survival in a series of patients treated at the Ochsner Clinic between 1945 and 1978.[5] Experience with embolization followed by delayed nephrectomy has been reported by three groups, two of which were multi-institutional. The overall complete and partial response rate in 164 treated patients was only 10%.[6-8] Although an additional 25 patients had stabilization of disease, median survival in these studies remained 6 to 7 months.

Nephrectomy has been suggested as a means to enhance the response rate to biologic therapy in renal cancer. It is theorized that reduction in the bulky primary lesion may allow immunotherapy to better control residual sites of disease. To date, definitive evidence supporting this concept is lacking.[9] The incidence of postoperative complications and perioperative mortality from nephrectomy in otherwise debilitated patients can be significant. The role of adjuvant nephrectomy remains to be defined, and should be confined to experimental protocols that specifically address this issue.

RESECTION OF METASTASES

Resection of solitary or even multiple pulmonary and other metastases may result in improved survival. Five-year survival in patients undergoing resection of isolated metastases ranges from 13 to 45%. Poorer results are obtained when metastatic sites other than lung are excised as noted by Dineen.[10] Although some authors report an improved prognosis for those with metastatic disease presenting after nephrectomy, this finding was not confirmed by a recent report in which survival for patients with and without metastases at diagnosis was identical.[10] It must be remembered that aggressive surgical management of isolated metastases is a palliative therapeutic modality since all patients eventually die of recurrent disease.

HORMONAL THERAPY

The possibility that hormonal therapy might induce regressions in metastatic renal cell cancer came directly from the model of estrogen-induced kidney tumors in male Syrian golden hamsters first described by Mathews in 1947.[11] By the early 1970s, Bloom reported a 15% response rate among 272 reviewed cases, including 80 of his own patients treated with progesterone or androgens.[12] In their 1977 review, Hrushesky and Murphy were unable to confirm these results. These authors collected 416 patients treated from 1971 to 1977, but noted only 8 responses (1.8%).[13] In general, response criteria and patient populations were poorly defined in the early reports of hormonal therapy. Harris has noted that subjective and objective responses were often combined to give a seemingly higher response rate.[14] The use of more stringent criteria for patient selection and response assessment most likely explains the poorer results of later trials.

Following reports that occasional renal cell carcinomas had low titers of estrogen and progesterone receptors, a number of trials were begun to test the effect of antiestrogens in advanced disease.[14] The results of these trials are summarized in Table 46-1. Among 192 patients treated with a wide range of daily doses, only 5% had objective responses. Combinations of hormonal agents with other hormones or chemotherapeutic drugs have not increased response rates. A review of the available literature by Harris noted only 12 objective responses in 179 patients (7%) treated with a variety of combinations.[14] In the only randomized trial, patients receiving either vinblastine or methyl-CCNU plus medroxyprogesterone acetate fared no better than those receiving these same drugs without the hormone.[17]

SINGLE-AGENT CHEMOTHERAPY

Numerous chemotherapeutic agents have been tested for activity in metastatic renal cell cancer. Among 33 drugs reviewed by Hrushesky and Murphy in 1977, vinblastine was most effective with a response rate of 25% (33 of 135 patients).[13] However, if stable disease is discounted as a positive

TABLE 46-1. *Antiestrogen Therapy in Metastatic Renal Cell Cancer*

DRUG	DAILY DOSE	NUMBER OF PATIENTS	NUMBER OF CR + PR*
Nafoxidine[14]	180 mg	20	1
Nafoxidine[15]	4 mg/kg	19	2
Tamoxifen[14]	20 mg	15	0
Tamoxifen[14]	20 mg	79	5
Tamoxifen[14]	20 mg	9	0
Tamoxifen[16]	30 mg	12	0
Tamoxifen[16]	40 mg	23	0
Tamoxifen[14]	80 mg	15	2
Totals		192	10

*CR = complete response; PR = partial response.

response, this result is decreased to 19%. Most of the other agents reported in this review were tested in too few patients to accurately assess potential activity. During the last decade, at least 43 antineoplastic drugs have been tested in adequately designed phase II trials. Although stabilization of disease or minor responses have been noted in 10 to 56% of patients receiving these drugs, the clinical utility of these results in terms of survival prolongation or even symptom palliation remains doubtful.

Many phase II drug trials reported since the review by Hrushesky and Murphy have noted occasional objective responses in metastatic renal cell cancer. In most studies, complete and partial response rates have been less than 10% and usually last for only a few months (Table 46-2). Of note is that activity for vinblastine is much less than previously reported. Five different trials employing intermittent (2 studies) or continuous (3 studies) infusion schedules have resulted in only 9 objective responses among 108 patients (8.3%).[14,17,19–21] Overall, results remain discouragingly poor, and no standard single-agent chemotherapy exists for this disease.

COMBINATION CHEMOTHERAPY

Despite the lack of activity with the use of single agents, a number of different combined chemotherapy regimens have been tested in metastatic renal cell cancer. Most of these have included vinblastine or a nitrosourea such as CCNU in a multidrug combination (Table 46-3). Overall, objective responses have been noted in only 14% of 445 patients treated with combination chemotherapy. Although 5 trials have reported response rates above 20%, 3 of these have included fewer than 20 patients.[14] No studies confirming the results of any of these regimens exist, except for the combination of vinblastine and CCNU. In this case, 4 trials employing essentially identical

TABLE 46-2. *Reported Responses to Single-Agent Chemotherapy in Metastatic Renal Cell Cancer**

DRUG	NUMBER OF EVALUABLE PATIENTS	NUMBER OF RESPONSES			% CR + PR
		CR†	PR†	STABLE	
FUDR (Cont. inf.)[18]	35	3	9	—	34
CCNU[14]	27	0	4	3	15
Vinblastine[14,17,19–21]	108	3	6	19	8.3
Hydroxyurea[14,15]	37	0	3	8	8.1
Ifosfamide[14,22]	39	0	3	1	7.7
Baker's antifol[16]	64	1	3	4	6.2
Methyl GAG[14,23]	187	2	9	30	5.9
Bisantrene[14,24–27]	123	1	5	24	4.9
Methyl CCNU[17]	45	0	2	8	4.4
Teniposide (VM-26)[16,28,29]	95	0	4	23	4.2
PALA[30,31]	58	0	2	0	3.4
Cyclophosphamide[16]	66	0	2	5	3.0
Deoxydoxorubicin[32,33]	36	0	1	22	2.8
Etoposide (VP-16-213)[16]	36	1	0	0	2.8
Diaziquone (AZQ)[34–36]	104	0	2	12	1.9
Actinomycin-D[16]	61	0	1	0	1.6
Amsacrine (mAMSA)[16,31,37]	127	0	2	12	1.6
Dianhydrogalactitol[14,16]	76	0	1	0	1.3

*Results limited to phase II trials reported since 1977.
†CR = complete response; PR = partial response (>50%).

doses have documented an overall response rate of 11% in 110 patients.[16,38] To date, there is no advantage of combination chemotherapy over single agents in this disease.

IMMUNOTHERAPY

Occasional reports of spontaneous regression of metastatic renal cell cancer have stimulated investigation of immunologic treatment approaches. Attempts have been made to transfer specific immunity to patients using RNA isolated from sheep or guinea pigs previously immunized to autologous tumor cells.[43] This xenogeneic RNA was injected directly into patients in one study and, in another trial, after incubation with autologous lymphocytes that were also injected. In 29 patients, 2 objective responses were reported.[43]

Tumor cell suspensions modified by chemicals or mixed with bacterial adjuvants to enhance immunogenicity have also been injected into patients with advanced renal cell cancer. Definite responses have been observed in 16% of 44 patients treated using these methods.[43] Modified renal tumor antigens admixed with an adjuvant such as tuberculin or phytohemagglutinin were given as a vaccine to 43 patients and compared

to the same number given hormone therapy with medroxyprogesterone acetate in a randomized trial.[44] A 9% response was observed for those patients undergoing the immunologic therapy, but none in the progesterone-treated group. Patients receiving the vaccine also had significantly longer time to disease progression (16 versus 9.2 weeks, P = 0.004).[44] This low response rate could not be confirmed by Fowler using a similar autologous or allogeneic tumor antigen preparation in 23 patients.[45]

INTERFERON

Interferons are a class of glycoproteins possessing antiviral, immunomodulatory, and antiproliferative activity. Three distinct antigenic types of interferon are designated α, β, and γ. Despite the difficulty in obtaining large amounts of partially purified interferon-α from virus-stimulated buffy-coat leukocytes, early studies using this preparation demonstrated clear antitumor activity in advanced renal cell cancer.[46] Between 1983 and 1985, five trials were published with an overall response rate of 18.4% in 141 patients (Table 46-4). Experience in 9 separate trials utilizing another partially purified

TABLE 46-3. *Combination Chemotherapy in Metastatic Renal Cell Cancer*

REGIMEN	NUMBER OF EVALUABLE PATIENTS	NUMBER OF OBJECTIVE RESPONSES (%)
VBL + CCNU[16,38]	110	12 (11)
VBL + CCNU + CYT + MPA[39]	37	7 (19)
VBL + CCNU + HU + MPA[40]	32	3 (9)
VBL + MethylCCNU[16]	13	1 (7.7)
VBL + Methyl GAG[14]	15	0
VBL + CYT + 5-FU[14]	10	0
VBL + CYT + HU + MPA + P[14]	42	8 (19)
VBL + Bleo[14]	15	2 (13)
VBL + Bleo + MTX (L) ± TAM[14]	33	10 (30)
VCN + HU[14]	15	0
CYT + VCN + MTX + 5-FU[14]	18	0
CYT + VCN + MTX (L) + Bleo[16]	12	2 (17)
CYT + VCN + Adria + Bleo +BCG[14]	13	3 (23)
CCNU + Bleo[14]	16	1 (6)
CCNU + Bleo + Adria[14]	14	3 (21)
CCNU + Megace + BCG + TF[14]	14	5 (36)
Adria + VBL + HU[14]	8	3 (37)
Adria + VCN + MPA + BCG[14]	28	10 (36)
Mitomycin C + Metronidazole[41]	12	3 (25)
CYT + Misonidazole [42]	30	1 (3.3)
Totals	487	74 (15.2)

VBL = vinblastine; CYT = cyclophosphamide; MPA = methylprednisolone acetate; 5-FU = 5-fluorouracil; HU = hydroxyurea; P = prednisone; Bleo = bleomycin; MTX (L) = methotrexate (leukovorin); TAM = tamoxifen; VCN = vincristine; Adria = adriamycin; BCG = Bacillus Calmette Guerin, TF = transfer factor.

interferon-α preparation from lymphoblastoid cells confirmed this activity. These results spurred the development of trials using purified interferons produced by recombinant DNA techniques. Response rates in renal cell cancer using recombinant interferon-α2a, -α2b, and -α2c have not differed significantly from the rates using impure preparations (see Table 46-4). These results are even more interesting because doses, schedules, and routes of administration have varied widely between studies. It does appear that interferon-γ may have less activity than either interferon-α or -β. This phenomenon may be related to increased toxicity observed at lower doses of interferon-γ.[57]

It has been suggested that intermediate doses of interferon (5 to 10 million units/day) may be more effective in renal cell cancer, but these data are difficult to interpret because of vary-

ing schedules, dose modification procedures, and small patient numbers.[46,50] Two randomized trials have demonstrated increased responses when higher doses were used.[46] A third larger trial concluded that a lower-dose subcutaneous regimen was as effective as a higher-dose regimen given intravenously.[46] All three studies utilized different interferon-α preparations, and additional trials will be necessary before a dose-response relationship for interferon is confirmed.

Schedule and route of administration appear to be independent of response to interferon. Although occasional trials report otherwise, there also appears to be no relation between likelihood of response in individual patients and pretreatment characteristics such as interval from nephrectomy to metastases, performance status, or prior treatment history.[46] Despite data from at least one large series showing that previous nephrectomy was associated with a favorable response to interferon, one review of the literature failed to confirm this conclusion.[60] Most patients entering interferon trials have already undergone nephrectomy, usually at different intervals prior to treatment for metastatic disease. This makes retrospective analysis of the effect of this procedure on response to biologic therapy extremely difficult. Until a well-designed randomized trial has been completed, all patients with metastatic disease should be considered candidates for interferon therapy, and none should undergo nephrectomy prior to treatment.

Unlike response, toxicity is clearly related to the prescribed dose of interferon, and includes flu-like symptoms of fever, chills, malaise, headache, and fatigue.[61] Occasionally, leukopenia, hepatic, cardiac, or central nervous system toxicity is observed. These more serious problems usually occur at higher doses. Usually, these side effects can be ameliorated pharmacologically or by dose reduction. Although some interferon preparations are known to induce antibody formation to the foreign protein, no clear association between development of anti-interferon antibodies and abrogation of response exists.[46]

Interferon and Chemotherapy

A number of reports have demonstrated potential in vitro synergy between interferons and chemotherapeutic agents.[46] Clinical trials have begun to address this issue in advanced renal cell cancer. Most studies have used vinblastine in combination with one of the subtypes of interferon-α. Overall, it appears that this combination may be more effective when recombinant interferon is utilized instead of partially purified preparations (Table 46-5). Preliminary reports of randomized trials testing whether vinblastine enhances the activity of interferon are now available. Fossa et al. noted a 21% response rate in 91 patients treated with 36 million units of intramuscular interferon-α2a thrice weekly plus vinblastine 0.1 mg/kg intravenously every three weeks compared to a 6% complete and partial response rate in 86 patients treated with interferon alone.[63] Median survival of responders also favored the combined regimen, 105 versus 66 weeks. No increased toxicity was observed in those receiving interferon plus vinblastine.

TABLE 46-4. *Summary of Interferon Trials in Metastatic Renal Cell Cancer*

IFN TYPE	NUMBER OF PHASE II TRIALS	NUMBER OF PATIENTS	CR	PR	MIN†	ST.†	% CR + PR
Le (partially purified)[46,47]	5	141	6	20	13	25	18.4
Ly (lymphoblastoid)[46,48,49]	9	383	7	57	13	73	16.5
α2a (Roferon)[46,50–54]	8	359	4	52*	42	90	15.6
α2b (Intron)[46]	3	184	3	20	2	35	12.5
α2c[55]	1	93‡	2	3	—	—	5.3
β[46,56]	2	36	1	5	4	7	16.7
γ[46,57–59]	5	170§	2	12	4	61	8.2
Totals	33	1366	25	169	78	291	14.2

*Degree of response in 18 cases not available; all assumed PR.
†No data given in 6 studies.
‡46 patients also given medroxyprogesterone acetate.
§One study included 10% stage I to III patients.

These results are in contrast to those of a multi-institutional trial of lymphoblastoid interferon-α given 5 consecutive days at doses of 3, 5, 20, 20, and 20 million units/m^2 every 2 weeks plus 10 mg/m^2 vinblastine every month versus interferon alone.[49] Unacceptable toxicity was encountered in the combination arm, and the vinblastine dose was halved after the first 20 patients. Even at the reduced dose, the combined regimen resulted in increased neutropenia, thrombocytopenia, and fatigue/malaise over that observed with interferon alone. Response in the 82 patients treated with interferon plus vinblastine was similar to that in the 80 patients receiving only interferon, 17% and 15% respectively.[49] In a smaller randomized trial, interferon-α did not enhance the 12% response rate observed in 16 patients treated with a four-drug combination chemotherapy regimen.[67] The possibility that chemotherapy may potentiate the effect of interferon in advanced renal cell cancer remains controversial. This is not entirely unexpected given the poor results generally observed with chemotherapy alone in this disease.

In vitro data suggesting antiproliferative synergy between interferon-α and interferon-γ have generated interest in the evaluation of combinations of these agents. Although de Mulder et al. reported a 28% response rate in 29 patients,[68] a randomized multi-institutional trial by Foon and colleagues failed to demonstrate any treatment differences between interferon-α2b, interferon-γ, and their combination.[69] Additional studies are needed since Quesada has suggested that response to combined therapy may be a function of the dose ratio of interferon-α to interferon-γ utilized.[70]

ADOPTIVE IMMUNOTHERAPY

The ability of interleukin-2 (IL-2) to induce activation of nonspecific cytotoxic lymphokine-activated killer lymphocytes (LAK cells) has led to a new wave of biologic therapy for metastatic renal cell cancer.[46] The LAK cells generated in vitro or in vivo by this 15,000-molecular-weight glycoprotein have the ability to lyse fresh or cultured, autologous or allogeneic renal tumor cell tissue.[71] The availability of pure interleukin-2 through the use of recombinant DNA technology has allowed clinical trials to be initiated.

Early studies showed that interleukin-2 had little activity when used alone in either bolus or continuous infusions (Table 46-6). Rosenberg et al. then developed a combined therapy in which patients were given a priming dose of inter-

TABLE 46-5 *Results of Combinaton Interferon Plus Chemotherapy in Metastatic Renal Cell Cancer**

INTERFERON + DRUG	NUMBER OF TRIALS	NUMBER OF PATIENTS	NUMBER OF RESPONSES†(%)
rIFN-α2a + VBL[46,62–65]	6‡	226	58 (25.7)
HUIFN (Le) + VBL[46]	1	23	3 (13)
HUIFN (Ly) + VBL[49,66]	2	92	10 (11)
rIFN-α2b + Adria[54]	1	15	0
rIFN-α2a + BCNU[54]	1	9	2 (22)
rIFN-α2b + CYT[46]	1	25	1 (4)
rIFN-α2c + MPA[55]	1	46	2 (4.3)

*Results of phase I or II trials with 9 or more patients.
†Complete + partial responses.
‡Type of IFN used not given in 9 patients (1 trial).
rIFN-α2a = recombinant IFN-α2a (Roferon®-A); HUIFN (Le) = human leukocyte IFN; HUIFN (Ly) = human lymphoblastoid IFN; rIFN-α2b = recombinant IFN-α2b (Intron®-A); rIFN-α2c = recombinant IFN-α2c; VBL = vinblastine; Adria = adriamycin; CYT = cyclophosphamide; MPA = medroxyprogesterone acetate.

TABLE 46-6 *Interleukin-2 ± LAK Cell Therapy in Metastatic Renal Cell Cancer*

TREATMENT REGIMEN	NUMBER OF PATIENTS	NUMBER OF RESPONSES		% CR + PR
		CR	PR	
IL-2[72]	21	1	0	5
IL-2[46]	17	0	3	18
IL-2[46]	20	0	1	5
Totals	58	1	4	8.6
IL-2/LAK[72]	36*	4	8	33
IL-2/LAK[46]	32*	2	3	16
IL-2/LAK[73]	6†	0	3	50
Totals	74	6	14	27

*Priming IL-2 given as bolus injection.
†Priming IL-2 given as continuous infusion.

leukin-2, followed by multiple leukophoretic procedures to obtain activated LAK cells.[72] These cells were further expanded in vitro in the presence of interleukin-2, and then reinfused into the patient, together with additional interleukin-2. In patients with metastatic renal cell cancer, this complex treatment regimen produced a response rate of 33% at the National Cancer Institute.[72] Responding patients appeared to maintain their remissions for prolonged periods, occasionally measured in years. An attempt to confirm these results by a multi-institutional trial using Rosenberg's identical regimen resulted in a 16% response rate, although equally prolonged remissions were noted (see Table 46-6). The initial enthusiasm generated by these reports has been tempered by the severe toxicity that commonly accompanies IL-2/LAK therapy. In addition to chills, nausea, vomiting, and diarrhea, life-threatening problems such as hypotension requiring pressors, respiratory difficulties, renal complications, and even myocardial infarction can occur.[46,72] Although treatment-related deaths have been reported, it appears that these become less frequent as experience with this complex regimen increases. Further trials of adoptive immunotherapy can be confidently expected in the future.

MISCELLANEOUS BIOLOGIC THERAPY

At least two trials have utilized thymosin fraction 5 to treat metastatic renal cell cancer.[54] Because this preparation is an extract of calf thymus containing 30 different polypeptides, a biologic mechanism of activity is presumed. Unfortunately, only 3 responses were observed among 35 patients treated with this agent. More exciting results have been reported for the combination of coumarin and cimetidine.[74] Coumarin is the parent compound of sodium warfarin, but does not itself possess anticoagulant properties. There is evidence that both these agents may be immune modulators, with direct antiproliferative activity also noted for coumarin. Marshall et al. observed a 33% response rate in 42 evaluable patients treated with daily coumarin, followed on day 15 by cimetidine.[74] All responses were in previously nephrectomized patients. Using a similar regimen, Herrmann and colleagues have reported no objective responses in 15 evaluable patients treated to date.[75] Further confirmatory trials using coumarin and cimetidine are awaited. Recently, the apparent in vitro antitumor activity of tumor necrosis factor has generated considerable interest in the therapeutic potential of this agent in renal cell cancer. This cytotoxic factor is now available in a purified recombinant form and phase II testing is underway. One preliminary report has noted no responses among 14 patients with metastatic renal cell cancer.[76]

CURRENT RECOMMENDATIONS

Over the last decade, it has become increasingly apparent that no standard chemotherapy exists for metastatic renal cell cancer. The previously recommended drug, vinblastine, has now been shown to have minimal activity in this disease. Similarly, hormonal therapy has little place in the management of advanced renal cell cancer. Surgical resection of isolated metastases should be attempted in appropriate patients. Although no cures can be expected, occasional prolonged disease-free intervals follow this procedure. For nonresectable or multiple metastatic foci, participation in cooperative group trials utilizing new drugs or biologic agents is strongly recommended. If this is not possible, a trial of interferon is warranted, provided the patient is aware of the palliative nature and relatively high cost of this agent. Progress in adoptive immunotherapy using interleukin-2 plus LAK cells may make this experimental treatment less toxic and more effective in the future.

REFERENCES

1. PATEL, N. P., and LAVENGOOD, R. W. Renal cell cancer: Natural history and results of treatment. J. Urol., *119*:722, 1977.
2. MONTIE, J. E., et al. The role of adjuvant nephrectomy in patients with metastatic renal cell carcinoma. J. Urol., *117*:272, 1977.
3. JOHNSON, D. E., KAESLER, K. E., and SAMUELS, M. L. Is nephrectomy justified in patients with metastatic renal carcinoma? J. Urol., *114*:27, 1975.
4. MIDDLETON, R. G. Surgery for renal cell carcinoma. J. Urol., *97*:973, 1967.
5. FUSELIER, H. A., et al. Renal cell carcinoma: The Ochsner Medical Institution experience (1945–1978). J. Urol., *130*:445, 1983.
6. SWANSON, D. A., WALLACE, S., and JOHNSON, D. E. The role of embolization and nephrectomy in the treatment of metastatic renal carcinoma. Urol. Clin. North Am., *7*:719, 1980.
7. KURTH, K. H., et al. Embolization and postinfarction nephrectomy in patients with primary metastatic renal adenocarcinoma. Eur. Urol., *13*:251, 1987.

8. GOTTESMAN, J. E., et al. Infarction-nephrectomy for metastatic renal carcinoma. Urology, *25*:248, 1985.

9. FLANAGAN, R. C. The failure of infarction and/or nephrectomy in stage IV renal cell cancer to influence survival or metastatic regression. Urol. Clin. North Am., *14*:757, 1987.

10. DINEEN, M. K., et al. Results of surgical treatment of renal cell carcinoma with solitary metastasis. J. Urol., *140*:277, 1988.

11. MATHEWS, V. S., KIRKMAN, H., and BACON, R. L. Kidney damage in golden hamster following chronic administration of diethylstilbesterol and sesame oil. Proc. Soc. Exp. Biol., *66*:195, 1947.

12. BLOOM, H. J. G. Hormone-induced and spontaneous regression of metastatic renal cancer. Cancer, *32*:1066, 1973.

13. HRUSHESKY, W. J., and MURPHY, G. P. Current status of the therapy of advanced renal carcinoma. J. Surg. Oncol., *9*:277, 1977.

14. HARRIS, D. T. Hormonal therapy and chemotherapy of renal-cell carcinoma. Semin. Oncol., *10*:422, 1983.

15. STOLBACH, L. L., et al. Treatment of renal carcinoma: A phase III randomized trial of oral medroxyprogesterone (Provera), hydroxyurea, and nafoxidine. Cancer Treat. Rep., *65*:689, 1981.

16. TORTI, F. M. Treatment of metastatic renal cell carcinoma. Recent Results Cancer Res., *85*:123, 1983.

17. HAHN, R. G., et al. Phase II study of vinblastine, methyl-CCNU, and medroxyprogesterone in advanced renal cell cancer. Cancer Treat. Rep., *62*:1093, 1978.

18. HRUSHESKY, W. J. M., et al. Effective safe outpatient treatment for progressive metastatic renal cell cancer (RCC). Proc. ASCO, *7*:133, 1988.

19. KUEBLER, J. P., et al. Phase II study of continuous 5-day vinblastine infusion in renal adenocarcinoma. Cancer Treat. Rep., *68*:925, 1984.

20. TANNOCK, I. F., and EVANS, W. K. Failure of 5-day vinblastine infusion in the treatment of patients with renal cell carcinoma. Cancer Treat. Rep., *69*:227, 1985.

21. CRIVELLARI, D., et al. Phase II study of five-day continuous infusion of vinblastine in patients with metastatic renal-cell carcinoma. Am. J. Clin. Oncol., *10*:231, 1987.

22. DEFORGES, A., et al. Phase II trial of ifosfamide/mesna in metastatic adult renal carcinoma. Cancer Treat. Rep., *71*:1103, 1987.

23. FUKS, J. Z., et al. Phase II trial of methyl-G (methylglyoxal bisguanylhydrazone) in patients with metastatic renal cell carcinoma. Cancer Clin. Trials, *4*:411, 1981.

24. ELSON, P. J., et al. Phase II studies of PCNU and bisantrene in advanced renal cell carcinoma. Cancer Treat. Rep., *71*:331, 1987.

25. SPICER, D., et al. Phase II study of bisantrene administered weekly in patients with advanced renal cell carcinoma. Proc. ASCO, *4*:101, 1985.

26. EVANS, W. K., et al. Phase II evaluation of bisantrene in patients with advanced renal cell carcinoma. Cancer Treat. Rep., *69*:727, 1985.

27. MYERS, J. W., et al. Phase II evaluation of bisantrene in patients with renal cell carcinoma. Cancer Treat Rep., *66*:1869, 1982.

28. OISHI, N., et al. Teniposide in metastatic renal and bladder carcinoma: A Southwest Oncology Group study. Cancer Treat. Rep., *71*:1307, 1987.

29. PFEIFLE, D., et al. Phase II trial of VM-26 in advanced measurable renal cell cancer. Proc. ASCO, *3*:162, 1984.

30. NATALE, R. B., et al. Phase II trial of PALA in hypernephroma and urinary bladder cancer. Cancer Treat. Rep., *66*:2091, 1982.

31. EARHART, R. H., et al. Phase II study of PALA and AMSA in advanced renal cell carcinoma. Am. J. Clin. Oncol., *6*:553, 1983.

32. KISH, J., et al. Phase II evaluation of deoxydoxorubicin for patients with advanced and recurrent renal cell cancer. Proc. ASCO, *5*:106, 1986.

33. WILLIAMS, R. D., et al. A phase II trial of 4'-deoxydoxorubicin (DXDX) in metastatic carcinoma of the kidney: A trial of the Northern California Oncology Group. Proc. ASCO, *5*:109, 1986.

34. NICHOLS, W. C., et al. A phrase II study of aziridinylbenzoquinone (AZQ) in advanced genitourinary (GU) cancer. Proc. ASCO, *1*:117, 1982.

35. HANSEN, M., et al. Phase II trial of diaziquinone in advanced renal adenocarcinoma. Cancer Treat. Rep., *68*:1055, 1984.

36. STEPHENS, R. L., et al. High dose AZQ in renal cancer. A Southwest Oncology Group phase II study. Invest. New Drugs, *4*:57, 1986.

37. AMREIN, P. C., et al. Phase II study of amsacrine in metastatic renal cell carcinoma: A Cancer and Leukemia Group B study. Cancer Treat. Rep., *67*:1043, 1983.

38. SOMMER, H. H., FOSSA, S. D., and LIEN, H. H. Combination chemotherapy of advanced renal cell cancer with CCNU and vinblastine. Cancer Chemother. Pharmacol., *14*:277, 1985.

39. PUCKETT, J. B., et al. Combination chemotherapy of advanced renal cell carcinoma with megestrol acetate, CCNU, vinblastine, and cyclophosphamide. Proc. ASCO/AACR, *21*:380, 1981.

40. BRUBAKER, L. H., TRONER, M. B., and BIRCH, R. Advanced adenocarcinoma of the kidney: Therapy with lomustine, vinblastine, hydroxyurea, and medroxyprogesterone acetate and regression analysis of factors relating to survival. Cancer Treat Rep., *67*:741, 1983.

41. STEWART, D. J., et al. Mitomycin-C and metronidazole in the treatment of advanced renal cell carcinoma. Am. J. Clin. Oncol., *10*:520, 1987.

42. GLOVER, D., et al. Phase II trial of misonidazole (MISO) and cyclophosphamide (CYC) in metastatic renal cell carcinoma. Int. J. Radiat. Oncol. Biol. Phys., *12*:1405, 1986.

43. MCCUNE, C. S. Immunologic therapies of kidney cancer. Semin. Oncol., *10*:431, 1983.

44. NEIDHART, J. A., et al. A randomized study of polymerized tumor antigen admixed with adjuvant (PTA) for therapy of renal cancer. Proc. ASCO, *2*:49, 1983.

45. FOWLER, J. E., JR. Failure of immunotherapy for metastatic renal cell carcinoma. J. Urol., *135*:22, 1986.

46. MUSS, H. B. The role of biological response modifiers in metastatic renal cell carcinoma. Semin. Oncol., *15*:30, 1988.

47. MAGNUSSON, K., et al. Interferon therapy in recurrent renal carcinoma. Acta Med. Scand., *213*:221, 1983.

48. EISENHAUER, E. A., et al. Phase II study of high dose weekly intravenous human lymphoblastoid interferon in renal cell carcinoma. Br. J. Cancer, *55*:541, 1987.

49. NEIDHART, J., HARRIS, J., and TUTTLE, R. A randomized study of wellferon (WFN) with or without vinblastine (VBL) in advanced renal cancer. Proc. ASCO, *6*:239, 1987.

50. KROWN, S. E. Therapeutic options in renal cell carcinoma. Semin. Oncol., *12*:13, 1985.

51. BUZAID, A. C., et al. Phase II study of interferon alfa-2a, recombinant (Roferon-A) in metastatic renal cell carcinoma. J. Clin. Oncol., *5*:1083, 1987.

52. FIGLIN, R. A., et al. Recombinant interferon alfa-2a in metastatic renal cell carcinoma: Assessment of antitumor activity and anti-interferon antibody formation. J. Clin. Oncol., *6*:1604, 1988.

53. SCHNALL, S. F., et al. Treatment of metastatic renal cell carcinoma (RCC) with intramuscular (IM) recombinant interferon alfa A (IFN, Hoffman-LaRoche). Proc. ASCO, *5*:227, 1986.

54. QUESADA, J. R. Biologic response modifiers in the therapy of metastatic renal cell carcinoma. Semin. Oncol., *15*:396, 1988.

55. Porzsolt, F., et al. Treatment of advanced renal cell cancer with recombinant interferon alpha as a single agent and in combination with medroxyprogesterone acetate. J. Cancer Res. Clin. Oncol., 114:95, 1988.

56. Kinney, P. Preliminary report of a phase II trial of interferon-beta serine in metastatic renal cell carcinoma. Proc. ASCO, 7:162, 1988.

57. Quesada, J. R., et al. Phase II studies of recombinant human interferon gamma in metastatic renal cell carcinoma. J. Biol. Response Mod., 6:20, 1987.

58. Koiso, K. Phase II study of recombinant human interferon gamma (S-6810) on renal cell carcinoma. Cancer, 60:929, 1987.

59. Kuebler, J. P., et al. Phase II study of continuous infusion recombinant gamma interferon in renal carcinoma. Invest. New Drugs, 1990 (in press).

60. Muss, H. B. Interferon therapy for renal cell carcinoma. Semin. Oncol., 14:36, 1987.

61. Quesada, J. R., et al. Clinical toxicity of interferon in cancer patients: A review. J. Clin. Oncol., 4:234, 1986.

62. Fossa, S. D., and DeGaris, S. T. Further experience with recombinant interferon alfa-2a with vinblastine in metastatic renal cell carcinoma: A progress report. Int. J. Cancer (Suppl.), 1:36, 1987.

63. Fossa, S. D., et al. Randomized study of Roferon-A (IFN) with or without vinblastine (VBL) in advanced or metastatic renal cell cancer (RCC). Proc. ASCO, 7:118, 1988.

64. Schornagel, J., et al. Phase II study of recombinant interferon alpha-2 (IFN) and vinblastine (V) in advanced renal carcinoma (ARC). Proc. ASCO, 6:106, 1987.

65. Cetto, G. L., et al. Phase I/II trial of recombinant alpha-2 interferon (IFN) and vinblastine (VBL) in metastatic renal cell carcinoma (MRCC). Proc. ASCO, 5:110, 1986.

66. Ravdin, P., et al. Phase I/II trial of human lymphoblastoid interferon (L-IFN, Wellferon^R) and continuous infusion vinblastine (VBL-c.i.) in advanced renal cell cancer. Proc. ASCO, 4:101, 1985.

67. Dexeus, F., et al. Phase III study in metastatic renal cell carcinoma (RCC) comparing combination chemotherapy (CT) versus interferon (IFN) alternating with combination chemotherapy. Proc. ASCO, 7:131, 1988.

68. de Mulder, P. H. M., et al. Recombinant (R) interferon (IFN) α and γ in the treatment of advanced renal cell carcinoma (RCC). Proc. ASCO, 7:131, 1988.

69. Foon, K., et al. A prospective randomized trial of α2B-interferon/γ-interferon or the combination in advanced metastatic renal cell carcinoma. J. Biol. Response Mod., 7:540, 1988.

70. Quesada, J. R., et al. Recombinant interferon alpha and gamma in combination as treatment for metastatic renal cell carcinoma. J. Biol. Response Mod., 7:234, 1988.

71. Belldegrun, A., Uppenkamp, I., and Rosenberg, S. A. Anti-tumor reactivity of human lymphokine activated killer (LAK) cells against fresh and cultured preparations of renal cell cancer. J. Urol., 139:150, 1988.

72. Rosenberg, S. A., et al. Progress report on the treatment of 157 patients with advanced cancer using lymphokine activated killer cells and interleukin-2 or high dose interleukin-2 alone. N. Engl. J. Med., 316:889, 1987.

73. West, W. H., et al. Constant infusion recombinant interleukin-2 in adoptive immunotherapy of advanced cancer. N. Engl. J. Med., 316:898, 1987.

74. Marshall, M. E., et al. Treatment of metastatic renal cell carcinoma with coumarin (1,2-benzopyrone) and cimetidine: A pilot study. J. Clin. Oncol., 5:862, 1987.

75. Herrmann, R., et al. Coumarin and cimetidine in the treatment of metastatic renal cell carcinoma. Proc. ASCO, 7:131, 1988.

76. Figlin, R., et al. Phase II study of recombinant tumor necrosis factor (rTNF) in patients with metastatic renal cell carcinoma (RCCa) and malignant melanoma (MM). Proc. ASCO, 7:169, 1988.

Immunotherapy of Bladder Carcinoma

Donald L. Lamm
Jacek T. Sosnowski

Transitional cell carcinoma of the bladder is one of the first human malignancies to consistently respond to immunotherapy, and is an ideal tumor for the evaluation and development of immunotherapy. Unlike most tumors, 75% of patients with bladder cancer initially present with superficial, resectable disease. After tumor resection, as many as 70% of patients will develop disease recurrence. We therefore have the opportunity to study agents not only for their ability to cause tumor regression, but also for their ability to prevent tumor recurrence. Bladder tumors are also easily accessible to topical or intralesional therapy, and the results of such treatments can be assessed and measured by direct transurethral inspection. The success of immunotherapy of bladder cancer confirms the work of multiple immunologists who have found evidence that this is an immunogenic tumor. Although bladder cancer presents most commonly at an age when the immune system is decreasing in strength, bladder cancer patients typically have neither the malnutrition nor the profound debilitation of the immune system that is common in patients with advanced malignancies.

The most successful form of therapy currently available for superficial bladder carcinoma, particularly carcinoma in situ, is immunotherapy with Bacillus Calmette Guerin (BCG).[1] BCG's remarkable success has prompted the study of other immunostimulants, many of which have been successfully used in animal models and recent human trials. Currently, multiple immune treatments have potential or proven clinical application in bladder carcinoma. These include various tumor vaccines, monoclonal antibodies, interferon and interferon inducers, tumor necrotic factor (TNF), interleukin-2 (IL-2), lymphokine-activated killer (LAK) cells, keyhole limpet hemocyanin (KLH), and maltose tetrapalmitate (MTP).

Immunotherapies can be classified into two broad categories: active, which induces in the host a state of immune responsiveness to tumor antigen, and passive, which directly delivers to the host immunologically active reagents that mediate an antitumor response. Each of these categories of im-

TABLE 47-1. *Categories of Immunotherapy*

ACTIVE IMMUNOTHERAPY

SPECIFIC
Tumor vaccines, e.g. tumor extracts, polymerized tumor
protein, and irradiated cells
NONSPECIFIC
Bacteria: BCG, *Corynebacterium parvum,* and bacterial
products, Streptococcal OK432, and MDP
Lymphokines: interferon, interleukin-2, and tumor necrosis
factor

PASSIVE IMMUNOTHERAPY

SPECIFIC
Monoclonal antibodies
NONSPECIFIC
LAK cells-generated by IL-2 expansion

---

munotherapies can be divided into specific and non-specific immunologic stimulants, depending on whether or not the response is directed only toward the host's tumor. Table 47-1 illustrates examples of the various types of immunotherapies available at this time.

The importance of the immune system in cancer is evidenced by multiple clinical observations. The spontaneous regression of tumors such as malignant melanoma, neuroblastoma, and renal cell carcinoma has long been considered to be mediated by immune mechanisms. The incidence of malignancy is increased in the very young and the aged, when immune defenses are weakest. Immune suppression as a result of inherited defects, viral infections, irradiation, or immunosuppressive drug therapies significantly increases the risk of malignancy.

Both cell-mediated and humoral responses are considered to be important in the defense against malignancy.[2] A subpopulation of thymus-derived (T) lymphocytes will lyse malignant cells after stimulation by tumor antigens. Antibodies, which are produced by bone marrow-derived (B) lymphocytes, lyse tumor cells by interaction with complement or a subset of T cells, killer (K) cells. The latter is termed antibody-dependent cellular cytotoxicity. Natural killer (NK) cells nonspecifically kill only malignant cells by direct interaction. Some investigators believe that NK cells have an important function in immune surveillance against the occurrence of malignancy. Macrophages, when activated by a specific macrophage-activation factor, are also potent tumor cell killers. BCG and *Corynebacterium parvum* are good examples of macrophage activators. After activation, macrophages produce immunomodulators such as interferon and tumor necrosis factor (TNF), as well as nonimmunomodulatory substances such as hydrolytic enzymes and oxidative substances, which have antitumor activity.

The immune system is incompletely understood and the interaction between host and tumor is extremely complex. A thorough understanding of these interactions may permit the effective application of the principles of immunotherapy, non-

specific activation of the host immune response by adjuvants, and elimination of tumor cells by active immunization or by passively transferred specific or nonspecific reagents in immunocompromised patients. This chapter will review the current successes and the future prospects for immunotherapy in bladder cancer.

BACILLUS CALMETTE-GUERIN

Bacillus Calmette-Guerin is an attenuated tuberculosis vaccine isolated through 13 years of serial subculture of a virulent strain of *Mycobacterium bovis.*[3] The first clinical use of this vaccine was in 1921 when oral BCG was given to protect a girl born in household with active tuberculosis infection. The child suffered no ill effects and did not contract tuberculosis.[3] Since that time, more than 1.5 billion BCG vaccinations have been given with little morbidity.[4]

BCG was found to be a potent stimulant of the immune system, particularly the reticulo-endothelial system.[5] Stimulation of the reticulo-endothelial system had been observed to be associated with the prevention of animal tumor growth. Therefore, investigation of the role of BCG in the treatment of cancer was initiated. Successful treatment of many animal tumors with BCG led to multiple clinical trials with human malignancies. Early reports in the 1970's touted the benefit of BCG treatment in numerous human tumors, but BCG fell into disrepute when multiple controlled trials revealed no significant advantage to BCG treatment. In the treatment of bladder cancer, however, consistently significant therapeutic benefit has been observed.

Though the efficacy of BCG cannot be denied, its mechanism of action remains largely undetermined. Intravesical BCG administration results in an intense inflammatory cell infiltration of the lamina propria. BCG affects a range of cell types including B cells, T cells, macrophages, killer (K) cells, and natural killer (NK) cells.[6] BCG also stimulates interferon and interleukin 2 levels.[7,8] The complexity of these immune responses suggests that multiple factors are involved in the antitumor response to BCG, and confirms the wisdom of early immunologists who termed BCG a nonspecific immune stimulant.[9] Indeed, BCG may well induce lymphokines and antitumor factors that are yet to be identified.

BCG Trials

The first clinical trial of intravesical BCG therapy was reported in 1976 by Morales and associates,[10] who observed a 12-fold reduction of tumor recurrence in nine patients given intravesical and percutaneous BCG. Since that time, numerous prospective randomized clinical trials have confirmed the benefit of BCG immunotherapy in preventing tumor recurrence. Lamm et al. randomized 94 patients to transurethral resection alone or with intravesical BCG.[11] Nineteen of 40 (47.5%) control patients had tumor recurrence compared with only 10 of 54 (18.5%) patients treated with BCG (P = 0.003 chi squared). The mean disease-free interval was prolonged from

31 months in controls to 58 months with BCG treatment (P = 0.0017). Another prospective randomized trial in high-risk patients reported a dramatic reduction in tumor recurrence from 2.37 tumors per patient-month in control to 0.7 tumors per patient-month in the BCG group.[12] Similar protection from tumor recurrence has been reported by Martinez-Peneiro,[13] Bastian,[14] Adolphs and Bastian,[15] Netto and Lemos,[16] Babayan and Krane,[17] deKernion and associates,[18] Haaff and associates,[19] Schellhammer,[20] and others.

Two studies failed to demonstrate benefit of BCG immunotherapy. Flamm and Grof observed a disappointing 59% recurrence rate in patients treated with Connaught BCG given intravesically.[21] This same strain has been highly effective in multiple other studies. The other negative study was reported by Stober and Peters, who used only percutaneous BCG after transurethral surgery, and compared this with surgery alone.[22] These studies suggest that the mode of administration is important and may be especially so when shorter courses of therapy are given.

Animal studies suggest that BCG is rarely effective when tumor burden exceeds 100,000 cells. Every effort should be made to completely resect all visible tumor prior to initiation of BCG immunotherapy. However, BCG has been remarkably effective in the treatment of patients with residual bladder cancer. Complete response rates have ranged from 36 to 83%, and compare favorably with those for intravesical chemotherapy (Table 47-2).[23]

In the prevention of tumor recurrence, BCG also compares favorably with current chemotherapy. Seventeen randomized prospective comparisons of intravesical therapy with surgical resection alone are available for review.[23] The average recurrence rate with surgical resection alone is 58% and ranges from 32 to 97%. Treatment with intravesical chemotherapy or BCG immunotherapy reduces tumor recurrence to 33% (range 7 to 65%). Statistically significant reduction in tumor recurrence at the p < 0.05 level occurred in 60% of 10

thiotepa studies, 50% of 2 doxorubicin and mitomycin C studies, and 100% of 3 BCG studies. All BCG studies (100%) were significant at the p < 0.001 level, compared with only 1 of 15 chemotherapy studies.

Varying entry criteria and risk factors preclude direct comparison of results from these studies, but relative benefit can be estimated by comparing the advantage observed in treatment groups over control groups. Average relative benefits are 13% for doxorubicin, 17% for thiotepa, 14% for mitomycin C, and 47% for BCG (Table 47-3).

BCG in Carcinoma in situ

BCG immunotherapy is perhaps most successful in carcinoma in situ (CIS) of the bladder. CIS is a poorly differentiated and, therefore, a presumably antigenic tumor. Although the disease may be diffuse, it involves only a few cell layers and, in the bladder, it is accessible to direct contact with BCG. CIS of the ureter or the urethra is less accessible and more difficult to manage. The complete response rate of 72% in a combined experience with 500 patients with CIS is higher than that reported with any other intravesical agent. Reported responses range from 40% to 100% (Table 47-4).

Ongoing randomized studies confirm the superior response rate of BCG in patients with CIS. Adriamycin, with a reported complete response rate in CIS of 59% in five series' totaling 76 patients,[23] has been compared with Connaught BCG in an ongoing Southwest Oncology Group trial.[40] Fifty-seven patients were randomized to Adriamycin, 50 mg weekly for 4 weeks and then monthly for 11 months, and 52 were randomized to BCG, 120 mg weekly for 6 weeks, at 3 months, 6 months, and every 6 months for 4 years. Complete response was seen in 27 patients (47%) treated with Adriamycin and 37 patients (71%) treated with BCG. Increasing extent of disease was found in 37% of patients in the Adriamycin group and only 15% of patients in the BCG group.[40] The high incidence of long-term, complete response of CIS to BCG treatment is changing our treatment strategy in this disease. Early cystectomy has previously been recommended for diffuse flat CIS associated with concurrent multiple superficial papillary tumors because of reported progression to muscle invasive disease in 40 to 80% of cases within 5 years.[41] Our preliminary data revealed that BCG treatment in high-risk patients, 69% of whom had lamina propria invasion, resulted in decreased risk for progression to muscle invasion when compared to untreated controls.[29] In this study, patients with CIS treated with BCG had a prognosis that was not different from those without CIS. It would therefore appear to be safe to reserve cystectomy for those CIS patients who fail BCG treatment, especially because cystectomy itself has significant morbidity and mortality.

BCG Immunotherapy Versus Chemotherapy

The most commonly used intravesical chemotherapies are alkylating agents. Resistance to one agent increases the likeli-

TABLE 47-2. *BCG Response Rates in Residual Tumor**

REFERENCE	NO.	RESPONSE	PERCENT
Doville et al. (1978)[24]	6	4	67
Morales et al. (1981)[25]	23	14	61
Lamm et al. (1982)[26]	10	6	60
Brosman (1982)[14]	12	10	83
deKernion et al. (1985)[18]	2	8	36
Kojima et al. (1985)[27]	29	16	55
Schellhammer et al. (1986)[32]	22	14	64
Kavoussi et al. (1988)[33]	27	11	41
TOTALS	145	79	55

*CIS only patients not included

TABLE 47-3. *Controlled Studies Versus Surgery Alone*

TREATMENT	TRIALS	RX (%)	SURGERY (%)	P < .05	<.001	ADVANTAGE (%)
Thiotepa	1009/10	62	45	4/10	1/10	17
Adriamycin	443/2	46	33	1/2	0	13
Mitomycin	379/3	51	37	1/3	0	14
BCG	192/3	82	35	3/3	3/3	47
AVERAGES	2023/18	60%	38%	9/18	4/18	23%

hood of resistance to the second. BCG has an advantage over intravesical chemotherapy in that its mechanism of action, although not completely defined, is clearly different from that of chemotherapy. Cross resistance has not been identified between chemotherapy and BCG, but cross resistance may be a future problem when additional immunotherapies are used. In our experience with 22 patients who failed intravesical chemotherapy, 82% responded favorably to BCG.[29] Fortunately, patients who fail BCG treatment will also commonly respond to intravesical chemotherapy.

Several direct comparisons of intravesical therapies, including two studies of BCG and thiotepa, have been conducted. In Brosman's study, 47% of patients treated with thiotepa had tumor recurrence and none of the patients treated with BCG had tumor recurrence.[14] Interestingly, although not an intra-

TABLE 47-4. *BCG Therapy for Carcinoma in Situ*

REFERENCE	NUMBER OF PATIENTS	COMPLETE RESPONSE	PERCENT
Morales (1980)[28]	7	5	71
Lamm (1985)[29]	14	11	79
Herr et al. (1983)[30]	47	34	72
Brosman (1985)[31]	33	27	82
Schellhammer et al. (1986)[32]	6	6	100
deKernion et al. (1985)[18]	19	13	68
Kavoussi et al. (1988)[33]	50	23	46
Rintala (1989)[34]	10	4	40
Brosman (1989)[35]	40	28	70
Steg et al. (1988)[36]	30	23	77
SWOG (1989)*	52	37	71
Pagano (1989)[37]	27	21	78
Prescott (1989)[38]	16	14	94
Reitsma (1989)[39]	153	107	70
TOTALS	513	368	72

*Current data from authors' ongoing study

vesical study, Netto and Lemos observed a 43% recurrence in patients treated with thiotepa compared with 7% recurrence in patients treated with high-dose oral Moreau RJ substrain.[16]

Preliminary evaluation of the EORTC comparison of BCG-RIVM given weekly for 6 weeks, with mitomycin C given weekly for 4 weeks and monthly for 6 months, showed no advantage for either treatment.[42] With 308 patients enrolled and an average follow-up of 12 months, 30% of patients treated with BCG have had tumor recurrence compared with 25% of patients treated with mitomycin C. However, concern has been raised about the efficacy of the RIVM preparation. BCG attaches to bladder cells by means of fibronectin receptors,[43] and such attachment is necessary for both immune stimulation and antitumor activity. BCG-RIVM, like Glaxo BCG, is grown in suspension rather than on the surface of the medium. The detergents required to keep BCG in suspension lower fibronectin receptor concentration. Clinical evidence supports the importance of fibronectin receptors because, in addition to a disappointing recurrence rate with BCG-RIVM, the incidence of BCG cystitis is a low 7%.

The Southwest Oncology Group has recently completed a prospective randomized comparison of Connaught BCG with doxorubicin. Two hundred thirty six patients are evaluable; 109 with carcinoma in situ and 127 with rapidly recurrent papillary carcinoma.[40] Complete resolution of carcinoma in situ occurred in 37 of 52 BCG-treated patients (71%) and 27 of 57 doxorubicin-treated patients (47%, p < 0.01). Papillary tumors recurred in 34 of 60 BCG-treated patients (57%) and 53 of 67 doxorubicin-treated patients (79%, p < 0.005).

Prevention of Disease Progression and BCG

Despite the extensive experience with multiple intravesical chemotherapies over the past 3 decades, evidence does not confirm that chemotherapy reduces the incidence of muscle invasion, metastasis, or even long-term tumor recurrence. Prout has reported a detailed 60-month follow-up of 90 patients randomized to thiotepa prophylaxis or no treatment.[44] One-third of these patients had previously responded to thiotepa and therefore demonstrated sensitivity to chemotherapy. Late recurrence occurred in 29 of 45 thiotepa-treated patients (64%) and 35 of 45 control group patients (78%, p < 0.05). Muscle invasion or metastasis occurred in six

TABLE 47-5. *Tumor Progression with BCG Versus TUR Treatment*

TREATMENT	NUMBER OF PATIENTS	PROGRESSION (%)	T2/METASTASIS (%)	CYSTECTOMY (%)	DEATH
TUR	43	41 (95%) 12 months	20 (46%)	18 (42%) 8 months	16 (32%)
BCG	43	23 (53%) 60 months	12 (28%) 36 months	11 (25%) 26 months	6 (14%)
p value:		0.0001	0.01	0.001	0.032

Herr, H. W., et al. Bacillus Calmette-Guerin therapy alters the progression of superficial bladder cancer. J. Clin. Oncol., 6:1450, 1988

thiotepa-treated patients and in only four control group patients. This multicenter trial, like that of Medical Research Council, suggests that no effect on long-term recurrence, disease progression, or patient survival results from intravesical thiotepa chemotherapy. Evidence for long-term benefit with other intravesical chemotherapies is similarly lacking.

We have compared progression to lamina propria invasion, muscle invasion, or metastasis in 90 patients on randomized BCG protocols.[41] Of 26 control patients, 65% had tumor recurrence, 23% progressed to invasion to or beyond the lamina propria, and 8% progressed to muscle invasion or metastasis. Of 64 BCG-treated patients, 16% had tumor recurrence (p < 0.001), 6% progressed to lamina propria invasion or beyond (p < 0.05), and 3% progressed to muscle invasion or metastasis (not statistically significant). Only 4% of BCG-treated patients progressed from stage T1 to T2 or greater. In patients followed for an average of 62 months, only 1 of 12 patients with CIS has had recurrent disease, 0 of 43 patients with stage 0 (Ta), and 2 of 32 patients (6%) with lamina propria invasion treated with BCG have had disease progression.[45]

In Herr's study of a much higher risk group of patients, the results are even more impressive. Progression was significantly reduced with BCG and, despite the earlier and more frequent use of cystectomy in the control group, mortality was reduced from 32% in control group patients to 14% with BCG treatment (Table 47-5).

BCG Treatment Techniques

The optimal protocol for BCG immunotherapy remains undefined and is somewhat controversial. Substrains that have demonstrated efficacy include Armand-Frappier, Connaught, Glaxo (Evans) in high dose, Pasteur, Japanese, RIVM, and Tice. Because treatments have been given empirically, the optimal dose of vaccine has not been firmly established. Commonly used and effective intravesical doses of these vaccines are 120 mg for Armand-Frappier, BCG-RIVM, Connaught, and Pasteur preparations, 50 mg for Tice, and 40 mg for Japanese BCG (Table 47-6).

Patients have been treated empirically at weekly intervals for 6 weeks. Uncontrolled series suggest that a single 6-week treatment course is suboptimal because significantly fewer patients have complete resolution of papillary or in situ disease or effective prophylaxis with a 6-week course than those given a second 6-week course at the time of recurrence.[46] It is critically important, however, that excessive BCG administration be avoided, because such treatment not only increases toxicity but can, as confirmed by animal studies, reduce antitumor effect. While Brosman has observed increasing antitumor activity with continuation of weekly treatments in patients with persistent CIS using 50 mg Tice BCG, Ratliff has observed a reduced immunoproliferative response and a discouraging clinical response effect in patients given 12 weekly treatments of 120 mg Armand Frappier BCG.[47]

The necessity of maintenance BCG immunotherapy remains debatable. Because it is known that the immune stimulation induced by BCG wanes with time, and the proclivity of the urothelium to tumor formation persists, in theory, periodic retreatment with BCG should improve long-term results. In our experience with previously randomized patients followed for at least 1 year or until tumor recurrence, maintenance BCG immunotherapy reduced the rate of tumor recurrence fourfold, from 1.9 to 0.49 tumors per 100 patient months.[29] In a randomized study of 42 evaluable patients, Hudson et al. found no difference in tumor recurrence between patients receiving a 6-week course of intravesical BCG and those receiving an additional BCG treatment every 3 months.[48] Similarly, Badalament et al. reported equal recurrence in 93 patients randomized to nonmaintenance or maintenance BCG at monthly intervals beginning at 3 months.[49]

TABLE 47-6. *Effective Vaccines and Doses*

VACCINE	DOSE
Armand-Frappier	120 mg
Connaught	120 mg
Pasteur	120 mg
Tice	50 mg
Japanese	40 mg
RIVM	10^9 CFU

These randomized studies document the remarkable effectiveness of a single 6-week course of BCG and cast serious doubt on the benefit of maintenance therapy. Maintenance therapy is, by definition, designed to sustain complete response after optimal induction therapy. Both of the randomized studies used a 6-week induction and did not initiate maintenance until the third month. Because a single 6-week course of BCG is highly effective and our controlled animal model studies have demonstrated that the protective effect of BCG is long-term, that is, persists for at least 8 months in mice without further BCG administration,[50] it is likely that more patients followed for longer periods of time will be needed to determine whether maintenance BCG therapy will further improve clinical results.

A randomized prospective study has confirmed that percutaneous BCG alone has no antitumor activity, but the added value of percutaneous BCG had not been adequately evaluated.[22] Excellent results can be obtained with intravesical BCG alone, but our early experience with Armand-Frappier BCG given only intravesically was disappointing: 40% of patients developed tumor recurrence, and no patient converted from skin test negative to positive with 6 weekly intravesical instillations.[29] With a subsequent course of intravesical plus percutaneous BCG, patients both converted skin test reactivity and remained free of tumor recurrence. To evaluate the role of percutaneous BCG, we conducted a randomized prospective comparison. Sixty-six patients with recurrent superficial bladder tumors were randomized to receive intravesical Tice BCG, 50 mg weekly for 6 weeks, at 8, 10, and 12 weeks, 6 months, and every 6 months for 4 years with or without simultaneous percutaneous BCG. Mean follow-up was 12 months for the intravesical only group (IVES) and 11 months for the intravesical plus percutaneous (IVPRC) group. Of the 30 evaluable patients randomized to IVES, only BCG 13 (43%) had biopsy-confirmed tumor recurrence at a mean of 5 months. Of the 36 patients who received intravesical plus percutaneous BCG, 15 (42%) had tumor recurrence at a mean of 7 months.

The use of oral rather than intravesical BCG has been even more controversial. Our experience,[50] as well as that of multiple investigators,[51] has demonstrated that juxtaposition of BCG and tumor antigens provides the best antitumor response. The reported dramatic reduction in tumor recurrence with oral BCG, as reported by Netto and Lemos, and the subsequent report of regression of muscle invasive disease with oral therapy were, therefore, surprising.[16,52] Oral BCG therapy has been reported to be virtually without side effects, and evaluation of this therapy is important because animal data from two independent laboratories have confirmed that high-dose systemic BCG does inhibit peripheral transitional cell carcinoma and,[53,54] if oral BCG inhibits transitional cell carcinoma in the bladder, it would be expected to be equally effective in inhibiting occult transitional cell carcinoma in the lung or pelvic lymph nodes. Such therapy could thus become that elusive effective adjuvant to cystectomy that is yet to be developed.

A randomized prospective comparison with standard intravesical and oral BCG was performed to evaluate the efficacy of oral BCG. In 88 evaluable, randomized patients, tumor recurrence was documented in 21 of the 33 (64%) treated with oral BCG and 18 of the 55 (32%) treated with intravesical BCG (p, 0.001, chi-squared). In fact, no antitumor activity of oral BCG could be demonstrated.

Complications of BCG Treatment of Bladder Cancer

Although most patients tolerate BCG well, life-threatening and even fatal complications of BCG therapy can occur.[55] Intravesical BCG produces a granulomatous cystitis with frequency and dysuria in 7% (with BCG RIVM) to over 90% of patients. Symptoms usually begin after the second or third instillation and persist for 2 days. Mild gross hematuria is not uncommon and about one-fourth of patients will have low-grade fever, malaise, or nausea. The most frequent major complication has been fever of over 39.5°C, which occurred in 3% of 2,473 patients we recently reviewed.[56] Granulomatous prostatitis occurred in 0.9% of patients. Although generally asymptomatic, the induration produced in the prostate is suggestive of carcinoma and requires biopsy. Systemic BCG infection with pneumonitis or clinically significant hepatitis occurred in 0.7%. Systemic BCG infection usually responds to isoniazid and rifampin, but acute septic or anaphylactic shock can occur. In these cases, multiple antituberculous agents should be initiated. Cycloserine inhibits BCG-growth within 1 day, isoniazid and other antibiotics take up to 1 week to act. Cycloserine at 250 to 500 mg twice daily should, therefore, be included in the early treatment of life-threatening infections. Shock may also be caused by hypersensitivity to BCG, and prednisone 40 ms daily has been used with apparent response.

Other complications included arthritis or arthralgia in 0.5%, hematuria requiring catheterization or transfusion in 1.0%, and skin rash or skin abscess from percutaneous inoculation in 0.3%. Ureteral obstruction secondary to cystitis or ureteritis occurred in 0.3%. Bladder contracture has occurred in 6 patients (0.2%), epididymo-orchitis in 10 patients (0.4%), hypotension in ten patients (0.4%), and cytopenia in 2 patients. The increased incidence of BCG sepsis observed in our most recent review, plus the four deaths from BCG sepsis that have occurred in the combined experience, is alarming. Those using BCG must be familiar with its toxicity and the use of antituberculous antibiotics including cycloserine. Isoniazid should *never* be avoided because of concern about reduction of antitumor activity because isoniazid does not effect antitumor activity, but excessive numbers of BCG organisms, as may occur with infection, clearly do inhibit antitumor immunity.

BCG is the most effective intravesical therapy currently available for superficial bladder cancer. However, in patients with rapidly recurrent disease, as many as 57% will have tumor recurrence.[23] The number of patients failing BCG, in addition to the significant toxicity of this treatment, indicate the need for more effective and less toxic treatments. The demonstrated immunosensitivity of bladder cancer suggests that immunotherapeutic agents are prime candidates for new, effective treatments. Several of these agents have already demonstrated clinical efficacy.

KEYHOLE LIMPET HEMOCYANIN

Keyhole-limpet hemocyanin (KLH), a high molecular weight protein, is the respiratory pigment (hemolymph) of a mollusc, Megathura crenulata,[57] and has been used for decades as an experimental antigen. KLH is among the most immunogenic of proteins, producing delayed-type hypersensitivity, antibodies, and specific lymphocytes that undergo a blastogenic response to KLH in vitro.[57] This antigen has been used extensively to evaluate cellular and humoral immune response to neoantigens, because prior exposure to Megathura crenulata is unlikely.

Surprisingly, in studies of immunologic reactivity in bladder cancer patients using KLH and other antigens, Olsson found a great reduction in tumor recurrence in patients immunized with subcutaneous KLH.[58] Before KLH immunization, 7 of 10 patients had recurrence and 13 recurrences were noted in 203 patient-months. After KLH, only 3 patients had recurrence and a total of only 4 recurrences were noted in 213 patient-months (p < 0.005). In a subsequent study, 19 patients were divided into KLH immunized and nonimmunized groups. Only one tumor occurred in the KLH group during the subsequent 204 patient-months. In the 10 control patients, 7 had tumor recurrence and the total recurrence rate was 18 per 228 patient-months (p < 0.005). No toxicity of KLH administration was seen.

On the basis of this notable observation, KLH was evaluated in the murine bladder cancer model MBT2.[59] Three weekly intralesional KLH injections significantly reduced tumor growth (p < 0.01) and prolonged survival (p < 0.01), compared to saline and immune RNA-treated animals.

Jurincic et al. compared KLH immunotherapy with mitomycin C in 44 randomized patients with recurrent superficial bladder cancer.[60] One mg of KLH was given intradermally followed by 10 mg intravesically on a monthly maintenance schedule for 2 years, versus 20 mg mitomycin C on a monthly maintenance schedule. With a mean follow-up of 20 months, 3 of 21 patients (14%) receiving KLH had recurrent tumor compared with 9 recurrences (39%) in 23 patients receiving mitomycin C (p < 0.07). The rate of tumor recurrence was 3.26 and 9.28 per 100 patient-months respectively. An additional 81 patients were treated with KLH without randomization. The rate of tumor recurrence in this group was a remarkably low 1.19 per 100 patient months. Again, as with previous studies, no KLH toxicity was noted.

Flamm recently presented a randomized prospective comparison of Epodyl and KLH in patients with stage pTO-pT1, grade 0-II transitional cell carcinoma of the bladder.[61] KLH was given in a dose of 1 mg intradermally followed by 30 mg in 30 cc saline intravesically weekly for 4 weeks and then monthly. Thirty patients were randomly assigned to KLH and

30 were assigned to Epodyl treatment groups. With a mean follow up of 9 months, two patients (7%) in the KLH group and eight (27%) in the Epodyl group have had tumor recurrence (p < 0.05).

KLH has, therefore, been found to be superior to mitomycin C, and Epodyl, the most effective intravesical agents. KLH has succeeded where BCG has failed in randomized comparison with mitomycin C, and so is potentially more effective than BCG. Moreover, KLH has no reported toxicity.

INTERLEUKIN-2

Interleukin-2 (IL-2), originally termed T-cell growth factor, is a 15,000 dalton glycoprotein.[62] This lymphokine is produced by helper T-lymphocytes (human phenotypic markers Leu3 and OKT4) after primary activation by specific antigen or mitogens, and is the second signal for lymphocyte proliferation. IL-2 has been shown to induce the proliferation of activated T lymphocytes, as well as improve the immune function of lymphocytes in patients with immunodeficient states associated with cancer, rheumatoid arthritis, and leprosy.[63–65] In vitro administration of IL-2 can improve the immunogenic response to weak antigens, and immunologic activity in cyclophosphamide-treated animals can be restored by in vivo injection of IL-2.[65]

In 1980, several workers observed that the incubation of normal lymphocytes in IL-2 supernatant induced proliferation of cytotoxic effector cells (now known as lymphokine-activated killer cells or LAK cells) that would lyse autologous tumor cells but not normal cells.[66,67] From the beginning of this fascinating discovery, LAK cells were distinguished from natural killer (NK) cells on the basis of differential function in vitro. LAK cells stimulated with IL-2 lyse fresh tumor cells. NK cells do not.

In addition to stimulating LAK cell expansion, IL-2 induces the release of several other lymphokines, including gamma-interferon and tumor necrosis factor.[68–71] More recently, a role of IL-2 in B-cell and macrophage function has been indicated by the discovery of IL-2 receptors on B cells and macrophages. The nature of this relationship is under investigation.[72]

Systemic administration of high doses of recombinant IL-2 (rIL-2) alone or rIL-2 plus LAK cells has resulted in the regression of experimental tumors as well as human malignancies, including renal cell carcinoma and melanoma.[73] In the mouse sarcoma model, the administration of LAK cells or rIL-2 alone had a minimal antitumor effect on the number of metastases. However, when LAK-cell and rIL-2 therapies were combined, over a 90% reduction in the number of metastases was observed.[73] In human malignancy, the combined treatment regimen of rIL-2 with LAK cells induced a response rate of 30% in renal cell carcinoma, 23% in melanoma, 12% in colorectal cancer, and 100% in two patients with non-Hodgkin's lymphoma.[74] Tumor regression was observed in multiple metastatic sites: lung, liver, bone, skin, lymph nodes, bone marrow, and circulating lymphoma cells.

Although these responses are encouraging, the clinical application of rIL-2/LAK cell treatment is limited by the toxicity of intravenous IL-2. Because IL-2 has a short, 7-minute half-life,[75] high doses of IL-2 are required for intravenous administration and serious, even fatal side effects may occur. The major side effect of IL-2 is increased capillary permeability, which shifts intravascular fluids to the extravascular compartment, decreases systemic vascular resistance, and leads to profound hypotension. Azotemia, oliguria, weight gain, interstitial pulmonary edema, myelosuppression, hyperbilirubinemia, arrhythmia, myocardial infarction, and changes in mental status (confusion, disorientation, combative behavior, and psychosis) have occurred,[76] and five patients have died as a result of treatment.[76,77]

Alternative routes of rIL-2 or rIL-2/LAK administration may be more effective and less toxic. Because many tumors spread through the lymphatic system and the activity of IL-2 is on lymphocytes, which are concentrated in the lymphatic system, the intralymphatic route of administration has been investigated.[78,79] Pizza et al. recently reported the results of a preliminary study of intralymphatic IL-2/LAK cell therapy in patients with advanced renal, oral, pancreas, breast, and testicular cancer.[79] With the exception of the patient with pancreatic cancer, all of the patients had liver and/or lung metastasis. They reported over 50% regression in six patients and four (57%) had complete response. No serious side effects were observed.

Intralesional injection may improve the antitumor response by increasing effective local concentration of IL-2 while reducing systemic toxicity. In 1976, Papermaster et al. reported that IL-2 could be safely injected intralesionally into human cutaneous metastases.[80] In 1984, Pizza et al. reported the successful therapy of bladder cancer using intralesional IL-2 in 10 patients.[81] Six of these patients received 2,000 to 4,000 units of intralesional xenogeneic lymphoblastoid IL-2 in two to three fractions given over intervals ranging from 7 to 54 days. Three patients had complete tumor regression, and the remaining three experienced more than a 50% reduction in tumor volume. In four other patients receiving 156 to 1400 units of IL-2, none had clinical or histologic improvement. None of the patients had adverse clinical side effects of treatment. Intralesional IL-2 therapy also induced necrosis of invasive bladder tumors. We have recently initiated a phase I-II trial of intralesional IL-2, and have confirmed the safety of multiple intralesional intravesical injections of 2,000 units of IL-2.

Interferon gamma (IFN-G) has been found to be synergistic with IL-2 in murine melanoma.[82] Using intralesional administration in the mouse bladder cancer model, MBT2, we have confirmed that interferon increases the antitumor activity of IL-2, decreasing tumor growth and increasing animal survival.[83] Intravesical IL-2 administration has been reported by Merguerin et al.,[84] who reported a successful trial of intermittent intravesical IL-2 administration in combination with BCG. Although this report confirms the relative safety of low-dose (3600 units) intravesical IL-2, confirmation of efficacy will require a phase-II trial using IL-2 alone. Ratliff et al. found, in

the murine model, that weekly intravesical IL-2 produced edema and inflammatory infiltration of the bladder, but no antitumor effect.[85] The absence of antitumor effect in this experiment may relate to the in-vitro observation that continuous IL-2 is required to maintain LAK cell activity. Using high-dose continuous infusion IL-2 administration, Huland et al. have demonstrated that such treatment can cause regression of carcinoma of the bladder.

In the murine bladder tumor model, systemic intraperitoneal IL-2 in high doses (5,000 units every 8 hours) has, as expected, inhibited transplanted tumor growth.[86,87] Interestingly, the combination of BCG and IL-2 was found to be more effective than either treatment alone.

Systemic IL-2, while effective, has major, life-threatening toxicity. Intralesional injection of IL-2 may be the preferable route of administration. Intralesional injection can effectively maximize the availability of IL-2 to immune cells within the tumor tissue, overcome local absorption barriers, reduce the effect of the short IL-2 half-life, minimize systemic toxicity, and potentially maximize the antitumor effects of IL-2. A second cell population that may be responsible for IL-2-induced antitumor responses are the tumor-infiltrating lymphocytes (TIL).[88] These cells are reportedly 50 to 100 times more potent than LAK cells, and unlike LAK or NK, they bear T-cell markers. We have recently confirmed the safety of weekly intralesional IL-2 injection in patients with bladder cancer who have failed BCG therapy, and hope to see responses similar to that reported by Pizza. The combination of IL-2 with other lymphokines such as tumor necrotic factor, IFN-alfa, or IFN-gamma may improve antitumor effects in human trials. Alternatively, preliminary treatment with BCG, KLH, or other nonspecific stimulants to attract lymphocytes to the tumor may augment response to intralesional IL-2. Our preliminary data in the mouse bladder model confirm that BCG pretreatment enhances the antitumor effect of intralesional IL-2.

INTERFERON

Interferons are a family of naturally-occurring glycoproteins with antiviral, antiproliferative, and cellular immunomodulating properties. Interferons can be classified into two major groups, class I (alpha and beta IFN) and class II (gamma IFN), based on antigenic and physico-chemical criteria, and modes of induction. They are synthesized by a variety of cells, including leukocytes (alpha IFN), fibroblasts (beta IFN), and T and NK cells (gamma IFN). Interferons with differing actions interact with target cells through specific high affinity receptors. IFN alpha and beta appear to share the same receptors, while IFN-gamma has a unique receptor.[89]

Interferons have direct cytotoxic and antiproliferative effects as well as indirect immunomodulatory antitumor effects. The antiproliferative effects of interferon are related to decrease in DNA, RNA, and protein synthesis required for proliferation. Interferon changes the cellular metabolism of virus-infected cells by inducing alternative enzymes such as:

$2',5'$ oligoadenylate synthetase, protein kinase, $2'5'$ phospho-diesterase, and indoleamine 2,3 dioxygenase.[90] Such changes may also be involved in the interaction of interferon with tumor cells.

Interferons modulate various components of the immune system, including antibody production, delayed type hypersensitivity, IL-2 and TNF synthesis, T and NK cell activity, and macrophage-mediated cytotoxicity. Activated macrophages have antitumor cytotoxic activity and selectively lyse a variety of tumor cell lines in vitro.[91] Macrophage cytotoxic antitumor activity can be increased by pretreatment with lymphokines, including interferons.[92] Macrophage activation and secretion of cytolytic factors and toxic substances such as hydrogen peroxide are responsible for tumor killing.[93] However, inhibition of macrophage activation and the resultant cytolytic activity can be suppressed by tumor products such as prostaglandin.[94]

Alpha interferon modulates NK cell cytotoxicity by stimulating NK cell maturation.[95] NK cells are thought to play an important role in antitumor defense mechanisms. NK cells mature in the presence of IL-2, and produce gamma IFN. In vivo, IFN has a negative feedback inhibition interaction with NK cell activity. An initial increase in NK cell cytotoxicity is followed by reduction in this cell's cytotoxic activity, suggesting the existence of NK suppressor cells or other regulatory mechanisms stimulated by IFN.[96]

The first interferon clinical trials were begun in Sweden and the USA in the early 1970's using crude IFN-alpha. Several different advanced malignancies responded with rates comparable to those achieved by chemotherapy.[97] Highly purified recombinant alpha IFN has been less effective, presumably because of the presence of other immunomodulatory lymphokines in the crude preparation that enhanced the antitumor response. Since that time, IFN-alpha has had the best responses rate in hematologic malignancies such as hairy-cell leukemia (100%), chronic myeloid leukemia (80%), and nodular lymphoma (50%).[98–100] Satisfactory responses are seen in other neoplasms such as Kaposi's sarcoma (34%), malignant melanoma (18%), and renal cell carcinoma (15%).[100–102] Excellent responses have been achieved with alpha IFN therapy in two very troublesome benign neoplasms; laryngeal papillomas and condyloma acuminata.[102]

As with IL-2, the efficacy and toxicity of interferons may be improved with local rather than systemic administration. The high response rate of local therapy of some neoplasms has encouraged the investigation of alpha IFN in the treatment of superficial and invasive carcinoma of the bladder.[101]

Christophersen et al., in 1978, were the first to report the successful treatment of superficial papillary bladder tumors with intramuscular injections of crude IFN alpha ($1-2 \times 10^6$ U) protein).[102] The therapy included daily injections of IFN-alpha for 2 months, followed by three injections per week for 5 months (two cases) and 16 months (one case). Two patients were treated, two with 1-cm tumors experienced a complete response, and a third patient's tumor remained stable. These results were confirmed by Hill et al., who observed a complete response in two patients with TCC of the bladder at the dose 3×10^6 IU IFN-alpha.[103] After daily treatment for 3 weeks, the patients remained free of tumor for at least 8 and 14 months.

In 1981, Ikic et al. reported encouraging results with 2×10^6 IU of crude IFN-alpha administered transurethrally into the tumor base daily for 3 weeks.[104] In this series, four of eight patients with recurrent bladder papillomatosis had complete tumor regression. In two patients, IFN was simultaneously given by intramuscular injection at a dose of 2×10^6 IU, in addition to intralesional injections. The treatment was repeated at monthly intervals until the tumor regressed. Patients remained free of tumor for 3 to 24 months. Scorticatti et al. reported partial responses (PR) to intramuscular administration in eight patients receiving 1×10^6 IU IFN-alpha every other day over a 6-month period.[105]

In 1984, Shortliffe et al. observed complete response in four of eight patients with CIS treated with high doses of alpha 2 IFN.[106] The treatment schedule included weekly intravesical instillation of recombinant alpha-2 IFN at doses of 50, 100, and 200 million U for 8 weeks. The remaining four patients had stable disease. Ackermann et al., using recombinant alpha-2 IFN in the same dosage and treatment schedule, observed one complete response and one partial response in 4 patients with CIS.[107] Two remaining CIS patients experienced progressive disease. Two of five patients with stage Ta TCC had partial response. Schmitz-Drager et al. reported similar results, and pointed out that although intravesical administration of interferon induced some antitumor activity, mainly in patients with carcinoma in situ, the evaluation of adequate alpha-2 IFN dosage and therapy intervals is needed to improve the efficacy of this therapy.[108]

Torti et al. recently reported a much more complete and encouraging study of the treatment of superficial bladder cancer with alpha-2 IFN.[109] Thirty-five patients with histologically documented recurrent grade I or II transitional cell carcinoma of bladder stage Ta, T1, and Tis were treated intravesically with alpha-2 IFN weekly for 8 weeks. The initial interferon dose was 50×10^6 IU/dose and was escalated to 1.000×10^6 IU. Six of 17 patients (32%) with CIS had complete a response to interferon therapy. Three of these six patients relapsed at 10, 14, and 17 months. The remaining three patients (16%) were disease-free, without maintenance therapy, for 18, 32, and 37 months. Five additional patients (26%) had a complete resolution of all evidence of CIS, but had persistently positive cytology and were designated as partial responses. Three of these five patients remain free of disease in the bladder with a minimum follow-up of 15 months. Sixteen patients with recurrent papillary tumors were also treated but only four had complete response (25%). In 12 patients without prior intravesical immunotherapy or chemotherapy, 67% responded. Only seven patients (30%) with prior intravesical treatment responded (Table 47-7). Alpha-2 interferon, which is now commercially available in the United States, is an important therapeutic alternative for carcinoma in situ.

TABLE 47-7. *Interferon Alfa Response Rate in Bladder Tumor*

AUTHOR	INTERFERON	SCHEDULE	N	RESULTS
Christophersen[102]	crude IFN alpha $1-2 \times 10^6$ IU	il. daily for 2 months then $3 \times$ week (5 to 16 months)	10	2 CR (20%)
Hill[103]	crude IFN alpha 3×10^6 IU	il. daily for 3 weeks	2	2 CR (100%)
Ikic[104]	crude IFN alpha 2×10^6 IU	il. daily for 3 weeks	8	4 CR (50%)
Scorticatti[105]	crude IFN alpha 1×10^6 IU	il. daily for 6 months	8	—8 PR (100%)
Shortliffe[106]	rIFN, alpha $50-200 \times 10^6$ IU	intravesical weekly for 8 weeks	8[cis]	4 CR (50%)
Ackerman[107]	rIFN alpha $50-200 \times 10^6$ IU	intravesical weekly for 8 weeks	4[cis]	1 CR and —1 PR (25%) (25%)
			5	—2 PR (40%)
Schmitz-Drager[108]	rIFN alpha 5×10^6 IU	intravesical $2 \times$ weekly for 6 weeks	10	2 CR (20%)
Torti[109]	rIFN alpha	intravesical weekly	17[cis]	6 CR —5 PR
			16	4 CR (25%)
Total			59	14 CR (24%) —10 PR (16%)
Total (cis)			29	11 CR (38%) —6 PR (21%)

il.—intralesional injection
ive.—intravesical injection
rIFN—recombinant IFN
CR—complete response
PR—partial response

TUMOR NECROSIS FACTOR

Spontaneous regression of cancer, often associated with bacterial infection, has been recorded by generations of investigators. A small group of physicians, including William B. Coley, attempted to induce infections in patients with advanced cancer.[110] Although antitumor responses were observed, the side effects of infection were severe. Therefore, in 1893, Coley initiated the use of killed bacteria, and the mixture of Streptococcus pyogenes and Serratia marcescens came to be known as Coley's toxins. At that time, Coley's toxins represented the only known systemic therapy for cancer in the western world.

Interest in toxin therapy diminished with advances in radiotherapy and chemotherapy, but laboratory studies of microbial products as antitumor agents proceeded. The majority of these studies concentrated on gram-negative bacteria, *Corynebacterium parvum,* and BCG. In 1952, Algire et al. reported a few cases of total tumor regression after systemic injection of lipopolysaccharide (LPS),[111] which had been described earlier as a major component of the cell wall of gram-negative bacteria. LPS have long been recognized as the agent causing endotoxic shock, which may be associated with hemorrhagic necrosis and tumor regression.

For many years it was believed that the action of LPS was indirect and mediated by the host. In 1975, Carswell et al. reported that hemorrhagic necrosis of tumors could be induced in mice by injection of LPS-induced shock sera derived from animals previously "primed" by administration of bacillus Calmette-Guerin.[112] The serum factor eliciting hemorrhagic tumor necrosis was named Tumor Necrotic Factor (TNF). It is now believed that T cells stimulate the proliferation of macrophages to induce their production of TNF.[113]

Human TNF is a 17,000-dalton polypeptide which has about 50% structural homology to interferon.[114] TNF, unlike endotoxin, has a direct effect on a variety of malignant cells in vitro and in vivo, but is less toxic or non-toxic to normal cells. The precise mechanism of TNF's cytostatic and cytolytic effects are unknown. TNF induces procoagulant activity in vascular endothelium and increases neutrophil adherence in ways that promote clot formation.[115,116] Most hemorrhagic necrosis in tumors occurs at the center rather than the periphery because the vascular structure of the center is more sensitive to hypotension. Therefore, peripheral tumor cells may regrow after the initial TNF-induced necrotic reaction. Excellent antitumor responses have been observed with recombinant TNF (rTNF) in animal model tumors including Colon 26, Meth A sarcoma, sarcoma 180, MM 46, Lewis lung carcinoma, and HMV-1.[117] In murine transitional cell carcinoma (MBT2), Lee et al.[118] evaluated the efficacy of intravesically administered TNF. Modest inhibition of tumor growth was observed after tumor transplantation but, as with most treatments in the MBT2 model, no reduction of established tumor occurred. Kadhim and Chin similarly reported that intravenous TNF inhibited subcutaneously transplanted MBT2 for a short time (2 weeks), but long-term benefit did not occur even with continued TNF treatment.[119] The demonstrated activity of TNF in the MBT2 tumor model and the minimal toxicity of TNF have prompted clinical trials. TNF antitumor activity has been confirmed in early clinical trials in the Southwest Oncology Group.[120]

MONOCLONAL ANTIBODY

Since the development of the hybridoma technique by the 1984 Nobel Prize laureates Kohler and Milstein,[121] a major limitation of passive immunotherapy, that is, the availability of sufficient quantity of immune reagents, has been eliminated. Passive immunotherapy with antibody or antibody-directed toxins has new potential. Currently, the major application of monoclonal antibodies (Mab) in clinical oncology is the identification of tumor-associated antigens or tumor markers such as alpha fetoprotein, beta human chorionic gonadotropin, or prostate-specific antigen.

In the last few years, a number of Mab directed against the tumor associated antigens of bladder carcinoma have been produced.[122-124] These provided a panel for the selection of Mab that could be used in clinical detection of tumor cells in bladder cancer (e.g., bladder washing).[124-127] A useful application of Mab is the study of the relationship between antigenic phenotype and biologic characteristics of bladder tumors, such as the properties of invasiveness and metastasis.[128] Such studies may eventually provide a basis for better selection of treatments and the use of Mab in the selective destruction of bladder tumor cells.

Monoclonal antibodies can lyse tumor cells by direct action or by activation of complement.[129,130] Murine Mab have been found to be cytotoxic to a human bladder cancer cell line, TSGH-8301.[131] Immunotherapy of xenografted tumors in nude mice using Mab has demonstrated that therapeutic efficacy is dose-dependent and closely related to tumor burden.

Unfortunately, animal model studies have demonstrated that enormous amounts of antibody are required to eliminate even small tumor masses. Therefore, alternative approaches are being studied to improve antitumor activity. Cytotoxic drugs, toxins, or radioisotopes can be conjugated with Mab to utilize the specificity of the antigen combining site to deliver a lethal hit directly to the tumor without requiring participation of host effector cells.

Theisen et al., in 1987, reported that monoclonal antibody 486P 3-12-1, raised against transitional cell carcinoma and conjugated to A and B chains of ricin, showed selective antitumor activity against human bladder cancer cells in vitro.[132] Recently, Yu et al. evaluated a murine IgG3 monoclonal antibody conjugated with doxorubicin in the treatment of human bladder cancer and suggested that such immunochemotherapy may offer advantages over chemotherapy or immunotherapy alone.[133] These findings suggest that cytotoxic drugs, toxin, or radioisotope therapy can be conjugated to Mab to reduce side effects and improve delivery of these therapies.

NONSPECIFIC IMMUNE ADJUVANTS

Maltose Tetrapalmitate

Maltose tetrapalmitate (MTP) is a synthetic glycolipid with a structure similar to the immunoadjuvant bacterial lipid A.[134] Unlike lipid A, MTP has no endotoxin activity and toxicity studies have shown no apparent side effects. MTP has been found to have antitumor activity in murine bladder cancer and has recently been effective in the prevention of bladder tumor recurrence in man.[135] In 47 patients randomized to transurethral resection only, resection plus MTP, or resection plus BCG, the recurrence rate (recurrence/100 patient months) was 11.3, 7.4, and 7.2 respectively ($p < 0.05$). Like KLH and interferon, intravesical MTP has minimal toxicity.

OK-432

OK-432 is a lyophilized preparation of attenuated streptococci.[136] Fujita et al. evaluated antitumor efficacy of OK-432 in 78 patients with stage Ta, T1, and T2 bladder cancer.[137] Thirty-six patients with primary disease and 42 patients with recurrent TCC were randomized to OK-432 or control groups. OK-432 was injected intralesionally three times before transurethral resection, and thereafter was given by intravesical instillation (0.5 mg once every 2 weeks for 6 months). The recurrence rate for patients with primary disease was 3.6 per 100 months for the OK-432 group and 9.1 per 100 months for the control group ($p < 0.05$). This study suggested that OK-432 was effective, and, surprisingly, was especially encouraging in high-risk patients with multiple, large, sessile, and high-grade tumors.

INTERFERON INDUCERS

Poly I:C

Poly I:C, an interferon inducer, has demonstrated efficacy in animal as well as human bladder cancer.[138,139] Kemeny et al.

evaluated the ability of poly I:C to decrease tumor recurrence after endoscopic resection.[139] Although there was no significant difference in recurrence rate in the 32 patients, a difference in survival favoring the poly I:C group was observed. The median time of survival was 170+ months for the poly I:C group as compared with 76+ months for the control group (p < 0.05).

Pyrimidinones

Another class of interferon inducers, pyrimidinones, have also been demonstrated to have antitumor activity in both animal and human bladder cancer. In the mouse bladder tumor model, we found both 2-phenyl-5-bromo-6-phenyl-4-pyrimidinol (ABPP) and the 5-iodo analog (AIPP) to significantly inhibit MBT2 growth.[140] Unlike most immunotherapy and chemotherapy in this model, the pyrimidinone interferon inducers caused regression of established tumor. Sarosdy et al. have confirmed this work and demonstrated that ABPP appears to potentiate the response to BCG in the animal model.[141] Phase I-II clinical trials have been initiated and are too early to report, but the drug appears to be well-tolerated and clinical response has already been documented.

ACTIVE SPECIFIC IMMUNOTHERAPY
Irradiated Tumor Vaccine

Autologous tumor cells have been used as specific active immunotherapy against various malignancies with varying, but limited, success.[142,143] The potential benefit of autologous irradiated tumor cell vaccine in combination with BCG has been evaluated as an adjuvant to colectomy in patients with adenocarcinoma of the colon. Hanna et al. have observed a 44% recurrence in 47 patients treated with surgery alone compared with an only 23% recurrence in patients treated with immunotherapy. Tumor deaths have been reduced from 4 to 1.[144] We have investigated the response of murine cancer (MBT2) to immunotherapy with irradiated cells (Ir-MBT2) with and without BCG.[145] Fresh, enzymatically dissociated, MBT2 was irradiated with 10,000 cGy and administered intralesionally. Surprisingly, the optimal dose (10^7) and ratio of tumor cell:BCG (1:1) used by Hanna in the guinea pig hepatocarcinoma model was found to increase tumor progression and death in the mouse bladder tumor model.[146] Significant reduction in tumor incidence relative to saline controls (93%) was observed only in BCG (27%, p < 0.005) treated animals, and the addition of irradiated tumor vaccine consistently reduced antitumor response in a dose-dependent manner. The use of autologous irradiated bladder tumor vaccines, alone or in combination with BCG, appears to have no immunotherapeutic advantage in this model. Concern is raised that the addition of irradiated tumor vaccine in bladder cancer may even *detract* from the results achievable with BCG alone.

Butanol-extracted Tumor Antigens

LaGrue et al., in an effort to extract antigen from tumor cells in tissue culture while maintaining their viability, used 1-butanol as solvent. Immunotherapy with butanol extracted antigens was highly effective and superior to 3M KCl extracted antigens in animal models.[147] We evaluated the antitumor activity of immunotherapy with butanol extracted antigens and documented significant long-term protection from transplantation of MBT2.[148] We observed in significant reduction in tumor growth and prolonged survival. No untoward reactions to butanol-extracted antigen immunotherapy were noted.

Ethylchlorformate Polymerized Tumor Protein

Soluble tumor antigens typically elicit a weak immune response and are more commonly associated with suppression of effective antitumor immunity. By polymerizing tumor proteins, ineffective soluble antigens can be converted to effective, particulate antigens. Tykka has reported regression of lung metastasis in 9 of 21 patients (43%) with renal cell carcinoma treated with ethylchlorformate polymerized tumor antigen plus PPD or *Candida albicans* antigen.[149] No serious side effects of treatment were observed. In the MBT2 mouse bladder cancer model, dose-dependent immunity was observed following immunotherapy with ethylchlorformate polymerized antigen. Protection from this therapy was long-term and the combination of vaccine plus BCG was superior to treatment with either agent alone.[150,151]

CONCLUSION

Immunotherapy has been remarkably effective in the treatment of superficial bladder cancer. A large number of agents are effective, and, unlike chemotherapy, immunotherapy appears to significantly alter the course of the disease, reduce progression, and improve survival. Although these new modalities are not always curative, they offer a more comprehensive approach than simple transurethral resection of visible bladder tumors. Immunotherapeutic agents have mechanisms of action that are different from commonly used, locally acting alkylating agents such as thiotepa, Epodyl, and mitomycin. BCG is currently the most effective treatment for superficial bladder cancer and has already significantly changed our management of carcinoma in situ.

Although BCG is highly effective, at least 30% of patients with carcinoma in situ or rapidly recurring papillary tumors will fail to respond to treatment. Moreover, BCG has significant and potentially fatal toxicity. Newer immunotherapies, which have largely been developed with the aid of animal tumor models, hold promise of increased efficacy as well as reduced toxicity. Promising new agents, such as KLH, vaccines, interleukin 2, and other lymphokines will be welcome additions to our clinical armamentarium.

REFERENCES

1. Lamm, D. L. BCG immunotherapy in bladder cancer. In *1987 Urology Annual*. Edited by S. N. Rous. Norwalk, Appelton and Lange, 1987, p. 77.

2. Friedman, R. M., and Vogel, S. N. Interferons with special emphasis on the immune system. In *Advances in Immunology*. Volume 34. Edited by F. J. Dixon and H. G. Kunkel. New York, Academic Press, 1983, p. 97.

3. Crispen, R. G. BCG vaccine in perspective. Semin. Oncol., *1:*311, 1974.

4. Lotte, A., et al. BCG complication: Estimated risks among vaccinated subjects and statistical analysis of main characteristics. Adv. Tuberc. Res., *21:*107, 1984.

5. Biozzi, G., et al. Granulopexique du systeme reticulo-endothelial au cours de l'infection tuberculeuse experimentale de la souris. Ann. Inst. Pasteur Microbiol., *87:*291, 1954.

6. Davies, M. Bacillus Calmette-Guerin as an antitumor agent. The interaction with cells of the mammalian immune system. Biochem. Biophys. Acta, *651:*143, 1982.

7. Winters, W. D., and Lamm, D. L. BCG-induced circulating interferon, antibody, and immune complexes in bladder cancer patients treated with intravesical BCG. J. Urol., *134:*40, 1985.

8. Haaf, E. D., Catalona, W. J., and Ratliff, T. L. Detection of interleukin-2 in urine of patients with superficial bladder tumors after treatment with intravesical BCG. J. Urol., *136:*970, 1986.

9. Freund, J. The mode of action of immunologic adjuvants. Adv. Tuberc. Res., *7:*130, 1956.

10. Morales, A., Eidinger, D., and Bruce, A. W. Intracavitary bacillus Calmette-Guerin in treatment of superficial bladder tumors. J. Urol., *116:*180, 1976.

11. Lamm, D. L., et al. Bacillus Calmette-Guerin immunotherapy of superficial bladder cancer. J. Urol., *124:*38, 1980.

12. Camacho, F., et al. Treatment of superficial bladder cancer with intravesical BCG. In Immunotherapy of Human Cancer. Edited by W. T. Terry and S. A. Rosenberg. New York, Elsevier, North Holland, 1982, p. 309.

13. Martinez-Peneiro, J. A. BCG Vaccine in the treatment of noninfiltrating papillary tumors of the bladder. In *Bladder Tumors and Others Topics in Urologic Oncology*. Edited by M. Pavonemacabew, P. H. Smith, and F. Edsmyr. New York, Plenum Press, 1980, p. 173.

14. Brosman, S. A. Experience with bacillus Calmette-Guerin in patients with superficial bladder cancer. J. Urol., *128:*27, 1982.

15. Adolphs, H. D., and Bastian, H. P. Chemoimmune prophylaxis of superficial bladder tumors. J. Urol., *129:*29, 1983.

16. Netto, N. R., Jr., and Lemos, C. G. A comparison of treatment methods for prophylaxis of recurrent superficial bladder tumors. J. Urol., *129:*33, 1983.

17. Babayan, R. K., and Krane, R. S. Intravesical BCG for superficial bladder cancer. Abstract 393. American Urological Association. 80th Annual Meeting. Atlanta, May, 1985.

18. deKernion, J. B., et al. The management of superficial bladder tumors and carcinoma in situ with intravesical Bacillus Calmette-Guerin. J. Urol., *133:*598, 1985.

19. Haaf, E. O., et al. Results of retreatment with intravesical BCG therapy for patients failing the initial BCG course. Abstract 289. American Urological Association. 80th Annual Meeting. Atlanta, May, 1985.

20. Schellhammer, P. F., and Ladaga, L. E. Bacillus Calmette-Guerin for therapy of superficial transitional cell carcinoma of the bladder. J. Urol., *135:*261, 1986.

21. Flamm, J., and Grof, F. Adjuvant local immunotherapy with Bacillus Calmette-Guerin (BCG) in treatment of urothelial carcinoma of the urinary bladder. Wien. Med. Wochenschr., *131:*501, 1981.

22. Stober, U., and Peters, H. H. BCG-immunotherapie zur rezidiuphylaxe bein harnblasenkarzinom. Therapiewoche, *30:*6067, 1980.

23. Kowalkowski, T. S., and Lamm, D. L. Intravesical therapy of superficial bladder cancer. In *Current Trends In Urology*. Volume 4. Edited by M. Resnick. Baltimore, Williams & Willkins, 1988.

24. Doville, Y., et al. Recurrent bladder papilomata treated with Bacillus Calmette-Guerin: A preliminary report (phase I trial). Cancer Treat. Rep., *62:*551, 1978.

25. Morales, A., Ottenhof, P., and Emerson, L. Treatment of residual, non-infiltrating bladder cancer with Bacillus Calmette-Guerin. J. Urol., *125:*649, 1981.

26. Lamm, D. L., et al. Bladder cancer immunotherapy. J. Urol., *128:*931, 1982.

27. Kojima, L., Ishida, Y., and Mori, C. Eradication of superficial transitional cell carcinoma of the bladder by intravesical instillation of Bacillus Calmette-Guerin (BCG). Abstract 395. American Urological Association. 80th Annual Meeting. Atlanta, May, 1985.

28. Morales, A. Treatment of carcinoma in situ of the bladder with BCG. A phase II trial. Cancer Immunol. Immunother., *9:*69, 1980.

29. Lamm, D. L. BCG Immunotherapy in bladder cancer. J. Urol., *134:*40, 1985.

30. Herr, H. W., et al. Effect of intravesical Bacillus Calmette-Guerin (BCG) on carcinoma in situ of the bladder. Cancer, *51:*1323, 1983.

31. Brosman, S. The use of Bacillus Calmette-Guerin in therapy of bladder cancer in situ. J. Urol., *134:*36, 1985.

32. Schellhammer, P. F., Ladaga, L. E., and Fillion, M. B. Bacillus Calmette-Guerin for superficial transitional cell carcinoma of the bladder. J. Urol., *135:*261, 1986.

33. Kavoussi, L. R., et al. Results of 6 weekly intravesical Bacillus Calmette-Guerin instillations on the treatment of superficial bladder tumors. J. Urol., *139:*935, 1988.

34. Rintala, M., et al. Mitomycin-C and BCG in intravesical chemotherapy and immunotherapy of superficial bladder cancer. In BCG in Superficial Bladder Cancer. Edited by F. M. J. Debruyne, L. Denis, Ad. P. M. van der Meijden. New York, Alan R. Liss, Inc., 1989, p. 271.

35. Brosman, S. The influence of Tice strain BCG treatment in patients with transitional cell carcinoma in situ. In BCG in Superficial Bladder Cancer. Edited by F. M. J. Debruyne, L. Denis, Ad. P. M. van der Meijden. New York, Alan R. Liss, Inc., 1989, p. 193.

36. Steg, A., Leleu, C., and Boccon-Gibod, L. Treatment des tumerus superficielles de la vessies par BCG-therapie intravesicale. Edited by F. Di Silverio and A. Steg. In Internation Workshop in Urology— New trends in bladder cancer chemotherapy. Rome: Acta Medica, p. 203, 1988.

37. Pagano, F. personal communication.

38. Prescott, S. et al. Immunopathological effect of intravesical BCG therapy. In BCG in Superficial Bladder Cancer. Edited by F. M. J.

Debruyne, L. Denis, Ad. P. M. van der Meijden. New York, Alan R. Liss, Inc., 1989, p. 93.

39. RETISMA, D.J. Long-term effect of intravesical Bacillus Calmette-Guerin (BCG) Tice strain on flat carcinoma in situ of the bladder. In BCG in Superficial Bladder Cancer. Edited by F. M. J. Debruyne, L. Denis, Ad. P. M. van der Meijden. New York, Alan R. Liss, Inc., 1989, p. 171.

40. LAMM, D. L., et al. *Adriamycin versus BCG in Superficial Bladder Cancer.* Edited by M. J. Frans and M. D. Debruyne. New York, Alan R. Liss. In press.

41. REYNOLDS, R. H., STODGILL, V. D., and LAMM, D. L. Disease progression in BCG-treated patients with transitional cell carcinoma of the bladder. A.U.A. Proc. 133:390 (392) April, 1985.

42. DEBRUYNE, F. M. J. Superficial bladder cancer intravesical therapy trials: An interim report. Evansville, Bristol-Meyers, 7, 1988.

43. RATLIFF, T. L., et al. Intravesical Bacillus Calmette-Guerin therapy for murine bladder tumors: Initiation of the response by fibronectin-mediated attachment of bacillus Calmette-Guerin. Cancer Res., 47:1762, 1987.

44. PROUT, G. R., et al. Long-term fate of 90 patients with superficial bladder cancer randomly assigned to receive or not receive thiotepa. J. Urol., 130:677, 1983.

45. SAROSDY, M. F., GRAU, D. G., and LAMM, D. L. Long term results of Bacillus Calmette-Guerin immunotherapy for superficial bladder cancer. J. Urol., 139l:299a (548), 1988.

46. TORRENCE, R. J., et al. Prognostic factors in patients treated with intravesical Bacillus Calmette-Guerin for superficial bladder cancer. J. Urol., 139:941, 1989.

47. RATLIFF, T. L., and CATALONA, W. J. Depressed proliferative response in patients treated with 12 weeks of intravesical BCG. J. Urol., 141:230 A, (244), 1989.

48. HUDSON, M. A., et al. Single course versus maintenance Bacillus Calmette-Guerin therapy for superficial bladder tumor: A prospective, randomized trial. J. Urol., 138:295, 1987.

49. BADALAMENT, R. A., et al. A prospective randomized trial of maintenance versus non-maintenance Bacillus Calmette-Guerin therapy of superficial bladder cancer. J. Clin. Oncol., 3:441, 1987.

50. REICHERT, D. F., and LAMM, D. L. Long term protection in bladder cancer following intralesional immunotherapy. J. Urol., 132:570, 1984.

51. BAST, R. C., and BAST, B. S. Critical review of previously reported animal studies of tumor immunotherapy with nonspecific immunostimulants. Ann. N.Y. Acad. Sci., 227:60, 1976.

52. NETTO, N. R., JR., and LEMOS, G. C. A comparison of treatment methods for prophylaxis of recurrent superficial bladder tumors. J. Urol., 129:33, 1983.

53. PANG, A. S., and MORALES, A. Immunoprophylaxis of a murine bladder cancer with high dose BCG immunization. J. Urol., 132:675, 1984.

54. DRAGO, J. R., and SIPIO, J. Characterization of the Nb rat bladder cancer model. Surg. Forum, 36:645, 1985.

55. RAWLS, W. H., LAMM, D. L., and EYOLFSON, M. F. Septic complication in the use of Bacillus Calmette-Guerin for non invasive transitional cell carcinoma. J. Urol., 139:300A (522), 1988.

56. LAMM, D. L., et al. Complications of Bacillus Calmette-Guerin Immunotherapy: Review of 2602 patients and comparison of chemotherapy complications. In BCG in Superficial Bladder Cancer. Edited by F. M. J. Debruyne, L. Denis, Ad. P. M. van der Meijden. New York, Alan R. Liss, Inc., 1989, p. 335.

57. CURTIS, J. E., et al. The human primary immune response to Keyhole limpet hemocyanin: Interrelationships of delayed hypersensitivity, antibody response and in vitro blast transformation. Clin. Exp. Immunol., 6:473, 1970.

58. OLSSON, C. A., CHUTE, R., and RAO, C. N. Immunologic reduction of bladder cancer rate. J. Urol., 111:173, 1974.

59. LAMM, D. L., REYNA, J. A., and REICHERT, D. F. Keyhole-limpet hemocyanin and immune ribonucleic acid immunotherapy of murine transitional cell carcinoma. Urol. Res., 9:227, 1981.

60. JURINCIC, CD., et al. Immunotherapy in bladder cancer with keyhole-limpet hemocyanin: Randomized study. J. Urol., 139:723, 1988.

61. FLAMM, O. A. personal communication, 1988.

62. MORGAN, D. A., RUSCETTI, F. W., and GALLO, R. Selective in vitro growth of lymphocytes from normal human bone marrows. Science, 193:1007, 1976.

63. ROOK, A. H., et al. Interleukin-2 enhances the depressed natural killer and cytomegalovirus specific cytotoxic activates of lymphokines from patients with the acquired immune deficiency syndrome. J. Clin. Invest., 72:398, 1983.

64. FLOMENBERG, N., et al. Immunologic effect of interleukin-2 in primary immunodeficiency disease. J. Immunol., 130:2644, 1983.

65. MERLUZZI, V. J., et al. Recovery of the in vivo cytotoxic T-cell response in cyclophosphamide-treated mice by injection of mixed-lymphocyte-culture supernatants. Cancer Res., 41:3663, 1981.

66. YORN, I., et al. In vitro growth of murine T cells. V. The isolation and growth of lymphoid cells infiltrating syngeneic solid tumors. J. Immunol., 125:238, 1980.

67. LOTZE, M. T., et al. In vitro growth of cytotoxic human lymphocytes. IV. Lysis of fresh and cultured autologous tumor by lymphocytes cultured in T cell growth factor (TSGF). Cancer Res., 41:4420, 1981.

68. VOSE, B. M., and BONNARD, G. D. Limiting dilution analysis of frequency of human T cells and large granular lymphocytes proliferating in response to interleukin-2. J. Immunol., 130:687, 1983.

69. KASAHARA, T., et al. Interleukin-2-mediated immune interferon (IFN-gamma) production by human T cells in T cell subsets. J. Immunol., 130:1784, 1983.

70. SVERDERSKY, L. P., et al. Interferon-gamma enhances induction of lymphotoxin in recombinant interleukin 2-stimulated peripheral blood mononuclear cells. J. Immunol., 134:1604, 1985.

71. NEDWIN, G. E., et al. Effect of interleukin-2, interferon-gamma, and mitogens on production of tumor necrosis factors alpha and beta. J. Immunol., 135:2492, 1985.

72. WALDMAN, T. A., GOLDMAN, C. K., and ROBB, R. J. Expression of interleukin-2 receptors on activated human B cells. J. Exp. Med., 138:185, 1984.

73. ROSENBERG, S. A., LOTZE, M. T., and MULE, J. J. New approaches to the immunotherapy of cancer using interleukin-2. Ann. Intern. Med., 108:6, 1988.

74. SIMPSON, S., SEIPP, C. A., and ROSENBERG, S. A. The current status and future applications of interleukin-2 and adoptive immunotherapy in cancer treatment. Semin. Oncol. Nurs., 4:2, 1988.

75. LOTZE, M. T., et al. In vivo administration of purified human interleukin-2: Half life and immunologic effects of the Jurkat cell line derived Il-2. J. Immunol., 134:157, 1985.

76. ROSENBERG, S. A., et al. A progress report of the treatment 157 patients with advanced cancer using lymphokine-activated killer cells and interleukin-2 or high dose of interleukin-2 alone. N. Engl. J. Med., 316:889, 1987.

77. West, H. W., et al. Constant-infusion recombinant interleukin-2 in adoptive immunotherapy of advanced cancer. N. Engl. J. Med., *316*:898, 1987.

78. Pulley, M. S., et al. Lymphokine Res., *5* (Suppl 1):157, 1986.

79. Pizza, G., et al. Intra-lymphatic administration of interleukin-2 (IL-2) in cancer patients: A pilot study. Lymphokine Res., *7*:45, 1988.

80. Papermaster, B. W., McEntire, J. E., and Gilliland, C. D. The biological immune response modifiers. In humans lymphokines. Edited by A. Khan and N. O. Hill. New York, Academic Press, 1982, p. 459.

81. Pizza, G., et al. Tumor regression after intralesional injection of interleukin-2 (IL-2) in bladder cancer. Preliminary report. Int. J. Cancer, *34*:359, 1984.

82. Silagi, S., Dutkowski, R., and Schaefer, A. Eradication of mouse melanoma by combined treatment with recombinant human interleukin-2 and recombinant murine interferon-gamma. Int. J. Cancer, *41*:315, 1988.

83. Sosnowski, J. T., et al. Treatment of murine transitional cell carcinoma with interleukin-2 and interferon. J. Urol., *141*:215A, (183) 1989.

84. Merguerin, P. A., Donahue, L. A., and Cocett, A. T. K. Intracavitary Bacillus Calmette-Guerin and interleukin-2 therapy for bladder cancer. J. Urol., *135*:121A, 1986.

85. Ratliff, T. L. personal communication.

86. Lee, K. E., et al. Reduction of bladder cancer growth in mice treated with intravesical Bacillus Calmette-Guerin and systemic interleukin-2. J. Urol., *137*:1270, 1987.

87. Lee, K. E., et al. Interleukin-2 suppression of a murine bladder cancer implanted into kidney, bladder and skin; Its organ specificity. J. Urol., *140*:840, 1988.

88. Rosenberg, S. A., Spiess, P. F., and Larfreniere, R. A. A new approach to the adoptive immunotherapy of cancer with tumor-infiltrating lymphocytes. Science, *223*:1318, 1986.

89. Orchansky, P., et al. Type I and II interferon receptors. J. Interferon Res., *4*:275, 1984.

90. Samuel, C. Molecular mechanism of interferon action. In *Clinical Applications of Interferons and Their Inducers.* Edited by D. Stringfellow. New York, Marcel Dekker, 1986, p. 1.

91. Adams, D. O. Effector mechanism of cytolytically activated macrophages. I. Secretion of neutral proteases and effect of protease inhibitors. J. Immunol., *124*:286, 1979.

92. Schultz, R. M., Papamatheakis, J. D., and Chirigos, M. A. Interferon: An inducer of macrophage activation by poly anions. Science, *197*:674, 1976.

93. Adams, D. O., et al. Hydrogen peroxide and cytolytic factor can interact synergistically in effecting cytolysis of neoplastic targets. J. Immunol., *127*:1973, 1981.

94. Russell, S. W., Doe, W. F., and Tozier McIntosh, A. Functional characterization of a stable noncytolytic stage of macrophage activation in tumors. J. Exp. Med., *146*:1511, 1977.

95. Schmitz-Drager, B. J., Marumo, K., and Ackerman, R. Kinetik der spontanen zellvermittelten Zytotoxizitat bei Patienten mit Prostatarzinom. In *Experimentelle Urologie.* Edited by R. Harzmann. Berlin, Springer, 1985, p. 495.

96. Santoni, A., et al. Suppression of activity of mouse natural killer (NK) cells by activated macrophages from mice treated with pyran copolymer. Int. J. Cancer, *26*:837, 1980.

97. Strander, H., et al. Interferon treatment of osteogenic sarcoma: A clinical trial. Conference on Modulation of Host Immune Resistance in the Prevention and Treatment of Induced Neoplasms. Washington, DC. US Government Printing Office, *28*:377, 1980.

98. Talpaz, M., et al. Hematologic remission and cytogenetic improvement induced by recombinant human interferon alpha A in chronic myelogenous leukemia. N. Engl. J. Med., *314*:1064, 1986.

99. Goldstein, D., and Laszlo, J. Interferon therapy in cancer: From imaginon to interferon. Cancer Res., *46*:4315, 1986.

100. Rios, A., et al. Treatment of acquired immunodeficiency syndrome-related Kaposi's sarcoma with lymphoblastoid interferon. J. Clin. Oncol., *3*:506, 1985.

101. Kirkwood, J. M., et al. Comparison of intramuscular and intravenous recombinant alpha-2 interferon in malignant melanoma and other cancers. Ann. Intern. Med., *103*:32, 1985.

102. Christophersen, I. S., et al. Interferon therapy in neoplastic disease. Act. Med. Scand., *204*:471, 1978.

103. Hill, N. O., Parude, A., and Khan, A. Phase II human leukocyte interferon trials in leucemia and cancer. J. Clin. Hemat. Oncol., *11*:23, 1981.

104. Ikic, D., et al. Application of human leukocyte interferon in patients with urinary bladder papillomatosis, breast cancer, and melanoma. Lancet, *1*:1022, 1981.

105. Scorticatti, C. H., et al. Systemic IFN alpha treatment of multiple bladder papilloma grade I or II patients-pilot study. J. Interferon Res., *3*:339, 1978.

106. Shortliffe, L. C., et al. Intravesical interferon therapy for carcinoma in situ and transitional cell carcinoma of the bladder. J. Urol., *131*:171, 1984.

107. Ackermann, D., et al. Treatment of superficial bladder tumors with intravesical recombinant interferon alpha-2a. Urol. Int., *43*:85, 1988.

108. Schmitz-Drager, B. J., Ebert, T., and Ackerman, R. Intravesical treatment of superficial bladder carcinoma with interferons. World J. Urol., *3*:218, 1986.

109. Torti, F. M., et al. Alpha-interferon in superficial bladder cancer: A Northern California Oncology Group Study. J. Clin. Oncol., *6*:475, 1988.

110. Old, L. J. Tumor necrotic factor. Science, *230*:630, 1985.

111. Algire, G. H., Legallaris, F. Y., and Anderson, B. F. Vascular reaction of normal and malignant tissues in vivo. V. Role of hypotension in action of bacterial polysaccharide. J. Natl. Cancer Inst., *12*:1279, 1952.

112. Carswell, E. A., et al. An endotoxin-induced serum factor that causes necrosis of tumor. Proc. Natl. Acad. Sci. U.S.A., *72*:3666, 1975.

113. Niitsu, Y., et al. T cell involvement in production of tumor necrosis factor: Reconstitution experiments with nude mice. Jpn. J. Cancer Res. (Gann), *76*:395, 1985.

114. Aggarwal, B. B., et al. Human tumor necrosis factor. Production, purification, and characterization. J. Biol. Chem., *260*:2345, 1985.

115. Bevilacqua, M. P., et al. Recombinant tumor necrosis factor induces procoagulant activity in cultured human vascular endothelium: Characterization and comparison with the actions of Interleukin-1. Proc. Natl. Acad. Sci. U.S.A., *83*:4533, 1986.

116. Pohlman, T. H., et al. An endothelial cells surface factor(s) induced in vitro by lipopolysaccharide, interleukin-1, and tumor necrosis factor alfa increases neutrophil adherence by a CDw18-dependent mechanism. J. Immunol., *136*:4548, 1986.

117. Haranaka, K., et al. Antitumor activity of murine tumor necrosis

factor against heterotransplanted human cancer cells in nude mice. In the Proceedings of the Japanese Cancer Association 41st Annual Meeting, 1985, p. 231.

118. LEE, K. E., et al. Effect of intravesical administration of tumor necrosis serum and human recombinant tumor necrosis factor on a murine bladder tumor. J. Urol., *138*:430, 1987.

119. KADHIM, S. A., and CHIN, J. L. Anti-tumor effect of tumor necrosis factor and its induction of tumor variant of MBT2 transitional cell carcinoma of the bladder. J. Urol., *139*:1091, 1988.

120. CRAWFORD, E. D. personal communication, 1988.

121. KOHLER, G., and MILSTEIN, C. Continuous culture of fused cells secreting antibody of predefined specificity. Nature, *256*:497, 1975.

122. GROSSMAN, H. B. Hybridoma antibodies reactive with human bladder carcinoma cell surface antigens. J. Urol., *130*:610, 1983.

123. MESSING, E. M., et al. Murine hybridoma antibodies against human transitional carcinoma-associated antigens. J. Urol., *132*:167, 1984.

124. CHOPIN, D. K., et al. Monoclonal antibodies against transitional cell carcinoma for detection of malignant urothelial cells in bladder washing. J. Urol., *134*:260, 1985.

125. YOUNG, D. A., PROUT, G. R., JR., and LIN, C-W. Production and characterization of mouse monoclonal antibodies to human bladder tumor-associates antigens. Cancer Res., *45*:4439, 1985.

126. HULAND, H., et al. Monoclonal antibody 486 P 3/12: A valuable bladder carcinoma marker for immunocytology. J. Urol., *137*:654, 1987.

127. CHI-WEI, L., et al. Detection of tumor cells in bladder washings by a monoclonal antibody to human bladder tumor-associates antigen. J. Urol., *140*:672, 1988.

128. FRADET, Y., et al. Cell surface antigen of human bladder tumors: Definition of tumors subsets by monoclonal antibodies and correlation with growth characteristics. Cancer Res., *46*:5183, 1986.

129. CAPONE, P. M., et al. Experimental tumoricidal effect of monoclonal antibody against solid breast tumors. Proc. Natl. Acad. Sci. U.S.A., *80*:7328, 1983.

130. HERLYN, D., et al. Inhibition of growth of colorectal carcinoma in nude mice by monoclonal antibody. Cancer Res., *40*:717, 1980.

131. YU, D. S., YEH, M. Y., and CHANG, S. Y. Immunotherapy of xenografted human bladder cancer in nude mice using monoclonal antibody. Eur. Urol., *13*:198, 1987.

132. THIESEN, H. J., JUHL, H., and ARNDT, R. Selective killing of human bladder cancer cells by combined treatment with A and B ricin antibody conjugates. Cancer Res., *47*:419, 1987.

133. YU, D-S., et al. Antitumor activity of doxorubicin-monoclonal antibody conjugate on human bladder cancer. J. Urol., *140*:415, 1988.

134. SKIDMORE, B. J., et al. Immunologic properties of bacterial polysaccharide (LPS): Correlation between the mitogenic, adjuvant and immunogenic activities. J. Immunol., *114*:770, 1975.

135. IBRANIEM, E. I., et al. Prophylactic maltose tetrapalmitate and Bacillus Calmette-Guerin immunotherapy of recurrent superficial bladder tumors: Preliminary report. J. Urol., *140*:498, 1988.

136. KIMURA, I., et al. Immunotherapy in human lung cancer using the streptococcal agent OK-432. Cancer, *37*:2201, 1976.

137. FUJITA, K. The role of adjuvant immunotherapy in superficial bladder cancer. Cancer, *59*:2027, 1987.

138. DROLLER, M. J., and GOMOLKA, D. Indonethacin and poly I:C in the inhibition of carcinogen-induced bladder cancer in an experimental animal model. J. Urol., *131*:1212, 1984.

139. KEMENY, N., et al. Randomized trial of standard therapy with or without poly I:C in patients with superficial bladder cancer. Cancer, *48*:2154, 1981.

140. SIMMONS, W. B., et al. Pyrimidinone interferon inducers in the treatment of murine transitional cell carcinoma. Abstract no 309, American Urological Association 78th Annual Meeting, Nevada, April 17–21, 1983.

141. SAROSDY, M. F., KIERUM, C. A., and MUNOZ, D. A. Potentiation of Bacillus Calmette-Guerin activity in bladder cancer by the pyrimidinone interferon inducer ABPP. J. Urol., *139*:300 (549), 1988.

142. CZAJKOWSKI, N. P., ROSENBLATT, M., and WOLF, P. L. A new method of active immunization to autologous human tumor tissue. Lancet, *27*:905, 1967.

143. ZBAR, B., et al. Immunoprophylaxis of syngeneic metylchloanthere-induced murine sarcomas with Bacillus Calmette-Guerin and tumor cells. Cancer Res., *40*:1036, 1980.

144. HOVER, H. C., PETERS, L. C., and BRANDHORST, J. S. Therapy of spontaneous metastases with an autologous cell vaccine in a guinea pig model. J. Surg. Res., *30*:409, 1981.

145. DEHAVEN, J., et al. Immunotherapy of murine bladder cancer by irradiated tumor vaccine. J. Urol., *141*:213a (248), 1989.

146. PETERS, L. C., and HANNA, M. G. The specific immunotherapy of established micrometastases: Effect of cryopreservation procedures on tumor cell immunogenicity in guinea pigs. J. Natl. Cancer Inst., *64*:1521, 1980.

147. LaGRUE, S. J., KAHAN, B. D., and PELLIS, N. R. Extraction of murine tumor-specific transplantation antigen with 1 butanol. 1. Partial purification be isoelectric focusing. J. Natl. Cancer Inst., *65*:191, 1980.

148. ROCHESTER, G. M., et al. Immunotherapy of murine transitional cell carcinoma with butanol-extracted antigens. J. Urol., *133*:618 (268a), 1984.

149. TYKKA, H. Active specific immunotherapy with supportive measures in the treatment of advanced palliatively nephrectomized renal adenocarcinoma: a control clinical study. Scand. J. Urol. Nephrol., *63*:7, 1981.

150. STOGDILL, B., et al. Ethylchloroformate polymerized tumor proteins and BCG in the immunotherapy of murine bladder cancer. J. Urol., *133*:615 (267a), 1984.

151. ROCHESTER, M. G., SAROSDY, M. S., and PICKETT, S. H. Tumor-specific immunotherapy of murine bladder cancer with butanol-extracted antigens and etylchoroformate polymerized tumor protein. J. Urol., *140*:647, 1988.

CHAPTER
48

Chemotherapy of Bladder Cancer

Ronald L. Stephens

The chemotherapy of patients with bladder cancer has evolved rapidly during the past decade. Whereas complete responses to chemotherapy were once rare, they are now being reported with increased frequency, usually from single institutions reporting their success with combination drug treatment. This chapter evaluates both single-agent and combination chemotherapy in patients with advanced bladder cancer, the combined use of radiation and chemotherapy, and the use of adjuvant chemotherapy in patients who have had or will have cystectomy.

SINGLE AGENTS IN METASTATIC DISEASE

As combinations become increasingly successful, new information on single agents in this disease becomes rare. Table 48-1 selectively summarizes published results of single-agent activity in the treatment of patients with advanced bladder cancer. This table and the supporting discussion refers only to reports of the most commonly seen bladder cancer in Western society, transitional cell carcinoma. No effort will be made in this chapter to discuss the rarer adenocarcinoma, squamous cell carcinoma, or to delve into the use of intravesical chemotherapy.

Only those studies that follow the modern criteria for response determination are listed in the table. A complete response is defined as a total disappearance of all measurable disease on physical exam and/or x-ray, whereas a partial response represents a 50% decrease in the product of two diameters of all measurable disease, which lasts for 4 weeks and takes place in the absence of new lesions.

5-Fluorouracil (5-FU), a drug tested during the 1960's, has not been included in Table 48-1. This is because the drug does not appear to have been tested against the modern response criteria mentioned above, although anecdotal responses have been mentioned. Although tested in a limited number of patients, it does represent one of the few instances where a double-blind placebo trial was conducted in cancer patients, and in the circumstance of bladder cancer, 5-FU failed to produce more tumor shrinkage than the placebo.[1] However, newer dose schedules such as continuous infusion 5-FU should be explored.

Adriamycin

Adriamycin (doxorubicin hydrochloride), an anthracycline antibiotic with dose-limiting cardiotoxicity, is recognized for

TABLE 48-1. *Single Agents*

DRUG	REFERENCE	DOSE RANGE mg/M²	COMPLETE RESPONSE	PARTIAL RESPONSE	RESPONSE (%)
Adriamycin	2	60–75	0/19	1/19	5.3
	3	30–90	0/35	5/35	13
	4	45–75	2/65	9/65	17
	5	50	0/40	8/40	20
	6	60–75	0/39	14/39	36
Cisplatinum	7	75	1/9	2/9	33
	8	50–65	0/24	8/24	33
	9	70	0/13	6/13	46
	10	40	1/14	7/14	57
Methotrexate	13	20–250	0/42	11/42	26
	14	50–200*	4/61	19/61	38
	11	NS+	1/23	9/23	44

*absolute dose
NS + not stated

its broad antineoplastic activity in almost all types of cancer except melanoma and adenocarcinoma of the lower gastrointestinal tract. Most of the phase-II data on Adriamycin as a single agent in bladder cancer derive from studies completed over a decade ago.[2–6] Table 48-1 illustrates a wide range of response rates for Adriamycin, with overall responses ranging from 5.3 to 36%. In one of the earlier studies by O'Bryan and his Southwest Oncology Group (SWOG) colleagues, a significant dose response relationship was observed in bladder cancer patients. While the overall response in the earlier SWOG study was 36%,[6] a later, more expanded data base demonstrated that response rates over 30% required a higher dose.[4] In patients described as "good-risk," the response rates to Adriamycin in bladder cancer by dose were as follows: at 75 mg/M² 6/15 (35%), at 60 mg/M² 2/7 (29%), and at 45 mg/M² 3/20 (15%). This compound remains an important agent in the treatment of advanced bladder cancer patients.

Cisplatinum

A substantially more tested, and consistently more active agent in bladder cancer is cisplatinum.[7–10] Table 48-1 demonstrates that overall response rates have exceeded 30%. In two separate studies, the British and WHO Collaborating Centre have published response rates for cisplatinum of 3/15 (20%) and 30/74 (41%), respectively.[11,12] The interpretation of both trials is difficult, as a "minimal" response criteria was used in the first study and the WHO trial included local disease patients. Although it may be the most active single agent available in this disease, its rate-limiting nephrotoxicity may often preclude its use in bladder cancer patients, many of whom already have impaired renal function. Nevertheless, if renal function can be preserved through proper stenting and hydra-

tion, among currently available drugs, this agent is clearly the first choice when treating bladder cancer patients.

Methotrexate

An antifolate antimetabolite, methotrexate has been reported to produce response rates ranging from 26 to 44% in patients with bladder cancer.[11,13] Although one of the oldest drugs to show any activity in this disease, some of the earlier studies were flawed by poorly defined dose and response criteria.[14] In its more standard or lower doses, methotrexate does not cause renal damage but it is dependent on normal renal function for timely elimination from the body. Consequently, many patients with bladder cancer and impaired renal function are not candidates for this agent.

Other Single Agents

Bleomycin, an antineoplastic antibiotic with dose-limiting pulmonary toxicity and elimination dependent on renal function, has been tested as a single agent in only a few patients. In those few reported series' with small patient numbers (ranging from 4 to 23 patients), the response rates have varied from the extremes of 0 to 100%,[15–17] suggesting that the drug has not undergone adequate phase-II testing. Exceptionally, the WHO Collaborating Centre reports a 23% response in 56 patients treated with bleomycin.[12]

Other agents with limited phase-II information include cyclophosphamide, where response rates in the three separate studies ranged from 17 to 52%,[12,17,18] and mitomycin C, where in two studies, one with 19 patients and another with 75 patients, the response rates were 21 and 33% respectively.[19,12] In recent years, another single agent to receive attention in this disease has been vinblastine. In 28 patients, the majority of whom had received prior chemotherapy, a once weekly intravenous regimen resulted in an 18% response rate.[20]

Several investigational drugs have shown mild to modest activity in bladder cancer patients. Deaza-aminopterin, a folate analog, has been associated with 3 out of 15 responses. Twelve of 15 patients had received prior chemotherapy.[21] m-AMSA was subjected to a phase-II trial in the Southwest Oncology Group, and one complete response and three partial responses were seen in 22 previously untreated patients for an overall response rate of 18%.[22] Oishi and associates observed about a 5% response rate for teniposide (VM-26), and reviewed the work of other investigators whose response rates ranged from 5 to 26%[23]

COMBINATION CHEMOTHERAPY IN METASTATIC DISEASE

One of the most rapidly evolving and newly encouraging areas in the systemic treatment of malignant disease is the use of combination chemotherapy in patients with bladder cancer. Combination drug therapies have been used in this disease for over a decade, and once again, there is a wide range in the percentage of patients who have responded.

Two Drug Combinations

Early combination trials often centered around Adriamycin, usually in combination with one other drug such as cyclophosphamide.[24,25] Response rates in about 20 patients per trial yielded results of 50 to 17% respectively.[18,24] Because cisplatinum had shown such excellent activity as a single agent, it was inevitable that it would be combined with cytotoxic agents. In one disappointing, early undertaking, the combination of cisplatinum and cyclophosphamide provided only two responses out of 10 patients.[25] In a randomized prospective study of cisplatinum and cyclophosphamide, the response rate was actually higher for the single agent cisplatinum (20% with 50% of the responses being complete) than for the combination (11.9%).[26] This resulted in a waning enthusiasm for cyclophosphamide in this disease, but continued interest in cisplatinum.

The combination of adriamycin and cisplatinum resulted in a response rate (43%) superior to Adriamycin alone (19%), but no statistically significant survival benefit was present.[27] Another recently tested, two-drug combination included vinblastine and methotrexate, where 19 of 47 patients (40%) responded with a significant number of complete responses.[28] The two most active single agents, cisplatinum and methotrexate, have also been tested together with an impressive complete response rate of 10/43 or 23% and an identical partial response rate of 10/43 or 23%.[29] Despite these attractive response rates, this particular study used a dose schedule that was associated with considerable toxicity in the form of muco-

sitis and myelosuppresion. Cisplatinum proceeded the Methotrexate in this trial, and it is possible that cisplatinum interferes with the prompt clearance of methotrexate by the kidneys.

Three or More Drug Combinations

One early three-drug trial on 10 patients showed a significant result, with 9 of the studied patients responding to a combination of cyclophosphamide, Adriamycin, and cisplatinum (CAP).[30] Several clinical investigators subsequently attempted to duplicate these favorable results. Unfortunately, a less impressive results of 38%[31] and 44%[22] response rates were observed. There were several complete responses in both of these series.

The combination of 5-fluorouracil, Adriamycin, and cyclophosphamide (FAC) has been evaluated by the Indiana Group where 18/39 (46%) responses were recorded.[32] There were no complete responders in this trial. In another, less common studied combination, the four drugs, Adriamycin, bleomycin, 5-fluorouracil, and methotrexate resulted in a 5/9 (56%) response.[33] Another uncommon combination of cyclophosphamide, doxorubicin, and bleomycin has demonstrated a 35% partial remission in only 23 patients.[34]

One Japanese trial of 5-fluorouracil, vincristine, bleomycin, cyclophosphamide, mitomycin, and methotrexate witnessed two complete responses and five partial responses in 22 patients (overall response rate: 32%).[35] A French study of Adriamycin, VM-26, 5-fluorouracil, and Mitomycin revealed only one significant response in 18 patients.[36]

Recent clinical trials of combination chemotherapy in advanced bladder cancer have shown increasing response rates, with a significant increase in reported complete responses. Using cisplatinum, methotrexate and vinblastine (CMV), the Northern California Oncology Group has reported their results in 50 evaluable patients where 14 (28%) were complete responses, and another 14 (28%) achieved partial responses.[37] In such a large group of patients, this overall 56% response rate is quite remarkable. At about the same time, equally excellent results emerged from the Memorial Sloan-Kettering Center, with the most recent update of their combination of methotrexate, vinblastine, doxorubicin and cisplatinum (M-VAC) revealing an overall response rate of 69% in 83 adequately treated and evaluable patients.[38] In this latter series, 17 of the 31 complete responders were surviving from 26+ to 49+ months. A prospective intergroup study currently exists which, when completed, will more widely test the notion of whether or not cisplatinum alone is inferior to the four-drug combination, M-VAC.

RADIATION AND CHEMOTHERAPY

Patients with locally advanced bladder cancer (muscle invasion, T_2 to T_4) represent the single greatest management challenge in this disease. In American texts, it is rare to see radiation mentioned as an alternative to cystectomy for this particular subset of patients. Even in prospective American trials, combined chemotherapy and radiation approaches appear to be reserved for patients "who were *not* candidates for cystectomy."[39] Conversely, the Europeans have been willing to utilize radiation earlier, and this section will examine those series in both the continents where radiation and chemotherapy are the primary treatment modalities.

There are no substantive randomized trials that compare radiation against cystectomy for T_2 to T_4 bladder tumors. One earlier, nonrandomized British study attempted to add Adriamycin and 5-fluorouracil within 3 months of definitive radiation and concluded that the addition of these two agents did nothing to improve survival over radiation alone.[40] Another British trial evaluated four cycles of cyclophosphamide, 5-fluorouracil, and methotrexate followed by definitive radiation, without seeing much improvement in survival over historic controls.[41]

It wasn't until radiation and chemotherapy were used together that more exciting results were seen. The notion that radiation and chemotherapy should be given together is not new in the field of oncology, but it is relatively new in the management of bladder cancer. The utility of chemotherapy agents such as radiosensitizers has been tested recently in patients with invasive bladder cancer. Havsteen and associates used cisplatinum alone to induce three complete responses in 22 patients and, while continuing cisplatinum, added radiation to increase the complete responses to a total of eight patients.[42] Ultimately, 10 patients of the original 22 (46%) responded, with followup ranging between 46 to 80 months, 7 of the 10 remain free of recurrence. In another nonrandomized American trial, concomitant continuous 5-fluorouracil and radiation was administered to 70 patients "not" candidates for cystectomy.[39] Sixty-two patients completed the planned radiation and 48 (77%) achieved a complete response. Most encouraging is that 30 patients (48%) remain free of disease, with a median response for all 70 original patients of 30 months. Another smaller American trial using concomitant 5-fluorouracil infusion, occasional mitomycin and radiation witnessed a complete response in 11 of the 18 (61%) with locally evaluable disease.[43] Another five patients, with less than complete chemotherapy-radiation regression, were locally controlled by transurethral resection and two patients required salvage cystectomy.

To date, the most impressive results are to be found in a West German trial where 41 patients with invasive bladder cancer were treated with simultaneous radiation and cisplatinum.[44] Although median followup is only 1 year, only 7 cystectomies have had to be performed, and 34 of 41 (83%) patients have remained free of cancer, retained their bladders, and have normal bladder function. Obviously more followup time is required to assess both freedom from relapse as well as bladder toxicity, but this early report represents a major contribution suggesting a possible alternative approach to cystectomy. It is worth emphasizing that in the trials that effectively used radiation and chemotherapy, the two modalities were utilized in a concurrent fashion.

SURGERY AND CHEMOTHERAPY

The substantial increase in the response rates associated with the combination chemotherapies has heightened interest in adding chemotherapy to standard surgical approaches for patients with invasive bladder cancer (T_2 to T_4). Surgery alone for this stage of the disease results in 5-year cure rates of less than 50%. The advantages of giving chemotherapy before (neoadjuvant) definitive surgery (cystectomy) include tumor reduction and a theoretical assistance to subsequent tumor removal, the enhanced ability of drugs to penetrate an unoperated unscarred tumor bed, the ability to conduct an in-vivo sensitivity to the chemotherapy selected, and the theoretical elimination of small undetectable metastatic foci. The advantages of delaying chemotherapy until definitive surgery (cystectomy and pathologic staging) include avoiding any delay in tumor removal because of the theoretical chance of tumor spread should the cancer be insensitive to chemotherapy, more accurate pathologic staging to better understand just which anatomic spread of the disease either needs the chemotherapy or ultimately benefits from drug treatment, and the avoidance of any possible nutritional disadvantage incurred secondary to chemotherapy while awaiting a major operative procedure.

All of the published series' in which surgery is the definitive local therapy, with either postoperative chemotherapy (adjuvant) or preoperative chemotherapy (neoadjuvant), are nonrandomized, uncontrolled trials.

The majority of reported trials using adjuvant chemotherapy are single institution studies in patients judged to be at high risk for postoperative failure. Occasionally these trials have even attempted to utilize transurethral resections as the only surgery used in conjunction with adjuvant chemotherapy. Such an undertaking was accomplished in Britain where eight adjuvant doses of methotrexate plus leucovorin resulted in 19/24 (79%) patients (T_2-T_{3b}) still free of invasive bladder cancer at two years of followup.[45] Although the authors were optimistic about this result, other adjuvant studies, where cystectomy was the surgical endpoint, resulted in conservative degrees of enthusiasm because of failure of the adjuvant chemotherapeutically treated groups to show any survival advantage over expectantly followed control groups.[46,47] One nonrandomized trial, with a concomitantly run control group of "high-risk" patients, demonstrated a statistically significant advantage for adjuvantly administered cyclophosphamide, Adriamycin and cisplatinum.[48] This trial's control population was not identical to the treated group, by virtue of refusal to take chemotherapy, failure to be referred for chemotherapy, or having medical contraindication to therapy. All of these reasons cast considerable doubt on the demonstrated differences between treated and control group patients in this study.

Some of the earlier, seemingly successful neoadjuvant trials have utilized up-front cisplatinum. In one such study, cisplatinum at 100 mg/m² dosage was given every 3 weeks, with 11/17 patients showing a partial response. Partial response apparently had a favorable effect on survival when definitive surgery was performed after the chemotherapy.[49] The most promising recent neoadjuvant trial is that of M-VAC, where investigators at Memorial Sloan-Kettering have recorded 26/41 responders (63%) in patients with T_{2-4} lesions when this combination is used as initial treatment.[50] Others have found similar favorable results of 50% complete responses and 69% overall response in 16 patients.[51] The true impact of this four-drug combination on disease-free survival, in patients with unfavorable local features who undergo cystectomy, will need to await the results of the current intergroup trial which compares neoadjuvant M-VAC and cystectomy to cystectomy alone.

CONCLUSION

Current prospective randomized intergroup trials with cisplatinum versus cisplatinum plus three other drugs for pa- tients with advanced disease, as well as the randomized neoadjuvant trial currently underway in patients with advanced local disease, will hopefully answer the questions regarding the true role of chemotherapy in the therapy of patients with bladder cancer. It is difficult to imagine that any group of cancer patients, in whom complete responses to drug treatment have improved so much in recent years, would not be benefited, but only time and these trials will provide convincing evidence. The European investigative community has helped to tantalize the larger medical community with regard to the importance of using radiation and chemotherapy together. It is imperative for us to re-evaluate the role of radiation and chemotherapy together. It is imperative for us to re-evaluate the role of radiation and chemotherapy in the treatment of certain stages of bladder cancer, which the American medical community currently treats by utilizing only surgery.

REFERENCES

1. PROUT, G. R., JR., et al. Carcinoma of the bladder, 5-fluorouracil and the critical role of a placebo: A cooperative group report. I. Cancer, 22:926, 1968.

2. WEINSTEIN, S. H., and SCHMIDT, J. D. Doxorubicin chemotherapy in advanced transitional cell carcinoma. Urology, 8:336, 1976.

3. YAGODA, A., et al. Adriamycin in advanced urinary tract cancer. Cancer, 39:279, 1977.

4. O'BRYAN, R. M., et al. Dose response evaluation of adriamycin in human neoplasia. Cancer, 39:1940, 1977.

5. GAGLIANO, R. Adriamycin versus adriamycin plus cis-platinum in transitional cell bladder carcinoma. A SWOG study. Proc. ACCR and ASCO, 21:347, 1980.

6. O'BRYAN, R. M., et al. Phase II evaluation of adriamycin in human neoplasia. Cancer, 32:1, 1973.

7. ROSSOF, A. J., et al. Phase II evaluation of cis-dichlorodiammineplatinum (II) in advanced malignancies of the genitorurinary and gynecologic organs: A Southwest Oncology Group study. Cancer Treat. Rep., 63:1557, 1979.

8. YAGODA, A., et al. Cis-dichlorodiammineplatinum (II) in advanced bladder cancer. Cancer Treat. Rep., 60;917, 1976.

9. SOLOWAY, M. D. Cis-diamminedichloroplatinum II in advanced urothelial cancer. J. Urol., 120:716, 1978.

10. MERRIN, C. Treatment of advanced bladder cancer with cis-diamminedichloroplatinum (II NSC 119875): A pilot study. J. Urol., 119:493, 1978.

11. OLIVER, R. T. D., et al. Methotrexate, cisplatin and carboplatin as single agents and in combination for metastatic bladder cancer. Br. J. Urol., 58:31, 1986.

12. EDSMYR, F., ANDERSSON, L., and ESPOSTI, P. Chemotherapy in advanced urinary bladder cancer. Urology, 23(Suppl):51, 1984.

13. NATALE, R. B., et al. Methotrexate: An active drug in bladder cancer. Cancer, 47:1246, 1981.

14. TURNER, A. G., et al. The treatment of advanced bladder cancer with methotrexate. Br. J. Urol., 49:673, 1977.

15. TURNER, A. G., DURRANT, K. R., and MALPAS, J. S. A trial of bleomycin versus adriamycin in advanced carcinoma of the bladder. Br. J. Urol., 51:121, 1979.

16. COSTANZI, J. J., et al. Intravenous bleomycin infusion as a potential synchronizing agent in human disseminated malignancies. A preliminary report. Cancer, 38:1503, 1976.

17. YAGODA, A. Future implications of phase II chemotherapy trials in ninety-five patients with measurable advanced bladder cancer. Cancer Res., 37:2775, 1977.

18. MERRIN, C., et al. Chemotherapy of bladder carcinoma with cyclophosphamide and adriamycin. J. Urol., 114:884, 1975.

19. EARLY, K., et al. Mitomycin C in the treatment of metastatic transitional cell carcinoma of urinary bladder. Cancer, 31:1150, 1973.

20. BLUMENREICH, M. S., et al. Phase II trial of vinblastine sulfate for metastatic urothelial tract tumors. Cancer, 50:435, 1982.

21. AHMED, T., et al. Phase II trial of 10 deaza-aminopterin in patients with bladder cancer. IND., 4:171, 1986.

22. AL-SARRAF, M., et al. Phase II trial of cyclophosphamide, doxorubicin, and cisplatin (CAP) versus Amsacrine in patients with transitional cell carcinoma of the urinary bladder: A Southwest Oncology Group study. Cancer Treat. Rep., 69:189, 1985.

23. OISHI, N., et al. Teniposide in metastatic renal and bladder cancer: A Southwest Oncology Group study. Cancer Treat. Rep., 71:1307, 1987.

24. YAGODA, A., et al. Adriamycin and cyclophosphamide in advanced bladder cancer. Cancer Treat. Rep., 61:97, 1977.

25. NARAYANA, A. S., LOENING, S. A., and CULP, D. A. Chemotherapy for advanced carcinoma of the bladder. J. Urol., 126:594, 1981.

26. SOLOWAY, M. S., et al. A comparison of cisplatin and the combination of cisplatin and cyclophosphamide in advanced urothelial cancer: A National Bladder Cancer Collaborative Group A study. Cancer, 52:767, 1983.

27. GAGLIANO, R., et al. Adriamycin versus adriamycin plus cis-diamminedichloroplatinum (DDP) in advanced transitional cell bladder carcinoma: A Southwest Oncology Group study. Am. J. Clin. Oncol., 6:215, 1983.

28. AHMED, T., et al. Vinblastine and methotrexate for advanced bladder cancer. J. Urol., 133:602, 1985.

29. STOTER, G., et al. Combination chemotherapy with cisplatin and

methotrexate in advanced transitional cell cancer of the bladder. J. Urol., *137*:663, 1987.

30. STERNBERG, J. J., et al. Combination chemotherapy (CISCA) for advanced urinary tract carcinoma. JAMA, *238*:2282, 1977.

31. TROPER, M. D., and HEMSTREET, G. P. Cyclophosphamide, doxorubicin, and cisplatin (CAP) in the treatment of urothelial malignancy: A pilot study of the Southeastern Cancer Study Group. Cancer Treat. Rep., *65*:29, 1981.

32. WILLIAMS, S. D., EINHORN, L. H., and DONOHUE, J. P. Cis-platinum combination chemotherapy of bladder cancer: An update. Cancer Clin. Trials, *2*:335, 1979.

33. HALL, R. R., et al. Combination chemotherapy for advanced bladder cancer. Br. J. Urol., *54*:16, 1982.

34. LEVI, J. A., ARONEY, R. S., and DALLEY, D. N. Combination chemotherapy with cyclophosphamide, doxorubicin, and bleomycin for metastatic transitional cell carcinoma of the urinary tract. Cancer Treat. Rep., *64*:1011, 1980.

35. KUBOTA, Y., et al. Combination chemotherapy for metastatic urinary bladder cancer with 5-FU, vincristine, bleomycin, cyclophosphamide, mitomycin and methotrexate. Cancer Treat. Rep., *68*:1167, 1984.

36. GARCIA-GIRALT, E., et al. Combination chemotherapy in the management of metastatic bladder cancer. Br. J. Urol., *53*:318, 1981.

37. MEYERS, F. J., et al. The fate of the bladder in patients with metastatic bladder cancer treated with cisplatin, methotrexate and vinblastine: A Northern California Oncology Group study. J. Urol., *134*:1118, 1985.

38. STERNBERG, C. N., et al. M-VAC (methotrexate, vinblastine, doxorubicin and cisplatin) for advanced transitional cell carcinoma of the urothelium. J. Urol., *139*:461, 1988.

39. SHIPLEY, W. V., et al. Treatment of invasive bladder cancer by cisplatin and radiation in patients unsuited for surgery. JAMA, *258*:931, 1987.

40. RICHARDS, B., et al. Adjuvant chemotherapy with doxorubicin (adriamycin) and 5-fluorouracil in T_3, N_x, M_o bladder cancer treated with radiotherapy. Br. J. Urol., *55*:386, 1983.

41. KAYE, S. B., et al. Chemotherapy before radiotherapy for T_3 bladder cancer: A pilot study. Br. J. Urol., *57*:434, 1985.

42. HAVSTEEN, H., et al. Cisplatin as a first-line treatment in T_2 and T_3 bladder carcinoma. Cancer Treat. Rep., *71*:1285, 1987.

43. ROTMAN, M., et al. Treatment of advanced bladder carcinoma with irradiation and concomitant 5-fluorouracil infusion. Cancer, *59*:710, 1987.

44. SAUER, R., et al. Preliminary results of treatment of invasive bladder carcinoma with radiotherapy and cisplatin. Int. J. Radia. Oncol. Biol. Phys., *15*:871, 1988.

45. HALL, R. R., et al. Treatment of invasive bladder cancer by local resection and high dose methotrexate. Br. J. Urol., *56*:668, 1984.

46. SKINNER, D. G., DANIELS, J. R., and LIESKOVSKY, G. Current status of adjuvant chemotherapy after radical cystectomy for deeply invasive bladder cancer. Urology, *24*:46, 1984.

47. CLYNE, C. A. C., et al. A trial of adjuvant chemotherapy for stage T_3 bladder tumors. J. Urol., *129*:736, 1983.

48. LOGOTHETIS, C. J., et al. Adjuvant cyclophosphamide, doxo-rubicin, and cisplatin chemotherapy for bladder cancer: An update. J. Clin. Oncol., *6*:1590, 1988.

49. FAGG, S. L., et al. Cis-diamminedichloroplatinum (DDP) as initial treatment of invasive bladder cancer. Br. J. Urol., *56*:292, 1984.

50. SCHER, H. I., et al. Neoadjuvant M-VAC (methotrexate, vinblastine, doxorubicin and cisplatin) effect on the primary bladder lesion. J. Urol., *139*:470, 1988.

51. ZINCKE, H., et al. Neoadjuvant chemotherapy for locally advanced transitional cell carcinoma of the bladder: Do local findings suggest a potential for salvage of the bladder? Mayo Clin. Proc., *63*:16, 1988.

Hormonal Therapy of Advanced Carcinoma of the Prostate

"We shall not cease from exploration
And the end of all our exploring
Will be to arrive where we started
And know the place for the first time"

T. S. ELIOT

Sakti Das
E. David Crawford

Adenocarcinoma of the prostate represents the quintessential paradigm of a human malignancy in which growth can be modified by hormonal manipulations. In 1939, Huggins conceived the idea of endocrine management of disseminated carcinoma of the prostate in the laboratory and subsequently observed that "in many instances a malignant prostatic tumor is an overgrowth of adult epithelial cells. All known types of adult prostatic epithelium undergo atrophy when androgenic hormones are greatly reduced in amount or inactivated. Therefore, significant improvements should occur in the clinical condition of patients with far-advanced prostatic cancer subjected to castration (or estrogen administration)".[1] Half a century later, Huggins' concept of biologic syllogism continues to prompt and promote the evolution of therapeutic maneuvers designed to interfere with the androgen-nurtured growth of prostatic carcinoma. The resultant modification of the biologic behavior of this neoplasm has provided some of the most spectacular palliative treatment known for metastatic carcinoma.

To understand the various levels where androgen ablation or interruption can be instituted, it is necessary to review the endocrinology of prostatic tissue growth and differentiation.

Biologic effects of testicular and adrenal androgens on the prostate depend on their conversion within the prostatic cells into dihydrotestosterone (DHT) by the enzyme 5-alpha-reductase. DHT then combines with the specific cytoplasmic receptor protein and is translocated to the cell nucleus, where it binds to the nuclear chromatin. At this level, DHT precipitates biochemical reactions leading to protein synthesis by the prostate cells.

The production of testosterone by the testes and adrenal is controlled by the hypothalamus and the anterior pituitary gland. Hypothalamus produces releasing factors that are transported to the anterior pituitary via the hypothalamus-pituitary portal venous system. The hypothalamic hormones with prostate cell specific effects include gonadotrophin releasing hormone (GnRH, also known as leutinizing hormone releasing hormones LHRH) and corticotrophin releasing factor (CRF). In response to these hypothalamic hormones, the anterior pituitary dispenses leutinizing hormone (LH) and adrenal corticotropic hormone (ACTH) to the testes and the adrenal cortices respectively. LH stimulates the testicular Leydig cell production of 90 to 95% of circulating testosterone, while ACTH stimulates the adrenal cortical production of andro-

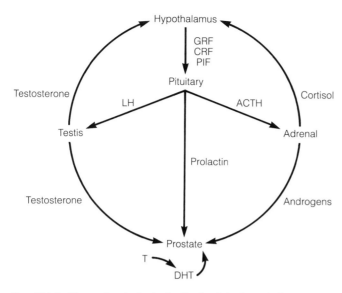

FIG. 49A-1. The endocrinologic feedback of the hypothalamus-pituitary-end organs circuit.

stenedione and dihydroepiandrosterone, which are subsequently converted to testosterone and dihydrotestosterone (Fig. 49A-1).

More than 95% of the circulating testosterone in the plasma is bound with high affinity to a specific plasma protein known as testosterone-estrogen binding globulin, and bound with lower affinity to plasma albumin. The unbound moiety is the biologically active form of circulating androgen as it effects the growth and metabolism of androgen-sensitive cells, including prostatic tissues.

The secretion of trophic hormones by the anterior pituitary are modified through feedback loops (Fig. 49A-1). Testosterone secreted by the testes, and exogenous estrogen, feed back to the hypothalamus and pituitary, thereby decreasing LH secretion. Similarly, cortisol secreted by the adrenal cortex, or exogenously administered glucocorticoids, feed back to the pituitary, affecting lower levels of ACTH secretion.

Based on the physiology of androgen production and utilization, the methods of antiandrogen therapies can be grouped as follows: (1) surgical ablation of androgen sources, (2) suppression of pituitary LH secretion, (3) inhibition of enzymes responsible for androgen synthesis, and (4) androgen blockade at the cellular level.

SURGICAL ABLATION OF ANDROGEN SOURCES

Bilateral Orchiectomy

Bilateral orchiectomy remains the gold standard for ablation of testicular androgen. Surgical removal of the testes results in a

95% reduction of circulating testosterone to about 10-50 ng/100 ml in approximately 3 hours with effective tumor regression and appreciable symptomatic improvement.[2] The advantage of this popular form of surgical ablation include efficacy, assured patient compliance, and cost effectiveness. Infection and bleeding are occasionally encountered. Rare contraindications to orchiectomy include chronic infection, immunosuppression, and bleeding dyscrasias. The major side-effects associated with bilateral orchiectomy are impotence (reported in 50 to 75% of previously potent patients), occasional breast tenderness, and mild to severe hot flashes.[2] After orchiectomy, symptomatic improvement ranging from relief of obstructive uropathy to significant relief from painful metastasis is commonly experienced. Psychologic trauma precipitated by the prospect of orchiectomy has been suggested.[3] In a survey of 147 patients with metastatic prostatic carcinoma, 78% selected a LHRH analog therapy as opposed to only 22% selecting orchiectomy as their initial therapy.[4]

Hypophysectomy and Adrenalectomy

Hypophysectomy in the form of surgical removal, cryodestruction, and interstitial radiation have been used to palliate metastatic carcinoma of the prostate in patients who have failed primary hormonal therapy. With ablation of the pituitary, the source of gonadotrophins and ACTH is removed. Androgen production, both in the testes and adrenals, is thereby suppressed. Subjective response rates of 63 to 91% have been reported, but objective responses ranged only from 0 to 37%. This discrepancy probably results from alteration in the levels of endorphins and enkephalins, which are endogenous opiate receptors that effect the subjective interpretation of pain after hypophysectomy. The subjective responses, therefore, may represent an alteration in the perception of pain rather than a favorable impact on the disease process itself.[3]

Likewise, adrenalectomy has been used for palliative therapy of disseminated cancer of the prostate. By removing the source of extratesticular androgen production, adrenalectomy serves to decrease already low levels of serum androgen in previously castrated males with carcinoma of the prostate. Testosterone levels determined by selective adrenal vein catheterization range from 16 to 217 ng/day. An additional 228 to 294 ng/day of testosterone is produced by direct conversion from androstenedione.[5] This represents only 0 to 3% of the total amount produced in intact males. The contribution of this small amount to the total androgen pool, with its potential effects on carcinoma of the prostate, is the crux of the debate about the rationale of combined androgen therapy. Brendler reported a 73% subjective improvement, but only a 6% objective response following adrenalectomy.[6] Most of these responses are of short duration with a median survival of only 6 to 12 months. Adrenalectomy is, at present, an infrequently used mode of therapy because the surgical procedure is quite formidable with associated morbidity, and the overall objective response rate is poor.

SUPPRESSION OF PITUITARY LEUTINIZING HORMONE SECRETION

Estrogens

Exogenous administration of estrogens is the most prevalent therapeutic modality that suppresses LH release from the pituitary, thereby eliminating the stimulus for testicular production of testosterone. Estrogens have also been shown to stimulate the production of increased levels of sex steroid binding globulin, thereby increasing the proportion of bound and metabolically inactive testosterone. Secondary immunoregulatory effects, including stimulation of phagocytic activity with a rise in gammaglobulin levels, may contribute to the therapeutic profile of estrogens. Estrogens in high concentration may exert direct inhibitory influences on testicular steroidogenesis and on the metabolism of prostatic cells. In-vitro estrogen inhibits DNA polymerase and 5-alpha-reductase activity, suggesting a direct nuclear site of inhibition. Clinical applicability of this effect is limited because of the high concentration required in the in-vitro experiment.

Estrogens promote prolactin release from the pituitary. Prolactin is known to enhance androgen utilization and transport into the prostatic cells. Prolactin effect of estrogen may prove deleterious to the orchiectomized patient in enhancing the utilization of the available androgen by the androgen-dependent carcinoma prostate cells.

Estrogen used in the treatment of cancer of the prostate can be natural or synthetic. Natural estrogens are not active orally unless modified, whereas synthetic estrogens are active orally, and are less expensive.

Diethylstilbestrol (DES) is the most widely used synthetic estrogen in the treatment of carcinoma of the prostate. The therapeutic dosage that is most effective, as well as safe, has not yet been convincingly determined. Various doses ranging from 1 to 5 mg daily have been explored primarily through the studies of the Veterans Administration Cooperative Urologic Research Group.[7] Predictable increased incidence of cardiovascular morbidity and mortality have been associated with higher doses. The daily, 3-mg dose of DES is more effective in suppressing plasma testosterone levels to the range seen after castration than is a 1-mg daily dose, with a similar cardiovascular risk profile, thus supporting its general use.[8]

Alternative natural synthetic estrogens, although less clinically effective than DES, can also reduce serum testosterone levels and have unique, individual therapeutic indications.

Premarin and Ethinyl Estradiol are as effective as DES in suppressing serum testosterone, but neither offers any significant advantage over DES. Cholotriansene (TACE), a synthetic estrogen, has produced clinical responses in patients without completely suppressing LH or testosterone levels. A dose of 12 mg twice a day, orally, yields a 40 to 60% suppression of serum testosterone. The drug is structurally different from DES and has fewer side effects; however it is not therapeutically superior.[8]

Polyestradiol phosphate (Estradurin) is a depot formulation of estrogen. Administered at a dose of 40 to 80 mg intramuscularly every 3 to 4 weeks, it may be helpful for patients with gastrointestinal intolerance to oral estrogens. Diethylstilbesterol diphosphate (Stilphostrol), an intravenously administered estrogen, has been reported to provide symptomatic relief to patients who are unresponsive to other modalities. The usual dose is 500 to 2000 mg daily, administered intravenously by bolus or drip infusion. Theoretically, enzymatic hydrolysis by prostatic acid phosphatase should liberate stilbesterol, therefore, a higher concentration of estrogen can be achieved at the target site.[9]

Estramustine phosphate (EMCYT) is a cytotoxic combination of nitrogen mustard linked to a phosphorylated estradiol. About 50% of patients with disseminated disease that are resistant to estrogen therapy have been reported to respond favorably to this drug.[10] This agent, however, does not appear to offer any survival advantage either in the previously untreated or patients failing prior hormonal therapy.

Side effects of estrogen therapy can be categorized under feminizing effects, cardiovascular complications, gastrointestinal disturbances, and edema. The feminizing effects include atrophy of genitalia, loss of libido, impotence, azospermia and gynecomastia associated with hypersensitivity, and tenderness and hyperpigmentation of the nipples. In most cases, the gynecomastia can be prevented by pretreatment with prophylactic irradiation of the breast with 800 to 1500 rads delivered in three divided fractions.

Progestational Agents

Progestational agents, including Depostat and megestrol acetate (Megace), act primarily by suppressing pituitary secretion of LH, while directly inhibiting steroidogenesis and weakly binding to androgen receptors in the prostate gland. With therapy, there is a transient reduction in plasma testosterone followed, however, by a gradual rise with chronic use. The mechanism of this escape is poorly understood. Progestational agents are usually administered concomitantly with other agents, such as DES, to prevent the escape.[11]

Prolactin Antagonist

As prolactin promotes pituitary mediated androgen activity, prolactin antagonists, including levodopa and bromocriptine, have demonstrated efficacy in relieving symptoms, especially pain, in some patients no longer responsive to the standard hormonal therapy.[12]

Leutinizing Hormone-Releasing Hormone Agonist

The naturally occurring LHRH has a short half-life. Synthetic analogs produced by substitution at the 6th, 9th, and 10th position of the decapeptide greatly increase the potency with prolonged retention in the circulation. Single injections of synthetic LHRH agonists cause transient elevation of serum testosterone, but paradoxical suppression occurs with repeated administrations.[13] The number of GnRH receptors in the pituitary diminishes with resultant pituitary depletion of LH and FSH. The end result is a chemically selective hypophysectomy causing suppression of testicular synthesis of testosterone.[14]

LHRH analog administration initially causes stimulation of the LH and FSH production, with a resultant rise in the level of testosterone to 140 to 170% of basal levels within several days, with a falling pattern demonstrated within 1 to 2 weeks and achievement of castrate levels in approximately 1 month. This low level of testosterone can be maintained with chronic administration. However, the initial surge of testosterone, referred to as the "flare phenomenon," may have clinical consequences. Temporary increases in the degree of bone pain and obstructive voiding symptoms have been noted within the first 72 hours of therapy. The presumed etiology is stimulation of prostatic tumor cells by the transiently raised level of testosterone.[15] Waxman and associates reported that 53% of their patients with bone pain experienced enhancement of their symptoms in the immediate period following institution of LHRH therapy. In 14 patients who were asymptomatic at presentation, 2 experienced subjective disease flare.[16] This has led to the recommendation that administrations of adjunctive drugs to neutralize the transiently elevated serum testosterone level during the period of flare should be considered. Crawford and Davis, in their review of literature on LHRH analog, advise that "LHRH analogs should not be used alone in patients who have neurologic symptoms or life-threatening metastatic disease."[17]

LHRH analogs are peptides and, therefore, are not active orally but are administered as nasal sprays or daily subcutaneous injections. More recently, a long-acting depot injection has been marketed. The depot formulations provide a better assurance of patient compliance.[18] Although the nasal spray is convenient, accurate quantification of drug administration is not possible with this route.

Several prospective randomized trials have compared LHRH agonists with standard forms of therapy, that is bilateral orchidectomy or DES in the control arms. Thus far, the LHRH agonists have shown comparable response rates and have not been proven to be more advantageous as measured by disease response and progression. The advantage of LHRH agonist therapy however, lies in its limited morbidity.[15,19] Side effects of LHRH analogs include atrophy of the reproductive organs, loss of libido, and impotence. The disadvantages relate to the cost and necessity of either daily or monthly parenteral administration. The medications do not cause many of the side effects associated with estrogen, namely gynecomastia, gastrointestinal disturbances, or cardiovascular and thromboembolic complications. The most commonly used LHRH agonists at present are leuprolide, buserelin acetate, and Zoladex. Leuprolide is administered as a daily subcutaneous injection, and a depot form of injection is available as a single, monthly, intramuscular injection. Buserelin can be administered by either intranasal insufflation or by daily subcutaneous injection. Zoladex is a depot formulation administered subcutaneously every 28 days.[20]

The Leuprolide study group has provided the largest clinical trial involving the use of LHRH analogs. This randomized multicenter trial compared Leuprolide 1.0 mg subcutaneously daily with DES 3 mg orally daily in 98 and 100 patients, respectively, with previously untreated Stage D2 carcinoma of the prostate. The objective results by NPCP criteria were similar in the Leuprolide and DES treated groups. Suppression of testosterone, DHT, and acid phosphatase were comparable in the two groups, although the reduction in acid phosphatase occurred earlier in the DES group. Actuarial survival rates at 1 year were 87% for the leuprolide group and 78% for the DES group. Side effects of painful gynecomastia, nausea, vomiting, and edema were more common in the DES treated group, whereas hot flashes were more common in the leuprolide group. There appeared to be no difference relative to major cardiovascular complications. The study group concluded that for the initial systemic management of disseminated prostate cancer, leuprolide was therapeutically equivalent to DES, with fewer side effects.[15]

INHIBITORS OF ANDROGEN SYNTHESIS

Androgen blockade, with inhibition of steroidogenesis mainly in the adrenal gland, can be an effective and well-tolerated regimen for the treatment of some cases of advanced refractory prostate cancer. Drugs that inhibit one or more essential enzymes necessary for androgen synthesis, thereby interrupting androgen production in the testes and/or adrenals, include ketoconazole, spironolactone, and aminoglutethimide. Aminoglutethimide predominantly inhibits the adrenal steroidogenesis whereas ketoconazole and spironolactone effect both testicular and adrenal steroidogenesis.

Ketoconazole, an orally administered, broad-spectrum antifungal agent, inhibits the cytochrome P-450 enzyme-dependent synthesis of testicular and adrenal androgen. It can cause a rapid decline of serum testosterone to castrate levels within hours. Side effects include weakness, lethargy, nausea, vomiting, decreased libido, and mild to severe hepatotoxicity.[21,22]

Spironolactone acts by inhibition of 17 alphahydroxylase and 17,20 desmolase. Walsh and Siteri demonstrated the drug's ability to depress the serum testosterone and dihydrotestosterone levels.[23]

Aminoglutethimide, originally introduced as an anticonvulsant therapy of epilepsy, had to be discontinued because of its profound inhibitory effect on adrenal steroidogenesis. It prevents the conversion of cholesterol to delta-5-pregnenolone by blocking the 20–24 desmolase enzyme with corresponding inhibition of synthesis of glucocorticoids, mineralocorticoids, and sex steroid. Resurgance of interest in this drug prompted clinical trials in hormonally sensitive tumors, primarily breast and prostate cancer.[24,25] Concomitant administration of hydrocortisone is necessary to prevent the development of Addison's syndrome as well as to prevent ACTH mediated override of the blockade. Crawford and associates, in their study of Aminoglutethimide therapy in 129 patients with Stage-D2 carcinoma of the prostate, reported a 10% partial response and a

39% stable response using the NPCP criteria. Subjective improvement was reported in 61% of the patients. Side effects of aminoglutethimide include occasional hypotension, nausea and vomiting, fatigue, anorexia, depression, edema, and skin rashes. Mineralocorticoid replacement along with glucocorticoid supplement may be necessary.[26]

ANTIANDROGENS

Nonsteroidal antiandrogens are a new and unique class of drugs that are neither hormone nor hormonal analogs, and their action does not result in reduction of serum levels of androgens. These compounds block the cellular action of androgens at the target organ by inhibiting the nuclear uptake of dihydrotestosterone.[6] The negative feedback of testosterone on the hypothalamus no longer registers, resulting in higher levels of LHRH and LH. The testes are thus stimulated to produce higher levels of testosterone. The high serum level of testosterone, however, is of no consequence because the androgen receptors in the prostate are insensitive or blocked. Higher levels of estrogen also result from the LHRH and LH stimulus. Attendant side effects such as gynecomastia commonly result. The available nonsteroidal antiandrogens include Flutamide, Anandron, and Casodex.

Cyproterone acetate (CPA) and megestrol acetate (Megace) are synthetic steroids with pronounced progestational and antiandrogenic properties. As steroidal antiandrogens, they block the gonadotrophin release from the pituitary. In addition, they inhibit the formation of dihydrotestosterone-receptor complex in the prostatic cells, as well as inhibiting the C21-19 desmolase enzyme, which is the key to the synthesis of adrenal androgens. Synthesis of testosterone in the leydig cells of the testes is also inhibited. CPA is well tolerated but requires reinforcement with low-dose DES to maintain serum testosterone levels in the castrate range.[27,28] CPA is not approved in the United States. Multiple reports in the European studies attest to the drug's effectiveness although it is no more effective than the standard estrogen therapy.

Flutamide is a nonsteroidal derivative of toluidine that inhibits uptake of testosterone or nuclear binding of testosterone and DHT to the androgen receptors. Flutamide does not inhibit the production of gonadotrophins by the pituitary. Gonadal and adrenocortical steroidogenesis continues unabated and, therefore, the patients maintain normal or elevated levels of serum testosterone.[14,29,30] Although most patients experience gynecomastia when the drug is utilized alone, the incidence is less common than that associated with estrogen therapy. Nausea, vomiting, diarrhea and, rarely, altered liver function tests are reported side effects. Because serum testosterone levels do not drop and often rise, most patients retain libido and sexual potency.[31]

Anandron is another synthetic nonsteroidal antiandrogen that has a similar mechanism of action as flutamide. In at least one study, visual disturbances in some patients caused its abandonment. Other side effects include alcohol intolerance and interstitial pneumonitis.[32,33]

TOTAL ANDROGEN SUPPRESSION WITH COMBINED THERAPY

Combined endocrine manipulation has been advocated to achieve total androgen suppression by the employment of means to suppress the effects of both adrenal as well testicular androgens. Although the concept itself is not new, emergence of new drugs have rekindled the interest.[34,35] In support of this concept, Labrie and associates point to the statistics that approximately 30% of patients with disseminated prostate cancer relapsing after orchiectomy or estrogen therapy respond to hypophysectomy or surgical and medical adrenalectomy.[36] In addition, it has been observed that after gonadal ablation, intracellular levels of DHT within the prostate remain disproportionately high, despite reduction of serum testosterone levels to castrate levels. This persistence of DHT may result from the continued conversion of adrenal androgen precursors (androstenedione and dihydroepiandrosterone) to testosterone and subsequently to dihydrotestosterone in the prostatic cells. Therefore, it has been hypothesized that after gonadal ablation there continues to be substantial androgenic stimulation of tumor growth by the androgens of adrenal origin.[37] Laboratory experiments, however, have provided contrasting opinion. Experiments performed with the Shionogi mammary cell line investigated the heterogenicity of androgen sensitivity of clones of tumor cell lines in vitro. The heterogenicity of androgen sensitivity may explain the clinical relapse that occurs after initially successful palliation achieved with hormonal therapy. It has been proposed that proliferation of tumor cells sensitive to low levels of androgens may be responsible for such clinical relapse.[38] However, Coffey and associates, working with the Dunning tumor model in rats, observed with kinetic studies that prostatic cancer can be heterogenically composed of a variety of phenotypically distinct cell clones.[39] The populations of cells of differing hormonal sensitivity are responsible for clinical relapses. These cells are unresponsive to hormonal manipulation and are androgen insensitive. In another series of experiments, the authors demonstrated that lowering the testosterone levels to a critical level (0.25 ng/ml) obtained maximal responses. Lowering the testosterone level below the critical level did not further retard tumor growth. The authors concluded that there was no benefit to complete androgen ablation in the treatment of prostatic adenocarcinoma in rats.[40]

The logical consequence of these experimental and clinical observations is the initiation of controlled clinical trials to elucidate any possible relevance of complete androgen suppression in the management of disseminated carcinoma of the prostate relapsing after initial hormonal therapy. The most enthusiastic advocate of combined therapy, Labrie and associates, published several reports in the 1980's demonstrating the benefit of combined therapy.[34–37] These studies, however, were uncontrolled and involved patient numbers ranging from 10 to 191. Instead of including a monotherapy treatment arm to compare the results of combined therapy, the study relied on historical data as a basis for comparison. The clinical studies unequivocally attested to the benefit of combined hormonal therapy.

In 1987, the Canadian investigators reported the results of a multicenter study in which 154 patients with Stage-D2 carcinoma of the prostate were treated with the combination of leuprolide and flutamide for an average of 22 months. The responses of these patients were compared with the average responses from five previously published studies employing monotherapy in the form of orchiectomy, DES, or leuprolide alone. The complete response rate of the patients receiving combined therapy was 29.2% compared to 4.6% response in patients having monotherapy. 18% of the patients on monotherapy did not respond in contrast to only 4.5% of the combined therapy patients that did not respond. Duration of response was longer in patients receiving combined therapy. They concluded, "the present data . . . clearly indicates that the use of combination . . . significantly increases the rate of objective response, the duration of response as well as survival."[37] In another study, the same workers administered combined therapy to patients who had received previous antiandrogen therapy (that is DES, castration, or flutamide alone). When compared to the results obtained with newly diagnosed patients, the responses were significantly decreased. They theorize that the previous partial hormonal therapy, by affecting incomplete androgen suppression, had permitted a population of low sensitivity cells to proliferate; thus, the inferior clinical results. Their conclusion was that "complete—androgen withdrawal should be performed as early as possible after diagnosis at least in advanced prostate cancer."[35,41]

Sander and associates compared the combined effect of orchiectomy plus cyproterone acetate (CPA) through a prospective randomized trial. Patients had locally advanced or disseminated prostatic adenocarcinoma. Two weeks following orchiectomy, 7 patients were given a placebo, 13 patients were given 50 mg CPA orally four times a day for 6 weeks, and 14 patients were given 2.5 mg Prednisone 18 mg orally four times a day for 6 weeks. Six of the 7 patients in the control group had objective responses, in comparison to 8 of the 13 patients in the CPA group and 13 of the 14 patients in the Prednisone group. Progression of disease in patients treated with CPA was felt to be secondary to increased prolactin levels. Thyrotrophin-releasing hormone (TRH) stimulation of CPA treated patients yielded prolactin levels higher than those noted after TRH stimulation of patients receiving the placebo and Prednisone. Also significant was the objective response in patients previously treated with CPA who were crossed over to Prednisone therapy. The good results obtained with Prednisone were felt to be secondary to the suppression of adrenal androgen secretion. This suppression was documented by the reduced excretion of adrenal androgens, particularly dihydroepiandrosterone, etiocholanolone, and androsterone. The authors concluded that orchiectomy should be the treatment of choice for patients with advanced prostatic carcinoma. They also recommend combined therapy to be instituted with Prednisone, should no clinical improvement be apparent within 6 weeks.[42]

In 1987, Schroeder and associates published a nonrandomized study involving 71 previously untreated patients with disseminated prostatic cancer treated with either buserelin (LHRH agonist) alone or buserelin plus CPA. Neither response rates nor rates of progression were more favorable in the combined therapy group. Thus, this small study did not demonstrate any superiority of total androgen suppression.[28]

Navratil and associates conducted a multicenter, double-blind, randomized study comparing the effects of combined therapy versus monotherapy. Forty-nine patients with stage-D2 carcinoma of the prostate were randomized to receive Buserelin and Anandron or Buserelin and placebo. National prostatic cancer projects (NPCP) criteria were used to evaluate patients at 6-month intervals. Forty-five percent of patients showed progression in the Buserelin and placebo group compared with 37% in the Buserelin and Anandrone group. Median time to progression was 13 months with the administration of Anandron compared to 10 months in the other group. The actuarial survival rate at 18 months favored the combined therapy group over monotherapy.[32]

The European organization for research on the treatment of cancer began a randomized study in 1981 to compare monotherapy to combined therapy. A total of 350 patients were entered into the study. The treatment of combined therapy consisted of orchiectomy plus the progestational antiandrogen CPA, the monotherapy consisted of orchiectomy and DES. Preliminary results as of 1987 do not show any benefit for combined therapy regarding time of progression or survival.[43] The use of CPA as an antiandrogen has been criticized because the drug has a progestational-like action that may have a stimulatory affect on the prostate.

Brisset and associates published the findings of another multicenter prospective randomized trial in France. A total of 195 patients with metastatic carcinoma of the prostate, who had received no prior treatment, were entered in the study to receive combined treatment versus monotherapy. The three treatment groups were orchiectomy plus placebo, orchiectomy and antiandrogen Anandron 150 mg orally, daily, and orchiectomy plus Anandron 300 mg orally, daily. Using the NPCP criteria, 61% of patients in both combined treatment groups, and 33% of patients in the monotherapy group had regression. The progression-free actuarial rate at 18 months was similar for all three groups as was the survival rate at 24 months. The authors concluded that the addition of the antiandrogen to orchiectomy enhances the quality of life and objective tumor regression rate. The survival however, is not changed.[33]

To critically evaluate the relative value of combined androgen therapy, a multiinstitutional clinical trial was begun in 1985 under the aegis of The National Cancer Institute. The study design was placebo-controlled, double-blinded, prospective, and randomized, including patients with disseminated, previously untreated prostate cancer (stage D2). Of the total 603 evaluable patients, 300 received leuprolide and placebo and 303 patients received leuprolide and flutamide. Both regimens were well tolerated, although a significantly increased incidence of diarrhea was noted in the combined therapy group (13.5% versus 5%). This side effect did not require discontinuance of therapy.

Analysis of certain variables such as performance status, level of pain, and acid phosphatase values for the first 12 weeks was carried out in order to discover if flutamide could ameliorate the flare phenomenon reported to occur with leuprolide alone. The data indicated that the patients receiving flutamide had relatively better odds for improvement.

Statistically significant differences in progression-free survival were observed in the group receiving Leuprolide and Flutamide. Median progression-free survival times were 16.5 months for patients in the leuprolide and flutamide arm and 13.9 months for the Leuprolide and placebo arm. Estimates of the median survival were 35.6 months for the leuprolide and flutamide arm and 28.3 months for the leuprolide and placebo arm. The difference in survival distributions favored the leuprolide and flutamide arm. The differences between the treatment groups in both progression-free survival and overall survival were particularly evident in patients with minimal disease. The number of patients in this subgroup of minimal disease was small however, and additional followup is planned before definitive conclusions can be made. The authors concluded that "combined androgen blockade with leuprolide and flutamide is more effective than leuprolide alone for patients with metastatic cancer of the prostate. Combination therapy produced small, but important improvement in both progression free survival and overall survivals. The therapeutic benefits may be greatest in patients with minimal disease but this issue should be evaluated in prospective randomized trials specifically designed for this subset of patients."[44]

CONCLUSIONS

Reviewing the preceding data, the following conclusions may be drawn regarding our understanding of the present state of the knowledge of hormonal therapy of advanced carcinoma of the prostate.

1. Bilateral orchiectomy still remains the gold standard for primary hormonal therapy of disseminated carcinoma of the prostate.
2. It is assumed that the clinical efficacy of LHRH analogs are equivalent to orchiectomy, but this is not yet been demonstrated conclusively.
3. Theoretical benefit of total androgen suppression is based on the conjecture that adrenal androgens may be clinically significant in the proliferation of carcinoma of the prostate cells. Presently, there are no clear objective data to either support this proposition or to deny it.
4. If an LHRH analog is chosen for the treatment of disseminated carcinoma of the prostate, the addition of the antiandrogen flutamide would offer a survival advantage over the LHRH agent alone.
5. A small subset of patients with minimal metastatic disease, treated with combined hormonal therapy, appears to have experienced a significant benefit, but further clinical trials are needed to further define the magnitude of this benefit.
6. Not all patients show survival advantage with combined therapy, and further studies of prognostic variables are necessary.
7. The question regarding initiation of hormonal therapy, whether immediately at the time of diagnosis of metastatic carcinoma of the prostate or delayed until the onset of symptoms, is still unsettled.

REFERENCES

1. HUGGINS, C., and HODGES, C. V. Studies on prostatic cancer I. The effect of castration, of estrogen and of androgen injection on serum phosphatases in metastatic carcinoma of the prostate. Cancer Res., 1:293, 1941.
2. GRAYHACK, J. T., KEELER, T. C., and KOZLOWSKI, J. M. Carcinoma of the prostate: Hormonal therapy. Cancer, 60:589, 1987.
3. SMITH, J. A. New methods of endocrine management of prostatic cancer. J. Urol., 137:1, 1987.
4. CASSILETH, B. R. et al. Patients' choice of treatment in Stage D prostate cancer. Urology, 33(Suppl. 5):57, 1989.
5. DRAGO, J. R. et al. Clinical effects of aminoglutethimide, medical adrenalectomy in the treatment of 43 patients with advanced prostatic carcinoma. Cancer, 53:1447, 1984.
6. BRENDLER, H. Adrenalectomy and hypophysectomy for prostatic cancer. Urology, 2:99, 1973.
7. Veterans Administration Cooperative Urological Research Group: Treatment and survival of patients with cancer of the prostate. Surg. Gynecol. Obstet., 124:1011, 1967.
8. RESNICK, M. I. Hormonal therapy in prostatic carcinoma. Urology, 24(Suppl. 5):18, 1984.
9. TRAFFORD, H. S. The place of Honvan (diethylstilbesterol diphosphate) in the treatment of prostatic cancer. Br. J. Urol., 37:317, 1965.
10. BENSON, R. C., WEAR, J. B., and GILL, G. M. Treatment of Stage D hormone resistant carcinoma of the prostate with estramustine phosphate. J. Urol., 121:452, 1979.
11. GELLER, J. et al. Medical castration of males with megestrol acetate and small doses of diethylstilbestrol. J. Clin. Endocrinol. Metab., 52:576, 1981.
12. VON ESCHENBACH, A. C. Cancer of the prostate. Curr. Probl. Cancer, 5:12, 1981.
13. WENDEROTH, U. K., and JACOBI, G. H. Gonadotropin-releasing hormone analogues for palliation of carcinoma of the prostate. World J. Urol., 1:40, 1983.
14. SOLOWAY, M. S. Newer methods of hormonal therapy for prostate cancer. Urology, 24(Suppl. 5):30, 1984.
15. The Leuprolide Study Group: Leuprolide versus diethylstilbestrol for metastatic prostate cancer. N. Engl. J. Med., 311:1281, 1986.
16. WAXMAN, J. H. et al. Treatment of advanced prostatic cancer with

buserelin, an analogue of gonadotropin-releasing hormone. Br. J. Urol., 55:737, 1983.

17. CRAWFORD, E. D., and DAVIS, M. A. Luteinizing hormone-releasing hormone analogues in the treatment of prostate cancer. In *Endocrine Therapies in Breast and Prostate Cancer.* Edited by C. K. Osborne. Boston, Kluwer Academic Publishers, 1988, pp. 25–52.

18. DEBRUYNE, F. M. J. et al. Long-term therapy with a depot luteinizing hormone-releasing hormone analogue (Zoladex) in patients with advanced prostatic carcinoma. J. Urol., 140:775, 1988.

19. SINGER, J. H. et al. A comparison of prostatic cancer treated with GnRH or DES. Proceedings of American Urological Association, Las Vegas, May 6–9, 1984.

20. AHMANN, F. R. et al. Zoladex: A sustained release luteinizing hormone-releasing hormone analogue for the treatment of advanced prostate cancer. J. Clin. Oncol., 5:912, 1987.

21. TRACHTEBERG, J., HALPERN, N., and PONT, A. Ketoconazole: A novel and rapid treatment for advanced prostatic cancer. J. Urol., 130:152, 1983.

22. JOHNSON, D. E. et al. Ketoconazole therapy for hormonally refractive metastatic prostate cancer. Urology, 31:132, 1988.

23. WALSH, P. C., and SIITERI, P. K. Suppression of plasma androgens by spironolectone in castrated men with carcinoma of the prostate. J. Urol., 114:254, 1975.

24. ROBINSON, M. R. G. Aminoglutethimide: Medical adrenalectomy in the management of carcinoma of the prostate. A review after five years. Br. J. Urol., 52:328, 1980.

25. WORGUL, T. J. et al. Clinical and biochemical effect of aminoglutethimide in the treatment of advanced prostatic carcinoma. J. Urol., 123:51, 1983.

26. CRAWFORD, E. D., AHMANN, F. R., and DAVIS, M. A. Aminoglutethimide in metastatic adenocarcinoma of the prostate. In Prostate Cancer Part A: Research, Endocrine treatment and Histopathology. Edited by G. Murphy et al. New York, Alan R. Liss, Inc., 1987, pp. 283–289.

27. BRACCI, U. Antiandrogens in the treatment of prostatic cancer. Eur. Urol., 5:303, 1979.

28. SCHROEDER, F. H. et al. Metastatic cancer of the prostate managed with buserelin versus buserelin plus cyproterone acetate. J. Urol., 137:912, 1987.

29. SUFFRIN, G., and COFFEY, D. S. Flutamide: Mechanism of action of a new nonsteroidal antiandrogen. Invest. Urol. 13:429, 1976.

30. NERI, R., and KASSEM, N. Biological and clinical properties of antiandrogens. In *Hormones and Cancer, 2: Proceedings of the Second International Congress on Hormones and Cancer. Progress in Cancer Research and Therapy.* Vol. 31. New York, Raven Press, 1984, pp. 507–518.

31. SOGANI, P. C., and WHITMORE, W. F., JR. Experience with flutamide in previously untreated patients with advanced prostatic cancer. J. Urol., 122:640, 1979.

32. NAVRATIL, H. Double-blind study of Anandron versus placebo in Stage D$_2$ prostate cancer patients receiving Buserelin. In *Prostate Cancer Part A: Research, Endocrine Treatment and Histopathology.* Edited by G. Murphy et al. New York, Alan R. Liss, Inc., 1987, pp. 401–410.

33. BRISSET, J. M. et al. Anandron (RU23908) associated to surgical castration in previously untreated Stage D prostate cancer: Multicenter comparative study of two doses of the drug and of a placebo. In *Prostate Cancer Part A: Research, Endocrine Treatment and Histopathology.* Edited by G. Murphy et al. New York, Alan R. Liss, Inc., 1987, pp. 411–422.

34. LABRIE, F. et al. New hormonal therapy in prostatic carcinoma: Combined treatment with an LHRH agonist and an antiandrogen. Clin. Invest. Med., 5:267, 1982.

35. LABRIE, F. et al. New approach in the treatment of prostate cancer: Complete instead of partial withdrawal of androgens. Prostate, 4:579, 1983.

36. LABRIE, F., DUPONT, A., and BELANGER, A. Complete androgen blockade for the treatment of prostate cancer. In *Important Advances in Oncology.* Edited by V. T. DeVita, Jr., S. Hellman, and S. A. Rosenberg. Philadelphia, J. B. Lippincott, 1985, pp. 193–217.

37. LABRIE, F. et al. Combination therapy with flutamide and (D-Trp^6) LHRH ethylamide in advanced (stages C and D) previously untreated prostate cancer. In *International Symposium on Hormonal Therapy of Prostatic Disease.* Edited by M. Motta, and M. Serio. London, Medicom, 1988.

38. LABRIE, F., and VEILLUX, R. A wide range of sensitivities to androgens develops in cloned Shionogi Mouse mammary tumor cells. Prostate, 8:293, 1986.

39. COFFEY, D. S. et al. Growth characteristic and immunogenicity of the R-3327 rat prostate carcinoma. NCI Monogr., 49:289, 1978.

40. ISAACS, J. T., and COFFEY, D. S. Adaptation versus selection as the mechanism responsible for the relapse of prostatic cancer to androgen ablation therapy as studied in the Dunning R-3327-H adenocarcinoma. Cancer Res., 41:5070, 1981.

41. LABRIE, F. et al. Treatment of prostate cancer with gonadotropin-releasing hormone agonists. Endocr. Rev., 7:67, 1986.

42. SANDER, S., NISSEN-MEYER, R., and AAKVAAG, A. Orchiectomy combined with cyproterone acetate or prednisone in the treatment of advanced prostatic carcinoma. Scand. J. Urol. Nephrol., 16:193, 1982.

43. ROBINSON, M. R. G. Complete androgen blockade: The EORTC experience comparing orchiectomy versus orchiectomy plus cyproterone acetate versus low-dose stilboesterol in the treatment of metastatic carcinoma of the prostate. In *Prostate Cancer Part A: Research, Endocrine Treatment and Histopathology.* Edited by G. Murphy et al. New York, Alan R. Liss, Inc., 1987, pp. 383–390.

44. CRAWFORD, E. D. et al. A controlled trial of Leuprolide with and without flutamide in prostatic carcinoma. N. Engl. J. Med., 321:419, 1989.

CHAPTER
49B

Chemotherapy in Prostate Cancer

Mario A. Eisenberger

ndrogen deprivation remains the main therapeutic approach for patients with disseminated cancer of the prostate. Despite the evidence that significant benefits can be accomplished in most patients with disseminated disease, this form of treatment remains primarily palliative. Evidence of tumor progression mostly unaffected by subsequent hormonal manipulations develops in an almost predictable fashion following first-line treatment. In tumor models, this phenomenon is associated with the development of various phenotypic changes that may represent evidence of mutation of previous sensitive tumor cell clones, expansion of pre-existing androgen independent cells unaffected by treatment or, most likely, both.[1–5] The development of endocrine resistance in this disease is a much more definitive and irreversible phenomenon than in breast cancer for example, where subsequent responses to second- and third-line endocrine manipulations can be observed in patients whose tumors are rich in estrogen and progesterone receptors. In cancer of the prostate, response to second-line hormonal approaches are uncommon and mostly short-lived. These data strongly support the need for continuing to focus vigorous efforts on the development of non-endocrine approaches.

EVALUATION OF THERAPEUTIC EFFICACY

The difficulty in assessing response to treatment in this disease by using conventional criteria is a well-recognized limitation.[6–16] The application of the usual criteria for response employed in most clinical trials may only be possible in a smaller proportion of patients with evidence of bidimensionally measurable disease. The main problem is that metastatic cancer of the prostate most frequently manifests itself by osteoblastic bone lesions or mixed "blastic" and "lytic" lesions, which are virtually impossible to quantitate prospectively in a reliable fashion. Evaluation of responses in bone metastasis are notoriously difficult to reproduce.

Table 49B-1 illustrates the most commonly employed methods to evaluate the effects of chemotherapy (or other systemic treatments) in patients with metastatic disease. Probably no more than 25% of patients with metastatic disease present with evidence of bidimensionally measurable disease that allows investigators to quantitate certain disease sites along with treatment. Not uncommonly, some patients demonstrate evidence of "mixed responses," that is, improvement of soft tissue disease sites but increased or persistent symptomatology in other areas, most commonly bones. Patients

TABLE 49B-1. *Objective Parameters Most Commonly Used to Assess Responses in Patients with Endocrine Resistant Prostatic Cancer*

METHOD	LIMITATIONS
Bone Radiographs	Lesions are predominantly blastic and usually will not change with treatment
Bone Scans	Quantitative assessments of positive areas are difficult in both directions. More useful to document progression
Serum Acid Phosphatase	Valuable only in rare occasions when high values return to normal. Significant variations may be observed independent of treatment
Serum Alkaline Phosphatase	Usually do not correlate with response or progression after treatment
Measurement of Prostatic Size	Measurements are frequently unidimensional (digital exam). The use of transrectal ultrasound and prostatic CAT scan or magnetic resonance imaging are still controversial for monitoring response to treatment

1. Data with prostatic-specific antigen is still lacking at this time (1989)
2. Modified from Eisenberger, M., Kennedy, P., and Abrams, J. Oncology, *1*:59, 1987.

TABLE 49B-2. *Overall "Objective Responses" Reported**

TOTAL NO. PATIENTS TREATED	COMPLETE AND PARTIAL RESPONSES	STABLE DISEASE
3184	202 (6.5%)	485 (15%)

*Extracted from all trials reviewed by Eisenberger et al. A re-evaluation of non-hormonal cytotoxic chemotherapy in the treatment of prostatic carcinoma. J. Clin. Oncol., *3*:827, 1985.

whose disease is progressing slower. Regardless of these well-recognized deficiencies, the NPCP criteria for response has been widely employed and this was particularly emphasized for studies involving patients without evidence of bidimensionally measurable disease. It should be recognized that including SD patients in the responding group may falsely inflate response rates. Table 49B-2 demonstrates that in a sizeable number of patients pooled from several phase II and phase III studies with chemotherapy in this disease, the overall average complete and partial response rate (CR + PR) is disappointingly low, whereas most of the "responders" are actually included on the SD category.

The efficacy data with chemotherapy in prostate cancer is usually described by using response rates, however, because of the above factors, urological oncologists should be critical when interpreting clinical trials in this disease. It is this author's opinion that methodological factors have a strong influence in the outcome of a study and that the variability of results observed with similar treatment programs are largely related to the application of different methods of disease assessment.

THE EXPERIENCE WITH SINGLE AGENTS AND MULTIDRUG COMBINATIONS IN UNCONTROLLED CLINICAL TRIALS

Table 49B-3 lists alphabetically the drugs thus far evaluated in metastatic "endocrine-resistant" prostate cancer patients. The experience with commonly used single agents is illustrated in Table 49B-4. In view of the methodological problems alluded to above, it is difficult to estimate the exact level of antitumor

with evidence of visceral organ involvement are frequently debilitated, have far-advanced disease with extensive bone involvement, and many times received significant prior palliative radiotherapy, all of which usually limit optimal use of cytotoxic drugs. Similarly, the issue of whether patients with visceral involvement represent a subset of patients with different prognosis from those with bone disease only, remains unclear. Although the subset of patients with measurable disease may be more appropriate for clinical trials, it is possible that they also represent a subgroup less likely to respond to any treatment.

For several years, the National Prostatic Cancer Project (NPCP) has utilized a criteria for response developed by their group, which includes a category of disease stabilization (SD) as evidence of response to treatment.[15] In their definition, SD reflects no evidence of disease progression (or worsening) during the initial 12 weeks of treatment. Survival analysis of SD patients appeared to be comparable to those who had evidence of tumor regression (partial responses) during that same 12-week period and SD and PR lived significantly longer than those that did not respond (NR). These observations prompted NPCP investigators to consider SD in the category of "responding" patients, together with those who demonstrated evidence of partial response. What remains unproven, however, is that stabilization of disease was caused by treatment. Similarly, it is possible that SD patients have a relatively indolent biology and slow progression rate, which is inherent in their disease and unrelated to treatment. It is quite conceivable that those that have demonstrated evidence of disease progression at 12 weeks will die sooner than those patients

TABLE 49B-3. *Single Agents Studied in Prostatic Cancer*

AMSA	Esorubicin	MGBG	Nitrogen Mustard
AZQ	Estracyt	ME-CCNU	Prednimustine
BCNU	Etoposide	Melphalan	Procarbazine
Bisantrene	5-FU	Methotrexate	Spirogermanium
CCNU	GANO$_3$	Mitomycin-C	Streptozotocin
Cyclophosphamide	HMM	Mitoxantrone	Vinblastine
Cisplatin	Hydrea	Neocarcinostatin	Vincristine
Doxorubicin	Ifosfamide		Vindesine

Modified from Eisenberger, M. et al. A re-evaluation of non-hormonal cytotoxic chemotherapy in the treatment of prostatic carcinoma. J. Clin. Oncol., *3*:827, 1985.
Abbreviations:
AMSA = Amsacrine
AZQ = Aziridinyl Benzoquinone
BCNU = Carmustine
CCNU = Lomustine
5-FU = 5-fluorouracil
GANO$_3$ = Gallium Nitrate
HMM = Hexamethylmelamine
MGBG = Mitoguazone

TABLE 49B-4. *Experience with Commonly Used Single Agents (Including Uncontrolled and Randomized Trials)*

DRUG/INVESIGATOR	CR + PR/ EVALUABLE	OTHER RESPONSE (INCLUDING SD)
Doxorubicin		
O'Bryan et al.[17]	2/9	NR
O'Bryan et al.[18]	5/15	NR
Torti et al.[19]	4/25	17/25
Scher et al.[20]	2/39	4/39
Eagan, Hahn, and Myers[12]	NR/19*[1]	5/19
Pavone-Macaluso et al.[21]	0/11*[1]	3/11
DeWys et al.[11]	15/61*[1]	0
Torti et al.[22]	1/13*[1]	8/20
Cyclophosphamide		
NPCP 100[6,23]	4/41*[1]	20/41
NPCP 300[24]	01/35*[1]	9/35
NPCP 700[25]	3/43*[1]	12/47
Chlebowski et al.[26]	0/15*[1]	8/15
Muss et al.[27]	0/17*	9/17
Cisplatin		
Yagoda et al.[10]	3/25	1/25
Merrin[28]	17/54	7/54
Rossof et al.[29]	4/21	0
Qazi and Khandekar[30]	0/17	0
NPCP 1100[31]	2/50*[1]	16/50
NPCP 1200[32]	0/42*[1]	9/42
Moore et al.[33]	0/29	3/29
5-Fluorouracil		
Moore et al.[34]	4/7	3/7
Ansfield, Shroeder, and Curreri[35]	1/7	NR
Weiss, Jackson and Carabasi[36]	1/4	NR
Hall and Good[37]	3/6	NR
NPCP 100[6,23]	4/33*[1]	14/33
Smalley et al.[38]	2/32*	5/32
Tejada et al.[39]	2/8*	1/8
DeWys et al.[11]	3/42*	0/51*
Estramustine Phosphate		
Mittleman, Shukla, and Murphy[40]	9/44	0/44
Fossa and Miller[41]	NR/17	6/17
Johnson, Hogberg, and Nilsson[42]	NR/91	28/91
Kuss et al.[43]	3/15	0/15
Leistenschneider and Nagel[44]	8/23	0/23
Edsmyr, Espositi and Anderson[45]	NR/90	19/90
Nilsson[46]	NR/91	28/91
Veronesi et al.[47]	3/27	17/27
NPCP 200[6,48]	3/46*[1]	11/46
NPCP 800[49]	1/27*[1]	6/27
NPCP 1100[31]	1/50*[1]	16/50
NPCP 1200[32]	0/40*[1]	7/40
Methotrexate		
NPCP 1100[31]	3/58*[1]	21/58
Hydroxyurea		
Lerner and Malloy[50]	15/30	4/30
NPCP 700[25]	2/28*[1]	2/28
Stephens et al.[51]	1/24*[1]	9/69

*One of the arms of a randomized study
[1]More than 10% (at times up to 50%) exclusions for inevaluability reasons or lack of bidimensionally measurable disease or both

activity of most drugs. This is particularly evident with drugs frequently employed in this disease, such as doxorubicin (Adriamycin) and others. As shown in Table 49B-4, there is a disturbing divergence in response rates reported with the use of this drug by different investigators. This variability most likely reflects differences in key issues such as criteria used for establishing response, patient selection factors, and the number of patients included in individual trials. Scher et al.,[20] using an every-3-week schedule of Doxorubicin, evaluated 39 patients with measurable disease and reported a 50% or more decrease in tumor mass in only 2 patients. Torti et al. reported 21/25 responses using the National Prostatic Cancer Project criteria for response with a weekly "low-dose" schedule of the same drug (the total dose over a three-week period was approximately the same as Scher et al.), however, only 4 had complete (CR) or partial responses (PR) by conventional criteria.[19] Cisplatin was reported by Merrin et al. to produce responses in 25/54 evaluable patients, 17 of whom fulfilled the investigators' criteria for objective responses.[28] Unfortunately, these initial, encouraging results with this drug have not been reproduced by others.[10,28–33] The true level of activity of cisplatin in this disease is most likely less than 20% (see Table 49B-4). Several years ago, Lerner et al., reported complete plus partial responses in 15/30 patients treated with single agent hydroxyurea.[49] Subsequent trials by Loening et al.[25] and Stephens, et al.[50] failed to substantiate these initial findings and, in fact, demonstrated the inefficacy of this drug.

In an attempt to improve the therapeutic results with single agents, and based on observations in other tumor types suggesting the superiority of drug combinations over single agents, various multidrug regimens have been developed. The development of such treatment regimens was based on various concepts, ranging from kinetic, pharmacologic, or simply additive effects. Table 49B-5 illustrates the combinations tested in this disease and Table 49B-6 illustrates the results with some of the most commonly used regimens. The incidence of actual complete plus partial responses with the combinations shown has been disappointingly low. In general, such programs are more toxic than single agents and this lim-

TABLE 49B-5. *Multidrug Combinations Studied in Prostatic Cancer*

CTX + 5 FU	Adria + DDP
CTX + 5 FU + Adria	Adria + 5 FU + Mito-C
CTX + 5 FU + MTX	Estracyt + DDP
CTX + 5 FU + MTX + VCR + Prednisone	Estracyt + VCR
CTX + Adria	
CTX + Adria + BCNU	Estracyt + Prednimustine
CTX + DDP + Prednisolone	Chlorambucil + Prednisone
CTX + Prednisolone	

From Eisenberger, M.
Abbreviations:
  CTX = cyclophosphamide
  5-FU = 5-fluorouracil
  Adria = Doxorubicin
  MTX = methotrexate
  VCR = vincristine
  DDP = cisplatin
  BCNU = carmustine

TABLE 49B-6. *Commonly Used Drug Combinations (Including Uncontrolled and Randomized Trials)*

DRUG/INVESTIGATOR	COMPLETE RESPONSE AND PARTIAL RESPONSE/ EVALUABLE	OTHER RESPONSE (INCLUDING SD)
Cyclophosphamide + Doxorubicin		
Izbicki, Amer, and Al-Sarraf[52]	3/20	5/20
Ihde et al.[9]	7/22	4/22
Merrin et al.[53]	0/19	5/19
Lloyd et al.[54]	2/11	0/11
Soloway, Shippel, and Ikard[55]	0/21	12/21
Stephens et al.[51]	6/19* (meas. disease)	18/68 (all pts)
Cisplatin + Doxorubicin		
Citrin et al.[13]	NR/21	10/21
Perloff et al.[56]	9/17	0/17
Torti et al.[22]	2/10* (meas. disease)	9/17
Doxorubicin + 5 FU + Mito-C		
Logothetis et al.[15]	NR/62	30/62
Kasimis et al.[57]	0/16	7/16
Hsu and Babaian[58]	1/14	8/14
Cyclophosphamide + MTX + 5 FU		
Muss et al.[27]	1/15	7/15
Herr[59]	3/20	4/20
Cyclophosphamide + Doxorubicin + 5 FU		
Smalley et al.[38]	2/39* (total entered 52)	4/39
Chlebowski et al.[26]	0/12	6/12
Other Combinations		
Cyclophosphamide + Prednisolone[60]	NR/83	7/83
BCNU + Cyclophosphamide + Doxorubicin[61]	7/27	4/27
Cyclophosphamide + MTX + 5 FU + VCR[62]	5/16	1/16
Estramustine Phosphate + 5 FU[63]	0/25	3/25

*More than 10% excluded or not analyzed either because of inevaluability or lack of measurable disease

its their use in patients with extensive prior radiation and bone marrow tumor involvement.

PROSPECTIVE RANDOMIZED STUDIES WITH CHEMOTHERAPY IN ENDOCRINE-RESISTANT PATIENTS

Tables 49B-9 and 49B-10 illustrate all prospective randomized studies reported in the English literature. Randomized studies are easier to evaluate because they provide the opportunity for assessing the effects of a treatment regimen relative to a concurrent control. They also serve for evaluating other endpoints such as survival and time to treatment failure.

In two earlier trials conducted by investigators of the National Prostatic Cancer Project, patients with stage-D2 endocrine resistant disease were randomized to various chemotherapeutic single agents or a no chemotherapy control arm

TABLE 49B-7. *NPCP #100 (Less than 20 Gy Pelvic RT)[6,23]*

Cyclophosphamide (CTX) ⟶ 5 FU
5-Fluorouracil ⟶ CTX
Standard Treatment ⟶
(No Chemotherapy)

	INITIAL			CROSSOVER			ALL TREATED		
	#	PR	SD	#	PR	SD	#	PR	SD
CTX	41	3	16	19	1	4	60	4	20
5 FU	33	4	8	20	0	6	53	4	14
ST	36	0	7	—	—	—	36	0	7

PR = Partial Response
SD = Stable Disease

TABLE 49B-8. *NPCP #200 (20 Gy or More Pelvic RT)*[6,48]

Estracyt ⟶ Streptozotocin
Streptozotocin ⟶ Estracyt
Standard Treatment ⟶
(No Chemotherapy)

	# EVALUABLE PATIENTS	PR	SD
Estracyt	46	3	11
Streptozotocin	38	0	12
Standard	21	0	4

PR = Partial Response
SD = Stable Disease

("standard" treatment), which consisted of various palliative measures such as corticosteroids, estrogenic compounds, analgesics, palliative radiation to symptomatic areas, or spironolactone. In the first trial (NPCP study 100), patients having had less than 20 Gy prior pelvic radiation were randomized to receive 5-fluorouracil, cyclophosphamide, or standard treatment (Table 49B-7 and Fig. 49B-1).[6,23] On NPCP study 200, patients having had more than 20 Gy prior pelvic radiation were randomized to receive estramustine phosphate, streptozotocin, or standard treatment (Table 49B-8 and Fig. 49B-1).[6,47] As illustrated on the tables, the number of responders (complete and partial responses) were small and most of the "responding" patients were actually included in the stable-disease category. On both studies, the Kaplan-Meier survival curves distribution was virtually identical and, although the numbers of patients in each arm may be considered sufficient to rule out only large differences between arms, smaller improvements would only reflect a prolongation of survival by weeks or a few months, which probably does not represent significant thera-

TABLE 49B-9. *National Prostatic Cancer Project: Randomized Trials In Prostatic Carcinoma*

TREATMENT (REF)	NUMBER EVALUABLE/ENTERED	CR + PR	SD	MEDIAN SURVIVAL (WEEKS)
NPCP Study 100[6,23]				
CTX	41	4	20	47
5FU	33	4	14	44
Standard*	36	0	7	38
NPCP Study 200[6,48]				
Estramustine Phosphate	46/54	3	11	26
Streptozotocin	38/46	0	12	25
Standard*	21/25	0	4	24
NPCP Study 300[24]				
CTX	35/39	0	9	27
DTIC	55/68	2	13	40
Procarbazine	39/58	0	5	31
				Mean:Survival
NPCP Study 400[64]				
Estramustine Phosphate + Prednimustine	54	1	6	37
Prednimustine	62	0	8	36
NPCP Study 700[25]				
CTX	43/47	3	12	41
MeCCNU	27/38	1	7	22
Hydroxyurea	28/40	2	2	19
NPCP Study 800[49]				
Estramustine Phosphate (E)	27/38	1	6	26
Vincristine (V)	29/42	1	4	22
E + V	34/41	0	7	32
NPCP Study 1100[31]				
Estramustine Phosphate	50/63	1	16	43
MTX	58/67	3	21	37
DDP	50/59	2	16	33
NPCP Study 1200[32]				
Estramustine Phosphate (E)	40/50	0	7	38
DDP	42/51	0	9	28
E + DDP	42/48	0	14	40

*Radiation therapy, prednisone, TACE, dexamethasone, testosterone, DES, stilbestrol, Aldactone, cryosurgery, dicorvin, estinyl

TABLE 49B-10. *Other Randomized Trials in Prostatic Carcinoma*

TREATMENT (REF)	NUMBER EVALUABLE/ ENTERED	CR + PR	SD	IMPROVEMENT	MEDIAN SURVIVAL	RESPONSE[2] CRITERIA
Smalley et al.[38]						
5-FU	32/49	2	5	—	34 weeks	A
CTX + Doxorubicin + 5-FU	39/52	2	4	—	25 weeks	
Eagan, Hahn, and Myers[12]						
Adriamycin	19	—	—	5	NR	B
CTX + 5-FU	18	—	—	2	NR	
Chlebowski et al.[26]						
CTX	15	0	8	—	7,2 mos	C
CTX + Doxorubicin + 5-FU	12	0	6	—	8,9 mos	
Muss et al.[27]						
CTX	17	0	9	—	8 mos	C
CTX + MTX + 5-FU	15	1	7	—	5 mos	
Herr[59]						
CTX + MTX + 5-FU	20	3	4	—	26 weeks	D
CCNU	20	0	6	—	24 weeks	
Tejada et al.[39]						
5-FU	8	2	1	—	NR	D
CCNU	10	4	2	—	NR	
Pavone-Macaluso et al.[21]						
Doxorubicin	11/22	0	3	—	NR	C
Procarbazine	14/24	1	0	—	NR	
DeWys et al.[11]						
Doxorubicin	96/112	15/61*	0	—	29 weeks	D
5-FU	51/54	3/42	0	—	24 weeks	
Stephens et al.[51]						
CTX + Doxorubicin	68	6/19*	18	—	27 weeks	D
Hydroxyurea	69	1/24*	9	—	28 weeks	
Torti et al.[22]						
Doxorubicin	20	1/13**	8	**	48 weeks	E**
Doxorubicin + Cisplatin	17	2/10**	9	**	43 weeks	

[1]Improvement reported but not quantitated, or some evidence regarded as treatment benefit (decrease in marker values, decrease in prostatic size)
[2]A Southeastern Cancer Study Group Criteria[26]
B Ancillary Scoring System (including crossed-over patients)[11]
C National Prostatic Cancer Project[12]
D Usual criteria for solid tumors, including a decrease in acid phosphatase
*Patients with "measurable disease" only (including bidimensionally measurable disease and elevation or presence of evaluable bony lesions). Figures include crossed-over patients
**Northern California Oncology Group criteria for response. Objective Responses are recorded separately according to their category of measurable versus evaluable (this also applies for the SWOG study reported by Stephens).[49] Ancillary responses included on the improvement section do not allow for a determination of an actual denominator
NR Not reported
5 FU 5-Fluorouracil
CTX Cytoxan

peutic advances. The same argument may be raised on other NPCP chemotherapy studies (see below and Table 49B-9). It may be argued that crossover treatment, as it was applied on both studies, may have influenced survival. This, however, can be considered highly unlikely in view of the relative inefficiency of chemotherapy in this disease. Furthermore, on studies 100 and 200, patients randomized to one of the chemotherapy arms were crossed over to receive the other drug, while those initially randomized to receive standard treatment were followed until death without other salvage treatment.

Based on the initial observations on studies 100 and 200, NPCP investigators conducted a number of other trials illus-trated in Table 49B-9 and Figure 49B-1. Various evaluations of NPCP trials have raised major criticisms and among those are: (1) common practice of excluding inevaluable patients from analysis, (2) high exclusion rates, (3) systematic inclusion of stable disease patients in the responding category, (4) conclusions of relative efficacy based primarily on observed response rates, (5) the use of suboptimal doses of chemotherapy, and (6) imprecise toxicity description. Despite the concerns regarding their studies, the group has made important contributions regarding basic observations of the course of this disease and elements of prognostic importance.[64] In all NPCP studies, the survival curves' distribution and median survival times are

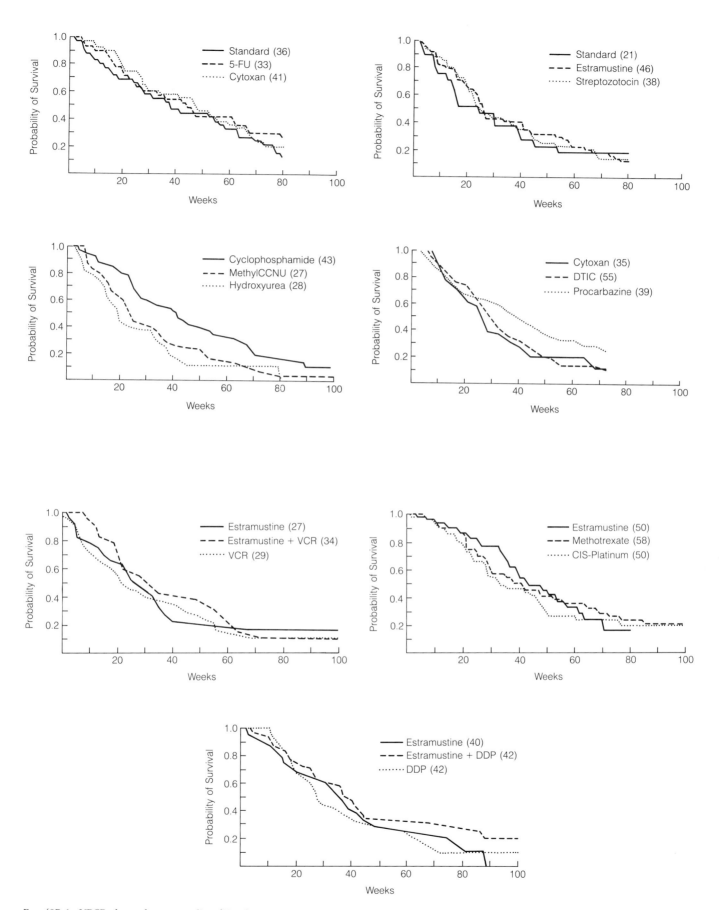

FIG. 49B-1. NPCP chemotherapy studies. (Numbers in parentheses indicate number of patients.)

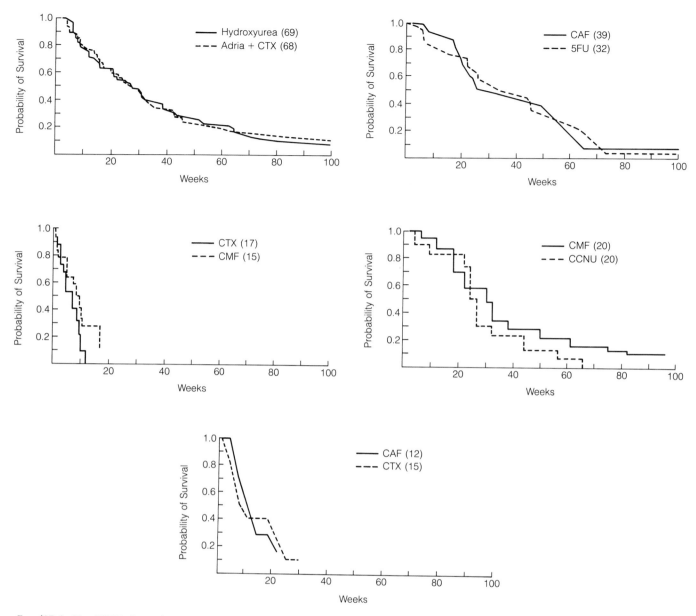

Fig. 49B-2. Non-NPCP chemotherapy studies. (Numbers in parentheses indicate number of patients.)

similar for all treatment regimens and these, in turn, were comparable to the standard treatment (no chemotherapy) control arms of studies 100 and 200. This suggests that the chemotherapy programs tested by NPCP have not been shown to prolong survival over a no chemotherapy control arm.

Table 49B-10 describes the results of various studies conducted by other groups. Like NPCP studies, these other trials failed to demonstrate a clear superiority of one treatment regimen over another. The survival curves on these studies are shown on Figure 49B-2, which again stresses the similarities between survival curves observed with the various treatment programs tested. It also stresses the point that survival of endocrine resistant remains uniformly poor.

The various standard chemotherapeutic drugs that have shown at least some activity in other human malignancies have resulted in disappointing overall order of activity in this disease. In situations where cytotoxic treatment is opted for, physicians should recognize that treatment produces only modest palliation and most likely does not affect survival. Thus, an agent with reasonable tolerance should be chosen with special attention to issues related to quality of life. In such rare situations, we have selected single alkylating agents given at proper doses for a short period of time and continued only when unequivocal benefits have been accomplished. In view of the data illustrated in this chapter, routine use of multidrug regimens cannot be supported at this time.

COMBINED CHEMO-ENDOCRINE TREATMENT AS THE INITIAL SYSTEMIC APPROACH

More recently, much attention has been focused to define the optimal timing for treatment with cytotoxic drugs in cancer of the prostate. Data derived from preclinical experiments in the Dunning adenocarcinoma tumor model indicate that this tumor is comprised of hormonally dependent and independent cell clones (tumor cell heterogeneity).[1-5] Experiments using androgen ablation and/or chemotherapy in this tumor model suggest that early combined therapy may be superior to treatment with either modality alone or applied in any other sequence.[66] Unfortunately, however, although antitumor mechanisms and effects with endocrine treatment in the Dunning tumor model are somewhat comparable with human prostate cancer, the same is not true with nonhormonal chemotherapeutic agents.[67] Extrapolation of data with chemotherapy between species should be cautiously undertaken primarily because the results with this modality in the Dunning tumor model have not been reproducible in prostate cancer in man.[67] Nonetheless, because tumor progression following gonadal ablation reflects to a great extent an expansion of previously existing endocrine independent clones, the use of combined endocrine and "nonendocrine" treatment as the initial approach has sound theoretical rationale, and early initiation of combined treatment may be more effective when the tumor burden is smaller.

This, however, has not been confirmed by existing clinical data. Clinical trials combining chemotherapy plus endocrine treatment have focused primarily on patients with stage-D2 disease without prior systemic treatment.

The National Prostatic Cancer Project conducted two randomized trials, one in newly diagnosed stage-D2 patients comparing diethylstilbestrol (DES) or orchiectomy versus DES plus Cyclophosphamide versus Cyclophosphamide plus Estramustine Phosphate (NPCP #500), and another comparing DES, DES plus cyclophosphamide, or DES plus estramustine phosphate on stable patients on initial hormonal therapy (NPCP #600). No response or survival (Fig. 49B-3) differences were observed in either study.[68,69]

The Southeastern Cancer Study Group conducted a trial comparing DES alone to DES plus Cyclophosphamide in newly diagnosed stage-D2 patients. Preliminary results of this study did not demonstrate an advantage for the combination arm.[70] A follow-up report has not been published at this time.

The Southwest Oncology Group has conducted a study comparing orchiectomy alone to orchiectomy plus the combination of cyclophosphamide and doxorubicin, however, the results of this trial are yet to be published.

The median survival curves on all randomized studies with combined endocrine/chemotherapy are comparable to those reported on the VA studies (VACURG) more than 2 decades ago and also to more contemporary studies with various endocrine treatment alone in patients with stage-D2 disease.[71,72]

The administration of exogenous testosterone for priming prostate cancer cells and therefore increasing their suscepti-

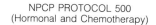

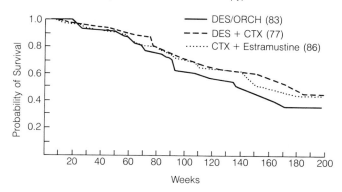

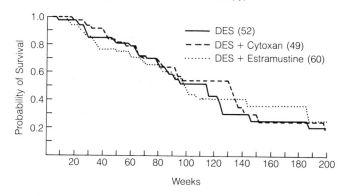

FIG. 49B-3. NPCP protocols 500 and 600 (hormonal and chemotherapy). (Numbers in parentheses indicate number of patients.)

bility to chemotherapy, has also been explored.[73,74] Manni et al. studied this approach in 85 patients with endocrine-resistant disease, all of whom had an orchiectomy followed by adrenal androgen suppression with aminoglutethimide and hydrocortisone.[74] All patients were randomized to receive exogenous androgen treatment with combination chemotherapy or combination chemotherapy alone and the results showed no advantage in response rates, time to progression, or survival. These negative results may be at least partly explained by the selection of patients with endocrine resistant (or androgen-independent) disease who may have been only minimally susceptible to exogenous androgenic stimulation even though some increase in toxicity on the stimulation arm was reported. Similarly, the lack of significant antitumor activity observed with chemotherapy in both arms suggests that this study did not constitute optimal conditions for testing this interesting approach.

More recently, Huben et al. reported on a trial in stage-D2 patients randomly allocated to receive treatment with DES or orchiectomy, buserelin (LHRH analogue) or DES, or orchiectomy plus methotrexate (MTX).[75] The authors report a significant difference in time to progression in favor of the DES/orchiectomy with and without MTX over the LHRH arm, but no differences in survival even though median survival figures had not been reached for all arms. They concluded that the shorter time to progression on buserelin may be explained by the initial "flare phenomenon" observed with LHRH analogue treatment. This phenomenon could result in a higher incidence of early progressions and therefore shorten the overall median time to progression for the entire group.

In summary, the results of these studies have not supported the usefulness of combined chemoendocrine approaches, however, it may be argued that this is not completely surprising in view of the lack of efficacy of the chemotherapeutic agents available this far. Although routine use of combined treatment with conventional cytotoxic drugs and endocrine manipulations can be justified at this time, this approach remains a viable option for future research with new systemic treatments for this disease.

IMPORTANT CONSIDERATIONS FOR FURTHER EVALUATION OF CHEMOTHERAPY

The data reviewed in this chapter illustrates that the palliative effects of chemotherapy for endocrine resistant prostate cancer are quite limited. Prospective randomized studies have failed to determine a clearcut impact on response rates and survival in favor of any treatment tested, furthermore in two studies, chemotherapy did not prolong survival compared to a "no chemotherapy" control arm. Current trials testing combinations of chemohormonal therapy have not shown any advantages over hormonal treatment alone in patients with newly diagnosed stage-D2 disease.

Despite the discouraging results, it is clear that a continued vigorous search for nonhormonal approaches is critical for progress in the treatment of this disease. Data in large numbers of patients treated with various androgen deprivation procedures indicate that major tumor responses and many times dramatic symptomatic improvement are achieved in the majority of patients with stage-D2 disease. The experience of others with patients with metastatic disease, entered onto large scale prospective randomized trials comparing different methods of endocrine manipulations, have shown comparable results between treatments and have not changed throughout the years. The median time to progression and median survival have ranged from approximately 12 to 18 months and 24 to 30 months respectively, regardless of the treatment employed.[68–72]

Although preclinical observations suggest that somatic mutations play an important role in the development of endocrine resistance, it is also true that "de novo" androgen-insensitive clones are already present during early stages of the disease.[1] It is unquestionable that better understanding of the mechanisms involved in the process of endocrine resistance will provide a new basis for discovering new and effective nonhormonal treatments for prostatic cancer.

Much has been written with regard to the disease process itself whereas the status of the host is also of major importance. The overwhelming majority of the patients included on the chemotherapy trials described in this review had been extensively pretreated and had far-advanced disease. Such characteristics, together with the host's performance status, are strong prognostic factors with regard to survival and chances for effective palliation. Despite these well-recognized limitations, urological oncologists still reserve chemotherapy for those patients who have become refractory to first-line and, many times, second- and third-line endocrine treatments, and are usually given palliative radiation to various painful areas. The experience derived from other more chemosensitive tumors strongly supports the view that extent of prior treatment, performance status, and extent of disease are among the strongest prognostic indicators for outcome in therapeutic trials. Thus, the poor results observed with chemotherapy thus far may, at least partly, be explained by the selection of a group of patients with adverse features unlikely to respond to any treatment.

The overall and long-term results with endocrine treatment in patients with far advanced stage-D2 are significantly worse than those observed in patients with lesser tumor burden and this probably reflects the presence of an already substantial proportion of androgen independent tumor clones. Although the poor response to cytotoxic treatment is largely a function of its relative inefficacy against this disease, some theoretical considerations, based on the lessons learned thus far, can be entertained. These include: (1) the mechanisms involved in the development of endocrine resistance may have an important role in the development of resistance to cytotoxic treatment, (2) as with endocrine treatment, response to cytotoxic chemotherapy may be less likely in more advanced and heavily pretreated patients, and (3) as in other more responsive tumor types (such as testis cancer, lymphomas, breast cancer, and small cell lung cancer), the magnitude of response to treatment may be proportional to the initial tumor burden. Such hypothetical considerations may be evaluated clinically by treating selected, newly diagnosed, stage-D2 patients (such as those described above with poor prognostic features and measurable disease) with chemotherapy prior to endocrine treatment. This should obviously be conducted in a strictly controlled and investigational setting. In a preliminary trial reported by Seifter et al., patients with newly diagnosed stage-D2 disease received a combination of cyclophosphamide, doxorubicin, and cisplatin before endocrine treatment was given.[76] This approach was shown to be feasible and to produce some responses. In our opinion, such investigational therapeutic intervention is ethically and scientifically justified because it has not been shown conclusively that early androgen ablation results in survival advantages over delayed treatment at the time patients become symptomatic with their disease. This is particularly the case of those patients with extensive stage-D2 disease in whom survival is usually short and significantly worse than those with relatively "limited metastatic disease," but could also include this latter group because overall survival may not be adversely reflected by this approach. This concept offers a new avenue for testing promising new agents under potentially more optimal conditions.

REFERENCES

1. ISAACS, J. T. et al. Genetic instability coupled to clonal selection as a mechanism for tumor progression in the Dunning R-3327 rat prostatic adenocarcinoma system. Cancer Res., *42*:2353, 1982.

2. ISAACS, J. T. et al. Models for development of non-receptor methods for distinguishing androgen-sensitive and insensitive prostatic tumors. Cancer Res., *39*:2657, 1979.

3. ISAACS, J. T., and COFFEY, D. S. Adaptation versus selection on the mechanism responsible for the relapse of prostatic cancer to androgen ablation therapy studied in the Dunning R-3327-H adenocarcinoma. Cancer Res., *41*:5070, 1981.

4. ISAACS, J. T. et al. Establishment and characterization of seven Dunning rat prostatic cancer cell lines and their use in developing methods for predicting metastatic abilities of prostatic cancer. Prostate, *9*:261, 1986.

5. CUNHA, G. R. et al. The endocrinology and developmental biology of the prostate. Endocr. News, *8*:338, 1987.

6. EISENBERGER, M. et al. A re-evaluation of non-hormonal cytotoxic chemotherapy in the treatment of prostatic carcinoma. J. Clin. Oncol., *3*:827, 1985.

7. YAGODA, A. Response in prostate cancer: An enigma. Semin. Urol., *1*:311, 1984.

8. SCHIMDT, J. D. et al. Chemotherapy of advanced prostatic cancer. Evaluation of response parameters. Urology, *7*:602, 1976.

9. IHDE, D. C. et al. Effective treatment of hormonally unresponsive metastatic carcinoma of the prostate with adriamycin and cyclophosphamide. Methods of documenting tumor response and progression. Cancer, *45*:1300, 1980.

10. YAGODA, A. et al. A critical analysis of response criteria in patients with prostatic cancer treated with cis-diaminedichloro platinum II. Cancer, *44*:1553, 1979.

11. DEWYS, W. D. et al. A comparative clinical trial of Adriamycin and 5-fluorouracil in advanced prostatic cancer: Prognostic factors and response. Prostate, *4*:1, 1983.

12. EAGAN, R. T., HAHN, R. G., and MYERS, R. R. Adriamycin (NSC-123127) versus 5-fluorouracil (NSC-19893) and cyclophosphamide (NSC-26271) in the treatment of metastatic prostate cancer. Cancer Treat. Rep., *60*:115, 1976.

13. CITRIN, D. et al. Systemic treatment of advanced prostatic cancer. Development of a new system for defining response. J. Urol., *125*:224, 1981.

14. SLACK, N. H. et al. The importance of the stable category for chemotherapy treated patients with advanced and relapsing prostate cancer. Cancer, *46*:2393, 1980.

15. LOGOTHETIS, C. J. et al. Doxorubicin, mitomycin-C and 5-fluorouracil (DMF) in the treatment of metastatic hormonal refractory adenocarcinoma of the prostate, with a note on the staging of metastatic prostate cancer. J. Clin. Oncol., *1*:368, 1983.

16. TORTI, F. M., and CARTER, S. K. The chemotherapy of prostatic adenocarcinoma. Ann. Intern. Med., *92*:681, 1980.

17. O'BRYAN, R. M. et al. Phase II evaluation of Adriamycin in human neoplasia. Cancer, *32*:1, 1973.

18. O'BRYAN, R. M. et al. Dose response evaluation of Adriamycin in human neoplasia. Cancer, *39*:1940, 1977.

19. TORTI, F. et al. Weekly doxorubicin in endocrine refractory carcinoma of the prostate. J. Clin. Oncol., *1*:477, 1983.

20. SCHER, H. et al. Phase II trial of Adriamycin in bidimensionally measurable prostatic adenocarcinoma. J. Urol., *13*:1099, 1984.

21. PAVONE-MACALUSO, M. et al. EORTC protocols in prostatic cancer. An interim report. Scand. J. Urol. Nephrol., *55*(Suppl):163, 1980.

22. TORTI, F. M. et al. A randomized study of doxorubicin versus doxorubicin plus cisplatin in endocrine—unresponsive metastatic prostatic carcinoma. Cancer, *56*:2580, 1985.

23. SCOTT, W. W. et al. The continued evaluation of the effects of chemotherapy in patients with advanced carcinoma of the prostate. J. Urol., *116*:211, 1976.

24. SCHMIDT, J. D. et al. Comparison of procarbazine, imidazole-carbamide and cyclophosphamide in relapsing patients with advanced carcinoma of the prostate. J. Urol., *121*:185, 1979.

25. LOENING, S. A. et al. A comparison of hydroxyurea, methyl-chloro-ethyl-chlorohexyl-nitrosourea and cyclophosphamide in patients with advance prostate cancer. J. Urol., *125*:812, 1981.

26. CHLEBOWSKI, R. T. et al. Cyclophosphamide (NSC 26271) versus the combination of Adriamycin (NSC 123127), 5-fluorouracil (NSC 19893) and cyclophosphamide in the treatment of metastatic prostatic cancer—a randomized trial. Cancer, *42*:2546, 1978.

27. MUSS, H. et al. Cyclophosphamide versus cyclophosphamide, methotrexate and 5-fluorouracil in advanced prostatic cancer—randomized trial. Cancer, *47*:1949, 1981.

28. MERRIN, C. E. Treatment of genitourinary tumors with cis-dichloro diammine platinum(II). Experience in 250 patients. Cancer Treat. Rep., *63*:1579, 1979.

29. ROSSOF, A. H. et al. Phase II evaluation of cis-dichloro diammine platinum(II) in advanced malignancies of the genitourinary and gynecological organs: A Southwest Oncology Group Study. Cancer Treat. Rep., *63*:1557, 1979.

30. QAZI, R., and KHANDEKAR, J. Phase II study of cisplatin for metastatic prostatic carcinoma. An Eastern Cooperative Oncology Group study. Am. J. Clin. Oncol. (CCT), *6*:203, 1983.

31. LOENING, S. A. et al. Comparison of estramustine phosphate, methotrexate, and cis-platinum in patients with advanced, hormone refractory prostate cancer. J. Urol., *129*:1001, 1983.

32. SOLOWAY, M. S. et al. A comparison of estramustine phosphate, versus cis-platinum alone versus estramustine phosphate plus cis-platinum in patients with advanced hormone refractory prostate cancer who had extensive irradiation to the pelvis or lumbosacral area. J. Urol., *129*:56, 1983.

33. MOORE, M. R. et al. Phase II evaluation of cisplatin for metastatic prostatic carcinoma. An Eastern Cooperative Oncology Group Study. Am. J. Clin. Oncol., *6*:203, 1983.

34. MOORE, G. E. et al. Effects of 5-fluorouracil (NSC-19893) in 389 patients with cancer. Eastern Clinical Drug Evaluation Program. Cancer Chemo. Rep. Part 1, *52*:641, 1968.

35. ANSFIELD, F. J., SCHROEDER, J., and CURRERI, A. R. Five years clinical experience with 5-fluorouracil. JAMA, *181*:295, 1962.

36. WEISS, A. J., JACKSON, L. G., and CARABASI, R. An evaluation of 5-fluorouracil in malignant disease. Ann. Intern. Med., *55*:731, 1961.

37. HALL, B. E., and GOOD, J. W. Treatment of far advanced cancer with 5-fluorouracil used alone and in combination with irradiation. Incidence and duration of remission and survival data in 223 patients. Cancer Chemo. Rep., *16*:369, 1962.

38. SMALLEY, R. V. et al. A phase II evaluation of a three drug combination of cyclophosphamide, doxorubicin and 5-fluorouracil and of 5-fluorouracil in patients with advanced bladder carcinoma or stage D prostatic carcinoma. J. Urol., *125*:191, 1981.

39. TEJADA, F. et al. 5-fluorouracil versus CCNU in the treatment of metastatic prostatic cancer. Cancer Treat. Rep., *6*:1589, 1977.

40. MITTLEMAN, A., SHUKLA, S. K., and MURPHY, G. P. Extended therapy of

stage D carcinoma of the prostate with oral estramustine phosphate. J. Urol., *115*:403, 1976.

41. Fossa, D. S., and Miller, A. Treatment of advanced carcinoma of the prostate with estramustine phosphate. J. Urol., *115*:406, 1976.

42. Jonsson, G., Hogberg, B., Nilsson T. Treatment of advanced prostatic carcinoma with estramustine phosphate (Estracyt). Scand. J. Urol. Nephrol., *11*:231, 1977.

43. Kuss, R. et al. Estramustine phosphate in the treatment of advanced prostatic cancer. Br. J. Urol., *52*:29, 1980.

44. Leistenschneider, W., and Nagel, R. Estracyt therapy of advanced prostatic cancer with special reference to control of therapy with cytology and DNA cytophotometry. Eur. Urol., *6*:111, 1980.

45. Edsmyr, F., Esposti, P. L., and Anderson, L. Estramustine phosphate therapy in poorly differentiated carcinoma of the prostate. Scand. J. Urol. Nephrol., *55*(Suppl):138, 1980.

46. Nilsson, T. Estracyt—clinical experiences. Scand J. Urol. Nephrol., *55*(Suppl):135, 1980.

47. Veronesi, A. et al. Estramustin phosphate (Estracyt) treatment of T_3-T_4 prostatic carcinoma. Prostate, *3*:159, 1982.

48. Murphy, G. P. et al. A comparison of estramustine phosphate and streptozotocin in patients with prostatic carcinoma who had extensive irradiation. J. Urol., *118*:288, 1977.

49. Soloway, M. S. et al. Comparison of estramustine phosphate and vincristine alone or in combination for patients with advanced hormone refractory previously irradiated carcinoma of the prostate. J. Urol., *125*:664, 1981.

50. Lerner, H. J., and Malloy, T. R. Hydroxyurea in stage D carcinoma of the prostate. Urology, *10*:35, 1977.

51. Stephens, R. L. et al. Adriamycin and cyclophosphamide versus hydroxyurea in advanced prostatic cancer. A randomized Southwest Oncology Group study. Cancer, *53*:406, 1984.

52. Izbicki, R. M., Amer, R. H., and Al-Sarraf, M. Combination of cyclophosphamide prednisone therapy in advanced prostatic carcinoma. Scand. J. Urol. Nephol., *55*:169, 1979.

53. Merrin, C. et al. Chemotherapy of advanced carcinoma of the prostate with 5-fluorouracil, cyclophosphamide, and Adriamycin. J. Urol., *115*:86, 1976.

54. Lloyd, R. E. et al. Combination chemotherapy with Adriamycin (NSC-123127) and cyclophosphamide (NSC-26271) for solid tumors: A phase II trial. Cancer Treat. Rep., *60*:77, 1976.

55. Soloway, M. S., Shippel, R. M., and Ikard, M. Cyclophosphamide, doxorubicin hydrochloride and 5-fluorouracil in advanced carcinoma of the prostate. J. Urol., *122*:637, 1979.

56. Perloff, M. et al. Adriamycin (ADM) and diammine dichloroplatinum (DDP) in advanced prostatic cancer. Proc. ASCO, Abstract C-265, 333, 1977.

57. Kasimis, B. S. et al. Treatment of hormone resistant metastatic cancer of the prostate with 5-FU, doxorubicin and mitomycin-C (FAM): A preliminary report. Cancer Treat. Rep., *67*:937, 1983.

58. Hsu, D. S., and Babaian, R. J. 5-Fluorouracil, Adriamycin, mitomycin-C (FAM) in the treatment of hormone-resistant stage D adenocarcinoma of the prostate. Proc. ASCO, Abstract C-520, 133, 1983.

59. Herr, H. W. Cyclophosphamide, methotrexate and 5-fluorouracil combination chemotherapy versus chlorethyl-cyclohexy-nitrosourea in the treatment of metastatic prostatic cancer. J. Urol., *127*:462, 1982.

60. Anderson, L. et al. Cyclophosphamide, prednisolone therapy in advanced prostatic carcinoma. Scand. J. Urol. Nephrol., *55*(Suppl):169, 1980.

61. Presant, C. A. et al. Chemotherapy of advanced prostatic cancer with adriamycin, BCNU and cyclophosphamide. Cancer, *46*:2389, 1980.

62. Buell, G. V. et al. Chemotherapy trial with COMP-F regimen in advanced adenocarcinoma of the prostate. Urology, *11*:247, 1978.

63. Kennealy, G. T. et al. Treatment of advanced carcinoma of the prostate with estramustine and 5-fluorouracil (5-FU). Proc. ASCO, Abstract C-351, 1978.

64. Murphy, G. P. et al. The use of estramustine and prednimustine versus prednimustine alone in advanced metastatic prostate cancer patients who have received prior irradiation. J. Urol., *121*:763, 1979.

65. Emrich, L. J., Priore, R. L., and Murphy, G. P. Prognostic factors in patients with advanced stage prostatic cancer. Cancer Res., *45*:5173, 1985.

66. Isaacs, J. T. The timing of androgen ablation therapy and/or chemotherapy in the treatment of prostatic cancer. Prostate, *5*:1, 1984.

67. Block, N. L., Canuzzi, F., and Denefrio, J. Chemotherapy of the transplantable adenocarcinoma (R-3327) of the Copenhagen rat. Oncology, *34*:110, 1977.

68. Murphy, G. P., Beckley, S., Brady, M. F., et al. and NPCP Investigators. Treatment of newly diagnosed prostate cancer patients with chemotherapy agents in combination with hormones versus hormones alone. Cancer, *51*:1264, 1983.

69. Gibbons, R. P. et al. The addition of chemotherapy to hormonal therapy for treatment of patients with metastatic carcinoma of the prostate. J. Surg. Oncol., *23*:133, 1983.

70. Moore, M. Chemohormonal therapy for stage D prostatic cancer. Preliminary results of a randomized trial. Proc. ASCO, Abstract C-461, 1982.

71. Byar, D. P. The Veterans Administration Cooperative Urological Research Group's studies of cancer of the prostate. Cancer, *32*:1126, 1973.

72. The Leuprolide Study Group: Leuprolide versus diethylstilbestrol for metastatic prostatic cancer. N. Engl. J. Med., *311*:1281, 1984.

73. Kedia, K. R., and Kellermeyer, R. W. Hormonal stimulation followed by multiagent chemotherapy in advanced prostatic cancer. Cancer Chemother. Pharmacol., *18*:261, 1982.

74. Manni, A. et al. Androgen priming and chemotherapy in advanced prostate cancer: Evaluation of determinants of clinical outcome. J. Clin. Oncol., *6*:1456, 1988.

75. Huben, R. P., Murphy, G. P., and NPCP investigators. A comparison of DES/orchiectomy with Buserelin and with methotrexate plus DES and orchiectomy in newly diagnosed patients with clinical stage D2 cancer of the prostate. Cancer, *62*:1881, 1988.

76. Seifter, E. et al. A trial of combination chemotherapy followed by therapy for previously untreated metastatic carcinoma of the prostate. J. Clin. Oncol., *4*:1305, 1984.

CHAPTER 50

Chemotherapy of Testicular Cancer

Craig R. Nichols

In the modern era of treatment of germ cell cancer, cure is the expectation for nearly all stages of the disease. Fulfillment of these expectations requires an integrated, expert approach to diagnosis, staging, and treatment. There is no room for the dilettante. To understand the role of chemotherapy in the management of nonseminomatous germ cell cancers, the clinical determinants of outcome in disseminated disease, the treatment of good- and poor-risk testicular cancer, and the role of chemotherapy as an adjuvant to retroperitoneal lymphadenectomy, will be reviewed. In addition, the emerging role of chemotherapy in the treatment of seminomatous germ cell cancer will be discussed.

HISTOLOGY AND STAGING

Clinical decisions in patients with germ cell cancer rely heavily on accurate determination of histologic subtype and precise measurement of serum beta-subunit human chorionic gonadotropin (HCG) and alpha-fetoprotein (AFP). From a clinician's viewpoint, the important distinction is whether the primary tumor is pure seminoma or has histologic or serologic evidence of nonseminomatous disease. Pure seminoma is most

frequently associated with normal tumor markers, but may have a low-level elevation of HCG (usually less than 100 mIV/ml). About 85% of patients with nonseminomatous disease will have elevated serum levels of either AFP or HCG. Unlike HCG, which can be slightly elevated in pure seminoma, an elevated AFP must be viewed as evidence of nonseminomatous disease, even in the presence of histopathologic findings of pure seminoma. Such patients are managed as if they have nonseminomatous disease.

The role of preorchiectomy determination of markers, as well as the role of serum tumor markers in determining the need for retroperitoneal lymphadenectomy, is limited. In early stage disease, as many as one-third of the patients with nonseminomatous disease are marker negative. Although it is important to determine serum markers before and after orchiectomy and retroperitoneal lymphadenectomy, the absolute value of these markers must not guide the decision to undertake these diagnostic and therapeutic options.

Modern clinical staging procedures have allowed for accurate assignment of the patients with testicular cancer to disseminated categories or those with clinically localized disease that may be amenable to surgery or radiotherapy. At Indiana

University, the clinical staging procedures are history and physical examination, determination of serum HCG, AFP, and LDH, and CT scans of the chest and abdomen. Head CT and other imaging procedures are performed only as indicated by the clinical presentation. The results of the initial staging allow assignment of patients to clinical categories—stage I, where disease is confined to the testis; resectable stage-II disease where radiographically apparent lymph nodes are smaller than 3 to 4 cm in greatest transverse diameter; unresectable stage-II disease with a larger than 3 to 4 cm nodal mass; or stage-III with disseminated disease. Those patients with clinical stage-I disease or resectable stage-II disease undergo retroperitoneal lymphadenectomy, and those with bulky abdominal disease or disseminated disease undergo initial chemotherapy without attempts at debulking surgery.

HISTORICAL PERSPECTIVE

Since the 1960's, combination chemotherapy has been the cornerstone of treatment for those patients with unresectable abdominal disease or disseminated disease. The initial breakthrough came with the demonstration of synergy between bleomycin and vinblastine.[1]

The discovery of the platinum coordination compound, cisplatin, and the significant activity of this compound in germinal neoplasms, led to the incorporation of this agent into regimens of vinblastine and bleomycin, both at Indiana University and Memorial Sloan-Kettering Cancer Center.[2,3] The initial trial at Indiana University of cisplatin, vinblastine, and bleomycin (PVB) produced complete remission in 70% of 47 patients. Doses of chemotherapy agents in this trial included cisplatin at 20 mg/M^2/day × 5, vinblastine at 0.4 mg/kg, and 30 units of bleomycin weekly. Maintenance vinblastine was given for 2 years.

Subsequent to these initial studies, serial randomized trials at Indiana University and the Southeastern Cancer Study Group (SECSG) demonstrated that equivalent results could be obtained with a lower dose of vinblastine (0.3 mg/kg) and with the elimination of maintenance therapy.[4,5]

Investigators at Memorial Sloan-Kettering Cancer Center began a series of trials with vinblastine, bleomycin, and cisplatin with the addition of other agents. Serial improvements were obtained with increases of cisplatin dose intensity, decrease in therapy duration, as well as elimination of doxorubicin and chlorambucil. The current program, VAB-VI, which includes vinblastine, actinomycin-D, bleomycin, cyclophosphamide, and cisplatin induces complete remission rates in greater than 80% of patients with disseminated germ cell cancer.[6] Although never compared in a randomized trial, these results appear comparable to the current program at Indiana University with the three-drug combination of cisplatin, etoposide, and bleomycin.

PROGNOSTIC FACTORS

The definition of prognostic factors for favorable outcome in disseminated germ cell tumors and the validation of these fac-

tors in clinical trials has provided a focus for further refinement of chemotherapy in this patient population. Most investigators agree that the extent of disease and the volume of disease are powerful prognostic factors. There is near concurrence that primary mediastinal nonseminomatous disease carries a poor prognosis. Also, most investigators view massive elevation of HCG as an adverse prognostic factor. Many of these factors are interrelated in a complex and poorly understood way and this had led to less unanimity regarding the prognostic impact of such factors as elevation of markers other than HCG, histologic subtype, or certain sites of metastatic disease.

The utility of identifying prognostic factors is demonstrated by the application of the classification system developed at Indiana University to a group of 180 patients entering the 1978 study of cisplatin, vinblastine, and bleomycin, with or without adriamycin, and subsequently randomized to receive or nor receive vinblastine maintenance.[7] The Indiana classification system is illustrated in Table 50-1.

This classification system was able to discriminate between a group of patients with minimal or moderate disease that had an excellent outcome (99% and 92% respectively), and a group of patients with advanced disease that had a relatively poor outcome, with just over 50% of patients surviving.

The classification system developed at Memorial Sloan-Kettering utilizes the absence or presence of extragonadal nonseminoma or the predicted probability of complete remission to classify nonseminomatous germ cell cancer patients as either good or poor risk. The probability of CR is determined by a mathematical model utilizing the serum LDH and HCG as continuous variables, and the number of sites of metastatic disease (TOTMET), as illustrated in Table 50-2.

This system, like the Indiana system, has been validated using a group of 118 patients treated with VAB-6 or etoposide plus cisplatin (good-risk patients), or VAB-6 alternating with etoposide/cisplatin (poor-risk patients).[8] Again, this classification system provided excellent discrimination of patients with a favorable outcome or poor results from therapy (95% of

TABLE 50-1. *Indiana Classification System for Disseminated Germ Cell Cancer*

	MINIMAL	MODERATE	ADVANCED
Abdominal	Unresectable and nonpalpable	Palpable (>10 cm) only	Palpable (>10 cm) plus supradiaphragmatic
Pulmonary Number of metastases and size	<5 per lung <2 cm	5–10 per lung largest <3 cm or solitary >2 cm	>10 per lung or multiple >3 cm
Other	Elevated markers Cervical ± abdominal		Mediastinal NSGCT* hepatic, osseous, CNS

*NSGCT: Nonseminomatous germ cell tumor

TABLE 50-2. *Memorial Sloan-Kettering Cancer Center Classification System for Disseminated Germ Cell Tumors*

$$hi = 8.514 - 1.973 \log (LDH + 1)$$
$$- 0.530 \log (hCG + 1) - 1.111 \; TOTMET$$
$$\text{where probability of CR} = e^{hi}/(1 + e^{hi})$$

good-risk patients and 38% of poor-risk patients achieved complete remission.)

DIMINISHING CHEMOTHERAPY TOXICITY IN GOOD-RISK PATIENTS

The ability to accurately assign probable outcome of chemotherapy has allowed for the development of therapeutic approaches with diverse goals. In the favorable group of patients with a predicted cure rate of 90 to 100%, the therapeutic goal has been achieved and subsequent advances will be diminishing the morbidity of chemotherapy. Several recently completed trials emphasize this switch in investigative focus in patients with a high probability of cure.

In a large cooperative group trial of the Southeastern Cancer Study Group and Indiana University, 261 patients were randomly allocated to receive either cisplatin, vinblastine, and bleomycin (PVB), or cisplatin, etoposide, and bleomycin (BEP).[9] Of the 244 patients evaluable for response, 121 received PVB and 74% obtained disease-free status. 123 patients received BEP and 83% achieved disease-free status. In the combined subgroups of patients with minimal and moderate disease, 90% achieved a disease-free status with no difference between treatment arms. Although PVB and BEP gave equally good therapeutic results, there was a significant difference in neuromuscular toxicity with the PVB treated patients experiencing more paresthesias, myalgias, and abdominal cramping. Because BEP had substantially less neuromuscular toxicity with equal or superior therapeutic effect, four courses of BEP became the new standard.

In an effort to further reduce toxicity, Indiana University and the Southeastern Cancer Study Group designed a trial comparing four courses of BEP to three identical courses of the same combination, in patients with minimal or moderate extent disseminated testicular cancer as determined by the Indiana classification system.[10] 184 of these favorable prognosis patients were randomized. 99% of minimal-stage patients and 95% of moderate-stage patients in both arms achieved disease-free status. Relapses were equally divided between the two arms, and over 90% of patients have been continuously disease free. Thus, at Indiana University, the current standard of therapy for patients with minimal or moderate extent disseminated disease is three courses of bleomycin, etoposide, and cisplatin for patients with minimal or moderate extent disseminated disease.

A trial in patients with good-prognosis germ cell tumors, recently conducted at Memorial Sloan-Kettering Cancer Center in New York, produced similar results.[11] 164 patients with good-prognosis germ cell cancer, as determined by the pre-

dicted probability of remission greater than 0.5 in the Memorial predictive model, were randomized to receive either five-drug combination of vinblastine, actinomycin-D, cyclophosphamide, cisplatin, and bleomycin (VAB-6), or the two-drug combination of etoposide plus cisplatin. This group of patients did equally well with either therapy, with approximately 95% obtaining disease-free status. As expected, there was a striking reduction of toxicity, with the two-drug arm showing significantly less myelosuppression, mucositis, nausea and vomiting, and pulmonary fibrosis. All of these studies, aimed at diminishing toxicity, herald the day when patients with good-risk testis cancer can be reliably cured with intense but brief, relatively nontoxic therapy.

TREATMENT FOR POOR-RISK PATIENTS

The one-third of patients disseminated testicular cancer who present with poor prognostic features, and those patients relapsing after initial chemotherapy, remain a therapeutic challenge. The current emphasis in the initial treatment of poor-risk patients is the exploration of platinum-intensive regimens and the use of etoposide in front-line therapy. An initial clue to the importance of etoposide in patients with advanced disease was found in the randomized comparison of BEP versus PVB.[9] Among the 72 patients with advanced disease by the Indiana classification system, 37 were randomized to receive PVB and 35 to receive BEP. There was a significant difference in disease-free survival, with 63% of patients receiving BEP remaining disease-free, compared to only 38% of patients receiving PVB (p = 0.06).

Preclinical models, as well as dose-intensity analysis of clinical trials, suggest a steep dose-response effect for cisplatin. This relationship has been exploited in the development of clinical trials of intensive cisplatin therapy for patients with poor prognostic features. Ozols and colleagues at the National Cancer Institute recently reported the results of a randomized trial of aggressive, high-dose cisplatin therapy versus PVB in poor-risk, testicular cancer patients.[12] In this trial, there was a 2:1 randomization of poor-risk patients to receive the aggressive arm with cisplatin 40 mg/M^2 on days 1 to 5 with vinblastine, bleomycin, and etoposide versus classic PVB with cisplatin 20 mg/M^2 on days 1 to 5 with vinblastine plus bleomycin. Thirty-four patients were randomized to receive the aggressive arm of treatment while 18 were given PVB. Eight-eight percent of the patients receiving the aggressive treatment obtained a complete remission compared to 67% of the patients receiving PVB. The PVB arm had a high incidence of relapse with 41% having disease recurrence compared to 17% of the PVBE treated group. Overall, 68% of the group randomized to the aggressive treatment are alive and disease-free, compared to only 33% of the patients treated with standard therapy. Unfortunately, accompanying this apparent improvement in therapeutic outcome was substantial increase in toxicity. There was a significant increase in myelosuppression and hearing loss in the patients receiving the high-dose cisplatin arm.

It is unclear whether the apparent superiority of the high-dose cisplatin regimen in this trial is due to the twice normal cisplatin dosage, the inclusion of etoposide, or to other factors. Again, the SEG trial of PVB versus BEP had a clear-cut advantage for the etoposide containing arm in patients with poor prognosis disease. Rigid testing of the impact of high-dose cisplatin is ongoing in the current advanced disease trial of Indiana University and the Southwest Oncology Group, which compares etoposide plus bleomycin plus either standard or double-dose cisplatin. Although results are still preliminary, there is no apparent therapeutic advantage to the double-dose cisplatin regimen to date and there is a significant difference in toxicity. Such results suggest that high-dose cisplatin therapies should only be given in the context of a clinical trial.

ADJUVANT THERAPY

The development of curative chemotherapy for metastatic germ cell cancer prompted investigation of similar chemotherapy in patients with a high risk of recurrent disease after retroperitoneal lymph node dissection. Modern chemotherapy principles suggest that the most effective adjuvant therapy would be intense but brief chemotherapy employing drugs known to be effective in metastatic disease. With these principles in mind, the Testicular Cancer Intergroup Study addressed the issue of adjuvant therapy.[13] Following surgery, 195 patients who could be fully evaluated and had completely resected stage-B disease, were randomized to either observation only or to two postoperative courses of cisplatin, vinblastine, and bleomycin, or similar intense cisplatin-based chemotherapy such as VAB-VI (vinblastine, dactinomycin, cyclophosphamide, bleomycin, and cisplatin). In this study, the relapse rate in the observation arm was the expected 48%. However, all but three of these patients were cured with appropriate chemotherapy administered at relapse. Among the patients randomized to receive two courses of postoperative cisplatin-based chemotherapy, one patient died related to recurrent cancer. Thus, the overall survival for the entire study was 96%, and not significantly different in either arm. Conclusions from the study were that two postoperative courses of cisplatin-based chemotherapy nearly always prevent disease recurrence. However, similar good results can be obtained with careful observation of patients after retroperitoneal lymph node dissection and reservation of chemotherapy for those patients who relapse. These results do not support the use of "adjuvant" chemotherapy as a supplement of an inadequate or "debulking" retroperitoneal lymph node dissection. Such patients with residual disease after surgery should be treated as if they have metastatic disease.

The approach to disseminated testicular cancer can be summarized as follows:

1. Patients with favorable prognostic features (Indiana classification—minimal/moderate disease or Memorial Sloan-Kettering classification—good risk) have an excellent expectation of cure with standard therapies. Ide-

ally, such patients should be entered onto protocols designed to investigate diminution of toxicity. We believe adequate standard therapy for such patients is *three* courses of cisplatin (20 mg/m^2 daily $\times$ 5), etoposide (100 mg/m^2 daily $\times$ 5), and bleomycin (30 units weekly $\times$ 9). These courses should be given every 3 weeks with as few dose adjustments and delays as possible.

2. Patients with unfavorable prognostic features (Indiana classification—advanced disease or Memorial Sloan-Kettering classification—poor risk) have an expected cure rate of 50 to 60% or less. In these patients, primary consideration should be enrollment into clinical trials using intense, untruncated treatments. Our current recommendations for such patients would be *four* courses of cisplatin (20 mg/m^2 daily $\times$ 5), etoposide (100 mg/m^2 daily $\times$ 5) and bleomycin (30 units weekly $\times$ 12) given every 3 weeks. Again, every effort should be made to give treatment on time and in full dose.

3. All patients completing chemotherapy for disseminated nonseminomatous germ cell cancer should be restaged. Those patients who obtain a serologic and radiographic complete remission should be followed closely without further treatment. Our current recommendations are that these patients should have monthly chest x-rays and serum AFP and HCG for the first year after diagnosis and every other month for the second year. Thereafter, patients are seen three to four times a year up to 5 years and then once yearly. Those patients obtaining complete serologic remission with residual radiographic abnormalities should be considered for aggressive resection of the residual disease. In those patients in whom necrosis or teratoma are found, no further therapy is indicated. It has been our practice to treat those patients in whom residual viable cancer is completely resected with two additional courses of induction chemotherapy. For those patients who have persistent elevation of markers after completion of four courses of induction therapy, further treatment with induction regimens are not useful and patients should be considered for an immediate switch to a salvage regimen. Aggressive resection for patients who remain with elevated markers is not indicated.

4. The use of adjuvant chemotherapy for those patients with completely resected abdominal disease is *not* mandated by the findings of recent trials. We believe that virtually all patients in this clinical category will be cured. The alternatives are close observation with chest x-ray and markers with chemotherapy for metastatic disease at time of relapse *or* brief but intense adjuvant therapy with cisplatin-based regimens. The excellent results of the recent Intergroup Trial cannot be guaranteed if less intense therapy is used. Likewise, the use of "adjuvant chemotherapy" cannot be endorsed for patients with incomplete resected abdominal disease and such patients should receive therapy for metastatic disease.

SEMINOMA

Until effective cisplatin-combination chemotherapy was developed, treatment of all stages of seminomatous germ cell tumors remained in the domain of the radiotherapists. Recent demonstration of effective chemotherapy for advanced seminoma has changed this approach to patients with disseminated seminoma. In addition, the demonstrated efficacy of combination chemotherapy has resulted in the rethinking of radiotherapy extent and indications in earlier-stage seminoma.

Cure of disseminated seminoma with chemotherapy has been amply demonstrated in several series. Investigators at Memorial Sloan-Kettering, Dana Farber Cancer Institute, Royal Marsden Hospital, and M. D. Anderson, treated patients with advanced or recent seminoma with cisplatin combination chemotherapy and reported long-term, disease-free survivals in 60 to 80% of patients.[14-18] Loehrer and colleagues reported the results of the Southeastern Cancer Study Group protocols.[19] Between 1978 and 1984, 62 patients with advanced seminoma were treated with combination chemotherapy. Patients received cisplatin plus bleomycin with either vinblastine (+/- doxorubicin) or etoposide. Overall, 41 of the evaluable patients (68%) had a favorable response with 37 of the 41 patients remaining alive and continuously free of disease. Univariant and multivariant analysis demonstrated prognostic significance of two factors; extent of disease and extent of prior radiotherapy. Using the Indiana staging system of disseminated germ cell cancer, 87% of patients with minimal disease, 81% with moderate disease, and 52% of patients with advanced disease achieved complete remissions. Patients receiving chest *and* abdominal radiotherapy prior to chemotherapy had a statistically significant diminution in survival.

In the past, patients with stage-II seminoma often received prophylactic, mediastinal irradiation. The emerging role of chemotherapy in seminoma, and the difficulty of using chemotherapy in patients who receive mediastinal radiotherapy in addition to infra-diaphragmatic radiation, has called for the review of the role of prophylactic mediastinal irradiation. For patients with less than bulky, stage-II disease, isolated mediastinal recurrences are rare. A Canadian series showed only eight of 197 patients with stage-IIA disease having an isolated mediastinal recurrence, and only two of these patients dying of seminoma.[20] In bulky, stage-II disease, isolated mediastinal failure is somewhat more common (15 to 20%), but the majority of these failures can be salvaged with further radiotherapy or chemotherapy. Because isolated recurrences within the mediastinum are rare events and prophylactic mediastinal radiotherapy significantly compromises chemotherapy dose and schedule, the treatment policy at Indiana University does not include prophylactic mediastinal irradiation for any stage of seminoma.

The management of bulky, stage-II seminoma remains controversial. Overall, about 40% of patients with bulky, stage-II seminoma will be not cured by radiation. For this reason, some investigators advocate initial chemotherapy for patients with bulky abdominal disease. There are no direct comparisons of these different modes of therapy. Currently, at Indiana University, initial chemotherapy is given for patients with far advanced abdominal disease. Comparable results should be obtained with infradiaphragmatic radiotherapy followed by close observation and cisplatin-based chemotherapy reserved for relapsing patients.

The role of postchemotherapy resection of residual disease in patients with seminoma likewise remains controversial. The experience at Indiana University and elsewhere suggests that surgery rarely produces findings that alter patient care. First, the surgeon often encounters a dense desmoplastic reaction that makes complete resection difficult. Second, these patients are prone to postoperative complications as a consequence of previous chemotherapy, radiation therapy, and age. Finally, the finding of residual viable cancer or unsuspected teratoma is rare (about 10%).

Motzer and colleagues, at Memorial Sloan-Kettering, report a different experience.[21] Forty-one patients with bulky, stage-II or III seminoma were treated with cisplatin-based chemotherapy. Twenty-three patients had residual disease after chemotherapy including 14 with masses larger or equal to 3 cm in diameter. Nineteen of these patients underwent biopsy or surgery and five were found to have abnormalities other than fibrosis (four viable seminoma, one teratoma). All positive surgical findings were in those patients with residual masses larger than or equal to 3 cm. This group recommends biopsy of the area of radiographic abnormalities in those patients with residual disease measuring larger than 3 cm.

In summary, the current approach to clinical staged patients with newly diagnosed seminoma at Indiana University is as follows:

Stage I	—orchiectomy plus infradiaphragmatic radiotherapy without prophylactic mediastinal irradiation
Stage IIA	—orchiectomy plus infradiaphragmatic radiotherapy without prophylactic mediastinal irradiation
Stage IIB (>5 cm nodel mass)	—cisplatin combination chemotherapy or infradiaphragmatic radiotherapy without prophylactic mediastinal irradiation
Stage III	—cisplatin combination chemotherapy

Subsequent to initial treatment, continued vigilance for relapse is required. We currently recommend monthly chest radiographs plus serum AFP, HCG, and LDH for the first year and every other month for the second year. Thereafter, observations can be reduced to several times each year. In those patients with residual radiographic abnormalities after chemotherapy or radiotherapy, close serial observations are required to detect early progression of disease.

CONCLUSION

The last decade has brought in a golden age in the treatment of germinal malignancies of the testis. Refinement of prognostic indicators has allowed for rational selection of treatment for patients with good and poor prognosis. Less toxic treatments with equal efficacy are now available for treatment of patients with a good prognosis. For patients with poor prognosis, the quest for more effective treatment continues. Promising new developments include the introduction of ifosfamide and the cisplatin analogues.

REFERENCES

1. SAMUELS, M. L., JOHNSON, D. E., and HOLOYE, P. Y. Continuous intravenous bleomycin (NSC-15066) therapy with vinblastine (NSC-49842) in stage III testicular neoplasia. Cancer Chemother. Rep., 59:563, 1975.

2. EINHORN, L. H., and DONAHUE, J. P. Cis-diamminedichloroplatinum, vinblastine, and bleomycin combination chemotherapy in disseminated testicular cancer. Ann. Intern. Med., 87:293, 1977.

3. CHENG, F. et al. Germ cell tumor VAB-II in metastatic testicular cancer. Cancer, 42:2162, 1978.

4. EINHORN, L. H., and WILLIAMS, S. D. Chemotherapy of disseminated testicular cancer. Cancer, 46:1333, 1980.

5. EINHORN, L. H., et al. The role of maintenance therapy in disseminated testicular cancer. N. Engl. J. Med., 305:727, 1981.

6. BOSL, G. J., et al. VAB-VI: An effective chemotherapy regimen for patients with germ cell tumors. J. Clin. Oncol., 4:1493, 1984.

7. BIRCH, R. et al. Prognostic factors for favorable outcome in disseminated germ cell tumor. J. Clin. Oncol., 3:400, 1986.

8. BAJORIN, D., et al. Comparison of criteria for assigning germ cell tumor patients to "good risk" and "poor risk" studies. J. Clin. Oncol., 5:786, 1988.

9. WILLIAMS, S. D., et al. Treatment of disseminated germ cell tumors with cisplatin, bleomycin and either vinblastine or etoposide. N. Engl. J. Med., 23:1435, 1987.

10. EINHORN, L. H. et al. A comparison of four courses of cisplatin, VP-16 and bleomycin ($PVB_{16}B$) in favorable prognosis disseminated germ cell tumors: A Southeastern Cancer Study Group (SECSG) Protocol. Proc. Am. Soc. Clin. Oncol., 7:120, 1988.

11. BOSL, G. J. et al. A randomized trial of etoposide plus cisplatin versus vinblastine plus bleomycin plus cisplatin plus cyclophosphamide plus dactinomycin in patients with good prognosis germ cell tumors. J. Clin. Oncol., 8:1231, 1988.

12. OZOLS, R. R. et al. A randomized trial of standard chemotherapy vs. a high-dose chemotherapy regimen in the treatment of poor prognosis non-seminomatous germ cell tumors. J. Clin. Oncol., 6:1031, 1988.

13. WILLIAMS, S. D. et al. Immediate adjuvant chemotherapy versus observation with treatment at relapse in pathological stage II testicular cancer. N. Engl. J. Med., 317:1433, 1987.

14. VUGRIN, D., and WHITMORE, W. The VAB-6 regimen in the treatment of metastatic seminoma. Cancer, 53:2422, 1984.

15. FRIEDMAN, E. L. et al. Therapeutic guidelines and results in advanced seminoma. J. Clin. Oncol., 3:1325, 1985.

16. PECKHAM, M. J., HORWICH, A., and HENDRY, W. F. Advanced seminoma: Treatment with cisplatinum based combination chemotherapy or carboplatin (JM8). Br. J. Cancer, 52:7, 1985.

17. SAMUELS, M. et al. Sequential weekly pulse dose cisplatinum for advanced seminoma. [Abstract]. Proc. Am. Soc. Clin. Oncol., 21:423, 1980.

18. SAMUELS, M. L., and LOGOTHETIS, C. J. Follow-up study of sequential weekly pulse-dose cisplatinum for far advanced seminoma. [Abstract]. Proc. Am. Soc. Clin. Oncol., 2:137, 1983.

19. LOEHRER, P. J. et al. Chemotherapy of metastatic seminoma: The Southeastern Cancer Study Group Experience. J. Clin. Oncol., 8:1212, 1987.

20. HERMAN, J., STURGEON, J., THOMAS, G. M., and the Canadian Testis Group. Mediastinal prophylactic irradiation in seminoma. Proc. Am. Soc. Clin. Oncol., 2:133, 1983.

21. MOTZER, R. et al. Residual mass: An indicator for further therapy in patients with advanced seminoma following systemic chemotherapy. J. Clin. Oncol., 7:1064, 1987.

CHAPTER
51

Chemotherapy and Radiation Therapy for Wilms' Tumor

Marilyn H. Duncan

Major contributions to success in the treatment of this rare childhood cancer have come from the organized study of multidisciplinary cancer treatment, including surgery, radiation therapy, and chemotherapy. Over the past four decades, the discovery of effective treatment for Wilms' tumor has dramatically improved long-term survival rates. The decreasing mortality rate observed among children with all stages of Wilms' tumor appears to have resulted directly from the use of more effective chemotherapy rather than from earlier detection of the disease or a change in incidence.[1-2] The longterm survival rate among children with Wilms' tumor has risen from approximately 30% with surgery alone to greater than 80% with current therapeutic regimens.[3-8,10-12]

The first National Wilms' Tumor Study (NWTS) trials began in 1969.[5] Participation in NWTS protocols is currently the standard management for most children with Wilms' tumor diagnosed in the United States. Sequential prospective randomized clinical trials conducted by the NWTS have addressed important questions regarding epidemiology,[13] histopathology,[14-18] and combined modality treatment including surgery, chemotherapy, and radiation therapy.[5-8,19-25] Infor-

mation gained from the NWTS trials has made significant contributions to the multidisciplinary management of patients with Wilms' tumor. Cooperative trials in Europe have also addressed important aspects of Wilms' tumor management.[10-12]

A major objective of current Wilms' tumor therapy is to refine treatment so that children with good-risk tumors have fewer complications while disease-free survival is improved for those with poor-risk tumors. The successful treatment of Wilms' tumor requires multidisciplinary cooperation among urologic surgeons, pathologists, pediatric oncologists, and radiation therapists. Chemotherapy is routinely given in all stages of Wilms' tumor to supplement surgery and to achieve control of both microresidual and overt metastatic disease.

CLINICAL STAGING AND HISTOLOGIC TYPE (NWTS)

Patients entering NWTS trials have been categorized by clinical stage and histologic type.[5-8] Clinical staging of Wilms' tumor must be accurate at the time of initial diagnosis, as this information is necessary for planning postoperative chemotherapy and radiation therapy. Clinical stage is ascertained by

TABLE 51-1. *National Wilms' Tumor Staging System*[*8]

STAGE I

Tumor is limited to kidney and is completely excised.
The surface of the renal capsule is intact. Tumor was not ruptured before or during removal. There is no residual tumor apparent beyond the margins of resection.

STAGE II

Tumor extends beyond the kidney but is completely excised.
There is regional extension of the tumor, i.e., penetration through the outer surface of the renal capsule into the perirenal soft tissues. Vessels outside the kidney substance are infiltrated or contain tumor thrombus. The tumor may have been biopsied or there has been local spillage of tumor confined to the flank. There is no residual tumor apparent at or beyond the margins of excision.

STAGE III

Residual nonhematogenous tumor confined to abdomen.
Any one or more of the following occur:
  a. Lymph nodes on biopsy are found to be involved in the hilus, the periaortic chains, or beyond
  b. There has been diffuse peritoneal contamination by tumor such as by spillage of tumor beyond the flank before or during surgery, or by tumor growth that has penetrated through the peritoneal surface
  c. Implants are found on the peritoneal surfaces
  d. The tumor extends beyond the surgical margins either microscopically or grossly
  e. The tumor is not completely resectable because of local infiltration into vital structures

STAGE IV

Hematogenous metastases.
Deposits beyond Stage III, e.g., lung, liver, bone, and brain.

STAGE V

Bilateral renal involvement at diagnosis.
An attempt should be made to stage each side according to the above criteria on the basis of extent of disease prior to biopsy.

*The clinicopathologic stage is determined by the surgeon and the pathologist who also determines whether the histologic features are favorable or unfavorable

the surgeon in the operating room and by the pathologist, who further establishes whether histology is favorable (FH) or unfavorable (UH). Wilms' tumor types with unfavorable histology, currently treated on NWTS protocols, include those with focal or diffuse anaplasia and sarcomatous features.[14,17,18] The NWTS clinicopathologic staging system is summarized in Table 51-1.[8]

HISTOPATHOLOGIC CONSIDERATIONS AND PROGNOSIS

The histologic classification system derived from analysis of NWTS data has good correlation with the clinical out-

come.[14,20,22,23] In NWTS-1, 11% of children had renal tumors with "unfavorable" histologic features. These children suffered a much higher tumor-related mortality rate than the other children with "favorable" histologic characteristics (57% vs. 7%).[14] Other pathologic findings that correlated with the increased risk of local and/or distant relapse included the following: large tumor mass, capsule penetration, direct extension to adjacent organs, and involvement of regional lymph nodes.[20] On the basis of these findings, staging and treatment protocols for subsequent NWTS protocols have been modified to intensify therapy for high-risk histologic types, regardless of stage, and to reduce therapy for patients with localized disease and favorable histologic types.[4,6–9,22,23]

SINGLE-AGENT CHEMOTHERAPY

Current therapy for children with Wilms' tumor includes radical nephrectomy, followed by combination chemotherapy with or without postoperative radiation therapy.[8,9,11,12] Three drugs have proven activity against Wilms' tumor: actinomycin D, vincristine, and Adriamycin. The development of effective chemotherapeutic regimens utilizing these drugs has led to dramatic improvement in the overall survival rate from Wilms' tumor.[4–8,10–12,26]

A number of other chemotherapy agents have activity against Wilms' tumor and are being tested in the treatment of children with high-risk or recurrent tumors.

Actinomycin D (dactinomycin)

In the late 1950's, Farber and colleagues reported that the antibiotic actinomycin D showed clinical activity against Wilms' tumor. Dramatic tumor regressions were observed in children with advanced metastatic disease. A prospective trial demonstrated improved survival in patients with Wilms' tumor who received nephrectomy followed by postoperative chemotherapy with actinomycin D and radiation therapy. Pulmonary metastases were also curable by chemotherapy and radiation.[27] Following confirmation of these results by other investigators,[28] cooperative group studies utilizing standardized protocols were organized to systematically answer questions regarding therapy.[29–31]

Leukemia Study Group B found that, following surgery and radiation therapy, children who also received chemotherapy with actinomycin D developed fewer metastases and had improved survival compared to children who received no chemotherapy.[29] The Children's Cancer Study Group A observed that children who received maintenance chemotherapy with single-agent actinomycin D had significantly fewer recurrences than those who were given only a single postoperative course of chemotherapy.[30,31]

Vincristine

Vincristine was identified as an active antitumor agent for the treatment of Wilms' tumor in the early 1960s.[32,33] When used as adjuvant chemotherapy following surgery and postoperative radiation therapy, vincristine gave survival rates comparable to those reported for actinomycin D.[33] Southwest Oncology Group investigators found that vincristine combined with radiation therapy was an effective treatment for metastatic disease in patients unresponsive to actinomycin D.[34]

Adriamycin (doxorubicin)

The anthracycline antibiotic Adriamycin is active against Wilms' tumor. Early clinical trials of Adriamycin demonstrated regression of metastatic disease in advanced, refractory Wilms' tumor.[35,36] The potential for cardiac toxicity in patients receiving Adriamycin has required that it be used cautiously in the management of children with Wilms' tumor. The NWTS-2 found that surgery and radiation therapy combined with three-agent chemotherapy (Adriamycin, actinomycin and vincristine) was better than two-agent chemotherapy (actinomycin D and vincristine) for patients with stages II, III and IV (FH) tumors.[6]

In NWTS-3, the survival for stage-III (FH) patients was best when three-agent chemotherapy with Adriamycin, actinomycin D, and vincristine was combined with low-dose radiotherapy.[8]

Other Drugs

Cyclophosphamide has some activity against Wilms' tumor in patients with metastatic disease.[37,38] Because cyclophosphamide was useful in the treatment of soft tissue sarcomas, the NWTS-3 trial added the drug to the combination chemotherapy regimen for patients with unfavorable histology tumors. In that study, patients with stages II through IV anaplastic tumors seemed to have better survival with four-drug combination chemotherapy including cyclophosphamide, Adriamycin, actinomycin D, and vincristine.[8]

Ifosfamide, a new alkylating agent, is a chemical analog of cyclophosphamide. Recent phase-II studies of high-dose ifosfamide with mesna bladder protection and hyperhydration have demonstrated promising antitumor activity and acceptable toxicity in patients with advanced and recurrent Wilms' tumor.[39] Cisplatin and etoposide (VP-16-213), used in combination, have shown good activity against high-risk Wilms' tumors.[40]

COMBINATION CHEMOTHERAPY

The use of effective combination chemotherapy has made a major impact on the relapse-free survival rates of children with Wilms' tumor. NWTS-1, completed in 1974 (Table 51-2), showed that combination chemotherapy with actinomycin D and vincristine was superior to the use of either agent alone in children with locally advanced tumors (stages II and III).[5]

NWTS-2, finished in 1979, (see Table 51-2) demonstrated that double-agent chemotherapy (vincristine and actinomycin D) improved the relapse-free survival for stage-I patients by

reducing the frequency of flank and distant recurrences. Furthermore, the length of treatment could be reduced from 15 months to 6 months without worsening the excellent (above 90%) survival. Triple-agent chemotherapy (Adriamycin, vincristine, and actinomycin D) was superior to double-agent chemotherapy (actinomycin D and vincristine) in Stage-II, III, and IV FH patients.[6,7]

The British Medical Research Council trial reported that maintenance chemotherapy with intensive vincristine was better than single-agent intermittent actinomycin D.[41]

The NWTS-3, completed in 1985, (see Table 51-2) found that survival (above 90%) for stage-I FH patients was similar whether double-agent chemotherapy (vincristine and actinomycin D) was given for 6 months or 10 weeks. Patients with stage-II FH tumors had excellent (about 90%) survival with double-agent chemotherapy (vincristine and actinomycin D) given for 15 months without radiation therapy. The addition of a third drug (Adriamycin) or radiation therapy (2000 cGy) made no difference in outcome. In stage-III FH patients, three-agent chemotherapy (vincristine, actinomycin D, and Adriamycin) with either 1000 cGy or 2000 cGy radiation therapy, gave slightly better relapse-free survival (84%) than double-agent chemotherapy (74%). For all high-risk patients (stage-IV FH or all stages UH), the addition of cyclophosphamide to standard three-agent chemotherapy (vincristine, actinomycin D, and Adriamycin) did not improve the survival rate. Only patients with stages II through IV anaplastic tumors did better (4-year survival, 82% versus 37%) on the four-agent regimen (cyclophosphamide, Adriamycin, vincristine, and actinomycin D). The subset of UH patients with stage-I anaplastic and clear cell sarcoma tumors did well (4-year survival of 89% and 75% respectively) with three-agent chemotherapy (Adriamycin, vincristine, and actinomycin D) and radiation therapy.[8]

NATIONAL WILMS' TUMOR STUDY-4

The NWTS-4, a randomized, prospective clinical trial started in 1985, is in progress and has the following objectives: (1) to simplify, shorten, and refine treatment methods for all children, (2) to test treatment hypotheses relating to chemotherapy dose intensity, schedule, and duration of treatment, (3) to collect epidemiologic data, (4) to correlate outcome with clinicopathologic stage and histologic type, and (5) to evaluate long-term effects of treatment.[9]

Patients are randomized both by stage and by whether the histology is "favorable" or "high risk" (anaplastic or clear cell sarcoma of kidney). Patients with stage-I FH and anaplastic tumors receive postoperative double-agent chemotherapy (actinomycin D and vincristine) for either 18 or 24 weeks without radiation therapy. In stage-II FH tumors, postoperative double-agent chemotherapy (actinomycin D and vincristine) is given for a short course (18 or 22 weeks) or a longer course (60 or 65 weeks) without radiation therapy. Stages III and IV FH, and stages I through IV clear cell sarcoma of kidney receive postoperative triple-agent chemotherapy (actinomycin D, vincristine, and Adriamycin) given for a short (26 weeks)

TABLE 51.2 *Survival Rates, National Wilms' Tumor Studies I-III*

GROUP/STAGE	THERAPY	SURVIVAL RATE AT 4 YEARS (%)	
		RELAPSE FREE	ALIVE
NWTS-1			
I (<2 years)	AMD × 15 months, RT	89	94
	AMD × 15 months, no RT	88	90
I (≥2 years)	AMD × 15 months, RT	76	98
	AMD × 15 months, no RT	57	81
II/III	AMD, RT	56	71
	VCR, RT	57	71
	AMD + VCR, RT	79	84
NWTS-2			
I	AMD + VCR × 6 months, no RT	96	97
	AMD + VCR × 15 months, no RT	90	91
II/III/IV	AMD + VCR × 15 months, RT	65	74
	AMD + VCR + ADR × 15 months, RT	79	84
NWTS-3+			
I FH	AMD + VCR × 10 weeks vs. 6 months, no RT	90	97
II FH	AMD + VCR ± ADR × 15 months, ± RT (2000 cGy)	88	92
III FH	AMD + VCR ± ADR × 15 months, RT (1000 vs. 2000 cGy)	79	87
IV FH	AMD + VCR + ADR × 15 months, vs. AMD + VCR + ADR + CPM × 15 months, RT*	75	83
I/II/III/UH	SAME	65	68
IV UH	SAME	56	55
All Patients		83	89

RT = radiation therapy; AMD = actinomycin D; VCR = vincristine; ADR = Adriamycin; CPM = cyclophosphamide; FH = favorable histology; UH = unfavorable histology; cGy = centiGray = 1 rad

All patients received nephrectomy and cyclic chemotherapy
*All stage IV FH patients received 2000 cGy flank RT and RT to other sites
UH patients of all stages received age-adjusted flank RT and RT to other sites
+Chemotherapy Dosage:

AMD = 15 mcg/kg/d × 5d (iv)   VCR = 1.5 mg/M^2/week (iv)
ADR = 20 mg/M^2/d × 3d (iv)   CPM = 10 mg/kg/d × 3d (iv)

or longer (65 weeks) course plus radiation therapy. Stages II through IV anaplastic tumors receive postoperative three- or four-agent chemotherapy (actinomycin D, vincristine, Adriamycin ± cyclophosphamide) for 65 weeks plus radiotherapy. The treatment regimens are also comparing the effectiveness and toxicity of a standard chemotherapy dose and schedule with a new "pulsed intensive" schedule (single day therapy given more frequently).[9]

SPECIAL MANAGEMENT PROBLEMS

Bilateral Wilms' Tumors

The prognosis for children with bilateral Wilms' tumors entered on the National Wilms' tumor studies has been good.

These children have had nearly 80% 3-year survival when managed on various treatment regimens including surgery, chemotherapy, and radiation therapy.[42,43] Treatment should be individualized to preserve as much renal parenchyma and function as possible while obtaining tumor control. Recommendations for the management of bilateral tumors on NWTS-4 include the following: (1) initial surgical exploration and complete excision when possible, bilateral biopsies and staging, and postoperative two-agent chemotherapy (vincristine and actinomycin D) given for approximately 15 weeks, (2) second-look operation and complete tumor excision when possible or biopsies of remaining tumor followed by postoperative chemotherapy for 65 weeks, (3) if persistent tumor is identified at the second-look operation, postoperative radiation therapy and more intensive three-agent chemotherapy (vincristine, actinomycin D, and Adriamycin) are given, (4) additional surgical procedures may be undertaken if there is evidence of persistent tumor and permitted by the clinical condition of the patient.[9]

Inoperable Tumors

Experience in NWTS trials and European studies have shown that preoperative chemotherapy and/or radiotherapy can often reduce tumor bulk and the risk of tumor rupture during nephrectomy.[5,6,8,10,11,44,45]

Overall survival rates have not been influenced significantly by preoperative therapy and accurate surgical staging information may be lost.[45] For these reasons, the current NWTS-4 recommendations for the management of inoperable tumors are as follows: (1) initial double-agent chemotherapy (vincristine and actinomycin D) given for about 4 weeks while observing for tumor shrinkage, (2) if there is no reduction in tumor size, radiation therapy is begun along with single-agent (vincristine) chemotherapy, (3) when adequate shrinkage has occurred, surgery should be performed. The NWTS studies assume that all patients receiving pre-operative chemotherapy are stage III. All children receiving preoperative chemotherapy are given postoperative radiation therapy and chemotherapy.[9]

The International Society of Paediatric Oncology studies have not routinely given radiation therapy if the tumor is confined to the kidney.[10,11,44]

Radiation Therapy

In the past, postoperative radiotherapy was given routinely to all children with Wilms' tumor, but its role in management has gradually been refined.

The results of the first three NWTS trials are summarized as follows: (1) routine, postoperative radiation therapy of the flank is not necessary for children with stage-I FH or anaplastic tumors, nor for stage-II FH tumors when postoperative double-agent chemotherapy with vincristine and actinomycin D is administered, (2) the prognosis for stage-III FH patients is best when three-drug chemotherapy with actinomycin D, vincristine, and Adriamycin is combined with low dose (1000 cGy) radiation therapy to the flank.[5,6,8]

Toxicity

In general, the therapeutic regimens currently used in the treatment of Wilms' tumor are well tolerated. The most significant toxicities have been noted in children receiving both chemotherapy and radiation therapy and include myelosuppression, hepatic toxicity, and enhanced radiation reaction from actinomycin D and Adriamycin.[19,24,25,46] The incidence of lethal treatment-related toxicity has been approximately 1 to 2% in the first three of NWTS trials.[5,8,21] Infants under 12 months of age are sensitive to chemotherapy and related toxicity. Chemotherapy dose reduction (50%) has significantly reduced the toxicity experienced by babies without loss of therapeutic efficacy.[24]

Radiation sequelae have resulted in cosmetic deformities and increased disease morbidity.[19,25] The potential for the development of radiation-associated second malignancies is being evaluated in long-term, follow-up studies of NWTS patients.

The current management of children with suspected or confirmed Wilms' tumor is complex. Once diagnosed, these patients should be treated by a multidisciplinary team of trained oncologists familiar with all aspects of surgery, radiation, and chemotherapy.

REFERENCES

1. EVERSON, R. B., and FRAUMENI, J. F., JR. Declining mortality and improving survival from Wilms' tumor. Med. Pediatr. Oncol., 1:3, 1975.
2. YOUNG, J. L., JR., et al. Cancer incidence, survival, and mortality for children younger than age 15 years. Cancer, 58:598, 1986.
3. LADD, W. E., and WHITE, R. R. Embryoma of the kidney (Wilms' tumor). JAMA, 117:1858, 1941.
4. D'ANGIO, G. J., et al. Wilms' tumor: An update. Cancer, 45:1791, 1980.
5. D'ANGIO, G. J., et al. The treatment of Wilms' tumor-results of the National Wilms' Tumor Study. Cancer, 38:633, 1976.
6. D'ANGIO, G. J., et al. The treatment of Wilms' tumor: Results of the Second National Wilms' Tumor Study. Cancer, 47:2302, 1981.
7. D'ANGIO, G. J. Wilms' tumor. Curr. Concepts Oncol., 4:3, 1982.
8. D'ANGIO, G. J., et al. The treatment of Wilms' tumor: Results of the Third National Wilms' Tumor Study. Cancer, 64:349, 1989.
9. D'ANGIO, G. J., (Chairman, National Wilms' Tumor Study Committee). Personal communication, 1989.
10. LEMERLE, J., et al. Effectiveness of preoperative chemotherapy in Wilms' tumor: Results of an International Society of Paediatric

Oncology (SIOP) clinical trial. J. Clin. Oncol., 1:604, 1983.
11. BURGER, D., et al. The advantages of preoperative therapy in Wilms' tumour. A summarized report on clinical trials conducted by the International Society of Paediatric Oncology (SIOP). Z. Kinderchir., 40:170, 1985.
12. PRITCHARD, J., et al. Preliminary results of the First United Kingdom Children's Cancer Study Group Wilms' Study [Abstract]. Proc. Annu. Meet. Am. Soc. Clin. Oncol., 6:A862, 1987.
13. BRESLOW, N. E., and BECKWITH, J. B. Epidemiological features of Wilms' tumor: Results of the National Wilms' Tumor Study. J. Natl. Cancer Inst., 68:429, 1982.
14. BECKWITH, J. B., and PALMER, N. F. Histopathology and prognosis of Wilms' tumor—results from the First National Wilms' Tumor Study. Cancer, 41:1937, 1978.
15. HAAS, J. E., et al. Ultrastructure of malignant rhabdoid tumor of the kidney. Hum. Pathol., 12:646, 1981.
16. BECKWITH, J. B. Wilms' tumor and other renal tumors of childhood: A selective review from the National Wilms' Tumor Study Pathology Center. Hum. Pathol., 14:481, 1983.
17. HAAS, J. E., BONADIO, J. F., and BECKWITH, J. B. Clear cell sarcoma of

the kidney with emphasis on ultrastructural studies. Cancer, 54:2978, 1984.

18. BONADIO, J. F., et al. Anaplastic Wilms' tumor: Clinical and pathologic studies. J. Clin. Oncol., 3:513, 1985.

19. TEFFT, M. Radiation related toxicities in National Wilms' Tumor Study Number 1. Int. J. Radiat. Oncol. Biol. Phys., 2:455, 1977.

20. BRESLOW, N. E., et al. Wilms' tumor: Prognostic factors for patients without metastases at diagnosis—results of the National Wilms' Tumor Study. Cancer, 41:1577, 1978.

21. JONES, B., BRESLOW, N. E., and TAKASHIMA, J. Toxic deaths in the Second National Wilms' Tumor Study. J. Clin. Oncol., 2:1028, 1984.

22. BRESLOW, N., et al. Prognosis for Wilms' tumor patients with non-metastatic disease at diagnosis—results of the Second National Wilms' Tumor Study. J. Clin. Oncol., 3:521, 1985.

23. BRESLOW, N. E., et al. Clinicopathologic features and prognosis for Wilms' tumor patients with metastases at diagnosis. Cancer, 58:2501, 1986.

24. MORGAN, E., et al. Chemotherapy-related toxicity in infants treated according to the Second National Wilms' Tumor Study. J. Clin. Oncol., 6:51, 1988.

25. THOMAS, P. R. M., et al. Acute toxicities associated with radiation in the Second National Wilms' Tumor Study. J. Clin. Oncol., 6:1694, 1988.

26. GREEN, D. M., and JAFFE, N. Wilms' tumor-model of a curable pediatric malignant solid tumor. Cancer Treat. Rev., 5:143, 1978.

27. FARBER, S. Chemotherapy in the treatment of leukemia and Wilms' tumor. JAMA, 198:826, 1966.

28. FERNBACH, D. J., and MARTYN, D. T. Role of dactinomycin in the improved survival of children with Wilms' tumor. JAMA, 195:1005, 1966.

29. BURGERT, E. O., JR., and GLIDEWELL, O. Dactinomycin in Wilms' tumor. JAMA, 199:464, 1967.

30. WOLFF, J. A., et al. Single versus multiple dose dactinomycin therapy of Wilms's tumor. N. Engl. J. Med., 279:290, 1968.

31. WOLFF, J. A., et al. Long-term evaluation of single versus multiple courses of actinomycin D therapy of Wilms' tumor. N. Engl. J. Med., 290:84, 1974.

32. SUTOW, W. W., THURMAN, W. G., and WINDMILLER, J. Vincristine (leurocristine) sulfate in the treatment of children with metastatic Wilms' tumor. Pediatrics, 32:880, 1963.

33. SULLIVAN, M. P. Vincristine (NSC-67574) therapy for Wilms' tumor. Cancer Chemother. Rep., 52:481, 1968.

34. VIETTI, T. J., et al. Vincristine sulfate and radiation therapy in metastatic Wilms' tumor. Cancer, 25:12, 1970.

35. TAN, C., et al. Adriamycin-An antitumor antibiotic in the treatment of neoplastic diseases. Cancer, 32:9, 1973.

36. PRATT, C. B., and SHANKS, E. C. Doxorubicin in treatment of malignant solid tumors in children. Am. J. Dis. Child., 127:534, 1974.

37. HADDY, T. B., et al. Clinical trials with cyclophosphamide (Cytoxan) in children with Wilms' tumor—Preliminary report. Cancer Chemother. Rep., 25:81, 1962.

38. SUTOW, W. W. Cyclophosphamide (NSC-26271) in Wilms' tumor and rhabdomyosarcoma. Cancer Chemother. Rep., 51:407, 1967.

39. TOURNADE, M. F., et al. Ifosfamide is an active drug in Wilms' tumor: A phase II study conducted by the French Society of Pediatric Oncology. J. Clin. Oncol., 6:793, 1988.

40. DOUGLASS, E. C., et al. Cis-platinum/VP-16 initial therapy in high risk Wilms' tumor [Abstract]. Proc. Annu. Meet. Am. Assoc. Cancer Res., 28:221, 1987.

41. MORRIS-JONES, P. H., PEARSON, D., and JOHNSON, A. L. Medical Research Council's Working Party on Embryonal Tumors in Childhood: Management of nephroblastoma in childhood. Arch. Dis. Child., 53:112, 1978.

42. BISHOP, H. C., et al. Survival in bilateral Wilms' tumor—review of 30 National Wilms' Tumor Study cases. J. Pediatr. Surg., 12:631, 1977.

43. BLUTE, M. L., et al. Bilateral Wilms' tumor. J. Urol., 138:968, 1987.

44. VOUTE, P. A., et al. Preoperative chemotherapy as first treatment in children with Wilms' tumor. Results of the SIOP nephroblastoma trials and studies [Abstract]. Proc. Annu. Meet. Am. Soc. Clin. Oncol., 6:A880, 1987.

45. D'ANGIO, G. J., SIOP and the management of Wilms' tumor [Editorial]. J. Clin. Oncol., 1:595, 1987.

46. GREEN, D. M., et al. Severe hepatic toxicity after treatment with single-dose dactinomycin and vincristine. Cancer, 62:270, 1988.

SECTION XI

RADIATION THERAPY

CHAPTER
52

Introduction to Radiation Therapy in the Management of Genitourinary Cancer

Jeffrey D. Forman
Allen S. Lichter

Radiation therapy is a local-regional treatment modality. Successful treatment is defined as local-regional tumor control with few complications. This is the therapeutic ratio of definitive radiation, which refers to the ability to deliver tumoricidal doses of radiation to a neoplasm without exceeding the tolerance of the surrounding normal tissues. Thus, a broad knowledge of the natural history of the disease, radiobiology, and physics is essential to the successful management of genitourinary malignancies.

THE NATURAL HISTORY OF GENITOURINARY CANCER

The natural history of genitourinary cancer may be defined as the clinical and pathologic manifestations of the disease in the untreated host. It provides the basis for selection of treatment and a framework on which to assess the success or failure of treatment. Unfortunately, for most urologic malignancies, this natural history is incompletely defined.

Achieving local-regional control of the primary tumor is a necessary step toward curing the patient. Decisions regarding the choice of therapy (local, regional, or systemic) are made difficult by the propensity for urologic malignancies to disseminate through lymphatic or hematogenous pathways. Understanding the natural history of these diseases will allow appropriate treatment, that is, treatment that will permit the patient a qualitatively and quantitatively normal life.

RADIOBIOLOGY OF GENITOURINARY MALIGNANCIES

Familiarity with the biologic principles of radiotherapy provides a better appreciation of the strengths and weaknesses of various techniques and a rational approach to new techniques. However, achieving a favorable therapeutic ratio can be viewed simply as avoiding under-irradiation of the tumor and over-irradiation of the normal tissues.

The primary reason for failure to control a tumor is a relative underdosage: there are probably no absolutely radio-resistant tumors. However, because of limitations on total dose and because of normal tissue tolerance, relative underdosage may occur. Tumor-related factors such as hypoxia, regeneration during treatments, and radio-resistance that may contribute to local failure, have been addressed by varying fractionation, daily dosage, and a variety of experimental techniques.

Modern radiobiology has clarified the mechanisms that explain the preferential effect of radiation on a tumor. Protraction of treatment has circumvented the problem of hypoxic cells by allowing the hypoxic cells to become fully sensitive, a process called reoxygenation. Normal cells have a greater ability to repair and repopulate after radiation damage than do tumors. The result is that the processes of repair, reoxygenation, and repopulation create a favorable therapeutic ratio for normal tissue.

RADIATION PHYSICS AND TREATMENT PLANNING

Careful treatment planning can ensure delivery of a homogeneous dose of radiation to the target volume. However, the extreme importance of encompassing all the tumor in the treatment volume is evidenced by the fact that if even a 1 mm^3 volume is not irradiated in a 4 to 5 cm tumor, the whole treatment has been wasted because the tumor will recur. A number of techniques have been utilized to improve the therapeutic ratio through physical means (improvement of radiation depositions, the use of highly ionizing irradiation, and hyperthermia), chemical forms of protecting normal tissues (WR.2721), and sensitizing tumors (misonidazole). Advances continue to be made.

Therefore, the use of radiation therapy in the management of urologic malignancies is based on a thorough understanding of the natural history of the disease, radiobiology, and physics. This ensures that local-regional treatment will be applied to the patients who will benefit most. The principles of radiobiology and physics can be exploited to improve the therapeutic ratio between local control and complications, which will then lead to the most favorable outcome.

CHAPTER
53

Radiation Therapy of Urinary Bladder Cancer

Kenneth J. Russell

Major changes in the management of both invasive and noninvasive bladder cancer are occurring as new treatment modalities and new sequencing of established modalities yield promising results. Although radiation therapy is an established treatment for bladder cancer, its role as a primary treatment is also undergoing a period of reassessment. With the advent of effective intravesical immunotherapy and chemotherapy for noninvasive tumors, improved surgical techniques for cystectomy, and aggressive adjuvant and neoadjuvant chemotherapy regimens, it would seem that the indications for radiotherapy are changing. However, despite progress in these areas, significant problems persist in the treatment of bladder cancer for which radiotherapy remains an indispensable part of the therapeutic armamentarium. Issues that will be addressed in the following review include

1. Patients with noninvasive cancers continue to recur after intravesical chemotherapy or immunotherapy. Radiotherapy can be curative for these patients and is an attractive alternative to cystectomy.
2. Continent urinary pouches or neobladders, while constituting major surgical advances in the management of

invasive cancers, are not wholly satisfactory substitutes for the removed bladder. Radiotherapy delivered with high-energy megavoltage equipment and modern techniques to appropriately selected patients remains a well-tolerated treatment that preserves normal bladder function in the majority of cured patients.
3. Although contemporary surgical techniques are associated with a low incidence of pelvic tumor recurrence, there remains a considerable body of clinical experience to suggest that combined preoperative radiation and surgery yields superior survival results to those obtainable with either modality alone.
4. At a time when treatments of widely different morbidity are available for the management of invasive bladder cancer, the response of bladder tumors to radiotherapy remains the best established predictor of patient prognosis for an individual patient. The capability to predict an individual patient's prognosis on the basis of tumor radioresponsiveness allows selection of a treatment or combination of treatments appropriate for that individual's tumor. This is a major consideration, given the lifestyle adjustments required by urinary diversion, the substantial toxicity of current combination chemotherapy,

and the frail medical condition of many elderly patients with bladder cancer.

RADIOTHERAPY OF NONINVASIVE TUMORS

Primary management of noninvasive transitional cell carcinomas of the urinary bladder involves transurethral resection of the tumor(s) followed by a course of intravesical chemotherapy employing one of a number of active agents, of which thiotepa, mitomycin C, doxorubicin, and bacillus Calmette-Guérin (BCG) are among the most widely used drugs. This approach can be expected to delay or prevent recurrence of bladder tumors in 60 to 81% of cases.[1-5] The acute side effects of intravesical treatment include myelosupression with thiotepa; chemical cystitis with doxorubicin; skin eruptions with mitomycin C; and cystitis, malaise, and fever with BCG. These side effects are largely self-limited to the time of treatment, and are overall quite acceptable. For those patients who prove refractory to such an approach and who recur with an increasing number of tumors or progressively anaplastic lesions, cystectomy is often indicated.

EXTERNAL BEAM

External beam radiation therapy has been employed in the treatment of noninvasive bladder cancer. The number of patients treated in most series has been few, and representative data are summarized in Table 53-1. The doses required to treat such tumors are in the same 6,500 to 7,000 cGy range required for the treatment of invading bladder tumors and achieve a durable complete response rate of 47 to 57%.[6-9] In by far the largest experience, reported by Quilty and Duncan, 48% of 190 patients attained a complete tumor response. Grade-3 tumors had a 55% tumor control rate at 5 years compared with 29% for grade-2 tumors and 16% for grade-1 tumors (p < .01). Patients with solid tumors appeared to fare better than patients whose tumors had a papillary morphology.[7,10] Although the survival results are as good or better than those achieved with other techniques, the 5-year recurrence-free rate was only 27.7%. At the present time, there is limited active clinical investigation using external beam irradiation by itself as the primary treatment of these tumors, as recent interest has focused on more localized techniques of radiation, as described below.

TABLE 53-1. *External Beam Radiotherapy for Nonmuscle-Invading Bladder Cancer T1(A)*

AUTHORS	NUMBER OF PATIENTS	5-YEAR SURVIVAL RATE (%)
Quilty and Duncan[10]	190	61
Goffinet et al.[30]	33	35
Finney[75]	29	24
Fish and Fayos[76]	16	51

INTRAVESICAL RADIOTHERAPY

The superficial nature of noninvasive bladder tumors has encouraged the use of radiation modalities with a limited range of penetration. Intracavitary or interstitial radiation are two such approaches, because a high dose can be delivered over a short period of time to bladder epithelium with a rapid attenuation of this dose in the uninvolved muscle layers and extravesical tissues. Such a relative localization of radiation allows the delivery of higher doses to the tumor resulting in more reliable eradication of tumor without concurrent increased complications for normal tissues.

Techniques for delivering such localized radiation are not new and a variety of methods have been developed for achieving optimal dose distributions. These include interstitial implants employing radioactive sources inserted via open cystotomy or transcystoscopically, intracavitary placement of a centrally located radiation source into the bladder via a transurethral catheter, and instillation of intravesical colloidal solutions of radioisotopes.

INTERSTITIAL IMPLANTS

Interstitial bladder irradiation was popularized by Williams, Trott, and Bloom at the Royal Marsden Hospital in England and Van der Werf-Messing and coworkers at the Rotterdam Radiotherapy Institute in The Netherlands. Patients with both noninvasive and invasive tumors have been treated, with tumor stages ranging from T1 to T3.

The Royal Marsden group employed gold-198 grains or tantalum-182 wires and ideally treated patients with solitary tumors less than 4 cm in size, with minimal undifferentiation, and with limited invasion. The treatment results for their 147 patients are presented in Table 53-2, where 5- and 10-year actuarial survival is correlated with both clinical tumor stage for the 147 patients and with pathologic tumor stage and tumor grade for the 123 patients for whom accurate assessment of histologic invasion and differentiation were possible. The presence of coexisting carcinoma in situ had no adverse

TABLE 53-2. *Royal Marsden Hospital Experience with Interstitial Irradiation for Carcinoma of the Bladder[11]*

	STAGE	NUMBER OF PATIENTS	5-YEAR SURVIVAL RATE (%)	10-YEAR SURVIVAL RATE (%)
Clinical	T1	47	69	40
	T2	76	41	21
	T3	24	21	11
Pathologic	Ta	34	73	45
	T1	39	57	29
	T2	50	33	15
Grade	G1	24	78	50
(T1 and T2 only)	G2	52	53	25
	G3	47	37	20

impact on the treatment results, and the rate of salvage cystectomy for the entire patient cohort was 7%. Complications of treatment included a 8.2% risk of suprapubic urinary leak and a 25% risk of ureteric reflux. For those patients who developed vesicoureteric reflux, less than 10% progressed to chronic, upper urinary tract infections.[11]

The Rotterdam Institute group selected patients with tumors smaller than 5 cm in size who underwent transurethral resection of the primary tumor. The implant procedure was carried out through a suprapubic cystotomy, with radium needles placed in parallel arrays through the area of the tumor. Depending on the tumor stage, the dose from the implants was supplemented with either preimplant or postimplant external beam irradiation. Patients with T1 lesions were treated with implants alone or preceded by 1,050 cGy external beam pelvic irradiation (350 cGy × 3 fractions) to reduce the risk of tumor implants in the cystotomy wound.[12] In recent years, patients with more advanced T2 to T3 lesions have received additional postimplant external beam pelvic irradiation to a total dose of 3,000 to 4,000 cGy, with the dose delivered by the implant reduced accordingly.[13,14]

The patients treated with T1 lesions were involved in a nonrandomized prospective study comparing primary treatment with transurethral tumor resection (TUR) to treatment combining TUR and radium implant. The results summarizing relapse-free survival and metastasis-free survival for the two groups of patients are summarized in Table 53-3 along with corresponding data about tumor morphology, differentiation, and relapse-free survival.

The results of treatment for patients with T2 and T3 tumors treated without postoperative external beam irradiation are summarized in Table 53-4, which includes clinical parameters that proved statistically significant in predicting a successful treatment outcome for each stage of tumor. Treatment complications for the patients with T2 to T3 tumors included a 16% incidence of asymptomatic necrosis at the implant site, a 7% incidence of bladder stone formation, and a 1% incidence of symptomatic necrosis or chronic radiation cystitis.[15]

TABLE 53-4. *Rotterdam Radiotherapy Institute Experience with Interstitial Implants for Muscle-Invading Bladder Cancer (T2, T3)*[15]

	NUMBER OF PATIENTS	10-YEAR SURVIVAL RATES (%)*
T2	328	69
Papillary	173	75 ⎱ †
Nonpapillary	149	62 ⎰
Well or moderately differentiated	194	75 ⎱ †
Poorly differentiated	133	60 ⎰
IVP normal	297	70 ⎱ †
IVP abnormal	20	34 ⎰
T3	63	59 ⎱
Papillary	19	86 ⎱ †
Nonpapillary	44	49 ⎰

*p < 0.05
†p < .05.

Whereas interstitial radium needle implants have proved to be highly efficacious in the management of selected patients with *solitary* tumors, this approach is not suitable for patients with multiple tumors scattered throughout the bladder. For these clinical situations, a homogeneous dose is required for the entire mucosal surface of the bladder. This has been achieved by intracavitary placement of centrally located radioactive sources or by instillation of colloidal solutions of radioisotope.

INTRACAVITARY IMPLANTS

Intracavitary irradiation of bladder cancer was first described by Friedman and Lewis in 1949. The technique involved the use of either radium or cobalt-60 sources inserted individually or in tandem into the tip of a catheter, which was subsequently inserted transurethrally into the bladder. Central positioning of the source(s) was confirmed both by radiographic

TABLE 53-3. *Rotterdam Radiotherapy Institute Experience with T1 Bladder Cancer Treated with TUR or TUR and Radium Implant*[77]

	TUR ALONE		TUR AND IMPLANT	
	NUMBER OF PATIENTS	5-YEAR BLADDER RELAPSE-FREE (%)	NUMBER OF PATIENTS	5-YEAR BLADDER RELAPSE-FREE (%)
Total	143	20	196	82
Tumor morphology				
Papillary	100	27	115	86
Solid or mixed	27	12	75	79
Tumor differentiation				
High	25	30	19	93
Medium	83	23	115	82
Low	18	12	56	84

visualization of contrast in the inflated catheter balloons and by direct inspection via open cystotomy. Cystotomy also permitted tumor debulking (in the era prior to routine transurethral resections) as well as suprapubic urinary drainage. Patients received two implants performed 5 to 10 days apart, delivering a total of 6,000 to 10,000 R. Fifty patients were treated with this technique, with a 5-year control rate of 56%. These 50 patients had a variety of tumors ranging in stage from noninvasive primary tumors to recurrent tumors with deep muscle invasion.[16]

More recently, 55 patients at the Cleveland Clinic have undergone a similar treatment employing intracavitary radium, with a complete response rate of 60% reported in patients with recurrent stage-A tumors following prior resections or resections followed by intravesical chemotherapy. Freedom from tumor recurrence was 39% in patients with stage-A, grade-I tumors; 44% for those patients with stage-A, grade-II tumors; and 62% for patients with carcinoma in situ. In contrast to the experience of Quilty and Duncan, well-differentiated tumors were felt to be more radioresponsive, and treatment was therefore limited to patients with low-grade tumors, only one patient with a grade-III histology included. A total of five patients incurred major symptoms of radiation cystitis of which 2 patients eventually required cystectomy.[17,18]

An intracavitary approach using cesium has been successfully used in combination with a modest dose of preimplant external beam irradiation. Treatment consisted of an initial 3,600 to 5,066 cGy external beam irradiation covering the bladder and the first-echelon, low-pelvic lymph nodes. The intracavitary implant delivered between 2,000 and 3,200 cGy over 2 to 3 days resulting in a combined implant and external beam dose of 6,500 to 7,500 cGy.

Seventeen patients have been treated using this approach, with eleven of the patients having had prior recurrent and multifocal superficial cancers and with eight of those patients having relapsed following prior intravesical chemotherapy. Of 15 evaluable patients with follow-up, 11 (73%) remain disease free, 3 (20%) have recurred in the bladder but have retained their bladders, and only 1 patient has required cystectomy. All 4 failures occurred in the subgroup of 8 patients who had recurred after intravesical chemotherapy, resulting in a 50% radiation therapy salvage of patients after failure of intravesical chemotherapy.[19]

Most recently, the intracavitary approach has been adapted so as to permit afterloading of high-activity sources through a modified cystoscope. The high-activity sources shorten the implant time, and the afterloading of the sources (i.e., sources are loaded and unloaded as needed using a shielded applicator and storage device) minimizes exposure of the medical staff.[20]

INTRAVESICAL RADIOCOLLOIDS

Solutions of radioactive isotopes have also been used in the past as a means of delivering a homogeneous distribution of dose to the urothelium. Direct instillation of yttrium-90 yielded a 72% "prolonged improvement" in 38 patients with multiple superficial papillary tumors.[21] Cobalt-60 in solution has also been employed, with the solution confined to a 75 mL catheter balloon within the bladder. Thirty-nine patients achieved a 41% complete response rate when treated in this fashion.[22]

Concerns about radiation safety for both patient and medical staff have curtailed the development of this approach, and there is no current active research using radiocolloids.

RADIOTHERAPY OF MUSCLE-INVADING TUMORS

A variety of radiotherapeutic modalities have been used to treat invasive bladder cancer. These include external beam irradiation with photons, fast neutrons or pi-mesons, interstitial irradiation, interstitial implants combined with external beam irradiation, and intraoperative irradiation. External beam photon irradiation is by far the most frequently used technique today.

TABLE 53-5. *External Beam Radiotherapy for Stage-T2 (B1) Tumors*

AUTHOR	NUMBER OF PATIENTS	5-YEAR SURVIVAL RATE (%)
Goffinet et al.[30]	68	42
Edsmyr[77]	80	34
Miller[37]	45	24
Fish and Fayos[75]	29	43
Yu et al.[33]	62	42

TABLE 53-6. *External Beam Radiotherapy for Stage-T3 (B2 and C) Tumors*

AUTHORS	NUMBER OF PATIENTS	5-YEAR SURVIVAL RATE (%) B2	B2 AND C	C
Miller[37]	71	21		
	66			18
Fish and Fayos[75]	19	26		
	23			13
Goffinet et al.[30]	123	35		
	95			20
Edsmyr[77]	106		25	
Yu et al.[33]	120	35		
	75			23
Morrison[79]	40		28	
Hope-Stone et al.[29]	194		34	
Bloom et al.[24]	91		29	

TABLE 53-7. *External Beam Radiotherapy for Stage-T4 (D) Tumors*

AUTHOR	NUMBER OF PATIENTS	5-YEAR SURVIVAL RATE (%)
Blandy et al.[28]	262	8
Miller[37]	136	9
Goffinet et al.[30]	65	8
Edsmyr[77]	82	7
Fish and Fayos[75]	40	11
Shipley et al.[80]	18	9

External Beam Photons

Multiple investigators have reported long-term control and survival rates for primary photon irradiation of invasive bladder cancer. The data are fairly consistent from one series to another and reveal a 5-year survival rate of 24 to 42% for stage-T2 (B1) tumors, 21 to 35% for stage-T3 (B2) tumors, 13 to 23% for stage-T3b (C) tumors, and 7 to 11% for stage-T4 (D) tumors. These data are summarized in Tables 53-5 to 53-7. As treatment is far from uniformly successful, particularly in the case of the locally advanced lesions, considerable efforts have been made to define patient and tumor parameters that permit selection of appropriate candidates for primary radiotherapy. Pretreatment clinical factors that have been reported to predict a successful response to radiotherapy include patient age, patient hemoglobin, tumor stage, tumor number, morphology, grade, size, transurethral resectability, lymphatic space invasion and the presence or absence of hydronephrosis on intravenous pyelography (IVP).[23–27] Unfortunately, except for a consensus that patients with lower stage tumors have a better outcome than patients with higher stage tumors, considerable differences exist among investigators as to the significance of each parameter. Representative data are provided in Table 53-8.

Despite the controversy about suitable pretreatment selection factors, there are ample data that the posttreatment factor of greatest prognostic significance is prompt tumor response. Patients with radioresponsive tumors that completely resolve within 3 to 6 months of treatment have a substantially better prognosis than those with incomplete responses or no responses. This information has been verified by a number of investigators, with representative data shown in Table 53-9.

Not surprisingly, the ability to determine which patient may have a result with radiotherapy comparable to that achieved with combined radiation and planned cystectomy (see results in "Preoperative Irradiation and Cystectomy") has led to the proposition that primary radiotherapy treatment be prescribed for all patients, with prompt cystectomy at 6 months for those without a complete tumor response. Patients with incomplete tumor responses at 6 months appear to benefit from a planned cystectomy at this time, because they have a 47% 5-year survival compared with an 18% 5-year survival for patients unable to undergo salvage cystectomy.[28,29]

Overall, the results of primary irradiation for invasive bladder cancer are suboptimal. This is partially due to inadequacy of radiotherapy to control the local tumor. Local tumor recurrences in patients with deeply invasive tumors (B2–C or T3) occur in as many as 47 to 65%[30–33] of patients treated with primary radiotherapy. Suboptimal survival results are also because of the 20 to 40% of patients who develop metastatic disease. There is, however, no question that *selected* patients with locally advanced but *radioresponsive* tumors enjoy a good survival, as high as 69%.[29] Were there clear-cut pretreatment characteristics that would predict an individual's successful result with radiotherapy, these parameters could guide the choice of treatment modalities. In the absence of clear-cut selection criteria, however, there remains considerable merit to the concept of testing the individual patient's tumor radiosensitivity by a trial of irradiation. The information obtained by

TABLE 53-8. *Pretreatment Clinical and Pathologic Factors of Patients with Invasive Bladder Cancer Predicting a Favorable Survival with Primary Radiotherapy*

	AUTHOR (NUMBER OF PATIENTS)			
	QUILTY AND DUNCAN[26] (899)	BLOOM ET AL.[24] (91)	BATATA ET AL.[23] (104)	SHIPLEY ET AL.[27] (55)
Morphology			Papillary tumor	Papillary tumor
Stage	Lower	Lower	Lower	Lower
Tumor size	<5 cm	<5 cm	<4 cm	
Hemoglobin	>12 gm/dl			
Patient age	<60 years	<60 years		
Histologic grade			I/II	
Tumor number			Multifocal	
TURB			Prior to radiation	Complete TURB
IVP				Normal

TABLE 53-9. *Survival after Primary Radiotherapy for Muscle-Invading Bladder Cancer in Relation to Initial Tumor Response*

AUTHOR	NUMBER OF PATIENTS	STAGE	5-YEAR SURVIVAL RATE (%)			
			TOTAL	COMPLETE RESPONSE	PARTIAL RESPONSE	NO RESPONSE
Quilty and Duncan[32]	272	T3	25.9	45	21	
Hope-Stone et al.[29]	194	T3	40.0	69	18	6
Bloom et al.[24]	91	T3	29.0	49	27	14

the tumor response to radiation can determine the need for further treatment, either cystectomy, chemotherapy, or both. This concept is currently being explored in separate clinical trials, and will be discussed more fully subsequently.

BLADDER TOLERANCE. The advantage of primary radiotherapy over cystectomy is the preservation of normal bladder function. It will be useful to review how successfully this is achieved in patients whose tumor is cured by radiotherapy. Bladder radiation injury is seen in the form of acute, subacute, or chronic manifestations, both from a symptomatic perspective as well as from histopathologic and functional changes. Acutely, radiation bladder injury manifests itself as cystitis, with urinary urgency, frequency, and burning beginning approximately 2,500 to 3,500 cGy into a fractionated course of external beam treatment, when doses to the entire bladder are given at 180 to 200 cGy per day. The bladder capacity is reduced, and cystoscopic findings vary from a diffuse hyperemia to varying degrees of desquamation or superficial ulceration. Edema of bladder mucosa is characteristically bullous and may persist for some months.[34,35] Although a secondary ureteritis and hydroureter can occur, these are rare complications. The acute cystitis generally subsides 2 to 4 weeks after the conclusion of treatment.

Subacute and chronic signs of bladder radiation injury most frequently take the form of bladder contracture and trigonal ulceration, although ureteral strictures and reversible hydronephrosis associated with bladder ulcerations and surrounding obstructive edema are less frequent complications. Late effects are usually manifest at 1 to 4 years following treatment. Patient symptoms are that of urinary frequency, nocturia, painless hematuria, and dribbling. Cystoscopic findings reveal bladder thickening, induration, and diminished capacity. Mucosal ulcers may contain crystalline urinary salts and fibrinous exudate. Telangiectatic blood vessels may persist for varying periods of time, are fragile, and can be the source of repeated hemorrhage. Collagen replaces muscle tissue, arterioles show myointimal proliferation, and atypical fibroblasts may be present in sufficient quantity to produce a pseudosarcomatous appearance in portions of the bladder wall.[34,35] The late effects of external beam irradiation of the bladder must be interpreted in the context of the fractionation schema employed. Daily fractions of 180 to 200 cGy in a continuous course, 5 days a week, is a widely used fractionation scheme, but varia-

tions including accelerated fractionation, large daily fractions, multiple daily fractions, and split-course treatments have been employed. As late tissue effects are strikingly dependent on fraction size, data reported from series using large daily fractions would be expected to have higher complication rates than those resulting from more protracted treatment.

In terms of acute effects during treatment, 70% of patients will typically develop dysuria and frequency by the conclusion of a course of radiotherapy.[30] The incidence of late complications, however, has varied considerably from one series to another. This likely reflects differences in patient selection and pretreatment bladder function, differences in radiotherapy technique, and fractionation (as above). In England, where primary radiotherapy has been a far more frequently employed alternative to cystectomy than in the United States, large radiation fractions are the rule for treatment of bladder cancer. In the United States, large fractions are uncommonly used. Table 53-10 summarizes the data on bladder tolerance to primary irradiation from representative series in the United States and abroad.

Goodman and colleagues[36] in Canada have reported probably the most complete data on bladder tolerance in a cohort of 470 patients with stage-B or stage-C tumors who received irradiation with large daily fractions: Fifteen equal daily fractions of 335 cGy were given over 3 weeks, using a three-field technique employing 10×8 cm portals or smaller. The 10-year survival rate was 34%, with evaluation of bladder function carried out in all 10-year survivors and with no survivor lost to follow-up. Approximately 68% of survivors had healthy functioning bladders, 3% had contracted disease-free bladders, 3% had both recurrent cancer and contracted bladders, 7% had recurrent cancer without late normal tissue sequelae, and 19% were without bladders. Those 19% had undergone cystectomy largely for salvage of recurrent disease.

In the M. D. Anderson Hospital, randomized trial comparing radiotherapy alone with preoperative radiotherapy plus cystectomy for clinical stage-T3 tumors, full toxicity information was obtainable on 494 patients and 10-year data were available on 280 patients.[37] The radiation fractionation employed varied with the clinical circumstances. To account for the differences in fractionation, doses were adjusted by time-dose-fractionation analysis[38] and major complications were scored at each dose level. These data have been fully analyzed by Moss,[39] and are reproduced in Table 53-11, where the data

TABLE 53-10. *Incidence of Late-Appearing Bladder Complications of Primary External Beam Photon Radiotherapy for Bladder Cancer*

AUTHOR	NUMBER OF PATIENTS	FRACTIONATION	SEVERE COMPLICATION
Duncan and Quilty[7]	963	275 cGy/fraction 20 fractions/4 weeks	11.5%
Hope-Stone et al.[29]	194	250–270 cGy/fraction 20 fractions/4 weeks	1.5%
Yu et al.[33]	356	200 cGy/Fx 30–33 Fx/6–6.5 weeks	2.0%
Goodman et al.[36]	470	335 cGy/Fx 15 Fx/3 weeks	6.0% *

*Three percent contracted, without tumor, three percent contracted, with recurrent tumor.

are presented as if all patients received 200 cGy fractions and continuous-course treatment.

Over a range of dose from 3,600 to 7,260 cGy, no clear-cut dose response for complications could be discerned for late bladder injury, although rectal injuries increased dramatically at the highest dose level. At 7,260 cGy, 5 out of 38 patients (13%) had a bladder complication, although only 5 out of 122 patients (4%) had problems at the 6,600 to 7,200 dose range.

It seems clear that continuous-course external beam photon irradiation delivering 5,000 cGy to the pelvis and 6,500 to 7,000 cGy to the bladder is a treatment that results in a low incidence of bladder contracture or chronic radiation cystitis.

TECHNIQUE. Although clinical trials have investigated the use of multiple fractions of radiation per day, or split-course treatment involving one or more weeks of rest between successive

TABLE 53-11. *Correlation of Bladder Dose and Incidence of Radiation-Induced Bladder Sequelae in Patients with Cancer of the Bladder**

	PERCENT PATIENTS WITH SEQUELAE IN PARTICULAR DOSE RANGE								
	3,600	3,660–4,170	4,228–4,800	4,860–5,400	5,460–6,000	6,066–6,620	6,680–7,200	7,260	TOTAL
Number of patients	27	52	18	63	93	81	122	38	533
Bladder (27)†			6	5	8	6	5	5	5
Rectum (13)				5	1	1	2	16	2
Kidney (10)	4	3		3	2	2		3	2
Small Bowel (8)		4			1	4		5	1.5
Subcutaneous tissue (1)								3	
Bladder and rectum (7)					1		3	5	1
Bladder and kidney (6)					3	2	1		1
Rectum and small bowel (1)								3	
Bladder and rectum and small bowel (1)							1		
Rectum, small bowel and bone (1)								1	
Bladder, subcutaneous tissue and bone (1)								1	
Total‡ (76)	4	6	6	13	16	16	12	42	14

*Modified from Miller, L. S. Cancer, *39*:973, 1977.
†Total number of patients with particular sequela(e) = number in parentheses.
‡Cardiovascular exlcuded.
From Moss, W. T., Brand, W. N., and Battifora, H. *Radiation Oncology, Rationale, Technique, Results.* St. Louis, C. V. Mosby Co., 1979.

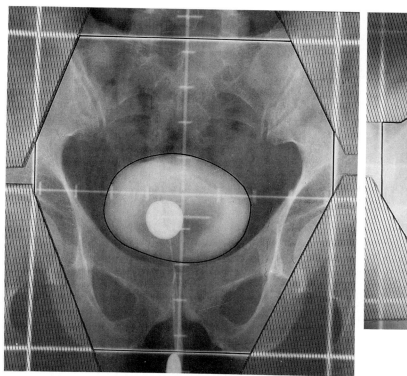

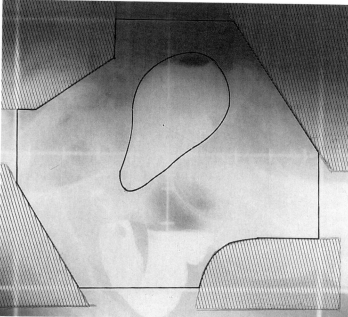

FIG. 53-1. Treatment planning films for megavoltage radiation treatment of invasive bladder tumors and the regional pelvic lymph nodes. *A*, Anterior/posterior ports. *B*, Right and left lateral ports. Radio-opaque dye has been inserted in the bladder, the balloon of the indwelling Foley catheter, and the rectum to assist in the initial treatment planning. Custom lead shielding spares uninvolved organs and bone marrow.

cycles of radiation, the great majority of patients treated with external beam irradiation have received continuous-course treatment, 5 days a week, one treatment per day. External beam photon irradiation is given through treatment portals that initially treat both bladder and regional pelvic nodes (Fig. 53-1*A,B*). By careful treatment planning with shaped radiation fields, by treating 4 portals per day (anterioposterior, posterioanterior, right and left lateral), and by using megavoltage photons (4 MeV energy or greater), radiation injury to adjacent bowel, rectum, and subcutaneous tissues can be minimized. After 5,000 cGy have been delivered (180 to 200 cGy/day), treatment fields are reduced to incorporate the whole bladder (Fig. 53-2*A,B*), or in some cases, just the portion of the bladder involved with tumor. This boost field delivers an additional 1,600 to 2,000 cGy for a total dose to the bladder of 6,600 to 7,000 cGy.

External Beam Photons Plus Implant

In addition to the use of implants alone for invasive tumors, the Rotterdam group has combined 1,050 cGy preoperative irradiation with an interstitial implant delivering 3,500 cGy by radium implant and an additional course of postoperative external irradiation to the pelvis consisting of 3,000 cGy. The results of treatment in this selected group of 41 patients with T3 tumors are among the best in the literature, regardless of

treatment modality, with a 74% 3-year survival rate and only 2 patients with late radiation complications (5%).[13,14]

Intraoperative Electron Beam Radiation

Intraoperative radiotherapy is a technique involving the delivery of a collimated radiation beam directly to a tumor during surgery, with the adjacent normal tissues displaced away from the radiation. This technique has the advantage of permitting high doses to the tumor with no morbidity to normal organs. Different types of radiation can be delivered by this technique, the most widely used being megavoltage electrons, which have the property of delivering all radiation within a defined depth of penetration determined by their energy.

A substantial experience exists in Japan using this technique for the treatment of T1 and T2 tumors. Electron doses of 2,500 to 3,000 cGy have been delivered with 4 to 6 MeV electrons to 116 patients with either solitary or multiple lesions that could be all confined within a 6 cm diameter or smaller treatment cone inserted into the bladder through a suprapubic cystotomy. Five-year survivals of 96% and 61% have been reported for patients with T1 and T2 tumors, respectively, with a bladder recurrence-free success rate of 81%. Five patients required salvage cystectomy for recurrent tumors, and only one patient for late radiation toxicity.[40] This approach is applicable for treating locally advanced tumors, and in the United States,

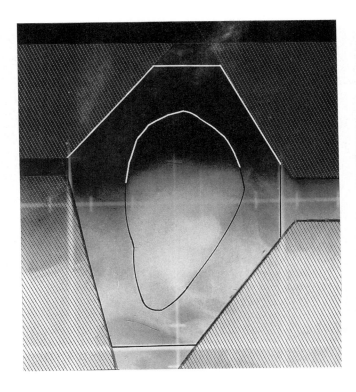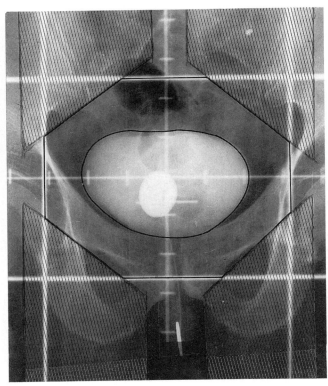

FIG. 53-2. Treatment planning films for megavoltage radiation boost treatment of the primary bladder tumor. A, Anterior/posterior boost ports. B, Right and left lateral ports.

it is currently being developed for clinical trials by the Radiation Therapy Oncology Group (RTOG).[41]

External Beam—Neutrons

Clinical trials employing fast neutrons in the treatment of bladder cancer evolved in an attempt either to improve on the results obtainable with primary photon radiation or to increase the percentage of tumor downstaging in combined modality approaches. The high linear energy transfer (LET, dose deposited per unit of tissue traversed) properties of neutrons relative to photons result in major radiobiological differences between neutrons and photons and a relative biologic effectiveness (RBE) for neutrons that is at least three-fold greater than photons per unit of dose. This theoretical advantage was the impetus to encourage clinical trials. In the United Kingdom two randomized trials have been completed comparing primary photons and primary neutron treatment. One trial was carried out at Christie Hospital in Manchester and the other at Western General Hospital in Edinburgh.

The Christie Hospital trial involved 99 patients with T2 or T3 staged bladder carcinomas. The 3-year survival for all groups was 43%, with no difference in survival between patients treated with photons or patients treated with either of two dose levels of neutrons. No differences in tumor control by treatment were observed on a stage-for-stage analysis. Seventy-eight patients had cystoscopic follow-up. A total of 22 out

of 41 (54%) photon-treated patients and 11 out of 29 (38%) neutron-treated patients had locally recurrent tumor (p = n.s.).[42]

In the Edinburgh study, 113 patients were stratified by tumor stage and randomized. Complete tumor regression was achieved in 64% of the neutron cohort and 62% of the proton cohort. Local tumor recurrences were observed in 31% of the patients in both arms. Again, no differences in tumor control by treatment were observed on a stage-for-stage analysis. Morbidity was assessed in both cohorts and judged to be substantially greater in the patients who received neutrons. A total of 19 patients died of neutron treatment complications and 2 patients died from photon complications. Overall survival rates reflected these treatment-related deaths as well as the inability to surgically salvage local tumor recurrences in neutron-treated patients because of excessive pelvic fibrosis. The 5-year survival for the photon-treated group was 45.3% (±11%) versus 12.0% (±6%) for patients receiving neutrons.[43,44]

In the United States, neutrons have been investigated in a nonrandomized phase I/II study by RTOG. Patients with muscle-invading tumors received either precystectomy radiation or definitive radiation, with surgery reserved for salvage of local recurrences. Most neutron-treated patients actually received "mixed-beam" therapy, in which alternating treatments of neutrons or photons were given such that the percentage of the dose contributed by neutrons was 40%. Mixed-beam therapy was employed to minimize potential neutron late tissue injury, although at the time the study was initiated, these complications were as yet unknown.

Mixed-beam treatment preoperatively followed by a cystectomy 4 to 6 weeks following completion of therapy was given to 13 patients, and 26 patients received definitive mixed-beam treatment alone. Of the patients treated in a combined modality fashion, 58% had no evidence of tumor in the cystectomy specimen. This is a higher percentage of complete tumor downstaging than results from conventional photon irradiation, in which a 25 to 35% incidence of complete downstaging has been observed.

Of the 26 patients treated with definitive mixed-beam radiation, 69% achieved tumor clearance at some time during their follow-up, but 44% who had initially achieved a complete response exhibited local relapse. The 5-year survival was 12% for the patients receiving mixed beam alone and 31% for the patients who underwent planned cystectomy. Locoregional pelvic tumor control at 5 years was 23% in the mixed-beam group and 61% in the combined modality group (p < .02).[45]

A summary of the results reported in these three trials is presented in Table 53-12. There has not proved to be an advantage for neutrons over photons as measured by survival or freedom from local tumor recurrence. The late complications in normal pelvic tissues following neutron irradiation with the then-available low-energy neutron beams have been substantial. A partial explanation for the neutron toxicity is no doubt due to the poorly penetrating beams of the original neutron equipment available at the time of the trials. This necessitated giving higher doses to the normal pelvic organs in order to deliver adequate neutron doses to the bladder tumor. Despite the advent of higher energy cyclotrons, which deliver beams of a comparably penetrating nature to megavoltage photons, it is unlikely that neutron trials will be continued for bladder tumors.

PREOPERATIVE IRRADIATION AND CYSTECTOMY

The concept of combined modality treatment developed in the setting of suboptimal results for either primary irradiation or primary cystectomy. While cystectomy alone is able to cure 45 to 53% of patients with T2 tumors[46-48] the results for patients with T3 tumors have been far less successful. Table 53-13 lists the survival results from surgical series reporting on the treatment of *clinically* staged T3 tumors. Because 37 to 53% of patients will have upstaging at surgery by the discovery of involved pelvic lymph nodes,[49-52] these data from institutions reporting results on the basis of clinical stage are the most appropriate to compare with primary radiotherapy results, as they incorporate the same uncertainties of tumor staging.

Additional considerations for combining preoperative radiation with cystectomy included a known 28% incidence of pelvic tumor failure after cystectomy alone[53] as well as a 7 to 14% incidence of tumor recurrences in surgical scars (from open cystotomy).[12,54] The theoretical contribution of radiotherapy would be to sterilize microscopic aggregates of tumor in regional lymph nodes as well as diminish the incidence of tumor seeding in the surgical wound. Doses of radiation required to control nodal micrometastases involve 4,500 to 5,000 cGy, whereas doses to reduce wound implantation have been shown to be as little as 1,050 cGy.[12] Combined modality trials have employed preoperative doses ranging from 2,000 cGy, delivered over 1 week immediately prior to cystectomy, to 5,000 cGy delivered over 5 weeks, with cystectomy performed 3 to 4 weeks after completion of radiation. The results of these trials are shown in Tables 53-14 to 53-16, and are grouped by the radiation doses employed.

The results obtained in these combined modality trials were consistently better than the results obtainable with either modality alone. Two randomized trials, carried out at the

TABLE 53-12. *Trials of Fast Neutrons for Bladder Cancer*

TRIAL	NUMBER OF PATIENTS	STAGE	TREATMENT	BLADDER DOSE (Gy or cGy)	SURVIVAL, % (YEARS)	LOCAL TUMOR RECURRENCE RESISTANCE (%)	SEVERE COMPLICATIONS (%)
Manchester[42]	20	T2, T3	Neutrons	16.5–17.0	43 (3)	29	15
	20	T2, T3	Neutrons	18.0–18.5	43 (3)	47	10
	59	T2, T3	Photons	52.5–55.0	43 (3)	54	5
Edinbergh[43,44]	53	T1, T2, T3	Neutrons	15.0–16.5	12 (5)	31	78
	60	T1, T2, T3	Photons	52.5–55.0	45 (5)	31	38
RTOG[45]	26	B1, B2, C, D1	Mixed beam	65–70*	12 (5)	77	55
	13	B1, B2, C, D1	Mixed beam and cystectomy	50*	31 (5)	39	23

*Photon Gy equivalent.

TABLE 53-13. *Five-Year Survival Results Following Total or Radical Cystectomy Alone for Clinical Stage B2–C (T3) Bladder Cancer*

AUTHOR	INSTITUTION	DATES PATIENTS ENTERED STUDY	CLINICAL STAGES	NUMBER OF PATIENTS	5-YEAR SURVIVAL RATE (%)
Jewett et al.[48]	Johns Hopkins	Not reported	B2–C	55	13
Poole-Wilson and Barnard[81]	Manchester	1950–1969	T1–T3 (previously untreated)	21	24
Stadie and Kuhne[82]	Halle/Saale, East Germany	1945–1965	B2–C	33	18
Brannan et al.[83]	Ochsner Clinic	1942–1968	B2–C	22*	18†
Varkarakis et al.[84]	Roswell Park	1961–1971	B2–C–D	26‡	20
Slack et al.[64]	NSABP trial	1964–1970	T2–T4	129§	32
Marshall and McCarron[85]	New York Hospital– Cornell	1960–1971	B2–C	163	26
Whitmore et al.[52]	Memorial Sloan- Kettering	1949–1958	B2–C	64	16
Vinnicombe and Abercrombie[86]	St. Mary's Hosp. (Portsmouth)	1966–1977	T3	17‖	35
Morabito et al.[87]	West Virginia University	1961–1978	B–C	29	24
Drago and Rohner[59]	Pennsylvania State University (Hershey)	1971–1981	Muscle invasive	13¶	31 (4/13)
Montie et al.[88]	Cleveland Clinic	1960–1975	T3AB, T4A	24**	40

*Some patients received radiation therapy.
†Five-year survival was 25% for ileal conduit group.
‡Includes 21 B2–C and 5 Stage D patients, of whom 18 B2–C and 4 D patients died of bladder cancer.
§Fifteen percent had partial cystectomy.
‖Seventeen patients had 5-year minimum follow-up; 4,000 rad preoperative irradiation was used in an unspecified number of these patients.
¶Excludes 7 patients treated by partial cystectomy.
**Some patients received postoperative radiation therapy.
From Parsons and Million.[69]

Institute of Urology in London and at the M. D. Anderson Hospital in Houston, directly addressed the question of whether combined modality treatment was superior to radiation alone. Both trials confirmed the superiority of the combined treatment, with the London trial demonstrating a 45% 5-year survival for male patients treated with combined modality treatment and a 29% 5-year survival for the comparable patients treated with radiation alone.[24,55] The Houston trial showed comparable 5-year survival rates of 46% and 16%, respectively, for patients with T3 tumors.[37]

A consistent finding in virtually all series employing preoperative radiation followed by cystectomy was the significant incidence of tumor downstaging found at the time of cystectomy. This was defined as less invasive tumor in the cystectomy specimen than observed in the original biopsy material. Between 14 and 43% of patients had no histologic evidence of

TABLE 53-14. *Five-Year Survival Results following 2,000 Rad Preoperative Irradiation Plus Cystectomy for Clinical Stage B2–C (T3) Bladder Cancer*

AUTHOR	INSTITUTION	DATES PATIENTS ENTERED STUDY	CLINICAL STAGE	NUMBER OF PATIENTS	TREATMENT	5-YEAR SURVIVAL RATE (%)
Batata et al.[89]	Memorial Sloan-Kettering	1966–1974	T3	106	2000 rad/1 week; immediate cystectomy; lymph node dissection	40

From Parsons and Million.[69]

TABLE 53-15. *Five-Year Survival Results Following 4,000 Rad Preoperative Irradiation Plus Cystectomy for Clinical Stage B2–C (T3) Bladder Cancer*

AUTHOR	INSTITUTION	DATES PATIENTS ENTERED STUDY	CLINICAL STAGE	NUMBER OF PATIENTS	TREATMENT	5-YEAR SURVIVAL RATE (%)
Bloom et al.[24]	Institute of Urology (London)	1966–1975	T3	77	4000 rad/4 weeks; cystectomy and lymph node dissection 4 weeks later	44*
Batata et al.[89]	Memorial Sloan-Kettering	1959–1965†	T3	50	4000 rad/4 weeks; radical cystectomy and lymph node dissection 4–12 weeks later	34
Van der Werf-Messing et al.[90]	Rotterdam Radiotherapy Institute	1966–1978	T3 (> 5 cm)	183	4000 rad/4 weeks; simple cystectomy as soon as possible	52
Timmer et al.[91]	State University Hospital Groningen, The Netherlands	1975–1980	T3	14‡	4000 rad/4 weeks; cystectomy 4 weeks later	56

*Determinate survival.
†Dates found in Whitmore et al.[52]
‡Four of the fourteen patients underwent cystoscopic re-evaluation after 4,000 rad and were found to have an unfavorable tumor response.
From Parsons and Million.[69]

TABLE 53-16. *Five-Year Survival Results Following 4,500 to 5,000 Rad Preoperative Irradiation Plus Cystectomy for Clinical Stage B2–C (T3) Bladder Cancer*

AUTHOR	INSTITUTION	DATES PATIENTS ENTERED STUDY	CLINICAL STAGE	NUMBER OF PATIENTS	TREATMENT	5-YEAR SURVIVAL RATE (%)
Slack et al.[64]	NSABP trial	1964–1970	T2–T4	70*	4,500 rad/4–4.0 weeks; cystectomy 4–8 weeks later	54
DeWeerd and Colby[92]	Mayo Clinic	1963–1966	T2–T4	45	4,800 rad; cystectomy; lymph node dissection	51
Chan and Johnson[93]	M. D. Anderson Hospital	1969–1975	T3	89	5,000 rad/5 weeks; cystectomy 6 weeks later	55
Tjabbes[94]	Gravenhage, The Netherlands	1968–1978	T3	48	4,500 rad; immediate cystectomy	45
Hall and Heath[95]	Freeman Hospital (Newcastle-upon-Tyne)	1964–1978	T3	102	4,000–4,500 rad/4–4.0 weeks; cystectomy 1–6 weeks later	50†

*Received radiation therapy, cystectomy, and "no drug" or "placebo"; 5-fluorouracil patients excluded.
†Overall 5-year survival figure not given in paper but was calculated from available data. Survival in the 74% of patients whose tumors were downstaged was 60% versus 30% in the 26% of patients whose tumors were not downstaged, which equals 50.4% 5-year survival overall.
From Parsons and Million.[69]

TABLE 53-17. *Pathological Findings in Cystectomy Specimens of Patients with Clinical Stage B2–C (T3) Bladder Cancer Following 4,000 to 5,000 Rad Planned Preoperative Irradiation*

AUTHOR	INSTITUTION	NUMBER OF PATIENTS	RADIATION DOSE (rad/number of weeks)	NO TUMOR IN CYSTECTOMY SPECIMEN (%)	TOTAL PERCENT DOWNSTAGED*	PATH N+
Blackard et al.[68]	VA trial	17	4,500/4–5	24	n.d.†	n.d.
Whitmore et al.[52]	Memorial Sloan-Kettering	50	4,000/4	14	44	10%‡
Slack et al.[64]	NSABP trial	138	4,500/4.5–5	34	51	n.d.
Miller[96]	M. D. Anderson Hospital	30	5,000/5	43	73	n.d.
Peeples et al.[97]	Eastern Virginia Medical School	10§	4,500/4.5	40	80	0%‡
Sagerman et al.[98]	Upstate Medical Center, SUNY	22	4,000–5,000/4–5	32	82	n.d.
Hall and Heath[95]	Freeman Hospital (Newcastle-upon-Tyne)	102	4,000–4,500/4–4.5	35	74	n.d.
Bloom et al.[24]	Institute of Urology (London)	74‖	4,000/4	31	49	20%‡
Van der Werf-Messing et al.[90]	Rotterdam Radiotherapy Institute	181	4,000/4	37	73	n.d.
Scanlon et al.[57]	Mayo Clinic	416	4,800–5,000/7	43	55	25%‡

*Pathologic stage less than clinical stage.
†n.d. = no data.
‡Pelvic lymphadenectomy was performed at time of cystectomy.
§All patients had histologic evidence of muscle invasion and were classified as stage B. Nine patients underwent lymphadenectomy.
‖Pathology not recorded in 3 patients.
From Parsons and Million.[69]

residual tumor following the preoperative radiation. These data are summarized in Table 53-17.

The prognostic importance of tumor radioresponsiveness in these patients, as in the patients treated with primary irradiation, was to predict a favorable survival outcome. Those patients with no residual tumor enjoyed a survival of 64 to 80% compared to 27 to 48% without downstaging.[24,25,56–58] Additionally, the incidence of pelvic failures for patients with downstaged tumors dropped to as low as 4% compared to 23% for comparable patients without downstaged tumors.[53] This improvement presumably occurred as a result of radiation sterilization of tumor deposits in pelvic lymph nodes. Support for this explanation can be found in the reduced incidence of nodal involvement with tumor in patients receiving preoperative irradiation, 10 to 25%, compared with the 40 to 50% normally found for comparable patients with locally advanced tumors treated with cystectomy alone.[52,59]

Patients treated with a short course of 2,000 cGy in 1 week followed by immediate cystectomy rarely exhibited downstaging, both because the radiation dose was lower and because less time elapsed between radiation and surgery in which tumor regression could occur. Not surprisingly, the incidence of pelvic nodal involvement following short-course radiotherapy is no different than following cystectomy alone.[52] However, it appears that *overall* survival of patients receiving either short-course or prolonged course (4,000 to 5,000 cGy) preoperative radiation are similar, as analyzed in two retrospective and nonrandomized series where these regimens have been compared. In the experience at Memorial Sloan-Kettering Hospital, 43% and 42% 5-year survivals were recorded for patients receiving long- (4,000 cGy) and short-course (2,000 cGy) treatment, respectively.[60] The equivalent figures from the Mayo Clinic, comparing 4,800 to 5,000 cGy treatment with 2,000 cGy treatment are 54% and 54%.[57] This conclusion about the relative efficacy of the two preoperative regimens is not uniformly shared by all investigators, with data from other institutions suggesting an improved result after high-dose radiotherapy (63% 5-year survival) than after low-dose or no preoperative radiation (21% 5-year survival).[61] The case for a radiation dose-response relationship in combined modality approaches has also been well presented by Miller.[62]

At a time when surgical techniques have improved such that pelvic tumor control approaches 85 to 95% following cystectomy alone,[63] the question is again being raised whether combined modality treatment remains the standard treatment for muscle-invading tumors.

Results from five completed randomized trials have reported, comparing combined modality treatment with cystectomy alone. These trials varied considerably in study design, with one (National Surgical Adjuvant Breast Project Study) incorporating adjuvant 5-fluorouracil,[64] two involving patients

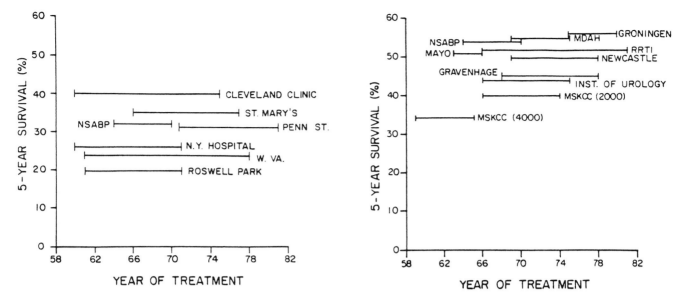

FIG. 53-3. *A*, Five-year survival (%) following total or radical cystectomy alone for 7 series of patients with clinical stage B2–C (T3) bladder cancer according to the year patients were treated. All patients were treated between 1960 and 1981. Five-year results for patients treated during this time period range from 20 to 40% survival (median = 32%). If the probability of 5-year survival (%) for each of the reported series is multiplied by the number of patients in each series and then divided by the total number of patients in all the series combined, an estimate of the probability of 5-year survival for the 401 patients can be determined. The estimate is 28.7% (115.4/401). *B*, Five-year survival (%) for preoperative irradiation plus total or radical cystectomy for 10 series of patients with clinical stage-B2–C (T3) bladder cancer according to the year patients were treated. All patients were treated between 1959 and 1981. Five-year results for patients treated during this time period range from 34 to 55% survival (median = 50%). The estimate of the probability of 5-year survival for the 784 patients (calculated as described for Figure 53-3*A*) is 48.3% (378.6/784). From Parsons and Million.[69]

with bilharzial bladder cancers (National Cancer Institute (NCI) of Egypt and NCI, Egypt—Memorial Hospital Cooperative Trial),[65,66] one involving 44 patients with a spectrum of T1 to T3 lesions,[67] and the last involving three treatment arms (combined, radiation alone, and surgery alone) and low patient accrual (Veterans Administration Hospital Trial).[68] Accordingly, there are controversial elements in each of these trials, which color the interpretation of their findings and are beyond the scope of this work. These controversies are well discussed in the review paper by Parsons and Million.[69] A capsule summary of the five randomized trials would be that three studies[64–67] confirmed a survival benefit for the combined treatment, one study[68] found no difference in outcome and one study[67] concluded that patients treated with combined modality treatment had a poorer survival than those treated with surgery alone.

More recently, a randomized trial of cystectomy versus 2,000 cGy radiation followed by cystectomy was carried out by the Southwest Oncology Group. Although the results are too preliminary to draw conclusions, there seems to be no survival advantage to the combined approach.[70] Potential criticisms of this study would be (1) the use of the 2,000 cGy dose, which most radiation oncologists do not believe to be the optimal regimen, and (2) the inclusion of a wide spectrum of tumor presentations ranging from carcinoma in situ and superficial tumors to locally advanced tumors with pelvic nodal involvement.

In order to synthesize the existing data about the relative efficacy of combined modality treatment versus cystectomy, Parsons and Million have summarized the results of a number of sentinel experiences involving either cystectomy alone or combined modality treatment and graphed survival results according to treatment modality and treatment era. This latter variable takes into account any changes in techniques over time that have led to improved results. These results are presented in Figure 53-3. The pooled results of these 1,185 patients suggests the continued survival benefits of combined modality treatment.

CURRENT AND FUTURE DIRECTIONS

Current clinical trials involving radiotherapy focus largely on two of the critical lessons learned from past experience: (1) patients with radioresponsive tumors treated with primary radiotherapy and salvage cystectomy, as needed, have a prognosis comparable to those treated with combined modality regimens and have a high percentage of functionally intact bladders and a low incidence of late radiation complications and (2) patients with locally controlled tumors continue to succumb to systemic metastases. Accordingly, these trials have incorporated (a) a decision point during treatment when response to radiotherapy can be assessed and the need for more aggressive local treatment (i.e., cystectomy) considered and (b) systemic treatment in the form of single-agent or combina-

TABLE 53-18. *Complete Response Rates Complete Histologic Downstaging (PO) Following Combined Chemotherapy and Irradiation*

AUTHOR	NUMBER OF PATIENTS	T STAGE	DRUGS	PO (%)	CLINICAL CR (%)
Sauer et al.[99]	41	T1–T4	Cisplatinum	77	77
Marks et al.[100]	19	T2–T4	MCV*	57	57
Shipley et al.[101]	62	T2–T4	Cisplatinum		77
Jakse et al.[102]	22	T3–T4	Cisplatinum		77
Rotman et al.[103]	19	T1–T4	5-Fluorouracil		61
Russell et al.[104]	14	T1–T4	5-Fluorouracil	71	71

*Methotrexate, cisplatinum, velban.

tion chemotherapy. Insofar as the effective single-agent chemotherapeutic drugs for bladder cancer are also believed to enhance radiation efficacy (radiation sensitizers), these trials also indirectly test the hypothesis that chemotherapy combined with radiation may yield a greater percentage of complete primary tumor clearance than achievable by irradiation alone. Because a goal of these trials is to avoid cystectomy when the tumors appear radioresponsive, assessment of complete tumor clearance to PO (no pathological evidence of tumor) status has generally been performed by cystoscopy and transurethral bladder wall biopsy. To the extent that a concerted effort is made to obtain multiple deep-muscle biopsies of representative areas, this approach is expected to yield comparable information to that obtained by pathologic examination of the entire cystectomy specimen. This may not be the case, as evidence suggests that this may underestimate the true residual tumor by 34%.[71] Conversely, favorable outcomes with radiotherapy have historically been reported by defining complete tumor responses as occurring within 6 months of treatment, and the current trials involve therapeutic decisions within a much shorter, and therefore stricter, time frame of 3 to 4 weeks after therapy. This should presumably select only the most responsive tumors for bladder-sparing treatment.

To date, most of these trials have only short-term survival data. However, the high incidence of complete histologic tumor clearance with combined chemoradiotherapy appears promising, and to the degree that complete downstaging predicts for a favorable survival rate and recurrence-free bladders, these trials are of great interest. The results of some of these ongoing efforts are summarized in Table 53-18.

CONCLUSION

With the advent of efficacious chemotherapy, which has a documented effect on both systemic metastases[72,73] and the primary tumor,[71,76] new possibilities arise to combine systemic and local modalities in the hope of improved outcomes. An opportunity exists to apply what has been learned from past experience to develop treatment strategies that are applied not solely on the basis of individual tumor or patient parameters, but rather on an assessment of the individual tumor's biological aggressiveness. This tailoring of treatment to the severity of the individual's problem can provide a rational framework for choosing one of a number of treatment alternatives, each of which has different toxicity and consequences for the patient.

REFERENCES

1. Brosman, S. A. The use of bacillus Calmette-Guérin in the therapy of bladder carcinoma in situ. J. Urol., *134:*36, 1985.
2. Herr, H. W. et al. Long-term effect of intravesical bacillus Calmette-Guérin on flat carcinoma in situ of the bladder. J. Urol., *135:*265, 1986.
3. Lamm, D. Bacillus Calmette-Guérin immunotherapy for bladder cancer. J. Urol., *134:*40, 1985.
4. Soloway, M. S. Intravesical and systemic chemotherapy in the management of superficial bladder cancer. Urol. Clin. North Am., *11:*623, 1984.
5. Torti, F. M., and Lum, B. L. The biology and treatment of superficial bladder cancer. J. Clin. Oncol., *2:*505, 1984.
6. Caldwell, W. L. Radiotherapy: Definitive, integrated, and palliative therapy. Urol. Clin. North Am., *3:*129, 1976.
7. Duncan, W., and Quilty, P. M. The results of a series of 963 patients with transitional cell carcinoma of the urinary bladder primarily treated by radical megavoltage x-ray therapy. Radiother. Oncol., *7:*299, 1986.
8. Sawczuk, I. S., Olsson, C. A., and deVere White, R. The limited usefulness of external beam radiotherapy in the control of superficial bladder cancer. J. Urol., *61:*330, 1988.
9. Whitmore, W. F., and Prout, G. R., Jr. Discouraging results for high dose external beam radiation therapy in low stage (O and A) bladder cancer. J. Urol., *127:*902, 1982.
10. Quilty, P. M., and Duncan, W. Treatment of superficial (T1) tumors of the bladder by radical radiotherapy. Br. J. Urol., *58:*147, 1986.
11. Williams, G. B., Trott, P. A., and Bloom, H. J. G. Carcinoma of the

bladder treated by interstitial irradiation. Br. J. Urol., *53*:221, 1981.

12. VAN DER WERF-MESSING, B. Carcinoma of the bladder treated by suprapubic radium implants. The value of additional external irradiation. Eur. J. Cancer, *5*:277, 1969.

13. VAN DER WERF-MESSING, B., MENON, R. S., HOP, W. C. J. Carcinoma of the urinary bladder category $T_3N_xM_0$ treated by the combination of radium implant and external irradiation: Second report. Int. J. Radiat. Oncol. Biol. Phys., *9*:177, 1983.

14. VAN DER WERF-MESSING, B., STAR, W. M. and MENON, R. S. T3NXMO carcinoma of the urinary bladder treated by the combination of radium implant and external irradiation. A preliminary report. Int. J. Radiat. Oncol. Biol. Phys., *6*:1723, 1980.

15. VAN DER WERF-MESSING, B., MENON, R. S., HOP, W. C. J. Cancer of the urinary bladder category T2, T3, (NXMO) treated by interstitial radium implants: Second report. Int. J. Radiat. Oncol. Biol. Phys., *9*:481, 1983.

16. FRIEDMAN, M., and LEWIS, L. G. Irradiation of carcinoma of the bladder by a central intracavitary radium or cobalt-60 source (the Walter Reed technique). Am. J. Roentgenol., *79*:6, 1958.

17. HEWITT, C. B., BABISZEWSKI, J. F., and ANTUNEZ, A. R. Update on intracavitary radiation in the treatment of bladder tumors. J. Urol., *126*:323, 1981.

18. HEWITT, C. B. et al. Intracavitary radiation in the treatment of bladder tumors. J. Urol., *107*:693, 1972.

19. RUSSELL, K. J. et al. Combined intracavitary and external beam irradiation for superficial transitional cell carcinoma of the bladder: An alternative to cystectomy for patients with recurrence after intravesical chemotherapy. J. Urol., *141*:30, 1989.

20. HARADA, T. et al. Trancystoscopic intracavitary irradiation for carcinoma of the bladder: Technique and preliminary clinical results. J. Urol., *138*:771, 1987.

21. DURRANT, K. R., and LAING, A. H. Treatment of multiple superficial papillary tumors of the bladder by intracavitary yttrium-90. J. Urol., *113*:480, 1975.

22. MULLER, J. H. Radiotherapy of bladder cancer by means of rubber balloons filled in situ with solutions of a radioactive isotope (Co^{60}). Cancer, *8*:1035, 1955.

23. BATATA, M. A. et al. Factors of prognostic and therapeutic significance in patients with bladder cancer. Int. J. Radiat. Oncol. Biol. Phys., *7*:575, 1981.

24. BLOOM, H. J. G. et al. Treatment of T3 bladder cancer: Controlled trial of preoperative radiotherapy and radical cystectomy versus radical radiotherapy: Second report and review. Br. J. Urol., *54*:136, 1982.

25. BOILEAU, M. A. et al. Bladder carcinoma. Results with pre-operative radiation therapy and radical cystectomy. Urology, *16*:569, 1980.

26. QUILTY, P. M., KERR, G. R., and DUNCAN, W. Prognostic indices for bladder cancer: An analysis of patients with transitional cell carcinoma of the bladder primarily treated by radical megavoltage x-ray therapy. Radiother. Oncol., *7*:311, 1986.

27. SHIPLEY, W. U., and ROSE, M. A. Bladder cancer. The selection of patients for treatment by full-dose irradiation. Cancer, *55*:2278, 1985.

28. BLANDY, J. P. et al. T3 bladder cancer—The case for salvage cystectomy. Br. J. Urol., *52*:506, 1980.

29. HOPE-STONE, H. F. et al. T3 bladder cancer: Salvage rather than elective cystectomy after radiotherapy. Urology, *24*:315, 1984.

30. GOFFINET, D. R. et al. Bladder cancer: Results of radiation therapy in 384 patients. Radiology, *117*:149, 1975.

31. MILLER, L. S., and JOHNSON, D. E. Megavoltage irradiation for bladder carcinoma: Alone, postoperative, or preoperative? Proc. Natl. Cancer Conf., *7*:771, 1973.

32. QUILTY, P. M., and DUNCAN, W. Primary radical radiotherapy for T3 transitional cell cancer of the bladder: An analysis of survival and control. Int. J. Radiat. Oncol. Biol. Phys., *12*:853, 1986.

33. YU, W. S. et al. Bladder carcinoma. Experience with radical and preoperative radiotherapy in 421 patients. Cancer, *56*:1293, 1985.

34. FAJARDO, L. F. *Pathology of Radiation Injury.* New York, Masson Publishing USA, 1982, pp. 103–107.

35. RUBIN, P., and CASARETT, G. W. *Clinical Radiation Pathology.* Philadelphia, W. B. Saunders, Co., 1968, pp. 334–374.

36. GOODMAN, G. B. et al. Conservation of bladder function in patients with invasive bladder cancer treated by definitive irradiation and selective cystectomy. Int. J. Radiat. Oncol. Biol. Phys., *7*:569, 1981.

37. MILLER, L. S. Bladder cancer: Superiority of preoperative irradiation and cystectomy in clinical stages B2 and C. Cancer, *39*:973, 1977.

38. ORTON, C. G., and ELLIS, F. A Simplification in the use of the NSD concept in practical radiotherapy. Br. J. Radiol., *46*:529, 1973.

39. MOSS, W. T., BRAND, W. N., and BATTIFORA, H. *Radiation Oncology Rationale, Technique, Results.* St. Louis, C. V. Mosby Co., 1979, pp. 396–404.

40. MATSUMOTO, K. et al. Clinical evaluation of intraoperative radiotherapy for carcinoma of the urinary bladder. Cancer, *47*:509, 1981.

41. Personal communication, William U. Shipley, M.D., Chairman. RTOG Genitourinary Committee.

42. POINTON, R. S., READ, G., and GREENE, D. A randomized comparison of photons and 15 MeV neutrons for the treatment of carcinoma of the bladder. Br. J. Radiol., *58*:219, 1985.

43. DUNCAN, W. et al. A report of a randomized trial of d(15) + Be neutrons compared with megavoltage x-ray therapy of bladder cancer. Int. J. Radiat. Oncol. Biol. Phys., *11*:2043, 1985.

44. DUNCAN, W. et al. An analysis of the radiation-related morbidity observed in a randomized trial of neutron therapy for bladder cancer. Int. J. Radiat. Oncol. Biol. Phys., *12*:2085, 1986.

45. LARAMORE, G. E. et al. Radiation therapy oncology group phase I-II study on fast neutron teletherapy for carcinoma of the bladder. Cancer, *54*:432, 1984.

46. CORDONNIER, J. J. Cystectomy for carcinoma of the bladder. J. Urol., *99*:172, 1968.

47. COX, C. E., CASS, A. S., and BOYCE, W. H. Bladder cancer: A 26-year review. J. Urol., *101*:550, 1969.

48. JEWETT, H. J., KING, L. R., and SHELLEY, W. M. A study of 365 cases of infiltrating bladder cancer: Relation of certain pathological characteristics to prognosis after extirpation. J. Urol., *92*:668, 1964.

49. KUTSCHER, H. A., LEADBETTER, G. W., JR., and VINSON, R. K. Survival after radical cystectomy for invasive transitional cell carcinoma of bladder. Urology, *17*:231, 1981.

50. MARSHALL, V. F. The relation of the preoperative estimate to the pathologic demonstration of the extent of vesical neoplasms. J. Urol., *68*:714, 1952.

51. RICHIE, J. P., SKINNER, D. G., and KAUFMAN, J. J. Radical cystectomy for carcinoma of the bladder: 16 years of experience. J. Urol., *113*:186, 1975.

52. WHITMORE, W. F., JR. et al. Radical cystectomy with or without prior irradiation in the treatment of bladder cancer. J. Urol., *118*:184, 1977.

53. Batata, M. A. et al. Patterns of recurrence in bladder cancer treated by irradiation and/or cystectomy. Int. J. Radiat. Oncol. Biol. Phys., 6:155, 1980.

54. Melicow, M. M. Tumors of the urinary bladder: A clinico-pathological analysis of over 2500 specimens and biopsies. J. Urol., 74:498, 1955.

55. Wallace, D. M., and Bloom, H. J. G. The management of deeply infiltrating T3 carcinoma. Controlled trial of radical radiotherapy versus preoperative radiotherapy and radical cystectomy: First report. Br. J. Urol., 48:587, 1976.

56. DeWeerd, J. H. et al. Cystectomy after radiotherapeutic ablation of invasive transitional cell cancer. J. Urol., 118:260, 1977.

57. Scanlon, P. W., Scott, M., and Segura, J. W. A comparison of short-course, low-dose and long-course, high-dose preoperative radiation for carcinoma of the bladder. Cancer, 52:1153, 1983.

58. Slack, N. H., and Prout, G. R., Jr. The heterogeneity of invasive bladder carcinoma and different responses to treatment. J. Urol., 123:644, 1980.

59. Drago, J. R., and Rohner, T. J., Jr. Bladder cancer: Results of radical cystectomy for invasive and recurrent superficial tumors. J. Urol., 130:460, 1983.

60. Whitmore, W. F. et al. A comparative study of two preoperative radiation regimens with cystectomy for bladder cancer. Cancer, 40:1077, 1977.

61. Spera, J. A. et al. A comparison of preoperative radiotherapy for bladder carcinoma. The University of Pennsylvania Experience. Cancer, 61:255, 1988.

62. Miller, L. S. T₃ bladder cancer. The case for higher radiation dosage. Cancer, 45:1875, 1980.

63. Wishnow, K. I., and Dmochowski, R. Pelvic recurrence after radical cystectomy without preoperative radiation. J. Urol., 140:42, 1988.

64. Slack, N. H., Bross, I. D. J., and Prout, G. R., Jr. Five-year follow-up results of a collaborative study of therapies for carcinoma of the bladder. J. Surg. Oncol., 9:393, 1977.

65. Awwad, H. et al. Pre-operative irradiation of T3 carcinoma in bilharzial bladder: A comparison between hyperfractionation and conventional fractionation. Int. J. Radiat. Oncol. Biol. Phys., 5:787, 1979.

66. Ghoneim, M. A., et al. Randomized trial of cystectomy with or without pre-operative radiotherapy for carcinoma of the bilharzial bladder. J. Urol., 134:266, 1985.

67. Anderstrom, D. et al. A prospective randomized study of pre-operative irradiation with cystectomy or cystectomy alone for invasive bladder carcinoma. Eur. Urol., 9:142, 1983.

68. Blackard, C. E., Byar, D. P., and Veterans Administration Cooperative Urological Research Group. Results of a clinical trial of surgery and radiation in stages II and III carcinoma of the bladder. J. Urol., 108:875, 1972.

69. Parsons, J. T., and Million, R. R. Planned preoperative irradiation in the management of clinical stage B2–C (T3) bladder carcinoma. Int. J. Radiat. Oncol. Biol. Phys., 14:797, 1988.

70. Crawford, E. D., Das, S., and Smith, J. A., Jr. Preoperative radiation therapy in the treatment of bladder cancer. Urol. Clin. North Am., 14:781, 1987.

71. Scher, H. I. et al. Neoadjuvant M-VAC (methotrexate, vinblastine, doxorubicin and cisplatin) effect on the primary bladder lesion. J. Urol., 139:470, 1988.

72. Logothetis, C. J. et al. Cyclophosphamide, doxorubicin and cis-platin chemotherapy for patients with locally advanced urothelial tumors with or without nodal metastases. J. Urol., 134:460, 1985.

73. Sternberg, C. N., et al. M-VAC (methotrexate, vinblastine, doxorubicin and cisplatin) for advanced transitional cell carcinoma of the urothelium. J. Urol., 139:461, 1988.

74. Finney, R. The treatment of carcinoma of the bladder by external irradiation: A clinical trial—Part II. Clin. Radiol., 22:225, 1971.

75. Fish, J. C., and Fayos, J. W. Carcinoma of the urinary bladder. Radiology, 118:179, 1976.

76. Meyers, F. J. et al. The fate of the bladder in patients with metastatic bladder cancer treated with cisplatin, methotrexate and vinblastine: A Northern California Oncology Group Study. J. Urol., 134:1118, 1985.

77. Edsmyr, F. Radiotherapy in the management of bladder cancer. In: *The Biology and Clinical Management of Bladder Cancer.* Edited by E. H. Cooper and R. E. Williams. Oxford, Blackwell Scientific, 1975, p. 229.

78. Van Der Werf-Messing, B., and Hop, W. C. J. Carcinoma of the urinary bladder (category T₁NₓM₀) treated either by radium implant or by transurethral resection only. Int. J. Radiat. Oncol. Biol. Phys., 7:299, 1981.

79. Morrison, R. The results of the treatment of cancer of the bladder—A clinical contribution to radiobiology. Clin. Radiol., 26:67, 1975.

80. Shipley, W. U. et al. Full dose irradiation for patients with invasive bladder carcinoma: Clinical and histologic factors prognostic of improved survival. J. Urol., 134:679, 1985.

81. Poole-Wilson, D. S., and Barnard, R. J. Total cystectomy for bladder tumours. Br. J. Urol., 43:16, 1971.

82. Stadie, G., and Kuhne, U. Late results of cystectomy in carcinoma of the urinary bladder. Int. Urol. Nephrol., 3:379, 1971.

83. Brannan, W. et al. Cystectomy and segmental resection for primary carcinoma of the bladder: Experience at Ochsner Clinic 1942–1968. South. Med. J., 66:241, 1973.

84. Varkarakis, M. J. et al. Prognosis of bladder carcinoma in patients treated with cystectomy. Int. Urol. Nephrol., 7:38, 1975.

85. Marshall, V. F., and McCarron, J. P., Jr. The curability of vesical cancer. Greater now or then? Cancer Res., 37:2753, 1977.

86. Vinnicombe, J., and Abercrombie, G. F. Total cystectomy—A review. Br. J. Urol., 50:488, 1978.

87. Morabito, R. A., Kandzari, S. J., and Milam, D. F. Invasive bladder carcinoma treated by radical cystectomy: Survival of patients. Urology, 14:478, 1979.

88. Montie, J. E., Straffon, R. A., and Stewart, B. H. Radical cystectomy without radiation therapy for carcinoma of the bladder. J. Urol., 131:477, 1984.

89. Batata, M. A. et al. Preoperative whole pelvis versus true pelvis irradiation and/or cystectomy for bladder cancer. Int. J. Radiat. Oncol. Biol. Phys., 7:1349, 1981.

90. Van Der Werf-Messing, B., et al. Carcinoma of the urinary bladder T3NXMO treated by preoperative irradiation followed by simple cystectomy. Int. J. Radiat. Oncol. Biol. Phys., 8:1849, 1982.

91. Timmer, P. R., Hartlief, H. A., and Hooijkaas, J. A. P. Bladder cancer: Pattern of recurrence in 142 patients. Int. J. Radiat. Oncol. Biol. Phys., 11:899, 1985.

92. DeWeerd, J. H., and Colby, M. Y., Jr. Bladder carcinoma treated by irradiation and surgery: Interval report. J. Urol., 109:409, 1973.

93. Chan, R. C., and Johnson, D. E. Integrated therapy for invasive bladder carcinoma. Experience with 108 patients. Urology, 12:549, 1978.

94. TJABBES, D. Surgical treatment of 81 deep infiltrating bladder tumours after preoperative irradiation. In: *Bladder Tumors and Other Topics in Urological Oncology.* Vol. 1. Edited by, M. Pavone-Macaluso, P. H. Smith, and F. Edsmyr. New York, Plenum Press, Ettore Majorana International Science Series (Life Sciences), 1980, p. 283.

95. HALL, R. R., and HEATH, A. B. Radiotherapy and cystectomy for T3 bladder carcinoma. Br. J. Urol., *53:*598, 1981.

96. MILLER, L. S. Preoperative irradiation for bladder cancer: The 2,000- versus 5,000-rad controversy. In: *Cancer of the Genitourinary Tract.* Edited by, D. E. Johnson and M. L. Samuels. New York, Raven Press, 1979, p. 81.

97. PEEPLES, W. J. et al. Pathological findings after preoperative irradiation for carcinoma of the urinary bladder. Radiology, *132:*451, 1979.

98. SAGERMAN, R. H. et al. Integrated preoperative irradiation and radical cystectomy. Int. J. Radiat. Oncol. Biol. Phys., *6:*607, 1980.

99. SAUER, R. et al. Preliminary results of treatment of invasive bladder carcinoma with radiotherapy and cisplatin. Int. J. Radiat. Oncol. Biol. Phys., *15:*871, 1988.

100. MARKS, L. B. et al. Invasive bladder carcinoma: Preliminary report of selective bladder conservation by transurethral surgery, upfront MCV (methotrexate, cisplatin, and vinblastine) chemotherapy and pelvic irradiation plus cisplatin. Int. J. Radiat. Oncol. Biol. Phys., *15:*877, 1988.

101. SHIPLEY, W. U. et al. Treatment of invasive bladder cancer by cisplatin and radiation in patients unsuited for surgery. JAMA, *258:*931, 1987.

102. JAKSE, G., FROMMHOLD, H., and ZUR NEDDEN, D. Combined radiation and chemotherapy for locally advanced transitional cell carcinoma of the urinary bladder. Cancer, *55:*1659, 1985.

103. ROTMAN, M. et al. Treatment of advanced bladder carcinoma with irradiation and concomitant 5-fluorouracil infusion. Cancer, *59:*710, 1988.

104. RUSSELL, K. J. et al. Transitional cell carcinoma of the urinary bladder: Histologic clearance with combined 5-FU chemotherapy and radiation therapy. Radiology, *167:*845, 1988.

Radiation Therapy of Prostate Carcinoma

Don R. Goffinet
Malcolm A. Bagshaw

Megavoltage radiation therapy has been used to treat prostate cancer for over 30 years. The techniques of treatment have evolved so that radiation doses of 7,000 rad or more may be safely given to the prostate gland, while, if indicated, at the same time delivering approximately 5,000 rad to the pelvic lymph nodes. With current radiation field-shaping techniques, severe complications from treatment are rare and sequellae during therapy are limited to fatigue, mild diarrhea, and dysuria.[1,2]

Other techniques of prostate irradiation have also been used less frequently. Isotopic radiation sources, such as ^{192}Ir, may be temporarily inserted transperineally into the prostate gland before or after external beam irradiation as a high-dose, limited-volume boost.[3,4] Permanent implants of radioactive sources, usually without concomitant external beam irradiation, using ^{125}I or [103]Pd seeds, may be performed via either the ultrasound-guided transperineal technique[5] or by the retropubic approach to the gland.[6,7]

An individual with newly diagnosed but localized prostate carcinoma is often faced with several choices of treatment, all of which may provide a high probability of local control. For urologic stage-A1, -A2, -B1, and -B2 prostate carcinomas, nerve-sparing radical prostatectomy,[8] external beam irradiation, (possibly with a removable ^{192}Ir implant boost), and permanent ^{125}I seed implantation yield similar results.[9]

PATIENT EVALUATION

In addition to the documentation of the usual urinary symptoms (frequency, nocturia, hesitancy, decreased stream, hematuria, and occasionally hematospermia), the history should include the presence or absence of erectile potency. A tumor drawing detailing the size and extent of the tumor and the prostatic dimensions should be made. The precise documentation of the area of tumor involvement is facilitated by the recent availability of multiple ultrasound-directed transrectal biopsies of the prostate gland.[10] A baseline bone scan, chest film, and computerized tomography (CT) scan of the pelvis and abdomen should be obtained. The prostate specific antigen (PSA) level should be determined. The latter sample should be taken prior to digital prostatic examination. The PSA, although frequently modestly elevated in association with benign prostatic hypertrophy, is an excellent disease-activity

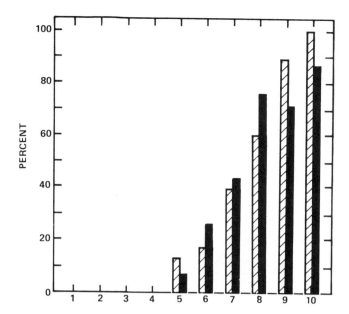

FIG. 54-1. Patients with lymph node metastases versus Gleason pattern score of primary tumor.

marker postoperatively or after a radiation therapy course.[11] Extraperitoneal lymph node sampling is less frequently performed prior to the management of prostate carcinoma by radiation therapy at present. Several reports are available that correlate prostatic cancer size and tumor (Gleason) grade with the risk of lymph node metastases (Fig. 54-1). A useful formula for predicting the incidence of lymph node metastases follows. Percent probability of pelvic or para-aortic lymphadenopathy = (combined Gleason pattern score − 4) × 15.[12]

If a transurethral prostate resection (TURP) is required, radiation therapy (XRT) should be delayed for 6 weeks to 3 months to avoid a possible postirradiation urethral stricture. In addition, ^{125}I seed implants in post-TURP patients may result in urinary seed loss, presumably due to loss of integrity of the urethral epithelium. The possible adverse effect of a TURP on survival and local control after XRT remains controversial.[13,14] In patients with high PSA values, a lymphangiogram may be useful in demonstrating enlarged pelvic or para-aortic lymph nodes with filling defects. Such lymph nodes are accessible to transcutaneous fine-needle aspiration cytologic biopsies without the need for a staging pelvic lymph node dissection. Determining prostate and seminal vesicle size by CT or magnetic resonance imaging (MRI) may be helpful in planning the radiation ports and field sizes.

RADIATION TREATMENT PLANNING

If external beam irradiation is to be performed, the prostate volume must be clearly defined and appropriately localized. The distal prostate (apex) may be well localized by a urethrogram: after topical anesthesia of the urethra with lidocaine, Hypaque is instilled, and a distal (Zipser) penile clamp is ap-

plied while the localizing radiographs are obtained. Orthogonal radiographs and a treatment planning CT scan are used to identify the width and superior extent of the prostate gland and the superior level of the seminal vesicles. In patients with stage-A1 and -B1 cancers, which have a low Gleason grade, a small prostatic portal is satisfactory, usually 8 × 7 or 9 × 7 cm. Such fields may be treated using 120° bilateral arcs at 180 to 200 rad per day for a total dose to the prostate gland of approximately 7,600 rad in 7.5 weeks. Alternatively, four fields may be used (AP-PA, right and left lateral) that are especially prepared with cerrobend collimators, which conform to the treatment volume (Fig. 54-2). A treatment plan is produced that documents the prostatic, rectal, and femoral head radiation doses. A more advanced or higher grade prostate neoplasm (A2, B2, C, or high Gleason grade) may require irradiation of both the pelvic lymph nodes and the prostate.

PELVIC-PROSTATE IRRADIATION

The prostate is localized as above by the use of a urethrogram and CT or MRI scan. An individually planned four-field radiation technique, consisting of anterior-posterior and specially shaped opposed lateral portals is used; all of the radiation ports are treated each day. The shaped fields extend from the superior margin of the fifth lumbar vertebra caudal to the bulbar urethra (Fig. 54-3). Posteriorly, the anus and posterior rectum are shielded, while much of the bladder is protected anteriorly. These radiation fields are treated five times per week (200 rad per day) to a total dose of 2,600 rad, at which time the four-field pelvic ports are discontinued and the prostate alone is treated (usually by bilateral 120° arcs) for the next 10 fractions over 2 weeks (Fig. 54-4). The large pelvic fields are then resumed, completing the treatment to the lymph nodes and the prostate. During this 7-week period, the pelvic lymph nodes receive 5,000 rad and the prostate 7,000 rad.

If there is extensive pelvic lymph adenopathy or proven para-aortic lymph node involvement, the para-aortic lymph nodes may also be irradiated. They are treated by anterior and posterior ports (two fields per day) for 4 weeks, beginning coincident with the start of the midcourse pelvic field reduction and continuing through the middle and final thirds of the pelvic treatment. A radiation dose of 4,000 rad is delivered through the AP-PA fields and the final booster dose of 1,000 rad is given through shaped opposed lateral ports.

SURVIVAL FOLLOWING X-IRRADIATION

The Stanford series is now approaching 30 years in scope and it continues to reflect the general experience following x-irradiation of prostatic cancer; the longest survivor is still living without clinically evident disease (NCED) at 29 years post-treatment. For example, similar long-term survival has been reported by Perez and coworkers for the Washington University series, and by Hanks and coworkers for the Patterns of Care experience.[15,16]

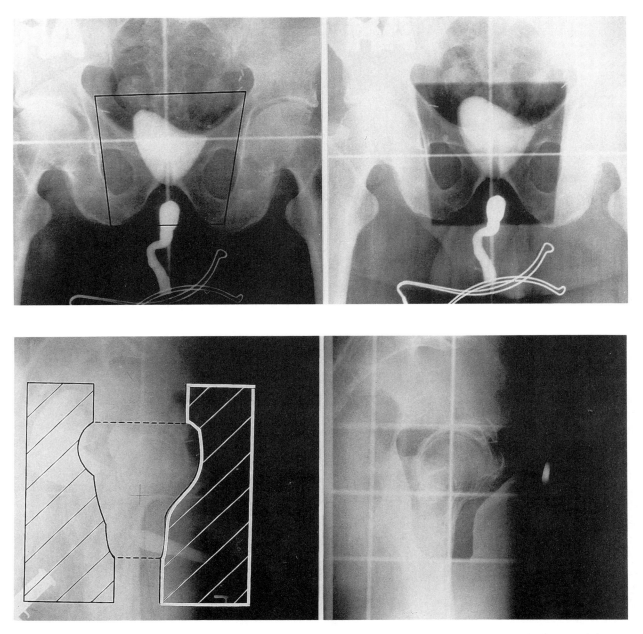

FIG. 54-2. *A,* Anterior-posterior opposed component of small four-field (keystone) prostate radiation technique. This is termed the *keystone technique* because of the trapezoidal shape of the anterior and posterior fields. The wide base of the trapezoid covers the superior region of the seminal vesicles. *B,* Left and right lateral fields of the four-port keystone treatment technique. These fields are individually shaped by cerrobend outboard collimators (hatched lines) to conform to the prostatic bed and protect the posterior wall of the rectum and the anterior cortex of the pubic bone. The bulbar urethra is identified by radio-opaque contrast (Hypaque) introduced through the meatus and held in place by a Zipser clamp placed across the penis. Before inserting the Hypaque, the urethra is anesthetized by inserting 2% lidocaine jelly. It is believed necessary to irradiate at least 1½ cm of the prostatic urethra in the postprostatectomy situation in order to sterilize potential residual tumor at the site of the prostatic apex.

The overall survival by clinical stage for the Stanford series is shown in Figure 54-5. The Stanford clinical staging system is presented in more detail elsewhere;[2] however, a comparison with more conventional urological systems is given in Table 54-1. The disease-specific survival, that is, counting death owing to prostatic cancer only, is presented in Figure 54-6. Freedom from relapse is shown in Figure 54-7. Local control, as determined by digital rectal examination (DRE), is presented in Figure 54-8.

Figure 54-9 demonstrates the survival following irradiation of patients who were comparable to those currently being selected for radical prostatectomy in many centers, with one powerful exception. That exception is adenopathy. Positive adenopathy is usually considered a contraindication to radical prostatectomy and, therefore, patients with biopsy-proven lymph nodes are excluded. The status of the lymph nodes is usually unknown in patients treated by radiation, as was the case for most of the patients included in Figure 54-9. All pa-

TABLE 54-1. *Nominal Comparison of American ABC Staging System and Stanford TNM System*

STAGING	
A, B, C, D	STANFORD TNM
A1, A2	T0f, T0d
B1, B2 ~ B3	T1a, T1b, T1c, T1d
~B3	T2a, T2b
C	T3a, T3b, T4
D	Any T + N

tients with the relevant primary tumor stages were included, irrespective of whether lymphadenopathy was known. Information gleaned from previous staging laparotomies indicates that at least 20% of the patients included in Figure 54-9 already had lymph node metastases.[17] Yet the 15-year survival value of 40% is only 8% less than that expected for an age-matched cohort. Moreover, in contrast to the surgical selection process in which patients are occasionally rejected for surgery due to medical reasons, there were no medical contraindications to radiotherapy. This figure also demonstrates the disease-specific survival in this group of patients, revealing that at 15 years only 30% of the patients have died because of prostate cancer.

OTHER RADIATION MODALITIES

Treatment with permanent ^{125}I implants and pelvic lymph node dissection has been used to treat localized prostate can-

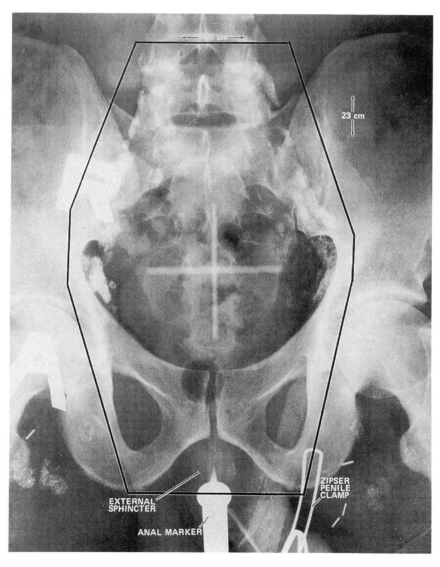

FIG. 54-3A. Parallel-opposed anterior and posterior fields in the large 4-field pelvis-prostate treatment technique. These are called *stopsign* fields because of the obvious similarity to the shape of a traffic stopsign.

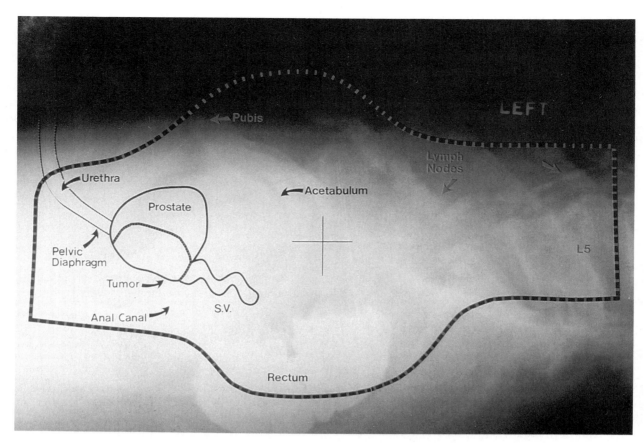

Fig. 54-3B. Left and right lateral fields in the large four-field treatment technique. As in the small four-field technique, the lateral fields are individualized by the preparation of collimators cast in cerrobend to protect the posterior wall of the rectum and anterior pubic bone.

cers at Memorial Hospital in New York City for the last 15 years.[6] The results in patients with stage-B1 and -B2 tumors, with and without pelvic lymph node involvement, are similar to those obtained with external beam irradiation at Stanford. A subgroup of patients with high Gleason pattern scores has been found to have a high local relapse rate after ^{125}I seed implants, suggesting that tumor cell repopulation occurred during the low rate of delivery of photon irradiation characteristic of ^{125}I radiation.[7] Perhaps [103]Pd sources, which have a shorter half-life (17 days) than [125]I (60 days) and therefore deliver radiation at a higher dose rate, will be a more suitable permanent implant source for patients with high Gleason grade neoplasms.

Apparently viable tumor cells have been noted in over 70% of postirradiation biopsies (more than 17 months after treatment) in patients who originally had extracapsular tumor extension, when such biopsies were performed prospectively.[18] For this reason, removable transperineal [192]I implants may be used to boost the prostate dose an additional 3,000 rad after a 5,000 rad external beam radiation course. Such combined treatment can deliver a higher radiation dose to the tumor volume, with lower normal tissue side effects, than can be obtained with external beam irradiation alone. The interstitial treatments may also be carried out with the adjuvant use of radiofrequency hyperthermia, but such treatments are experi-

mental at present and should be limited to centers performing clinical trials for prostate cancer.

In a previous study, external beam radiotherapy appeared useful in certain patients after radical prostatectomy (Fig. 54-10). More recently, 23 patients at Stanford had detectable levels of serum PSA after prostatectomy and prior to radiotherapy. A total of 20 patients had detectable serum PSA after surgery as the only evidence of recurrent or residual neoplasm (biochemical disease), while three patients had biopsy-proven palpable local recurrences. If a bone scan, physical examination, chest radiograph, and CT or MRI scan of the prostatic fossa fails to demonstrate a recurrence, it may be assumed that a subclinical prostatic bed relapse has occurred. The PSA values prior to radiotherapy ranged from 0.5 to 72.0, with a mean of 7.3 ± 15.8 ng/mL. Within 6 months of prostatectomy, 17 patients were irradiated to the prostatic bed; 6 received radiotherapy from 7 to 40 months after surgery. PSA values diminished in 18 of the 19 patients (determined serially post irradiation). The PSA remains detectable in the serum of 11 patients; in 4 of these, the PSA decreased to 0 after radiotherapy, but subsequently rose to detectable levels. The PSA value remains 0 in 6 patients. To date none of the patients has developed clinically apparent local recurrence or distant metastases. These data suggest that (1) any detectable level of PSA after radical prostatectomy is an indication of persistent or recur-

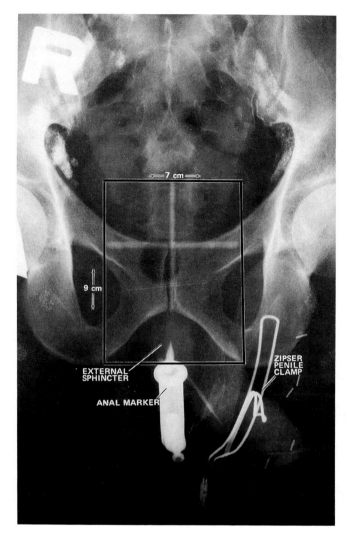

Fig. 54-4. Coned-down volume for delivery of radiation booster dose to the prostate and seminal vesicles. Either bilateral right and left 120° arcs or the four-field keystone technique may be used for the prostate-seminal vesicle boost.

rent carcinoma and (2) some patients may be cured of residual cancer by the addition of radiotherapy after prostatectomy.

MORBIDITY

In the most recent decade, morbidity attributed to radiation treatment has significantly decreased. In comparing the decade 1965 through 1974 with the decade 1975 through 1984, it was found in the Stanford series that severe intestinal sequellae dropped from 6.5 to 2.4%, and urologic sequellae decreased from 10.9 to 7.2%, representing a statistically significant overall reduction of morbidity.[2] In this analysis, there was no attempt to differentiate between the complications produced by the radiation and those produced by persistent or recurrent tumor. The numbers, therefore, overstate the true incidence of sequellae attributed to radiation alone.

Preservation of potency is an important consideration for patients undergoing treatment for prostatic cancer. In this

study, approximately one half, or 434 patients claimed erectile potency prior to irradiation. Of these, 86.4% remained potent at 15 months following treatment (Fig. 54-11). From that time onward, there was a gradual diminution of potency with advancing age. Nevertheless, 50% of the patients remained potent at the seventh postirradiation year and more than 30% maintained sexual performance for the duration of their survival.

Finally, there is concern as to whether the radiation exposure in the treatment of prostatic cancer can induce a second carcinoma. Table 54-2 demonstrates that 10.8% of the patients surviving prostatic cancer develop a second neoplasm. However, this was found to be nearly identical in incidence to the male population at large, and the spectrum of second cancers observed was essentially identical to that which would be expected in an age-matched population. There appears to be no additional risk for the development of a second neoplasm that can be attributed to irradiation.

CONCLUSION

The above data demonstrate that radiation therapy is a viable alternative to surgery in the treatment of patients with prostatic cancer. Actuarial survival rates of 81%, 60%, and 34% at 5, 10, and 15 years, respectively, have been achieved for patients with disease limited to the prostate and 60%, 35%, and 17% at 5, 10, and 15 years, respectively, for those with extracapsular extension. Higher survival rates can be achieved for patients with more restricted nodular disease and in patients with known absence of lymphadenopathy.

Evaluation of the histopathology by the Gleason method permits a reasonable estimate of the probability of both lymph

TABLE 54-2. *Incidence of Second Cancers Following Prostate Cancer* (914 Patients at Risk for More Than 7,000 Person-Years, 1956–1985)

TYPE OF CANCER*	OBSERVED	EXPECTED	P-VALUE
Lung	28	29.3	0.81
Colon	15	15.2	0.96
Bladder	11	10.2	0.80
Stomach	6	5.4	0.80
Rectum	4	7.4	0.21
Leukemia	4	3.8	0.92
Lymphoma	3	4.1	0.65
Pancreas	3	4.6	0.27
Kidney	1	2.9	0.26
Other	24	(24.0)	
Total	99 (10.8%)	106.9	0.48

*Observed second cancers versus expected incidence as calculated by the method of Monson from SEER Program data for San Francisco Bay Area white males.

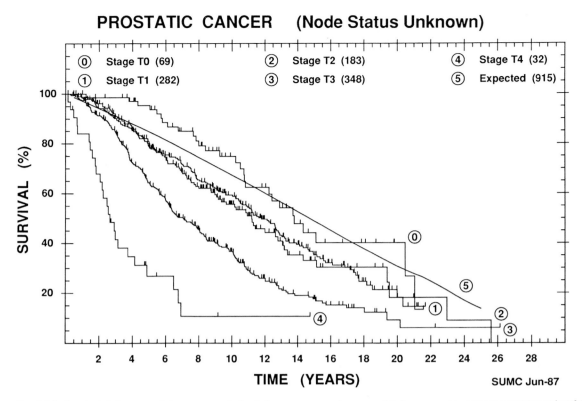

PROSTATIC CANCER   (Node Status Unknown)

⓪ Stage T0 (69)   ② Stage T2 (183)   ④ Stage T4 (32)
① Stage T1 (282)   ③ Stage T3 (348)   ⑤ Expected (915)

FIG. 54-5. Survival. A downward step represents death from any cause. An upward tick represents a patient surviving at last follow-up and censored at the time indicated by the abscissa. The patient may or may not have residual or metastatic cancer.

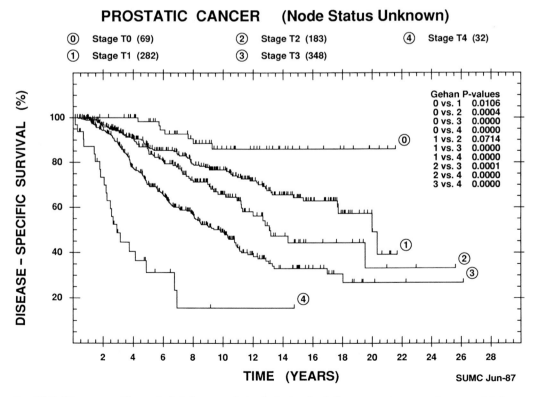

PROSTATIC CANCER   (Node Status Unknown)

⓪ Stage T0 (69)   ② Stage T2 (183)   ④ Stage T4 (32)
① Stage T1 (282)   ③ Stage T3 (348)

Gehan P-values
0 vs. 1   0.0106
0 vs. 2   0.0004
0 vs. 3   0.0000
0 vs. 4   0.0000
1 vs. 2   0.0714
1 vs. 3   0.0000
1 vs. 4   0.0000
2 vs. 3   0.0001
2 vs. 4   0.0000
3 vs. 4   0.0000

FIG. 54-6. Disease-specific survival. A downward step indicates death from prostate cancer. An upward tick represents a patient who either died because of intercurrent disease or was alive at the time of last follow-up. The patient may or may not have cancer.

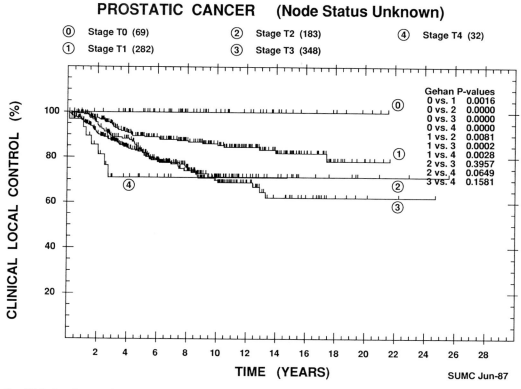

PROSTATIC CANCER (Node Status Unknown)

⓪	Stage T0 (69)	②	Stage T2 (183)	④	Stage T4 (32)
①	Stage T1 (282)	③	Stage T3 (348)		

Gehan P-values
0 vs. 1 0.0005
0 vs. 2 0.0000
0 vs. 3 0.0000
0 vs. 4 0.0000
1 vs. 2 0.0009
1 vs. 3 0.0000
1 vs. 4 0.0000
2 vs. 3 0.0001
2 vs. 4 0.0000
3 vs. 4 0.0001

FREEDOM FROM RELAPSE (%)

TIME (YEARS)

SUMC Jun-87

FIG. 54-7. Freedom from relapse. A downward step indicates the first evidence of recurrence, either at the primary site or at a metastatic site as detected by either clinical observation or by a positive biopsy. An upward tick represents a patient who was either observed disease free or died disease free at the time of last observation.

PROSTATIC CANCER (Node Status Unknown)

⓪	Stage T0 (69)	②	Stage T2 (183)	④	Stage T4 (32)
①	Stage T1 (282)	③	Stage T3 (348)		

Gehan P-values
0 vs. 1 0.0016
0 vs. 2 0.0000
0 vs. 3 0.0000
0 vs. 4 0.0000
1 vs. 2 0.0081
1 vs. 3 0.0002
1 vs. 4 0.0028
2 vs. 3 0.3957
2 vs. 4 0.0649
3 vs. 4 0.1581

CLINICAL LOCAL CONTROL (%)

TIME (YEARS)

SUMC Jun-87

FIG. 54-8. Local control. A downward step indicates clinical evidence of local regrowth after initial regression of tumor or after initially showing no evidence of local neoplasm. An upward tick represents a patient who demonstrated either no clinical evidence of local tumor at last follow-up or died without clinical evidence of local neoplasm. The patient could have had evidence of metastatic tumor either while living or at death.

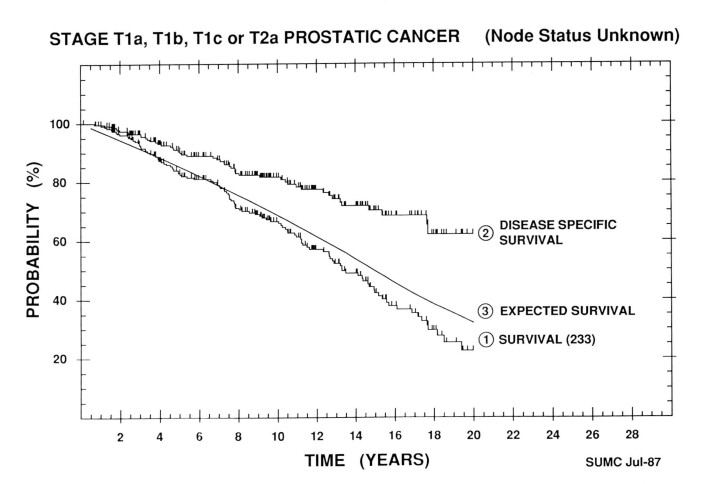

FIG. 54-9. Stage T1a, T1b, T1c, or T2a prostatic cancer (node status unknown). Survival and disease-specific survival for patients with nodular lesions, either apparently confined to 1 lobe (T1a, T1b, and T1c) or confined to 1 lobe with distortion of the capsule (T2a).

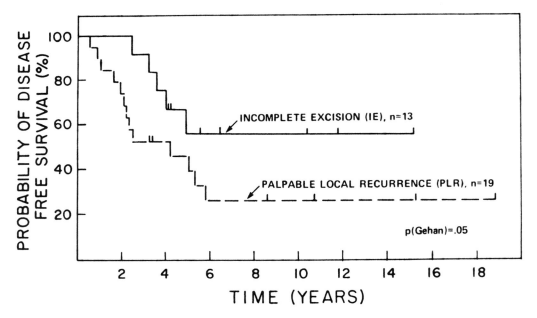

FIG. 54-10. Actuarial disease-free survival (freedom from relapse) in patients receiving radiation therapy for salvage after radical prostatectomy. Reprinted with permission from International Journal of Radiation Oncology Biology Physics, vol. 12, Bagshaw, Current conflicts in the management of prostatic cancer, 1986, Pergamon Press plc.

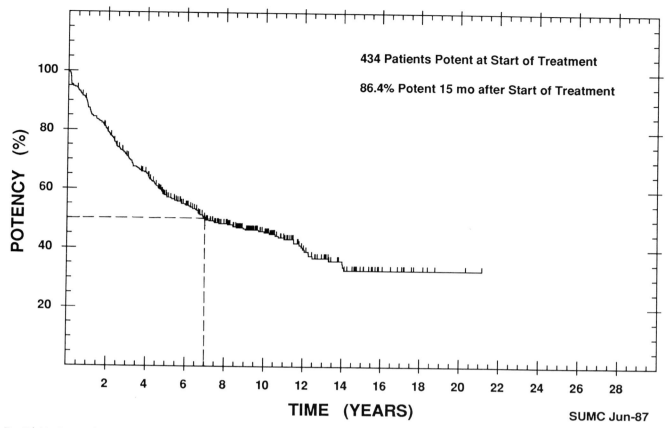

PROSTATIC CANCER (Node Status Unknown)

434 Patients Potent at Start of Treatment

86.4% Potent 15 mo after Start of Treatment

POTENCY (%)

TIME (YEARS)

SUMC Jun-87

FIG. 54-11. Status of erectile potency after external beam irradiation. A total of 50% of those patients who were initially potent retained the ability to have an erection at 7 years postirradiation (dotted line).

node involvement and ultimate survival. The morbidity of radiation therapy has been significantly reduced in the past decade, and all but a few patients tolerate the treatment without difficulty or significant morbidity.

Erectile potency is preserved in many patients; however, as might be expected, it diminishes with advancing age.

Radiation therapy is well tolerated after radical prostatectomy and should be administered in patients with frankly transected extracapsular disease, as in postprostatectomy patients in whom the PSA is rising but who have no other evidence of metastases.

REFERENCES

1. BAGSHAW, M. A. The role of radiation therapy in the management of prostate carcinoma. Probl. Urol., *1:*181, 1987.
2. BAGSHAW, M. A., COX, R. S., and RAY, G. R. Status of radiation treatment of prostate cancer at Stanford University. NCI Monogr, 7:47, 1988.
3. KHAN, K., CRAWFORD, E. D., and JOHNSON, E. L. Transperineal percutaneous iridium-192 implant of the prostate. Int. J. Radiat. Oncol. Biol. Phys., 9:1391, 1983.
4. TANSEY, L. A., SHANBERG, A. M., SYED, A. M. N., and PUTHAWALA, A. Treatment of prostatic carcinoma by pelvic lymphadenectomy, temporary iridium-192 implant, and external irradiation. Urology, *21:*594, 1983.
5. BLASKO, J. C., RADGE, H., and SCHUMACHER, D.: Transperineal percutaneous iodine-125 implantation for prostatic carcinoma using transrectal ultrasound and template guidance. Endocurie. Hypotherm. Oncol., *3:*131, 1987.
6. DEBLASIO, D. S. et al. Permanent interstitial implantation of prostatic cancer in the 1980's. Endocurie. Hypertherm. Oncol., *4:*193, 1988.
7. KUBAN, D. A., EL-MAHDI, A. M., and SCHELLHAMMER, P. F. I-125 interstitial implantation for prostate cancer: What have we learned 10 years later? Cancer, *63:*2415, 1989.
8. EGGLESTON, J. C., and WALSH, P. C. Radical prostatectomy with preservation of sexual function: Pathological findings in the first 100 cases. J. Urol., *134:*1146, 1985.
9. FREIHA, F. S., BAGSHAW, M. A., and TORTI, F. M.: Carcinoma of the prostate: Pathology, staging, and treatment. Curr. Probl. Cancer, *12:*1, 1988.

10. TORP-PEDERSEN, S. et al. Transrectal biopsy of the prostate guided with transrectal US: Longitudinal and multiplanar scanning. Radiology, *170*:23, 1989.

11. STAMEY, T. A. et al. Prostate-specific antigen as a serum marker for adenocarcinoma of the prostate. N. Engl. J. Med., *317*:909, 1987.

12. WOO, S., KAPLAN, I., ROACH, M., and BAGSHAW, M. Formula to estimate risk of pelvic lymph node metastasis from the total Gleason score for prostate cancer. J. Urol., *140*:387, 1988.

13. MCGOWAN, D. G. The effect of transurethral resectional on prognosis in carcinoma of the prostate: Real or imaginary? Int. J. Radiat. Oncol. Biol. Phys., *15*:1057, 1988.

14. SANDLER, H. M., and HANKS, G. E. Analysis of the possibility that transurethral resection promotes metastasis in prostate cancer. Cancer, *62*:2622, 1988.

15. PEREZ, C. A. et al. Definitive radiation therapy in carcinoma of the prostate localized to the pelvis: Experience at the Mallinckrodt Institute of Radiology. NCI Monogr., 7:85, 1988.

16. HANKS, G. E. External-beam radiation therapy for clinically localized prostate cancer: Patterns of care outcome studies. NCI Monogr., 7:75, 1988.

17. PISTENMA, D. A., BAGSHAW, M. A., FREIHA, F. S. Extended-field radiation therapy for prostatic adenocarcinoma: Status report of a limited prospective trial. In: *Cancer of the Genitourinary Tract.* Edited by D. E. Johnson and M. L. Samuels. New York, Raven Press, 1979, p. 229.

18. FREIHA, F. S., and BAGSHAW, M. A. Carcinoma of the prostate: Results of post-irradiation biopsy. Prostate, 5:19, 1984.

Radiation Therapy of Testicular Seminoma

William T. Sause

M alignant tumors of the testes constitute 1% of all cancers in North American men. The age-specific incidence reaches a high of 9.7 cases per 100,000 in men from 25 to 29 years of age and falls to 1.1 cases per 100,000 in men 65 to 69 years of age. Testicular neoplasms are the most common form of cancer in men between the ages of 20 and 34 years of age in the United States. Testicular seminoma represents a distinctive neoplasm constituting approximately 30 to 40% of all testicular tumors. Seminoma generally occurs in an older age than the nonseminomatous germ cell tumors. The peak incidence of seminomas ranges from approximately 30 to 40 years of age while the peak incidence for nonseminomatous tumors is from approximately 19 to 30 years of age.[1-3]

Histologically, seminomas have been divided into classic, anaplastic, and spermatic seminomas. Although the spermatic seminomas generally occur in an older age group, the prognosis and clinical behavior of seminoma based on histologic subclassification is not clinically useful. Stage for stage, these tumors behave in a similar fashion.[2-4]

Serum tumor markers are less important in the management and evaluation of seminomatous tumors than the nonseminomatous germ cell tumors of the testicle. Although small elevations in the human chorionic gonadotropin (HCG) levels are seen in pure seminomas, elevations of alpha-fetoprotein should never be seen in patients with pure seminoma.[2,4,5] The presence of alpha-fetoprotein in testicular tumors signifies the presence of yolk sac differentiation even when this is undetected histologically. Those patients should be treated as nonseminomatous germ cell tumors of the testicle. HCG is a glycoprotein produced by the syncytiotrophoblastic cells of choriocarcinoma, placenta, embryonal carcinoma, and seminoma. HCG is composed of an alpha and a beta chain, the latter being sufficiently dissimilar from the beta chains of other tropic hormones to be measured by radioimmunoassay. The development of sensitive beta chain HCG assays has revealed elevation in somewhere between 40 and 60% of patients with testicular neoplasms.[4] Approximately 5 to 10% of patients with pure seminoma will have elevated beta HCG levels. In most instances the levels are less than 100 mg/mL.[5] Little evidence exists however, that those patients respond differently to standard therapy than patients with no elevation of these HCG subunits. Although the prognosis is not altered by elevated HCG, it does allow the opportunity to determine the effectiveness of therapy with serial levels.

Several clinical staging systems are used for testicular neoplasms. The Walter Reed General Hospital System, Royal Marsden, the UICC, and the American Joint Committee are common staging systems for the management of testicular neoplasms (Table 55-1). The radiographic evaluation of patients with seminoma has undergone a substantial evolution during the past 25 years. Initially, only chest x-rays and intravenous pyelograms were utilized to stage patients with testicular neoplasms. Obviously, the inaccuracy of these studies resulted in a substantial understaging. Most series of any size report treatment results of patients staged with only chest

TABLE 55-1. *Staging Systems for Tumors of the Testis*

WALTER REED GENERAL HOSPITAL	UICC	AMERICAN JOINT COMMITTEE	ROYAL MARSDEN HOSPITAL
Stage IA: tumor confined to one testis; no clinical or roentgenographic evidence of spread by excretory or retrograde urography, lymphangiography, inferior venacavography, or chest roentgenography Stage IB: histologic evidence of metastases to the iliac or periaortic lymph nodes Stage II: clinical or roentgenographic evidence of metastases to femoral, inguinal, iliac, or periaortic lymph nodes with no evidence of metastases to lymphatics above the diaphragm or to visceral organs Stage III: clinical or roentgenographic evidence of metastases above the diaphragm or to visceral organs	T: primary tumor Tx: the minimum requirements to assess fully the extent of the primary tumor cannot be met T0: no evidence of primary tumor T1: tumor limited to the body of the testis T2: tumor extending beyond the tunica albuginea T3: tumor involving the rete testis or epididymis T4: tumor invading the spermatic cord and/or scrotal wall T4a: invasion of spermatic cord T4b: invasion of scrotal wall N: regional and juxtaregional lymph nodes Nx: the minimum requirements to assess the regional lymph nodes cannot be met N0: no evidence of involvement of regional lymph nodes N1: involvement of a single homolateral regional lymph node, which, if inguinal, is mobile N2: involvement of contralateral or bilateral or multiple regional lymph nodes, which, if inguinal, is mobile N3: a palpable abdominal mass is present or there are fixed inguinal lymph nodes N4: involvement of juxtaregional lymph nodes M: distant metastasis Mx: the minimum requirements to assess the presence of distant metastases cannot be met. M0: no evidence of distant metastases M1: distant metastases present	T: primary tumor Tx: minimum requirement cannot be met (in the absence of orchiectomy, Tx must be used) T0: no evidence of primary tumor T1: limited to body of testis T2: extends beyond the tunica albuginea T3: involvement of the rete testis or epididymis T4: invasion of spermatic cord T4a: invasion of spermatic cord T4b: invasion of scrotal wall N: nodal involvement Nx: minimum requirements cannot be met N0: no evidence of involvement of regional lymph nodes N1: involvement of a single homolateral regional lymph node which, if inguinal, is mobile N2: involvement of contralateral or bilateral or multiple regional lymph nodes which, if inguinal, are mobile N3: palpable abdominal mass present or fixed inguinal lymph nodes N4: involvement of juxtaregional nodes M: distant metastases Mx: not assessed M0: no (known) distant metastasis M1: distant metastasis present	I: lymphogram negative, no evidence of metastases II: lymphogram positive, metastases confined to abdominal nodes, 3 subgroups recognized A: maximum diameter of metastases 2 cm B: maximum diameter of metastases 2–5 cm C: maximum diameter of metastases 5 cm III: involvement of supradiaphragmatic and infradiaphragmatic lymph nodes; no extralymphatic metastases; abdominal status: A, B, C as for stage II IV: extralymphatic metastases

x-ray and intravenous pyelography and this makes comparison to modern treatment difficult. The development of the bipedal lymphangiography was a substantial improvement in the detection of retroperitoneal disease. Lymphangiography has an accuracy of 80%, however it will not detect occult metastases in approximately 15 to 20% of patients. Lately lymphangiography has been largely replaced by computerized tomography (CT). The accuracy of CT scanning is not appreciably better than lymphangiography, and in some instances the studies may be complimentary.[6,7] However, the noninvasive nature and technical ease of the CT scanning have resulted in its widespread acceptance.

The surgical cure rate for seminoma prior to the institution of radiation therapy was approximately 40%.[8] Postoperative radiation therapy to lymph nodes beyond radiographically detected disease has improved overall cure rates to 80 to 90%.[9-14] Although the cure rate is high, some areas of controversy have developed in the management of seminoma. Analysis of failure patterns and the development of successful systemic treatment for germ cell neoplasms have resulted in re-evaluation of our standard treatment policies. The routine use of postorchiectomy irradiation for stage-I patients, the necessity of mediastinal irradiation in patients with stage-II disease, and the optimal management of patients with bulky abdominal disease represent major areas of controversy.

Approximately 80% of patients with seminoma present with stage-I disease.[11,15,16] The cure rate with modern megavoltage radiation therapy in those patients with radiographic stage-I disease should exceed 95%.[12,15]

Traditional irradiation fields have included the para-aortic lymph nodes and ipsilateral iliac nodes. The primary areas of testicular lymphatic drainage are in the upper lumbar area and by extending the field to T11, the majority of potentially involved nodes will be encompassed (Fig. 55-1). The inguinal nodes and scrotum are not routinely treated unless violation of the scrotum occurs by tumor or at biopsy. Modern urologic intervention with high inguinal exploration should make scrotal biopsy an unusual event (see Chap. 33).

Doses as low as 2,500 cGy delivered in 20 fractions to the retroperitoneal lymph nodes have resulted in essentially 100% tumor sterilization.[8,10,15,17] The acute morbidity associated with this dose is related to mild nausea and diarrhea but long-term morbidity is virtually nonexistent.

Iatrogenic infertility following standard irradiation for stage-I seminoma is a concern. When the radiation portal does not extend below the obturator foramen, transient oligospermia may occur lasting 2 to 8 months but in most instances spermatogenesis is retained. When the field extends to the scrotum or inguinal area, permanent azospermia may occur.[18]

Several investigators have recommended surveillance in stage-I nonseminomatous tumor.[1] A surveillance policy spares the majority of patients retroperitoneal surgery and cytotoxic chemotherapy. Salvage chemotherapy is usually successful in case of relapse. A similar policy of observation has been advocated in stage I-seminoma.[19,20] Surgical data suggest that ap-

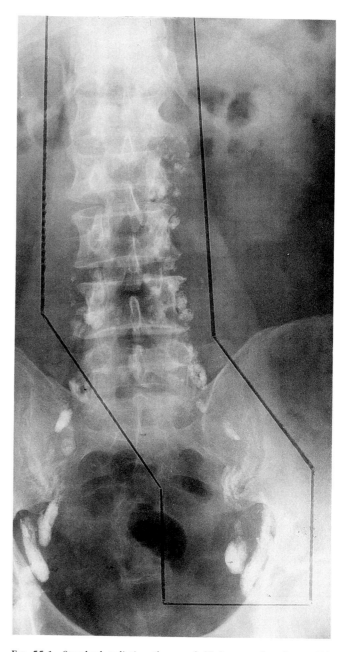

FIG. 55-1. Standard radiation therapy field for stage-I and stage-IIA seminoma.

proximately 20% of radiographic stage-I patients will have retroperitoneal disease and a surveillance policy would spare 80% of patients unnecessary irradiation. Several studies are currently in progress in an attempt to answer this question.[8]

Several factors make an observation policy in seminoma less attractive than in nonseminomatous tumors. Current radiotherapy policies are extremely effective with minimal morbidity. Relapses in seminoma may occur at a later time than nonseminomatous tumors and serum markers are generally not helpful. The cost and compliance with follow-up studies may be more difficult than routine adjuvant irradiation, and a bulky relapse may jeopardize the opportunity for cure. Standard therapy for stage-I seminoma should include routine retroperitoneal irradiation.

Traditionally in stage-IIA disease, radiation therapists have treated the subdiaphragmatic lymphatics as in stage-I disease. Standard treatment policy has been irradiation to the next echelon of uninvolved lymph nodes. In stage-II disease this represents the mediastinal and supraclavicular lymph nodes.[10,13,15] Local control and cure of patients with subdiaphragmatic disease less than 5 cm has been achieved in 89 to 100% of the patients utilizing standard treatment policies.[21]

The treatment policy of mediastinal irradiation was developed in an era prior to the development of effective systemic treatment for seminoma. Isolated mediastinal and supraclavicular relapses do occur in patients with stage-IIA disease. However, this relapse pattern is unusual and does not occur with a greater frequency than other systemic or abdominal relapses in patients with stage-IIA disease. Compiled data from Thomas and coworkers reveal that only 8 of 250 patients with stage-IIA disease treated with infradiaphragmatic irradiation therapy exhibited mediastinal relapse.[8,10,11] With effective systemic salvage therapy, routine mediastinal/supraclavicular radiation therapy is difficult to recommend in stage-IIA disease.

The major controversy in the treatment of testicular seminomas is in the management of stage-IIB disease. Patients with bulky retroperitoneal disease (>5 cm) can be cured with irradiation alone but many series have reported a high relapse rate.[5,21–23] Peckham reported a recurrence rate of 28% in patients with disease greater than 5 cm.[24] Thomas reported a cure rate of 62% with palpable abdominal disease.[8] Conversely, Smalley was able to obtain a cure rate of 100% in 16 patients with greater than 5 cm in diameter retroperitoneal disease.[25,26] These patients were treated with modern radiation therapy and the benefit of CT scanning. Although patients with stage-IIB disease represent a small number of patients, they do pose a difficult management problem.

Prophylactic mediastinal irradiation in patients with stage-IIB disease is discouraged. Although mediastinal relapses may occur in approximately 20% of patients with stage-IIB disease, they often occur in conjunction with abdominal and other systemic relapses.[11,24] With effective combination chemotherapy, the additional bone marrow irradiated by a prophylactic mediastinal field is probably unjustified, as cure rates (with or without mediastinal irradiation) in stage IIB are in the range of 75 to 80%.

Modern systemic therapy in advanced seminoma has produced response rates of 60 to 90%, with two thirds of those patients maintaining the response.[20,27–32] Some authors have advocated combination chemotherapy/irradiation in patients with stage-IIB disease.[33–35] The recommendation is based on the generally poor results reported in the radiation therapy literature and the effectiveness of chemotherapy. Whether combination chemotherapy/irradiation would be preferable with modern diagnostic imaging and irradiation is an unanswered question.[36]

Stage-III and -IV disease at presentation is unusual. Only 4% of those patients seen at the Princess Margaret Hospital between 1977 and 1981 presented with stage-III or -IV disease.[8] Cure rates for stage-III disease utilizing radiation therapy alone are approximately 30%.[8,37] Systemic chemotherapy should be more effective than irradiation in the management of stage-III and -IV disease. Radiation therapy may play a role in further sterilization of residual masses (>3 cm) following induction chemotherapy. Viable tumor can be found when residual disease is greater than 3 cm following chemotherapy.[38]

CONCLUSIONS

STAGE-I DISEASE: External beam irradiation to the retroperitoneum should be 95% effective and rarely cause complications. Although an observation policy is being tested, it is not yet recommended as standard therapy.

STAGE-IIA DISEASE: Radiation therapy as delivered in stage-I disease should be utilized in patients with minimal (<5 cm) retroperitoneal disease. Routine prophylactic mediastinal radiation therapy is not recommended.

STAGE-IIB DISEASE (>5 cm): The management of bulky retroperitoneal disease is controversial. Combined therapy utilizing chemotherapy and irradiation may be indicated although modern radiation therapy produces high cure rates.

STAGE-III AND -IV DISEASE: Cytotoxic chemotherapy is the treatment of choice with irradiation reserved for sterilization of residual disease following systemic therapy.

REFERENCES

1. DAHL, O. Testicular carcinoma—A curable malignancy. Acta Radiol. Oncol., 24:3, 1985.
2. LOEHRER, P. J., SLEDGE, G. W., and EINHORN, L. H. Heterogeneity among germ cell tumors of the testis. Semin. Oncol., 12:304, 1985.
3. DEL REGATO, J. A., SPJUT, H. J., and COX, J. D. Testis. In: Ackerman & del Regato's Cancer—Diagnosis, Treatment, & Prognosis. 6th Ed. Edited by S. Harshberger, and R. Kasper. St. Louis: C. V. Mosby Company, 1985, p. 705.
4. MOSTOFI, F. K. Tumor markers and pathology of testicular tumors. In: Progress and Controversies in Oncological Urology. Edited by K. H. Kurth, F. M. Dedruyne, and F. H. Schroeter. New York: Alan R. Liss, Inc., 1984, p. 69.
5. THOMAS, G. M. Controversies in the managment of testicular seminoma. Cancer, 55:2296, 1985.
6. TAYLOR, R. E., DUNCAN, W., BEST, J. J. K. Influence of computed tomography scanning and lymphography on the management of testicular germ-cell tumors. Clin. Radiol., 37:539, 1986.

7. Samuelsson, L., Forsberg, L., Olsson, A. M. Accuracy of radiological staging procedures in non-seminomatous testis cancer compared with findings from surgical exploration and histopathological studies of extirpated tissue. Br. J. Radiol., *59*:131, 1986.

8. Thomas, G. M., and Herman, J. G. The role of radiation in the management of seminoma. In: *Progress and Controversies in Oncological Urology.* Edited by K. H. Kurth, F. M. Dedruyne, and F. H. Schroeter. New York, Alan R. Liss, Inc., 1984, p. 91.

9. Hamilton, C., Horwich, D. E., and Peckham, M. J. Radiotherapy for stage I seminoma testis: Results of treatment and complications. Radiother. Oncol., *6*:115, 1986.

10. Sause, W. T. Testicular seminoma—Analysis of radiation therapy for stage II disease. J. Urol., *130*:702, 1983.

11. Thomas, G. M., et al. Seminoma of the testis: Results of treatment and patterns of failure after radiation therapy. Int. J. Radiat. Oncol. Biol. Phys. *8*:165, 1982.

12. Babaian, R. J., and Zagars, G. K. Testicular seminoma: The M. D. Anderson experience. An analysis of pathological and patient characteristics and treatment recommendations. J. Urol., *139*:311, 1988.

13. Maier, J. G., and Sulak, M. H. Radiation therapy in malignant testis tumors—Part I: Seminoma; Part II: Carcinoma. Cancer, *32*:1212, 1973.

14. Doornbos, J. F., Hussey, D. H., and Johnson, D. E. Radiotherapy for pure seminoma of the testis. Radiology, *116*:401, 1975.

15. Willan, B. D., and McGowan, D. G. Seminoma of the testis: A 22-year experience with radiation therapy. Int. J. Radiat. Oncol. Biol. Phys., *11*:1769, 1985.

16. Hanks, G. E., Herring, D. F., and Kramer, S. Patterns of care outcome studies: Results of the national practice in seminoma of the testis. Int. J. Radiat. Oncol. Biol. Phys., *7*:1413, 1981.

17. van der Werf-Messing, B. Radiotherapeutic treatment of testicular tumors. Int. J. Radiat. Oncol. Biol. Phys. *1*:235, 1976.

18. Fossa, S. D. Fertility after radiotherapy for testicular cancer. In: *Testicular Cancer.* Edited by S. Khoury, R. Kuss, and G. P. Murphy. New York: Alan R. Liss, Inc., 1985, p. 703.

19. Oliver, R. T. D. Limitations to the use of surveillance as an option in the management of stage I seminoma. Int. J. Androl., *10*:263, 1987.

20. Giannone, L., and Wolff, S. Recent progress in the treatment of seminoma. Oncology, *2*:21, 1988.

21. Gregory, C., and Peckham, M. J. Results of radiotherapy for stage II testicular seminoma. Radiother. Oncol., *6*:285, 1986.

22. Laukkanen, E., Olivotto, I., and Jackson, S. Management of seminoma with bulky abdominal disease. Int. J. Radiat. Oncol. Biol. Phys., *14*:227, 1988.

23. Huben, R. P., et al. Seminoma at Roswell Park, 1970 to 1979—An analysis of treatment failures. Cancer, *53*:1451, 1984.

24. Ball, D., Barrett, A., and Peckham, M. J. The Management of Metastatic seminoma testis. Cancer, *50*:2289, 1982.

25. Smalley, S. R., et al. Radiotherapy as initial treatment for bulky stage II testicular seminomas. J. Clin. Oncol., *3*:1333, 1985.

26. Green, N., et al. Radiation therapy in bulky seminoma. Urology, *21*:467, 1983.

27. Loehrer, P. J., et al. Chemotherapy of metastatic seminoma: The Southeastern Cancer Study Group experience. J. Clin. Oncol., *5*:1212, 1987.

28. Einhorn, L. H. Radiotherapy in seminoma: More is not better. Int. J. Radiat. Oncol. Biol. Phys., *8*:309, 1982.

29. Mendenhall, W. L., Williams, S. D., Einhorn, L. H., and Donohue, J. P. Disseminated seminoma: Re-evaluation of treatment protocols. J. Urol., *126*:493, 1981.

30. Fossa, S. D., et al. The treatment of advanced metastatic seminoma: Experience in 55 cases. J. Clin. Oncol. *5*:1071, 1987.

31. Einhorn, L. H. Testicular cancer as a model for a curable neoplasm: The Richard and Hinda Rosenthal Foundation Award Lecture. Cancer Res., *41*:3275, 1982.

32. Roth, B. J., et al. Cisplatin-based combination chemotherapy for disseminated germ cell tumors: Long-term follow-up. J. Clin. Oncol., *8*:1239, 1988.

33. Crawford, E. D., Smith, R. B., and DeKernion, J. B. Treatment of advanced seminoma with pre-radiation chemotherapy. J. Urol. *129*:752, 1983.

34. Motzer, R. J., et al. Advanced seminoma: The role of chemotherapy and adjunctive surgery. Ann. Intern. Med. *108*:513, 1988.

35. Daniels, J. R. Chemotherapy in seminoma: When is it appropriate initial treatment? J. Clin. Oncol., *10*:1294, 1985.

36. Sause, W. T., Hanks, G. E., and Trump, D. L. RTOG/SWOG/ECOG Protocol: Randomized phase III intergroup study of supradiaphragmatic irradiation in stage II-A seminoma. March 7, 1986–January 22, 1988.

37. Dosoretz, D. E., et al. Megavoltage irradiation for pure testicular-seminoma—Results and patterns of failure. Cancer, *48*:2184, 1981.

38. Motzer, R., et al. Residual mass: An indication for further therapy in patients with advanced seminoma following systemic chemotherapy. J. Clin. Oncol., *5*:1064, 1987.

Radiation Therapy of Penile, Urethral, and Renal Cell Carcinoma

Jorge C. Paradelo

CARCINOMA OF THE PENIS

Carcinoma of the penis is relatively rare in the United States, with an estimated incidence of one case per 100,000 per year. Higher rates have been linked to racial differences, lack of circumcision, and lower socioeconomic status. Arising from the lining of the glans, coronal sulcus, or prepuce, penile carcinoma is invariably epidermoid and metastasizes in a significant number of cases to the inguinal nodes, but distant metastases are rare. Thirty-five to 60% of patients have palpable inguinal nodes at presentation, but one-third of them have no evidence of metastasis at surgery. Large tumor size, high histologic grade, and involvement of the scrotum, root of the penis, corpus cavernosum, or inguinal nodes are all clinical prognostic indicators of poor 5-year survival rates ranging from 0 to 30%.[1]

In American centers, surgical intervention is the prevailing method of treatment, resulting in 5-year survival rates of 84 to 90% for stage-I disease and 51 to 64% for stage-II disease.[2,3] In Europe, where radiotherapy is widely used in initial management, similar results are obtained without mutilating surgery and with preservation of organ function. Surgical procedures are often employed in the treatment of radiotherapy failure, without compromising the ultimate cure rate.[4-6]

The radiotherapy management of cancer of the penis entails eradication of the primary tumor and of metastatic disease when present. Treatment is usually tailored to the patient's age, the extent of tumor involvement, and the presence or absence of metastatic involvement of inguinal nodes or distant metastasis. Radical radiotherapy can effectively cure early cases with minimal local side effects and preservation of a functional organ.[7] The lesser the degree of local involvement, the higher the chances for local control. Circumcision prior to irradiation is recommended to improve tolerance to treatment and to prevent synechia and phimosis.[9]

Several techniques can be adapted to the extent of the disease. Radioactive moulds, delivering doses in the range of 6000 to 8000 rads and given in 5 to 14 days at a rate of 1000 rads per day, are capable of achieving an excellent cure rate with satisfactory functional results and few complications.[8,10] This technique, effective for the treatment of superficial lesions, takes advantage of the localized delivery of radiation while affording relative protection to the urethra, thus decreasing the incidence of stricture to less than 5%. More extensive lesions can be treated by orthovoltage or megavoltage external radiotherapy, with a homogeneous dose distribution ensured by the use of specially designed treatment aids.

Doses in the range of 5500 rads, delivered over a period of 3 weeks, can control early tumors in 90% or more of cases, but the incidence of stricture is slightly higher than with moulds.[11]

In the absence of lymphadenopathy, treatment of the inguinal nodes is not recommended.[4] Careful and close follow-up is mandatory to detect suspicious nodes at an early date, and immediate and definitive radical surgical treatment is then indicated if suspicious nodes are found. In debilitated patients and in those for whom surgical intervention is contraindicated, a course of radiotherapy is effective in 25 to 50% of the cases, depending on the extent of involvement.[12-14]

CARCINOMA OF THE FEMALE URETHRA

Urethral carcinoma, which comprises 0.02% of all female malignant tumors, is twice as common in females as in males.[15] Chronic irritation, inflammation, trauma, and leukoplakia have been implicated in the development of this invasive carcinoma, more commonly seen in older, postmenopausal females. The majority of these tumors are epidermoid with transitional cell and adenocarcinoma constituting the remaining 10 to 15%. Prognosis depends primarily on stage and is not strongly influenced by histologic characteristics, which in turn are not related to radiosensitivity.[16,17]

Small lesions of the meatal and distal urethra, usually exophytic or ulcerative, present at a lower stage, which makes them amenable to local treatment,[18-21] with local control obtained in 63 to 88% of the patients.[16,17,22] Radiotherapy for these lesions is administered in the form of interstitial implants of radium, cesium, or iridium. Through single-plane, double-plane, or volume implants, doses of 5500 to 7000 rads are delivered in 5 to 10 days.[16,17] For larger lesions, a successful combination of external megavoltage irradiation in a dose of 4000 to 6000 rads over 4 to 5 weeks has been used, followed by an implant delivering 3000 to 4000 rads.[23]

The more extensive lesions involving the entire urethra, vagina, vulva, or the neck of the bladder have poor prognoses. Therapy with either surgical intervention or radiotherapy alone is discouraging. Combined therapy in the form of preoperative megavoltage irradiation, followed in 4 to 6 weeks by surgical treatment, appears to give the best results.[17,18]

Surgical treatment is required in cases of inguinal or pelvic lymphadenopathy. For meatal or distal tumors, without clinical adenopathy, conservative management is possible because only 10 to 15% of patients with primary local control will develop metastasis to the inguinal nodes.[2] Prophylactic irradiation is not indicated.

RENAL CELL CARCINOMA

Renal cell carcinoma accounts for 3% of all malignant tumors in adults and for approximately 80% of primary malignant tumors of the kidney. It occurs most commonly in the 5th decade and is three times more frequent in males. Surgery is the primary modality of treatment with 5-year survival rates of 65 to 76% for stage-I disease and 47 to 65% for stage-II disease. Conversely, untreated patients' survival at 5 years was 1.7% in a series of 443 patients by Riches and associates.[24] Regional node involvement, invasion through renal capsule, and extension to contiguous organs adversely affect outcome, decreasing survival to 50%. The role of radiation therapy, however, has not been definitely established, but several reports suggest that selected groups may benefit from radiotherapy.

Preoperative Radiotherapy

In 1951, Sir Eric Riches recognized the value of preoperative radiotherapy in the treatment of advanced carcinoma of the kidney.[24] He found that a dose of 3000 rads would facilitate the operation and could be used in selected cases without detrimental effects. His results, and those of Flocks and Kadesky, appeared to demonstrate an improvement in survival.[25] Others have endorsed the use of preoperative irradiation based on anecdotal but consistent findings of better resectability of tumors and unexpectedly long survival.[26-28]

In 1973, van der Werf-Messing reported the experiences of the Rotterdam group in treating carcinoma of the kidney.[29] In this trial, there appeared to be no advantage with the use of medium-dose radiotherapy for all patients clinically diagnosed as having carcinoma of the kidney. It was pointed out, however, that for the P3 category (tumors infiltrating intra- and extrarenal veins and/or lymph vessels), the incidence of complete removal was higher, the incidence of distant metastasis was significantly lower, and the prognosis of this subgroup was considerably better.

Paces and associates, from the Radiotherapy Institute in Prague, reported a randomized study in 1977.[30] Patients in this study received either nephrectomy alone, or preoperative cobalt irradiation in doses of 4000 to 5000 rads followed by nephrectomy. Six patients in the group randomized to nephrectomy alone received preoperative irradiation because of unresectability. In three of these, the tumor became resectable, and two patients survived for 2 and 4 years respectively. Improvement in survival was seen at 8 years in the preoperative group.

The advantage of preoperative radiotherapy, however, becomes lost in randomized studies when all patients are included and does not translate into survival benefits for the entire group. Theoretically, those advantages are: (1) the sterilization of tumor cells that could become disseminated at the time of the operation, (2) the sterilization of cells that may seed the operative bed, (3) shrinkage of tumor and decreased vein ingurgitation (which increase the resectability), and (4) alteration of immunity.[24,28,29] Recent studies suggest that cell-mediated immune responses exist in these patients.[31,32] Furthermore, preoperative irradiation appears to enhance this response in vivo and in vitro.[33]

Further studies in a selected group of patients with locally advanced cancer of the kidney appear warranted. New equipment and techniques in diagnostic radiology for the accurate preoperative staging of these patients could facilitate the selection of those who can benefit from preoperative irradiation.[34,35] Sophisticated treatment planning, simulators, computers, and megavoltage equipment, have improved the radiotherapist's ability to maximize treatment delivered to the tumor and to diminish the volume of normal tissue irradiated, resulting in an improved therapeutic ratio.

Postoperative Irradiation

After completion of the surgical procedure, one of several clinical possibilities exists:

No Residual Disease. In stage I there is no indication for irradiation regardless of tumor size or histology as these do not appear to influence local control. Patients with evidence of lymph node involvement or renal vein invasion have not benefited from postoperative radiotherapy following complete resection.

Microscopic Residual Disease. Tumors with perinephric extension or renal pelvis involvement, even when completely resected, are presumed to harbor microscopic disease and may require postoperative treatment. Improvement in survival with postoperative radiotherapy, under these circumstances, has been reported by Flocks and Kadesky, Rafla, Riches, and Bratherton and Chir.[25,36–39] Megavoltage doses of 4000 to 5000 rads are administered over a period of 4½ to 5 weeks, with careful planning minimizing the amount of normal tissue irradiated.

Macroscopic Residual Disease. The potential benefit of local treatment is limited here by the tolerance of normal tissue. However, doses of 5000 rads can achieve local control in some cases without undue toxicity, depending on the amount of residual tumor. In unresectable cases, effective palliation can be obtained with similar doses. The role of radioprotectors, intraoperative treatment, and new modalities such as biologic response modifiers remains experimental.[40]

REFERENCES

1. Baker, B., et al. Carcinoma of the penis. J. Urol., 116:458, 1976.
2. Hardner, G., et al. Carcinoma of the penis: Analysis of therapy in 100 consecutive cases. J. Urol., 108:428, 1972.
3. Dean, A. L., Jr. Epithelioma of the penis. J. Urol., 33:252, 1935.
4. Marcial, V., Figueroa-Colon, J., Marcial-Rojas, R., and Colon, J. Carcinoma of the penis. Radiology, 79:209, 1962.
5. Knedsen, O. S., and Brennhovd, I. O. Radiotherapy in the treatment of the primary tumor in penile cancer. Acta. Chir. Scand., 133:69, 1967.
6. Engelstad, R. B. Treatment of cancer of the penis at the Norwegian Radium Hospital. Am. J. Roentgenol., 60:801, 1948.
7. Murrell, D. S., and Williams, J. L. Radiotherapy in the treatment of carcinoma of the penis. Br. J. Urol., 37:211, 1965.
8. Jackson, S. M. The treatment of carcinoma of the penis. Br. J. Surg., 53:33, 1966.
9. Bloedorn, F. G. Penis and male urethra. In Textbook of Radiotherapy. 3rd Edition. Edited by G. H. Fletcher. Philadelphia, Lea & Febiger, 1980, p. 886.
10. Alexander, L., et al. Radium management of tumors of the penis. NY State J. Med., 8:1946, 1971.
11. Duncan, W., and Jackson, S. M. The treatment of early cancer of the penis with megavoltage x-rays. Clin. Radiol., 23:246, 1972.
12. Staubitz, W. J., Lent, M. H., and Oberkircher, U. J. Carcinoma of the penis. Cancer, 8:371, 1955.
13. Newaishy, G. A., and Deeley, T. J. Radiotherapy in the treatment of carcinoma of the penis. Br. J. Urol., 41:519, 1968.
14. Vaeth, J., Green, J., and Lowy, R. Radiation therapy of carcinoma of the penis. Am. J. Roentgenol., 108:130, 1970.
15. Fagan, G. E., and Hertig, A. T. Carcinoma of the female urethra: Review of literature report of 8 cases. J. Obstet. Gynecol., 6:1, 1955.
16. Antoniades, J. Radiation therapy in carcinoma of the female urethra. Cancer, 24:70, 1969.
17. Bracken, R. B., et al. Primary carcinoma of the female urethra. J. Urol., 116:188, 1976.
18. Grabstald, H. Tumors of the urethra in men and women. Cancer, 32:1236, 1973.
19. Rhamy, R. K., Boldurs, R. A., Allison, R. C., and Tapper, R. I. Therapeutic modalities in adenocarcinoma of the female urethra. J. Urol., 109:638, 1973.
20. Desai, S., Libertino, J. A., and Zinnan, L. Primary carcinoma of the female urethra. J. Urol., 110:693, 1973.
21. Howe, G. E., Prentiss, R. J., Mulenix, R. B., and Fenny, M. J. Carcinoma of the urethra: Diagnosis and treatment. J. Urol., 89:232, 1963.
22. Chu, A. M. Female urethral carcinoma. Radiology, 107:627, 1973.
23. Taggart, C. G., Castro, J. R., and Rutledge, F. N. Carcinoma of the female urethra. Am. J. Roentgenol., 114:145, 1972.
24. Riches, E., Griffiths, I. H., and Thackray, A. C. New growths of the kidney and ureter. Br. J. Urol., 23:297, 1951.
25. Flocks, R. H., and Kadesky, M. C. Malignant neoplasms of the kidney: An analysis of 353 patients followed five years or more. J. Urol., 79:196, 1958.
26. Bixler, L. C., Stenstrom, W., and Creevy, C. D. Malignant tumor of the kidney: Review of 117 cases. Radiology, 42:329, 1944.
27. Rubenstein, M. A., Walz, B. J., and Bucy, J. G. Transitional cell carcinoma of the kidney: 25 years' experience. J. Urol., 119:594, 1978.
28. Cox, C. E., Lacy, S. S., Montgomery, W. G., and Boyce, W. H. Renal adenocarcinoma: 28-year review, with emphasis on rationale and feasibility of preoperative radiotherapy. J. Urol., 104:53, 1970.
29. Van der Werf-Messing, B. Carcinoma of the kidney. Cancer, 32:1056, 1973.
30. Paces, V., Doleckova, V., and Zamecnik, J. Preoperative irradiation of renal carcinoma in adults (controlled clinical trial). Int. Urol. Nephrol., 10(2):77, 1978.
31. Stjernsward, J., et al. Tumor-distinctive cellular immunity to renal carcinoma. Clin. Exp. Immunol., 6:963, 1970.
32. DeKernion, J. B., and Berry, D. The diagnosis and treatment of renal cell carcinoma. Cancer, 45:1947, 1980.
33. Schwarze, G., Dietz, R., and Pappas, A. Studies on cellular immunity

in patients with renal carcinoma: Radiation-induced inhibition of leukocyte migration. Eur. J. Cancer, *15:*205, 1979.

34. EVANS, J. The accuracy of diagnostic radiology. JAMA, *204:*131, 1968.

35. KAHN, P. C., WISE, H. M., and ROBBINS, A. H. Complete angiographic evaluation of renal cancer. JAMA, *204:*95, 1968.

36. RAFLA, S. Renal cell carcinoma: Natural history and results of treatment. Cancer, *25:*26, 1970.

37. RAFLA, S. (quoted): Renal cell carcinoma: Does it resist radiation therapy? Urology, *2*(4):1980.

38. RICHES, E. The place of radiotherapy in the management of parenchymal carcinoma of the kidney. J. Urol., *95:*313, 1966.

39. BRATHERTON, D. G., and CHIR, B. The place of radiotherapy in the treatment of hypernephroma. Br. J. Radiol., *37:*141, 1964.

40. YUHAS, J., SPELLMAN, J. M., and CULO, F. The role of WR-2721 in radiotherapy and/or chemotherapy. Cancer Clin. Trials, *3:*211, 1980.

Palliative Irradiation for Genitourinary Carcinoma

Mark B. Hazuka

In 1989, the American Cancer Society estimates that there will be approximately 180,000 new cases of genitourinary (GU) cancer in the United States. Over 90% of these cases will be prostate, bladder, and kidney cancer with prostatic carcinoma accounting for more than 50% of all GU malignancies.[1] A significant proportion of these patients either present with or develop metastatic disease during the course of their illness. At that stage, the disease process is usually no longer considered curable and, therefore, treatment is given with palliative intention.

The development of metastases signifies systemic spread of disease. Consequently, treatment emphasis is frequently placed on systemic modes of therapy such as hormone therapy or chemotherapy, and because of this, the local benefits of radiation therapy are often overlooked.

The goal of palliative irradiation is to improve the quality of life. It may prolong life, but it should never be used to prolong death. When effectively employed, it may provide analgesia, improve function, alleviate obstruction, and control hemorrhage. The ability to achieve palliation depends on the extent of the disease, functional status of the patient, and, to a lesser degree, the tumor tissue structure.[2]

Before recommending palliative irradiation to patients with incurable cancer, the radiation oncologist must consider several important factors. These include the patient's expected survival time, likelihood of improvement, length and severity of possible side effects, discomfort encountered during transportation, and treatment costs to the patient. In addition, prior anticancer therapy may also influence treatment decisions (i.e., prior radiation therapy may limit normal tissue tolerance to further treatment or extensive prior chemotherapy and/or irradiation may suppress bone marrow function thus limiting the extent of or precluding further treatment). Palliative irradiation should not be recommended if the anticipated side effects greatly outweigh the potential gains. For example, a 3 to 4 week course of irradiation that causes daily nausea and vomiting in a patient whose life expectancy is measured in weeks is unacceptable. Likewise, radical irradiation to doses that exceed normal tissue tolerance (including retreatment) should be avoided because the complications are often greater than the symptoms that need alleviation. Conversely, irradiation to doses within tolerance of the surrounding normal tissues should be considered in patients with symptomatic metastases and at least 2 months expected survival. Once the decision has been made to treat, the treatment should be delivered in such a way as to maximize the potential benefits and at the same time, minimize the possible complications or side effects.

PATTERNS OF DISSEMINATION

Prostate

Prostate cancer spreads via hematogenous and lymphatic routes as well as through direct extension to seminal vesicles or bladder. Dissemination may progress from local to regional to distant lymph nodes, followed by or concurrent with spread to pelvic and distant bones. Bone metastases may also develop first, sometimes without lymph node involvement. However, once lymph node involvement occurs, bone metastases usually follow.[3] The incidence of metastases is directly related to the size of the gland (or clinical stage) and degree of differentiation of the tumor.[4,5]

About 50% of all patients who present with prostate cancer eventually develop bone metastases. Dissemination to bone by far represents the most common site of distant spread. Other sites of involvement include liver, lung, distant lymph nodes, and, less frequently, brain. Autopsy studies reveal that virtually no body organ or tissue is exempt from the possibilities of metastases.[6]

Prostatic carcinoma has long been theorized to preferentially metastasize to the bones of the pelvis and spine. Batson first proposed that the distribution of skeletal metastases in prostate cancer was unique, caused by dissemination of tumor through the vertebral system of veins, thus bypassing the vena cava and lungs.[7,8] This concept, however, was tested in a recent study by Dodds et al.[9] The study consisted of a review of 179 bone scans from 136 patients with bone metastases, of which 73 cases were metastatic prostate cancer. The authors found that the bony sites of involvement in patients with prostatic and nonprostatic tumors were similar. In addition, 25% of the patients with prostatic carcinoma had bone scan lesions exclusively outside the region comprising the pelvis, sacrum, and lumbar spine. The authors concluded that these findings did not support Batson's hypothesis and instead, metastases to the axial skeleton and long bones may be a function of regional arterial blood flow, with metastases most often found in skeletal regions containing active, well-vascularized bone marrow. Although the distribution of bone metastases was similar between the two groups, spine (74%) closely followed by ribs (70%) and pelvis (60%) were the most common involved bony sites with disseminated prostate cancer, with lumbar spine (49%) the most frequent involved spinal subdivision.

Bladder

Bladder cancer metastasizes by lymph, blood, and direct invasion. It tends to spread first to regional lymph nodes and then to distant sites such as liver, lungs, and bone. Patients with high-grade tumors are more apt to develop metastatic disease.[10]

Early clinical surveys reported that distant metastases occurred in only 4 to 17% of patients with bladder cancer.[11] At autopsy, however, approximately two-thirds of patients have metastatic disease. In a postmortem study of 107 patients with transitional cell carcinoma of the bladder, the most common sites of metastases were lymph nodes (78%), liver (38%), lung (36%), bone (27%), and adrenal gland (21%), with brain metastases occurring in only 7%. Metastases were limited to the pelvic region in one-third of patients and involved multiple-organ sites in another one-third of patients. Of 11 patients with radiographically identified bone metastases, 9 patients had osteolytic lesions and 2 had osteoblastic lesions.[10] In a larger study of 21 patients, however, Goldman et al. reported a 47% incidence of either osteoblastic or a mixed osteolytic-osteoblastic pattern.[12]

Kidney

Renal cell cancer spreads by way of direct contiguous extension into surrounding structures and by hematogenous and lymphatic pathways. The tumor itself is vascular and dissemination may occur to any organ although lungs, lymph nodes, liver, bone, adrenal, contralateral kidney, brain, heart, spleen, bowel, and skin are the most common. Metastases usually appear within 3 years of the primary, however, later occurring metastases are not uncommon with 5 of 35 patients in one study developing first metastases more than 8 years after the initial presentation.[13]

Other GU Cancers

Testicular cancers metastasize predominantly to retroperitoneal lymph nodes and then to the lungs. Hematogenous spread to other visceral organs occur less often. In an autopsy study of 154 men with germ cell tumors of the testis, Bredael and associates reported that lung, liver, brain, and bone (89%, 73%, 31%, and 30%, respectively) were the most common bloodborne metastatic sites.[14] Bony metastases generally occur late and represent advanced disease.[15]

Advanced cancers of the urethra and penis may spread to adjacent structures by direct invasion, or to the inguinal or pelvic lymph nodes by lymphatic routes. Hematogenous spread to lungs and liver, although less common, may also occur.

TREATMENT PLANNING

Careful treatment planning is essential prior to beginning a course of palliative irradiation. This process entails a thorough review of all pertinent findings obtained from the history and physical and diagnostic studies performed. For example, in a patient with painful bone metastases from metastatic prostate cancer, this would include a review of a recent bone scan or

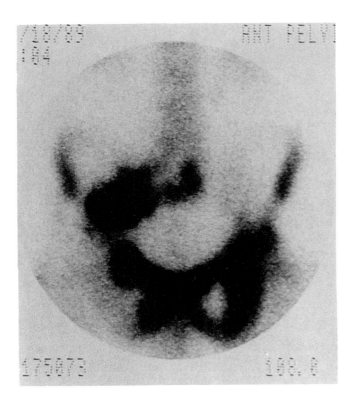

radiographs. These radiographic abnormalities are then correlated with painful areas either described by the patient during the interview or elicited by palpation or percussion on physical examination.

Bone scans are helpful to the radiation oncologist in planning field design because these studies are more sensitive than plain radiographs (Fig. 57-1). Asymptomatic metastases within close proximity to symptomatic sites are usually included in the field of irradiation because these areas may become symptomatic in the future thus requiring treatment. In patients with vertebral metastases from breast cancer, Bagshaw proposed that the entire spine should be treated since prolonged control was best achieved when metastases were small or asymptomatic.[16] In addition, potential overlap difficulties could also be avoided with this approach. If patients are to receive systemic chemotherapy, however, one may want to restrict the size of the radiation fields to include only the area of involvement plus a surrounding margin. Bone marrow ablation from large field irradiation may compromise the delivery of adequate doses of chemotherapy.

Modern radiation oncology departments are equipped with megavoltage treatment machines, a simulator with fluoro-

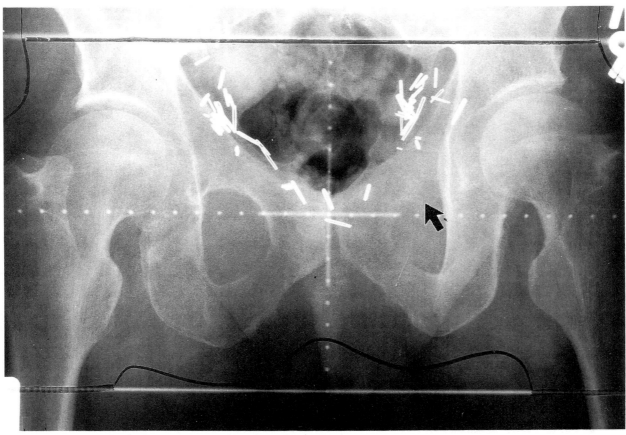

FIG. 57-1. Sixty-four-year-old man presented with severe left hip and pelvic pain. The patient underwent radical cystectomy with urinary diversion (Koch's pouch) for invasive transitional cell carcinoma of the bladder 2 years prior. *A*, Bone scan shows multiple areas of increased uptake in the pubic rami, ischia, and left acetabulum consistent with metastatic disease (increased activity in the right upper pelvis represents collection of the radioisotope in the Koch's pouch). *B*, AP/PA pelvic fields used in this patient. (Compare with Fig. 57-1A.) Areas of metastatic involvement are more clearly seen on bone scan than with the plain radiograph. However, the radiograph reveals a pathologic fracture of the right pubic ramus (arrow). Customized blocking is used to shield the perineum and other uninvolved soft tissues of the pelvis.

scopic capabilities, and a computerized treatment planning system. All treatment fields are simulated and shielding is designed on the simulator film. Customized blocking constructed from low-melting-temperature alloys (cerrobend) enables the radiation oncologist to selectively shield uninvolved, normal tissues thus lessening morbidity from treatment (Figs. 57-1B, 57-2). In some circumstances, a treatment planning computed tomography (CT) scan is obtained with the patient in the treatment position (i.e., flat tabletop) for more precise localization of the tumor volume and surrounding normal structures. This information is entered into the computer and various treatment plans are constructed (Fig. 57-3). This process entails dose optimization so that the maximum dose is delivered to the tumor while dose to the normal structures is minimized. Finally, the radiation oncologist will select what he/she considers as the most ideal plan for the patient.

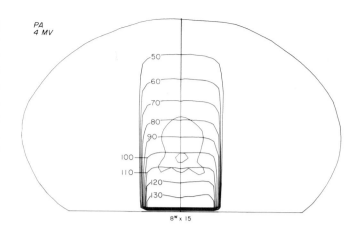

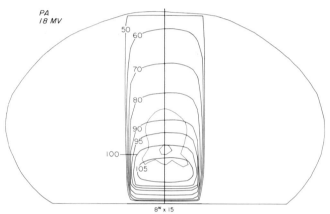

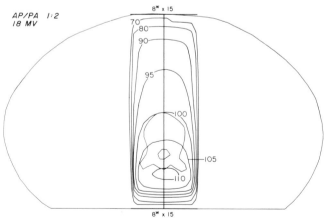

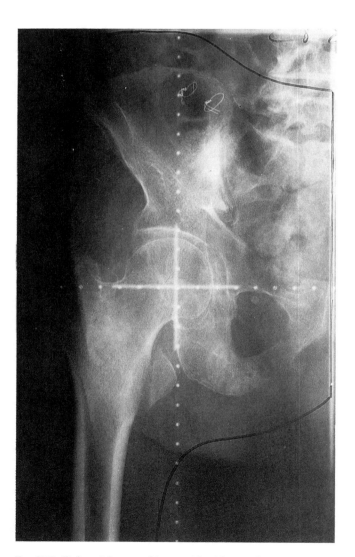

Fig. 57-2. Eighty-eight-year-old man with widespread metastatic prostate cancer who presented with pain in his right hip. Note avulsion fracture (pathologic) of the lesser trochanter. Entire right hemipelvis and proximal femur were treated with AP/PA fields.

Fig. 57-3. Computerized cross-sectional treatment plans for the lumbar spine. A, Isodose distribution for a single posterior (PA) field using 4 MV x rays. B, Isodose distribution for a single posterior field using 18 MV x rays. Note the improved homogeneity in dose throughout the vertebra and excellent sparing of the superficial, soft tissues of the back. C, Isodose distribution for opposed anterior-posterior (AP/PA) fields using 18 MV x rays with 2:1 weighting from the posterior. Again, note further improvement in dose homogeneity. (Compare with Figs. 57-3A and 57-3B.)

Common problems encountered in patients with bone metastases include disabling pain, forced immobility, and occasional pathologic fractures. Pain is the most frequent symptom associated with bone metastases. Pain generally has a gradual onset and becomes progressively more severe. This pain can often be localized by percussion tenderness over the involved site and often is more severe at night.[17] Bone pain secondary to osseous metastases results from stretching or destruction of the periosteum through either direct tumor expansion or mechanical stress of the weakened bone at the tumor site.[18] Bone pain occurring over weight-bearing areas should be evaluated with radiographs to rule out pathologic fracture. Bone involvement may also cause pain by nerve entrapment, which results from compression or direct invasion of nerves by tumor. This type of pain most often occurs with metastases to vertebral bodies or sacrum and is characterized by its radicular nature. These patients should also have a careful neurological examination to evaluate the possibility of concomitant epidural spread of tumor, which may lead to spinal cord compression. Further diagnostic studies such as a myelogram, CT, or magnetic resonance (MR) scan of the spine may be indicated in patients with back pain and neurological findings, because early treatment intervention may prevent progression or even reverse symptoms of spinal cord compression, which may lead to paralysis.

Radiation therapy is the most effective local means for palliating symptomatic bony metastases. Treatment goals often include relief of pain, reducing requirements for narcotic medication, increasing ambulation, and preventing pathologic fractures. About 80 to 90% of patients with painful osseous lesions experience significant relief of pain with irradiation[19-21] and more than 50% obtain complete relief.[21] Such pain relief is usually achieved during treatment and is complete within 1 month following completion of irradiation. Furthermore, in one study, more than 70% of patients who experienced relief of pain did not relapse in the field before death.[21]

Some controversy exists regarding the optimum dose and scheduling of irradiation for bone metastases. The Radiation Therapy Oncology Group (RTOG) conducted a prospective randomized trial to determine the palliative effectiveness of several different fractionated schedules for bone metastases (solitary metastases—4,050 cGy/3 weeks versus 2,000 cGy/ 1 week; multiple metastases—3,000 cGy/2 weeks versus 1,500 cGy/1 week versus 2,000 cGy/1 week versus 2,500 cGy/1 week). The authors concluded that the low-dose, short-course schedules were as effective as the high-dose protracted programs.[21] However, in a recent reanalysis of the RTOG data, Blitzer's conclusion differed in that the more highly fractionated regimens, which delivered higher total doses, were significantly associated with an improved outcome and better pain relief than the lower dose, short-course regimens.[22] At the University of Colorado Health Sciences Center (UCHSC), we prefer the more protracted, highly fractionated schedules to

higher total doses (e.g., 3,000 cGy/2 to 3 weeks to 5,000 cGy/ 5 to 5.5 weeks), especially when treating weight-bearing areas such as femur, acetabulum, or pelvis or where long-term survival is expected.

Pathologic fractures can occur when there is greater than 50% destruction of the bony cortex.[2] This is especially true for weight-bearing areas and an orthopedic consultation should be obtained. Pathologic fractures are more frequently seen with metastatic kidney and bladder cancer (Fig. 57-1B), because these metastatic bone lesions are more often osteolytic than osteoblastic. Pathologic fracture from metastatic prostate cancer is less likely yet may develop in patients with extensive bone involvement and in one series,[23] occurred in 5 of 75 patients with osseous metastases from prostate cancer (see Fig. 57-2). For those who present with fracture, internal fixation followed by radiation therapy after adequate wound healing is recommended to suppress progression of the underlying tumor.

Although most patients with bone metastases have a limited, short life expectancy, some patients may live for years (e.g., prostate and kidney) and thus normal tissue tolerance should be kept in mind when selecting dose schedules. Total dose, fraction size, time interval over which dose is delivered, and volume of irradiation all have bearing on the incidence of complications. This is especially true when the irradiated volume contains critical structures such as spinal cord. In these instances, large daily fractions given over short courses (2,000 cGy in 5 fractions in 5 days) should be avoided.

Various tumor tissue structures differ in their degree of radiosensitivity. Pure seminoma is highly radiosensitive and doses as low as 2,000 to 3,000 cGy are usually adequate. In contrast, renal cell carcinoma has long been considered radioresistant. However, in a study by Halperin and Harisiadis, bone pain secondary to metastatic renal cell carcinoma responded to irradiation at 77% of the treated sites. These investigators found no correlation between total dose and frequency of palliative response.[13] Onufrey and Mohiuddin, on the other hand, reported significantly better results with higher total doses, with 67% of patients achieving complete or near complete relief of pain.[24] Prostate and bladder (transitional cell) cancer are moderately radiosensitive malignancies. In the previously mentioned RTOG study of bone metastases, prostate along with breast primaries had more frequent complete relief of pain than other primaries as well as more frequent minimal relief.[21]

In patients with severe, diffuse pain and multiple sites of bone involvement, the use of half-body irradiation (HBI) may be beneficial. This technique has primarily been used in terminally ill patients with advanced disease and has been termed "systemic" irradiation. Large single doses (600 to 1,000 cGy) are delivered sequentially to both halves of the body with a 5-week rest period between treatments to allow for bone marrow recovery. A comprehensive premedication program is required for management of acute toxicity (acute radiation syndrome) and hospitalization is often necessary particularly when upper HBI is used. Because the major delayed toxicity is pulmonary for upper HBI, the middepth lung dose should not exceed 700 cGy (corrected for lung transmission).[25] Fitzpatrick and Rider initially reported that pain relief occurred in 70 to 80% of patients within 24 to 48 hours of HBI.[26] The RTOG studied this technique in 168 patients of whom all had advanced disease, with 59% of patients having an initial Karnofsky performance score of less than 50%. A total of 73% of patients improved with 19% completely, and 40% of patients responded within 48 hours. Of patients treated with HBI, however, 10% experienced severe to life-threatening toxicities, and these were generally seen in patients who had received prior intensive therapies. Those patients with prostate primaries had more frequent complete responses (26%) than did other primary sites.[27] Rowland et al. also reported on the use of sequential HBI (750 cGy upper HBI without lung correction followed in 4 to 5 weeks by 1,000 cGy lower HBI) in patients with metastatic prostate cancer. In this report, 80% of patients experienced immediate pain relief and 67% maintained relief until death.[28]

Also used to treat diffuse bone metastases has been [32]P. This radionuclide is taken up by proliferating neoplastic tissue and this uptake is enhanced by the administration of testosterone before, during and after treatment in metastatic prostate cancer. During the initial testosterone therapy, exacerbation of pain and spinal cord compression can occur.[29] A single dose of up to 10 mCi or 10 to 12 mCi in divided doses is given intravenously over a period of 1 week.[30] Approximately 75% of the patients respond to ^{32}P with about 45 to 50% achieving complete pain relief.[29–31] Pain relief is not immediate. It usually occurs within 3 to 5 days of the first injection of ^{32}P and lasts an average of 6 months.[30] Besides the possibility of exacerbation of pain and spinal cord compression from testosterone "priming," toxicity is generally mild and consists of transient myelosuppression and hypercalcemia.

SPINAL CORD COMPRESSION

Spinal cord compression is a neurologic emergency that requires prompt diagnosis and treatment. If not treated, progression of symptoms to complete loss of spinal cord function below the compression site is imminent. In a recent Memorial Hospital series, prostate followed by kidney were the third and fourth most common primary tumors causing epidural spinal cord compression.[32]

Epidural metastases can cause spinal cord compression by either local extension from metastatic tumor involving a vertebra or extension of tumor through the intervertebral foramens to compress the spinal cord. Pain is the most common symptom; it occurs in more than 90% of patients and is often localized over the involved site. Pain may also be radicular in nature, especially when the tumor is located in the cervical or lumbosacral regions. Pain is usually present weeks to months prior to the development of neurological signs such as sensory changes, motor weakness, or loss of sphincter function. Once neurologic signs begin, they usually progress rapidly to total paraplegia in a matter of hours to days.[33]

Myelography is indicated in all patients with suspected spinal cord compression. If a complete block is encountered on lumbar myelogram, contrast needs to be reintroduced above the block in order to determine the cephalocaudal extent of the lesion and to ascertain if other areas of involvement exist. This information will assist the radiation oncologist in defining field boundaries. CT scanning with metrizamide myelogram[34] and, recently, MR scanning have also been shown to be useful tests in the early diagnosis of epidural spinal cord compression.[35]

Once the diagnosis has been established, dexamethasone should be started immediately (usually 10 mg IV initially followed by 16 mg daily in divided doses).[33] Some investigators have recommended a high initial dose of 100 mg of dexamethasone daily for 3 days with rapid tapering as tolerated.[32] Steroids may act by decreasing spinal cord edema caused by overlying epidural tumor.

Decompressive laminectomy should be considered in the following instances: uncertain diagnosis (i.e., histologic diagnosis of the primary not established, neurologic progression during irradiation; known radioresistant tumor tissue structure; and relapse of tumor in an area previously treated to radiation tolerance. Following adequate healing (usually 5 to 7 days), patients should be considered for postoperative irradiation because epidural tumor usually grows circumferentially around the spinal cord and thus complete removal of the tumor is impossible.

For most patients, radiation therapy alone is the treatment of choice for spinal cord compression. Treatment should be initiated immediately after the diagnosis is made. Some investigators have recommended large fraction sizes (e.g., 400 cGy) for the first two to three fractions followed by conventional fractionation (e.g., 180 to 200 cGy) to 3,000 to 4,000 cGy total. This is based on experimental and clinical evidence that suggest that rapid reduction in tumor volume and greater cell kill is best achieved with high initial fractions of irradiation.[36,37] The field of irradiation should encompass the site of block plus an adequate margin such as 2 vertebral bodies above and below the block. Usually a single posterior field is used; however, when treating the lumbar region (lumbar spine is almost a midline structure), parallel opposed anterior-posterior fields may deliver a more homogeneous dose of irradiation to the tumor volume than a single posterior field (see Fig. 57-3). The best treatment results are obtained in those patients with mild neurologic dysfunction and conversely, the worse results in those who are already paraplegic. Less than 10% of patients with paraplegia at diagnosis become ambulatory. However, three-quarters of patients who are ambulatory at the time of diagnosis of spinal cord compression remain so after treatment and about 45% of those with mild to moderate weakness recover to an ambulatory state[32] (Fig. 57-4).

BRAIN METASTASES

Brain metastases are an ominous sign in a cancer patient. Because most patients have multiple brain lesions or disease else-

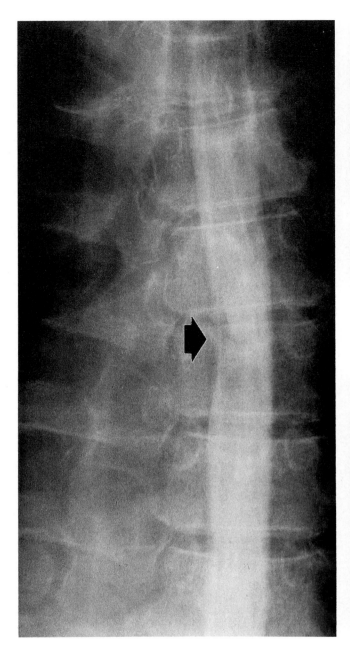

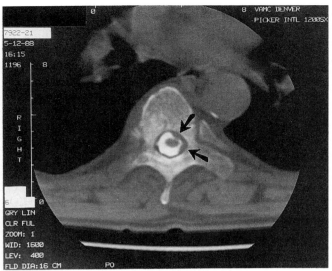

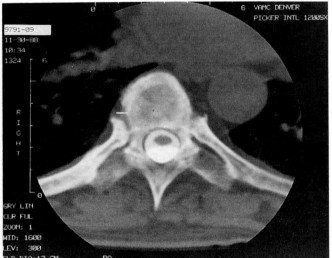

FIG. 57-4. Sixty-three-year-old man with metastatic prostate cancer who presented with back pain, right leg weakness, and decreased sensation. *A*, Myelogram demonstrates partial obstruction at the T6-T7 interspace (arrow). *B*, Postmyelogram CT scan through T7 shows extensive epidural metastases and blastic involvement of the vertebrae (arrows). *C*, Postmyelogram CT scan through T7 obtained 7 months after receiving 4,000 cGy shows blastic changes in the spine without epidural compromise. The patient was able to walk without significant back pain.

where, treatment is usually palliative. Radiation therapy is the mainstay of treatment for brain metastases. Surgery may also be indicated in selected patients with solitary metastasis and controlled primaries.

The most common presenting symptoms and signs of brain metastases are headaches, motor deficits, disorientation, and seizures.[38] All symptomatic patients should be started on dexamethasone prior to initiating radiation therapy unless there exists a medical contraindication to steroids. Posner reported that between 60 to 75% of patients experienced significant temporary relief of their symptoms with corticosteroids.[33] Usually 16 mg of dexamethasone daily in divided doses is suffi-

cient, however, sometimes higher doses (e.g., 100 mg or more of dexamethasone per day) may be necessary. Because of the known side effects of steroids, the steroid dose should be tapered during irradiation to the lowest dose possible that relieves symptoms.

The RTOG has studied various fractionated whole-brain schedules (ranging from 1,000 cGy/1 fraction to 5,000 cGy/4 weeks) in prospective, randomized trials to determine their palliative effectiveness in patients with brain metastases.[39–41] The ultrarapid, high-dose schedules (1,000 cGy/1 fraction and 1,200 cGy/2 fractions) were found not to be as effective as the more protracted schedules.[41] Improvement in neurologic function occurred in approximately 50% of all patients with the best improvement seen in those patients who were least ill at the start of irradiation. The duration of improvement lasted a median 10 to 12 weeks. The median survival ranged between 15 and 18 weeks with ambulatory patients surviving longer (21 weeks) than nonambulatory patients.[39]

At UCHSC, we generally recommend 3,000 cGy/2 to 3 weeks up to 5,000 cGy/5 to 5.5 weeks to the whole brain. The higher dose, more protracted schedules are given to those patients who are likely to have long-term survival. We don't recommend retreatment of brain metastases if metastases progress or recur. These recommendations are based on our prior experience with retreatment of brain metastases. We reviewed the results of reirradiation in 44 patients who failed whole-brain irradiation.[42] Retreatment was found to be of no value in these patients with only 27% showing neurologic improvement. Survival was also poor with a median of 8 weeks. In addition, there was no correlation between response to reirradiation and survival. Because of these unsatisfactory results and the fact that about one-half of all patients with brain metastases die from its manifestations, we recommend higher, and thus more durable, doses of irradiation for patients initially presenting with brain metastases.[43]

As mentioned, renal cell carcinoma is thought to be the most radioresistant GU malignancy. However, dramatic responses to radiation therapy are occasionally seen. In general, surgical removal followed by whole-brain irradiation should be considered in these patients with accessible metastases and extended disease-free intervals (usually of 1 year or more). Surgery may also be indicated in patients with a brain lesion of uncertain diagnosis and no known systemic spread and sometimes in patients who fail irradiation and steroids, particularly in those with symptomatic, surgically accessible metastases.

HEMORRHAGE AND OBSTRUCTION

Radiation therapy is sometimes effective in controlling moderate GU bleeding secondary to regionally advanced renal cell carcinoma or progressive pelvic neoplasms. Reduction in tumor bulk thereby facilitating mucosal healing through reepithelialzation and scar formation is thought to be the underlying mechanism of action for radiation-induced hemostasis.[2] Massive hemorrhage, however, caused by tumor erosion of a major vessel rarely responds to emergent irradiation. In these instances, surgery or intra-arterial embolization are more likely to produce hemostasis.

Bladder neck and ureteral obstruction from regionally advanced GU malignancies can at times be effectively managed with palliative irradiation. In the case of locally advanced prostatic carcinoma, especially with distant metastases, hormonal manipulation first with irradiation reserved for nonresponding lesions may be the most ideal order. In my experience, complete obstruction by tumor is rarely relieved by irradiation and instead, palliation is best achieved by surgical diversion or intraureteral stent. In contrast, partial urinary obstruction is more likely to respond to irradiation and doses of 4,000 to 5,000 cGy in 4 to 5 weeks are usually necessary.

PROPHYLAXIS OF GYNECOMASTIA

Gynecomastia and mammalgia are side effects frequently associated with the administration of estrogens in male patients. In fact, breast tenderness is often severe enough to warrant discontinuation of therapy. Prophylactic breast irradiation is an effective means of reducing these troublesome side effects. Larsson and Sundbom first demonstrated that gynecomastia could be prevented with a single dose of 1,000 R or 1,500 R given 2 weeks prior to starting estrogen therapy, with 4 of 6 unirradiated breasts developing gynecomastia.[44] If breast irradiation is started 1 or more months after beginning hormone therapy or after the development of breast symptoms, the treatment is not as successful. In a recent series of 87 patients with a minimum follow-up of 1 year and mean follow-up of 4 years, Fass et al. reported that prophylactic breast irradiation was effective in 77 and 83% of patients in preventing gynecomastia and mammalgia, respectively. In addition, only 2 acute reactions were noted during treatment and no long-term sequela. All patients in this series were treated with doses of 1,200 to 1,500 cGy in 3 fractions.[45] At UCHSC, we usually recommend 1,200 cGy in 3 fractions/1 week to the breast parenchyma with an electron beam centered over the nipple–areolar complex.

REFERENCES

1. Silverberg, E., and Lubera, J. A. Cancer statistics, 1989. CA, *39*:3, 1989.
2. Richter, M. P., and Coia, L. R. Palliative radiation therapy. Semin. Oncol., *12*:375, 1985.
3. Varkarakis, M. J. et al. Lymph node involvement in prostatic carcinoma. Urol. Clin. North Am., *2*:197, 1975.
4. Flocks, R. H., Culp, D., and Porto, R. Lymphatic spread from prostatic cancer. J. Urol., *115*:89, 1976.
5. Fowler, J. E., Jr., and Whitmore, W. F., Jr. The incidence and extent of pelvic lymph node metastases in apparently localized prostatic cancer. Cancer, *47*:2941, 1981.
6. Whitmore, W. F., Jr. The natural history of prostatic cancer. Cancer, *32*:1104, 1973.
7. Batson, O. V. The function of the vertebral veins and their role in the spread of metastases. Ann. Surg., *112*:138, 1940.
8. Batson, O. V. The role of the vertebral veins in metastatic processes. Ann. Intern. Med., *16*:38, 1942.
9. Dodds, P. R., Caride, V. J., and Lytton, B. The role of vertebral veins in the dissemination of prostatic carcinoma. J. Urol., *126*:753, 1981.
10. Babaian, R. J., et al. Metastases from transitional cell carcinoma of urinary bladder. Urology, *16*:142, 1980.

11. FETTER, T. R., et al. Carcinoma of the bladder: Sites of metastases. J. Urol., *81:*746, 1959.

12. GOLDMAN, S. M., et al. Metastatic transitional cell carcinoma from the bladder: Radiographic manifestations. AJR, *132:*419, 1979.

13. HALPERIN, E. C., and HARISIADIS, L. The role of radiation therapy in the management of metastatic renal cell carcinoma. Cancer, *51:*614, 1983.

14. BREDAEL, J. J., VUGRIN, D., and WHITMORE, W. F., JR. Autopsy findings in 154 patients with germ cell tumors of the testis. Cancer, *50:*548, 1982.

15. SAGALOWSKY, A. I., McCONNELL, J. D., and ADMIRE, R. Uncommon sites of recurrent seminoma and implications for therapy. Cancer, *57:*1060, 1986.

16. BAGSHAW, M. A. Presumptive palliative irradiation in metastatic carcinoma of the breast. Cancer, *28:*1692, 1971.

17. HENDRICKSON, F. R., and SHEINKOP, M. B. Management of osseous metastasis. Semin. Oncol., *2:*399, 1975.

18. MAUCH, P. M., and DREW, M. A. Treatment of metastatic cancer to bone. In: *Cancer Principles and Practice of Oncology.* Edited by V. T. DeVita, S. Hellman, S. A. Rosenberg. Philadelphia, J. B. Lippincott Co., 1985, p. 2132.

19. ALLEN, K. L., JOHNSON, T. W., and HIBBS, G. G. Effective bone palliation as related to various treatment regimens. Cancer, *37:*984, 1976.

20. HENDRICKSON, F. R., SHEHATA, W. M., and KIRCHNER, A. B. Radiation therapy for osseous metastasis. Int. J. Radiat. Oncol. Biol. Phys., *1:*275, 1976.

21. TONG, D., GILLICK, L., and HENDRICKSON, F. R. The palliation of symptomatic osseous metastases: Final results of the study by the Radiation Therapy Oncology Group. Cancer, *50:*893, 1982.

22. BLITZER, P. H. Reanalysis of the RTOG study of the palliation of symptomatic osseous metastasis. Cancer, *55:*1468, 1985.

23. GRAVES, R. C., and MILITZER, R. E. Carcinoma of prostate with metastases. J. Urol., *33:*235, 1935.

24. ONUFREY, V., and MOHIUDDIN, M. Radiation therapy in the treatment of metastatic renal cell carcinoma. Int. J. Radiat. Oncol. Biol. Phys., *11:*2007, 1985.

25. RUBIN, P., et al. Systemic hemibody irradiation for overt and occult metastases. Cancer, *55:*2210, 1985.

26. FITZPATRICK, P. J., and RIDER, W. D. Half body radiotherapy. Int. J. Radiat. Oncol. Biol. Phys., *1:*197, 1976.

27. SALAZAR, O. M., et al. Single-dose half-body irradiation for palliation of multiple bone metastases from solid tumors: Final radiation therapy oncology group report. Cancer, *58:*29, 1986.

28. ROWLAND, C. G., et al. Half-body irradiation in the treatment of metastatic prostatic carcinoma. Br. J. Urol., *53:*628, 1981.

29. CORWIN, S. H., et al. Experiences with ^{32}P in advanced carcinomas of prostate. J. Urol., *104:*745, 1970.

30. AZIZ, H., et al. Comparison of ^{32}P therapy and sequential hemibody irradiation (HBI) for bony metastases as methods of whole body irradiation. Am. J. Clin. Oncol. (CCT), *9:*264, 1986.

31. MAXFIELD, J. R., MAXFIELD, J. J. G., and MAXFIELD, W. S. The use of radioactive phosphorus and testosterone in metastatic bone lesions from breast and prostate. South. Med. J., *51:*320, 1958.

32. GILBERT, R. W., KIM, J. H., and POSNER, J. B. Epidural spinal cord compression from metastatic tumor: Diagnosis and treatment. Ann. Neurol., *3:*40, 1978.

33. POSNER, J. B. Management of central nervous system metastases. Semin. Oncol., *4:*81, 1977.

34. CACAYORIN, E. D., and KIEFFER, S. A. Applications and limitations of computed tomography of the spine. Radiol. Clin. North Am., *20:*185, 1982.

35. SARPEL, S., et al. Early diagnosis of spinal-epidural metastasis by magnetic resonance imaging. Cancer, *59:*1112, 1987.

36. RUBIN, P. Extradural spinal cord compression by tumor part I: Experimental production and treatment trials. Radiology, *93:*1243, 1969.

37. RUBIN, P., MAYER, E., and POULTER, C. Extradural spinal cord compression by tumor part II: High daily dose experience without laminectomy. Radiology, *93:*1248, 1969.

38. ZIMM, S., et al. Intracerebral metastases in solid-tumor patients: Natural history and results of treatment. Cancer, *48:*384, 1981.

39. BORGELT, B., et al. The palliation of brain metastases: Final results of the first two studies by the radiation therapy oncology group. Int. J. Radiat. Oncol. Biol. Phys., *6:*1, 1980.

40. KURTZ, J. M., et al. The palliation of brain metastases in a favorable patient population: A randomized clinical trial by the radiation therapy oncology group. Int. J. Radiat. Oncol. Biol. Phys., *7:*891, 1981.

41. BORGELT, B., et al. Ultra-rapid high dose irradiation schedules for the palliation of brain metastases: Final results of the first two studies by the radiation therapy oncology group. Int. J. Radiat. Oncol. Biol. Phys., *7:*1633, 1981.

42. HAZUKA, M. B., and KINZIE, J. J. Brain metastases: Results and effects of re-irradiation. Int. J. Radiat. Oncol. Biol. Phys., *15:*433, 1988.

43. HAZUKA, M. B., KINZIE, J. J., and KANTOROWITZ, D. A. La re-irradiation des metastases cerebrales est-elle efficace? Cancer Commun., *2:*181, 1988.

44. LARSSON, L. G., and SUNDBOM, C. M. Roentgen irradiation of the male breast. Acta. Radiol., *58:*253, 1962.

45. FASS, D. et al. Radiotherapeutic prophylaxis of estrogen-induced gynecomastia: A study of late sequela. Int. J. Radiat. Oncol. Biol. Phys., *12:*407, 1986.

SECTION XII

RADIOLOGIC EVALUATION

Diagnostic Imaging Evaluation of Genitourinary Neoplasms

Robert Rosenberg
Fred A. Mettler, Jr.
Michael Williamson

O ver the last decade, multiple new imaging methods have become available for evaluation of patients who have malignant genitourinary tumors. Ultrasonography, computerized tomography (CT), and specialized nuclear scintigraphy are noninvasive techniques that have become commonplace. In the last 5 years, magnetic resonance imaging (MRI) has become available in most centers and provides an additional technique.

This chapter addresses the current applications of diagnostic imaging procedures and their relative advantages and limitations. The final choice of which test should be used to evaluate a patient depends not only on the accuracy of the various diagnostic tests, but also on the available equipment and the expertise and experience of those performing and interpreting the new imaging examinations.

ADRENAL TUMORS

Adrenal neoplasms are usually identified on the basis of a clinical syndrome or by visualization on computed tomography.

Occasionally, neoplasms may be seen on an intravenous pyelogram or on a plain film because of internal calcifications. Approximately 15% of large adrenal tumors contain some internal calcification and the pattern of calcification is not specific for tumor types.[1]

Large adrenal masses that cause caudal displacement of the kidney may be seen on intravenous pyelography (Fig. 58-1). Small adrenal masses are usually missed on conventional excretory urogram even if tomograms are obtained. Retroperitoneal pneumography is no longer utilized. Gray-scale ultrasonography was popular for examination of the adrenals 5 to 10 years ago and, even though accuracy rates of 95% were reported by some authors, others were unable to obtain this degree of accuracy,[2] and at the present time computed tomography is the preferred diagnostic technique. Both normal adrenal glands are seen in over 90% of patients when CT scans are done at 1-cm intervals (Fig. 58-2). It is also possible to do thinner sections (5 mm) (see Fig. 58-2) to obtain finer detail. At the present time adrenal visualization may be best achieved either through the use of CT or possibly MRI.

Glazer et al. reviewed progress in clinical radiology and summarized current applications relative to adrenal imaging.[3]

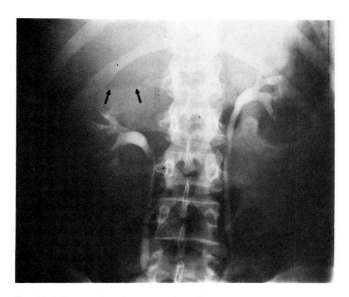

Fig. 58-1. Large adrenal mass on the right causing indentation on the superior pole (arrows) and caudal displacement of the right kidney.

Overall, CT is felt to be more sensitive than MRI even though CT is somewhat nonspecific. Specificity may be achieved through the use of various radionuclide examinations. The only adrenal masses that can be specifically identified by CT are adrenal cysts and an adrenal myelolipoma. Cysts are typically smooth in outline and have water densities ranging from 0 to 5 HU. Myelolipomas usually contain a significant amount of fat. CT is not specific in the differentiation between abnormalities such as adenoma, metastatic deposits, lymphoma, hemorrhage, and pheochromocytomas. Berland et al. tried to differentiate between small benign and malignant adrenal masses using dynamic incremental CT. Features that suggested a benign diagnosis were homogeneous low attenuation, a gland that retained its adrenal configuration, a thin or absent rim, round or oval shape, and diffusely homogeneous attenuation equal to or greater than that of muscle. Features used to suggest malignancy were thick enhancing rim, invasion of adjacent structures, poorly defined margins, and nonhomogeneous attenuation. Positive predictive values utilizing these criteria were reported to be about 90%.

Patients with Cushing's syndrome have bilateral adrenal hyperplasia in approximately 85% of cases, although the adrenals usually appear normal on CT. In patients with Conn's syndrome (primary hyperaldosteronism) CT detects the responsible benign adrenal adenoma in only about 60% of cases.

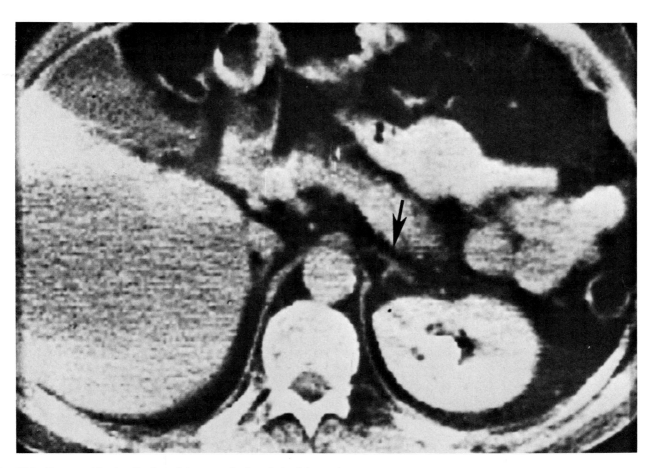

Fig. 58-2. Tomographic visualization of the normal adrenal gland (arrow).

Although early reports suggested that MRI could distinguish adrenal cortex from adrenal medulla, this has not been confirmed. Adrenal medullary hyperfunction is most commonly caused by pheochromocytomas and neuroblastomas. Although CT can be used (Fig. 58-3), imaging with newly developed agents such as iodine-labeled metaiodobenzalquanadine (MIBG) for detection of both extra-adrenal and recurrent pheochromocytoma is probably the test of choice with 90 to 95% sensitivity and specificity. If MIBG is not available, CT is the primary method of choice. MRI apparently has the capability to distinguish pheochromocytoma from nonhyperfunctioning adenoma. The latter tend to be isointense or slightly hyperintense compared with the liver on moderately T2-weighted pulse sequences (TR 2,000 and TE 60), while pheochromocytomas are markedly hyperintense.[3]

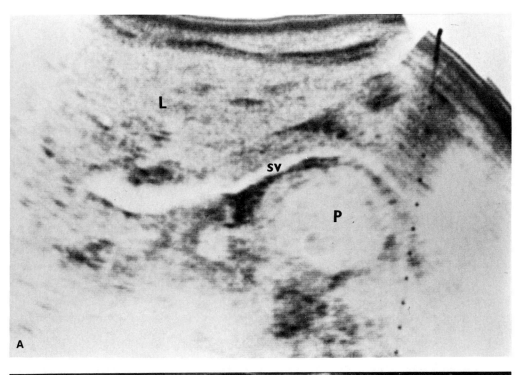

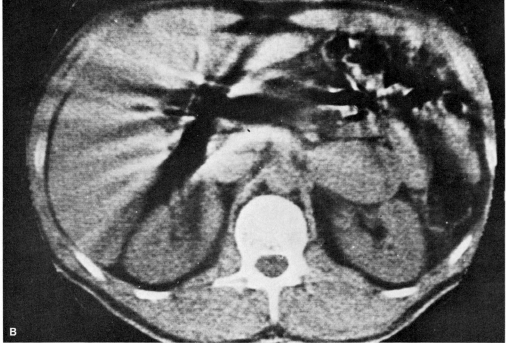

Fig. 58-3. *A*, Transverse sonogram demonstrating left adrenal pheochromocytoma (P). Other normal structures such as the liver (L), splenic vein (sv), and portal vein are easily identified. *B*, The CT scan easily identifies the same lesion.

One of the most common problems regarding adrenal imaging is the patient with normal adrenal function and an adrenal mass that is serendipitously found on CT. Even in patients with malignancy, such lesions are more likely to represent an adenoma than a metastatic deposit. The frequency of adenomas reported from various autopsy series ranges from 2 to 65%. About 1% of patients undergoing abdominal CT will be found to have an incidental adrenal mass larger than 1 cm. With normal serum biochemistry, major differential diagnosis is adenoma versus adrenal corticocarcinoma with adenoma being much more common. Some authors recommend that these lesions be conservatively followed with CT scanning to establish lack of growth.[4]

Lesions larger than 5 cm with irregular margins are usually removed at initial detection. Bernardino pointed that, in patients who do not have a malignancy, serendipitous lesions less than 3 cm in diameter can be watched.[5] There is some debate about lesions that are 3 to 5 cm, but with lesions greater than 5 cm the likelihood of silent carcinoma increases significantly.

It should be noted that in patients with small-cell carcinoma of the lung approximately 17% of patients with morphologically normal adrenal glands were found to have malignant cells in the adrenal and approximately 40% of patients who have large-cell carcinoma of the lung and solitary adrenal masses of 3 cm or smaller were found to have malignant or metastatic disease. In such a setting, percutaneous biopsy of asymptomatic lesions can be performed. Recent experience suggests that utilization of MRI reveals that most metastatic lesions are hyperintense compared to the liver, although hypointense lesions simulating adenomas have been described. Thus it appears that biopsy at this point is still necessary in order to make a clear distinction between a small metastatic lesion and an adrenal adenoma.

TUMORS OF THE KIDNEY

Parenchymal neoplasms, whether benign or malignant, in excess of 3 to 4 cm are usually visualized on a high-quality intravenous urogram. Larger renal neoplasms may be detected on plain film by visualization of renal displacement or abnormal configuration of the kidney. Nephrotomography provides some information about whether the mass is predominantly cystic or solid. Unfortunately, a number of renal cell carcinomas may be predominately cystic and nephrotomography cannot easily identify or differentiate between benign and malignant lesions.

Renal cysts are seen in approximately 50% of people over the age of 60. Because it is neither practical nor cost-effective to perform CT or cyst puncture on all these patients, most clinicians are willing to either ignore or follow lesions that meet ultrasound criteria for a benign cyst. These criteria are a thin smooth wall, no evidence of internal echoes, and enhanced acoustical through transmission.

Patients who present with lesions that do not meet the ultrasound criteria for benign swellings usually are referred for CT. CT criteria for a benign cystic lesion are (1) a homogeneous attenuation value at near water density, (2) no enhancement with intravenous contrast material, (3) no measurable thickness of the cyst wall, and (4) a smooth interface with the renal parenchyma. Warshaur et al. performed a prospective blind study on 201 patients to determine relative sensitivities and specificities of CT, urography, linear tomography, and ultrasound.[6] CT was used as the gold standard. As expected, the sensitivities of the various modalities are dependent on lesion size. Excretory urography and linear tomography permitted detection of 10% of CT-confirmed masses that were cystic or solid and less than 1 cm in size, 21% of lesions larger than or equal to 1 cm but smaller than 2 cm, and 52% of lesions greater than or equal to 2 cm but smaller than 3 cm. Ultrasound permitted detection of 26% of CT-confirmed lesions smaller than 1 cm and 60% of lesions larger than or equal to 1 cm but smaller than 2 cm. There was relative insensitivity, therefore, with both excretory urography and linear tomography for masses smaller than 3 cm in diameter and with ultrasound for lesions smaller than 2 cm in diameter.

Benign Tumors of the Renal Cortex

Prior to the advent of CT, most small benign tumors of the renal cortex were found incidentally during autopsy. The most common tumors are adenomas, lipomas, myomas, and fibromas. Most renal adenomas are smaller than 3 cm in size. CT and ultrasound provide information regarding the solid nature of these lesions but can do little to differentiate between them. Mesenchymal tumors such as fibromas, lipomas, connective tissue tumors, and angiomas can arise in various portions of the renal substance. Leiomyomas can be multiple or solitary and small or large. Approximately 50% of these cases of tumors will undergo sarcomatous change. They may also contain irregular calcification. Renal fibromas usually produce distortion of the calyceal system with few other radiographic findings. Hemangiomas are congenital lesions that are radiographically identified as intramedullary masses with possible calyceal deformity, separation of intrarenal arteries, hypovascularity, and poorly defined margins.

Angiomyolipomas, or hamartomas, are tumors composed of blood vessels, smooth muscle, and adipose tissue. These lesions may be multiple and bilateral in 80% of patients with tuberous sclerosis (Fig. 58-4). These benign neoplasms will deform the collecting system and may be identifiable because of their fat density. Calcification can occur in these lesions but is rare. Use of angiography to differentiate angiomyolipomas from renal cell carcinomas has been difficult. Both lesions may have vessels with a sacular appearance and demonstrate an onion-peel appearance in the venous phase. Arteriovenous shunting usually is not seen with angiomyolipomas. CT scans are probably the most useful because attenuation values of fat can easily be identified in the angiomyolipoma (Fig. 58-5A). Bosniak et al. indicated that some angiomyolipomas have a minimal amount of fat in them and the detection of this is crucial to the diagnosis.[7] The authors therefore suggested that

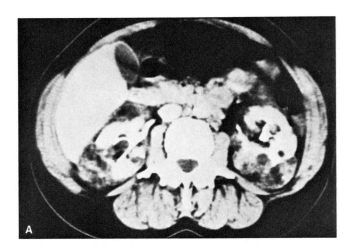

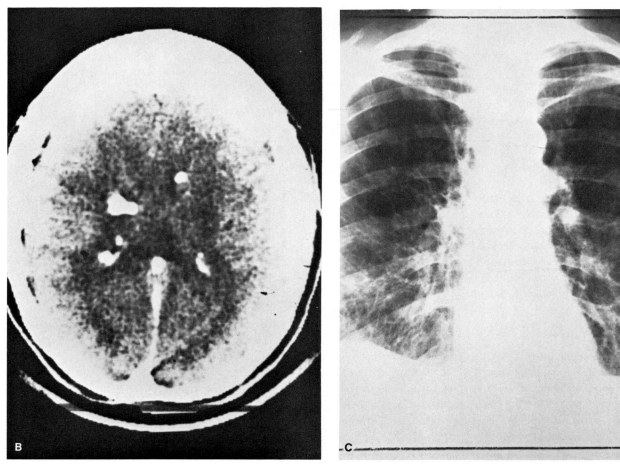

Fig. 58-4. Renal lesion in a patient with tuberous sclerosis. *A*, CT scan demonstrates bilateral fat containing angiomyolipoma with distortion of both kidneys. *B*, Other findings of intracranial calcification can also be identified on the CT scan. *C*, The chest roentgenogram demonstrates bronchiectasis. (Case courtesy of Robert S. Seigel, M.D.)

doing thin section nonenhanced CT may be necessary to differentiate an angiomyolipoma from a renal cell carcinoma. Uhlenbrock et al. compared CT, ultrasound, and MRI in the diagnosis of angiomyolipoma of the kidney.[8] A total of 5 of the 6 patients examined showed an MRI pattern with high signal intensity owing to fat on T1-weighted images and low signal on T2-weighted images (Fig. 58-5*B*). In four of the five patients examined with ultrasonography, the tumor could be recognized by the echodense pattern of fat. Arenson et al. recently reported a single case of an angiomyolipoma extending into the inferior vena cava.[9] CT, however, did indicate areas of fat within the tumor, confirming the diagnosis.

Renal oncocytomas are benign neoplasms that have commonly been misdiagnosed as renal adenomas, carcinomas, or other tumors. Because they often exceed 3 cm, there has been a tendency to perform radical nephrectomy rather than

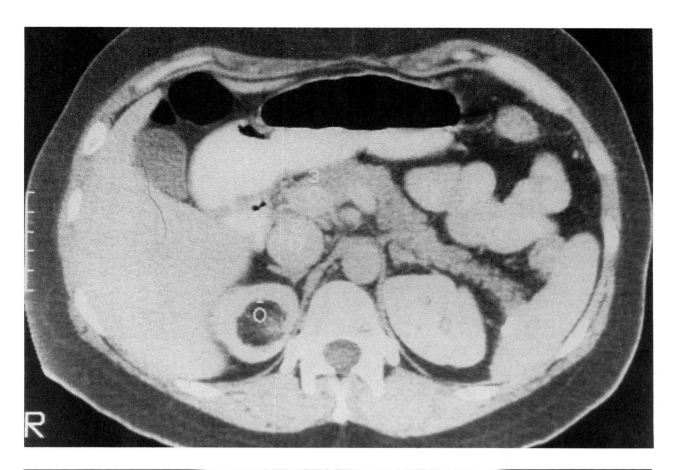

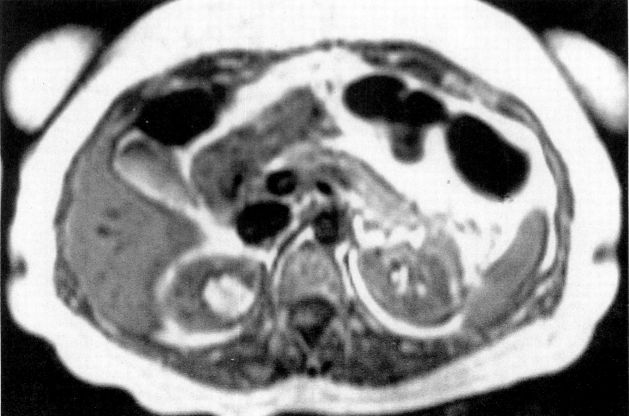

FIG. 58-5. Angiomyolipoma of right kidney with central fat seen as dark low density area on CT (*A*) and bright high signal on a transverse T1-weighted MRI (*B*).

enucleation. Angiographically, renal oncocytomas may show a "spoke-wheel" phenomenon, although this is not seen in all cases. Differentiation of oncocytomas from small renal cell carcinomas is not reliable using angiography. Central, stellate, low-attenuation "scars" have been described as a feature seen on CT, although they are only present in approximately one third of cases. CT is probably the most valuable way of making the diagnosis at the present time, although in many cases it is still not possible to make a differentiation.[10] Remark et al. described two cases of renal oncocytoma studied by MRI.[11] One of the reported cases contained a central scar that appeared as an area of high signal intensity, greater than that of the renal cortex on a T1-weighted sequence. Inversion recovery images (T1-weighted) showed the majority of the mass to be intermediate or of low signal, whereas on T2-weighted images, the intensity was either intermediate or high. The authors suggested that a low-intensity capsule is characteristic if it surrounds the entire periphery of the neoplasm.

McKeown et al. described radiologic findings in carcinoid of the kidney.[12] This is a rare neoplasm that may present with a hyperechoic mass on sonography and a hypovascular mass at angiography. No characteristic findings have been identified.

Malignant Tumors of the Renal Parenchyma

Calcification and large retroperitoneal masses owing to renal cell carcinoma may be visualized on plain films of the abdomen, whereas small lesions are usually only identified on the conventional excretory urogram or CT. The urographic features of these tumors include enlargement or irregularity of the renal outline, abnormal calyceal configuration, defects in the renal pelvis, and disruption of normal renal architecture (Fig. 58-6). Calcification of a mass lesion strongly suggests the possibility of a malignant tumor and, in fact, if the calcification is within the mass rather than at its periphery, there is a high probability that the lesion is malignant. Even with peripheral, curvilinear, or eggshell types of calcification, the incidence of renal carcinoma is at least 20%.[13] CT scans and ultrasonograms provide significant information concerning extrarenal extension or metastases of the tumor, both through the capsule and into the lymphatic system, liver, or vascular structures.

Warshauer et al. pointed out that renal cell carcinomas represent only 2% of all cancers.[6] They tend to be 7 to 8 cm on the average at the time of presentation. The prevalence of renal cell carcinoma in patients with hematuria is about 3 to 6%. The authors also pointed out that probably 6% of renal cell carcinomas are not visualized at the initial excretory urogram or at linear tomography and they suggested that using CT in a population with hematuria, but a negative excretory urogram, may be reasonable.

As might be expected, there is an immense volume of literature concerning renal cell carcinomas. One of the most interesting aspects of this literature is the diagnostic dilemma of small renal cell carcinomas. Work in the 1950s suggested that renal cortical tumors smaller than 3 cm in diameter could be

classified as benign cortical adenomas whereas tumors larger than this were renal adenocarcinomas. Amendola et al. reviewed 338 patients with renal cell carcinoma; 39 patients with pathologically proven renal cell carcinomas smaller than 3 cm were examined.[14] The overall prevalence of small renal cell carcinomas was about 10%. Intravenous urography has a sensitivity of 67% for these lesions whereas ultrasound was 79%, angiography 74%, and CT 94%. Although it is still not possible to distinguish grossly or microscopically or even ultrastructurally between subcortical adenomas and renal carcinomas, most authors support the view that these lesions are really small adenocarcinomas that have not yet metastasized. CT-guided, fine-needle aspiration biopsy of such lesions is warranted but because of the small size of the lesions, open biopsy often is required.

Staging of renal cell carcinomas using CT has been reported by many authors. Ueda et al. compared angiography with CT in staging of 59 patients with renal cell carcinoma[15] (Fig. 58-7). Overall, CT accuracy for tumor extension ranges between 85 and 95%. Accuracy for determination of regional lymph node involvement and venous involvement was in excess of 90%. Similar results were reported by Zeman et al.[16]

Use of MRI in staging and detection of renal neoplasms was reported by Hricak et al.[17] Initial reports by these authors suggested that staging accuracy with MRI was 96%.[18] In their recent reports, the authors used MRI on over 100 patients with renal cell carcinoma. MRI demonstrated all tumors larger than 3 cm. The staging, however, is now reported to have an accuracy rate of only 82%. The authors used both a 0.35 and a 1.5 Tesla magnet. Most of the lesions demonstrated intermediate signal intensity between that of renal medulla and cortex or greater than that of renal cortex on T1-weighted images (Fig. 58-8). On T2-weighted images, the lesions demonstrated varying degrees of signal intensity less than, equal to, or greater than that of renal cortex. At this point, CT should be considered the primary imaging and staging modality in patients with suspected renal masses although MRI may be complementary particularly for evaluation of the inferior vena cava. The incidence of caval involvement is approximately 14% on the right side and 4 to 5% on the left side. At the present time most institutions are utilizing CT for the staging although an inferior vena cavagram may still be clinically indicated. Most renal cell carcinomas are highly vascular and can easily be visualized on selective renal arteriograms (Fig. 58-9). In some instances, differentiation between tumor vessels and normal intrarenal vessels is not obvious and an epinephrine-enhanced arteriogram will aid in the diagnosis. The normal vessels will constrict, whereas the neoplastic vasculature may not (see Fig. 58-9A). The arteriogram is limited in that it gives less overall anatomic information than does the CT scan. It does, however, provide a useful vascular road map for the surgeon.

From 6 to 25% of primary renal cell carcinomas are either hypovascular or avascular.[19] As discussed earlier, some of these avascular tumors exhibit necrosis and cystic change in the central portion. A thickened wall suggests a cystic hyper-

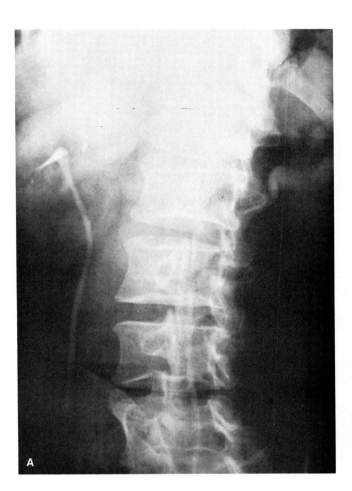

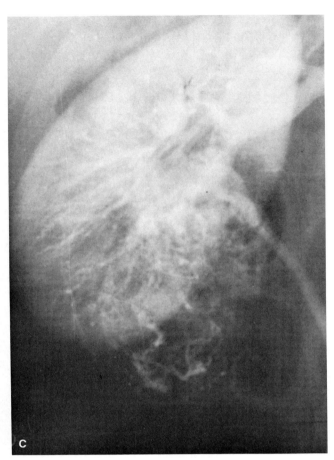

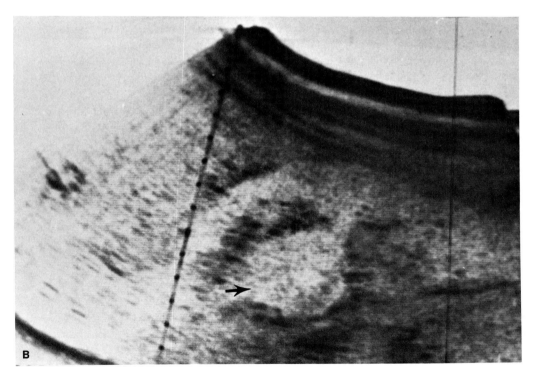

FIG. 58-6. *A,* A relatively small renal cell carcinoma was identified only on an oblique view of an excretory urogram by distortion of the normal renal contour. *B,* The longitudinal sonogram demonstrates the solid nature of this lesion (*arrow*). *C,* The arteriogram demonstrates the neovascularity of a renal cell carcinoma.

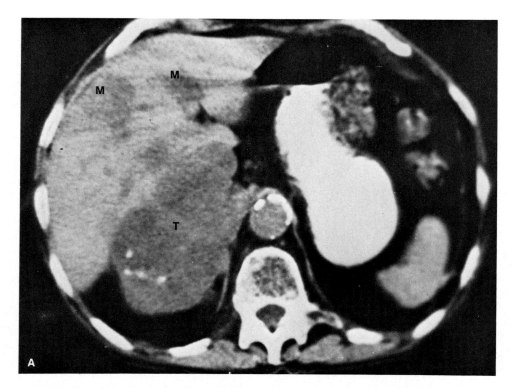

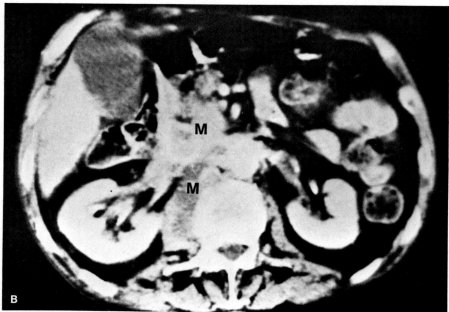

FIG. 58-7. *A*, CT scan adequately demonstrates the extensive nature of a large renal cell carcinoma in the upper pole of the right kidney, extension to the inferior vena cava, and liver metastases. *B*, At a lower level, the aorta and inferior vena cava, as well as the right psoas, are involved with retroperitoneal metastases. (Case courtesy of Robert S. Seigel, M.D.) M = metastases; T = tumor.

nephroma rather than a benign cyst. High-dose renal pharmacoangiograms combining a renal vasodilator, acetylcholine, or tolazoline hydrochloride (Priscoline) with a high dose of contrast medium may improve the visualization of tumor vessels and the tumor stain.[20]

Recently, embolization of vascular tumors has been employed preoperatively to reduce the vascularity of the lesion and to facilitate removal (Fig. 58-10). Gas formation may be observed in infarcted tissue of patients after embolization in

the absence of clinical evidence of abscess.[21] This is postulated to be part of the postinfarction syndrome, although occasionally a true abscess will ensue. In addition to studies previously mentioned, the staging of renal cell carcinomas should include a chest roentgenogram, CT scan of the chest, and other studies directed by the symptoms.

Optimal evaluation of the patient will include imaging evaluation of the contralateral kidney. Bilateral carcinomas, with second primary tumors or metastases, occur in 2 to 4% of

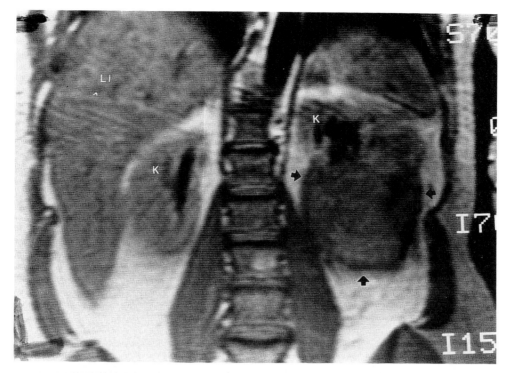

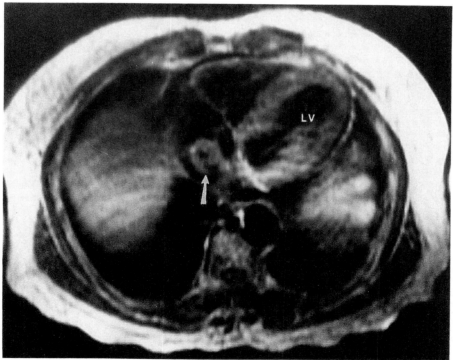

FIG. 58-8. MRI of renal cell carcinoma. *A,* Large tumor in inferior aspect of left kidney with almost the same signal intensity as surrounding normal kidney (T2-weighted image). *B,* Tumor thrombus extending into right atrium or transverse MRI through LV (left ventricle) (arrow).

patients. Autopsy studies indicate contralateral renal metastases occurring in 4 to 30% of patients. CT is probably the best noninvasive way for evaluating postnephrectomy patients for complications and tumor recurrence. Sonography has been advocated in the past, although scarring can simulate tumor in some cases and there is a major diagnostic problem with the bowel, which often lies in the renal bed and may mimic recurrence at sonography.

Many other types of neoplasm, including leukemia, lymphoma, lymphosarcoma, and multiple myeloma, may involve the renal parenchyma. Commonly these neoplastic processes cause generalized renal enlargement with stretching of the calyces rather than expansile focal renal masses. Even though there may be nodular involvement, the kidney often retains its normal shape when greatly enlarged (Fig. 58-11). Excretory urography, ultrasonography, and CT are all appropriate for

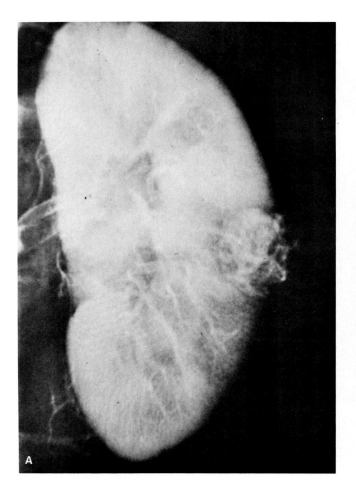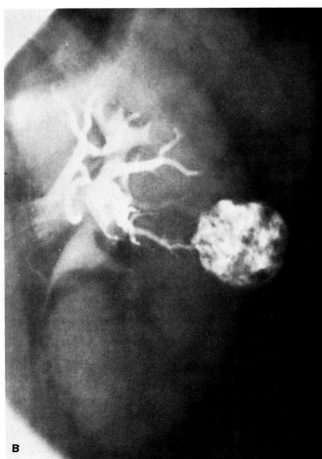

FIG. 58-9. *A*, A small left renal cell carcinoma is seen on the routine selective angiogram; however, the tumor vasculature does not constrict following infusion with epinephrine (*B*).

detecting these lesions and may demonstrate para-aortic, hepatic, splenic, or mesenteric involvement in addition to renal abnormalities. It should be remembered that metastases to the kidney are twice as common as primary tumors. The most common primary tumor locations responsible for renal metastases are carcinoma of the bronchus, breast, and stomach. The angiographic and CT picture of metastases is usually nonspecific and may vary from hypervascular to avascular in appearance, although most are hypovascular.

TUMORS OF THE RENAL PELVIS AND URETER

Benign tumors of the renal pelvis and ureter are generally considered to be of nonepithelial origin. The epithelial tumors are felt to be potentially malignant. Initially, most benign tumors of the ureter usually are thought to be ureteral polyps. They are found because of the mobility of the polyp, which causes obstruction of the ureter. The obstruction is easily identified on a conventional urogram; however, visualization of the pedunculated tumor itself may be difficult. In general, this is best visualized on retrograde examinations.

Most malignant tumors of the renal pelvis and ureter are of epithelial origin. There are two main types: transitional cell carcinoma and squamous cell carcinoma. Transitional cell tumors may be either papillary or nonpapillary, whereas squamous cell tumors are almost always nonpapillary. Approximately 80% of all epithelial tumors are papillary and are multiple in more than 40% of the cases.[22] Multiple papillary tumors frequently involve both the pelvis and ureter. Multicentric origin rather than metastatic spread is currently the more accepted explanation for multiple tumors.

Yousem et al. reported on the prevalence, incidence, and radiographic detection of synchronous and metachronous transitional cell carcinomas.[23] They retrospectively examined 645 patient records. Synchronous transitional cell carcinomas were found in 2.3% of patients with bladder transitional cell carcinoma, 39% who had ureteral transitional cell carcinoma, and 24% with renal transitional cell carcinoma. Among the 600 patients with transitional cell carcinoma of the bladder, 4% developed upper tract lesions after a delay of approximately 61 months. Metachronous upper tract tumors developed in 13% of 38 patients with primary ureteral transitional cell carcinoma and 11% of 63 patients with renal transitional

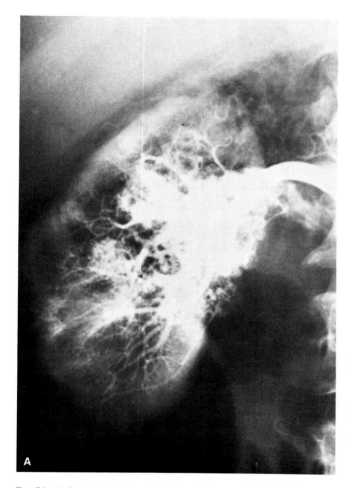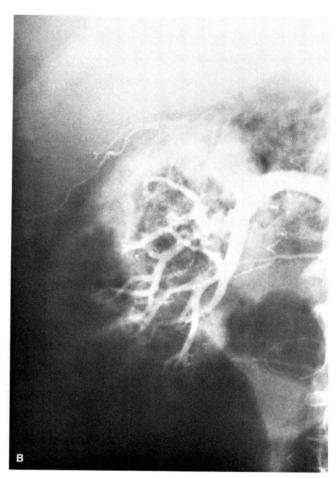

FIG. 58-10. Preoperative embolization of a tumor. *A*, The initial arteriogram demonstrates a hypervascular tumor in the medial portion of the right kidney. *B*, Following embolization, the vascularity of the neoplasm is reduced.

cell carcinoma. The authors recommend annual radiologic evaluation of the upper urinary tract for 2 years after initial diagnosis and treatment of either an upper tract or bladder transitional cell carcinoma.

Although epithelial carcinomas may cause hydronephrosis, this is not a consistent finding; therefore, they must be considered in differential diagnosis of an uncomplicated filling defect of the renal pelvis (Fig. 58-12). The neoplasms may have calcification present but this is unusual. Interestingly enough, transitional cell carcinomas often grow in an expansile fashion producing a mass while confined to the collecting system of the kidney, but they may convert to an infiltrative pattern when they actually invade the renal parenchyma.

Squamous cell carcinomas are rather difficult to demonstrate on imaging examinations, particularly because they often occur in the presence of renal calculi and chronic infection. There is usually minimal intrarenal abnormality caused by the tumor, which makes preoperative urographic diagnosis difficult. The CT appearance of renal pelvic tumors is variable.[24] Filling defects within the renal pelvis may be seen. In addition, the role of ultrasonography and angiography for tumors of the renal pelvis is limited. The imaging modality of choice at this time appears to be retrograde urography for

intraluminal visualization of the lesion and CT for assessment of extrinsic spread.

The diagnosis of small tumors of the ureter is often limited because of incomplete filling of the entire ureter either on the standard urogram or on the retrograde urogram.

An obstructed ureter may be the result of a nonopaque calculus or a neoplasm (Fig. 58-13). One observation that could help in the differential diagnosis is Bergman's sign. This sign indicates that there is often local dilatation of the ureter distal to a neoplasm that obstructs the ureter. The ureter immediately distal to a calculus is usually collapsed because of spasm. Although this sign is helpful, it is not pathognomonic.

CT scanning typically demonstrates the ureteral obstruction; however, if a periureteral mass is present, CT cannot distinguish between a primary ureteral neoplasm and obstruction caused by direct involvement of the ureter by tumors from other sources or even from an entity such as an endometrioma. CT can be used to diagnose obstruction as a result of calculi because most calculi have Houndsfield values on CT in excess of 50.[25,26]

Involvement of the ureter, either by direct extension or by metastases is not uncommon. In general, the cause of the lesions is usually retroperitoneal neoplasms, hypernephroma, or

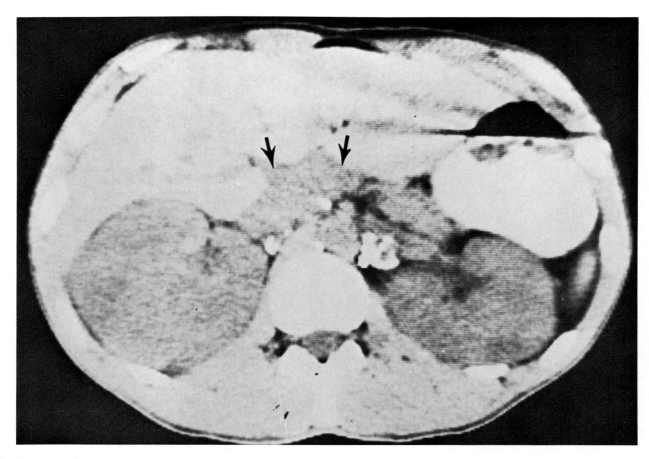

FIG. 58-11 Lymphoma involving both kidneys. CT scan in this case demonstrates nonspecific bilateral renal enlargement, although periaortic lymphadenopathy is often identified also in these cases (arrows).

melanomas. Carcinomas of the colon, bladder, prostate, and cervix may also involve the distal ureter by direct extension. In cases of metastases, the lesions are often multiple and produce bilateral negative defects. With direct extension encasement of the ureter is usually found. Ultrasound has little role to play, with the exception of demonstration of hydronephrosis and hydroureter. Although ultrasound can occasionally visualize a ureteral stone, it usually is obscured by overlying bowel gas.

BLADDER NEOPLASMS

As with tumors of the renal pelvis and calyces, all neoplasms of the bladder of transitional and squamous cell origin are regarded as malignant. The gross pathologic term "papillary" is generally applied to transitional cell neoplasms. This should not be confused with the term "pedunculated" neoplasms. Almost all squamous cell neoplasms are nonpapillary, with extension into the bladder wall, infiltration, and a resulting poor prognosis.

In general, the urogram is of limited value in the assessment of bladder tumors, with the exception of determining ureteral obstruction and tumors elsewhere in the upper urinary tract (Fig. 58-14). Generally, cystoscopic examination with biopsy

or cytologic studies is the most valuable primary diagnostic tool. In the past, investigators used the urogram to assess the thickness of the bladder wall as an indication of tumor extent. However, the diagnostic method of choice at the present time is CT scanning (Fig. 58-15) or MRI.

Reported accuracy rates for staging of bladder tumors utilizing transabdominal sonography have varied between 60 and 95%. Needless to say, MRI has been examined for its accuracy and usefulness in staging bladder carcinoma. Barentsz et al. examined 24 patients and reported accuracy rates between 55 and 80%.[27] Hosband et al. reported on a comparison of CT and MRI in staging bladder tumors in 30 patients.[28] Results did not show any significant differences between the accuracies of the two techniques for staging bladder carcinoma.

Ultrasonic examination of the bladder by means of an intravesicular transducer is accurate but the probes are not generally available and extensive infiltration of tumor to surrounding pelvic structures is not easily determined. Transabdominal ultrasonography is 80% accurate but tumors in the bladder outlet are difficult to evaluate. Extension into seminal vesicles or prostate is also difficult to evaluate using this method.

In general, CT cannot distinguish between stages A, B1, and B2 bladder carcinomas because CT is unable to differentiate

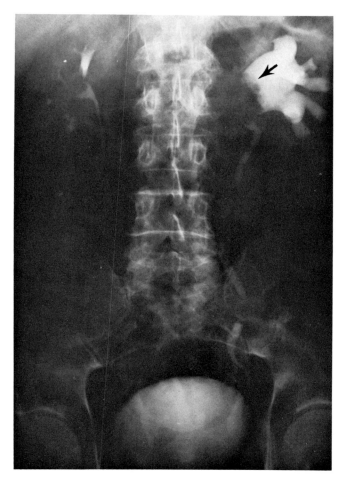

Fig. 58-12. Papillary transitional cell carcinoma of the left renal pelvis (arrow).

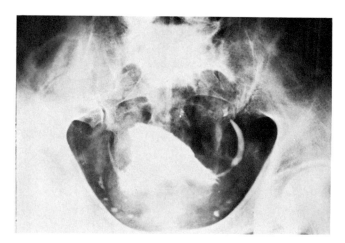

Fig. 58-14. Extensive involvement of the bladder by transitional cell carcinoma.

the various layers of the wall of the urinary bladder.[29] Reported accuracy rates for staging bladder carcinoma by CT are 64 to 90%.[30,31] CT is able to accurately depict spread of tumor to seminal vesicles but extension to prostate is difficult to appreciate.

Reported accuracy rates of lymphangiography in detecting lymph node metastases from bladder tumor is approximately 90% and about 75% for CT evaluation of lymph node metastases.[32,33] The staging of choice at this point is CT scanning initially and, if abnormal lymphadenopathy is identified, no further evaluation is usually performed. If CT is negative, lymphangiography is performed in some institutions.

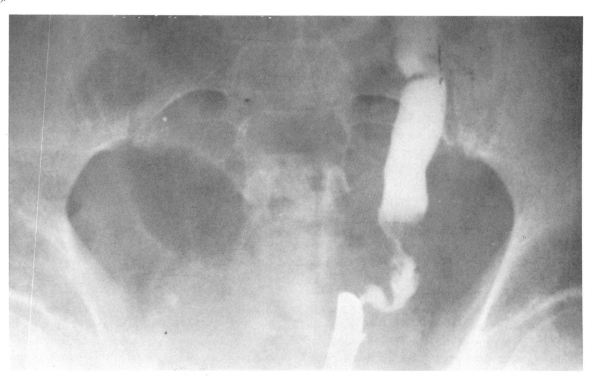

Fig. 58-13. Retrograde urogram of a transitional cell neoplasm of the distal left ureter.

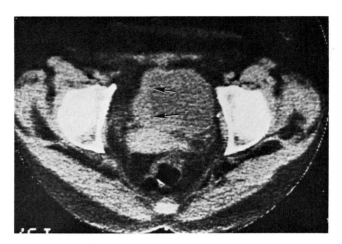

FIG. 58-15. Bladder wall thickening (arrows) can be demonstrated by the CT scan.

Buy et al. recently reported on MRI staging of bladder carcinoma in 40 patients.[34] All patients subsequently had total cystectomy as well as pelvic node dissection. Extension to deep muscle of the bladder wall was present in half of the patients and was diagnosed with sensitivity and specificity of 95%. Extension to perivesical fat was present in 18 of 40 patients and was diagnosed with a sensitivity of 66% and specificity of 100%. Invasion of adjacent organs was diagnosed with a sensitivity of 44% and specificity of 96%. The tumor was correctly staged according to the TNM classification in 60% of the patients, was overestimated in 7.5% and was underestimated in 32.5%. It appears at this time that MRI may be equal to CT in staging of bladder neoplasms.

Currently, arteriograms, lymphangiograms, and staging using ultrasonography are not commonly performed prior to surgery. Preoperative evaluation of patients with transitional cell carcinomas of the bladder should include a chest radiograph. Radionuclide bone scan and perhaps studies of the liver may be used as clinically indicated. Goldman and colleagues found metastases in 10 to 30% of patients with the most common sites being bone, lung, mediastinum, and liver.[35] Although most previous authors described the osseous metastases from bladder as being lytic in relation to bone, these authors found that many of the metastases were sclerotic or mixed lytic and sclerotic lesions.

Postoperative complications of bladder operations such as urine leaks can be evaluated on urograms or cystograms. CT scanning can easily demonstrate other problems such as lymphocele, seroma, urinoma, and abscess. Ultrasonography may also be utilized and percutaneous aspiration and drainage may be directed either utilizing ultrasonography or CT.

In the last several decades, urinary diversions have been accomplished by construction of an ileal conduit. Such a system drains continuously into a collecting device and allows free reflux into the collecting systems. Recently, continent urinary reservoirs with clean, intermittent catheterization have been developed. Most of the newer diversions open onto the abdominal wall although some are adaptable for bladder replacement. Amis et al. and Kruyt et al. reviewed the current radiologic imaging of these diversionary techniques and their articles are recommended reading for radiologic techniques related to the various diversions.[36,37]

Rose and coworkers described plain radiographic evaluation of artificial urinary sphincters.[38] In patients with bladder outlet incompetence, continence can be achieved with a hydraulically operated urinary sphincter. Occasionally, such sphincters malfunction. Approximately half of these malfunctions are the result of loss of water-soluble and radiopaque hydraulic fluid. If the hydraulic fluid is opacified and there is a slow leak, it is almost impossible to visualize radiographically because the fluid is water soluble and there is rapid absorption of the contrast material. Loss of the spherical shape of the balloon reservoir or a decrease in diameter of the reservoir are signs of fluid leakage.

PROSTATIC NEOPLASMS

An excretory urogram has little to offer in the staging of prostatic carcinoma, particularly in early neoplasms. Its primary value is in documenting the possible degree and site of urinary obstruction. Osteoblastic metastases may often be discovered through a radiograph, although a more sensitive indicator is a radionuclide bone scan. Although lymphangiograms have a reported accuracy of 90% in detecting nodal spread of disease, a more reasonable figure may be 70%. The limitations are the same as those applicable to the bladder—the primary drainage route by the obturator and hypogastric or internal iliac nodes are not visualized on lymphangiograms. At this point, lymphangiograms are not routinely used preoperatively. CT scanning has also been examined for use in staging of prostatic carcinoma. Unfortunately, there is a 40% incidence of false-negative findings in detection of lymph node metastases. This is because prostate and bladder carcinomas tend to enlarge lymph nodes only late in disease. The CT scan is unable to detect early metastases with only small peripheral defects in normal-size nodes and it is also unable to differentiate between hyperplasia and nodal involvement by tumor. There is a significant role for use of CT scanning in planning of radiation therapy for assessment of the depth and treatment volumes.

The high prevalence of prostatic carcinoma has prompted a continuing search for accurate screening and staging techniques. Transrectal sonography and early results with MRI have proved interesting but are not clinically impressive. There is a significant debate at the present time concerning the role of endorectal ultrasound and of the significance of small peripheral hypoechoic lesions that can be identified in the prostate. Rifkin et al. biopsied 80 lesions in 79 patients who had either normal or questionably abnormal digital examinations.[39] Twenty-one percent of the lesions were malignant. The authors felt that this was an insufficient percentage to recommend use of endorectal ultrasound as a screening tool. A similar study was performed by Lee et al., but in patients who also had prostatic specific antigen assayed.[40] The positive predictive value for transrectal ultrasound for cancer was only 24% if the digital rectal examination was normal and 12% if the prostate specific antigen was normal. The authors concluded that biopsy of small suspicious lesions may not be indicated if digital rectal and prostatic specific antigen studies are normal. Lee et al. also reported on 669 biopsies with 225 cancers diagnosed.[41] All cancers were hypoechoic relative to the normal peripheral tissue. A recent paper by Rifkin indicated that only about two thirds of carcinomas are hypoechoic, and these are, in general, the better differentiated lesions.[42] Approximately one third of lesions are either isoechoic, hyperechoic, or of mixed echogenicity. These latter lesions are usually poorly differentiated.

Resnick and coworkers questioned whether an ultrasound-guided prostatic biopsy is necessary if a distinct nodule is palpable.[43] They studied 45 patients with palpable nodules, and the results indicate that when a distinct nodule is palpable, ultrasound-guided biopsy is probably not necessary. Ultrasound-guided biopsies can be performed with a number of types of needle. Approximately 40% of patients will have blood in the urine after the biopsy procedure, 10% blood in the stool, and 5% blood in the ejaculate. Approximately 1% will have transient fever. Many authors at this time are giving prophylactic antibiotics at the time of the procedure. In general, core biopsies are detecting approximately 50% more cancers than aspiration biopsies.

MRI of the prostate has received a significant amount of attention. The zonal anatomy of the prostate is appreciated on T2-weighted images. On the T2-weighted images there is a bright signal in the peripheral zone and a relatively lower signal in the transitional and central zones, anterior and lateral to the prostate. The periprostatic venous plexus shows an intense signal. The zonal anatomy is usually more clearly defined in older patients than in the younger patients. Benign prostatic hypertrophy usually shows a mixed intermediate to high signal in an enlarged transitional zone. Unfortunately, separation of benign from malignant processes has been limited because they have similar MRI characteristics. Bezzi et al. reported on the staging of 81 patients with known disease, and MRI had an accuracy of 78% in differentiation of stage A or B from stage C or D disease.[44] Friedman et al. reported on 27 patients with biopsy proven carcinoma who had MRI, transrectal endosonography, and CT.[45] The authors reported that sonography was superior to MRI for detection of intraglandular carcinoma and capsular disruption but that MRI was superior to both sonography and CT for detecting seminal vesicle invasion. At the present time, a five-center National Cancer Institute–funded study to evaluate MRI and endorectal ultrasound is underway. The preliminary data on the first 100 patients indicate that MRI has about a 70% accuracy for staging A and B patients and endorectal sonography has a slightly (but not significantly) lower accuracy. To date, it does not appear that any modality has an accuracy for staging prostatic carcinoma in excess of 80%.

SCROTUM AND TESTICLE

Radiographic examination of patients with malignant testicular neoplasms has been of value in demonstrating metastases. Sonographic techniques permit detailed visualization of the normal and abnormal testicle (Fig. 58-16). Neoplasms are generally manifested as areas of decreased echogenicity within the testicle. A sonogram can differentiate cystic masses from solid testicular neoplasms and can aid in differentiating testicular from extratesticular processes. Benign cysts can occur within the testicle, although they are often nonpalpable and located near the mediastinum testis and are usually solitary. Malignant cysts tend to be multiple and are primarily formed by teratomas and occasionally by seminomas. Martin et al. reported on the role of scrotal ultrasound when physical examination of the scrotal sac was normal.[46] In a retrospective study of 520 patients, they found 15 patients who had either gynecomastia, abdominal lymphadenopathy, or male infertility. Seven testicular tumors were found and confirmed at surgery. At this point, however, no author is advocating routine screening in asymptomatic patients with a normal physical examination.

Testicular nuclear isotope scans have been available for at least a decade and are predominantly useful in differentiating the hypervascularity of epidydimitis from hypovascular entities such as hydrocele and testicular torsion. The sonographic pattern of testicular neoplasms is usually mixed, and the procedure seems of little value for differentiating the type or presence of tumor.

Thurnher et al. compared imaging of the testis utilizing MRI and ultrasound.[47] These authors concluded that ultrasound should continue to be the primary modality for imaging of testicular abnormalities.

Staging of patients with testicular tumors should include a chest radiograph and an excretory urogram (Fig. 58-17). Evaluation of lymphatic metastases is usually performed at this time through the use of CT (Fig. 58-18). Previously reported accuracy of lymphangiograms ranges between 50 and 90%. The use of the CT scan as the initial imaging study for lymphatic metastases is common because many testicular tumors produce nodal enlargement early in the disease. Although some authors have recommended a negative CT examination be followed by a lymphangiogram, Burney and Klatte compared excretory urograms, CT scans, lymphangiograms, and ultrasonograms in 136 patients and concluded that lymphangiography is no longer indicated in patients with testicular tumors.[48] Chest radiography and CT scans are usually the modalities employed for evaluation of tumor response.

TUMORS OF THE PENIS AND URETHRA

In general, urethral carcinoma is rare and the radiographic evaluation of the primary lesion is of little practical value. Furthermore, distant metastases are uncommon. As with some neoplasms of the bladder, cystoscopic examination is the procedure of choice for a definitive diagnosis. Urethrograms provide only minimal help in assessment of tumor extent. Utiliza-

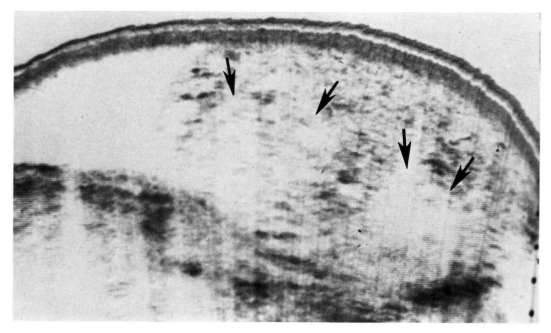

FIG. 58-16. Longitudinal testicular sonogram demonstrating nonhomogeneity and areas of relative sonolucency (arrows) throughout the testicle, in a patient with embryonal cell carcinoma.

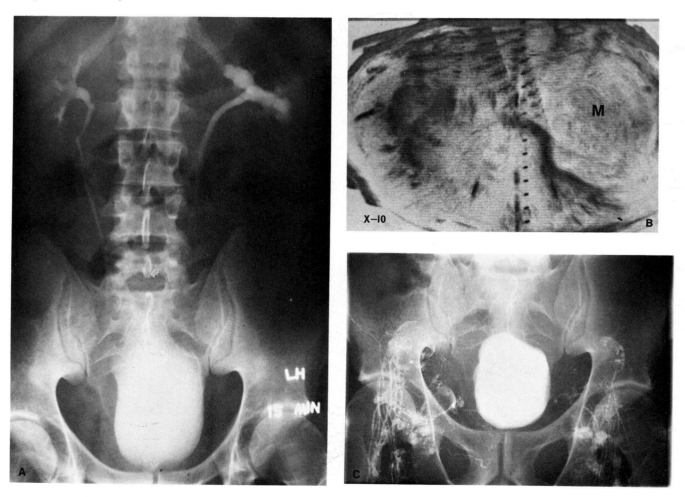

FIG. 58-17. Retroperitoneal and pelvic adenopathy in a patient with seminoma. *A*, The urogram demonstrates medial and anterior deviation of the left ureter, as well as bilateral compression of the bladder. *B*, The transverse sonogram 10 cm below the xiphoid demonstrates a large left-upper-quadrant retroperitoneal mass. *C*, The lymphangiogram demonstrates lymphatic obstruction bilaterally in the pelvis. M = mass.

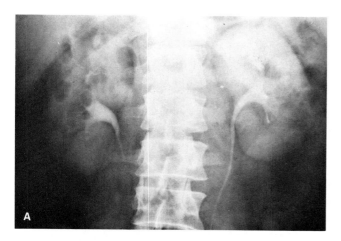

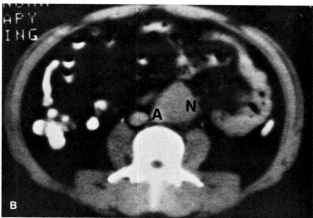

FIG. 58-18. *A*, The staging work-up of a patient with seminoma included an excretory urogram, which demonstrates slight lateral deviation of the proximal left ureter. *B*, The CT scan clearly demonstrates the mass of an enlarged node adjacent to the aorta. N = node; A = aorta.

tion of lymphangiography and arteriography have not been felt to be particularly useful. Some early data on utilization of MRI in evaluation of penile anatomy are available.[49] It does appear that MRI can provide useful images for a number of abnormalities, although its exact role in tumor evaluation remains unclear.

FEMALE REPRODUCTIVE SYSTEM

Evaluation of vaginal, uterine, and adnexal structures have primarily been the province of physical examination and the major imaging modalities used at this time are sonography, CT, and MRI. Recently, transvaginal ultrasound probes have been developed, and multiple studies comparing transvaginal and transabdominal sonography have been concluded. It appears that transvaginal sonography provides more information, particularly regarding the architecture and anatomy of pelvic masses.[50] The reason for this is that transvaginal sonography has somewhat improved spatial resolution compared to transabdominal sonography.

Tumors of the vagina are best delineated by visual inspection. Sonography and CT have played a limited role in tumor evaluation. There have been some recent papers in regard to MRI of the vagina. Chang et al. reported on use of MRI for evaluation of vaginal neoplasms in 87 patients.[51] Reported accuracy for detection of metastatic disease was 92% and accuracy for detection of recurrent vaginal cancer was 82%. Many authors have reported on the use of MRI staging of cervical carcinoma. The overall accuracy of CT staging in patients with cervical carcinoma ranges between 65 and 80%. Rubens et al. used MRI to stage 27 patients with 1B cervical carcinoma.[52] The authors pointed out that tumors are usually identified as high signal on T2-weighted MR images. In their study, in 6 of 10 patients the extent of disease was underestimated by clinical examination under anesthesia and these patients would have received radiation therapy prior to surgery if the MRI information had been used. Hricak et al. pointed out that clinical staging results in errors 23% of the time in patients with stage-2B disease and 64% of the time in patients with stage-3B disease.[53] This is primarily because of inaccurate assessment of the parametrial and pelvic sidewalls as well as the lymph nodes. The overall reported accuracy of MRI staging is approximately 80%.

For stage-1B to stage-2A tumors clinical staging by experienced gynecologists appears to have a higher accuracy (70 to 92%) than CT (30 to 58%).[52] CT is usually performed on stage-3B and -4 tumors. Limitations of CT are that the normal cervix and cervical carcinoma have similar attenuation values. On CT, carcinoma of the endometrium is usually demonstrated as enlargement or a focal mass in the uterine wall. MRI is better able to delineate normal from neoplastic tissue in this regard. Owing to the ease with which CT can be performed over the entire abdomen and pelvis, it is premature to replace CT with MRI for stage-2B to stage-4 tumors.

Evaluation of the uterus in regard to benign neoplasms such as leiomyomas was performed in the past with sonography. Dudiak et al. recently used MRI and compared it with ultrasound and hysterosalpingography. Specificity of all modalities was equal although the accuracy for MRI (94%) was slightly better than that for ultrasound (87%) (Fig. 58-19). The authors suggested that MRI be used for patients for whom myomectomy is contemplated and for whom sufficient myometrium will remain after reconstruction so that childbearing may be possible.

CT evaluation of lesions is usually performed for malignancies and evaluation of extrauterine extent. Trerotola et al. described the CT appearance of uterine sarcomas.[55] These are rare lesions and represent only 2% of uterine malignancies. In 12 of their 14 reported cases, CT characteristically demonstrated a low-density mass within the uterine cavity measuring between 4 and 30 cm.

Carcinoma of the endometrium is the fourth most common site of malignancy in American women. Hysterosalpingography is hardly ever used in this evaluation of these lesions. MRI is unable to distinguish endometrial carcinoma from blood clot or adenomatous hyperplasia, and its primary use is

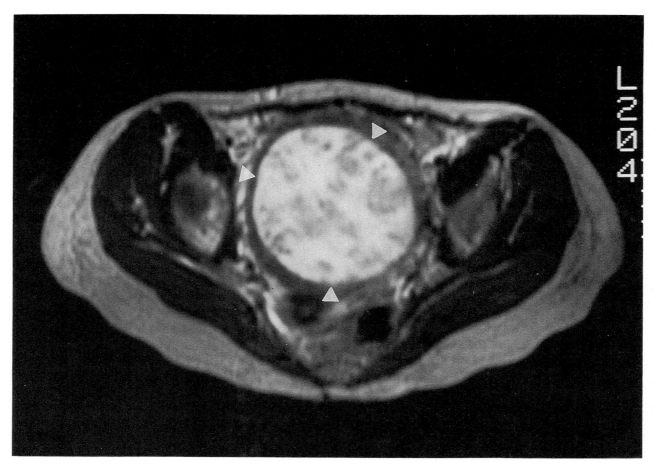

Fig. 58-19. MRI of degenerated uterine leiomyoma showing mixed signal intensity.

the local staging of the disease after the diagnosis has been histologically documented. On MRI, endometrial carcinoma is seen as an abnormality in the central endometrial cavity with widening of the endometrium or the presence of endometrial masses. Disruption of the low-intensity junctional zone located between the endometrium and myometrium represents myometrial invasion. Tumors are usually identified as high-intensity signal on T2-weighted images. Overall accuracy for staging is about 90% and overall accuracy demonstrating depth of myometrial invasion is about 80%.[56] Demonstration of adnexal, peritoneal metastases, or lymphadenopathy in general is suboptimal.

Sonography probably remains the imaging modality of choice for adnexal lesions. There is relatively accurate anatomic information with demonstration of either solid or cystic components. Unfortunately, although the sensitivity is high, specificity remains low with the exception of lesions such as cystadenocarcinomas. Sonographically appearing "solid lesions," which may represent a wide range of abnormalities such as complicated cysts, endometrioma, or a malignant neoplasm, are difficult to evaluate. In most cases, surgical exploration is necessary.

Most common malignant ovarian primary tumors are adenocarcinomas, serous or mucinous cystadenocarcinomas, and endometrioid carcinoma. The majority of patients with ovarian carcinoma present with stage-3 or -4 disease and the 5-year survival rate for ovarian cancer is only about 20 to 30%. Cystadenocarcinomas appear predominantly as cystic tumors either on CT or with sonography. Usually other ovarian tumors are mixed solid and cystic or predominantly solid masses.

Detection of both solid and cystic ovarian tumors with ultrasonography is 95% accurate. Although accurate staging for malignant ovarian tumors is about 50%.

It is not clear at the present time that use of MRI has significant advantages for evaluation of adnexal abnormalities compared with CT and ultrasound. All of the imaging modalities can easily detect the presence of ascites in a patient with ovarian carcinoma but have great difficulty in evaluation of peritoneal implants. CT scan detects peritoneal implant in slightly more than half the patients in whom they are present.

RETROPERITONEAL TUMORS

Primary retroperitoneal neoplasms involve the urinary tract either by direct invasion or displacement, often causing obstruction that is readily apparent on excretory urograms. The tumors may be generally classified as those of mesodermal, neural, or embryonic origin. The most common malignant tumors are lymphomas, liposarcomas, and leiomyosarcomas. There are several benign lesions that occur in the retroperitoneum such as pancreatic pseudocysts, dermoid cysts, and neurofibromas. Occasionally retroperitoneal fibrosis can simulate tumor involvement in the retroperitoneum.

In general, retroperitoneal tumors are difficult to assess accurately by standard urographic method. Involvement of the kidney or ureter may be surmised, but determination of the extent of the tumor and of the possible site of origin usually require a CT scan (Fig. 58-20). Sonography is of more limited value and angiograms are of little practical value in assessment of these tumors. It should be noted that CT demonstration of hypervascularity in a well-defined retroperitoneal tumor, particularly in the pelvis, is more suggestive of a hemangiopericytoma than a liposarcoma or malignant fibrous histiocytoma.[57]

PEDIATRIC TUMORS

Wilms' Tumor

The most common malignant tumor in infants and children is Wilms' tumor. This is the second most common intra-abdominal tumor in children. Patients who have these tumors usually present with palpable abdominal mass. The incidence of bilateral disease ranges from 5 to 12% in most series. Children with hemihypertrophy or sporadic aniridia have an increased incidence of Wilms' tumor. Excretory urography and CT are the most commonly used diagnostic imaging procedures. With excretory urography, a disturbance of the normal collecting system is seen in most cases because Wilms' tumor is an intrinsic renal lesion. Wilms' tumors may occasionally occur in adults and calcification is present in about 10 to 15% of tumors. CT is valuable in determining the size and extent of tumor as well as indicating the presence of liver metastases. CT scanning is of particular value in cases where the tumor is large enough to cause nonvisualization of the kidney on an intravenous pyelogram (Fig. 58-21). A preoperative chest roentgenogram is usually performed and estimates of pulmonary involvement at time of initial diagnosis range from 9 to 30%.

Most stage-1 Wilms' tumors previously reported in patients less than 6 months old have been found to be congenital mesoblastic nephromas. As with Wilms' tumor, these tumors demonstrate distortion of the collecting system of the kidney on urograms.

Neuroblastoma

Neuroblastoma is the most common malignant retroperitoneal tumor in childhood. These tumors may arise from the adrenal

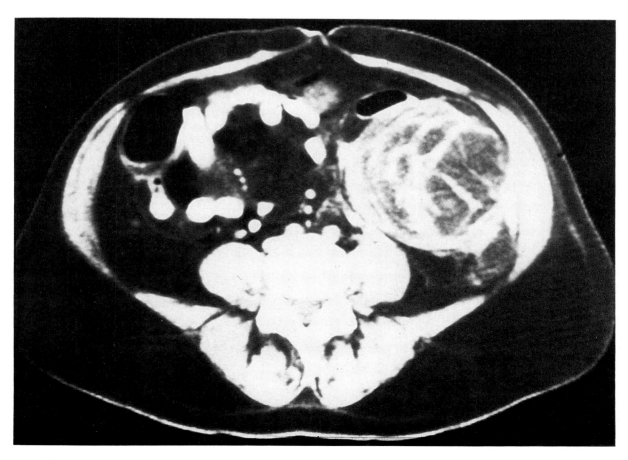

FIG. 58-20. CT scan of left retroperitoneal liposarcoma.

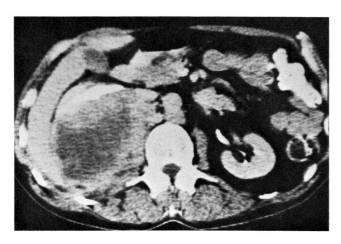

FIG. 58-21. Wilms' tumor occurring in an adult. The CT scan clearly demonstrates an intrinsic lesion of the right kidney with anterior displacement and distortion of the right collecting system. (Case courtesy of Robert S. Seigel, M.D.)

medulla or in sympathetic ganglia. Large, soft tissue masses may be identified on plain film, and an abdominal mass or distention is one of the most common presenting complaints. There are several important radiographic points that allow differentiation of these tumors on both plain films and excretory urograms. Calcification of neuroblastomas is common, occurring in about 50% of tumors. Tumors are extrarenal, usually displacing the kidney rather than causing an abnormal calyceal appearance.

The extent of disease at the time of diagnosis is significantly different from that of Wilms' tumor. Only 20% of Wilms' tumor patients have identifiable metastases, whereas 70% of patients with neuroblastoma will have distant disease. The predominant route of tumor spread is also different. The most common site of metastases from neuroblastoma is bone, whereas in Wilms' tumor pulmonary metastases are more common. In the evaluation of bony metastases, the use of plain film skeletal surveys and radionuclide bone scans are complementary. Arteriograms and venograms usually have little to offer in the staging work-up unless the surgeon requires this for a vascular road map. Evaluation of extent of neuroblastoma within the abdomen is usually performed by CT scanning.

REFERENCES

1. PICKERING, R. S., et al. Excretory urographic localization of adrenal cortical tumors and pheochromocytomas. Radiology, *114*:345, 1975.
2. SAMPLE, W. F. Adrenal ultrasonography. Radiology, *127*:461, 1978.
3. GLAZER, G., FRANCIS, I., and QUINT, L. Imaging of the adrenal glands. Invest. Radiol., *23*:3, 1988.
4. BERLAND, L. L. et al. Differentiation between small benign and malignant adrenal masses with dynamic increment at CT. AJR *151*:95, 1988.
5. BERNARDINO, M. E. Management of the asymptomatic patient with a unilateral adrenal mass. Radiology, *166*:121, 1988.
6. WARSHAUER, D. et al. Detection of renal masses: Sensitivities and specificities of excretory urography/linear tomography, ultrasound and CT. Radiology, *169*:363, 1988.
7. BOSNIAK, M. A., MEGIBOW, A. J., and HULNICK, G. H. CT diagnosis of renal angiomyolipoma: The importance of detecting small amounts of fat. AJR *151*:497, 1988.
8. UHLENBROCK, D., FISCHER, C., and BEYER, H. K. Angiomyolipoma of the kidney: Comparison between magnetic resonance imaging, computed tomography and ultrasonography for diagnosis. Acta Radiol., *29*:523, 1988.
9. ARENSON, A. et al. Angiomyolipoma of the kidney extending into the inferior vena cava: Sonographic and CT findings. AJR, *151*:1159, 1988.
10. NEISIUS, D. et al. Computed tomographic and angiographic findings in renal oncocytoma. Br. J. Radiol., *61*:1019, 1988.
11. REMARK, R. R. et al. Magnetic resonance imaging of renal oncocytoma. Urology, *31*:176, 1988.
12. MCKEOWN, D., et al. Carcinoid of the kidney: Radiologic findings. AJR, *150*:143, 1988.
13. WITTEN, D. M., MYERS, G. H., and UTZ, D. C. *Clinical Urography.* 4th Ed. Philadelphia, W. B. Saunders, Co., 1977.
14. AMENDOLA, M. A., et al. Small renal cell carcinoma: Resolving a diagnostic dilemma. Radiology, *166*:637, 1988.
15. UEDA, T., NISHITANI, H., and KUDO, H. Comparison of angiography and computed tomography using new morphologic criteria in staging renal cell carcinoma. Urology, *32*:459, 1988.
16. ZEMAN, R. K. et al. Renal cell carcinoma: Dynamic thin section CT assessment of vascular invasion and tumor vascularity. Radiology, *167*:393, 1988.
17. HRICAK, H. et al. Magnetic resonance imaging in the diagnosis and staging of renal and perirenal neoplasms. Radiology, *154*:709, 1985.
18. HRICAK, H. et al. Detection and staging of renal neoplasms: A reassessment of MR imaging. Radiology, *166*:643, 1988.
19. WATSON, R. C., FLEMING, R. J., and EVANS, J. A. Arteriography in the diagnosis of renal carcinoma: Review of 100 cases. Radiology, *91*:888, 1968.
20. CHUANG, V. T., and FRIED, A. M. High dose renal pharmacoangiography in the assessment of hypovascular renal neoplasms. Am. J. Roentgenol., *131*:807, 1978.
21. RANKIN, R. N. Gas formation after renal tumor embolization without abscess: A benign occurrence. Radiology, *130*:317, 1979.
22. KAPLAN, J. H., MCDONALD, J. R., and THOMPSON, G. J. Multicentric origin of papillary tumors of the urinary tract. J. Urol., *66*:792, 1951.
23. YOUSEM, D. et al. Synchronous and metachronous transitional cell carcinoma of the urinary tract: Prevalence, incidence and radiographic detection. Radiology, *167*:613, 1988.
24. POLLACK, H. M. et al. Computed tomography of renal pelvic filling defects. Radiology, *138*:645, 1981.
25. BOSNIAK, M. A. et al. Computed tomography of ureteral obstruction. AJR, *138*:1107, 1982.

26. FEDERLE, M. P., et al. Computed tomography of urinary calculi. AJR, *136*:255, 1981.

27. BARENTSZ, J. O. et al. Carcinoma of the urinary bladder: MR imaging with double surface coil. AJR, *151*:107, 1988.

28. HOSBAND, J. E. et al. Comparison of CT and MR imaging for staging bladder cancer. Presented at the Seventy-fourth Scientific Assembly and Annual Meeting of the Radiological Society of North America, Chicago, November 27–December 2, 1988.

29. MORGAN, C. L., CALKINS, R. F., and CAVALCANTI, E. J. Computed tomography in evaluation, staging and therapy of carcinoma of the bladder and prostate. Radiology, *140*:751, 1981.

30. JEFFREY, R. B., PALUBINSKAS, A. J., and FEDERLE, M. P. CT evaluation of invasive lesions of the bladder. J. Comput. Assist. Tomogr., *5*:22, 1981.

31. COSS, J. C. et al. CT staging of bladder carcinoma. AJR, *137*:359, 1981.

32. WALSH, J. W. et al. Computed tomographic detection of pelvic and inguinal lymph node metastases from primary and recurrent pelvic malignant disease. Radiology, *137*:157, 1980.

33. LEE, J. K. et al. Accuracy of CT in detecting intra-abdominal and pelvic lymph node metastases from pelvic cancers. AJR, *131*:675, 1978.

34. BUY, J. et al. MR staging of bladder carcinoma: Correlation with pathologic findings. Radiology, *169*:695, 1988.

35. GOLDMAN, S. M. et al. Metastatic transitional cell carcinoma from the bladder: Radiographic manifestations. Am. J. Roentgenol., *132*:419, 1979.

36. AMIS, E. S., NEWHOUSE, J. H., and OLSSON, C. A. Continent urinary diversions: Review of current surgical procedures in radiologic imaging. Radiology, *168*:395, 1988.

37. KRUYT, R. H., KUMS, J. J., and KOCH, K. Pouch urinary diversion: Follow-up by ultrasound. Br. J. Radiol., *61*:811, 1988.

38. ROSE, S. et al. Artificial urinary sphincters: Plain radiography of malfunctions and complications. Radiology, *168*:403, 1988.

39. RIFKIN, M., and CHOI, H. Implications of small peripheral hypoechoic lesions in endorectal ultrasound of the prostate. Radiology, *166*:619, 1988.

40. LEE, F. et al. Hypoechoic lesions of the prostate: Clinical relevance of tumor size, digital rectal examination and prostate specific antigen. Radiology, *178*:29, 1989.

41. LEE, F. et al. Prostate cancer: Comparison of transrectal ultrasound and digital rectal examination for screening. Radiology, *168*:389, 1988.

42. RIFKIN, M. D., McGLYNN, E. T., and CHOI, H. Echogenicity of prostate cancer correlated with histologic grade and stromal fibrosis: Endorectal ultrasound studies. Radiology, *170*:549, 1989.

43. RESNICK, M. I. Transrectal ultrasound guided vs. digitally directed prostatic biopsy: A comparative study. J. Urol., *139*:754, 1988.

44. BEZZI, M. et al. Prostatic carcinoma: Staging with MR imaging at 1.5 T. Radiology, *169*:339, 1988.

45. FRIEDMAN, A. C. et al. Relative merits of MRI, transrectal endosonography and CT in the diagnosis and staging of carcinoma of the prostate. Urology, *31*:530, 1988.

46. MARTIN, B., BELAISCH, J., and TUBLINA, J. M. What is the role for scrotal ultrasound when physical examination of the scrotal sac is normal? Presented at the Seventy-fourth Scientific Assembly and Annual Meeting of the Radiologic Society of North America, Chicago, November 27–December 2, 1988.

47. THURNHER, S. et al. Imaging of the testis: Comparison between MR imaging and ultrasound. Radiology, *167*:631, 1988.

48. BURNEY, D. G., and KLATTE, E. C. Ultrasound and computed tomography of the abdomen in the staging and management of testicular carcinoma. Radiology, *132*:415, 1979.

49. HRICAK, H. et al. Normal penile anatomy and abnormal penile conditions: Evaluation with MR imaging. Radiology, *169*:683, 1988.

50. LEIBMAN, A. J., KRUZE, B., and McSWEENEY, M. B. Transvaginal sonography: Comparison with transabdominal sonography in diagnosis of pelvic masses. Am. J. Roentgenol., *151*:89, 1988.

51. CHANG, Y. et al. Vagina: Evaluation with MR imaging. Part II. Neoplasms. Radiology, *169*:175, 1988.

52. RUBENS, D. et al. Stage 1B cervical carcinoma: Comparison of MR and pathologic staging. AJR, *150*:135, 1988.

53. HRICAK, H. et al. Invasive cervical carcinoma: Comparison of MR imaging and surgical findings. Radiology, *166*:623, 1988.

54. DUDIAK, C. M. et al. Uterine lyomyomas in the infertile patient. Radiology, *167*:627, 1988.

55. TREROTOLA, S. O., FISHMAN, E. K., and KUHLMAN, J. E. CT of uterine sarcomas. Presented at the Seventy-fourth Scientific Assembly and Annual Meeting of the Radiologic Society of North America, Chicago, November 27–December 2, 1988.

56. HRICAK, H. et al. Endometrial carcinoma staging by MR imaging. Radiology, *162*:297, 1987.

57. GOLDMAN, S. M., DAVIDSON, A. J., and NEAL, J. Retroperitoneal and Pelvic Hemangio-pericytomas: Clinical radiologic and pathologic correlations Radiology, *168*:13, 1988.

Transrectal
Ultrasonography

Glenn Gerber
Gerald Chodak

HISTORICAL PERSPECTIVE

The interest in prostatic ultrasonography has increased significantly since the 1960's. Initially, transabdominal, transvesical, and transrectal scanning were developed for imaging the pelvic structures.[1,2] A-mode imaging was originally used, but the multitude of interfaces in the pelvis made interpretation difficult.[1] Prostate ultrasound was developed with the aim of providing a safe, reliable method for determining the size of the prostate. The differential diagnosis or early detection of prostatic lesions were also deemed possible.[3] Beginning in the late 1960s, largely through the work of Watanabe et al., transrectal imaging of the prostate became increasingly effective.[4,5] A major advance was the use of B-mode imaging displayed on a black-and-white screen.[6] During the 1970s and early 1980s, several developments enhanced prostate imaging. These included the use of gray scale imaging, first reported by Boyce et al. in 1976,[7] as well as the introduction of real time imaging and high frequency transducers. Early studies were performed using 3.5 mHz transducers that rotated 360° at right angles to the probe yielding transverse serial sections of the prostate.

Recently, 4.0, 5.0, and 7.0 mHz transducers with phased array and linear array scanners have improved image quality and allowed the addition of sagittal views of the prostate.[8] As the ability to delineate the structure and outline of the prostate improved, the interest in developing and refining the clinical applications of transrectal ultrasound grew. Several investigators reported the use of ultrasound in screening, staging, and assessment of tumor response in prostate cancer.[9–22] In addition, the use of ultrasonography to enhance the accuracy of prostate biopsy was developed.[23–26] Although several controversies exist regarding these uses, the ability to reliably and safely image the prostate has made transrectal ultrasonography an increasingly useful part of the urologic diagnostic armamentarium.

GENERAL METHODS

To perform transrectal sonography, a transducer is coupled to an endorectal probe. The probe may be either chair mounted or hand held. The hand-held probes enable the physician to have greater control during the exam and they allow for ultrasound-guided biopsy of the prostate.

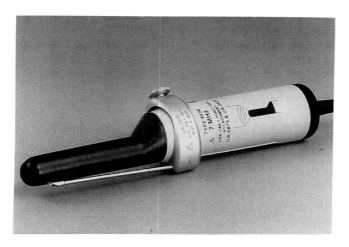

FIG. 59-1. Transrectal probe with needle guide attachment permits ultrasonically guided transrectal core biopsy.

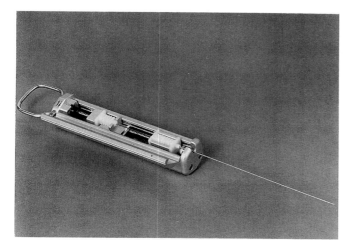

FIG. 59-2. Biopty instrument (Bard) fitted with an 18-gauge needle for core biopsy of the prostate.

A thorough examination of the prostate requires axial and longitudinal views. This can be accomplished using a single endorectal probe with either two transducers or a single rotating transducer. Alternatively, two different probes with differently oriented transducers can be employed.[27] Prior to transrectal insertion, the instrument is covered with a condom that is inflated with water. Some probes now have a built-in water bath. This provides a coupling mechanism between the transducer and the tissues. All air is aspirated from within the condom to prevent interference with ultrasonic visualization. Rather than a water-filled condom, a disposable latex cuff may be used. The patient may be positioned in the lateral knee-chest position, standing bent over the examining table, or in the dorsal lithotomy position. A sodium biphosphate (Fleet) enema is the only preparation required. In the lateral position, any air in the balloon will not distort the study.

The axially oriented image yields right-left symmetry as the probe is moved to visualize the structures from the seminal vesicles proximally to the prostatic apex distally. Longitudinal orientation images the prostatic urethra, base, and apex simultaneously. The probe is rotated to evaluate the lateral prostate and seminal vesicles.

Transrectal ultrasound may be used to biopsy the prostate. The needle may be inserted either transrectally or transperineally. With the latter method, once the suspicious area is located, the needle is passed into the perineum parallel to the probe after local infiltration with lidocaine. Continuous sonographic visualization is used as the needle is advanced into the lesion and a core is obtained.[23,24] Other investigators have used a grid with multiple needle holes placed against the perineum. With this method, the site of the needle entry corresponds to a grid appearing on the viewing screen.[25] Along similar lines, a puncture attachment mounted on the rectal probe may be used to facilitate needle placement.[26]

Alternatively, transrectal biopsy may be performed. This requires the use of a cleansing enema. The need for prophylactic antibiotics with transrectal biopsy is debated and may depend on whether aspiration or core biopsies are to be performed. The latter employs a larger needle and has been shown to have a higher complication rate, even with the routine use of antibiotics.[28] A variety of patient positions may be used for transrectal biopsy. Specially produced guides are placed over the insertable portion of the endorectal probe and are used to facilitate needle placement into the suspicious area (Fig. 59-1). The value of ultrasonically guided prostate biopsy and a comparison of biopsy techniques will be discussed in a later section. Recently, rapid-fire biopsy instruments have been developed for transrectal use with an 18-gauge needle (Fig. 59-2). This method appears to have a lower infection rate than previous core biopsy methods.

CLINICAL FINDINGS

Anatomically, the glandular prostate is divided into three zones (Figs. 59-3 and 59-4).[29] The transition zone is adjacent to the proximal urethra and the central zone is located posteriorly and comprises the base of the gland. The ejaculatory ducts are located in this zone. The peripheral zone contains approximately 70% of the glandular tissue of the prostate. It is located posteriorly, laterally, at the apex of the prostate, and to some extent anteriorly. In addition, fibromuscular stroma is present along the anterior surface of the urethra.

Transrectal sonography is usually not able to distinguish between the central and peripheral areas. Both appear homogeneous and isoechoic in the posterior portion of the gland. In the midline and the anterior-superior aspect of the prostate, a relatively hypoechoic area is seen. This represents the internal sphincter, the transition zone, and the periurethral glandular tissue and extends from the base of the prostate to the verumontanum.[27] The normal prostate is characterized by sharp contours, symmetry, and a semilunar shape (Fig. 59-5). Benign hyperplasia causes an increase in the anteroposterior diameter, giving the gland a more globular shape (Fig. 59-6). The symmetry is preserved, however, and the contours remain

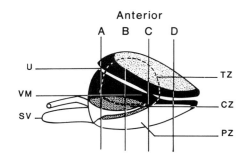

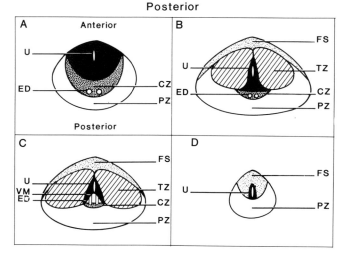

FIG. 59-3. Schematic drawing of axial images of prostate. (U = urethra, ED = ejaculatory duct, SV = seminal vesicle, VM = , TZ = transition zone, CZ = central zone, PZ = peripheral zone, and FS = fibromuscular stroma.)

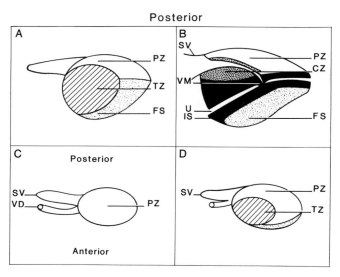

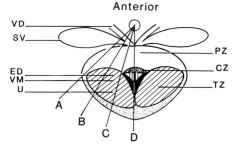

FIG. 59-4. Schematic drawing of sagittal images of prostate. (U = urethra, ED = ejaculatory duct, SV = seminal vesicles, IS = internal sphincter, TZ = transition zone, CZ = central zone, PZ = peripheral zone, and FS = fibromuscular stroma.)

sharp. The echo pattern of adenomatous tissue is fine and homogeneous and a plane of demarcation may be visible between the periurethral glandular tissue and the peripheral zone surgical capsule (see Fig. 59-6).[30] (Hyperplastic nodules may cause bulging of the capsule, but they should never cause infiltration or disruption.)

Prostatitis may cause a heterogeneous echo pattern or the echoes may be symmetrically decreased. This decrease is presumed to be secondary to edema.[31] Prostatic calculuses are usually brightly echogenic in one of two patterns (Fig. 59-7). Type A is characterized by discrete, small echoes and type B is seen as a large mass of multiple echoes.[32] Prostatitis may give the same echo appearance as cancer.

The normal seminal vesicles are sausage shaped and are generally more hypoechoic than the prostate. They may have unusual shapes, but are generally symmetrical and homogeneous (Fig. 59-8).

PROSTATE CARCINOMA

Prostate cancer may show a variety of sonographic appearances. Early reports noted cancer to be hyperechoic, hypoechoic or a mixture of both.[33] Further work, however, has demonstrated that hypoechoic lesions are the most common, particularly in small cancers (Fig. 59-9). Lee et al. reported a series of histologically proved cancers detected by

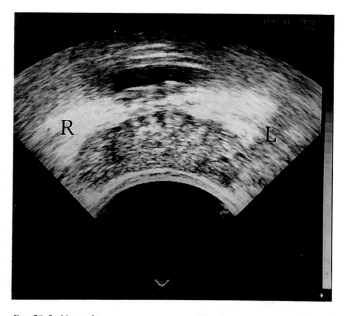

FIG. 59-5. Normal transverse sonogram. Gland appears sausage shaped with small anterior-posterior diameter. Echo pattern appears homogeneous. (R = right and L = left.)

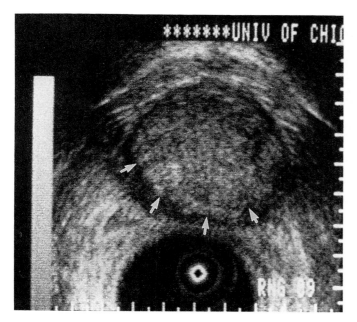

FIG. 59-6. Transverse sonogram showing marked BPH with increased anterior-posterior diameter of transitional zone and compressed peripheral zone. Surgical capsule indicated by arrows.

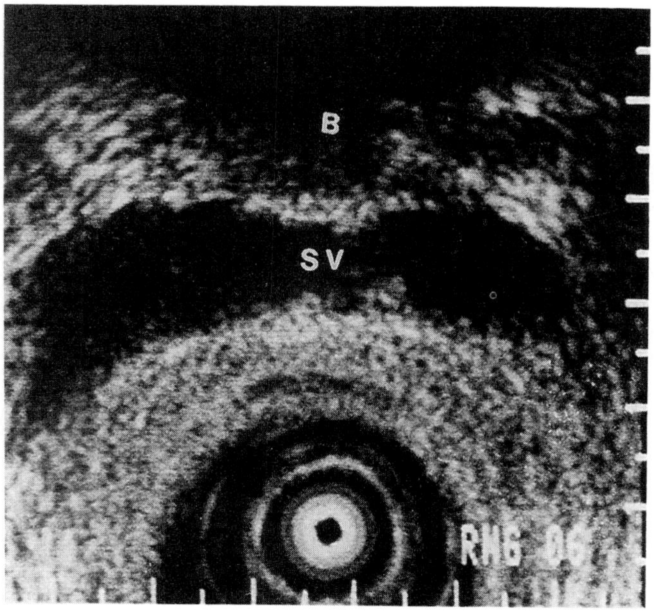

FIG. 59-8. Normal seminal vesicles (SV) seen on axial scan. No prostate is visualized proximally, but bladder (B) is present.

ultrasound, all of which were hypoechoic.[34] A group of over 200 cases of prostate cancer reported by Griffiths et al. revealed that 92% of confined tumors and 100% of unconfined tumors were hypoechoic.[35] One difficulty is that chronic bacterial prostatitis may also yield hypoechoic images. Overall, 20 to 25% of peripheral hypoechoic lesions are malignant.[27]

As lesions enlarge, they may appear more echogenic than surrounding prostatic tissue or they may show a mixed appearance. This is possibly caused by infiltration of normal or

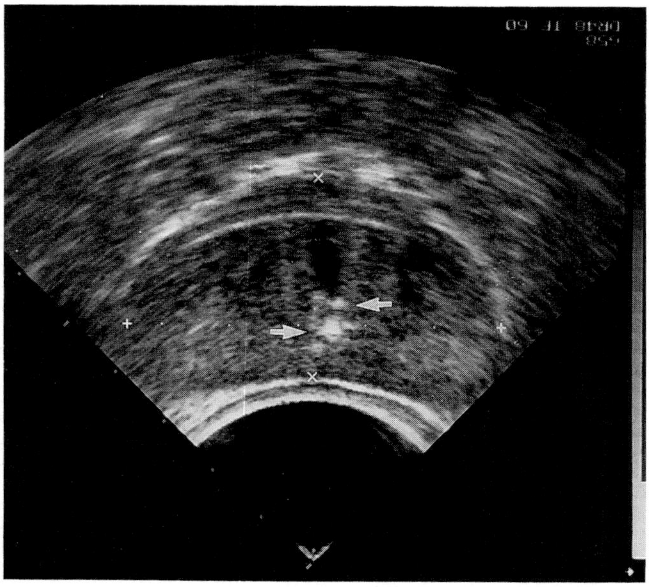

FIG. 59-7. Prostatic calculuses near posterior portion of peripheral zone. Calculuses produce shadow distal to the probe (see arrows).

benign hyperplastic tissues by cancer.[27] One study suggested that 25% of cancers are isoechoic and thus are not seen by ultrasound.[36] The etiology of changes in echogenicity has not been fully elucidated. Cellular differentiation, tumor size and desmoplastic or fibrous reaction have been postulated to play a role.[37,38] Salo et al. reported that anaplastic tumors show mixed or hyperechoic images, moderately differentiated tumors are isoechoic and well-differentiated tumors, in general, are hypoechoic.[38] This has been disputed by others.

In summary, prostate cancer is suggested by several characteristic ultrasonographic findings. These include asymmetrical or abnormal echogenic foci, asymmetry in the size or shape of the prostate, capsular disruption, and the loss of normal differentiation between the central tissues and the peripheral zone.[27]

ROLE OF ULTRASOUND IN STAGING PROSTATE CANCER

The determination of stage-B versus stage-C disease is usually a critical step in therapeutic decision making. Traditionally, digital rectal examination has been the primary means of making this differentiation. However, this approach is highly subjective and often unreliable.[39] As a result, transrectal sonography has become increasingly studied to determine if the staging accuracy can be improved. The additional information provided by the sonogram may enable the physician to offer better counseling to the patient regarding the optimum treatment. If tumor has spread to periprostatic tissues or into the seminal vesicles, the chance for local cure by surgery alone is small. Some patients might be reluctant to undergo surgery if they will also need to receive radiation as part of the treat-

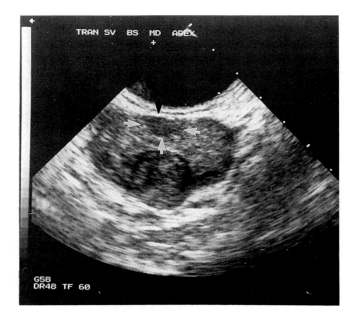

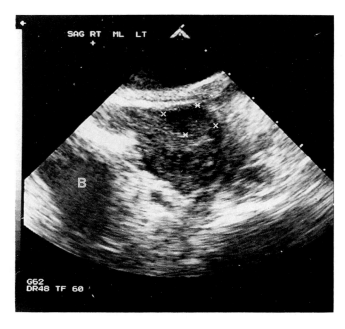

FIG. 59-9. *A,* Transverse scan showing hypoechoic lesion near midline of peripheral zone (shown by arrow). Patient had clinical tumor measuring approximately 13 × 8 mm. *B,* Sagittal image of same patient. Hypoechoic tumor is demonstrated and extends from apex to beyond midgland (tumor outlined by crosses, B = bladder).

ment. In these cases, radiation therapy may be a better option than radical prostatectomy. Conversely, if sonography confirmed that disease was confined within the prostatic capsule, the choice of radical prostatectomy could be made with greater confidence that cure could be obtained.

Several investigators have reported on the accuracy of transrectal sonography in staging prostate cancer. In 1980,

Resnick et al. showed that the stage of tumor determined by ultrasound corresponded exactly to the pathologic stage in 23 radical prostatectomy specimens. This included four patients, who had stage-B disease by digital examination, but spread to the seminal vesicles was noted sonographically.[10] Pontes et al. reported the sensitivity of ultrasound in detecting capsular and seminal vesicle involvement to be 89 and 100%, respectively. However, the specificity was only 50% for extracapsular spread. They speculated that the latter result was secondary to the inability of ultrasound to detect microscopic disease.[11] In a study by Fujino and Scardino, 8 of 18 patients, whose tumor appeared confined to the prostate by rectal examination had extension beyond the prostate by ultrasonography, which was also suggested by operative findings.[12] Recently, the value of magnetic resonance imaging (MRI), transrectal sonography, and computerized tomography (CT) scanning were evaluated in the staging of prostate cancer.[13] Ultrasound was deemed superior in detecting capsular disruption, but MRI was better in evaluating seminal vesicle invasion. No comparison was made with digital examination.

The major problem with staging by transrectal sonography is the difficulty in identifying microscopic invasion of the capsule. One study reported that 9 of 31 tumors that were confined to the prostate by ultrasound had capsular involvement in the prostatectomy specimen.[11] In addition, ultrasound demonstrated apparent capsular penetration that was not confirmed pathologically in two patients. The authors felt that these false-positive findings were the result of capsular distortion secondary to recent transurethral resection, which suggests that caution should be used in interpreting the scans in patients who had previous prostate surgery.

Detection of small volume seminal vesicle involvement may be even more difficult. Only 30% of tumors with spread to the seminal vesicles could be detected by ultrasound in two studies.[11,13]

The sonographic criteria for capsular and seminal vesicle invasion are still evolving. Spread to periprostatic tissues is determined sonographically by disruption of the normally well-defined echogenic capsule (Fig. 59-10). Seminal vesicle involvement by tumor may be suspected by asymmetry of the vesicles, alterations in echo texture (Fig. 59-11) and obliteration of the tissue planes in the angle between the seminal vesicles and the prostate (Fig. 59-12).[9] A major criticism of almost all of these studies is that there has been no correlation of the location of extracapsular tumor as assessed by ultrasound with that assessed by histology. Before ultrasound can be used reliably for these purposes, additional studies are clearly needed.

In summary, the initial studies suggest that transrectal ultrasonography is more effective than the digital examination in differentiating stage-B and stage-C prostate cancer. This differentiation is of great importance in determining therapy in the individual patient. The limitation of sonography lies in its inability to detect microscopic invasion of either the capsule or the seminal vesicles. Despite this shortcoming, staging by transrectal sonography may eventually be one of the most useful roles for this new modality.

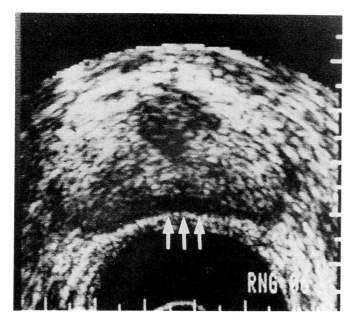

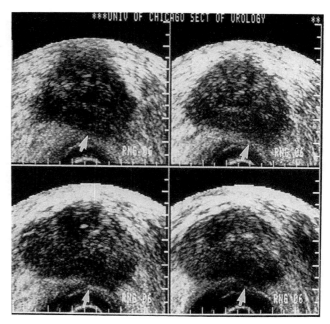

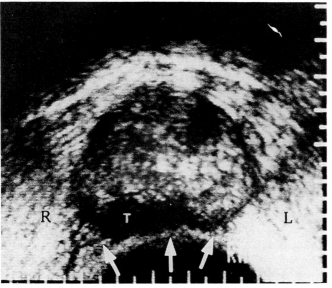

FIG. 59-10. *A,* Hypoechoic lesion (t) in peripheral zone (indicated by arrows) abuts capsule, but does not distort it. Patient had no extracapsular tumor following radical prostatectomy. *B,* Irregular hypoechoic lesion occupies posterior portion of peripheral zone with marked irregularity of capsule (shown by arrows) indicative of extracapsular tumor (R = right, L = left, and T = tumor). *C,* Four axial images of patient with metastatic tumor capsule is grossly distorted primarily at left posterior area (indicated by arrows).

ROLE OF ULTRASOUND IN ASSESSING RESPONSE TO THERAPY

For patients treated by hormonal manipulation or radiotherapy, criteria for assessing response of the primary tumor have been difficult to define. Transrectal ultrasonography has proven to be accurate in determining the size of the prostate with a variance of less than 5%.[4] In addition, prostatic sonography is reproducible and inexpensive with minimal morbidity, thus allowing serial examinations. The value of assessing reduction in prostate volume in response to treatment has been investigated (Fig. 59-13).

Carpentier et al. reported on 55 patients treated by orchiectomy for various stages of prostate cancer. Ten patients showed progression of distant metastases within 1 year of treatment. The initial volume reduction of the prostate in these 10 patients was significantly less than in the remainder of the patients. Also, of patients whose prostatic volume decreased to at least 50% of the pretreatment volume after 3 months, none developed distant progression within 1 year. Finally, 78% of patients whose prostatic volume decreased by less than 30% progressed before or after 1 year.[14] Other studies using luteinizing hormone-releasing hormone (LHRH) agonists, rather than orchiectomy, have confirmed that a rapid decline in prostate volume (greater than 50% in 3 to 4 months) portends a much better prognosis.[15,16]

Radiotherapy also leads to a reduction in prostate volume in most cases. However, at 3 months, the average volume decrease is significantly less than with castration.[12,17] One study noted that 5 of 24 patients treated with radiation showed an increased prostatic volume 3 to 9 months after initiation of therapy. All 5 patients developed pronounced acute proctitis;

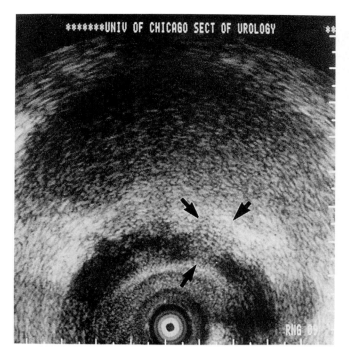

FIG. 59-11. Asymmetric seminal vesicles demonstrated by echogenic area on left infiltrating hypoechoic seminal vesicles (shown by arrows).

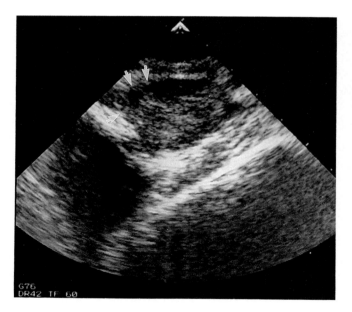

FIG. 59-12. Sagittal scan of patient with stage-C carcinoma. Hypoechoic lesion in peripheral zone extends into base of seminal vesicles distorting normal angle between prostate and seminal vesicles.

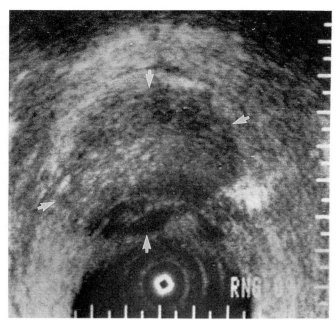

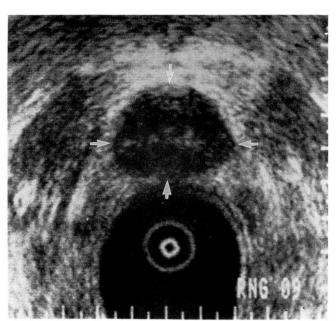

FIG. 59-13. *A*, Axial image of patient with metastatic prostate cancer taken prior to treatment. Image is 6.5 cm from anus and measures approximately 5.5 × 4 cm. *B*, Axial image of same patient approximately 6 months following bilateral orchiectomy. Scan is also 6.5 cm from anus and now measures 3.5 × 2.5 cm.

1 patient needed fecal diversion.[12] This early increase in volume was associated with heavy edema. It is unclear whether some degree of edema occurs in all or most patients as a normal effect of radiotherapy. This may make volume measurements of limited value in assessing early response to radiotherapy. A correlation of disease progression with volume changes in the prostate has not been defined for radiation. Fujino and Scardino noted that after radiation treatment the prostate typi-

cally assumed a more normal, symmetrical shape, a thickening and reformation of the prostatic capsule, a decrease in the volume of extracapsular disease, and a normalization of the seminal vesicles.[12]

These limited studies suggest that transrectal sonography appears to be accurate in assessing prostatic volume changes after therapy. The prognostic significance of these changes has been established for hormonal manipulation, but not for radiotherapy. Despite these observations, however, routine sonograms are not presently worthwhile after either of these two treatments because the sonographic findings will have little, if any, impact on clinical management. Few physicians would recommend additional treatment for men whose prostate volume has decreased only slightly but who are otherwise stable. For now, prostate specific antigen will be far more useful for identifying which patients are developing progressive disease.

An additional problem is the lack of information about changes in the tumor itself rather than the prostate as a whole. If a tumor represents 30% of the gland, it is quite likely that the normal prostate could shrink significantly while the tumor remained constant. Thus the change in volume may not reflect changes within the tumor. Until this is clarified, routine sonograms for monitoring are not appropriate.

ROLE OF ULTRASOUND IN DIAGNOSIS

The diagnosis of prostate cancer is most commonly established by biopsy of the prostate gland. Tissue for pathologic study may be obtained by transrectal or transperineal core biopsy or by transrectal aspiration biopsy (Fig. 59-14). The latter method has been popular in Sweden since 1960, but only recently has it been recommended in the United States. In one comparative study, transperineal core biopsy had a false-negative rate of 19% versus 2% for aspiration biopsy.[40] Other factors that make fine-needle aspiration biopsy more attractive include a lower cost, no anesthetic requirement, and a diminished complication rate. Recently, the use of ultrasonically guided rather than the traditional digitally guided biopsy for palpable nodules has been debated. Liddell et al. biopsied 55 men with suspected malignancy with and without ultrasound assistance. Prostate cancer was diagnosed in 15 patients. Only 9 of these were proved by digitally directed biopsy, whereas all 15 showed adenocarcinoma with a sonographically guided technique.[23] Rifkin et al. reported that biopsies of prostatic nodules were more accurate when ultrasound was employed.[24] However, only 13 patients with suspicious lesions were biopsied and the data were inconclusive. An opposite conclusion was obtained by Resnick. Using a study design similar to that of Liddell et al., Resnick reported that the accuracy of prostate biopsy was not enhanced by the use of ultrasonography. He concluded that routine use of sonographically guided biopsies for distinct nodules was not indicated.[25]

Although improved results with the routine use of sonographically guided biopsies for suspicious prostatic lesions has not been shown conclusively, there are roles for this modality. An ultrasonically guided biopsy is probably justified for patients in whom digitally directed biopsies have been negative, but malignancy is still strongly suspected. In addition, residual cancer following radiation therapy may be assessed more accurately by ultrasound than by palpation.[8]

ROLE OF ULTRASOUND IN PROSTATE CANCER SCREENING

The most controversial use of transrectal sonography is for routine screening for prostate cancer. Traditionally, digital rectal examination has been the procedure of choice for detection of prostate cancer. Recently, it has been demonstrated that transrectal sonography can detect nonpalpable, potentially curable tumors.[18,19] For ultrasonography to be deemed superior as a screening device, two requirements must be satisfied. First, it must be able to detect potentially curable lesions that are imperceptible to the examining finger, and second, the mortality from prostate cancer must be reduced in the group of men who are screened. To date, no long-term studies have been performed that assess the impact of screening on mortality from prostate cancer. Until those data are available, routine screening by transrectal sonography is not justified.

Another argument against screening is that this test has a low positive and negative predictive value. In one study, the positive and negative predictive values of transrectal sonography were 36 and 89%, respectively.[22]

For now, screening by transrectal ultrasonography must be considered experimental.[41] If the appropriate studies are performed, however, this diagnostic method may eventually be as important to men as the mammogram is to women.

ROLE OF ULTRASOUND IN RADIOACTIVE SEED IMPLANTATION

Another role for transrectal ultrasonography is for transperineal insertion of ^{125}I seeds in patients with prostate cancer.[42] A significant problem with this approach is the inhomogeneity of radiation within the tumor that results from difficulty in needle placement.[43] Shipley et al. demonstrated that a rela-

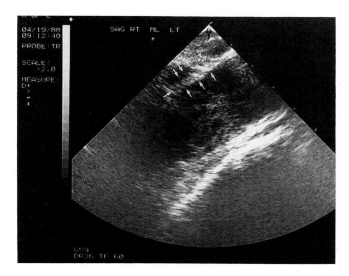

FIG. 59-14. Sagittal image of patient with hypoechoic lesion in posterior peripheral zone. Transrectal biopsy performed using ultrasound guidance and biopsy instrument. Scan taken immediately after needle passed into lesion. Needle is visualized as radiolucent linear area (shown by arrows).

tively inhomogeneous dose distribution predicted poorer regression of tumor.[44] Sonography can be used to guide seed insertion using a template over the perineum and a modification of the ultrasound-guided biopsy technique. The advantages of this method are an improvement in radioactive dose calculations, easier and more precise seed placement, and the lack of an open procedure.[42] Although these advantages are presently acknowledged, there are no data available concerning long-term results in patients treated with ultrasound-guided radioactive seed placement. Further studies are needed to substantiate that this method has improved efficacy compared to the previous approach.

SUMMARY

Transrectal ultrasonography of the prostate is a recent addition to the urologic armamentarium for which several uses have been suggested. The detection of extracapsular spread of tumor and the monitoring of response to endocrine therapy have been shown to be feasible. The routine use of ultrasound-guided biopsy is controversial, although in selected instances, it is useful. The role of sonography in prostate cancer screening and in the follow-up of patients treated with radiation is unclear. It is anticipated that advances in technology will improve prostatic imaging during the next few years, so that the role of ultrasound in prostate cancer will be better defined.

REFERENCES

1. MIZUNO, S. Diagnostic application of ultrasound in obstetrics and gynecology. In *Diagnostic Ultrasound.* Edited by C. C. Grossman. New York: Plenum Press, 1966, p. 452.

2. VON MICKY, L. I. Gynecologic ultrasonography. In *Diagnostic Ultrasound.* Edited by D. L. King. St. Louis: C. V. Mosby, 1974, p. 207.

3. KING, W. W. et al. Current status of prostatic echography. JAMA, *266*:444, 1973.

4. WATANABE, H. et al. Development and application of new equipment for transrectal ultrasonography. J. Clin. Ultrasound., *2*:91, 1974.

5. WATANABE, H. et al. Transrectal ultrasonography of the prostate. J. Urol., *114*:734, 1975.

6. WATANABE, H., KAIHO, H., TANAKA, M., and TERASAWA, Y. Ultrasonographic diagnosis of the prostate (II). Sagittal tomography of the prostate by means of B-mode scanning. Med. Ultrasonics, *9*:26, 1971.

7. BOYCE, W. H. et al. Ultrasonography as an aid in the diagnosis and management of surgical disease of the pelvis: Special emphasis on the genitourinary system. Ann. Surg., *184*:477, 1976.

8. RESNICK, M. I. Prostate ultrasound. Med. Instrum., *22*:74, 1988.

9. LEE, F. et al. Transrectal ultrasound in the diagnosis of prostate cancer: Location, echogenicity, histopathology, and staging. Prostate, *7*:117, 1985.

10. RESNICK, M. I., WILLARD, J. W., and BOYCE, W. H. Transrectal ultrasonography in the evaluation of patients with prostatic carcinoma. J. Urol., *124*:482, 1980.

11. PONTES, J. E. et al. Preoperative evaluation of localized prostatic carcinoma by transrectal ultrasonography. J. Urol., *134*:289, 1985.

12. FUJINO, A., and SCARDINO, P. T. Transrectal ultrasonography for prostate cancer: Its value in staging and monitoring the response to radiotherapy and chemotherapy. J. Urol., *133*:806, 1985.

13. FRIEDMAN, A. C. et al. Relative merits of MRI, US and CT in the diagnosis and staging of carcinoma of the prostate. Urology, *31*:530, 1988.

14. CARPENTIER, P. J., SCHROEDER, F. H., and SCHMITZ, P. I. M. Transrectal ultrasonometry of the prostate: The prognostic relevance of volume changes under endocrine management. World J. Urol., *4*:159, 1986.

15. DRAGO, J. R., NESBITT, J. A., and CIRCILLI, C. Effect of long-acting LHRH analog (Zoladex) on prostate cancer: Evaluation by transrectal ultrasonography. Urology, *32*:285, 1988.

16. KOJIMA, M. et al. Kinetic evaluation of the effect of LHRH analog on prostate cancer using transrectal ultrasonotomography. Prostate, *10*:11, 1987.

17. CARPENTIER, P. J., SCHROEDER, F. H., and BLOM, J. H. M. Transrectal ultrasonography in the follow-up of prostatic cancer patients. J. Urol., *128*:742, 1982.

18. COONER, W. H., EGGERS, G. W., and LICHTENSTEIN, P. Prostate cancer: New hope for early diagnosis. Ala. Med., *56*:13, 1987.

19. LEE, F. et al. The use of transrectal ultrasound in the diagnosis, guided biopsy, staging, and screening of prostate cancer. Radiographics, *7*:627, 634, 1987.

20. ROSENBERG, S., SOGANI, P. C., PARMER, E. A., and MULLER, D. G. Screening of ambulatory patients for prostate cancer by transrectal ultrasonography. J. Urol., *137*:241A, 1987.

21. KUDOW, C., GINGELL, J. C., and PINRY, J. B. Prostatic ultrasonography: A useful technique? Br. J. Urol., *5*:440, 1985.

22. CHODAK, G. W., et al. Comparison of digital examination and transrectal ultrasonography for the diagnosis of prostate cancer. J. Urol., *135*:951, 1986.

23. LIDDELL, H. T., MCDOUGAL, W. S., BURKS, D. D., and FLEISCHER, A. C. Ultrasound versus digitally directed prostatic needle biopsy. J. Urol., *135*:716, 1986.

24. RIFKIN, M. D., KURTZ, A. B., and GOLDBERG, B. B. Sonographically guided transperineal prostatic biopsy: Preliminary experience with a longitudinal linear array transducer. AJR, *140*:745, 1983.

25. RESNICK, M. I. Transrectal ultrasound guided versus digitally directed prostatic biopsy: A comparative study. J. Urol., *139*:754, 1988.

26. HOLM, H. H., and GAMMELGAARD, J. Ultrasonically guided precise needle placement in the prostate and seminal vesicles. J. Urol., *125*:385, 1981.

27. RIFKIN, M. D. Prostate ultrasound. Semin. Ultrasound CT MR, *9*:352, 1988.

28. DAVIDSON, P., and MALAMENT, M. Urinary contamination as a result of transrectal biopsy of the prostate. J. Urol., *105*:545, 1971.

29. STAMEY, T. A., HODGE, K. K. Ultrasound visualization of prostate anatomy and pathology. Monogr. Urol., *9*:55, 1988.

30. PEELING, W. B., and GRIFFITHS, G. J. Imaging of the prostate by ultrasound. J. Urol., *132*:217, 1984.

31. DEVONEC, M., CHAPELON, J. Y., and CATHIGNOL, D. Comparison of the diagnostic value of sonography and rectal examination in cancer of the prostate. Eur. Urol., *14*:189, 1988.

32. HARADA, K., IGARI, D., and TANAHASHI, Y. Gray scale transrectal ultra-

sonography of the prostate. J. Clin. Ultrasound, 7:45, 1979.

33. RIFKIN, M. D., KURTZ, A. B., CHOI, H. Y., and GOLDBERG, B. B. Endoscopic ultrasonic evaluation of the prostate using a transrectal probe: Prospective evaluation and acoustic characterization. Radiology, 149:265, 1983.

34. LEE, F., et al. Transrectal ultrasound in the diagnosis of prostate cancer. Location, echogenicity, histopathology and staging. Prostate, 7:117, 1985.

35. GRIFFITHS, G. J., et al. The ultrasound appearances of prostatic cancer with clinical correlation. Clin. Radiol., 38:219, 1987.

36. DAHNERT, W. F., et al. The echogenic focus in prostatic sonograms with xeroradiographic and histopathologic correlation. Radiology, 159:95, 1986.

37. RIFKIN, M. D., FRIEDLAND, G. W., and SHORTLIFFE, L. Prostatic evaluation by transrectal endosonography: Detection of carcinoma. Radiology, 158:85, 1986.

38. SALO, J. O., et al. Echogenic structure of prostatic cancer imaged in radical prostatectomy specimens. Prostate, 10:1, 1987.

39. JEWETT, H. J., EGGLESTON, J. C., and YAWN, D. H. Radical prostatectomy in the management of carcinoma of the prostate: Probable causes of some therapeutic failures. J. Urol., 107:1034, 1972.

40. CHODAK, G. W., et al. The role of transrectal aspiration biopsy in the diagnosis of prostatic cancer. J. Urol., 135:299, 1986.

41. CHODAK, G. W. Transrectal ultrasonography: Is it ready for routine use? JAMA, 259:2744, 1988.

42. HOLM, H. H., et al. Transperineal ^{125}Iodine seed implantation in prostatic cancer guided by transrectal ultrasonography. J. Urol., 130:283, 1983.

43. ROSS, G., et al. Preliminary observations on the results of combined ^{125}Iodine seed implantation and external irradiation for carcinoma of the prostate. J. Urol., 127:699, 1982.

44. SHIPLEY, W. U., et al. Preoperative irradiation, lymphadenectomy and ^{125}Iodine implant for patients with localized prostatic carcinoma: A correlation of implant dosimetry with clinical results. J. Urol., 124:639, 1980.

S E C T I O N
XIII

ANCILLARY SURGICAL PROCEDURES AND TECHNIQUES

60

Pelvic Exenteration in the Female

Even in medicine, though it is easy to know what wine, hellibore, cautery and surgery are, to know how and to whom and when to apply them so as to effect a cure is no less an undertaking than to be a physician.

ARISTOTLE
NICHOMACHEAN ETHICS IX

Ely Brand

Few operations demand as much of the surgeon in skill and judgement as pelvic exenteration. Often the patient and physician have exhausted all therapeutic modalities in treating a pelvic malignancy, leaving extended surgery as the only hope of cure. Occasionally, a patient may require exenteration to extend the quality of remaining life even though the hope of cure has passed.[1] The operation is technically demanding and requires constant vigilance for many hours. Anterior exenteration consists of removal of the para-aortic and pelvic lymph nodes, bladder, distal ureters, vagina, uterus, fallopian tubes, ovaries, and tumor with adjacent parametria and levator muscles. Posterior exenteration is rare and requires removal of the anus and rectosigmoid, while sparing the bladder and ureters. Total exenteration encompasses all of the pelvic viscera and may occasionally include the vulva and inguinal lymph nodes.[2] Often, the most challenging reconstructive phase begins only after a long day removing the tumor and adjacent viscera. Therefore, the procedure should be performed by two experienced surgeons operating in tandem. The well-thought-out exenteration begins with appropriate selection and counseling of the patient.

SELECTION OF THE PATIENT

The major indication for pelvic exenteration is centrally recurrent carcinoma of the cervix, particularly after pelvic irradiation, but occasionally after radical hysterectomy and irradiation. The central recurrence rate for stage-I disease after radiation is only 2%, but this increases to 17% for stage-III disease. Stage-IVA disease involving the bladder or rectal mucosa is not usually suitable for exenteration because of the high incidence of extrapelvic disease. After radiation or chemotherapy, some patients with residual disease in stage IVA may be salvaged by exenteration or they may require urinary or fecal diversion because of fistulae. Although the use of hydroxyurea (or cisplatin/5-FU) as radiosensitizers for advanced cervical carcinoma may improve survival, in a large Gynecologic Oncology Group study, the incidence of central pelvic recurrence was not diminished.[3] Persistence of cervical carcinoma 8 to 12 weeks following radiotherapy is generally considered an indication for exenteration. The use of radical hysterectomy after full pelvic irradiation is fraught with complications, particularly fistulae requiring diversions that the physician sought to avoid by doing the radical hysterectomy.[4]

Primary carcinomas of the vagina or urethra are best managed by radiotherapy, but may occasionally require exenteration. Extensive vulvar carcinoma (stages III and IV) may require pelvic exenteration, although recent advances in preoperative radiotherapy, with or without chemotherapy, often allow more conservative surgery. Sarcoma botryoides is no longer managed by exenteration because of excellent response rates to vincristine, actinomycin D, and cyclophosphamide. Recurrent uterine sarcoma has been treated by exenteration. Recurrent carcinoma of the endometrium is best treated with radiotherapy and progestational agents, although a rare patient may be managed surgically. Extensive or recurrent carcinoma of the bladder, anus, or rectum may also be managed by pelvic exenteration.

Occasionally, a patient develops carcinoma of the lower genital tract following pelvic irradiation. For instance, the patient radiated for cervical carcinoma who develops a vaginal primary many years later will require exenteration. Advanced stage DES related clear cell carcinoma of vagina or cervix may require exenteration. Vulvo-vaginal or urethral melanoma may require exenteration and radical vulvectomy as a primary procedure because of the lack of effective chemotherapy or radiotherapy. By far the majority of exenterations are undertaken for centrally recurrent postradiation cervical cancer.

After reviewing the initial histology and treatment, including radiation dosage, the surgeon should confirm that recurrent carcinoma is indeed present. The classic triad of sciatica, leg edema, and hydronephrosis is virtually pathognomonic for inoperability. In general, the shorter the interval from primary treatment to recurrence, the lower the likelihood of survival after exenteration. A diligent metastatic survey should follow. As a minimum, this includes CT scans of the abdomen and pelvis with fine-needle cytology of any suspicious lymph nodes, chest x-rays, and liver function tests. CT scanning of the chest may disclose occult lesions in patients with adenocarcinoma or sarcoma. Magnetic resonance imaging may be helpful in assessing whether tumor extends to the pelvic sidewall, although retroperitoneal detail is not necessarily improved with this modality. Preoperative intravenous pyelogram and barium enema facilitate surgical planning and rule out coexistent pathology. Hydronephrosis implies pelvic disease that is not resectable, but occasionally it results from obstruction of the distal or intravesical ureter and may allow exenteration. An upper gastrointestinal series with small bowel follow-through are important if small intestinal anastomosis or continent ileal diversion are planned.

The next step is counseling the patient about therapeutic options. This should not be undertaken in one session but is best staged in order to guide the patient through the defenses that accompany the diagnosis of recurrent carcinoma. We have found that women who have previously undergone exenteration are among the best support sources in newly diagnosed patients. Frank discussion of sexual rehabilitation is essential, and even abstinent patients are recommended a neovagina because of decreased postoperative morbidity in the reconstructed pelvis.

The patient should understand that a decision as to whether to complete the exenteration and the final decision as to type of exenteration can only be made intraoperatively. Approximately 50% of patients undergoing exploration will be found unresectable. The mortality from exenteration remains approximately 5% in most centers, however, the major morbidity is as high as 60%. The patient should have the psychologic fortitude to undergo a postoperative program of close follow-up and long-term rehabilitation.

PREOPERATIVE PREPARATION

Advanced age alone is not a contraindication to surgery, but careful selection of patients free from significant cardiopulmonary or renal disease is required. Routine spirometry and a baseline arterial blood gas are suggested. A chest x-ray and electrocardiogram are mandatory. Patients with serum albumin less than 3.0 or other signs of malnutrition benefit from preoperative parenteral hyperalimentation. Central venous access, at least 12 hours prior to surgery, will reduce the operative time and enable detection of complications, such as pneumothorax, while the patient is still awake. Pulmonary artery catheterization is preferred to central venous catheters because left atrial pressure correlates poorly with left ventricular end-diastolic pressure after pelvic exenteration.

Some authors routinely remove scalene nodes at a separate operation prior to laparotomy, but the yield of this approach in most hands remains relatively low. A 3-day bowel preparation is undertaken with clear liquids, enemas and cathartics. Polyethylene glycol (Go-Lytely), 2 to 3 L on the afternoon prior to surgery, is an excellent cathartic that results in minimal electrolyte imbalance. Neomycin and erythromycin base (1 gm) at 1 P.M., 2 P.M., and 11 P.M. are given orally. An enema of 2% neomycin (200 ml) is given on the morning of surgery. Potential stoma sites should be marked with methylene blue the day before surgery, with the patient both supine and sitting upright. Broad-spectrum prophylactic antibiotics are administered at least 1 hour prior to the skin incision, reinfused after 4 hours of surgery, and continued for 24 to 48 hours postoperatively. The patient takes hexachlorophene showers for 3 nights prior to surgery to reduce the bacterial skin count and uses a Betadine douche as well. Subcutaneous heparin, 5000 units every 8 hours, is started the night before surgery and timed so that no dose is given within 2 hours of surgery. It is helpful to begin intravenous fluids the day before surgery to allow slight hemodilution at the time of the operation. The preoperative hematocrit should exceed 35%, with transfusion if needed.

POSITIONING THE PATIENT

After satisfactory induction of general anesthesia, the patient should be positioned by the surgeon in Allen stirrups allowing exposure of the perineum, vagina, and abdomen. Pneumatic compression stockings are placed. The abdomen is prepped to the nipple line and the thighs should be prepped to the knees

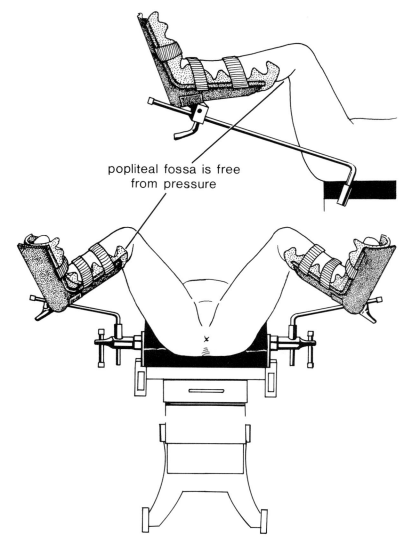

popliteal fossa is free
from pressure

FIG. 60-1. Proper positioning of the patient in stirrups for the combined abdominoperineal approach.

for access to gracilis myocutaneous flaps or split-thickness skin grafts. Great care is taken to avoid pressure on the peroneal nerves at the fibulae and to pad the soles of the foot, avoiding excessive dorsiflexion at the ankles.[5] The hips should be flexed at approximately 30 to 35° and abducted no more than 45°. The knees can be extended or slightly flexed and the hips internally rotated (Fig. 60-1).

SELECTION OF THE TYPE OF EXENTERATION

Examination under anesthesia is the first critical test of operability. The tumor should be free from the pelvic sidewall. At times, it may be difficult to distinguish radiation fibrosis from recurrent tumor, though the former tends to be smooth, regular, and symmetric. If there is a possibility of resectability, the patient should be explored. Cystoscopy and proctosigmoidoscopy are performed to visualize tumor spread and as a last check if bladder or rectal conservation are planned. Bullous edema of the bladder heralds muscular infiltration and mandates cystectomy. Very low rectal anastomosis can be accom-

plished if 3 to 5 cm of tumor clearance is possible above the anal sphincter. Involvement of the lower vagina will require a wider perineal phase (vulvectomy) and levator resection. Urethral or labial involvement will require vulvectomy as well. Having assessed the gross spread of tumor and the degree of resection required, the surgeons prepare for exploratory laparotomy.

OPERATIVE PROCEDURE

Exploratory Laparotomy

Most surgeons favor a midline incision for adequate exposure and exploration of the upper abdomen, high para-aortic lymphadenectomy, use of a transverse colon conduit, and omental lid. However, a midline incision does not provide as much exposure in the pelvis, especially at the sidewalls, as does a transverse incision. Our preference is to use a Cherney incision (division of the rectus muscles at their tendinous insertion into the pubic symphysis) or Mallard (rectus cutting) incision. This allows for more facile pelvic surgery at the expense of limiting the aortic node sampling to below the inferior mesenteric takeoff.

After thorough evaluation of the upper abdomen for metastatic spread, the para-aortic nodes are palpated and any enlarged nodes submitted for frozen section histology. Metastatic disease in the para-aortic nodes is an absolute contraindication to pelvic exenteration. In the absence of suspicious lymph nodes, formal para-aortic lymphadenectomy is begun.

Para-aortic Lymphadenectomy

The retroperitoneum is entered by dividing the round ligaments bilaterally. The incision extends cephalad, parallel to the infundibulopelvic ligaments. Usually, the cecum is mobilized along the line of Toldt and the ureter retracted medially. This will expose the common iliac vessels and lower inferior vena cava. Some surgeons continue lymphadenectomy to the level of the renal vessels. This may be easier to accomplish by a transmesenteric approach. The technical details of para-aortic lymphadenectomy are described in Chapters 34 and 35. Para-aortic node metastases contraindicate further surgery. Patients with centrally recurrent cervical carcinoma will have aortic node metastases in about 15% of cases, with no long-term survivors in this group.

Pelvic Exploration

In order to ascertain resectability in the pelvis, the pararectal and paravesical spaces are developed bluntly. Inability to develop free spaces at the pelvic sidewalls contraindicates pelvic exenteration, except in highly selected cases performed for palliation. After suture ligation and division of the round ligament near the canal of Nuck, the paravesical space can be developed with the back of a long DeBakey forceps or a straight Heaney retractor. Two forceps are placed against each other at the pelvic sidewall below the external iliac vessels, caudad to the round ligament and lateral to the ureters and the superior vesical artery. The angle of inclination is about 30°, pointing toward the apex of the vagina. With gentle spreading motions, the avascular potential space develops, pushing the vagina and bladder medially and the cardinal ligament posteriorly. In about 10% of patients an aberrant obturator artery or vein, arising from the external iliac will be noted and avoided. Exposure of the obturator nerve requires dissection more medially to avoid the obturator vein. The levator ani muscles form the floor of the paravesical space with the obturator internus muscle inferolaterally.

Next, the pararectal space is developed posterior to the cardinal ligament and lateral to the rectum. Staying close to the hypogastric vessels laterally will prevent incidental injury to the sigmoid and hemorrhoidal vessels medially on the left side. Inferiorly, the middle hemorrhoidal vessels should be avoided as they traverse the floor of the pararectal space. Aiming slightly caudally will avoid the gluteal branches of the hypogastric vessels. The intervening tissue between the pararectal and paravesical spaces constitutes the cardinal ligament, referred to as the vascular "web" by Meigs (Fig. 60-2). Although tumor extending to the levator or obturator muscles at the sidewall contraindicates exenteration, a frozen section is

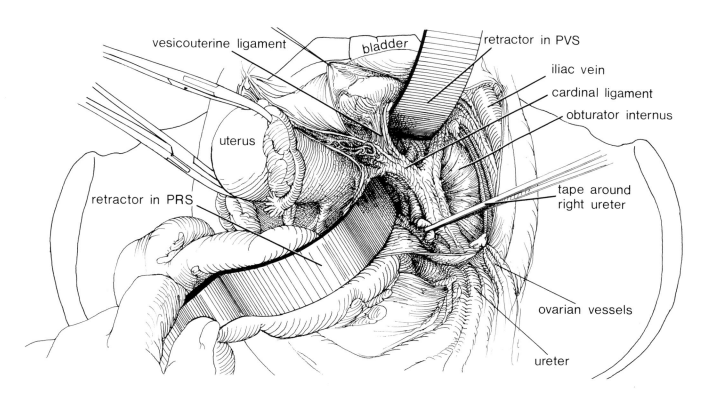

FIG. 60-2. Development of the paravesical (PVS) and pararectal (PRS) spaces with the intervening cardinal ligament between the spaces.

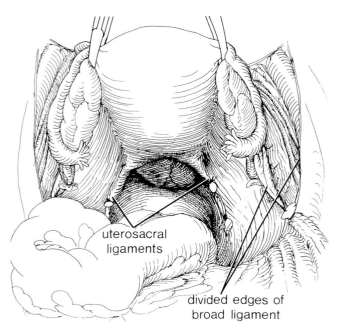

FIG. 60-3. Development of the rectovaginal septum and division of the uterosacral ligaments.

necessary to distinguish between radiation fibrosis and carcinoma.

Anterior Exenteration

The patient in whom anterior instead of total exenteration can encompass the tumor is one with a small central recurrence confined to the cervix and/or bladder. Parametrial extension is generally a contraindication to rectal preservation. The posterior vaginal fornices and posterior vagina should be free of disease on biopsy. Sigmoidoscopy and barium enema should be normal. Lesions larger than 3 cm are generally treated by total exenteration. Paradoxically, in a review from the University of Alabama, patients who had bladder invasion had only a 23% 5-year survival, compared to 70% if disease was confined to the cervix.[6] This may simply reflect the inadvisability of modified exenteration in patients with large lesions.

Anterior exenteration begins by ligating the uterine arteries at their origin from the hypogastric or superior vesical arteries. The superior vesical artery, the first branch of the anterior division of the hypogastric artery, is also ligated. Next the rectovaginal septum is developed by incising the peritoneum across the posterior cul-de-sac below the ureters. With firm elevation and caudal retraction of the uterus, the operator places a hand above the rectum and gently pushes it posteriorly in the midline. The volar surfaces of the fingers hold the vagina anteriorly. The dissection continues toward the inferior pubic ramus with the hand parallel to the floor. Induration or gross cancer here necessitate total exenteration. The uterosacral ligaments are divided between Heaney or Zeppelin clamps

and suture ligated near the sacrum, taking care to avoid the rectum medially (Fig. 60-3). The ureters may be divided before or after this step. The lower the ureteral division, the greater mobility for later anastomosis, but the higher the radiation dose to the ureter. The ureters should not be dissected out of the cardinal ligaments. The ureters are mobilized with preservation of a sheath of peritoneum and then divided. Vascular clips may be placed to prevent drainage of urine in the operative field, or ureters may be stented, with the ends placed in a bag, to measure urine output until a conduit is formed. If significant bleeding is encountered the hypogastric arteries can be isolated and ligated. Because most patients have received pelvic irradiation, the nonfunctioning ovaries should be removed. The infundibulopelvic ligaments are isolated above the ureters at the pelvic brim, ligated and divided.

The bladder is detached from the lateral vesical ligaments in the space of Retzius using electrocautery. The filmy retropubic attachments are lysed and the urethra is exposed for resection from below (Fig. 60-4).

The cardinal ligaments are divided between serial clamps at the pelvic sidewall avoiding the hypogastric veins (Fig. 60-5). In a fully irradiated pelvis, resection of the pelvic lymph nodes is controversial because disease here is unlikely to allow survival. Some surgeons remove the common, external and internal iliac, and obturator nodes for frozen section, proceeding with exenteration only if the nodes are negative. However, in a subgroup of patients with only unilateral microscopic involvement lymphadenectomy may have therapeutic benefit, with up to 25% alive at 5 years.[7] Clearly, morbidity increases after pelvic lymphadenectomy in a radiated pelvis, while the benefit is debatable. The availability of intraoperative radiotherapy

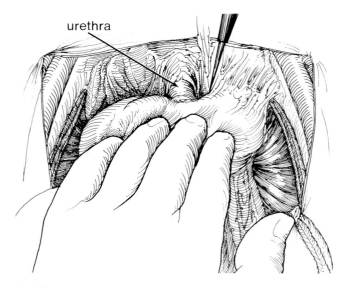

FIG. 60-4. Anteriorly, the urethra is defined and the bladder is detached by division of the lateral vesical ligaments.

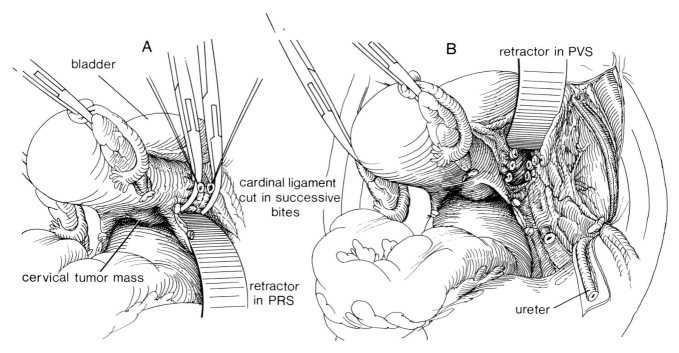

FIG. 60-5. *A & B.* Uterus is retracted laterally and the cardinal ligament is divided and ligated in successive pedicles at the pelvic sidewall.

may improve the prognosis in patients with sidewall disease. The details of pelvic lymphadenectomy are covered in Chapter 16.

Perineal Resection

The perineal phase of surgery can be started during this time. The second surgical team makes an incision below the clitoris if possible, and extending circumferentially around the vagina (Fig. 60-6*A*). Resection of the vulva requires a larger circumference. With Allis clamps at 4 and 8 o'clock positions, an incision is made at the mucocutaneous border of the vagina and perineum. The rectovaginal septum is developed sharply with Metzenbaum scissors. Moderate bleeding is common because of vascular attachments between the lower vagina and rectum. The internal pudendal vessels are ligated in Alcock's canal. The vagina is mobilized laterally and then anteriorly to expose the urogenital diaphragm. Detachment of the vagina and urethra from the pubic bone is one of the last steps because bleeding from the inferior pubic ramus may be difficult to control with the specimen in place. The inferior fascia of the urogenital diaphragm is divided with the electrocautery. The intervening superficial transverse perineal muscles are clamped laterally near the ischium below the pubic rami. If the abdominal surgeons divide the superior fascia of the urogenital diaphragm this guides the perineal team. The pubococcygeus portions of the levator ani can be divided by either team. Lastly, the urethra is freed from ligamentous attachments to the pubis. If bleeding is difficult to control, a 2-0 polyglactin suture on a Keith needle is passed from below under the pubis and back

again on the opposite side. The puborectalis portion of the levators are then approximated with 2-0 polyglactin sutures to support the perineum.

Posterior Exenteration

Posterior exenteration is performed for recurrent cervical cancer in the posterior vagina or rectovaginal septum. The

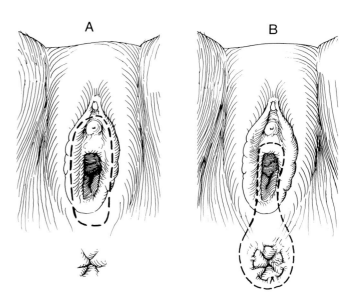

FIG. 60-6. Perineal incision for anterior (A) and posterior (B) exenteration.

operation is not appropriate if disease extends to the anterior vagina. In cases with cervical involvement or parametrial extension, total exenteration should be chosen because of occult spread anteriorly into the bladder pillars and to avoid any ureteral dissection in the parametria. Although the ureters could be divided at the pelvic brim and reimplanted into the bladder, this is not advisable because parametrial extension often goes hand in hand with vesicouterine extension. The posterior exenteration proceeds as described for anterior exenteration except that the rectovaginal septum is not dissected. Because the bladder is conserved, the anterior peritoneal incision extends from the round ligaments along the vesicouterine reflection in the anterior cul de sac. With the uterus firmly retracted cephalad, the bladder is developed sharply off of the cervix and upper vagina. This is best done in the relatively avascular midline. The uterine vessels are ligated and the superior vesical artery preserved. The ureter is dissected from the parametria using a right angle clamp and gently spreading directly on top of the ureter. The dissection continues to free the ureter in the vesicouterine pillar or "tunnel" as it enters the bladder. The smaller posterior vesicouterine ligament beneath the ureter is ligated separately. The ureters are then retracted laterally to allow resection of the lateral cardinal and uterosacral ligaments in successive pedicles replaced with 0 polyglactin sutures (Fig. 60-7). To this point, the technique resembles that of a radical hysterectomy, except for more careful attention to ureteral vascularity after irradiation.

The mesentery of the sigmoid colon is divided in an avascular area and the colon divided below the pelvic brim using the GIA stapler. The mesentery and inferior sigmoid vessels are then serially ligated. The surgeon separates the rectosigmoid from loose retrorectal attachments to the sacrum with the electrocautery. Care is taken not to injure the middle sacral vessels. The rectal stalks and proximal uterosacral ligaments are divided close to the sacrum. The rectum is freed from the puborectalis muscle posteriorly by blunt dissection with the hand insinuating toward the pubis in the presacral space (Fig. 60-8). The middle rectal artery is sacrificed near the hypogastric artery. The anococcygeal ligament is ligated and divided. The perineal phase of the procedure encompasses the rectum as in an abdominoperineal resection and continues anteriorly to circumscribe the vagina (Fig. 60-8B).

The disadvantage of posterior exenteration is the high degree of bladder atony and neurogenic incontinence because of sacrifice of the nervi erigentes in the uterosacral and rectal stalks. In addition, the ureteral dissection in the parametria, when the patient has received pelvic irradiation, is associated with a fistula rate of at least 5 to 10%. For these reasons, posterior exenteration is uncommonly performed for recurrent cervical carcinoma but may be utilized in certain cases of vaginal carcinoma not amenable to, or failing, radiotherapy. Occasionally modified posterior exenteration is used to clear the pelvis for optimal tumor reduction of ovarian carcinoma.

Total Exenteration

Total pelvic exenteration is required in at least half the cases of recurrent cervical carcinoma. The technique combines procedures outlined in the sections on anterior and posterior exenteration and may be performed with resection of the levator

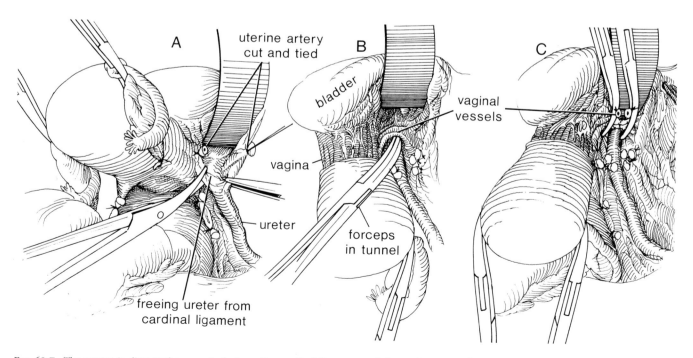

FIG. 60-7. The ureter is dissected successively from the cardinal ligament and the vesicouterine ligament.

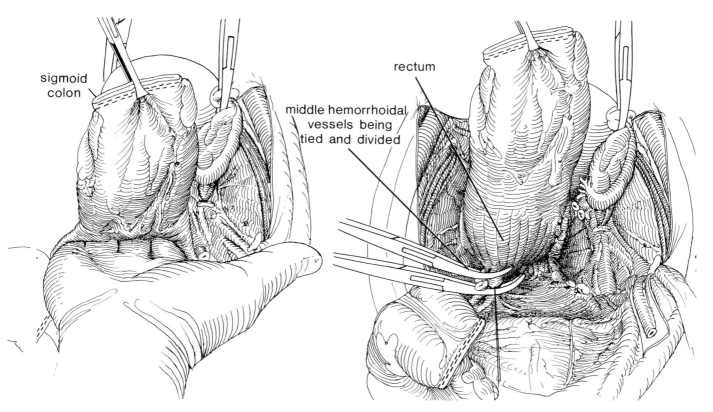

FIG. 60-8. *A*, Sigmoid colon is divided and the retrorectal space is developed. *B*, Rectal stalks are divided and ligated close to the sacrum.

plate (Fig. 60-9) or in a supralevator fashion (Fig. 60-10). As in posterior exenteration when the rectosigmoid colon is resected, the proximal sigmoid can be used for a urinary conduit in order to avoid use of the small bowel and enteroenterostomy. The perineal phase of total pelvic exenteration encompasses the urethra, vagina, perineum and anus. The gracilis myocutaneous flap with an overlying omental pedicle is the procedure of choice for vaginal and pelvic floor reconstruction.[8] Extended resections, as have been employed by Pearlman, Wanebo, and others for recurrent rectal carcinoma, may have a role in selected patients with symphysis and sacral recurrences.[9] These cases should be highly individualized. As experience accumulates with internal sacral resections, the pelvic surgeon may wish to consider these procedures.

Supralevator Exenteration

In certain patients with carcinoma above the lower vagina, the perineal phase of the operation may be omitted and the surgery undertaken abdominally to the levator plate (Fig. 60-10). The levator ani are preserved. The vagina is resected as low as possible without division of the urogenital diaphragm or distal puborectalis at the pelvic floor. The vaginal cuff is closed with interrupted sutures of 2-0 polyglactin. The rectum is transected at the levator muscles using the thoraco-abdominal stapler with a rotating head to facilitate acute angulation in the pelvis (TA-55). Preservation of the puborectalis and rectum

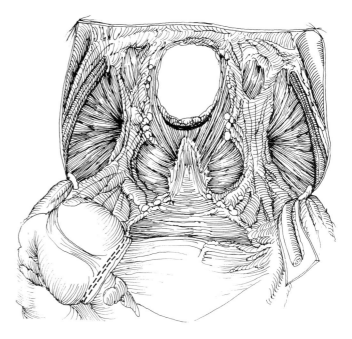

FIG. 60-9. Pelvis, viewed from above, following total exenteration.

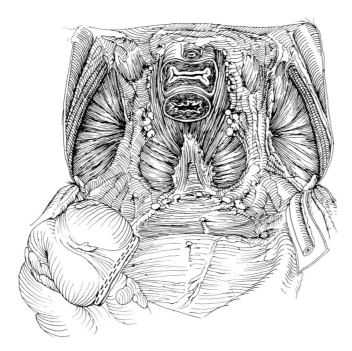

FIG. 60-10. Pelvis, viewed from above, following supralevator total exenteration.

allows reanastomosis of the rectosigmoid colon to the rectum using the end-end stapler (EEA) because carcinoma of the cervix rarely involves the anus or distal 5 cm of rectum. The distal urethra is not excised but resected at the superior fascia of the urogenital diaphragm. The supralevator exenteration usually does not require a perineal resection and allows the greatest flexibility in reconstructive options, though only small recurrences are appropriate for this type of exenteration. Frozen sections of the vaginal, urethral, and rectal margins are important in supralevator exenteration. Occasionally, a perineal resection facilitates total vaginectomy and still allows preservation of the urogenital diaphragm or puborectalis in selected cases.

Pelvic Reconstruction

After removal of the tumor, the surgeon begins the more arduous phase of attempting to minimize morbidity and allow functional restoration for the patient. The most common form of urinary diversion is the Bricker pouch or uretero-ileal conduit.[10,11] This procedure is described in Chapter 28. If the patient has undergone total exenteration, the sigmoid colon provides a conduit that may eliminate the need for small bowel anastomosis. However, because the sigmoid colon and ileum have often received significant irradiation, the transverse colon conduit may have to be considered. As surgical technique has improved, several centers have adopted techniques of continent urinary diversion such as the modified Kock pouch or the ileo-colonic pouch. Any grey-white discoloration of the small bowel that might signify radiation enteritis

would preclude use of these segments of bowel. Technical details can be found in Chapters 27–31.

Coloproctostomy

If the distal 3 to 8 cm of rectum are preserved, low or very low rectal anastomosis allows the patient to avoid colostomy.[12] However, in the heavily irradiated patient, the surgeon should opt for a temporary diverting colostomy. If possible, the anastomosis should be checked by filling the pelvis with saline and injecting air through a Toomey syringe placed in the anus. If bubbles are seen there is a leak. The anastomosis should be repaired or taken down entirely and redone. If there is tension on the anastomosis or inadequate repair, a diverting colostomy is necessary.

Most of the defects in low rectal anastomosis are posterior because of difficulty directly observing this part of the bowel. This can be checked by rotating the EEA stapler after firing and before releasing it. A newer type of stapler (CEEA, Autosuture Corp) allows a simpler solution since the head is easily detached. If there is enough mobility of the sigmoid colon, an end-to-side anastomosis (Strasbourg-Baker) may allow the formation of a rectal pouch which serves as a reservoir, as in the normal rectal ampulla.[13] The distal TA-55 staple line can be punctured with the shaft of the EEA. The proximal sigmoid is punctured using an adapter (CEEA) along the antimesenteric side 5 to 7 cm from the previously resected end (Fig. 60-11). The head of the CEEA is replaced onto the shaft through the colotomy in the proximal bowel segment. No purse strings are needed and firing of the stapler creates the end-side anastomosis. The proximal sigmoid is then closed with the TA-55 stapler. Although all of these maneuvers can be directly accomplished by hand, the use of the automatic stapling device shortens operative time, decreases complications, and allows for improved blood flow to the anastomosis.[13]

Neovagina

After rectal anastomosis, the vagina is reconstructed using a split thickness skin graft. A myocutaneous flap is generally not required because the rectum forms a suitable posterior vaginal plate. The Brown air-driven dermatome or Padgett dermatome is then set to 12 to 16/1000ths of an inch and the donor site prepared with mineral oil. Generally the anteromedial thigh is most accessible, although some patients prefer a lateral buttock site. The size of the graft should be 10 to 15 centimeters. The donor site is dressed with scarlet red and loose fluffy gauze.

The split thickness skin graft is meshed at a 2:1 or 3:1 ratio and sewn over a loose obturator such as a Heyer-Schulte stent or large syringe barrel that has been opened at both ends, using interrupted 4-0 polyglactin. The end that will become the proximal vagina is closed over the end of the stent (Fig. 60-12). The graft is then inserted into the vaginal cavity. Meticulous hemostasis is imperative because bleeding will separate the graft from the neovaginal bed. Evans has suggested the

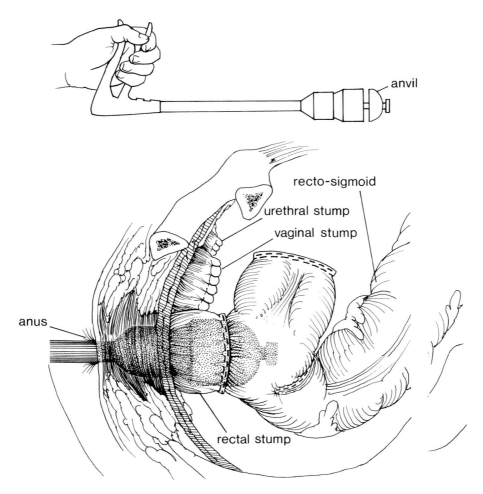

FIG. 60-11. Anastomosis of the rectal stump to the side of sigmoid colon using the CEEA stapler.

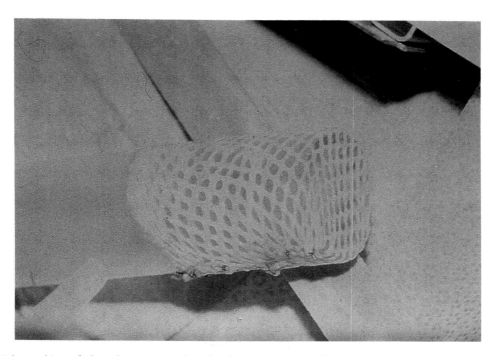

FIG. 60-12. Split thickness skin graft draped on a syringe barrel and sewn over one end.

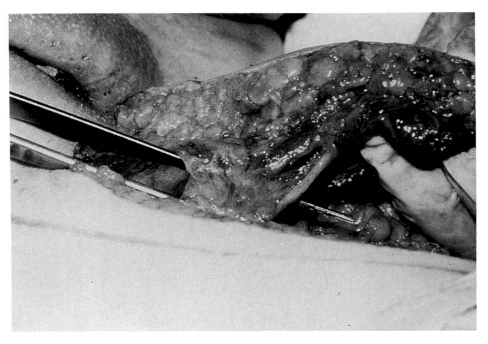

Fig. 60-13. Gracilis myocutaneous flap dissected with its intact neurovascular supply.

use of topical thrombin sprayed on the graft bed.[15] Serum will escape without separating the graft if it has been properly meshed or "pie-crusted." Several interrupted sutures are used to anchor the skin graft to the rectum and circumferentially to the labia at the introitus. As one team prepares the neovagina, the omental J-pexy is then brought into the pelvis anteriorly to support the neovagina and is sewn to the anterior and lateral rectum and the inferior pubic symphysis. The neovagina is then snugly packed, withdrawing the plastic obturator as the packing is laid. A Heyer-Schulte stent need not be removed at surgery. At 7 days, the packing or stent is removed and the vagina examined for percent engraftment.

Gracilis Myocutaneous Neovagina

If the levator plate has been resected and a colostomy performed, the capacious space in the pelvis is best filled with bilateral gracilis myocutaneous flaps. Unlike skin grafts, this type of neovagina achieves excellent sensation for coitus and, using omentum, prevents small bowel from adhering to the pelvic floor with possible perineal herniation or obstruction.

A line is drawn with a sterile surgical marker from the pubic tubercle to the medial tibial epicondyle using a straight edge. The gracilis muscle is just inferior to this line where a pedicle 10 to 15 cm long, and half as wide, is outlined in elliptical fashion. The myocutaneous flap is supplied by a neurovascular bundle emerging from the adductor longus muscle, superior to the adductor magnus. The neurovascular bundle is usually 6 to 9 cm from the pubic tubercle. Injury to this narrow and precarious pedicle may result in flap necrosis. Dissection of the pedicle flap continues with care not to separate the

skin from the underlying gracilis. The skin and gracilis are transected distally using electrocautery. It is not advisable to divide the gracilis near its insertion at the pubis. The skin and muscle are mobilized and the areolar attachments divided parallel to the neurovascular bundle (Fig. 60-13). It is usually necessary to secure the skin to the gracilis with interrupted 2-0 polyglactin proximally and distally. The pedicle flap is then rotated using Babcock clamps and brought under the skin bridge consisting of the superomedial thigh and vulva to lie perpendicularly at the introitus (Fig. 60-14). A continuous suture of 3-0 polyglactin is started superiorly and attaches the right and left flaps. This continues to the distal flap and then up to the proximal portions to form a pouch with skin inside and fatty tissue on the outside (Figs. 60-15 and 60-16). The grafts are then rotated 90° to fill the vaginal bed. The superior portion is attached by the abdominal team to the sacral periosteum, the pubis, the levator muscles and, finally, from below, to the introitus at the labia using 2-0 interrupted polyglactin sutures (Fig. 60-17). A stent or pack is usually not necessary. The incisions on the thigh are closed in 2 layers, the first with continuous 3-0 polyglactin and the skin with metal clips or mattress sutures. Closed suction drains are placed in the incision, exiting through stab wounds on the thigh. Other methods of neovaginal construction have been described, such as the use of the vascular but short vulvobulbocavernosus pedicle or a pedicle of rectus abdominis muscle.

Pelvic Floor

The omentum is detached from the transverse colon in the avascular plane and divided using the LDS stapler below the

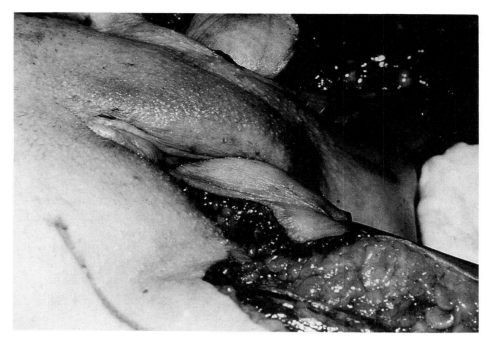

FIG. 60-14. The myocutaneous flap is brought onto the perineum underneath the bridge of the medial thigh and labia.

greater curvature of the stomach from the right side. The branches of the right gastroepiploic vessels are sacrificed and the J-shaped lid is fashioned with the left gastroepiploic vessels intact (Fig. 60-18A, B). The pedicle flap is carpeted over the pelvis to exclude the small bowel and is attached to the pelvis at the sidewalls and over the neovagina (Fig. 60-18C). If the omentum is not available or is inadequate, then a pelvic lid is fashioned with a double layer of absorbable mesh.[16] The major morbidity of exenteration remains small intestinal fistulae and obstruction.[17,18] Therefore, thoughtful pelvic floor reconstruction can avert disaster.

With the use of reconstructive procedures for the bladder, vagina, and rectum, it is possible for the first time to perform total pelvic exenteration without the use of any stomata except the continent urostomy stoma, thereby avoiding external appliances. Furthermore, vaginal reconstruction enables the preservation of sexual function and limits the psychologic debilitation that accompanies such radical resections.

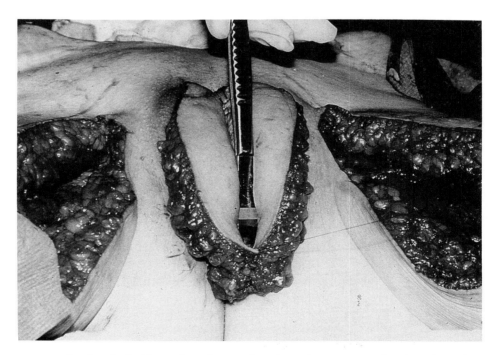

FIG. 60-15. The myocutaneous flap from both sides are brought onto the vulva and are sewn together from above downwards.

POSTOPERATIVE CARE AND COMPLICATIONS

In modern series, intraoperative mortality should be less than 2%. The total postoperative death rate remains between 3 to 5% in the first 90 days after surgery. The typical exenteration patient requires 3 to 5 days of intensive care, during which massive fluid and electrolyte shifts, hemorrhage, cardiopulmonary instability, and nutritional imbalance are corrected. The average blood loss is about 1500 to 2500 ml in the first 5 days. Even the young and otherwise healthy patient is best managed with Swan Ganz catheterization for 48 to 72 hours. When third space fluids re-enter the intravascular and intracellular compartments, one must vigilantly watch for pulmonary edema. This most common occurs between the second and fourth postoperative day.

Major operative morbidity is high after pelvic exenteration. Approximately one-third to one-half of the patients who undergo exenteration will experience some complications.[3,12] By far, the vast majority of these will need a blood transfusion or experience postoperative fever. Life-threatening postoperative complications are much less common, with fistulas and bowel obstruction leading the list.[17,20] Pelvic cellulitis and pelvic abscess are not unusual.

Febrile morbidity is the rule after exenteration.[21] However, rather than employ broad-spectrum triple antibiotics reflexively, a careful search for underlying causes, often pulmonary or renal, is more rewarding. The injudicious use of antibiotics may mask intra-abdominal abscess formation, delaying life-saving drainage. Supervening candidemia after prolonged courses of multiple antibiotics may be fatal. The use of CT

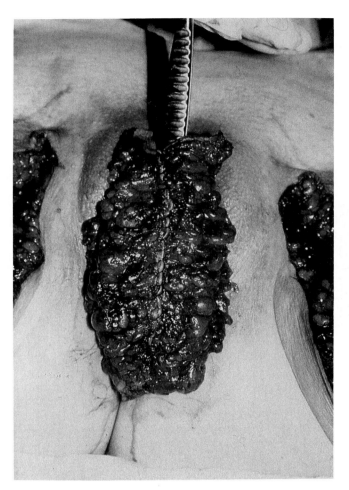

FIG. 60-16. The suturing is continued upward to create the neovaginal pouch.

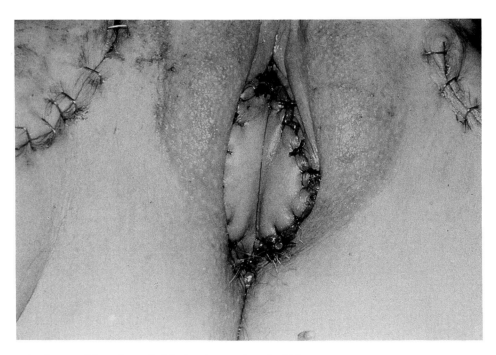

FIG. 60-17. The neovagina is rotated into the vaginal bed and sutured to the labia.

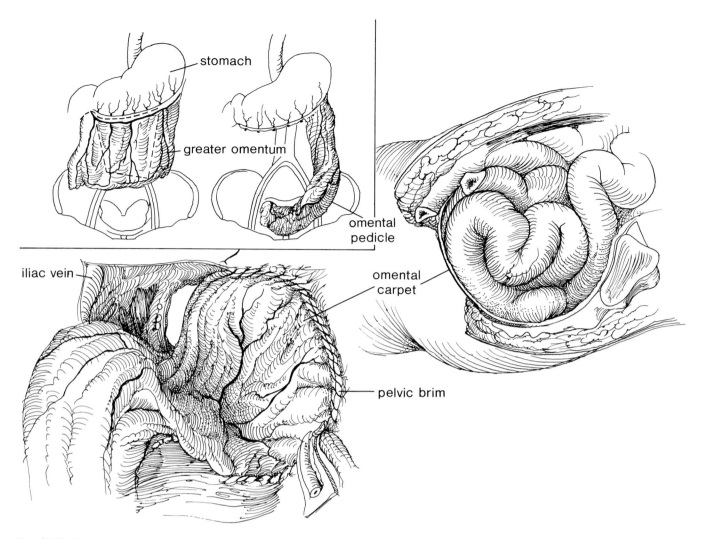

FIG. 60-18. Construction of the greater omental carpet. The greater omentum is detached from the transverse colon and the greater curvature of stomach by ligature and division of the right gastroepiploic vessels (A). The detached omentum is fashioned into a J-shaped lid with intact left gastroepiploic vessels (B). The pedicled flap is carpeted over the neovagina in the pelvis and attached to the pelvic parieties (C).

scanning or labelled white blood cell scans has not been particularly helpful in diagnosing abscesses because of the extensive anatomic changes and inflammation. Fungal blood cultures should be obtained in patients on broad-spectrum antibiotics. Often, colonization of the urinary tract with candida may be the first clue to fungal sepsis.

Occasional deleterious events include stomal necrosis or prolapse, urinary leakage from the conduit or ureter, hematoma, perineal or incisional hernia or dehiscence, and cardiovascular events, such as myocardial infarction and pulmonary embolism. Persistent sinus tachycardia is common and EKGs will rule out treatable supraventricular arrhythmias.

Prolonged ileus is managed with intestinal intubation, and there may be difficulty ruling out a small bowel obstruction. If the patient remains stable, continued expectant care is preferable to a hasty return to the operating room. In patients undergoing total exenteration with multiple small and large intestinal anastomoses, a gastrostomy tube placed in a Witzel fashion

at surgery avoids the discomfort of 7 to 21 days of nasogastric intubation. If a fistula is suspected, gastrograffin GI series are employed to define the anatomy. Ureteral obstruction should be evaluated with renal ultrasound or IVP. Most of these serious complications will resolve with continued parenteral nutrition. Obstructed ureters often result from edema at the anastomosis and temporary nephrostomies or antegrade endoscopic stents will often obviate surgical repair. Elective reoperations should be delayed for 4 to 6 weeks to allow the patient condition to improve and the associated edema and inflammation to subside.

Long-term complications include recurrent pyelonephritis, hyperchloremic acidosis, intestinal stricture or fistula, lymphedema, and lymphocysts. Lymphocysts can be avoided by drainage of the pelvic and para-aortic lymphadenectomy sites until the daily output is less than 30 cc. Chronic lymphedema occurs in less than 5% of patients. The risks of lymphatic complications must be weighed in deciding whether to perform a thorough pelvic lymphadenectomy at the time of exenteration in the irradiated pelvis.

PROGNOSIS AND LONG-TERM FOLLOW-UP

Of patients explored for pelvic exenteration, about one-half will be candidates for completion of the operation. Between 30 and 60% of exenteration patients will become long-term survivors.[22-25] Approximately 80% of recurrences manifest in the first 2 years. Progressive radiation fibrosis may be difficult to distinguish from recurrent tumor, though asymmetry in the pelvis suggests tumor. Fine-needle aspiration is often definitive. Tumor markers, including CEA and squamous cell carcinoma antigen, are useful adjuncts to clinical examination. A chest x-ray is obtained every 6 months for 2 years. CT or MRI scanning is relatively insensitive and nonspecific but may be helpful on an annual basis, particularly to rule out progressive hydronephrosis because of strictures. If native vagina remains, annual cytologic smears are indicated. In at least nine cases, squamous cell carcinoma has developed in a neovagina. Adenocarcinoma and transitional cell carcinoma have occurred in the urinary conduits. The treatment of recurrent disease remains unrewarding, with a mean survival of 3 to 6 months. Meticulous follow-up and continuing psychologic support allow most patients to resume healthy and productive lives free from disease.

ACKNOWLEDGEMENTS

Great appreciation is extended to Dr. Leo D. Lagasse for thoughtful and constructive review of this manuscript.

REFERENCES

1. STANHOPE, C. R., and SYMMONDS, R. E. Palliative exenteration—What, when, and why? Am. J. Obstet. Gynecol., *152*:12, 1985.
2. BRUNSCHWIG, A. Complete excision of the pelvic viscera for advanced carcinoma. Cancer, *1*:177, 1948.
3. HRESCHYSHYN, M. M., et al. Hydroxyurea or placebo combined with radiation to treat stages IIIB and IV cervical cancer confined to the pelvis. Int. J. Radiat. Oncol. Biol. Phys., *5*:317, 1979.
4. RUBIN, S. C., HOSKINS, W. J., and LEWIS, J. L. Radical hysterectomy for recurrent cervical cancer following radiation therapy. Gynecol. Oncol., *27*:316, 1987.
5. HOFFMAN, M. S., ROBERTS, W. S., and CAVANAUGH, D. Neuropathies associated with radical pelvic surgery for gynecologic cancer. Gynecol. Oncol., *31*:462, 1988.
6. HATCH, K. D., et al. Anterior pelvic exenteration. Gynecol. Oncol., *31*:205, 1988.
7. RUTLEDGE, F. N., and McGUFFEE, V. B. Pelvic exenteration: Prognostic significance of regional lymph node metastasis. Gynecol. Oncol., *26*:374, 1987.
8. BEREK, J. S., HACKER, N. F., and LAGASSE, L. D. Vaginal reconstruction performed simultaneously with pelvic exenteration. Obstet. Gynecol., *63*:318, 1984.
9. PEARLMAN, N. S., et al. Pelvic and sacropelvic exenteration for locally advanced or recurrent anorectal cancer. Arch. Surg., *122*:537, 1987.
10. BRICKER, E. M., KRAYBILL, W. G., LOPEZ, M. J., and JOHNSTON, W. D. The current role of ultraradical surgery in the treatment of pelvic cancer. Curr. Probl. Surg., *23*:871, 1986.
11. ORR, J. W., SHINGLETON, H. M., and HATCH, K. D. Urinary diversion in patients undergoing pelvic exenteration. Am. J. Obstet. Gynecol., *142*:883, 1982.
12. LAGASSE, L. D., et al. Use of sigmoid colon for rectal substitution following pelvic exenteration. Am. J. Obstet. Gynecol., *116*:106, 1973.
13. WHEELESS, C. R., and DORSEY, J. H. Use of the automatic stapler for intestinal anastomosis associated with gynecologic malignancies. Gynecol. Oncol., *11*:1, 1981.
14. KARLEN, J. R., and PIVER, M. S. Reduction of morbidity and mortality associated with pelvic exenteration. Gynecol. Oncol., *3*:154, 1975.
15. EVANS, T. N., POLAND, M. L., and BOVING, R. L. Vaginal malformations. Am. J. Obstet. Gynecol., *141*:910, 1981.
16. CLARKE-PEARSON, D. L., SOPER, J. T., and CREASMAN, W. T. Absorbable synthetic mesh (polyglactin 910) for the formation of a pelvic "lid" after radical pelvic resection. Am. J. Obstet. Gynecol., *198*:158, 1988.
17. LIFSHITZ, S., JOHNSON, R., ROBERTS, J. A., and BUCHSBAUM, H. J. Intestinal fistula and obstruction following pelvic exenteration. Surg. Gynecol. Obstet., *152*:630, 1981.
18. SYMMONDS, R. E., PRATT, J. H., and WEBB, M. J. Exenteration operations: Experience with 198 patients. Am. J. Obstet. Gynecol., *121*:907, 1975.
19. ROBERTS, W. S., et al. Major morbidity after pelvic exenteration: A 7-year experience. Obstet. Gynecol., *69*:617, 1987.
20. ORR, J. W., et al. Gastrointestinal complications associated with pelvic exenteration. Am. J. Obstet. Gynecol., *145*:325, 1983.
21. MORGAN, L. S., DALY, J. W., and MONIF, G. R. G. Infectious morbidity associated with pelvic exenteration. Gynecol. Oncol., *10*:318, 1980.
22. AVERETTE, H. E., LICHTINGER, M., SEVIN, B. U., and GIRTANER, R. E. Pelvic exenteration. A 15-year experience in a general metropolitan hospital. Am. J. Obstet. Gynecol., *150*:179, 1984.
23. BARBER, H. R. K. Pelvic exenteration. Cancer Invest., *5*:331, 1987.
24. CURRY, S. L., et al. Pelvic exenteration: A 7-year experience. Gynecol. Oncol., *11*:119, 1981.
25. MORLEY, G. W., and LINDENAUR, S. M. Pelvic exenterative therapy for gynecologic malignancy-An analysis of 70 cases. Cancer, *38*:581, 1976.

Intestinal Surgery for the Urologic Oncologist

Robert A. Read
Greg Van Stiegmann

This chapter will focus on selected aspects of intestinal surgery as they relate to urologic oncology. An overview of intestinal physiology and anatomy is discussed in the context of bowel operations germane to urologic disease. Several techniques for the repair, resection, and re-establishment of bowel continuity will be described as well as standard principles of perioperative management for patients undergoing intestinal surgery.

PHYSIOLOGY OF THE INTESTINAL TRACT

Digestion

The primary functions of the small and large intestine are digestion and absorption of water, nutrients, vitamins, and minerals. Fluid and electrolyte transport occur along the entire length of the small intestine. The net driving force for the movement of water and electrolytes represents the combined effects of active, passive, and solvent drag transport processes.[1] The majority of the estimated 9 L of daily intestinal fluid is absorbed in the jejunum by passive and solvent drag processes secondary to monosaccharide absorption.[2] Utilizing

these mechanisms, the jejunum absorbs large volumes of essentially isotonic fluid. The duodenum and ileum, although essential for the digestion and absorption of nutrients, play a relatively minor role in the balance of fluid and electrolytes and serve mainly to alter the qualitative composition of intestinal fluid.

The digestion and absorption of nutrients and vitamins, unlike the absorption of fluids and electrolytes, is complex and relies on sequential processes throughout the intestine, which are unique for each major nutrient category.[3] The majority of these processes occur in the proximal small bowel; however, bile salts are conserved through a high-efficiency reabsorption system in the distal ileum. The enterohepatic circulation recycles the entire bile salt pool approximately 6 times each day and limits the daily bile salt losses in the feces to only 500 mg.[4] With distal ileal resections of less than 100 cm, hepatic synthesis is usually able to adequately compensate for the resultant bile salt losses; however, the unabsorbed bile salts that pass to the colon often lead to a net colonic fluid secretion and bile salt diarrhea. Ileal resections greater than 100 cm may result in both bile acid malabsorption and steatorrhea (fecal fat greater than 20 gm/day). If the resultant steatorrhea exceeds 40 gm/

day, patients suffer from significant nutritional deficiencies and weight loss.[5] The majority of fat, carbohydrate, and protein digestion and absorption occur in the duodenum and jejunum. The ileum appears to be responsible for only a limited amount of normal nutrient digestion and absorption.[6–8]

The absorption of vitamins depends on their lipid solubility. Fat-soluble vitamins (A, D, E, and K) are metabolized and absorbed in the proximal intestine in a manner similar to the absorption of dietary fat. Water-soluble vitamins, with the exception of vitamin B12, are metabolized and transported across the intestinal brush boarder by way of vitamin-specific transport mechanisms. Vitamin B12 absorption is a complex process that requires gastric pepsin, intrinsic factor, pancreatic proteases, optimum intestinal pH, and ileal receptors specific for intrinsic factor–cobalamine complexes.[9]

Motility

Intestinal motility influences many aspects of intestinal function. At rest, the intestine displays a periodic pattern of bursts of propagated contractions. These begin in the stomach (sometimes as high as the distal esophagus) and migrate slowly through the length of the intestine approximately every 90 minutes.[10] Oral feedings temporally abolish these "migrating motor" complexes and induce a series of irregular contractions that persist for three to four hours after each meal. The irregular pattern of contraction then slowly reverts to the migrating pattern as digestion proceeds.[11,12]

Paralytic ileus, a relatively common form of functional intestinal obstruction that may follow abdominal operations, is thought to represent an imbalance between the sympathetic and parasympathetic nervous systems (i.e., a relative sympathetic hyperactivity). Animal studies have demonstrated elevated systemic catecholamine levels associated with paralytic ileus.[13] Postoperative ileus may be prevented in animals by chemical sympathectomy.[13,14] The clinical causes of paralytic ileus include all forms of peritonitis, retroperitoneal hematomas, ureteral colic, pneumonia, rib fractures, and myocardial infarction. The current mainstays of treatment are elimination of the cause, nasogastric decompression and time.

Microbiology

The rate of postoperative infectious complications following abdominal operations increases significantly if the intestine is opened. Although the polymicrobial nature of the intestinal microflora was described as early as the 1930s,[15] only recently, with improvements in collection and culture techniques, has the importance of anaerobic microflora been appreciated (Table 61-1).

The normal microflora of saliva includes aerobic streptococci, staphylococci, *Neisseria, Hemophilus,* and many anaerobes at a concentration of approximately 10^6 to 10^8 per mL. Large quantities of bacteria are ingested daily but few survive the acidic environment of the normal human stomach. The bacterial population of the stomach is directly related to its acidity and patients taking H2 antagonists or those who have undergone antiulcer procedures have a consistently higher bacterial load.[16] The proximal small intestine normally contains few gram-negative and anaerobic organisms. Except in disease states causing bacterial overgrowth, the bacterial count in the proximal small intestine is between 10^1 and 10^2 per mL.[17] The distal small bowel is a transition zone between the relatively sterile proximal bowel and the colon. Here, under normal conditions, there are relatively equal numbers of aerobic and anaerobic organisms (approximately 10^4 to 10^7 per mL). In contrast, the colon contains predominantly anaerobic organisms (10^9 to 10^{11} per mL). Disease states or alterations in the normal continuity of the bowel may result in dramatic alterations in the quality and quantity of intestinal microflora.

ANATOMY OF THE INTESTINAL TRACT

The entire small bowel, with the exception of the duodenum and occasionally the last few centimeters of ileum, is anchored to the posterior peritoneum by a mesentery that extends from the ligament of Treitz inferolaterally to the ileocecal valve in the right iliac fossa. The length of this segment of bowel measures 600 to 800 cm at autopsy. In the living state, however, this figure is closer to 300 cm, the discrepancy representing a reflection of the smooth muscle tone of the intestinal wall. The small bowel is supplied by the superior mesenteric artery (SMA), which originates from the abdominal aorta approximately 1 to 1.5 cm inferior to the celiac trunk. The initial branches of the SMA are the middle colic and inferior pancreaticoduodenal arteries; however, numerous aberrant branches have been described including right hepatic (16%), gastroduodenal (10%), and common celiomesenteric trunk (1%)[18] (Fig. 61-1). The superior mesenteric vein drains the jejunum, ileum, cecum, and ascending and transverse colon. Its branches roughly parallel the branches of the SMA.

The length of the colon is variable, measuring approximately 90 cm. The partial circumferences of both the ascending and descending colon are retroperitoneal, whereas the transverse and sigmoid colon are intraperitoneal. The transverse mesocolon extends from the junction of the first and second portion of the duodenum and across the pancreas and forms the inferior wall of the lesser peritoneal sac. Anteriorly, the transverse colon is covered by the omentum, which extends from the greater curvature of the stomach, draping the bowel, and forms the anterior wall of the lesser sac. Unlike the small bowel, the longitudinal muscle layer of the colon forms three distinct longitudinal bands, the tenia coli. These bands foreshorten the colon, drawing it into a series of sacculi or haustra along its length (Fig. 61-2).

The arterial supply of the colon arises from both the inferior and superior mesenteric arteries. A rich network of anastomoses between all of the principle vessels provides abundant collateral blood flow. Occasionally the anastomotic network is incomplete, most frequently at the watershed area of the splenic flexure between the left colic and branches of the middle colic arteries (Fig. 61-2).

TABLE 61-1. *Human Endogenous Gastrointestinal Microflora*

REGION	PREDOMINANT MICROFLORA	CONCENTRATION (per g or mL of aspirate)		AEROBES	ANAEROBES
		AEROBES	ANAEROBES		
Oropharynx	Slight predominance of anaerobic organisms	10^4–10^5	10^5–10^7	*Streptococcus, Hemophilus, Neisseria,* Diphtheroids	*Peptostreptococcus, Fusobacterium, Bacteroides melaninogenicus, Bacteroides oralis, Peptococcus*
Esophagus	Slight predominance of anaerobic organisms	10^4–10^5	10^5–10^7	———————— Same as oropharynx ————————	
Stomach	Both aerobic and anaerobic organisms	Microflora is absent or minimal if normal gastric acidity and motility are present		*Streptococcus, Escherichia coli, Klebsiella, Enterobacter, Enterococcus*	*Peptostreptococcus, Bacteroides oralis, Bacteroides melaninogenicus*
Proximal small intestine	Slight predominance of aerobic organisms	10^2	10–10^2	*Streptococcus, Escherichia coli, Klebsiella, Enterobacter, Enterococcus*	*Peptostreptococcus, Bacteroides oralis, Bacteroides melaninogenicus*
Distal ileum	Slight predominance of aerobic organisms	10^4–10^6	10^5–10^7	*Escherichia coli, Klebsiella, Enterobacter, Enterococcus*	*Bacteroides fragilis, Peptostreptococcus, Clostridium*
Colon	Great predominance of anaerobic organisms	10^5–10^8	10^9–10^{11}	———————— Same as distal ileum ————————	

From Adinolfi, M. F., Cerise, E. J., and Nichols, R. L. Microbiology of the small intestine. In: *Surgery of the Small Intestine.* Edited by R. L. Nelson and L. M. Nyhus. Norwalk, CT: Appleton and Lange, 1987.

PERIOPERATIVE MANAGEMENT

Both mechanical and chemical methods have been developed for the preoperative preparation of the intestinal tract. These have resulted in lowered postoperative infectious complication rates. The methods available for debulking intestinal stool include prolonged preoperative fasting on elemental diets, Mg-citrate, mannitol, and polyethylene glycol cathartics, in addition to various laxatives and enemas. Most of these methods are effective and can be used in combination, depending on the nature of the proposed operation and the tolerance of the patient. Antibiotic preparations, if used properly, reduce the bowel microflora to a minimum. Such regimens include oral administration of nonabsorbable neomycin and erythromycin prior to the planned operation. The typical large bowel preoperative regimen used at the University of Colorado consists of the oral administration of polyethylene glycol, with or without oral antibiotics, the day prior to the planned operation augmented as necessary with tap water enemas.

Nutritional Support

Many patients presenting with long-standing disease are physiologically malnourished. The key to optimal perioperative management is appropriate nutritional assessment and support. Consultation from a nutrition team should be sought early.

Adequate nutrition can be delivered by either enteral or parenteral routes. Feeding should begin 7 to 14 days preoperatively in the patient who has lost more than 10% of his lean-body mass. The choice of delivery route depends on the functional integrity of the bowel and the relative risks of potential aspiration and intravenous line complications. Various enteral formulas differ in protein, residue, fat, and caloric content. Parenteral formulas are complex mixtures of concentrated dextrose solutions together with amino acids, vitamins, and minerals, supplemented with hydrolyzed vegetable oils. These solutions are considerably more expensive than enteral formulas but are useful in patients with limited bowel function or severe nutritional deficits.

PERIOPERATIVE COMPLICATIONS

Complications unique to intestinal operations occur with an overall frequency of 6%.[19] Perioperative antibiotics together with meticulous operative technique have reduced the wound infection rate of abdominal operations without enterotomy to

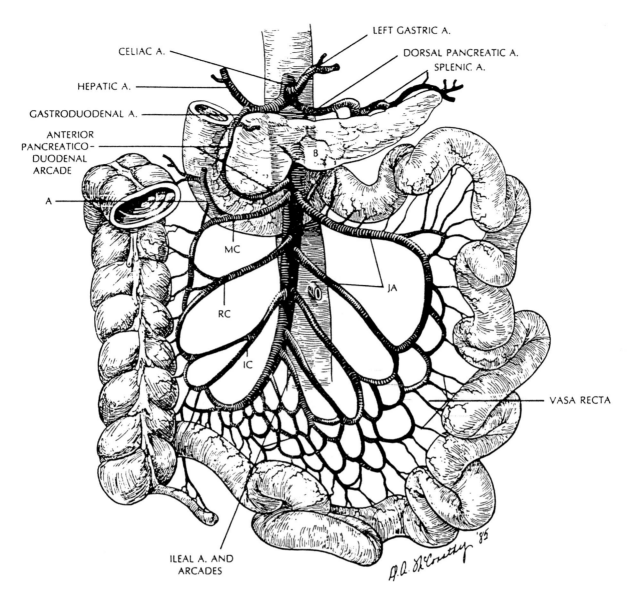

FIG. 61-1. Superior mesenteric artery and branches (A = left branch of middle colic artery, IC = ileocolic artery, JA = jejunal arteries, MC = middle colic artery, and RC = right colic artery). (From Monsen, H. Anatomy of the jejunum and ileum. In: *Surgery of the Small Intestine.* Edited by R. L. Nelson and L. M. Nyhus. Norwalk, CT: Appleton and Lange, 1987.

less than 2%. Enterotomies and resections without gross spillage (clean contaminated) are associated with a wound infection rate of approximately 6%, and gross spillage of intestinal contents increases this rate to 20 to 50%.[19]

Most postoperative intra-abdominal abscesses result from errors in surgical technique, commonly spillage of intestinal contents. The detection of an abscess is based on clinical suspicion supplemented with diagnostic studies. Most patients with intraperitoneal abscesses develop fever and leukocytosis and a progressive paralytic ileus. The diagnosis is confirmed with ultrasonography, computed tomography, or exploratory laparotomy. Therapy consists of aggressive drainage, antibiotics, and physiologic support. The mortality associated with an ineffectively treated intra-abdominal abscess remains high.

Enterocutaneous fistula may occur as a result of Crohn's disease or cancer; however, most follow abdominal operations in which the bowel is injured or an anastomosis fails. Management of a controlled fistula consists of skin protection and fluid and electrolyte replacement. Complete bowel rest and parenteral alimentation may be needed. Fistulas associated with inflammatory bowel disease, cancer, distal obstruction, foreign bodies, or abscesses rarely resolve with conservative therapy and usually require operative intervention.[20]

Paralytic ileus occurs frequently after intestinal operations and usually lasts for 24 to 72 hours. Prolonged paralytic ileus may result from ongoing peritonitis and mesenteric or retroperitoneal hematomas following extensive dissections. Prolonged or recurrent ileus typically produces silent, painless distension, whereas mechanical bowel obstruction is associated with colicky abdominal pain and characteristic high-pitched bowel sounds. Frequently, the distinction between prolonged ileus and mechanical obstruction is difficult. A meg-

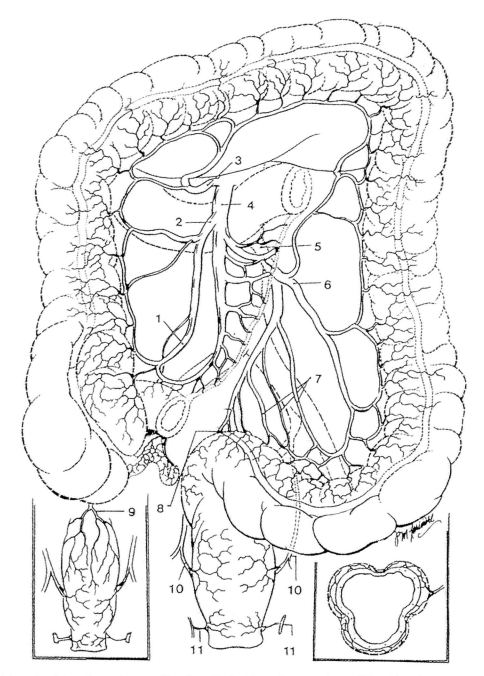

Fig. 61-2. The arterial supply of the colon and rectum (1 = ileocolic, 2 = ileocolic artery giving off the right colic artery, 3 = middle colic artery, 4 = superior mesenteric artery, 5 = inferior mesenteric artery, 6 = left colic artery, 7 = sigmoidal branches of the inferior mesenteric artery, 8 and 9 = superior hemorrhoidal artery, 10 = middle hemorrhoidal artery, and 11 = inferior hemorrhoidal artery). (From Ellis, H. Resection of the colon. In: *Maingot's Abdominal Operations.* Edited by S. Schwartz and H. Ellis. Norwalk, CT: Appleton-Century-Crofts, 1985.)

lumine diatrizoate (Gastrografin) contrast study may be helpful in delineating slow bowel transit from mechanical obstruction.

Anastomotic leaks are uncommon following properly conducted bowel operations. Colonic anastomoses are more prone to leakage because of the presence of virulent bacteria, the thin muscle wall, and less luxuriant blood supply of the colon. Rectal anastomoses may be associated with a nearly 20% leakage rate even though only about 5% of these are clinically significant. The latter may manifest as intra-abdomi-

nal abscesses and require laparotomy with a colostomy and wide drainage.[21]

OPERATIVE TECHNIQUES

Inadvertent Enterotomy

Inadvertent bowel lacerations may occur during lysis of adhesions commonly associated with previous operations or peritonitis. Multiple full-thickness bowel lacerations in close proximity are best treated by segmental resection of the affected bowel and primary reanastomosis. Small enterotomies in healthy bowel can be treated by primary repair. The edges of the enterotomy are debrided of any nonviable tissue. The enterotomy is then closed transversely using a two-layer technique with a running 3-0 absorbable suture full-thickness inner layer followed by an outer layer of interrupted 3-0 silk or absorbable suture material Lembert inverting seromuscular sutures (Fig. 61-3).

End-to-End Anastomosis

Segmental bowel resections are usually completed with primary end-to-end reanastomosis. Many techniques have been described. The most widely used in the United States is a two-layer open technique. Following placement of noncrushing bowel clamps proximal and distal to the limits of resection, the bowel is divided along with the intervening mesentery.

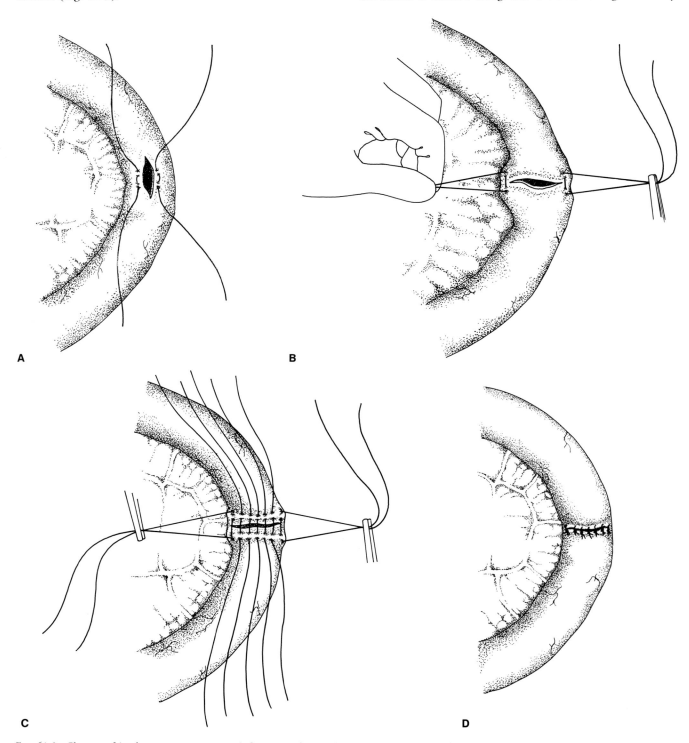

A

B

C

D

FIG. 61-3. Closure of inadvertent enterotomy. *A*, Seromuscular Lembert sutures placed on the mesenteric and antimesenteric aspects of the enterotomy. *B*, Tension applied to sutures to set up a transverse closure. *C*, The closure is completed with the placement of additional Lembert sutures between the initial corner sutures. *D*, The sutures are tied and cut; the enterorrhaphy is completed.

The edges of the bowel are carefully inspected for adequacy of blood supply and viability and approximated to ensure that an anastomosis can be constructed under no tension.

The initial step involves placement of a series of interrupted 3-0 Lembert sutures to approximate the posterior wall beginning with the corner sutures. Next, the inner layer is begun using two full-thickness 3-0 running absorbable sutures starting at the midpoint of the posterior wall and continued around the circumference of the bowel using a Connell or baseball stitch on the anterior wall. The anastomosis is then completed with a series of interrupted Lembert sutures forming the outer layer of the anterior wall. The patency of the lumen is checked and the mesenteric defect is closed (Fig. 61-4).

Side-to-Side Anastomosis

The chief utility of the side-to-side anastomosis is to bypass areas of obstruction secondary to malignant disease or radiation, resection of which would involve extensive or prolonged dissection. To employ this technique, normal areas of bowel proximal and distal to the point of obstruction are identified and arranged in an isoperistaltic fashion prior to the construction of the anastomosis. The common hand-sewn form of this technique utilizes two layers in a manner similar to the end-to-end anastomosis. Initially, 3-0 silk corner sutures are placed at either end of the proposed stoma, halfway between the mesenteric and antimesenteric borders of the bowel. The outer layer of the posterior row is then constructed with a series of interrupted 3-0 silk Lembert sutures. Longitudinal enterotomies twice the diameter of the bowel are made in each loop of bowel along the posterior row of sutures. The running inner layer of full thickness 3-0 absorbable suture is started at the midpoint of the posterior row and continued anteriorly with a Connell or baseball stitch. The anterior wall of the anastomosis is completed with a series of interrupted 3-0 silk Lembert sutures. The patency of the lumen is checked and the mesentery closed to prevent internal herniation of bowel (Fig. 61-5).

End Colostomy

A colostomy may be necessary when the colon or rectum is inadvertently entered, for decompression of distal obstruction, or diversion of the fecal stream from a segment of previously irradiated or otherwise compromised bowel. The colon is divided between bowel clamps or with a GIA stapling device and the mesentery mobilized to allow approximately 5 cm of viable bowel to extend through the abdominal wall at the site selected for the colostomy. The distal colonic segment is resected and closed in two layers and if possible sutured to the anterior abdominal wall near the colostomy site to facilitate future mobilization for colostomy takedown. A 2 to 3 cm diameter circle of skin is excised at the site selected for the colostomy. The abdominal wall muscles are divided and the fascia opened widely to avoid constriction of the bowel. The colon, still closed, is then passed through the abdominal wall

defect and anchored to the external fascia with four quadrant seromuscular 3-0 absorbable sutures. Any internal hernia is closed by attaching the colonic mesentery to the anterior and lateral abdominal wall and the operation completed and the incision closed prior to maturing the colostomy. The colostomy can be matured following closure of the abdomen or 24 to 48 hours later with a series of interrupted full thickness 3-0 sutures between the cut edge of the colon and the skin edge of the colostomy (Fig. 61-6).

Staple Techniques

The ease and speed of stapling devices for bowel operations has increased their popularity in recent years. The principles governing intestinal anastomoses are the same for staple and suture techniques. Adequate blood supply, meticulous anastomotic technique, and lack of tension are essential for the success of any bowel anastomosis. Common errors in staple techniques include failure to overlap suture lines leaving gaps in the anastomotic line, and failure to include the full thickness of the bowel wall within the jaws of the stapler creating weak points in the anastomosis and potentiating leaks.

A standard staple technique for an end-to-end anastomosis is the triangulation method. Preparation of the intestine for anastomosis includes mesenteric clearance of a more liberal margin of intestine at the points to be anastomosed to ensure that staples are placed through full thickness of the entire circumference of the bowel. Because excess bowel is ultimately excised, there is usually adequate vascularity to ensure healing of the anastomotic site.

With the aid of full-thickness stay sutures at the mesenteric and antimesenteric edges of the bowel to be anastomosed and with an Allis clamp grasping the full thickness of both bowel walls, the posterior row of staples is applied to the full thickness of both bowel walls, and the excess is excised from within the lumen. An additional stay suture placed anteriorly triangulates the bowel, and two additional applications of staples are made anteriorly to include the full thickness of the bowel wall. The lines of staples should overlap to avoid gaps in the anastomotic lines. The mesenteric defect is then closed (Fig. 61-7).

The use of the GIA stapling instrument provides a quick method of side-to-side anastomosis to bypass obstructed intestine. The loops are arranged in isoperistaltic fashion and approximated with full-thickness stay sutures placed a distance of 2 to 3 cm greater than the proposed stoma. One fork of the GIA instrument is inserted into each loop via an enterotomy; and the instrument is fired, thus making the entire anastomosis. After removal of the GIA, the twin enterotomies are closed with the TA 30, taking care that no gaps remain (Fig. 61-8).

Gastrostomy

The Stamm gastrostomy is one of several techniques commonly used to establish tube enterostomy access to the gastrointestinal tract for decompression or long-term enteral feeding.

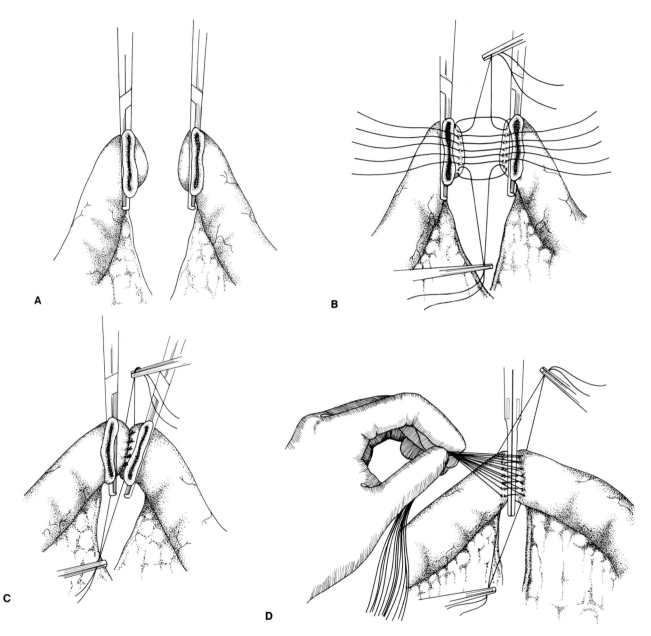

A

B

C

D

Fig. 61-4.

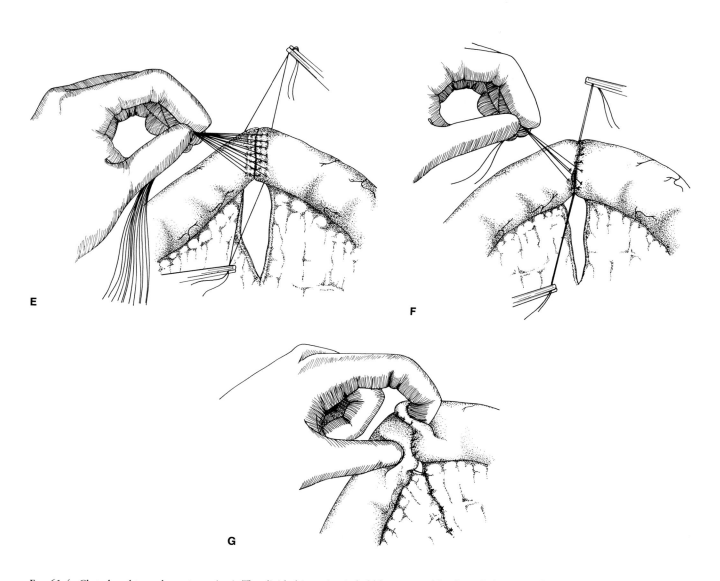

E

F

G

FIG. 61-4. Closed end-to-end anastomosis. *A,* The divided intestine is held by noncrushing bowel clamps. *B,* Corner sutures are placed in the mesenteric and antimesenteric edges and tagged. The back row of seromuscular Lembert sutures are placed. *C,* The posterior row is completed; the sutures are tied and cut. *D,* The anterior row of seromuscular Lembert sutures is placed after the excess bowel has been trimmed and the clamps approximated under no tension. *E* and *F,* The bowel clamps are removed and the anterior row of sutures is tied. *G,* The patency of the anastomosis is checked by palpation. The mesenteric defect is closed with interrupted sutures.

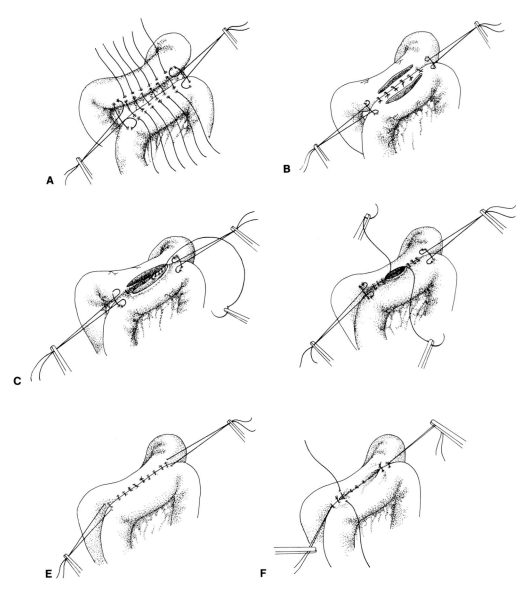

FIG. 61-5. Side-to-side two-layer anastomosis. *A,* The posterior layer of seromuscular Lembert sutures is placed first. *B,* The posterior sutures are tied and cut. The enterotomies are made and hemostasis secured with electrocautery. *C,* The inner layer of 3-0 absorbable suture is begun at the center of the posterior row and run as an over-and-over stitch toward each corner. *D* and *E,* The anterior inner layer is completed with a Connell or baseball stitch. *F,* The anastomosis is completed with the anterior outer layer of seromuscular Lembert sutures.

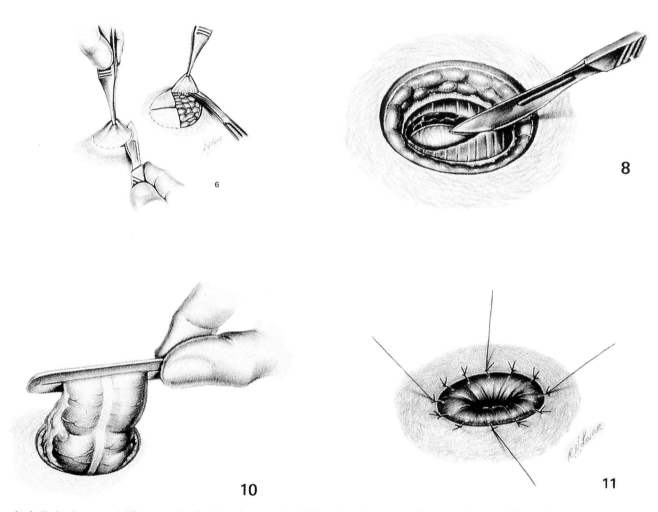

FIG. 61-6. End colostomy. *A*, The exact site for the colostomy should be selected to ensure that an appliance will fit satisfactorily away from the umbilicus. *B*, Fascia, muscle, and peritoneum are divided to create a generous opening for the colostomy. *C*, The colon is delivered through the anterior abdominal wall. *D*, Once the abdominal incision has been closed, a mucocutaneous suture is used to mature the colostomy. (From Thomson, J. P. S. Colostomy; end iliac and loop transverse 1. In: *Rob and Smith's Operative Surgery; Alimentary Tract and Abdominal Wall, Colon, Rectum, and Anus.* Edited by I. P. Todd and L. P. Fielding. London: Buttersworth, 1983.)

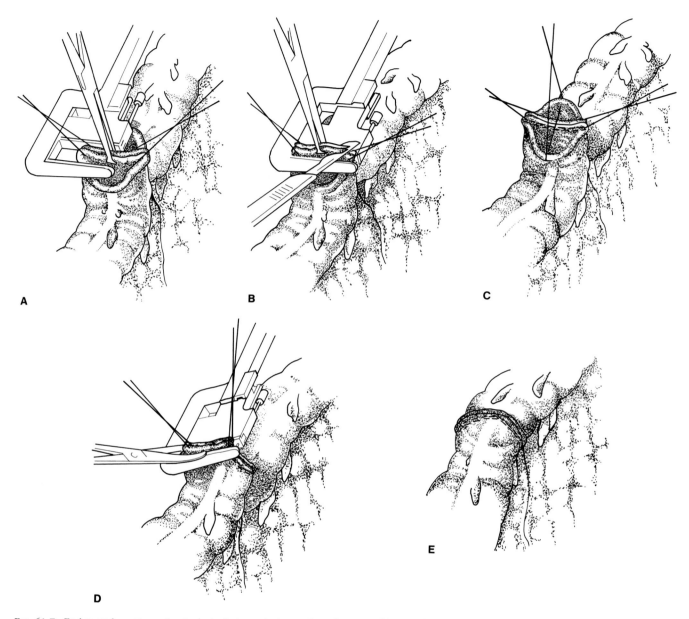

FIG. 61-7. End-to-end anastomosis, staple technique. *A*, Approximately 1 cm of bowel should be cleared of mesentery. This length will allow secure application of staples with the TA 55 and is not excessive, since the excess bowel will be trimmed. Full-thickness sutures of 2-0 silk are placed at the mesenteric and antimesenteric edges of the bowel to be anastomosed, and the full thicknesses of both posterior walls are held in the center with an Allis clamp. The jaws of the TA 55 are placed to include the full thickness of both posterior walls beneath the sutures and clamp. *B*, After the posterior row of staples is placed, the excess bowel is shaved above the TA 55 between the stay sutures, which are retained. *C*, An additional full-thickness stay suture of 2-0 silk is placed anteriorly, midway between the corner sutures. *D*, Taking care to overlap the previously placed posterior row of staples, the full thickness of each remaining half of the anterior wall is alternately placed between the jaws of the TA 55, and the anterior rows of staples are placed. The excess is shaved above the instrument, retaining the center suture until the final anterior row of staples has been placed. Retention of the suture at the midpoint anteriorly insures that the rows of staples overlap and that no gap exists between the anterior lines of staples. *E*, The anastomosis is completed and the mesenteric defect is closed. The anastomosis should be checked again to ensure that no gaps exist between the line of previously placed staples.

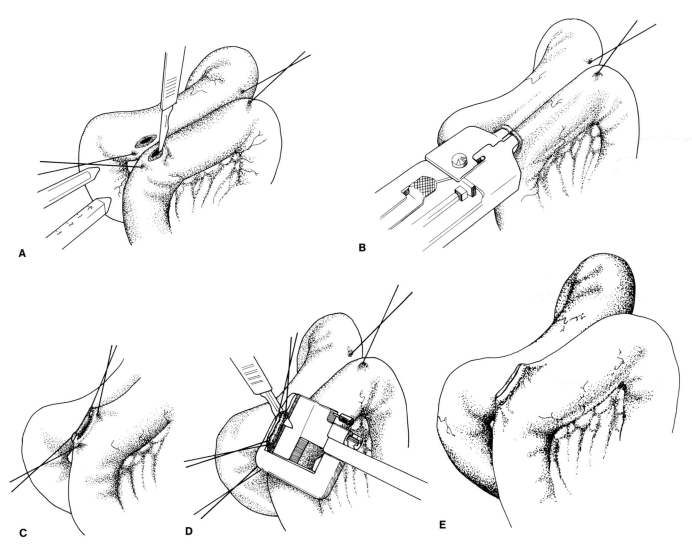

Fig. 61-8. Stapled side-to-side anastomosis. *A,* Stay sutures are used to the bowel. Small enterotomies are made to allow insertion of the GIA instrument. *B,* The side-to-side anastomosis is performed with the GIA instrument. *C,* The edges of the now-common enterotomy are separated with stay sutures. *D,* The enterotomy is closed with a TA instrument in line with the longitudinal axis of the intestine. *E,* The completed side-to-side stapled anastomosis.

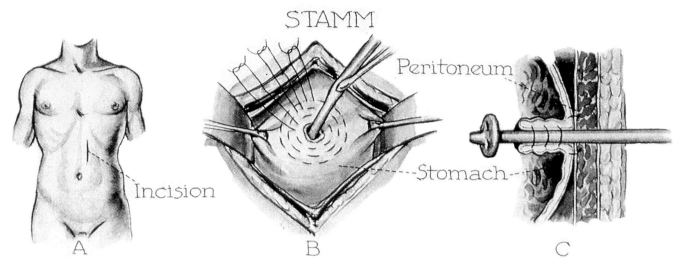

FIG. 61-9. Stamm gastrostomy. *A*, Insertion site identified in the body of the stomach through abdominal incision. *B*, A Foley or mushroom catheter is inserted within concentric purse-string sutures. *C*, Stomach sutured to the peritoneum after purse-string sutures are tied. (From Thorek, P. *Atlas of Surgical Techniques*. Philadelphia: J. B. Lippincott Co., 1970.)

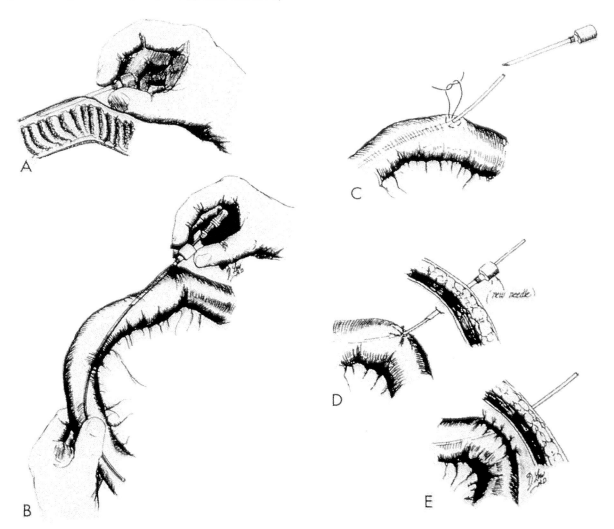

FIG. 61-10. Needle-catheter jejunostomy. *A*, Insertion of the needle within the jejunal wall. *B*, Insertion of the catheter with stylet through the needle into the jejunal lumen. *C*, Removal of the needle and placement of anchoring suture. *D*, Insertion of the needle through the abdominal wall for the catheter's exit. *E*, Jejunopexy. (From Rombeau, J. L., Barot, L. R., Low, D. W., and Twomey, P. L. Feeding by tube enterostomy. In: *Enteral and Tube Feeding*. Vol. 1. Edited by J. L. Rombeau and M. D. Caldwell. Philadelphia: W. B. Saunders, Co., 1984.)

A site in the body of the stomach along the greater curvature of the stomach is selected. Two concentric purse-string sutures are placed in the anterior surface of the stomach. The stomach is opened in the center of the purse-string sutures. The gastrostomy tube (usually a 24-French or larger Foley catheter) is placed within the stomach and the inner purse-string suture secured. A portion of the stomach wall is invaginated as the second purse-string suture is tied. The gastrostomy tube is brought out the abdominal wall through a separate incision. Several interrupted sutures are placed to fix the stomach to the abdominal wall and skin at the catheter exit site. Malecot, Foley, and mushroom catheters have all been used successfully as gastrostomy tubes. One advantage of the Stamm gastrostomy technique, is that once the need for enterostomy feeding has passed, the tube can simply be removed and the ostomy will generally seal promptly without the need for operative closure[22] (Fig. 61-9).

Needle-Catheter Jejunostomy

Another commonly used technique for enteral feeding is the needle-catheter jejunostomy. A thin-wall, 14-gauge needle is used to make a 3- to 5-cm seromuscular tunnel along the antimesenteric border of the jejunum 15 to 20 cm distal to the ligament of Treitz. A 16-gauge polyvinyl catheter is inserted through the thin-wall needle and fed 10 to 20 cm distally in the jejunum. The catheter is secured to the jejunal wall with a single 3-0 purse-string suture. A separate 14-gauge needle is passed through the abdominal wall and the catheter fed outside the abdomen. The jejunum, 5 to 10 cm proximal and distal to the insertion site, is secured to the abdominal wall and the catheter secured to the skin[23] (Fig. 61-10). Feeding may start at 24 to 48 hours following operation.

REFERENCES

1. BINDER, H. J. Absorption and secretion of water and electrolytes by small and large intestine. In: *Gastrointestinal Disease: Pathophysiology, Diagnosis, Management.* 3rd Ed. Edited by M. H. Sleisenger and J. S. Fordtran. Philadelphia, W. B. Saunders, Co., 1983, p. 844.

2. FORDTRAN, J. S. Stimulation of active and passive sodium absorption by sugars in the human jejunum. J. Clin. Invest., *55:*728, 1975.

3. GRAY, G. M. Mechanisms of digestion and absorption of food. In: *Gastrointestinal Disease: Pathophysiology, Diagnosis, Management.* 3rd Ed. Edited by M. H. Sleisenger and J. S. Fordtran. Philadelphia, W. B. Saunders, Co., 1983, p. 844.

4. HOFMANN, A. F., and POLEY, J. R. Role of bile acid malabsorption in the pathogenesis of diarrhea and steatorrhea in patients with ileal resection. Gastroenterology, *62:*918, 1972.

5. HOFMANN, A. F. Bile acid malabsorption caused by ileal resection. Arch. Intern. Med., *130:*597, 1972.

6. GRAY, G. M. Carbohydrate digestion and absorption: Role of the small intestine. N. Engl. J. Med., *292:*1225, 1975.

7. FORDTRAN, J. S., RECTOR, F. C., and CARTER, W. The mechanisms of sodium absorption in the human small intestine. J. Clin. Invest., *47:*884, 1968.

8. ADIBI, S. A., and KIM, Y. S. Peptide absorption and hydrolysis. In: *Physiology of the Gastrointestinal Tract.* Edited by L. R. Johnson. New York, Raven Press, 1981, p. 325.

9. DONALDSON, R. M. Intrinsic factor and the transport of cobalamin. In: *Physiology of the Gastrointestinal Tract.* Edited by L. R. Johnson. New York, Raven Press, 1981.

10. DENT, J. et al. Interdigestive phasic contractions of the human lower esophageal sphincter. Gastroenterology, *84:*452, 1983.

11. WEVER, I. D., et al. Disruptive effect of test meals on interdigestive motor complex in dogs. Am. J. Physiol., *235:*E661, 1978.

12. WOOD, J. D. Intrinsic neural control of intestinal motility. Annu. Rev. Physiol., *43:*33, 1981.

13. SMITH, J., KELLY, K. T., and WEINSHILBOUM, R. M. Pathophysiology of postoperative ileus. Arch. Surg., *112:*203, 1977.

14. HEIMBACH, D. M., and CROUT, J. R. Treatment of paralytic ileus with adrenergic neuronal blocking drugs. Surgery, *69:*582, 1971.

15. ALTEMIER, W. A. The bacterial flora of acute perforated appendicitis with peritonitis. Ann. Surg., *107:*517, 1938.

16. BROOKS, J. R., SMITH, H. F., and PEASE, F. B. Bacteriology of the stomach immediately following vagotomy; the growth of candida albicans. Ann. Surg., *179:*859, 1974.

17. BORNSIDE, G. H., WELSH, J. S., and COHN, I. Bacterial flora of the human small intestine. JAMA, *196:*109, 1966.

18. DERRIK, J. R., and FADHLI, H. A. Surgical anatomy of the superior mesenteric artery. Am. Surg., *31:*545, 1965.

19. McGUIRE, H. H. Complications of intestinal surgery. In: *Complications in Surgery and Trauma.* Edited by L. J. Greenfield. J. B. Lippincott Co., Philadelphia, 1984, p. 447.

20. REBER, H. A. et al. Management of external gastrointestinal fistulas. Ann. Surg., *188:*460, 1978.

21. BEART, R. W., and KELLY, K. A. Randomized prospective evaluation of the EEA stapler for colorectal anastomoses. Am. J. Surg., *141:*143, 1981.

22. RANDALL, H. T., and CALDWELL, M. D. Enteral nutrition: Nasoenteric and ostomy feeding. In: *Surgery of the Stomach, Duodenum, and Small Intestine.* Edited by H. W. Scott and J. L. Sawyers. Boston, MA, Blackwell Scientific Publications, 1987.

23. DELANY, H. M., CARNEVAL, N. J., and GARVEY, J. W. Jejunostomy by a needle catheter technique. Surgery, *73:*786, 1973.

Vascular Surgery for the Urologic Oncologist

Edward J. Bartle
W. Sterling Edwards

V ascular surgical techniques of some sophistication were introduced and widely applied in the early 1950s. Much of this advance was based on early investigation by Alexis Carrel, who demonstrated the methods of direct arterial and venous repair as well as the use of autogenous vein grafts in arterial repair and replacement.[1] Refinements in these technical strategies have been made over the years especially with the introduction of prosthetic materials for vascular reconstruction in the last three decades.

With these refinements in these vascular repairs, applications of these techniques for all types of surgical complications to the vascular system became practical. Besides vessel injury, other perioperative vascular problems include thrombophlebitis and pulmonary embolism. There have been many methods over the years in an attempt to reduce these complications, but this is still a major problem, unresponsive to most measures. Recently, there have been other measures that may prove to be beneficial such as sequential compression limb stockings and low-molecular-weight heparin.

VENOUS INJURIES

Radical pelvic surgical procedures for cancer of the bladder and prostate may involve injuries to pelvic veins or the removal of segments of vein involved in tumor. Laceration or excision of deep pelvic branches of the hypogastric veins during these procedures may result in hemorrhage that is difficult to control. Injuries to the external or common iliac veins or inferior vena cava are easier to control, but chronic leg edema may result if the venous repair is not meticulously performed or if the veins are ligated.

Surgical Technique

It is important to have sound knowledge of venous anatomy in the pelvis to avoid venous injury or to correct any injury or reconstruct or ligate any necessary operative removal of a venous segment. The major veins include the internal iliac veins (hypogastric) draining the pelvic venous plexus and the external iliac veins combining with the hypogastric and forming the

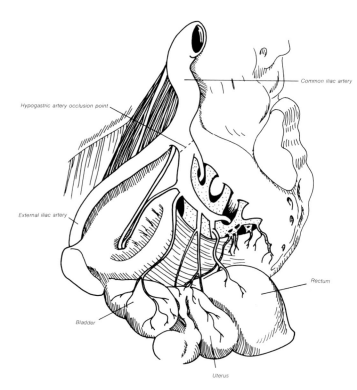

FIG. 62-1. Lateral view of the pelvic wall, showing the iliac arteries and their branches to deep pelvic organs. Hypogastric veins (not shown) accompany and usually lie behind each arterial branch. Dotted lines show the proper location of temporary or permanent clamping or ligation of the hypogastric artery for deep pelvic bleeding that cannot be directly controlled.

common iliac veins, which join posterior and usually lateral to the right iliac artery to form the inferior vena cava. Owing to the incidence of anomalous venous development, the possibility of duplication of the inferior vena cava or left transposition of the cava must be kept in mind.[2]

The internal iliac veins drain the pelvic venous plexuses, which are networks of thin-walled veins adjacent to and receiving the venous drainage from the bladder, prostate, uterus, and rectum. Hemorrhage after injury to this pelvic plexus (Fig. 62-1) is difficult to control, because exposure of these short friable structures for proximal and distal control is not easily obtained. Vision is often limited by continued hemorrhage, and clamping attempts may only further injure arteries and additional veins.

Elevation of the lower body and legs in a steep Trendelenburg position will often empty the pelvic veins sufficiently to allow precise clamping or suturing of the venous opening with a 5-0 monofilament suture. If good exposure is still not obtained, temporary occlusion of one or both internal iliac arteries with a vascular clamp at their origin from the common iliac artery (Fig. 62-1, Fig. 62-2) will often suffice. When venous bleeding cannot be directly controlled, a gauze pack can be left in the wound to provide enough pressure for indirect hemorrhage control. The abdominal incision is then closed completely over the pack, which can be removed 48 hours after the operation, with minimal risk of recurring hemorrhage.

Arteriovenous fistula formation is another complication of suture-ligature of pelvic veins as a result of poor exposure. If the needle punctures or tears an opening in adjacent arteries and veins, they may bleed into a common hematoma, which can later form an arteriovenous connection. Elective surgical closure may prove difficult, although the technique of occluding these fistulae with selective embolization through an arterial catheter has been developed and used with some success.

The common and external iliac veins drain the entire leg and many collateral veins are available through connections with the hypogastric and pelvic veins as well as through the lumbar branches of the vena cava. These collaterals can dilate in a few days after acute occlusion of the common or external iliac vein. Although injury to the larger vessels is more dangerous than injury to the hypogastric and pelvic veins, exposure and control of the larger vessels are facilitated because of their superficial location. Direct pressure should be maintained over the area of injury while the proximal and distal veins are dissected and clamped with an atraumatic clamp. Trendelenburg tilt and proximal common iliac artery occlusion may be used but are seldom necessary.

Injuries to the inferior vena cava are complicated by the location of the cava just to the right and behind the abdominal aorta (Fig. 62-2), making proximal and distal control difficult. When caval injuries occur, direct pressure over the vein using

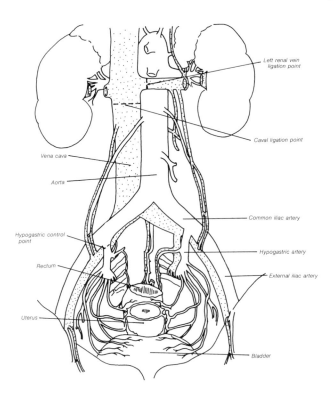

FIG. 62-2. Frontal view showing abdominal and pelvic vessels that may sustain injury during urologic procedures. Note that at the level of the renal arteries, the vena cava lies to the right of the aorta, but at the aortic bifurcation and beyond, the cava and iliac veins lie behind the arteries.

sponge sticks proximal and distal to the bleeding point will usually reduce bleeding enough to allow direct suture. If this is not successful, pressure over the bleeding point is maintained while the cava on either side is dissected and ligated. Reconstructive vein grafting of the cava is not necessary, but postoperative heparin may be required.

The lumbar veins entering the vena cava are easily injured. These thin-walled veins are short and friable, and if divided, the cut ends may retract into the vertebral interspaces. Direct suture control of both ends of the vein is necessary unless the area is packed until bleeding stops. Packing will control low-pressure venous bleeding when other measures fail, but direct control should be achieved as soon as possible to avoid hemorrhagic shock.

After hemorrhage is controlled, the vein can either be ligated or repaired. Ligation is indicated in the case of (1) an elderly patient in whom prolongation of the operation would be a considerable risk, (2) a patient with a poor long-term prognosis, and (3) extensive resection or injury of the vein, which would require a graft. Venous repair would be indicated (1) if the repair could be done rapidly, without significant additional loss of blood, (2) if a good chance exists for the repair remaining patent, and (3) in selected injuries as follows.

Venous repair is recommended if there is a longitudinal or transverse laceration or complete division of the vein and if the repair can be performed without constricting the vein, without creating tension, and without leaving ragged ends protruding into the lumen. If the existing deficit requires a graft to connect the two ends, ligation is recommended because grafts in the venous system have dismally short patency period. However, Dalton and Mulholland recommended saphenous replacement grafts when necessary.[3] Experience has shown that chronic edema will seldom develop after iliac occlusion if stasis thrombosis of the femoral and popliteal veins has been prevented by anticoagulation in the immediate postoperative period. The only exception to this rule is when extensive pelvic dissection has disrupted a number of important venous collateral branches.

After proximal and distal control has been obtained and inspection demonstrates a clean longitudinal, tangential, or transverse laceration (Fig. 62-3A), this laceration should be carefully sutured with 5-0 or 6-0 monofilament sutures, using a continuous over-and-over stitch, taking small bites no more than 1 to 2 mm deep and 1 mm apart (Fig. 62-4). An attempt should be made not to constrict the lumen with the repair, because stagnant flow in the area of the injury can cause thrombosis. If constriction does occur after laceration repair (Fig. 62-3B), the procedure should be repeated, using a patch of saphenous vein taken from the opposite leg.

A section of saphenous vein at the groin is removed, the vein is opened longitudinally, and valve tissue is excised. The vein patch is fashioned to fit one end of the tear (Fig. 62-3C), then sutured to that end with a double-armed monofilament suture. The midportions of the patch are sutured to the edges of the laceration, and the distal end of the patch is trimmed

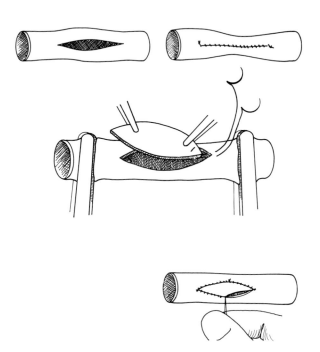

FIG. 62-3. A, Longitudinal laceration. Direct suture of a longitudinal venous laceration is preferred, unless this narrows the lumen of the vein (B). In that case, the lumen of the vein is enlarged by a vein patch constructed from a segment of long saphenous vein from the opposite leg (C and D).

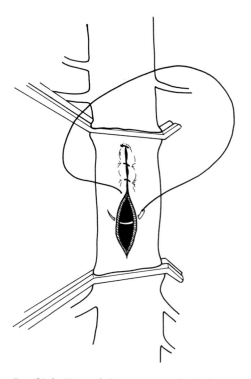

FIG. 62-4. View of the proper method of controlling an arterial or venous laceration, with vascular clamps and direct, continuous, over-and-over sutures.

and anchored at the distal end of the laceration. The patch anastomosis is completed using a continuous mattress stitch (Fig. 62-3D). The placement of stay sutures is particularly important in venous anastomosis (see Fig. 62-3D), because it avoids the traumatic use of tissue forceps on the edges of the cut vein, which promotes platelet deposition and thrombosis.

If constriction of the repair occurs after tangential or transverse laceration repair, the area of laceration should be excised, saving as much vein as possible (Fig. 62-5A). The 2 ends should be mobilized until they meet, if possible without tension, and are approximated using the technique shown in Figures 62-5B and 62-5C. If tension is unavoidable, the veins should be ligated. Attempts to spatulate the ends of the vein to obtain a greater circumference than the normal vein are not recommended, because this causes more tension on the repair.

If a vein graft is necessary because of disruption of pelvic collateral branches, the saphenous vein in the opposite leg is exposed, and several centimeters are dissected and excised after careful ligation of all branches. A segment much longer than the defect is removed to allow for vein contraction, and the proximal end is marked with a suture to indicate the direction of the valves. The saphenous vein is much smaller in caliber than the iliac vein. It is not used as a direct graft because of the risk of physiologic constriction (Fig. 62-6A). The vein is opened longitudinally with Pott's vascular scissors, and the two sections are sutured together snugly over a stent such as a Hegar dilator or a catheter of the approximate size of the iliac vein to be replaced (Fig. 62-6B). A good alternative at this point, especially if time is essential, is a patch of Gore-Tex, which is readily available in place of the saphenous vein patch.

The resulting paneled graft should not be significantly larger or smaller than the proximal or distal iliac because either condition can cause thrombosis. The graft is then sutured in place, using the same technique at both ends as described for the end-to-end repair (Fig. 62-6C). This repair is rarely used, however, because the rate of thrombosis seldom warrants the additional time required. This should only be attempted if near-total venous occlusion threatens a potential loss of the limb. Swan states that 50 to 60% of iliac grafts thrombose and thrombectomy is rarely successful in restoring patency.[4]

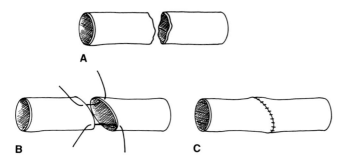

FIG. 62-5. If a ragged tear has transected a vein (A), its ends should be neatly trimmed and an end-to-end anastomosis performed (B and C).

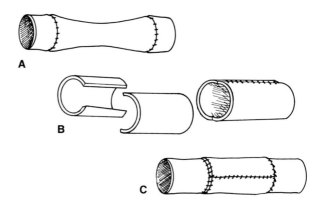

FIG. 62-6. If the ends of the divided vein cannot be approximated without tension, they are ligated. When venous collateral branches in the pelvis have been destroyed, a vein graft is recommended. A, Use of an intact saphenous vein as a graft is usually not satisfactory, since the reduction in caliber reduces venous flow and results in thrombosis. A composite tube graft made of two segments of saphenous vein is the graft of choice (B and C). It is important to remove all venous valves or to make certain that they point cephalad.

POSTOPERATIVE MANAGEMENT

Postoperative heparin administration can result in dangerous bleeding if a large bare area is left after extensive pelvic dissection. Experience has demonstrated that heparin only slightly improves the chances of a venous repair or graft remaining open. When lateral sutures are used, the repair has an excellent chance of remaining open without the use of heparin. If an end-to-end repair or a graft has been used, small doses of heparin, 5,000 units given subcutaneously every 8 hours, should be started 8 hours after completion of the operation if there is no evidence of oozing or bleeding. If there is evidence of bleeding, heparin can be promptly reversed with protamine.

If massive edema and cyanosis of the leg occur within days or weeks of the operation, heparin in full doses is required, starting with a constant intravenous drip of 800 to 1,000 units per hour, regulating the infusion rate to keep the partial thromboplastin time at one and one-half to two times the patient's normal value. This is continued for 10 days, followed by warfarin given orally for 3 to 6 months. Massive unilateral edema indicates occlusion of the repair or graft. Heparin is urgently indicated in this case to prevent proximal extension of the clot into the vena cava, with the accompanying possibility of pulmonary embolus, and to prevent distal propagation of the clot from stasis, which will interfere with collateral venous circulation from the femoral vein. After vena caval or iliac ligation, chronic edema occurs only in those who have secondary femoral and popliteal venous occlusion from distal propagation of the clot, which again can be prevented by the use of heparin.

Other postoperative measures, such as the use of supportive stockings or pressure bandages for several months postoperatively, raising the foot of the bed, early ambulation or avoiding sitting with the legs dangling, may be helpful in preventing venous stasis, but little data exist to support these measures. Currently, segmental limb compression with specially designed stockings are essential in all of these cases and should be started 12 hours preoperatively.

If heparin and warfarin have been effective in the prevention of femoral thrombosis postoperatively, and if the neoplastic process is under control but the patient still has significant edema 6 to 12 months after the operation, a saphenous vein cross-over graft from the opposite leg often can be used. This procedure, reported by Dale and Harris, transfers femoral venous flow across the pubis to the venous system of the opposite leg and up the unobstructed iliac veins on that side. It is effective in relieving edema from isolated iliac venous occlusion.[5]

ARTERIAL INJURIES

The two principle arterial complications that occur during urologic surgical procedures are iatrogenic laceration and neoplastic involvement. Arterial anatomy follows that of the venous structures previously elucidated but has the mild advantage of usually being located ventral to their venous counterparts. This may make control easier, but one must be aware of the possibility of venous injury associated with arterial control.

Arterial Laceration

Branches of the hypogastric arteries are those most likely to be lacerated during pelvic node dissection and can be controlled by clamping and ligation without the risk of ischemia. Traumatic laceration of the abdominal aorta or the common or external iliac artery must be repaired to avoid the potentially disastrous effects of irreversible ischemia of the legs. If there is massive arterial bleeding deep in the pelvis and accurate visualization of the cut vessel is impossible, the abdominal aorta is temporarily occluded just above the bifurcation or compressed against the vertebral bodies. This will reduce the arterial hemorrhage enough to allow visualization and control of the lacerated artery.

If hemorrhage from a lacerated artery is difficult to control, exposure is generally inadequate. While hemostasis is maintained by compression over the bleeding point, the injured artery is dissected for several centimeters proximal and distal to the point of injury. Arterial control can then be directly obtained using atraumatic clamps, which are closed only enough to prevent blood flow. This is especially important when clamping severely calcified arteries, as there is danger of dislodging a friable arterial plaque, resulting in embolization of local thrombosis.

If there is either a longitudinal or transverse tear, direct closure of the laceration with a 4-0 or 5-0 synthetic suture can be performed using a running over-and-over stitch (Fig. 62-4). If the laceration is tangential or if the edges are irregular, the artery can be completely divided, the ragged edges trimmed, and an end-to-end anastomosis performed. A gap of 1 cm can be closed by gently pulling the edges together with the vascular clamps. After flow is restored, there should be a strong pulse and no palpable thrill. If the pulse is weak or a notable thrill is present, the anastomosis should be redone or an arterial graft should be used. An iliac laceration, unless extensive, will seldom require a graft.

Extensive hemorrhage can result from a tie or clamp slipping off the renal artery during nephrectomy, which is a possibility especially in a transplant-donor nephrectomy in which a long section of renal artery is removed. If the left kidney is being removed through a flank or abdominal incision, emergency compression is placed on the bleeding pedicle area, while the aorta is quickly exposed and clamped at the diaphragm. The stump of the renal artery then can be identified and clamped. If the right kidney is being removed through the flank, proximal control of the aorta at the diaphragm is blocked by the liver. Thus, when removing the right kidney with as much as artery as possible, the vena cava is dissected away from the aorta, which is carefully exposed and controlled proximally and distally before the renal artery itself is clamped. As in all surgical procedures, adequate exposure of the bleeding vessels is the vital component of hemorrhage control.

Arterial Involvement in Tumor

Extensive pelvic lymph node metastasis or direct tumor extension occasionally may require the resection of a segment of external or common iliac artery or aorta. The tumor is resected as widely as necessary, including the involved iliac arteries, followed by graft replacement. A knitted Dacron graft that approximates the size of the artery to be replaced (10 mm inside diameter for the common iliac and 8 mm inside diameter for the external iliac) is selected and preclotted by being dipped in the patient's blood drawn from a convenient vein or artery, allowing the blood to clot around the graft. Blood is carefully aspirated from the lumen of the graft immediately before use.

The more difficult anastomosis is performed first with a continuous 4-0 monofilament suture, while the other end of the graft is left unattached. Before performing the second anastomosis, the graft should be gently stretched until all crimps are flattened in order to cut the graft to the proper length. When the graft is pressurized with arterial flow, these crimps essentially will be eliminated.

The second anastomosis is begun on its back side, working around toward the front, again performing the more difficult part first. Before completing the front of the anastomosis, each clamp should be temporarily released, allowing flushing of any fresh thrombi or other debris that could cause distal embolization down the leg. The anastomosis is then completed and flow is restored by releasing the distal clamp first, followed by the proximal clamp.

Additional anastomotic sutures may be necessary for gaps at the suture lines or for bleeding through the graft. In both situations, the artery is reclamped for approximately 1 minute to allow clotting of the graft wall to occur or for small spurts to stop at the anastomosis. An intraluminal clot may occur if the graft is clamped for longer than 1 minute. Again, a strong distal pulse without a palpable thrill should be present over the distal artery for indication of adequate restoration of blood flow.

Prosthetic arterial grafts are not used in an operative field that is actually or potentially infected, because disruption of the suture line with massive fatal hemorrhage may result. If tumor involves the artery that must be removed in an infected field, the arterial ends are carefully sutured closed. Blood flow can then be restored to the involved extremity by an extra-anatomic pathway such as transpubic femoral-femoral graft in a clean field, but this type of reconstructive procedure is more complicated.

POSTOPERATIVE THROMBOPHLEBITIS AND PULMONARY EMBOLISM

A century ago, the main causes of surgical mortality were infection, hemorrhage, and pulmonary embolism. The first two have been largely controlled, but the third remains a challenge, with little change in incidence. It has been recognized for some time that venous thrombi begin on the operating table and that prophylactic measures initiated in the recovery room are already too late. Advanced age, venous trauma from retractors used in pelvic operations, and the acute hip and knee flexion while in stirrups for certain procedures all contribute the development of thrombophlebitis. General and spinal anesthesia also may be factors, eliminating the venous pump mechanism in the leg veins by paralyzing leg muscles for several hours.

Three methods are currently being used to reduce intraoperative venous thrombosis: elastic stockings, low-dose heparin, and pneumatic leg pumps. Stockings theoretically work to reduce thrombosis by compressing superficial veins, thus increasing flow through deep veins; but they have never been shown statistically to decrease the incidence of thrombophlebitis. Low-dose heparin in a number of studies has reduced the incidence of both phlebitis and emboli, but often at the cost of increasing intraoperative or postoperative bleeding.[6] Intermittent calf compression with pneumatic boots also seems to be effective in decreasing thrombophlebitis complications without any ill effects (Fig. 62-7) and may be used increasingly in the next decade, especially in urologic patients.[7]

Currently, intermittent pneumatic leg compression with or without low-dose heparin is the prophylactic therapy of choice in higher risk patients and should be started prior to the operation because of the potential of increased fibrinolytic activity.[8,9]

If a patient is of extremely high risk, one may consider intraoperative caval interruption. Prophylactic caval interruption has not proven beneficial when broadly applied to groups of patients categorized as being at increased risk of embolism, but may occasionally be warranted in selected high-risk individuals undergoing abdominal surgery. In this group, operative application of the Moretz clip is the preferred method of prophylaxis.

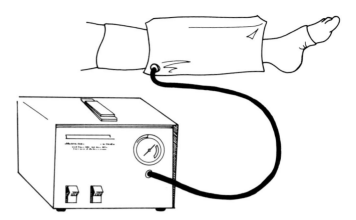

FIG. 62-7. Pneumatic leg pump is used during surgery and postoperatively to massage the calf veins to prevent stasis, which may lead to thrombophlebitis.

Patients who develop signs and symptoms of thrombophlebitis postoperatively should have the diagnosis confirmed by a noninvasive technique such as the impedance plethysmograph or the Cranley phleborrheograph or by venogram if these are not available.[10,11] If the diagnosis is positive, intravenous heparin should be given for 7 to 10 days, followed by several months of oral warfarin therapy. Plication or ligation of the inferior vena cava may be indicated under the following circumstances: development of a pulmonary embolus in a patient while on adequate anticoagulant therapy, development of a pulmonary embolus in a patient who cannot be given anticoagulants (usually because of the high risk of bleeding), development of recurrent pulmonary emboli months apart, patients who have complications (GI bleeding, hemarthrosis, etc.) on anticoagulants and patients who cannot or will not follow a proper anticoagulation regimen.

The history of surgical attempts to bar the passage of emboli to the lungs began with femoral vein ligation but changed to caval ligation with the realization that two-thirds of pulmonary emboli originated proximal to the femoral vein. Dissatisfaction with stasis sequelae after caval ligation then spawned a wide variety of partial interruption procedures; and, in turn, a desire to reduce the mortality associated with these procedures has stimulated the development of ingenious caval interruption devices that can be introduced via remote cutdown sites under local anesthesia. Initial devices include the Mobin-Uddin umbrella[12] but this has lost favor to the Greenfield filter. This filter can now be placed percutaneously via the femoral or jugular route with low morbidity and mortality reported in large series.[13]

The role of surgical procedures for iliofemoral thrombectomy or pulmonary thromboembolectomy is a limited one. Phlegmasia cerulea dolens is the main reason for iliofemoral thrombectomy. Despite the high incidence of late rethrombosis, thrombectomy here significantly reduces acute morbidity and the risk of venous gangrene.[14]

The practical clinical role of pulmonary embolectomy has proven to be a very limited one, not because the operation is not effective, but because so few patients who would die without it can be diagnosed with certainty, then brought to the operating theater and placed on a cardiopulmonary bypass in time. Most of those who recover hemodynamically deserve a caval interruption procedure rather than embolectomy. Although two large experiences have documented that the majority of patients with massive pulmonary embolism can be salvaged by an *ever-ready* team response, few hospitals have adopted this approach. Until they do, experience with pulmonary embolectomy will continue to be primarily anecdotal, as it has in the past.

As an alternative, catheter embolectomy may be performed with good results reported in experienced hands.[15]

REFERENCES

1. CARREL, A., and GUTHRIE, C. C. Uniterminal and biterminal venous transplantations. Surg. Gynecol. Obstet., 2:266, 1906.

2. BARTLE, E. J. Venous anomalies complicating AAA repair, recognition and management. In: *Seminars in Vascular Surgery.* Edited by R. Rutherford. Philadelphia, W. B. Saunders, Co., 1988, p. 145.

3. DALTON, J. R., and MULHOLLAND, S. G. Venous injury in major urological surgery. J. Urol., 22:508, 1979.

4. SWAN, K. G. *Venous Surgery in the Lower Extremity.* St. Louis, Green, 1974, p. 134.

5. DALE, W. A., and HARRIS, J. Cross-over vein grafts for iliac and femoral venous occlusions. Ann. Surg., 168:319, 1968.

6. HIRSH, J. Venous thromboembolism, diagnosis and treatment and prevention. Hosp. Pract., 10:53, 1975.

7. COE, N. P. et al. Prevention of deep vein thrombosis in urological patients: A controlled randomized trial of low-dose heparin and external pneumatic compression boots. Surgery, 83:230, 1978.

8. IMADA, K. et al. Effects of intermittent pneumatic leg compression for prevention of postoperative deep venous thrombosis with special reference to fibrinolytic activity. Am. J. Surg., 115:602, 1988.

9. SCHWARTZ, S. I. Prevention of deep venous thrombosis. Curr. Surg., 32:105, 1988.

10. WHEELER, H. B., et al. Impedence phlebography—technique, interpretation and results. Arch. Surg., 104:165, 1972.

11. CRANLEY, J. J., et al. Phleborrheographic technique for diagnosis of deep venous thrombosis of the lower extremities. Surg. Gynecol. Obstet., 141:331, 1975.

12. MOBIN-UDDIN, K., UTLEY, J. R., and BRYANT, L. R. The inferior vena cava umbrella filter. Prog. Cardiovasc. Dis., 17:391, 1975.

13. GREENFIELD, L. S., and ALEXANDER, L. Current status of surgical therapy for deep venous thromboses. Am. J. Surg., 150:64, 1985.

14. LANSING, A. M., and DAVIS, W. M. Five year follow-up study of iliofemoral venous thrombectomy. Ann. Surg., 168:620, 1968.

15. GREENFIELD, L. J., STEWART, J., and GRUTE, S. Results of surgical management of pulmonary thromboembolism. J. Clin. Surg., 1:194, 1982.

MEDICAL AND PSYCHIATRIC ASPECTS OF THE CANCER PATIENT

63

Presurgical Medical Evaluation

Richard M. Smith

Donald C. Fischer

John W. Vester

The first question that must always be asked in regard to a surgical procedure advocated for a patient is still: "If the surgical procedure is performed and the results are good, will the patient's health status enable him to enjoy life and be productive for a significant time in the future?" Simply put, this query is a request for a definition of the risk to benefit ratio. Once the hoped for benefit is defined, the role of the consulting internist in a presurgical evaluation is that of defining the risk. The purpose of this discourse is that of presenting methodologic and analytical approaches for the medical consultant who is called on to define that risk. Risk, of course, means the likelihood that the patient will die or suffer permanent disability as a result of the stress imposed by the operative procedure itself.

The key word here is still "stress." If the patient has sufficient physiologic reserves to adapt to the stress imposed by the operative procedure and all that it entails, he should survive the procedure without disability. Preoperative medical evaluation of the surgical patient thus involves identification of those indicators of diminished physiologic reserve that sig-

nify an increased risk of death or permanent disability as a direct consequence of the surgical procedure. The medical history, the physical examination and the routine laboratory work are, not surprisingly, the basis of such an analysis. An orderly, system by system, approach is the most efficient plan to follow.

Current regulations concerning health-care delivery now require that this evaluation be performed, wherever possible, on an out-patient basis prior to hospitalization for the procedure. Constraints imposed by concerns about the cost of health care now require that investigative procedures be precisely tailored to fit the needs of the individual patient as determined by the medical history and physical examination.

CARDIOVASCULAR SYSTEM

As indicated in the introduction, the routine history and physical examination are the cornerstone of evaluation. This history must inquire about previous diagnosis of cardiovascular disease and symptoms such as chest pain, especially exertional, that induced by emotional distress, and pain that wakes a patient from sleep. Shortness of breath, fatigue, palpitations, orthopnea, history of dependent edema, and paroxysmal nocturnal dyspnea are important indicators of pump inadequacy. Exercise tolerance (which can be defined as the ability to climb two flights of stairs without stopping because of shortness of breath) is an excellent indicator of a patient's ability of withstand the stress of a major operative procedure. In addition, diabetes, hypertension, and cigarette smoking are known risk factors. If a patient has none of the above complaints but gives a history of calf pain on walking (intermittent claudication), consideration should be given to further evaluation of the adequacy of myocardial blood supply.

On physical examination, one should concentrate on evidences of congestive heart failure. Jugular venous distention, inspiratory rales that do not clear on coughing, an enlarged liver, and peripheral edema are, of course, the cardinal signs to be sought. Evaluation of the peripheral pulses and listening for bruits may provide clues to peripheral vascular disease. When present, these findings should be followed up and the cause determined.

In the absence of any evidence of cardiovascular disease on the history and physical examination, routine preoperative laboratory evaluation is limited. Over the age of 40, an electrocardiogram should be performed. Under age 40, no routine laboratory investigation of cardiovascular status is necessary.

Any indication of the possible presence of coronary artery disease must be fully evaluated prior to the operative procedure. If a patient has sustained a myocardial infarction, there is a higher incidence of reinfarction during general anesthesia in the first 6 months after the infarction. This risk is higher in the first 3 months, is less over the next 3 months, then levels off at 6 months to a rate of 2 to 5%. Evidence is now accruing suggesting that a subset of patients with recent myocardial infarction can be operated safely more quickly after the myocardial infarction. These are patients who have had an uncomplicated clinical course after myocardial infarction, have no evidence of left ventricular dysfunction and have had a normal postmyocardial infarction low-level stress test. Weitz and Goodman believe that patients can be operated 4 to 6 weeks after myocardial infarction if surgery is important.[1]

For patients with angina pectoris, the situation is not quite as straightforward. Clearly, patients with unstable symptoms need immediate cardiologic evaluation. Patients with New York Heart Association (NYHA) class I (Table 63-1) symptoms can be operated on safely without further study or intervention. Patients with class III or IV angina, that is, marked limitation of normal activity or symptoms at rest, need further cardiac evaluation prior to surgery and may need myocardial revascularization or coronary angioplasty prior to surgery as part of preoperative management. Patients with class II angina pectoris, mild limitation of ordinary activity, have been controversial. Some would proceed with surgery if symptoms have been stable.[2] Others would prefer further investigation up to and including coronary arteriography prior to a major procedure.

TABLE 63-1. *New York Heart Association's Classification of Angina*

I. *Ordinary physical activity does not cause angina,* such as walking or climbing stairs; angina with strenuous or rapid prolonged exertion at work or recreation or with sexual relations
II. *Slight limitation of ordinary activity;* walking or climbing stairs rapidly, walking uphill, walking or stair climbing after meals, or in cold, or in wind, or under emotional stress, or only during a few hours after awakening; walking more than 2 blocks on the level or more than 1 flight of stairs at a normal pace and in normal conditions
III. *Marked limitation of ordinary physical activity;* walking 1 or 2 blocks on the level and climbing 1 flight of stairs in normal conditions and at a normal pace; "comfortable at rest."
IV. *Inability to carry on any physical activity without discomfort—anginal syndrome may be present at rest*

From Roizen, Michael F. Anesthetic implications of concurrent diseases. In: *Anesthesia.* Vol. I. Edited by Ronald D. Miller. New York: Churchill Livingstone. 1986, p. 287.

Congestive heart failure is a major risk factor for perioperative morbidity and mortality during major noncardiac surgery. Specifically, the presence of jugular vein distention, rales in the chest, or a ventricular gallop (S_3) should be looked for. In these patients, evaluation of LV function by means of echocardiography and/or radionuclide imaging should be performed to elucidate the etiology of the congestive heart failure. Systolic or diastolic dysfunction is an important determinant of the etiology of congestive heart failure. Clearly, the risk of postoperative pulmonary edema increases with the severity of preoperative symptoms. Although no controlled studies have been reported, it is reasonable to conclude from clinical experience that preoperative control of congestive heart failure substantively reduces postoperative morbidity. However, one should be cautioned about overdiuresis as vasodilation during anesthesia induction can lead to hypotension and complication from the abrupt pressure decrease. When the clinical picture is unclear or tenuous, preoperative insertion of a Swan-Ganz catheter to guide optimal hemodyamic management may be wise.

For patients suspected of valvular heart disease, echocardiograms with the doppler technique may be necessary to evaluate valvular function fully. Up to 20% of patients with valvular heart disease, especially those with aortic stenosis, will have new or worsening congestive heart failure after major noncardiac surgery. Again, Swan-Ganz catheter monitoring may be helpful here. Patients with hypertension should be evaluated for evidence of end-organ damage, especially to the central nervous system, blood vessels, and kidneys. While perfect control is not necessary prior to surgery, it is probably prudent to maintain diastolic blood pressures at less than 110 mm Hg prior to surgery. Arrhythmias should also be controlled prior to surgery. The impact of the arrhythmia relates to the underlying cardiac disease rather than the effect of the arrhythmia itself.

Asymptomatic vascular disease found at physical examination, such as decreased peripheral pulses, carotid or femoral bruits should be evaluated. Studies of asymptomatic carotid disease have shown a high perioperative morbidity and mortality from coronary artery disease.[3] The existence of asymptomatic carotid bruits did not predict the site of stroke or greatly influence the incidence of perioperative stroke. Therefore, unless the carotid artery disease is symptomatic, i.e., with transient neurological deficits, one may proceed with the planned surgery.

Cardiac prognosis in noncardiac surgery is related to all the above considerations. Gerson et al. studied prognosis in geriatric patients undergoing major noncardiac surgery.[4] They concluded that inability to perform 2 minutes of exercise with an appropriate increase in heart rate was the single best predictor of perioperative complications. Although their study only included geriatric patients, the conclusion is reasonable and practical, as exercise requires a fully functional individual. Those who are marginal or cannot complete this exercise certainly need further careful investigation and treatment prior to major noncardiac surgery.

RESPIRATORY SYSTEM

The respiratory system is highly susceptible to the development of such complications as atelectasis, pneumonia, and respiratory insufficiency in the perioperative period. The goal of presurgical medical evaluation of the respiratory system is identification of risk factors that lead to complications, as well as development of a plan to minimize the perioperative morbidity. The history and physical examination identify high-risk patients who need further evaluation.

Historically, one should look for dyspnea on exertion, cough, sputum productivity, a history of smoking, and chronic lung disease. Physical examination may reveal stigmata of chronic lung disease, such as clubbing, cyanosis, hyperinflation, crackles, wheezes, or prolongation of the expiratory phase. Identification of any of these factors should prompt complete pulmonary evaluation including chest x ray, pulmonary function tests, and arterial blood gases. All patients over 70 years of age, even without any evidence of chronic lung disease, should have a forced vital capacity curve. Further pulmonary evaluation here depends on the outcome of that study. Several studies have confirmed the identification of high-risk patients by pulmonary function testing alone.[5] Those at high risk should be entered into a preoperative program designed to promote cough and secretion clearance and discontinuance of cigarette smoking for at least 2 weeks prior to surgery. Antibiotics and bronchodilators can be administered if indicated. Often this can be accomplished as an out-patient through a pulmonary rehabilitation program designed to work closely with physicians. Preoperative teaching of proper cough techniques and the importance of lung expansion after surgery is extremely helpful in preventing postoperative complications.

It is clear that significant pulmonary disease carries an increased risk of postoperative complications, primarily atelectasis, pneumonia, and respiratory failure. However, no study has found an absolute level of lung function below which surgery is contraindicated. The urgency and importance of the surgery must be weighed against the possible risks. Patients with severe lung dysfunction should be considered for postoperative mechanical ventilation for 24 to 48 hours after surgery, until pulmonary mechanics begin to improve. An elevated P_{CO_2}, greater than 45 mm Hg, also identifies a high-risk group of patients who should be carefully followed and considered for postoperative ventilation. There is no difference in pulmonary risk of surgery between spinal versus general anesthesia. Prolonged anesthesia for longer than 3 hours is associated with an increased incidence of postoperative complications.[6]

KIDNEY AND ELECTROLYTE

The urologic surgeon is appropriately concerned about the risk of perioperative deterioration of renal function. Urological surgery patients have a relatively high incidence of compromised renal function, for whatever cause. Preservation of renal function is paramount, as most reports indicate a mortality rate of 50 to 60% when acute renal failure develops in the perioperative period.[7]

The most important factor in estimating the surgical risk of perioperative deterioration of renal function is the degree of pre-existing reduction in glomerular filtration rate (GFR). As the GFR declines, the risk of worsening renal function in the postoperative period increases. Even mild renal insufficiency (a reduced GFR that is still greater than 50 mL/min) is associated with a notable increase in risk. It follows that the patient with advanced renal failure (GFR lower than 10 mL/min) poses the greatest challenge to the surgeon and the internist. Although the blood urea nitrogen is routinely measured, it is not the best index of renal function, as the test lacks both sensitivity and specificity. The serum creatinine concentration is a more useful index of renal function but this value depends somewhat on the muscle mass of the patient. A serum creatinine concentration of 1.5 mg/dL may occur with a normal GFR in a young muscular male but would reflect a significant reduction of GFR in an elderly and malnourished patient. Generally, though, a serum creatinine level of 0.6 to 1.0 mg/dL in females and 0.8 to 1.3 mg/dL in males indicates an adequate degree of GFR reserve.

A more sensitive and specific estimate of GFR can be determined with measurement of the creatinine clearance. This, however, requires a timed urine collection. Nonetheless, if there is a history of frequency, nocturia, dysuria, or abnormal results in the routine urinalysis, measurement of creatinine clearance is indicated for estimation of surgical risk. Patients with nephrotic syndrome may already have a decreased circulating blood volume as a consequence of decreased colloid oncotic pressure and are more prone to hypotension and hypovolemic assaults on renal function.

The common practice of prohibiting oral intake the night before a major surgical procedure can contribute significantly to dehydration and diminished circulating blood volume. Any suggestion that there is already diminished circulating blood volume, such as the presence of nephrotic syndrome or the detection of an orthostatic drop in blood pressure on physical examination, should indicate consideration of intravenous fluid maintenance of normal blood volume during the time of restriction of oral fluid intake. Patients who are being treated with potent diuretics such as furosemide are also potentially at risk because of a pre-existing decrease in circulating blood volume. Patients with chronic renal insufficiency may have impaired concentrating mechanisms and therefore vascular volume may be poorly controlled. In these situations, strict attention should be paid to management of the circulating intravascular volume. When the situation is unclear, hemodynamic monitoring including possibly, the use of pulmonary artery catheterization should be employed.

Hyponatremia occurs in patients with salt-wasting renal disease states and/or diuretic therapy and its presence should be noted. The patient with preoperative impairment of renal function is at risk from potassium balance disturbance as well. In the surgical patient, rhabdomyolysis, tissue trauma, and hemolysis may result in an increased endogenous release of potassium. Exogenous sources include intravenous or oral potassium supplements, potassium penicillin, salt substitutes, red blood cell transfusion, and total parenteral nutrition.

If renal failure is present to the degree that the GFR is below 10 mL/min, potassium loads can produce serious hyperkalemia. The small group of patients with hyporeninemic hypoaldosteronism also has a risk of hyperkalemia as a consequence of potassium loads. Pre-existing hypokalemia can also be present and its most common cause is diuretic therapy. Vomiting and nasogastric suction are commonly associated with hypokalemia owing to increased renal excretion of potassium as a consequence of the induced metabolic alkalosis; therefore, both hyperkalemia and hypokalemia must be watched for and judiciously managed.

ENDOCRINE SYSTEM

A systematic review of indicators of abnormalities in all the endocrine glands is required. The indicators that should raise suspicion in this area are the presence of tachycardia, atrial fibrillation, or unexplained cardiac arrhythmias. If masked thyrotoxicosis is suspected (a finding more common in older patients), measurements of T_4, T_3 resin uptake, and free T_4 are generally sufficient as the next line of evaluation. Diagnosis of the presence of hyperthyroidism requires preoperative endocrine consultation and management.

Hypothyroidism is generally easier to identify clinically. If laboratory data confirm its presence, it should be treated preoperatively. Operations in patients with untreated hypothyroidism have been reported to result in hypotension on induction of anesthesia, increased sensitivity to sedatives and anesthetic agents, cardiac arrest, and myxedema coma.

Any suggestion from the medical history, physical examination, or laboratory data of the presence of diminished adrenal cortical function requires measurement of morning and evening serum cortisol levels for further evaluation. The patient who is deficient in adrenal cortical steroid function must be given corrective therapy once the diagnosis is made. Patients with a history of steroid therapy have a greater risk of hypoadrenocortical crisis as a consequence of the surgical procedure because of suppression of the pituitary-adrenal axis. These patients should likewise receive adrenocortical steroid supplementation.

Patients with diabetes mellitus require careful evaluation prior to surgery. One should achieve stable preoperative fasting blood sugars of 250 mg/dL or less, whether by diet, oral agents, or insulin. Higher levels result in a higher risk of infection and/or predispose patients to poor wound healing. Diabetics who are found to have metabolic acidosis should have their surgery postponed and the acute medical problem addressed prior to rescheduling.

In patients who are taking insulin, it is not clear as to whether tight control (i.e., blood sugars between 80 and 200) in the immediate postoperative period improves wound healing or decreases the incidence of infection. It is necessary, however, to follow blood sugars closely in the postoperative period until a stable status is attained.

LIVER

Any patient with pre-existing disease will worsen as a consequence of a major surgical procedure. A history of alcoholism, hepatitis, or jaundice is critical and physical examination for jaundice, hepatomegaly, ascites, and cutaneous indicators of liver disease is essential. Elective surgery in patients with acute hepatitis, either viral or alcoholic, should be postponed. In patients with cirrhosis, the perioperative morbidity and mortality increases with increasing severity of hepatic insufficiency. Preoperatively, one should determine the severity of hepatic disease, which is best done by Child's classification (Table 63-2). Liver disease patients who would be class A by Child's classification have a total serum bilirubin less than

TABLE 63-2. *Child's or Pugh's Class and Operability*

CLASS	OPERABILITY
A	No limitations
	Normal response to all operations
	Normal ability of liver to regenerate
B	Some limitations to liver function
	Altered response to all operations, but good tolerance with preoperative preparation
	Limited ability of the liver to regenerate new hepatic parenchyma; therefore, all sizable liver resections are contraindicated
C	Severe limitations to liver function
	Poor response to all operations regardless of preparatory efforts
	Liver resection regardless of the size is contraindicated

From Friedman, L., and Maddrey, W. Med. Clin. North Am., 71:3, 1987.

2.0 mg/dL, plasma albumin greater than 3.5 gm/dL, no ascites or encephalopathy, and in excellent nutritional status.[8] Class-B patients have a total bilirubin greater than 2.0 mg/dL but less than 3.0, a plasma albumin greater than 3.0 gm/dL but less than 3.5 gm/dL, ascites that is easily controllable, encephalopathy that is no more than mild, and good nutritional status. Liver disease patients in Child's class C have a total bilirubin greater than 3.0 mg/dL, plasma albumin less than 3.0 gm/dL, ascites that is difficult to control, significant encephalopathy, and poor nutritional status. For patients with Child's classes A, B, and C, mortality rates with abdominal surgery were 10, 31, and 76%, respectively. In addition, a full coagulation profile should be obtained. Patients with a prothrombin time prolonged more than 3 seconds have a greater risk of postoperative complications attributable to hepatic dysfunction. Complications of cirrhosis, such as encephalopathy and ascites, should be fully evaluated and treated prior to surgery.

HEMOSTATIC CONSIDERATIONS

Impairment of the ability of the blood to coagulate is a major hazard to the surgical patient. Here again, a routine history and physical comprise the initial approach. A history of excessive bleeding from any previous surgical or dental procedure indicates the need for further evaluation. Unexplained hematuria, excessive bruising, or epistaxis have a similar significance. If the history and physical examination do not indicate the presence of a bleeding disorder, a blood smear estimate of platelet numbers, prothrombin time, and an activated partial thromboplastin time are the only tests required for further evaluation. If an abnormality is detected in any of these parameters, the services of a specialist in coagulation disorders would be required.

NUTRITIONAL STATUS

Obesity is the most common nutritional disorder in the United States. Obese patients have greater risks of pulmonary complications, postoperative thrombophlebitis, and pulmonary embolism. If the surgical procedure is not an emergent one, the available data strongly suggest that an improvement in surgical morbidity and mortality can be expected with a return to normal or near-normal weight. Malnutrition also adds to the risk of a major surgical procedure. Because of impairment of immune status in the nitrogen-deprived patient, the risk of sepsis is increased and wound healing is impaired.

A history of weight status, appetite, and food intake and physical examination for evidence of recent or chronic weight loss are the basic data required for assessment of nutritional status. Laboratory indicators include levels of plasma albumin and plasma transferrin. The lower limit of normal for albumin is approximately 3.5 g/dL; levels lower than that strongly suggest protein malnutrition if protein loss is excluded. Another indicator is the serum transferrin level. A value of less than 150 mg/dL indicates moderate protein depletion. Values of less than 100 mg/dL are seen only in states of severe protein depletion. In patients who are significantly malnourished and whose surgery can be delayed, 10 days of nutritional repletion with enteral or parenteral nutrition may be indicated to decrease the risk of postoperative infection and improve wound healing.

GENERAL CONSIDERATIONS

Anemia and polycythemia are identified by routine laboratory data and require appropriate management. Patients undergoing urologic surgical procedures have a distinctly greater risk of deep venous thrombosis and consequential pulmonary embolism.[9] Preoperative and daily postoperative phleborrheograms can be used in identifying this risk until the patient is fully mobile. Management of such hazards requires the judicious evaluation of the relative dangers of thrombophlebitis versus induced bleeding disorders.

Routine laboratory evaluation of the asymptomatic patient remains controversial. Many sets of recommendations may be found in the literature and likely will undergo revision in the future. As a general guideline, the history and physical examination are adequate for patients under the age of 35. Between the ages of 35 and 60, one should obtain an electrocardiogram, complete blood count, blood sugar, and creatinine. Above the age of 60, one should add a chest x ray as well as a complete chemical profile. As stated earlier, all patients 70 years of age or older should also have a routine forced vital capacity curve.

Geriatric patients present a unique and increasing problem in preoperative evaluation. In general, the risk is related to underlying disease states. Physiologic age/reserve may not correlate with chronological age. One should not preclude surgery merely on the basis of age. A careful estimation of risk versus benefit, including estimations of expected life span is needed. If a person has reached age 70, an average expected life span is greater than 80 years. Unfortunately, evaluation of physiologic reserve is difficult. Clinical research is sorely needed in this area.

REFERENCES

1. WEITZ, H. H., and GOLDMAN, L. Noncardiac surgery in the patient with heart disease. Med. Clin. North Am., 71:413, 1987.
2. GOLDMAN, L. Cardiac risks and complications of noncardiac surgery. Ann. Intern. Med., 98:504, 1983.
3. ROIZEN, MICHAEL F. Anesthetic implications of concurrent diseases. In: Anesthesia. Vol. I. Edited by Ronald D. Miller. New York: Churchill Livingstone. 1986, p. 287.

4. GERSON, M. C. et al. Cardiac prognosis in noncardiac geriatric surgery. Ann. Intern. Med., *103:*832, 1985.

5. JACKSON, C. V. Preoperative pulmonary evaluation. Arch. Intern. Med., *148:*2120, 1988.

6. REHDER, K., JESSLER, A., and MARSH, H. M. General anesthesia and the lung. Am. Rev. Respir. Dis., *112:*541, 1975.

7. BURKE, J. F., and FRANCOS, G. C. Surgery in the patient with acute or chronic renal failure. Med. Clin. North Am., *71:*489, 1987.

8. FREIDMAN, L. S., and MADDREY, W. C. Surgery in the patient with liver disease. Med. Clin. North Am., *71:*453, 1987.

9. CRAWFORD, E. D. et al. Deep venous thrombosis following transurethral resection of the prostate: A new method of diagnosis. J. Urol., *120:*438, 1978.

Pre- and Postoperative Nutritional and Metabolic Care of Genitourinary Cancer Patients

Robert C. Flanigan

It is essential for the urologist to understand the basic physiology of nutrition and the metabolic abnormalities that are common to urologic cancer patients. In this chapter, both of these areas are reviewed individually, with special attention paid to the most common clinical problems seen in these patients.

NUTRITION

Malnutrition is a frequent secondary diagnosis in hospitalized adult cancer patients.[1,2] Malnutrition occurs in 40 to 50% of patients with advanced pelvic malignancies, including bladder cancer.[3] This is partly because anorexia is a common symptom of patients with malignancy and a major determinant of cancer cachexia.[4] Although the spectrum of symptoms of cachexia (anorexia, early satiety, weight loss, anemia, and asthenia) are typically associated with advanced cancers, lesser degrees of malnutrition are not uncommon in less-advanced cancer patients.

Malnutrition is basically an imbalance between the intake and expenditure of nutrients. This imbalance may be second- ary to inadequate dietary intake, impaired digestion, external nutrient loss, tumor host competition for nutrients, and increased energy expenditures of the host. In urothelial cancers, the additional problem of impaired renal function caused by urinary obstruction or direct involvement of the kidneys by the neoplasm adds to the difficulty in caring for these complicated patients.

METABOLIC CHANGES

Basal metabolic rates in patients with metastatic cancer have been consistently reported to be elevated.[5] In fact, in contradistinction to the situation with healthy subjects, cancer patients have an increased basal metabolism even in the face of decreased alimentation.[6,7]

Changes Specific to Cancer Patients

CARBOHYDRATE METABOLISM. A decreased sensitivity to insulin has been documented in a significant number of cancer patients who may also display a diabetic glucose tolerance curve.[8,9] Furthermore, cancer patients with a progressive weight loss caused by metastatic cancer often manifest an increase in Cori cycle activity associated with an increased glucose turnover, glucose oxidation, and total caloric expenditure.[10] This leads to a depletion of liver glycogen and a blunted glycogen response to glucagon.[5]

LIPID METABOLISM. The endpoint of cancer cachexia with regard to lipid metabolism is a progressive depletion of body fat.[7] This loss of body lipid, caused by mobilization of free fatty acids from adipose tissue, occurs in the cancer patient at a time of elevated caloric expenditures, resulting in an unbalanced caloric deficit.[11]

PROTEIN METABOLISM. Cachexia and negative nitrogen balance have been shown to result in a loss of skeletal muscle mass in patients with cancer.[11] This muscle loss may continue despite adequate nitrogen intake. Hypoalbuminemia, which is a prominent feature of cachexia in cancer patients, results from a decreased rate of albumin synthesis and an increased fractional catabolic rate.[12] Throughout the time of cancer growth and treatment, protein catabolism typically accounts for a relatively high percentage of total energy expenditures (15 to 20%) compared to the 5% or less that is seen in starvation-adapted individuals.

NUTRITIONAL ASSESSMENT

Nutritional status is critical for the cancer patient's ability to withstand therapy, including surgery, radiation therapy, or chemotherapy. Often, nutritional status is directly related to the mortality rate of the cancer patient. Harvey and colleagues demonstrated that the mortality rate of patients who were initially anergic but later became immunocompetent with nutritional therapy was 11%, as compared to 100% in patients who remained anergic.[14]

In determining nutritional status, three general areas of nutritional assessment have been evaluated. These include, anthropometric parameters, immune competence, and visceral protein status. Anthropometric parameters, including triceps skinfold, arm-muscle circumference, creatinine-height index, and weight-to-height ratio, are measurements of fat stores and muscle mass. Immune competence can be estimated by measurements of cell-mediated immunity, including total lymphocyte count, delayed hypersensitivity, skin-antigen testing with recall antigens (Candida ablicans, mumps, purified protein derivative, and Trichophyton). Visceral protein status may be determined by measurements of serum albumin, transferrin, and retinal binding protein (Table 64-1).

Nutritional assessment based on the above-mentioned factors typically demonstrates that approximately 20% of hospitalized patients are moderately malnourished and 5% are severely malnourished. In advanced urothelial cancers, 40 to 50% of the patients are severely malnourished. A recent study of 500 patients admitted to a New Jersey hospital indicated that:[15]

1. 7.6% had an abnormal serum protein (less than 3.5 g/dl).
2. 30.2% had an abnormal total lymphocyte count (less than 1,500 mm²).
3. 34% had either an abnormal albumin level or an abnormal lymphocyte count.
4. An abnormal albumin level was associated with a four-fold increase in complications and a sixfold increase in deaths.
5. When both serum albumin and total lymphocyte count were abnormal, an almost fourfold increase in complications and twentyfold increase in deaths were noted.

TABLE 64-1. *Indices of Malnutrition*

TEST	MILD	MODERATE	SEVERE
Weight loss/last 3 months	10 lbs	10–20 lbs	>20 lbs
Lymph ct/mm³	1200–2000	800–1200	<800
Albumin (gm/dl)	3–3.5	2.5–3	<2.5
Skin Recall Antigens	—	—	unresponsive
Transferrin (mg/dl)	150–200	100–150	<100

Another, potentially more accurate, nutritional assessment tool, currently available in many centers, is the technique of indirect calorimetry. This system measures the patient's oxygen consumption ($\dot{V}O_2$) and carbon dioxide production ($\dot{V}CO_2$). The respiratory quotient (RQ) is then calculated from the CO_2/O_2 volume ratio.[16] Using these values, the patient's basal energy expenditure can be determined and the proper number of calories needed to achieve a positive nitrogen balance can be estimated. The percentage of those calories derived from carbohydrate and fat can also be determined and, in fact, adjusted so as to achieve an optimal respiratory quotient.

NUTRITIONAL THERAPY

Anorexia commonly occurs in patients with malignancy and may be related to tumor volume and site of metastases, the emotional turmoil that the cancer has created in the patient, and the therapies that have been designed to treat the cancer.[17,18] Because of these factors, dietary evaluation should be initiated early and continued throughout therapy. It has been demonstrated that the counseling and nutritional assessment skills of a dietician on the oncology team can improve the care of the cancer patient.[19]

Enteral Nutrition

Enteral calories should be administered at a rate of 150% of basal energy expenditure with a protein intake of 1.2 to 1.5 g/kg of body weight per day.[14] When these caloric and protein

TABLE 64-2. *Enteral Formulas**

PRODUCT	CALORIE DENSITY (cal/ml)	% PROTEIN	% CARBO-HYDRATE	% FAT	OSMOLALITY mOsm/Kg H_2O	MANUFACTURER
General Use: Lactose-Free Products						
Ensure	1.06	14.0	54.5	31.5	470	Ross
Ensure plus	1.5	14.7	53.3	32.0	690	Ross
Sustacal	1.0	24.0	55.0	21.0	625	Meade-Johnson
Isocal	1.0	13.0	50.0	37.0	300	Meade-Johnson
Travasorb	1.0	14.0	54.5	31.5	488	Travenol
Elemental Diets (for patients requiring low residue only; require virtually no digestion)						
Vivonex	1.0	8.2	90.5	1.3	550	Eaton
Vivonex-TEN	1.0	17.7	81.5	0.8	630	Eaton
Travasorb-HN	1.0	18.0	70.0	12.0	560	Travenol
Travasorb-STD	1.0	12.0	76.0	12.0	560	Travenol
Chemically Defined Diets (bulk-free; require some digestion)						
Precision-LR	1.1	9.5	89.2	1.3	525	Doyle
Precision-HN	1.0	16.7	82.2	1.1	557	Doyle
Travasorb-MCT	1.0–2.0	20.0	50.0	30.0	312–590	Travenol
Vital	1.0	16.7	74.0	9.3	460	Ross
Specialized Formulas						
Amin-Aid (renal failure formula; essential amino acids only)	2.0	4.0	74.8	21.2	900	McGaw
Hepatic-Aid (hepatic failure formula)	1.6	10.4	69.8	19.8	900	McGaw
Travasorb-Renal (renal failure formula; essential and non-essential amino acids)	1.35	6.9	81.1	12.0	590	Travenol
Traumacal (trauma-formula; 23% branched-chain amino acids)	1.5	22.0	38.0	40.0	550	Meade-Johnson

*Reprinted with permission from Flanigan, R. C., Rapp, R. P., and McRoberts, J. W. Nutritional assessment and therapy in advanced urothelial cancer. Urol. Clin. North Am., *11:*671, 1984.

needs cannot be met through a regular diet, a variety of dietary supplements are available as additional sources of nutritional support (Table 64-2). These supplements must be titrated to the patient's taste and needs as well as to the complications of their therapy, including stomatitis and diarrhea.

If alimentary function is adequate but the patient's compliance with oral intake is less than satisfactory, a small silastic feeding tube may be used to assist in providing sufficient intake. When such a measure is undertaken, it is critical to avoid overdistention of the stomach with subsequent reflux and possible aspiration. In this sense, serial measurements of retained gastric volume are critical.

Total Parenteral Nutrition

Over the past 20 years, the use of total parenteral nutrition has increased dramatically. Balanced formulas are now available that are capable of providing protein, carbohydrate, and lipid calories in readily useable forms. When employing total parenteral nutrition formulas, a total nitrogen intake of 1 to 2 g/kg

body weight per day and carbohydrate caloric intake of no more than 175% of basal energy expenditure are suggested. Table 64-3 provides examples of nonrenal failure parenteral nutrition formulas, as well as a breakdown of their constituents. Recent clinical trials using formulations enriched in branched chain aminoacids (valine, leucine, and isoleucine) have demonstrated decreased skeletal muscle breakdown, improved nitrogen balance, and a normalization of serum aminoacid profiles.[20,21] Daly et al. reported that cumulative nitrogen balance was improved significantly by using a 45% enriched solution of branch-chain amino acids for patients with bladder cancer undergoing cystectomy.[22]

Intravenous fat emulsions are currently available as a caloric source and have been proven to be safe and effective.[23] Positive nitrogen balance can be achieved with a parenteral regimen consisting of up to 50% of the nonprotein calories provided as fat. Because clinical complications attributable to fat emulsions are rare, the only absolute contraindication to this treatment is a patient with type-IV hyperlipidemia.[24] Treatment with fat emulsions is typically begun slowly with a

TABLE 64-3. Formulas for Nonrenal Failure Patients*

Formula I

Synthetic amino acids	42.5 gm/L	⎫
Dextrose (12.5%)	125 gm/L	⎪
Potassium	50 mEq/L	⎪
Sodium	50 mEq/L	⎬ 3 liters per day
Calcium	6 mEq/L	⎪
Magnesium	6 mEq/L	⎪
Phosphate	15 mm/L	⎪
Chloride	45 mEq/L	⎭
Vitamins and trace elements		

20% fat emulsion, 500 ml/day

This formula will provide the following:
Protein—127.5 gm (20.4 gm of nitrogen) per day
Carbohydrate calories—1275 per day
Fat calories—1000 per day
Total non-protein calories = 2275 per day
Calorie:Nitrogen ratio = 111:1

Formula II

Synthetic amino acids	42.5 gm/L	⎫
Dextrose (25%)	250 gm/L	⎪
Potassium	50 mEq/L	⎪
Sodium	50 mEq/L	⎬ 2.4 liters per day
Calcium	6 mEq/L	⎪
Magnesium	6 mEq/L	⎪
Phosphate	15 mm/L	⎪
Chloride	45 mEq/L	⎭
Vitamins and trace elements		

10% fat emulsion, 500 ml/day

This formula will provide the following:
Protein—102.0 gm (16.3 gm of nitrogen) per day
Carbohydrate calories—2040 per day
Fat calories—550 per day
Total non-protein calories = 2590 per day
Calorie:Nitrogen ratio = 158:1

*Reprinted with permission from Flanigan, R. C., Rapp, R. P., and McRoberts, J. W. Nutritional assessment and therapy in advanced urothelial cancer. Urol. Clin. North Am., 11:671, 1984.

dose of 0.5 g/kg body weight per day given at a rate of 1 ml/min (10% emulsion). It is possible then to increase the dose in a stepwise fashion, to reach a total of 1.5 to 2 g/kg/day for adults and 4 g/kg/day for infants. When fat emulsions are used as a caloric source, they should not exceed 60% of the non-protein calories that the patient is receiving. A baseline serum triglyceride should be obtained and repeated at least once a week during therapy to ensure proper serum clearance of emulsified fat particles.

The most common complications of total parenteral nutrition are shown in Table 64-4.

Parenteral Nutrition and Renal Failure

A special problem confronting the urologic oncologist is the patient whose cancer has caused impairment of renal function.

In order to provide adequate nutrition to these patients, modification of the techniques, solutions, and monitoring procedures typically used for total parenteral nutrition is necessary. Several facets of therapy become extremely critical, including the careful control of volume, protein source, electrolyte intake, glucose intake, and the risk of infection.

Beginning in the 1940's, patients with renal failure were treated with diets that were low in protein and high in carbohydrates, in order to slow the rise in serum levels of urea nitrogen.[25] Although fats were added at a later date, this diet proved to be extremely unpleasant, tasteless, and did not lead to the desired anabolic state with preservation of lean body mass. With the introduction of hemodialysis and peritoneal dialysis in the 1960's, small amounts of protein were allowed back into the diet with a consequent improvement of patient's well-being and dietary acceptance.[26] Protein intake, however, was still limited (40 to 60 g/day) so that the production of nitrogenous metabolic waste products could be kept to a minimum.

In a landmark work, Rose and coworkers not only established and characterized the amino acids as either essential or nonessential, but also observed that in normal patients, as little as 1.42 g of essential amino acids along with small amounts of nonessential acids were capable of establishing nitrogen equilibrium.[25] Further research indicated that in patients fed pre-

TABLE 64-4. Complications of Total Parenteral Nutrition*

COMPLICATION	CAUSE
Sepsis	*Staphylococus aureus* *Candida albicans* Gram-negative (rare)
Metabolic	
Hyperosmolar nonketotic coma	Blood glucose 800–1500 mg% secondary to glucose intolerance (present in 15–25% of patients)
Hyperchloremic metabolic acidosis	Excess Cl⁻ in solution Renal failure resulting in inability to excrete acid urea Gastrointestinal or renal losses of base
Hyponatremia	Mild inappropriate ADH secretion with water retention
Abnormal liver functions (SGOT, SGPT, alkaline phosphatase, bilirubin)	Essential fatty acid deficiency Excess carbohydrate administration
Catheter insertion Pneumothorax Hemothorax Arterial injuries Air embolism	Technique

*Reprinted with permission from Flanigan, R. C., Rapp, R. P., and McRoberts, J. W. Nutritional assessment and therapy in advanced urothelial cancer. Urol. Clin. North Am., 11:671, 1984.

TABLE 64-5. *Renal Failure Formulas**

Nephramine (essential amino acids only)
  L-Amino acids

Isoleucine	1.4 gm
Leucine	2.2 gm
Lysine	2.0 gm
Methionine	2.2 gm
Phenylalanine	2.2 gm
Threonine	1.0 gm
Tryptophan	0.5 gm
Valine	1.6 gm
Dextrose (47%)	350 gm
Calories (nonprotein)	1190
Total nitrogen	1.4 gm
Volume	750 ml

Aminosyn RF (essential amino acids plus arginine and histidine)
  L-Amino acids

Isoleucine	1.4 gm
Leucine	2.2 gm
Lysine	1.6 gm
Methionine	2.1 gm
Phenylalanine	2.1 gm
Threonine	1.0 gm
Tryptophan	0.5 gm
Valine	1.6 gm
Arginine	1.8 gm
Histadine	1.3 gm
Dextrose (47%)	350 gm
Calories (nonprotein)	1190
Total nitrogen	2.4 gm
Volume	800 ml

*Reprinted with permission from Flanigan, R. C., Rapp, R. P., and McRoberts, J. W. Nutritional assessment and therapy in advanced urothelial cancer. Urol. Clin. North Am., 11:671, 1984.

dominantly essential amino acids, the nitrogen byproducts of urea could serve as a source of synthesis for nonessential amino acids.[25] In this setting, urea must be broken down into ammonia and carbon dioxide by intestinal bacteria, recycled in the biliary system, and transformed into nonessential amino acids.[27]

This concept has been incorporated into current day intravenous renal formula total parenteral nutrition solutions. These solutions typically contain 1.4 to 1.5 g of nitrogen as essential amino acid and 47% dextrose in 750 ml of solution. Flow rates for this solution should begin at approximately 30 ml/hr to a maximum of 75 to 80 ml/hr (Table 64-5).

Although the rationale for the use of essential amino acids in renal failure is to reduce the rate of urea production by eliminating nonessential amino acids, much controversy still exists regarding whether or not the use of essential amino acid solutions in this patient population is, in fact, necessary. Formulas containing both essential and nonessential amino acids in reduced quantities have also been tested in patients with renal failure. Freiend and associates demonstrated a decreased BUN and creatinine as well as decreased mortality in patients receiving only essential amino acids.[28] Conversely, in a prospective randomized trial, Mirtallo and associates found no dif-

ference in serum creatinine or survival.[29] For this reason, the use of essential amino acid in renal failure formulas remains questionable. Certainly if patients are receiving dialysis, these solutions are not mandatory.

RESULTS OF NUTRITIONAL THERAPY

Most patients with significant malnutrition present with advanced disease, therefore, the initiation of definitive treatment (surgery, chemotherapy, or radiotherapy) is relatively urgent. This urgency often does not allow for the time needed to rectify the malnutrition status.

Although theoretically appealing in concept, the idea that malnourished cancer patients benefit from perioperative parenteral nutrition remains unproven. In fact, a single prospective randomized 10-day trial of preoperative total parenteral nutrition compared to oral dietary therapy alone demonstrated a significant decrease in postoperative abscess formation, peritonitis, anastomotic leakage, and ileus in patients with gastrointestinal cancer.[30] In contrast, other trials in malnourished patients with gastrointestinal malignancies who received preoperative parenteral nutrition given for 72 hours[31] or for 5 or more days[32] and continued postoperatively until oral intake was resumed, failed to demonstrate any reduction in surgical morbidity or mortality rates compared to nutritionally unsupported patients. We have previously demonstrated that although malnourished patients with bladder cancer had a greater operative mortality and morbidity rate than their nutritionally normal counterparts, longterm survival rates in these two groups did not seem to be affected.[33] In our study of 33 patients with advanced bladder cancer, treated by radical cystectomy and carefully monitored from a nutritional viewpoint, we could find no evidence that nutritional support in the immediate perioperative period reduced perioperative complications or decreased mortality. Fundamental questions remain to be answered in this area, including whether or not aggressive nutritional therapy can, in fact, reliably restore malnourished patients to nutritionally normal status and, if so, will these patients enjoy the same low operative morbidity and mortality rates that their nutritionally normal counterparts enjoy? The corollary of this question is whether the time required to achieve a normal nutritional status and perhaps then, a decrease in the risk of morbidity and mortality in patients with advanced urologic malignancy, justifies the delay of definitive therapy with its attendant risk of cancer progression.

METABOLIC ABNORMALITIES

Although a vast variety of metabolic abnormalities can occur in the pre and postoperative periods in urologic cancer patients, only three major interrelated areas will be discussed in this chapter. These include special metabolic changes associated with renal failure, problems of volume and electrolyte abnormalities associated with urologic cancer surgery, and acid-base imbalances resulting from the construction of continent urinary diversions.

Renal Dysfunction

The diseased kidney producing azotemia or uremia results in abnormalities of protein metabolism, electrolytes, pH and acid balance, and water metabolism. Disturbances of cation concentration typically associated with uremia include potassium, sodium, calcium, and magnesium abnormalities.

POTASSIUM. Serum potassium is usually increased in uremia. This elevation can result from a dietary increase in potassium, from protein breakdown, and from acidosis. In acidosis, hydrogen ions are buffered by intracellular proteins, resulting in a release of intracellular potassium. Because potassium is secreted primarily by the distal tubules of the nephron, when urine output is low, as in severe renal failure, hyperkalemia occurs primarily because of the failure of the distal tubules to secrete potassium. If urine output is less than 500 to 1000 mL/day, the distal tubules do not secrete adequate potassium and the potassium concentration in the blood may rise to dangerous levels.[33]

Hyperkalemia produces symptoms of muscle weakness and paralysis with loss of reflexes. The most important toxic effects are cardiac, manifested by high-peaked T waves and later prolonged P-R intervals. These cardiac changes may result in complete heart block or atrial asystoles, especially in patients treated with digitalis.[34] Hyperkalemia may be treated in several ways. Dietary intake of potassium, including drugs that contain potassium or diuretics that "spare" potassium (spironolactone) should be strictly limited. Ion exchange resins (Kayexalate) may be given on an emergency basis. These compounds, which are not absorbed from the gastrointestinal tract, exchange sodium for potassium, which is then excreted in the feces. Kayexalate may be given orally or as a retention enema, the usual dose being 15 g one to four times per day. This dose will typically reduce the serum potassium by 1 to 2 mEq/L over 24 hours. Dialysis may be indicated. In situations where a potassium level is dangerously high and cardiac arrhythmias are imminent, intravenous calcium gluconate or calcium chloride may be given as an emergency measure. Calcium protects the heart from the effects of hyperkalemia but does not reduce serum potassium.

Sodium bicarbonate provides a second method of reducing hyperkalemia in an emergency situation. Because the renal failure patient is acidotic, intracellular proteins help buffer the hydrogen ion with the release of intracellular potassium. Sodium bicarbonate serves to force this potassium back into the cell, thus lowering the serum potassium level. The administration of insulin and glucose is a third emergency measure for the treatment of hyperkalemia. Insulin causes glucose to be driven into the cell taking potassium with it and reducing serum potassium.

Decreased serum potassium, only occasionally seen in renal failure, is most commonly associated with significant diuresis (as in the diuretic phase of acute renal failure or diuresis induced by drugs) or gastrointestinal loss from vomiting or diarrhea.[35] Hypokalemia is treated with oral or parenteral potassium supplements. Potassium should not be replaced at a rate greater than 10 to 15 mEq an hour without careful electrocardiographic monitoring.

SODIUM. Serum sodium may be either increased or decreased in renal failure. In severe renal failure with resultant diminution of the glomerular filtration rate and decrease in urine output, the kidney is unable to secrete sufficient sodium, resulting in hypernatremia.[34] This hypernatremia may be further aggravated by high dietary intake of salt. Hypernatremia usually occurs when the patient is oliguric and is suggested by the signs of fluid retention, weight gain, systemic edema, congestive heart failure, pulmonary edema, and hypotension. This entity is best treated by limiting sodium intake and by the administration of diuretics. Conversely, a decreased sodium concentration can occur in renal failure in association with significant diuresis as mentioned previously. Hyponatremia is more commonly seen in the urologic patient because of the absorption of large amounts of electrolyte-free solutions during transurethral resection (of the prostate or bladder tumors). It is characterized by a decreased blood pressure, listlessness, confusion, anorexia, and nausea. In severe cases, muscle cramps and generalized muscle twitching, convulsions, and coma may develop. Symptomatic hyponatremia is best treated with intravenous replacement with normal saline and diuretic (lasix) therapy. In severe cases, replacement with hypertonic saline or dialysis may be necessary.[37]

CALCIUM. Serum calcium is typically reduced in the uremic patient and is associated with an elevated phosphate level. This hypocalcemia, which is associated with a decreased absorption of calcium from the GI tract, may cause parathyroid dysfunction (secondary hyperparathyroidism) with subsequent normalization of the serum calcium. Derangements in calcium and phosphorous metabolism are interrelated. Hypocalcemia may be associated with EKG changes, the characteristic sign being prolonged QT intervals with a normal T-wave. Calcium lactate and calcium citrate can be given in doses of 1 to 2 g/day orally to raise serum calcium.[38] In the case of a cardiac emergency, 0.5 to 1.0 g IV calcium chloride or 1.0 to 2.0 g IV calcium gluconate may be given every 10 minutes. In addition, aluminum hydroxide gels may be given to retard absorption of phosphate from the gut, thus reducing serum phosphate and increasing serum calcium. A correction of the associated acidosis combined with the use of vitamin D may allow for the healing of some bone lesions.

MAGNESIUM. An increase in serum magnesium occurs in acute and chronic renal failure associated with low urine output. This phenomenon is caused by a decreased excretion of magnesium by the kidneys and by the use of magnesium containing drugs, especially antacids and cathartics. Serum levels greater than 3 mEq per L are associated with an increased risk of cardiac arrhythmias, respiratory paralysis, and prolonged muscle relaxation after anesthesia.[35]

ACIDOSIS. Because the diseased kidney is unable to excrete the normal acid waste load, an accumulation of nonvolatile acids result.[35] Although this is mild in acute renal failure, metabolic acidosis is nearly always present and may be severe in chronic renal failure. In most cases of chronic renal failure, the major abnormality is the patient's inability to excrete normal quantities of ammonium, although renal ability to reabsorb bicarbonate may also be impaired. Laboratory tests indicate a low plasma pH (below 7.35) and a normal to low level of plasma bicarbonate (CO_2) which results from the respiratory compensation of the patient to the metabolic acidosis.

Chronic acidosis is not generally treated unless the patient becomes symptomatic. Acidosis is treated with sodium bicarbonate or sodium lactate given orally or intravenously. Significant acidosis is also an indication for dialysis. It is important to remember that patients with chronic metabolic acidosis compensate by chronic hyperventilation. This hyperventilation must be maintained during anesthesia to prevent worsening of the metabolic acidosis and subsequent hyperkalemia with cardiac complications.[39]

PERIOPERATIVE VOLUME PROBLEMS

Volume Overload

Volume overload occurs frequently in the postoperative period and is often the result of the injudicious overuse of intravenous fluids in the operating or postoperative recovery rooms. This occurs most significantly in older patients with underlying cardiac disease. Congestive heart failure (with decreased renal perfusion), perioperative ischemia, and acute tubular necrosis may result in decreased urine output and aggravate the problem of volume overload. In such cases, careful perioperative monitoring with central venous or Swan-Ganz catheterization is particularly useful. With clinical signs of fluid overload, diuretic therapy and restriction of water and sodium intake is essential.

In addition to the previously mentioned electrolyte and acid-base abnormalities associated with renal insufficiency, these patients are particularly prone to develop volume imbalance.[34] Many renal failure patients have diminished capacity to excrete free water. This may be further aggravated by the release of antidiuretic hormone during anesthesia or surgery (see below) and may result in fluid overload and congestive heart failure. In contrast, certain renal failure patients may display an inability to concentrate urine, raising the risk of volume depletion.

Diuretics should be administered prophylactically in patients with renal insufficiency who are to undergo surgery in order to reduce the risk of further renal deterioration.[34] Both mannitol and furosemide may be useful in stabilizing renal function.[40,41] We prefer to use mannitol at a dose of 0.75 g/kg IV slowly during surgery with careful monitoring of the central venous pressure. Furosemide may be given by continuous infusion combined with mannitol or as a bolus (typically 100 mg). Urine volume is replaced with 0.45% saline with

potassium replacement as determined by serial urine and serum electrolyte measurements.[34]

Volume Depletion

Patients with severe renal insufficiency may have a decreased ability to concentrate their urine, leading to volume depletion. Volume depletion may also occur because of inadequate replacement of blood loss, third spacing of fluids, unrecognized insensible losses from fever, hyperventilation, or gastrointestinal sources, injudicious use of diuretics, or diabetic osmotic diuresis. Two disorders commonly associated with volume depletion that occur in urologic cancer patients are postobstructive diuresis and hypercalcemia.

POSTOBSTRUCTIVE DIURESIS. This can occur following relief of urinary tract obstruction and can cause a significant loss of fluid and electrolytes. The mechanisms responsible for this diuresis include an impaired renal concentrating ability, tubular defects with impaired reabsorption of sodium and water, and an osmotic effect because of the loss of urea and glucose.[42]

After release of *unilateral* obstruction of 5 hours or more, the lowered renal blood flow and filtration rate are associated with slightly decreased rates of solute reabsorption and impairment of concentrating ability. The result is typically a normal flowrate of *dilute* urine and no salt loss.[43] Occasionally, a significant diuresis can occur associated with unilateral obstruction, probably secondary to a normal glomerular filtration rate (GFR) in the face of distal tubular damage.[44]

BILATERAL URETERAL OBSTRUCTION. This produces a decreased renal blood flow but is not associated with the shifts in intrarenal blood distribution (to the inner cortex and medulla) as seen with unilateral obstruction.[45,46] A defect in concentrating ability occurs and the impairment of sodium absorption is great enough to cause diuresis and natriuresis despite a lowered GFR.

Treatment of a significant postobstructive diuresis is best accomplished using 0.45% normal saline with potassium replacement based on urinary and serum potassium levels. Although volume replacement may initially be at levels equal to urinary losses, replacement can be titrated downward gradually (with careful monitoring of vital signs, serum and urine Na, and osmolality) to 50 to 60% of urinary output. Glucosuria, or a potentiating factor in the diuresis, should be ruled out by a urine dip-stick test. A urine specific gravity of 1.010 suggests a solute diuresis.

Hypercalcemia

This may also cause a defect in renal concentrating ability resulting in polyuria.[29] The mechanism of this condition is unclear. All attempts to correct hypercalcemia preoperatively in any patient should be made not only for reasons of volume depletion but, more importantly, for reasons of anorexia, dehydration, prerenal azotemia, mental status changes, and cardiac abnormalities including shortening of the Q-T interval.

Inappropriate ADH Release

Hyponatremia occurring in the face of an inappropriately concentrated urine concentration (sodium concentration of greater than 20 mEq/L) may result from inappropriate release of antidiuretic hormone. This syndrome has been associated with a large number of underlying diseases and urologic cancer surgeries.[47,48] The resultant hyponatremia is rarely symptomatic unless sodium concentration is less than 125 mEq/L but levels between 100 to 120 mEq/L can cause severe CNS symptomatology including seizures, coma, and death.[49]

Treatment is generally directed at a gradual restoration of sodium concentration using normal saline intravenous therapy with diuresis using furosemide. In the presence of acute symptoms, hypertonic saline (3%) may be infused. Careful monitoring of vital signs and cardiac status is mandatory. Demeclocyline (600 to 1200 mg/d) has been shown to be effective in the management of chronic inappropriate ADH secretion.[50]

METABOLIC DERANGEMENTS CREATED BY URINARY DIVERSION WITH INTESTINAL SEGMENTS

The syndrome of hyperchloremic acidosis is characterized by fatigue, diarrhea, weight loss, thirst, and polydipsia. It is characterized metabolically by a depletion of bicarbonate and an elevation of chloride, hydrogen, and sulfate. The degree of hyperchloremic acidosis depends on the total surface area of bowel exposed to urine, the length of exposure time, renal function, and the type of bowel segment incorporated. The pathophysiology of this syndrome has been more clearly defined by Koch and McDougal.[51] They demonstrated that active transport of chloride across the mucosa was the primary impetus for the acidosis and that hydrogen, potassium, and ammonium ions were reabsorbed in equal amounts to chloride. Bone demineralization (osteomalacia) also occurs, occasionally even in the presence of normal electrolyte values.[51] Management in the past has been empiric titration of the acidosis with bicarbonate or citrate salts and restriction of dietary chloride. Intestinal cyclic-AMP inhibitors (nicotinic acid and chlorpromazine) have recently been proposed because chloride absorption and secretion by the intestinal mucosal cell is a cyclic-AMP mediated process.[52,53]

CONCLUSION

The nutritional and metabolic derangements associated with urologic malignancies are common and may be severe. Superimposed renal disease can potentiate these problems and necessitate adjustments in standard pre and postoperative care. A thorough understanding of the pathophysiologic processes involved in these derangements is important in the therapeutic planning of these often complex clinical problems.

REFERENCES

1. MEGUID, M. M., and MEGUID, V. Preoperative identification of the surgical cancer patient in need of postoperative supportive total parenteral nutrition. Cancer, 55:258, 1985.

2. BRISTRIAN, B. R., et al. Protein status of general surgical patients. JAMA, 230:858, 1974.

3. MOHLER, J. L., and FLANIGAN, R. C. The effect of nutritional status and support on morbidity and mortality of bladder cancer patients treated by radical cystectomy. J. Urol., 137:404, 1987.

4. DeWYS, W. D. Anorexia as a general effect of cancer. Cancer, 43:2013, 1979.

5. THEOLOGIDES, A. Cancer cachexia. Cancer, 43:2004, 1979.

6. GRANDE, F., ANDERSON, J. T., and KEYES, A. Changes of basal metabolic rate in men in semi-starvation and re-feeding. J. Appl. Physiol., 12:230, 1958.

7. THEOLOGIDES, A. Cancer cachexia in nutrition and cancer. In: Current Concepts in Nutrition. Volume 6. Edited by M. Winick. New York, John Wiley, 1977, p. 75.

8. MARKS, P. A., and BISHOP, J. S. Studies on carbohydrate metabolism in patients with neoplastic disease II. Response to insulin administration. J. Clin. Invest., 38:668, 1959.

9. SCHEIN, P.S., et al. Cachexia of malignancy: Potential role of insulin in nutritional management. Cancer, 43:2070, 1979.

10. HOLROYADE, C. P., et al. Altered glucose metabolism in metastatic carcinoma. Cancer Res., 35:3710, 1975.

11. KRALOVIC, R. C., ZEPP, E. A., and CENEDELLA, R. J. Studies of the metabolism of carcass fat depletion in experimental cancer. Eur. J. Cancer., 13:1071, 1977.

12. ROSSING, N. Albumin metabolism in neoplastic diseases. Scand. J. Clin. Lab. Invest., 22:211, 1968.

13. FLANIGAN, R. C., RAPP, R. P., and McROBERTS, J. W. Nutritional assessment and therapy in advanced urothelial cancer. Urol. Clin. North Am., 11:671, 1984.

14. HARVEY, K. B., BOTHE, A., JR., and BLACKBURN, G. L. Nutritional assessment and patient outcome during oncological therapy. Cancer, 43:2065, 1979.

15. GULLINO, P., et al. Studies on the metabolism of amino acids and related compounds in vivo: I. Toxicity of essential amino acids individually and in mixtures, the protective effect of L-arginine. Arch. Biochem. Biophys., 64:314, 1956.

16. CALDWELL, F. T. Measurement of oxygen consumption and CO_2 production in clinical nutritional assessment. In: Nutritional Assessment Present Status, Future Direction and Projects. Edited by S. Levenson. Columbus, Boss Conference on Medical Research, 1981, p. 19.

17. SHIH, V. E. Urea cycle disorders and other congenital hyperammonemic syndrome. In: The Metabolic Basis of Inherited Disease. 4th Edition. Edited by J. B. Stanbury and J. B. Wyngarden. New York, McGraw-Hill Book Co., 1979.

18. THEOLOGIDES, A. Weight loss in cancer patients. CA, *27*:205, 1977.

19. AKER, S. N. Oral feedings in the cancer patient. Cancer, *43*:2103, 1979.

20. BLACKBURN, G. L., et al. Branched chain amino and administration and metabolism during starvation, injury, and infection. Surgery, *86*:307, 1979.

21. KERN, K. A., et al. The effect of a new branched chain enriched amino acid solution on postoperative catabolism. Surgery, *92*:780, 1982.

22. DALY, J. M. Use of branched chain amino acids in surgical patients. Presented at the Eighth Clinical Congress. American Society for Parenteral and Enteral Nutrition. Las Vegas, January 30, 1984.

23. BIVINS, B. A., et al. The effect of ten and twenty percent safflower oil emulsion given as thirty to fifty percent of total calories. Surg. Gynecol. Obstet., *156*:433, 1983.

24. RAPP, R. P., DONALDSON, E. S., and BIVINS, B. A. Parenteral nutrition in a patient with familial Type IV hypertriglyceridemia: A dilemma. Drug Intell. Clin. Pharm., *17*:458, 1983.

25. ROSE, W. C., and WIXONI, R. L. The amino acid requirements of man. XVI. The role of the nitrogen intake. J. Biol. Chem., *217*:997, 1955.

26. MAHLER, J. F., and SCHREINER, G. E. Metabolic problems related to prolonged dialytic maintenance of life in oliguria. JAMA, *176*:399, 1961.

27. SCHBOERB, P. R. Essential L-amino acid administration in uremia. Am. J. Med. Sci., *252*:650, 1960.

28. FREIEND, H. R., and FISCHER, J. E. Parenteral nutrition in acute renal failure using essential and non-essential amino acids. Presented at the Fourth Clinical Congress. American Society of Parenteral and Enteral Nutrition. Chicago, January 30, 1980.

29. MIRTALLO, M. S., et al. A comparison of Nephranine and Freamine-II in the nutritional support of patients with compromised renal function. Presented at the Fourth Clinical Congress. American Society of Parenteral and Enteral Nutrition. Chicago, January 30, 1980.

30. MULLER, J. M., et al. Preoperative parenteral feeding in patients with gastrointestinal carcinoma. Lancet, *1*:68, 1982.

31. HOLTER, A. R., and FISCHER, J. E. The effects of perioperative hyperalimentation on complications in patients with carcinoma and weight loss. J. Surg. Res., *23*:31, 1977.

32. THOMPSON, B. R., JULIAN, T. B., and STREMPLE, J. F. Perioperative total parenteral nutrition in patients with gastrointestinal cancer. J. Surg. Res., *30*:497, 1981.

33. KASISKE, B. L., and KJELLSTRAND, C. M. Perioperative management of patients with chronic renal failure and postoperative acute renal failure. Urol. Clin. North Am., *10*:35, 1983.

34. ETTINGER, P. O., REGEN, T. J., and OLDEWORTH, H. A. Hyperkalemia, cardiac conduction and the electrocardiogram. A review. Am. Heart J., *88*:360, 1974.

35. BURKE, G. R., and FULYASSY, P. F. Surgery in the patient with renal disease and related electrolyte disorders. Med. Clin. North Am., *53*:1191, 1979.

36. HARRINGTON, J. D., and BRENNER, E. R. Conservative treatment of renal failure. In: *Patient Care in Renal Failure.* Philadelphia, W. B. Saunders, 1973, p. 65.

37. HANTMAN, D., et al. Rapid correction of hyponatremia in the syndrome of inappropriate secretion of antidiuretic hormone: An alternative treatment to hypertonic saline. Ann. Intern. Med., *78*:870, 1973.

38. PITTS, R. F. The uremic syndrome. In: *Physiology of the Kidney and Body Fluids.* Chicago, Year Book Medical Publishers, 1974, p. 286.

39. GOGGIN, M. J., and JOEKES, A. M. I. Dangers of hyperkalemia during anesthesia. Br. Med. J., *2*:244, 1971.

40. DAWSON, J. L. Post-operative renal function in obstructive jaundice. Effect of a mannitol diuresis. Br. Med. J., *1*:82, 1965.

41. NUUITNEN, L. S., et al. The effect of furosemide on renal function in open heart surgery. J. Cardiovasc. Surg., *19*:471, 1978.

42. GUGGENHEIN, S. J., and SCHRIER, R. W. Obstructive nephropathy: Pathophysiology and management. In: *Renal and Electrolyte Disorders.* Edited by R. W. Schrier. Boston, Little, Brown & Co., 1980, p. 443.

43. GILLENWATER, J. Y., WESTERVELT, F. B., JR., VAUGHAN, E. D., JR., and HOWARDS, S. S. Renal function after release of chronic unilateral hydronephrosis in man. Kidney Int., *7*:179, 1975.

44. SCHLOSSBERG, S. M., and VAUGHAN, E. D., JR. The mechanism of unilateral post-obstructive diuresis. J. Urol., *131*:534, 1984.

45. McDOUGAL, W. S., and WRIGHT, F. S. Defect in proximal and distal sodium transport in post-obstructive diuresis. Kidney Int., *2*:304, 1972.

46. JAENIKE, J. R. The renal functional defect of post-obstructive nephropathy: The effects of bilateral ureteral obstruction in the rat. J. Clin. Invest., *51*:2999, 1972.

47. BARTTER, F. C., and SCHWARTZ, W. S. The syndrome of inappropriate secretion of antidiuretic hormones. Am. J. Med., *42*:790, 1967.

48. HARRINGTON, J. T., and COHEN, J. J. Clinical disorders of urine concentration and dilution. Arch. Intern. Med., *131*:810, 1973.

49. LEAF, A. The clinical and physiologic significance of the serum sodium concentration. N. Engl. J. Med., *267*:24, 1962.

50. FORREST, J. N., JR., et al. Superiority of demeclocycline over lithium in the treatment of chronic syndrome of inappropriate secretion of antidiuretic hormone. N. Engl. J. Med., *298*:173, 1978.

51. KOCH, M. O., and McDOUGAL, W. S. The pathophysiology of hyperchloremic metabolic acidosis after urinary diversion through intestinal segments. Surgery, *98*:561, 1985.

52. KOCH, M. O., and McDOUGAL, W. S. Nicotinic acid: Treatment for the hyperchloremic acidosis following urinary diversion through intestinal segments. J. Urol., *134*:162, 1985.

53. KOCH, M. O., and McDOUGAL, W. S. Chlorpromazine: Adjuvant therapy for the metabolic derangements created by urinary diversion through intestinal segments. J. Urol., *134*:165, 1985.

CHAPTER
65

Psychosexual Support for Genitourinary Cancer Patients

"The Most Fundamental Principle of Medicine Is Love"
—PARACELSUS (1493–1541)

Marilyn Davis
Sakti Das

I n the practice of urology, informing the patient of the diagnosis of a genitourinary cancer is a disturbingly common scenario. With the increasing life expectancy patterns of both males and females, the incidence of genitourinary cancers will undoubtedly escalate as diagnoses of high-incidence tumors, such as prostate and bladder cancer, dramatically escalate with age. Advancements in diagnostic maneuvers, including the newer imaging and biopsy techniques, histologic confirmatory studies, computerized tumor models, and flow cytometry, are generating considerable excitement. Refinements in chemotherapy, laser therapy, radiation therapy, and surgical techniques, such as potency-preserving radical prostatectomy and cystectomy, and retroperitoneal lymph node dissections modified to preserve ejaculatory function, have expanded therapeutic horizons while decreasing morbidity. New endeavors in bone marrow protection and granulocyte-macrophage stimulation permit intensification of chemotherapy and radiation therapy. Finally, the elucidation of numerous compounds with the ability to enhance or modify host and tumor biologic behavior offers considerable promise in the design, delivery, and evaluation of therapy. This chapter will review principles and practices in the continuing communication and supportive maneuvers in the management of urologic malignancies with special emphasis on sexual concerns and interventions.

GENERAL CONSIDERATIONS

In the initial and subsequent discussions between the physician and patient, promoting and maintaining psychological preparation defined as "the emotional perspective that the patient and family will adopt to manage the diagnosis, treatment and related deficits" are imperative.[1] In today's media-saturated society, patients have become increasingly aware of the various manifestations of cancer as well as the available diagnostic and treatment modalities. Therefore, in planning physician-patient encounters, three major themes are suggested:

1. Continuous acknowledgment of the individuality of each patient
2. Awareness of the generality of predictable stressful points

3. Maintenance of a patient-centered focus rather than a disease-centered focus

In meeting the challenge of adapting to a cancer diagnosis, each patient responds with a complex, and frequently distorted array of facts, deficits, perceptions, and fears, as well as socioeconocultural biases. An understanding of the individual's experiential conditioning is critical in planning treatment. This may be facilitated by encouraging the patient to view his disease process as unique to himself, unlike that experienced by anyone else. Response to therapy can similarly be viewed as a unique phenomenon with the individual himself being the best barometer of subjective response. Encouraging the consideration of a cancer diagnosis as the identification of a chronic rather than a terminal condition allows the patient to direct his thinking toward living well rather than anticipating a process of dying.

A number of predictable phases or points in the continuum of cancer are associated with the precipitation or exacerbation of stress. These pivotal points include the workup and subsequent diagnosis phase, initiation of therapy, completion of therapy, evaluation of objective response, introduction of a new treatment modality, discovery of metastatic or recurrent disease, and, finally, the exhaustion of all viable treatment options.[2,3] It is suggested that the degree and intensity of stress may be directly proportional to the time interval between complete response and subsequent recurrence.[4]

In order to facilitate a patient-related rather than disease-related focus and to maximize psychological preparedness in clinician-patient dialogues, the following suggestions are offered.

1. Allow the presence of support individuals as chosen by the patient
2. Set a specific place and allow ample time for discussion
3. Use language and descriptions that are easily comprehended
4. Write down key words or descriptions
5. Provide diagrams or models to review involved anatomic structures and physiologic functions
6. Use a strategy to assess the patient's degree of comprehension such as asking the patient's recall of the information as heard and processed
7. Encourage the patient to write down questions and concerns as they arise for subsequent discussions

As the initial discussion may be accompanied by an overwhelming shutdown of sensory-receptive mechanisms, repetition at serial intervals may be necessary. It is not uncommon for patients to suggest a knowledge deficit in terms of diagnosis and treatment in subsequent interactions with other health-care providers. This may be a conscious or unconscious behavior designed to elicit congruity or incongruity and assess level of comfort and degree of continuity among various practitioners. Meticulous medical record documentation is paramount in maintaining a consistent, comprehensive approach.

Finally, a discussion of universal concerns along with the individual's specific concerns, although time-consuming, may be beneficial in the psychological adaptation process so essential for the patient's successful maintenance of a functional emotional outlook. The negativity with which all individuals react to the diagnosis of cancer is universal. Concerns regarding the impact, side effects, and costs associated with cancer treatment, loss of independence, as well as anger, confusion, fear of pain, and anticipation of death are commonly experienced. The establishment of effective communication patterns will enhance the patient's psychologic preparation, thereby facilitating treatment planning and promoting compliance.

AGE CONSIDERATIONS

Development Issues

Genitourinary cancers suggest special considerations for young, middle-aged, and older adults. Developmentally, each group has predictable tasks with early adulthood characterized by selecting and adapting to a mate, starting a family, developing work expertise, and expanding community and civic roles.[5] The middle-aged adult from 35 to 55 years of age is mastering an occupation, achieving civic and social maturity, experiencing physiologic changes, and adjusting to aging parents and older children, while developing leisure and volunteer activity patterns.[5]

With aging, intellectual function is usually maintained, although short-term memory may gradually decline. Sociologically, the transition from mid-life to older adulthood is characterized by role change as one eases into retirement and adjusts to declining economic opportunities and gradually shifting family responsibilities. As defined by Erickson, the major developmental challenge for the older adult is achieving ego integrity or a comfortable acceptance of one's achievements and limitations.[6] Havighurst summarized tasks challenging the aging adult as follows: adjusting to the process of physiologic aging, retirement, reduced income, loss of spouse, and the deaths of relatives and friends while affiliating with one's age group, and maintaining a safe and solvent environment.[5]

With genitourinary cancers accounting for 25% of all malignancies and the majority of these tumors being expressed in individuals over age 50, general values of the aging population are considered.[7] More than half of all cases of cancer are diagnosed after the age of 65, although this population accounts for approximately 12% of the U.S. population.[8] Prior to age 50, the incidence of cancer is higher in women, whereas after age 60, the incidence of cancer in men is significantly higher.[9] The probability of developing cancer within 5 years is 1 in 700 at the age of 25, at the age of 65 it is 1 in 14.[9,10]

The older patient with Medicare coverage has adequate insurance for acute care but does not have comprehensive coverage for preventative or maintenance care, including screening. The aggressive pursuit of symptoms is not seen in older patients. The older person himself may feel less comfortable in health-care facilities, thereby setting the stage for a delay in diagnosis. In general, the older person is concerned about finances, losing independence, placing a burden on family or society, and is more likely to approach the health-care system with a series of preconceived notions regarding a potentially negative outcome from the encounter. A conscious effort to psychologically prepare and support the older patient diagnosed with cancer is clearly in order so that myths can be dispelled and a positive attitude promoted.

SEXUAL CONSEQUENCES

Consideration of sexual consequences of cancer is essential not only in the diagnostic phase but also in the continuing-care phases to recognize frustrations peculiar to inability to fulfill age-specific developmental tasks. Sexuality is inextricably woven into the fabric of one's individual profile of developmental task challenge and achievement. For example, the young adult with cancer may experience an exaggerated sense of guilt, particularly with respect to abandoning the spouse or children, while the older adult may grieve the loss of intimacy with a spouse. Clarification of these issues will greatly enhance adjustment to disease and treatment.

Self-Image and Self-Esteem

Two closely related concepts, self-image (defined as a mental mirror image of oneself) and self-esteem (how valuable a person feels to himself and to others) are subject to actual physical changes, such as aging in general and cancer in specific, along with a host of external factors including employment, finances, socialization, and family. With the diagnosis of a malignancy, there is a potential impact on an individual's self-image. Specifically, the loss of any body part or function may have both positive and negative connotations. The loss or change in function will have a different meaning for each individual experiencing it. It has been suggested that women undergoing cystectomy may be more traumatically affected than men undergoing cystectomy. The expression of grief associated with loss is a normal reaction. However, persistence of grief or exacerbation of depression after removal of a body part or organ or loss of physiologic function accompanied by withdrawal, increasing dependency, or pronounced depression may signal the need for psychologic intervention. Other feelings may accompany the loss, including relief and hope, which spur an individual to master new challenges thereby expanding his inner resources. In general, if an individual cannot incorporate the physical changes into his self-image within 6 months to a year after surgery, outside support and counseling may be indicated.

The individual challenged by the diagnosis of a genitourinary malignancy and subsequent treatment has an equally difficult challenge; that is, maintaining his self-esteem. Enhancement or support of one's self-esteem is facilitated by encouraging the individual to accept his uniqueness and value as an individual. In promoting self-esteem, patients need to be encouraged to:

1. Share anxieties and fears along with dreams and joys with others
2. Respond to the challenges of the tumor diagnosis and treatment with courage
3. Take responsibility for what is happening to oneself

Sexuality

Closely associated with the concepts of self-image and self-esteem is the more global concept of sexuality, which can be defined as the "physical, emotional, intellectual, and social aspects of an individual's personality, which expresses maleness or femaleness."[11] Sexuality is an integral part of every individual's nature. Nonreproductive sexuality with its key component, sensuality, or the awareness and appreciation of the messages delivered to us by our senses—sights, sounds, touches, smells, tastes, and rhythms in life—is a continuing need in human beings throughout the life span.

As the genitourinary tract exists in tandem with the reproductive system in both males and females, changes in fertility and sexual function may often be associated with cancer treatment. Correspondingly, changes chemically mediated by chemotherapy and medications designed to alleviate the side effects of chemotherapy may alter mood as well as body image. Hormonal therapy and biologic response modifier therapy additionally may affect mood, body image, and energy levels.

Sexual function as a component of sexuality is often overlooked or avoided by physicians based on varying degrees of comfort with the topic as well as implied or direct messages received from the patient or from the patient's family members. Medical or surgical interventions designed to focus on the disease itself may be highlighted and concerns related to sexuality de-emphasized. In general, any time an individual's self-image or self-concept have been challenged by treatment modalities, sexuality also has been affected.

Quality of Life

Traditional end points in clinical trials for cancer have emphasized overall survival, progression-free survival, and tumor response. Philosophically, the benefits of therapy should outweigh the risks. Components of quality of life including physical, emotional, and global functioning and symptoms are now recommended for inclusion in selected therapeutic trials. Historically, measures of physical functioning have been applied universally in the clinical setting. For example, the Karnofsky performance status assigns a percentage score based on the physician's judgment of a patient's performance status. Quality of life measures, therefore, will allow for another perspective; that is, the patient's perspective.

Guidelines adopted by the Southwest Oncology Group for quality-of-life assessment in multimodality, multidisciplinary clinical trials are pertinent to urologic oncology in studies when:

1. Different treatment modalities are employed with equivalent survival expectations where quality of life may show treatment differences
2. Adjuvant therapy is instituted for patients at risk of recurrence[12]

Currently, Southwest Oncology Group quality-of-life companion studies are proposed for two prostate cancer clinical trials. One trial, for stage-A and stage-B prostate cancer, compares radical prostatectomy alone to definitive radiotherapy. The other trial contrasts radical prostatectomy to radical prostatectomy followed by radiotherapy for pathologic stage-C disease where the side effects of adjuvant therapy can be assessed along with traditional end points. As equivalent survival expectations are anticipated on both arms, quality of life may be the primary end point. Quality-of-life data may help in the assessment of risk to benefit ratios while promoting an integrated patient-focused approach to care and evaluation.

Baseline Sexual Evaluation

Cancer and sexuality are not mutually exclusive. In general, an individually or mutually satisfactory pattern of sexuality prior to a cancer diagnosis facilitates the continuation of an equally or acceptably satisfactory pattern after diagnosis. A troubled pattern prior to diagnosis predictably may remain troubled postdiagnosis. Sexuality concerns are not gender or age specific. Expressions of sexuality do not exist in a vacuum. Pain, fatigue, worry, and debility, as well as the symptom complex associated with the individual's disease, can profoundly affect libido and sexual performance. Assessment of patterns of sexuality expression prior to diagnosis greatly enhances the clinician's ability to predict the impact of therapy and institute interventions that may optimize continuation of a satisfactory sexual pattern. Guidelines for obtaining a brief sexual history include

1. Elicit information regarding degree of interest and physiologic function including
   a. Libido
   b. Ability to achieve and maintain an erection
   c. Ability to ejaculate
   d. Ability to experience orgasm
2. Allow expression of concerns via a technique of permission-granting general statements followed by individual specific questions regarding body image, intimacy, maintenance of work and family roles; for example, "some people report feeling tired and not interested in sexual activity; has this been the case with you?"
3. Review treatment-associated changes in physiologic function such as dry orgasms after removal of prostate and seminal vesicles, maintenance or loss of erectile functioning, and physical and physiologic changes associated with hormonal manipulation
4. Set the stage for continuing discussion by introducing general and specific recurring sexuality themes; general

themes are associated with age, sex, disease type, and treatment modalities, whereas specific sexuality concerns focus on the individual's perception of cancer and the impact of therapy on one's own life-style
5. Allow for the possibility of nontraditional partner and/or nontraditional expressions of sexuality

Masters and Johnson describe the physiologic changes of vasoconstriction and myotonia essential to the process of arousal and maintenance of physical capacity for sexual intercourse.[13] All treatment modalities for genitourinary malignancies can temporarily or permanently affect these physiological processes.

Specific disease sites, including bladder, prostate, testis, penis, and kidney, will be reviewed with particular emphasis on psychosexual concerns and necessary support.

BLADDER CANCER

Both males and females with a history of bladder cancer have undergone repetitive cystoscopies frequently accompanied by biopsies along with local therapies including transurethral resection, laser therapy, and instillation of anticarcinogens to prevent recurrences. The results from these procedures and interventions may include a decreased desire for intimate sexual experience. Some men report pain with erection or ejaculation and women may experience pain with intercourse. Additionally, the partners of individuals being treated for superficial bladder tumors may have concerns regarding tumor contagiousness. In this older population, cardiovascular disease and antihypertensive medication may impact on erectile status. In a series of 112 men interviewed prior to cystectomy, 35% reported at least mild erectile dysfunction unrelated to their cancer diagnoses and 20% were no longer sexually active with a partner. In the 73 men from the same series who provided follow-up data on sexual function after cystectomy, 50% remain sexually active, although 91% experienced some degree of erectile dysfunction. Intensity of orgasm was unchanged for 35%, reduced for 53%, and reported as more pleasurable for 11%. Twelve percent of the original sample, however, elected to have surgical implantation of a penile prosthesis.[14] Recent trends of bladder-preserving therapies for carcinoma of the bladder with intensive regimens of chemotherapy, radiotherapy, and local resection, as well as the newer surgical techniques of cavernous nerve-sparing cystoprostatectomy, address the overwhelming concern of sexuality and self-image especially in the potent and sexually active males.

Women undergoing radical cystectomy additionally have their ovaries, fallopian tubes, uterus, cervix, and anterior portion of the vaginal wall removed in order to get surgical margins completely free of tumor involvement. Oophorectomy decreases circulating estrogens, which, coupled with the anterior vaginal wall removal, decreases vaginal lubrication and flexibility. If the woman's postoperative expression of sexuality includes penile-vaginal intercourse, initial dyspareunia may be alleviated with a water-soluble vaginal lubricants or estrogen creams. As the pudendal nerve is not damaged in radical cystectomy, the orgasmic capacity is retained in both males and females.

PROSTATE CANCER

Therapeutic modalities for cancer of the prostate, including radical prostatectomy, transurethral resection, definitive radiotherapy, brachytherapy, and hormonal therapies such as orchiectomy, estrogens, progestins, medical or surgical adrenalectomy, hypothesectomy, and luteinizing hormone-releasing hormone antagonists/agonists all are accompanied by varying degrees of organic sexual dysfunction. Additionally, these therapies decrease or abrogate fertility. Generally speaking, this is not a compelling concern of the older man with prostate cancer. Historically, impotence has been a major complication of radical prostatectomy with 85 to 90% of men being incapable of sustaining an erection adequate for vaginal penetration postoperatively. With the new surgical technique popularized by Walsh, the cavernous nerves are spared allowing for preservation of the neural pathways required to maintain potency. Erectile dysfunction after external beam radiotherapy has been estimated to range from 22 to 84%. Interstitial irradiation is reported to have a more favorable side-effect profile as gauged by maintenance of erectile function. Goldstein hypothesized that radiotherapy accelerated arteriosclerotic changes in pelvic arteries thereby reducing blood flow to the penis.[15] Subsequent studies employing baseline and serial penile blood pressures and flow examinations have not sustained this hypothesis. Among the available hormonal therapies, the newer antiandrogen agents such as flutamide claim the distinct advantage of not interfering with sexual potency.

Patients with established iatrogenic impotence following treatment of cancer of the prostate may seek help and information from the urologist regarding their sexual dysfunction. Available therapeutic options include a whole spectrum of aids from constriction devices and pharmacologic erection programs employing self-injection of vasodilator substances such as papaverine, phentolamine, or prostaglandin, to the ultimate choice of a variety of rigid, mechanical, and inflatable penile prostheses. The physician should also bear in mind that many of these patients, by virtue of their age or secondary to therapy, may lose their libido and not be interested in coital sex. Instead of provocation or allurement of such patients into a quandary of irrational choices, the physician should carefully explore and inquire about, by a pragmatic as well as humane dialogue and discourse, their true needs.

TESTIS CANCER

Many of the patients successfully treated for testes tumors are interested in parenthood. The effects of therapy, including surgery, radiation, and chemotherapy, on fertility have been extensively addressed. In a prospective study of 41 patients prior to therapy, 77% were oligospermatic, 17% azoospermatic, and only 6.6% could meet the requirements for sperm banking.[16] In this same group of patients, 96% were azoospermic after 2 months of therapy. Retrospective review of a group of 28 patients indicated normal sperm counts in 46% of patients after chemotherapy.[16] Reviews also indicate that combination chemotherapy does affect fertility, rendering most patients azoospermic. However, a high degree of recovery of spermatogenesis is experienced after chemotherapy, usually within 2 to 3 years after initiation of therapy. This recovery, as measured by spermatogenesis, is indeed encouraging. Subsequent to successful pregnancy, no fetal abnormalities have occurred in the children of this group of patients. Treatment-specific correlations emerge, with men who have received radiotherapy to the retroperitoneum reporting higher rates of erectile dysfunction, difficulty reaching orgasm, and reduction in intensity of orgasm. The higher dose of irradiation to the periaortic field in men with seminoma was predictive of problems with erection and orgasm. Preservation of antegrade ejaculation is one of the principle reasons why several major centers no longer employ routine retroperitoneal lymphadenectomy for men with stage-I nonseminomatous tumors. In the event of recurrence, salvage chemotherapy can be successfully initiated in a satisfying percentage of these patients. Loss of seminal emission and/or retrograde ejaculation often result from damage to retroperitoneal sympathetic innervation following node dissection resulting in infertility. Modification of the retroperitoneal lymphadenectomy to preserve the sympathetic ganglia and preaortic plexus retains antegrade ejaculation in 45 to 81% of men. After standard bilateral retroperitoneal lymphadenectomy, 18% of men can be anticipated to recover antegrade ejaculation.

CANCER OF THE PENIS

In patients with cancer of the penis, the primary disease itself and the mutilating effects of various therapies can be devastating to self-image and sexuality. Because the majority of penile cancers occur distally on the penis, a functional phallus for the purpose of coitus and micturition in standing posture can often be achieved without vitiating adequate cancer excision. One should carefully plan for partial penectomy whenever feasible and if necessary combine it with a penile-lengthening procedure to gain extra length of the penile stump. A patient with an inadequate phallus after partial or total penectomy may be considered for phallic reconstruction for successful sexual rehabilitation.

RENAL CELL CANCER

Although the average age at diagnosis of a kidney cancer is 55, a number of younger patients are also encountered in clinical practice. The majority of patients with metastatic disease experience rapid progression; however, some patients do survive for long periods of time. The prognosis for metastatic kidney cancer is tempered by its lack of sensitivity to existing chemotherapy and radiation therapy programs. In the event the tumor is not amenable to complete surgical eradication, concerns of sexuality often are overlooked in the clinician's generalized view that a prolonged survival is unlikely. However, considerable emphasis may be placed on improving the quality of survival. As patients are well aware of the gradual nature of their declining process, offering unrealistic hope for a long-term survival is not prudent. However, the optimism surrounding the rapid advancements in the general field of biologic response modifiers may offer encouragement and hope for the individual faced with the challenge of living with metastatic renal cell carcinoma. Symptom control and promotion of intimacy may offer patients and their partners the opportunity to give and receive pleasure while communicating deeply with one another.

CONCLUSION

As all individuals are capable of deriving joy and satisfaction from everyday messages that are delivered through the senses, life is made infinitely more enjoyable through these messages, which are inherently sensual and often sexual. The urologist plays a pivotal role in supporting patients in the promotion and maintenance of a patient's healthy expression of sexuality.

"To the bee a flower is a fountain of life, And to the flower a bee is a messenger of love, And to both, bee and flower, the giving and receiving of pleasure is a need and an ecstasy."

—Kahlil Gibran

REFERENCES

1. Cassileth, B. R., and Steinfield, A. D. Psychological preparation of the patient and family. Cancer, 60:547, 1987.
2. Weisman, A. D., and Worden, J. W. The existential plight in cancer: The significance of the first 100 days. Int. J. Psychiatry Med., 7:1, 1976.
3. Schmale, A. H. Psychological reactions to recurrences, metastases, or disseminated cancer. Int. J. Radiat. Oncol. Biol. Phys., 1:1515, 1976.
4. Dansak, D. A. Psychiatric oncology. In: Genitourinary Cancer Surgery. Edited by E. D. Crawford and T. A. Borden. Philadelphia, Lea & Febiger, 1982, p. 517.
5. Havighurst, R. Developmental Tasks and Education. 3rd Ed. New York, David McKay Co., 1972.
6. Erikson, E., Ed. Adulthood. New York, W. W. Norton & Co., 1978.
7. Silverberg, E., and Lubera, J. A. Cancer statistics, 1989. CA, 39:3, 1989.
8. Sondik, E. J., et al. 1986 Annual Cancer Incidence Review. USPHS National Cancer Institute, NIH Publication No. 87-2789, 1987.
9. Kennedy, B. J. Aging and cancer. J. Clin. Oncol., 6:1903, 1988.
10. Yancik, R. Frame of reference: Old age as the context for prevention and treatment of cancer. In: Perspectives on the Screening and Treatment of Cancer in the Elderly. Edited by R. Yancik, et al. New York, Raven, 1983, p. 5.
11. Cornelius, D. A., et al. Who Cares? A Handbook on Sex Education and Counseling Services for Disabled People. Baltimore, University Park Press, 1982.
12. Moinpour, C. M., et al. Quality of life end points in cancer clinical trials: Review and recommendations. J. Natl. Cancer Inst., 81:485, 1989.
13. Masters, W. H., and Johnson, V. Sexual Response. Boston, Little, Brown, 1966.
14. Schover, L. R., Evans, R. B., and Von Eschenbach, A. C. Sexual rehabilitation and male radical cystectomy. J. Urol., 136:1015, 1986.
15. Goldstein, I., et al. Radiation-induced impotence: A clinical study of its mechanism. JAMA, 251:903, 1989.
16. Draga, R. E., et al. Fertility after chemotherapy for testicular cancer. J. Clin. Oncol., 1:37, 1983.

C H A P T E R
66

Supportive Care for the Patient with Terminal Genitourinary Cancer

S. L. Librach

Patients with advanced genitourinary cancer require a palliative and supportive approach to their care. It is often difficult to determine when a patient becomes "terminally ill." For those patients who have advanced genitourinary cancer, treatment with radiation and/or chemotherapy is usually palliative, i.e., not designed to cure but only to control disease and prolong life. Many of these patients have a steady downhill course leading to death. They are "dying" but not "terminal." Unfortunately, these patients are often deprived of adequate early supportive palliative care that could improve the quality of their life and that of their families. Such considerations for a palliative approach governed by considerations for quality of life may be forgotten in the pressure to prolong life and cure. Many studies have documented unmet psychosocial and physical needs of dying patients. This chapter reviews a comprehensive, supportive approach for patients with advanced and terminal cancer and their families, an approach best embodied by palliative or hospice care.

WHAT IS PALLIATIVE OR HOSPICE CARE

There is no universally accepted definition of palliative care or hospice care. A recent Canadian task force developed the following definition:

Palliative Care is a program of active compassionate care primarily directed towards improving the quality of life for the dying. It is delivered by an interdisciplinary team that provides sensitive and skilled care to meet the physical, psychosocial and spiritual needs of both patient and family.[15]

CARE FOR PHYSICAL NEEDS

Pain and Symptom Control

The patient with advanced genitourinary cancer will present a variety of physical symptoms for management. Pain and other symptoms need to have as high a priority for treatment as the disease itself. Many patients have died suffering needlessly from uncontrolled symptoms. Pain and many other symptoms can be controlled or at least ameliorated significantly if the physician takes an active and comprehensive approach.

GENERAL GUIDELINES. An adequate history is the important first step in attempting to control symptoms. The list of symptoms is often forgotten in the quest to obtain information about the tumor. The history of symptoms should be detailed, particularly in regard to pain because such a comprehensive history may provide significant clues to the cause of pain and, therefore, specific treatment. Other important symptoms such as constipation should not be dismissed as insignificant, because they often contribute greatly to patient suffering.

A pain history should cover the development of pain and the usual questions of location, radiation, quality, duration, severity, timing, and aggravating and relieving factors. The physician should also inquire about analgesic use, the effects and side effects of those medications, and the fears the patient and family have in regard to the pain and its treatment. Many cancer patients have more than one type of pain, and not all pain reported by cancer patients is directly related to the tumor. This is also the time to ensure that a psychosocial history is done, because psychosocial issues may be a factor in the expression and treatment of pain.

The assessment of pain remains an unclear area for many physicians. Failure to take into account the differences in the manifestations of acute and chronic pain, worry about addiction, and a variety of other biases lead to a mistrust in patient reports of pain. There is no direct way to measure pain. The best judge of a patient's pain is the patient.

PAIN CONTROL

The causes of pain in advanced genitourinary cancer. Table 66-1 lists the causes of pain in cancer in general.[1] These mechanisms all play a role in genitourinary cancers. Bone pain is, of course, a particular problem for prostatic cancer. Pelvic pain from invasive tumors is also quite common in advanced genitourinary cancer. This pain comes from sacral nerve root pressure and destruction, from invasion of soft tissues and from local bony invasion. Pelvic pain can be particularly resistant to treatment because of these multifactorial causes.

TABLE 66-1. *Causes of Pain in Cancer Patients*

CAUSED BY CANCER	RELATED TO CANCER
Bone infiltration, with or without muscle spasm	Muscle spasm
Nerve compression/infiltration	Constipation
Visceral involvement	Lymphedema
Soft tissue infiltration	Candidiasis
Ulceration, with or without infection	Herpetic neuralgia
Raised intracranial pressure	Deep-vein thrombosis pulmonary embolus

RELATED TO THERAPY	UNRELATED TO CANCER THERAPY
Postoperative acute pain	Musculoskeletal
Postoperative neuralgia	Headache
Phantom limb pain	Arthritis
Postradiation inflammation/fibrosis	Cardiovascular
Postradiation myelopathy	
Postchemotherapy neuropathy	
Bone necrosis	

From Scott.[1]

TABLE 66-2. *Nonopioid Analgesics*

Acetaminophen
Acetylsalicylic acid
NSAIDs

Pain is common in advanced cancer of any type. Approximately 65 to 85% of such patients in a number of studies were found to have pain.[2] Genitourinary cancers, particularly prostatic and renal cancers, have high incidences of pain.

Non-narcotic analgesics. Table 66-2 lists the most useful non-narcotic (non–opioid) analgesics. These drugs are appropriate for mild to moderate pain, but have little use in more severe pain unless there are specific indications for their use in combination with other drugs for conditions such as bone pain. Acetylsalicylic acid should be given in enteric-coated formats. Acetaminophen should be used in full doses of 1,000 mg every 4 hours. Both these agents are used in combinations with codeine but no added analgesic effect is seen above the base drug until 60 mg of codeine is added.

A variety of nonsteroidal anti-inflammatory drugs (NSAIDs) are available. All may have some analgesic effect but they are most useful as adjuncts in the treatment of pain due to bony metastases.

The Use of Opioids in the Treatment of Cancer Pain

Opioid drugs (also called narcotics or opiates) are the most effective drugs in relieving cancer pain. Unfortunately, the proper use of these analgesics is clouded by groundless fears and myths. Addiction is not a problem in cancer patients receiving opioids. Inadequate understanding of the origin and management of the predictable side effects of these agents also contributes to their underutilization and consequent undertreatment of pain. It is worthwhile to note that most pain suffered by cancer patients is severe pain and therefore treatment should begin with potent drugs except in circumstances where the patient says the pain is mild. The following section will describe a practical approach to the use of opioids.

GENERAL PRINCIPLES FOR THE USE OF OPIOIDS

Opioids and other analgesics are just one part of comprehensive pain-treatment plan. The term "total pain" has been used to describe the pain experience of cancer patients and others with chronic pain.[3] Pain and suffering involve many emotional, familial, spiritual, and cultural factors that need to be addressed by a multidisciplinary team. There should be no hesitation in involving others to help in addressing those needs.

Match the severity of the pain to the strength of the drug. There is little point in starting with weak drugs for severe pain. The stepped approach from weaker to stronger agents just leaves the patient suffering unnecessarily for a longer period of time. Do not persist in giving weak opioids if the pain is not rapidly controlled.

Give medication orally whenever possible. In most patients, opioids can be given orally to control pain. The physician must be aware of the parenteral to oral ratios as demonstrated in Tables 66-3 and 66-4, but the approach must be flexible.

Give medication regularly and never prn. Cancer pain, particularly severe pain, is constant, and such constant pain requires continuous around-the-clock administration of analgesics. The medication chosen should be given according to the duration of its analgesic effect. A double dose of the medication may be given at bedtime to avoid waking the patient in the middle of the night. This will not have any detrimental effect on the patient.

Anticipate and prevent side effects. Opioids have a number of frequent and predictable side effects. The best approach to these is a preventive one. Constipation is almost universal among patients who are on opioids. Nausea and associated vomiting will occur in up to 70% of patients on opioids, particularly when the medication is first administered or the dose is increasing. Treatment of these side effects is covered in "Other Symptoms." Sedation is the other common side effect, one that usually improves quickly on chronic administration of the opioid. The best treatment of this is to ignore it for the first few days. Respiratory depression, the most feared of potential side effects of opioids, is, in fact, rarely seen with appropriate oral regimens. Although many patients say they are allergic to opioids, true allergy is quite rare. Patients often interpret previous encounters with opioid side effects, such as nausea, as an "allergy."

Always leave an order for a "breakthrough" dose. The order for constant regular administration of an opioid should always be accompanied by a PRN "as required" dose to handle any uncontrolled pain. Monitoring of the number of breakthrough doses will indicate the need for an adjustment in the regular dose.

Explain what you are doing to patient and family and give them some control. Careful explanation to patient and family

TABLE 66-3. *Useful Weak Opioid Analgesics*

| DRUG | EQUIVALENT DOSE TO MORPHINE 10 mg s.c. | | ORAL DURATION OF ACTION |
	S.C.	PO	
Codeine	120 mg	200 mg	3–4 hours
Oxycodone*	n/a	10–15 mg	2–3 hours

*Available only in combination with acetylsalicylic acid or acetaminophen.

TABLE 66-4. *Useful Strong Opioid Analgesics*

| DRUG | EQUIVALENT DOSE TO MORPHINE 10 mg s.c. | | ORAL DURATION OF ACTION |
	S.C.	PO	
Morphine	10 mg	20–30 mg	3–4
Hydromorphone	2 mg	4 mg	3–4
Diamorphine (heroin)	6 mg	10–15 mg	3–4
Meperidine*	75 mg	300 mg	2–3
Anileridine	25 mg	75 mg	2–3
Methadone	10 mg	20 mg	6–8
Oxymorphone	1.5 mg	5 mg (supp)†	3–4
Levorphanol	2 mg	4 mg	4–6
Pentazocine*	60 mg	180 mg	3–4

*Not recommended for chronic pain or p.o. use.
†Available only in suppository form for nonparenteral use.

about the opioid medication, its purpose, effects, and side effects is important. This is also an opportunity to explore the patient and family's fears about taking "narcotics." Patients and families should be trusted to monitor medication use and response and be given a range of dosage over which they can exercise some control.

Be flexible. There is no one dose of medication that will suit all patients when it comes to treating severe pain with opioids. Fixed dosage limits will only promote uncontrolled pain. There, in fact, seems to be no firm upper limit to the amount of opioid required, and doses of morphine greater than 100 mg every 4 hours are common. A high dose is not an indicator of addiction.

Use adjuvant drugs and other pain-relieving modalities as appropriate. In bone pain, physicians should also consider the use of NSAIDs. Pain as a result of nerve compression and destruction may respond to corticosteroids or tricyclic antidepressants. These drugs are rarely effective alone and should be given with opioids. Radiotherapy and chemotherapy may also provide relief from pain but patients should be covered with opioids until those modalities have demonstrated effect. Hypnotherapy, relaxation therapy, and other modalities of pain control of that type are rarely effective when used alone but can be of value in combination with analgesic medication.

Monitor response to treatment frequently. Severe pain requires at least daily monitoring until pain is controlled. Pain diaries are useful to monitor response to analgesics, record doses, and list side effects.

The most appropriate parenteral route is the subcutaneous route. If parenteral opioids must be administered, use them subcutaneously and not intramuscularly. This is more comfortable for patients especially those who are quite cachectic. If long-term parenteral opioids are required, then constant subcutaneous infusion of opioids should be considered.

Do not be afraid to ask for help from palliative care consultants. For difficult pain problems or in cases where the physician is unsure of the use of particular analgesics, involve palliative care or pain consultants early on in the management of pain.

WEAK OPIOIDS. Table 66-3 lists the weak opioids and their appropriate dose ranges. Codeine is the drug of choice in this class because of the flexibility of its dosage forms. Oxycodone is available only in fixed combinations with acetaminophen or acetylsalicylic acid and it is no more effective than codeine. Dextropropoxyphene should not be used because of inconclusive evidence of its potency above placebo.

STRONG OPIOIDS. Table 66-4 lists the more potent opioids. Morphine is the gold standard and the drug of choice. Although other drugs such as hydromorphone and methadone are more potent on a milligram per milligram basis they are not in fact more effective. Long-acting, slow-release preparations of morphine are now available, and these reduce the need for longer acting drugs such as methadone.[4] Hydromorphone and diamorphine, if available, are the best choices for a parenteral agent if high doses are required. Meperidine (Demerol) is a good choice for patients in acute pain, for example, postoperative pain, but, it is a poor choice for chronic pain because of its poor oral absorption and short duration of action. Pentazocine also has limited usefulness because of poor oral absorption and frequent psychotomimetic side effects.

The initial oral dose of a potent opioid depends on the severity of the pain, the previous daily amount of parenteral opioid administered, and the cause of the pain. However, a usual starting dose of morphine in patients receiving as-required doses of opioids or patients who have not received potent opioids is 10 to 15 mg every 4 hours with a 5 mg breakthrough dose. The dose can be increased every 12 hours if necessary. The dose can be increased by 5 mg increments initially, but as the dose goes above 50 to 60 mg, increments of 10 mg are appropriate. Many patients will be controlled with doses of morphine less than 30 mg every 4 hours but there are patients, particularly those with nerve compression or destruction who will require much higher doses. Again, a flexible approach is required. Some adjustment of the dose may be required after the first 2 or 3 weeks to account for drug tolerance but many patients remain on a stable dose for a long time.

Morphine is available as an oral liquid in a variety of concentrations up to 100 mg/mL. This liquid is likely the preferred dosage form to begin with. Once the dose of morphine is stabilized, then a switch may be indicated to the long-acting, slow-release forms on a q12h or q8h basis. Some patients will prefer the immediate-release tablets to the oral liquid. Breakthrough doses should be in the immediate-release liquid or tablet form. Rectal suppositories are available as well, although there is limited flexibility in dosage. Sublingual preparations may be available shortly.

OPIOID-RESISTANT PAIN. Certain types of pain may be resistant to opioids. Pain resulting from nerve destruction and damage may not respond to opioids or may only respond to large doses of opioids. Such patients often require a combination of drugs and analgesic modalities as discussed later on in this chapter.

OTHER METHODS OF ADMINISTERING OPIOIDS. There are methods of controlling pain using opioids administered by a number of parenteral techniques. Continuous infusions of potent opioids by intravenous or subcutaneous route[5] and epidural administration[6] may have particular application in some patients.

Continuous intravenous infusions may be successful for short periods of time but resistance to this route often develops quickly. Such chronic intravenous therapy may preclude home care.

Continuous subcutaneous infusion is the best method of administering opioids parenterally. The advent of modern syringe drivers and pumps has made this technique more feasible. Continuous subcutaneous infusion of potent opioids may be indicated when there is complete bowel obstruction, dysphagia-limiting oral administration, uncontrolled opioid side effects such as nausea, the occurrence of bolus side effects seen in conjunction with peak serum levels with intermittent administration, the need for home care, overwhelming pain, and the need for large doses of oral analgesics. This method of administering opioids should be reserved for the above indications and not used indiscriminately for its high-tech approach.

The choice of opioid for continuous subcutaneous infusion relates to potency and solubility. Morphine is much less soluble than hydromorphone or diamorphine and therefore has limited use in this technique unless patients are on relatively small doses of morphine. Hydromorphone seems to be the preferred drug in North America because diamorphine is not readily available. In the UK, diamorphine seems to be the drug preferred because hydromorphone is not available. Longer acting drugs such as methadone are probably unsuitable for long-term infusions.

The patient, family and home-care nurses can be taught to monitor continuous subcutaneous infusion at home easily. Helpful teaching guides are available from infusion-device manufacturers and from cancer and palliative centers using this technique.

Epidural administration of opioids may be needed for pelvic pain that is resistant to large doses of analgesics.[6] The epidural catheter needs to be permanently implanted for best results. Resistance to epidural opioids may develop rapidly.

Use of Analgesic Adjuncts

There are a number of agents that can be used as adjuncts in the treatment of cancer pain. Bone pain from metastases should usually involve the use of NSAIDs unless there are contraindications to these agents. These drugs should be used at full dose.

The pain of nerve compression may respond to corticosteroids such as prednisone 20 to 60 mg per day or dexamethasone 4 to 16 mg daily.

The deafferentation pain of nerve destruction may respond to tricyclic antidepressants such as amitriptyline. These drugs have a constellation of frequent side effects, which may limit use. Small doses should be tried at first and the dose gradually increased until pain relief is improved or side effects intervene.

If anxiety and depression are thought to be factors in the production of pain, then psychotropic drugs such as the benzodiazepines, phenothiazines, and antidepressants may be used to supplement the effects of analgesics. Caution must be used in using these psychotropic drugs as substitutes for analgesics like opioids.

For the patient in overwhelming pain that does not respond to opioids well, high doses of dexamathasone up to 100 mg daily for 3 or 4 days may be effective in helping to control pain.

The Use of Other Modalities of Pain Control

Neurosurgical lysis of spinal cord pathways is best reserved for the patients with unilateral lower limb pain. Hypnosis and acupuncture are rarely effective for any length of time as sole measures. Hypnosis or relaxation techniques may be used as adjuncts in some patients with good effect. Transcutaneous electrical nerve stimulation can be effective particularly using the new types of stimulator, which stimulate a larger number of points randomly.[7]

Nerve blocks such as caudal blocks using neurolytic agents like phenol or alcohol may be helpful in patients with pelvic pain that is resistant to other measures.[8]

The use of radiation as a palliative treatment for pain should not be ignored. However, treatment with analgesics should be not be delayed and should be maintained until the full effect of the radiation is obtained. This may take more than 2 weeks.

Other Symptoms

CONSTIPATION. Constipation is a common symptom in patients who are terminally ill. There are a number of causes of constipation as outlined in Table 66-5. Untreated constipation may lead to other problems such as nausea and vomiting and may increase pain particularly if patients have to strain considerably. The approach to treatment of constipation depends to an extent on the cause.

TABLE 66-5. *Causes of Constipation*

General weakness and debility
Poor nutrition: decreased intake, low-fiber diet, and poor fluid intake
Medications: opioids, antidepressants, and many others
Metabolic: hypercalcemia, dehydration, and hypothyroidism
Intestinal obstruction

Dietary manipulation to include more fiber and fruits may be successful depending on the cause of the constipation. However, this regimen is rarely sufficient alone in patients because high-fiber diets may be unpalatable for ill and anorexic patients and because the mild peristaltic stimulation provided may not be sufficient to counteract the cause of the constipation. This is particularly true of opioid-induced constipation. Bulk-forming agents such as psyllium mucilloids may not be effective for similar reasons.

It is safe to make the assumption that every patient on opioids will develop constipation. This constipation usually requires the use of a combination of laxatives including

stool softener, e.g., docusate sodium 100 mg bid
stimulant laxatives, e.g., senna, cascara, or bisacodyl
osmotic agents, e.g., lactulose

The dose range for these agents in treating constipation induced by opioids is often considerably higher than normal. The aim should be for a bowel movement every 2 or 3 days. It is prudent to use suppositories or enemas if there is no movement after this time period. It may also be prudent to keep the stools of a patient with widespread cancer in the pelvis soft to prevent constipation, possible obstruction from fecal material, and increased pain.

NAUSEA AND VOMITING. The physician needs to understand both the physiology of nausea and vomiting as well as the cause of nausea and vomiting in patients with cancer. The vomiting center located in the reticular formation of the medulla close to the respiratory center receives input from gastrointestinal nervous system afferents, from the chemoreceptor trigger zone, from the cerebral cortex, and from the vestibular nucleus. The complex reflex that leads to vomiting may involve inputs from one or more of these sites.[8] The action of antiemetics also differs as to site of action and this must be taken into account. Table 66-6 lists the causes of nausea in patients with cancer.

For opioid-induced nausea, the best drugs are those that bind to dopamine receptor sites in the chemoreceptor trigger zone where opioids mainly act to produce nausea. Haloperidol, a butyrophenone drug, is particularly useful in such nausea. It can be given once daily orally in a dose up to 15 mg daily but most patients require only 1 or 2 mg daily. It is relatively free of side effects at these low dosages. Phenothiazine drugs such as prochlorperazine are also quite useful in opioid induced nausea. For prochlorperazine the dose is 5 to 10 mg

TABLE 66-6. *Causes of Nausea in Patients with Cancer*

Other treatment
    Radiation
    Chemotherapy
Abdominal cancer
    Gastric cancer
    Hepatic enlargement
    Involvement of celiac axis plexus
    Diffuse abdominal carcinomatosis
    Intestinal obstruction
Drugs
    Opioids
    NSAIDs
    Other drugs
Constipation
Metabolic
    Renal failure
    Other metabolic imbalances

---

every 4 to 6 hours. In the higher dose ranges there may be considerable sedation and extrapyramidal side effects may limit use. Chlorpromazine in a dose of 25 mg every 4 to 6 hours may also be effective.

Antihistamine drugs, such as dimenhydrinate, that act on the vomiting center have little use in opioid-induced nausea despite the popularity of use of these drugs. They may be effective if there is a distinct but uncommon vestibular component of the nausea but they should not be used routinely.

Opioids and the cancer itself may induce gastric and bowel hypomotility leading to nausea and vomiting. If this is suspected, drugs such as metochlopramide and domperidone that stimulate gastric emptying and bowel motility are useful. Domperidone in a dose of 10 to 30 mg 4 times a day is probably the drug of choice because of a more favorable side effect profile as compared to metochlopramide.

If patients have overwhelming nausea and the cause is not evident or resistant to usual therapy, then dexamethasone in a dose of 16 to 60 mg daily for 3 or 4 days may be useful.

If the cause of nausea and vomiting is from bowel obstruction as it may be in patient with pelvic and abdominal disease from genitourinary cancer, then therapeutic options must be carefully considered. Surgery should still be considered as the first option if the patient's general condition warrants this. Long-term use of nasogastric suction and intravenous fluids beyond 2 weeks should be avoided because of the discomfort to the patient. If the patient is close to death, treatment should be aimed at the use of opioids and antispasmodics to reduce pain, the use of antiemetics to reduce nausea, and the tolerance of 2 or 3 episodes of vomiting without panic by patient, family, or staff. The patient and family as well as nursing staff require considerable support and education if this latter approach is used. In some cases obstruction may be intermittent

in nature and simple measures as described above may be all that is needed.

ANOREXIA AND CACHEXIA. Many patients with advanced cancer have anorexia and cachexia.[9] Certainly as the disease progresses toward its terminal phase these symptoms become almost universal. Anorexia is distressing to patient, family, and staff because of the symbolic importance of food and eating to us all. "If only he would eat, he would feel better" is a common complaint. Patients with cancer develop anorexia and cachexia for a number of complex and interrelated factors related to the cancer itself, related to the cancer treatment, and related to the psychological impact of cancer on the patient.

Expensive, commercial nutritional supplements are often promoted as the answer to anorexia and cachexia, but there is in fact little evidence to support their extensive use. The use of small frequent feedings that cater to the patient's food preferences and that make use of high-calorie foods may be enough to maintain caloric intake at a reasonable level. Prednisone at a dose of 15 to 20 mg daily may help to stimulate appetite. Careful counseling and support of the patient, family, and health-care staff may help to minimize unnecessary pressure on the patient.

When the patient stops taking oral fluids, there is always a temptation to start intravenous therapy so that the patient does not become dehydrated. Dehydration by itself is not terribly uncomfortable as long as mouth care is rigorous. Intravenous therapy provides no nutrients of any significance and may be prolonging suffering rather than helping to prevent it. Patients and families need to be counseled and supported appropriately if the decision is made not to start intravenous therapy.

DRY AND SORE MOUTH. A dry and sore mouth is a relatively common symptom which is often multifactorial. It may be caused by decreased fluid intake; by drug side effects from agents such as opioids, anticholinergics, and antidepressants; by chemotherapeutic agents; and by a variety of infections. Oral candidiasis is a commonly overlooked infection. It rarely presents with the classic findings of the thrush seen in infants but often presents as generalized hyperemia. Candidiasis will respond to oral nystatin administered as a mouth rinse or in stubborn cases it will respond to a short 1-week course of ketoconazole. In patients with dry and sore mouths, mouthwashes containing alcohol (most commercial mouthwashes) should be avoided. Frequent mouth cleansing with aqueous solutions containing salt and sodium bicarbonate are effective and much less irritating.

OTHER SYMPTOMS. There are many other symptoms that can be problematic for the patient with advanced genitourinary cancer. A number of references are available for further information.[10–13]

CARE FOR PSYCHOLOGICAL NEEDS

Patients with advanced cancer and their families have psycho-social needs that must be addressed. Patients and families should be assessed early on in the course of the illness by the multidisciplinary team. Such assessment is not only important as a prelude to supporting persons who are undergoing tremendous stress and suffering but also important to help physicians plan for care appropriately.

Dying patients and their families present a host of emotional reactions including sadness, guilt, anger, and anxiety. Families require help from understanding health-care professionals who can help mobilize the family's own resources to deal with this time of crisis and loss and who can provide continuing support. Such support is critical to the task of improving the quality of the remaining life for the patient. The physician should be able to provide such support at times but most surgeons usually rely on their colleagues in other professions such as social work and psychology to provide such support. The family physician should not be forgotten as an important resource in managing patients and families. Dying is not a psychiatric illness and psychiatric consultation for such patients should be reserved for those patients and families with serious dysfunction.

Although psychotropic agents such as anxiolytics and antidepressants can be useful in managing psychological distress, they should be used as adjuncts to adequate support and counseling provided by knowledgeable care givers.

The unit of care in palliative care is the family. Support can be provided to family members on an individual basis as needed but emphasis should be placed on working with the family. The patient and family must have sufficient information about the illness in order to cope with the tasks engendered by this life crisis. Truth telling is important but the truth must be communicated with sensitivity and with repetition so that the patient and family understand clearly what is happening. The patient and family have an absolute right to participate in decision making around the illness. The onus is on the physician to present information clearly and honestly and to avoid pressuring the patient unnecessarily to accept suggested treatment. The patient and family should be given time to make decisions because few treatment options can be considered emergency situations.

Patients with genitourinary cancers may be very susceptible to psychological problems induced by altered body and self-image and loss of function.[14] All surgical and chemotherapeutic procedures in patients with genitourinary cancer should be explained carefully and fully to the patient and then to the family. Sensitive areas of urinary function, disfigurement, or loss of sexual organs and sexuality should be sensitively and confidentially probed by the physician and other team members.

In patients with genitourinary cancers, sexuality is a topic that must be raised with patients and their partners. Sexual counseling of these patients requires adequate knowledge and sensitivity. Many of the surgical and hormonal treatments may be detrimental to sexual functioning. Patients must be informed that there are options available to them regarding sexual functioning and fulfillment that extend beyond the act of intercourse. Care should be taken to involve the usual sexual partner in the counseling. One should also avoid assuming that the elderly patient is not interested in sexual functioning.

After the patient dies, the family may require assessment and support during the period of bereavement. Families should be clearly informed of the resources available for such support.

Care for Social Needs

Dying patients and their families also present with a variety of social needs that require exploration. The physician should ensure that these needs are adequately explored by social workers on the team.

Care for Spiritual Needs

In facing the crisis of dying, all patients and families will have spiritual concerns and needs. Religious issues are not the same as spiritual issues. Although patients and their families may profess that religion is not important to them, they may have significant spiritual questions about the meaning and purpose of life and death. These concerns can best be dealt with by clergymen who have special training and expertise. Spiritual support must be individualized and recognize differences in faith and culture. Physicians need to be aware of this important area and ensure that spiritual counseling is available to their patients.

Care at Home

A cornerstone of palliative care is home care. Patients have a need and a right to be maintained at home as long as possible. Home care requires a dedicated multidisciplinary team with a flexible approach and 24-hour service. The aim is to keep patients at home as long as possible and to allow patients to die at home if this is their wish. Often patients are maintained in hospitals far too long because adequate consideration has not been given to home care. Community-based palliative care or hospice programs can provide this home-care expertise. The patient's family physician should play a key role in the home management.

CONCLUSION

All patients with advanced genitourinary cancer should receive multidisciplinary care that emphasizes the quality of life. Control of pain and other symptoms is of prime importance if this goal is to be achieved. The physician also needs to be aware of the variety of psychosocial and spiritual needs of patients and families and to ensure appropriate treatment so that patients can live and die with support, love, and dignity.

REFERENCES

1. SCOTT, J. F. *Cancer Pain: A Monograph on the Management of Cancer Pain.* Health and Welfare Canada, Ottawa, Canada, 1984.

2. TWYCROSS, R. G., and LACK, S. A. *Symptom Control in Advanced Cancer: Pain Relief.* London: Pitman, 1983, p. 3.

3. SAUNDERS, C. M. *The Management of Terminal Disease.* London: Edward-Arnold, 1978, p. 193.

4. KHOJASTEH, A., et al. Controlled release oral morphine sulphate in the treatment of cancer pain with pharmacokinetic correlation. J. Clin. Oncol., 5:956, 1987.

5. PORTNOY, R. Continuous infusion of opioid drugs in the treatment of cancer pain. J. Pain Symptom Control, 1:223, 1986.

6. SHETTER, A. G., et al. Administration of intraspinal morphine sulfate for the treatment of intractable cancer pain. Neurosurgery, 18:740, 1986.

7. LIBRACH, S. L., and RAPSON, L. TENS: Its role in palliative care. Palliative Med., 2:15, 1988.

8. FERRER-BRECHNER, T. Anesthetic management of cancer pain. Semin. Oncol., 12:431, 1985.

9. DEWYS, W. Management of cancer cachexia. Semin. Oncol., 12:452, 1985.

10. DOYLE, D., Ed. *Palliative Care: The Management of Far-Advanced Illness.* Philadelphia: The Charles Press, 1984.

11. LEVY, M., and CATALANO, R. B. Control of common physical symptoms other than pain in patients with terminal disease. Semin. Oncol., 12:411, 1985.

12. LEVY, M. Pain management in advanced cancer. Semin. Oncol., 12:394, 1985.

13. TWYCROSS, R. G., and LACK, S. A. *Control of Alimentary Symptoms in Far Advanced Cancer.* New York: Churchill Livingstone, 1986.

14. MOUNT, B. M. Psychological impact of urologic cancer. Cancer, 45:223, 1980.

15. Report of the Subcommittee on Institutional Programme Guidelines for Establishing Standards; Palliative Care Services. Health and Welfare Canada. Ottawa, Canada, 1989.

retroperitoneal tumors and, 129
testicular carcinoma and, 309–310, 316, 319,
    342, 348, 457, 519, 520, 563–564
See also Monoclonal antibody; Tumor
    markers
HVA. *See* Homovanillic acid
Hydrocortisone, androgen inhibition and, 502
Hydromorphone, for pain, 677t, 678
Hydronephrosis:
    bladder carcinoma and, 217, 222, 226
    as complication from radiation therapy, 539
    compromising of kidney by, 51
    Indiana continent reservoir urinary diversion
        and, 290
    inoperable carcinoma and, 617
    pediatric, diagnosis of carcinoma and, 402
    renal pelvic carcinoma and, 89
    ureterosigmoidostomy and, 263
Hydroureteronephrosis:
    bladder carcinoma and, 222
    distal ureterectomy and, 112
11-Hydroxylation, Cushing's syndrome and, 10
17-Hydroxyprogesterone, virilizing tumors and,
    10
Hydroxyurea:
    for cervical carcinoma, 630
    for prostatic carcinoma, 461t, 508t, 509, 509t
    for metastatic renal cell carcinoma, 471t,
        472t
Hyperaldosteronism:
    computerized tomography for, 583
    secretory adrenal cortical adenomas and, 10
Hypercalcemia:
    complications from, 666–667
    renal cell carcinoma and, 23, 26
    upper urinary tract carcinoma and, 117
Hyperchloremic acidosis:
    characteristics of, 667
    as complication from female pelvic
        exenteration, 630
    following ureterosigmoidostomy, 258, 259,
        263
    Indiana continent reservoir urinary diversion
        and, 291
Hyperkalemia:
    causes of, 665
    characteristics of, 665
    prevention of, 666
    surgery for aldosteronism and, 13
    treatment for, 665
Hypernatremia:
    aldosteronism and, 8
    causes of, 665
    treatment for, 665
Hyperparathyroidism, primary, familial
    pheochromocytoma and, 12
Hyperplasia:
    adrenal, virilizing tumors and, 10
    benign prostatic (BPH). *See* Benign prostatic
        hyperplasia
    renal tubular, renal cell carcinoma and, 22
    of zona glomerulosa cells, aldosteronism
        and, 8
Hypertension:
    aldosteronism and, 8, 11
    Cushing's syndrome and, 9
    neuroblastoma and, 404, 417
    pheochromocytoma and, 11
    renal cell carcinoma and, 23
    ureteral carcinoma and, 107
    Wilms' tumor and, 440
Hyperthyroidism, examination for, in presurgical
    medical evaluation, 657
Hypervolemia:
    aldosteronism and, 8

retroperitoneal lymphadenectomy and, 332
Hypnosis, for pain, 677, 679
Hypoalbuminemia, cancer patients and, 661
Hypocalcemia:
    characteristics of, 665
    treatment for, 665
Hypokalemia:
    aldosteronism and, 8
    treatment for, 665
Hyponatremia:
    characteristics of, 665, 667
    corticosteroids and, 13
    examination for, in presurgical medical
        evaluation, 657
    treatment for, 665
Hypophysectomy, for metastatic prostatic
    carcinoma, 500, 503
Hypotension:
    as complication from,
        adoptive immunotherapy, 474
        aminoglutethimide, 503
        bacillus Calmette-Guérin, 482
        corticosteroids, 13
        retroperitoneal lymphadenectomy and, 332
        surgery for pheochromocytoma and, 18, 19
Hypothermia:
    during partial nephrectomy, renal
        preservation and, 54–55, 56, *56*
    vena caval extension of renal cell carcinoma
        and, 83–84
Hypoxanthine, levels of, renal preservation and,
    55
Hypoxia, of tumor cells, radiobiology and, 533

^{125}I. *See* Iodine-125
^{192}Ir. *See* Iridium-192
Ifosfamide:
    for metastatic renal cell carcinoma, 471t
    for testicular carcinoma, 458, 459
    for Wilms' tumor, 527
Ileal interposition, ureteral carcinoma and, 107
Ileal reservoir, without valve urinary diversion,
    298–299, *299*
Ileocecal reservoir, without valve urinary
    diversion, 301–302
Ileocecal segment, bladder substitution using,
    299–302, *300, 301, 302*
Ileocolonic pouch (Le Bag) urinary diversion,
    302, *302*
    female pelvic exenteration and, 624
Ileocolostomy, Indiana continent reservoir
    cutaneous diversion and, 284–287,
    285, 286, 287
Ileostomy, in radical cystectomy, 236. *See also*
    Urinary diversion, ileal conduit
Ileum:
    ileal conduit urinary diversion, 265–271, *266,
        267, 268, 269, 270, 271, 272*
    Kock pouch cutaneous urinary diversion and,
        276–279, *276, 277, 278, 279, 280*
Imidazolecarboxamide, for rhabdomyosarcoma,
    404
Imipramine, to control urination, 258
Immunotherapy:
    active, 477–478, 478t, 488
        bacillus Calmette-Guérin (BCG), 477, 478–
            483, 479t, 480t, 481t
        interferon, 463, 463t, 471–473, 473t, 484–
            485, 486t, 487–488
        interleukin-2, 477, 483–484
        keyhole-limpet hemocyanin, 477, 483
        maltose tetrapalmitate, 477, 487
        OK-432, 487
        pyrimidinones, 488

tumor necrosis factor (TNF), 477, 486–487
adoptive, 473–474, 474t
    for bladder carcinoma, 477, 478–484, 479t,
        480t, 481t, 484–488, 486t
    passive, 477–478, 478t
        interleukin-2, 477, 483–484
        monoclonal antibody (Mab), 487
    for renal cell carcinoma, 463, 463t, 471–474,
        473t, 474t
Impotence:
    as complication from,
        hormonal therapy, 501, 502
        radiation therapy, 155
        radical prostatectomy, 154, 171
    treatment for prostatic carcinoma and, 673
    See also Sexual function
Incontinence:
    following radical prostatectomy, 154
    following total perineal prostatectomy, 199
    ileocolonic pouch urinary diversion and, 302
    Khafagy modified ileocecal cystoplasty urinary
        diversion and, 300
Indiana continent reservoir cutaneous urinary
    diversion:
    conversion from ileal conduit urinary
        diversion, 290
    ileal conduit urinary diversion versus, 287–
        288
    patient selection for, 287–288, 290
    postoperative care for, 290–291
    preoperative preparation for, 290
    results of, 285
    surgical technique for, 284–287, *285, 286,
        287, 288, 289, 290*
Indigo carmine:
    in partial nephrectomy, 58–59, *59, 60, 61*
    in total perineal prostatectomy, 197–198
Inferior vena cavography:
    for renal cell carcinoma, 72, *73,* 588
    for retroperitoneal tumors, 129, *137*
    for Wilms' tumor, 440
Insulin, sensitivity to, 660–661
Interferon therapy:
    for bladder carcinoma, 477, 484–485, 486t,
        487–488
        interleukin-2 and, 484
    for renal cell carcinoma, 463, 463t, 471–473,
        473t
    side effects of, 472
Intergroup Rhabdomyosarcoma Study (IRS),
    445, 446, 447, 448
Interleukin, metastatic renal cell carcinoma and,
    26
Interleukin-2:
    for bladder carcinoma, 477, 483–484
    interferon therapy and, 484
    See also Cytokines; Lymphokine-activated
        killer (LAK) cells
Internal iliac nodes, in lymphatic drainage from
    prostate, 164, *164*
Interstitial irradiation. *See* Irradiation, interstitial
Intestinal surgery:
    anatomical considerations for, 631–632, 633t,
        634, 635
    bowel resection and, 636–637, *638–639,
        640, 642, 643*
    colostomy and, 637, *641*
    complications from, 633–635
    gastrostomy and, 637, *644,* 645
    inadvertent enterotomy and, 635–636, *636*
    needle-catheter jejunostomy and, *644,* 645
    preoperative management for, 633
    staple techniques for, 637, *642, 643*
    technique for, 635–637, *636, 638, 639, 640,
        641, 642, 643, 644, 645*

complications with, 331t, 340–341
dissection between great vessels in, 335–338, *340, 341, 342, 343, 344*
fertility and, 347–349, *348*
historical perspectives on, 328–330, *330*
margins of dissection in, 331, *332,* 333, 335, *339*
morbidity and mortality following, 331t
nerve-sparing,
anterior transabdominal incision for, 349, *349*
bilateral and suprahilar, 355, *355*
closure for, 356
dissection boundaries for, 347–348, *348*
left-sided, 354, *354, 355*
patient evaluation for, 348
postoperative care for, 356
preoperative preparation for, 348–349
right-sided, 349–354, *351, 352, 353, 354*
surgical technique for, 349–355, *349, 350, 351, 352, 353, 354, 355*
orchiectomy and, 330
for paratesticular rhabdomyosarcoma, 448
peritoneal mobilization in, 333, 337, *338, 339*
position for, 333, *334*
postoperative care following, 339–340
preoperative preparation for, 332
rationale for, 328, 330–331, 331t
surgical technique for, 332–333, *334,* 335–338, *335, 336, 337, 338, 339, 340, 341, 342, 343, 344*
thoracoabdominal incision for, 331, 333, *335, 336*
for Wilms' tumor, 441
for ureteral carcinoma, 94
for urethral carcinoma, 391
Lymphangiogram, high PSA levels and, 553
Lymphangiography:
accuracy of, 565
for bladder carcinoma, 595
for metastatic penile carcinoma, 374
pedal, for pelvic lymph nodes, 163
for prostatic carcinoma, 152, 596
for retroperitoneal tumors, 129, *598*
for testicular carcinoma, 311, 313, 597
for urethral carcinoma, 363, 395, 597, 599
Lymphangioma, cystic, pediatric testicular carcinoma and, 434t, 435
Lymphedema, as complication from:
female pelvic exenteration, 630
ilioinguinal lymphadenectomy, 361
inguinal lymphadenectomy, 379
radiation therapy, 155
Lymphocysts, as complication from female pelvic exenteration, 630
Lymphokine-activated killer (LAK) cells, interleukin-2 stimulation of, 463–464, 483–484
Lymphoma:
interferon therapy for, 485
pediatric testicular carcinoma and, 433
Lyphadenectomy, retroperitoneal, chemotherapy and, 522

Magnesium, renal dysfunction and, 665
Magnetic resonance imaging (MRI):
for adrenal tumors, 582, 583, 584, 585
for bladder carcinoma, 235, 594, 596
for bone metastases, 576
for endometrial carcinoma, 599–600
for female pelvic carcinoma, 617
following female pelvic exenteration, 630
FLASH pulse sequence, 71

GRASS pulse sequence, 71
for neuroblastoma, 404, 417, *418,* 419, 423
for pediatric carcinoma, 403
for pelvic lymph nodes, 163
for prostatic carcinoma, 152, 153, 553, 556, 596, 597, 608
for renal cell carcinoma, 23, *24,* 45, 53, 54, 71, *71, 72,* 586, *587,* 588, *591*
for retroperitoneal tumors, 129, *133*
for spinal cord compression, 577
for testicular carcinoma, 597
for urethral carcinoma, 383, 384, *386,* 391, 395, *396*
for uterine carcinoma, 599, *600*
for vaginal tumors, 599
for Wilms' tumor, 403
Mainz pouch cutaneous urinary diversion, *292, 293,* 300–301, *301*
Malnutrition:
consideration of, in presurgical medical evaluation, 658
indices of, 661t
See also Metabolism; Nutrition
Maltose tetrapalmitate, for bladder carcinoma, 477, 487
Mammalgia, radiation therapy for, 579
Mannitol:
in partial nephrectomy, 54, 56, 58, 60
renal function and, 54, 55, 666
in retroperitoneal lymphadenectomy, 335, 340
Marcaine. *See* Bupivacaine hydrochloride
Meatotomy, penile carcinoma and, 359
Meconium peritonitis, pediatric testicular carcinoma and, 434t, 435
Mediastinal tumors, pediatric, surgery for, 422
Medical evaluation, presurgical:
cardiovascular system assessed in, 654–656, 655t
electrolytes assessed in, 656–657
endocrine system assessed in, 657
hemostatic considerations in, 658
liver assessed in, 657–658, 657t
nutritional status assessed in, 658
purpose of, 654
renal function assessed in, 656–657
respiratory system assessed in, 656
special considerations in, 658
Medroxyprogesterone, for renal cell carcinoma, 462
Medroxyprogesterone acetate, for metastatic renal cell carcinoma, 26, 470, 471, 473t
Medullary thyroid carcinoma, familial pheochromocytoma and, 12
Medulloblastoma, tumor cell markers for, 414
Megestrol acetate (Megace), for prostatic carcinoma, 461t, 501, 503
Meglumine diatrizoate (Gastrografin) contrast study, for bowel obstruction, 634–635
Melanoma, malignant, interferon therapy for, 485
Melphalan (L-PAM), for neuroblastoma, 425, 425t
Meperidine, for pain, in cancer patients, 677t, 678
Metabolism:
abnormalities in, 664–666, 667
of carbohydrates, 660–661
changes in, 660–661
of lipids, 661
of protein, 661
See also Malnutrition; Nutrition
Metaiodobenzylguanidine (MIBG):
for detection of adrenal tumors, 584
for pediatric carcinoma, 403

pheochromocytoma and, 11, 12
for radioisotope scan, 418–419, *418,* 426
Metanephrine(s), in urine, pheochromocytoma and, 11
Methadone, for pain, 677t, 678
Methotrexate (leucovorin):
for bladder carcinoma, 165–166, 219, 453, 453t, 454, 455t, 494, 494t, 495, 496
for metastatic renal cell carcinoma, 472t
for penile carcinoma, 361
for prostatic carcinoma, 157, 461, 461t, 508t, 509t, 510t
for retroperitoneal tumors, 138
for rhabdomyosarcoma, 444
for urethral carcinoma, 391, 392
See also CMV; MVAC
Methyl CCNU:
for metastatic renal cell carcinoma, 470, 471t, 472t
retroperitoneal tumors and, 138
Methylprednisolone acetate, for metastatic renal cell carcinoma, 472t
Metochlopramide, for nausea, 680
Metronidazole, for patient preparation, in radical nephrectomy, 46
Metyrapone, Cushing's syndrome and, 10
Metyrapone stimulation test, Cushing's disease and, 10
MIBG. *See* Metaiodobenzalquanadine
Micturition:
pheochromocytoma and, 11
urethral carcinoma and, 362
Mineralocorticoids, surgery for aldosteronism and, 13
Mini-VAB (vinblastine, actinomycin-D, and bleomycin), for testicular carcinoma, 313
Mitomycin C:
for bladder carcinoma, 218, 226, 479, 480t, 483, 494, 495, 496, 535
for metastatic prostatic carcinoma, 508t, 510t
side effects of, 227
for upper urinary tract carcinoma, 121
for ureteral carcinoma, 113
for urethral carcinoma, 397
Mitosis-karyorrhexis index (MKI), histology of neuroblastoma and, *412,* 413
Moh's micrographic surgical technique, for penile carcinoma, 361, 369
Monoclonal antibody (Mab), for bladder carcinoma, 487. *See also* Tumor markers
Morphine:
catecholamine release by, pheochromocytoma and, 11
for pain, 677t, 678
Motility, as function of intestinal tract, 632
Mouth, control of dryness and soreness in, with cancer patients, 680
MRI. *See* Magnetic resonance imaging
Mucositis, as side effect of chemotherapy, 495
Multiple endocrine adenomatosis type I (MEA-I), familial pheochromocytoma and, 12
Multiple endocrine adenomatosis type II (MEA-II), familial pheochromocytoma and, 12
MVAC (methotrexate, vinblastine, adriamycin, and cisplatinum):
for bladder carcinoma, 165–166, 219, 454, 455, 455t, 495, 497
for urethral carcinoma, 391
Myasthenia, neuroblastoma and, 417
Mycobacterium bovis, production of bacillus Calmette-Guérin and, 478

Myelography:
    for bone metastases, 576
    for spinal cord compression, 577, *578*
Myelosuppression, as side effect of
        chemotherapy, 227, 495, 535
Myocardial revascularization, for class III or IV
        angina, 655
Myoclonus-opsoclonus syndrome,
        neuroblastoma and, 417

N-myc oncogene, prognosis of neuroblastoma
        and, 413–414, 413t
Nafoxidine, for metastatic renal cell carcinoma,
        470t
Naphtylamine, urinary tract carcinoma and, 88,
        116
Narcotics. *See* Opiates; Pain
National Wilms' Tumor Study-4 (NWTS-4), 527–
        528, 529
Nausea, control of, 679–680, 680t
Nd.:YAG laser. *See* Laser, neodymium:YAG
NE. *See* Norephinephrine
Neck tumors, pediatric, surgery for, 422
Neoloid, for patient preparation:
    in female pelvic exenteration, 617
    in radical cystectomy, 236, 249
    in surgery for Kock pouch cutaneous urinary
        diversion, 275
Neomycin:
    ileal conduit urinary diversion and, 264
    intestinal surgery and, 633
    Kock pouch cutaneous urinary diversion and,
        275
    radical cystectomy and, 236, 249
    radical nephrectomy and, 46
Neovagina:
    gracilis myocutaneous, female pelvic
        exenteration and, 626, *626, 627, 628*
    skin graft, female pelvic exenteration
        and, 624, *625*
Nephrectomy:
    adjuvant, metastatic renal cell carcinoma and,
        26
    bilateral, incision for, 30
    control of hemorrhaging during, 650
    historical perspectives on, 29, 39–40
    metastatic renal cell carcinoma and, 470
    palliative, for renal cell carcinoma, 26, 33, 40
    partial,
        for compromised contralateral kidney
            patients, 51–52
        for diagnostic purposes, 52–53
        extracorporeal, 56–57
            autotransplantation and, 64–66, *66*
            rationale for, 64
            technique for, 64–65
        historical perspectives on, 50
        in situ, 57–64, *57, 58, 59, 60, 61, 62, 63*
            closure for, 64
            incision for, 57–58
            kidney reconstruction following, 59–60,
                61, 62, 63, 64, 65
            renal preservation for, 58
            surgical principles for, 57, *57*
            technique for, 58–60, *58, 59, 60, 61,* 62,
                62, 63, 64
        incision for, 39
        indications for, 51–53
        non-cancer indications for, 53
        postoperative problems with, 66–67
        preoperative preparation for, 54
        prognosis for, 51

    radical nephrectomy versus, 24, 30, 53
    renal ischemia and, 54–56
    renal preservation and, 51, 54–57
    for simultaneous bilateral renal cell
        carcinoma, 26
    for transitional cell tumor patients, 52
    for Wilms' tumor, 52
    radical,
        for adrenal neuroblastoma, 405
        anterior transabdominal approach for, 45–
            49, *46, 47, 48, 49*
            lymphadenectomy and, 48
            vena caval extension and, 48
        anterior transperitoneal approach, rationale
            for, 29–30
        eleventh-rib supracostal extrapleural
            transperitoneal, 30, *30*
        following supradiaphragmatic-
            intrapericardial surgery, 80
        localized renal cell carcinoma and, 24
        rationale for, 30
        simple/partial nephrectomy versus, 24, 30,
            53
        for simultaneous bilateral renal cell
            carcinoma, 26
        in solitary kidney, incision for, 30, *31*
        surgical objectives of, 29–30
        tenth-intercostal-space approach, rationale
            for, 30
        thoracoabdominal extrapleural approach
            for, 29–38, *30, 31, 32, 33, 34, 35, 36,
            37, 38*
            left radical nephrectomy in, 31–34, *31,
                32, 33, 34, 35, 36*
            right radical nephrectomy in, 34, 37, *37,
                38*
        thoracoabdominal intrapleural approach for,
            39–44, *41, 42, 43, 44*
            rationale for, 29–30, 39
        for Wilms' tumor, 403, 441
    in radical nephroureterectomy, 101
    for renal pelvic carcinoma, 91, 97
    for ureteral carcinoma, 94, 97
Nephroblastoma. *See* Wilms' tumor
Nephroma, pediatric congenital mesoblastic,
        402
Nephrostolithotomy, defined, 120
Nephrostomy, percutaneous:
    complications following, 121
    future perspectives for, 121, 123
    indications for, 120
    patient selection for, 120
    postoperative care for, 121
    technique for, 120–121, *122*
Nephrotomography, for renal cell carcinoma,
        23, 585
Nephroureterectomy:
    incision for, 39
    for pediatric ureteral carcinoma, 403
    radical, 97–103
        adrenalectomy in, 101
        closure in, 102–103
        distal ureterectomy versus, 106–107
        history of, 98
        incision in, 98–99, *98, 99*
        nephrectomy in, 101
        postoperative care for, 103
        preoperative preparation for, 98
        rationale for, 97–98
        renal pedicle controlled in, 99–101, *100,
            101*
        upper ureterectomy in, 101
        ureteral dissection in, 101–102, *101, 102,
            103*

    rationale for, 106
    for upper urinary tract transitional cell
        carcinoma, 52
    for ureteral carcinoma, 94
    Wilms' tumor and, 440
Nephroureteroscopy:
    defined, 120
    for renal pelvic carcinoma, 91–92
Nerves:
    blocking of, for pain, 679
    stimulation of, for pain, 679
Neuroblastoma:
    adrenal, 9t, 12
        radical nephrectomy for, 405
    chemotherapy for, 424–426, 425t, 426t
    chromosome analysis and, 413–414, 413t
    diagnosis of, 404, 417, *418,* 419–420, *419*
    diagnostic imaging of, 601–602
    hematologic studies for, 420
    histology of, 412–413, *412,* 426t
    incidence of, 407
    intraspinous extension of, 423
    late stages of, treatment for, 423–424
    locations of, 404, 407, 409, 409t
    metastases from, 410–411, 416–417, 434t,
        435, 602
    olfactory, catecholamine excretion and, 407
    as pediatric carcinoma, 402
    prognosis for, 404
    radiation therapy for, 426, 426t
    resectability of, 412
    spontaneous regression of, 408–409
    staging of, 404–405, 409–412, 410t, 411t,
        426t
    surgical procedure for, 420–424, *421,* 426t
    survival rates for, 407–416, *408,* 409t, 410t,
        411t, 413t, 423–424
    symptoms of, 416–417
    syndromes associated with, 417
    total body irradiation (TBI) for, 425–426, 426t
    treatment options for, 405, 420–426, *421,*
        425t, 426t
    tumor cell markers for, 414–416, *415,* 416t
        426t
Neurofibromatosis:
    neuroblastoma and, 417
    pediatric testicular carcinoma and, 429, 434t,
        435
Neuron-specific enolase (NSE). *See* Enolase,
        neuron-specific
Neutrons, external beam, radiation therapy, for
        bladder carcinoma, 542–543, 543t
Neutropenia, as complication from interferon/
        chemotherapy regimen, 473
Nichol's bowel preparation, modification of,
        prior to cystectomy, 249
4-Nitrobiphenyl, as occupational carcinogen, 88
Nitrofurazone, opening of bladder and, in
        nephroureterectomy, 98
Nitroprusside, in surgery for retroperitoneal
        tumors, 134
Nitrosamine, urothelial carcinoma and, 88
Nitrosoureas, for prostatic carcinoma, 461
Nomogram, in interstitial brachytherapy, 206,
        207
Nonseminomatous testicular carcinoma, 308
Norepinephrine (NE):
    neuroblastoma and, 414–415, *415*
    pheochromocytomas and, 10–11
NSAIDs (nonsteroidal anti-inflammatory drugs),
        for pain, 676, 676t, 677, 679
NSE. *See* Enolase, neuron-specific
Nuclear isotope scan, for testicular carcinoma,
        597

Renal function:
assessment of, in presurgical medical
evaluation, 656–657
failure in, symptoms and treatment of, 663–
664, 664t, 665–666
urinary diversion and, 259, 260
Renal pedicle, control of, in radical
nephroureterectomy, 99–101, *100, 101*
Renal pelvis, carcinoma of:
bladder carcinoma versus, 97t
causes of, 88, 116
diagnosis of, 89, *89, 90*
diagnostic imaging of, 592–594, *595*
incidence of, 88, 116
partial nephrectomy and, 52
pathology of, 89–90
prognosis for, 92, *92*
staging of, 90–91, *90,* 117
nephrostomy for, 120–121, *122,* 123
nephroureterectomy, radical for. *See*
Nephroureterectomy
ureteroscopy for, 89, *90,* 118–120
symptoms of, 89
treatment of, 91–92, 91t
ureteral carcinoma versus, 91t, 97t, 104
See also Urinary tract, upper, carcinoma of
Renal preservation:
extracorporeal, 56–57
history of, 54–55
in situ, 56
ischemia and, 55–56
pharmacology for, 55–56
Renin:
Cushing's syndrome and, 9
plasma, aldosteronism and, 8
renal, in aldosteronism, 8
Reoxygenation, of tumor cells, radiobiology and,
533
Reproductive system, diagnostic imaging
evaluation, 599–600, *600*
Resectoscope:
in fulguration for bladder carcinoma, 225
in transurethral resection, 222
ureteroscopic loop, upper urinary tract
carcinoma and, 119, *121*
Retinoblastoma:
neuroblastoma versus, 412
tumor cell markers for, 414
Retroperitoneal connective tissue. *See*
Connective tissue, retroperitoneal
Retroperitoneal tumors, 128–138
benign, 129
chemotherapy for, 133, 138
classification of, 128–129
complications from, 137–138
diagnosis of, 129–130, 130t, *131, 132, 133*
diagnostic imaging evaluation of, *598,* 600–
601, *601*
pediatric, surgery for, 422
postoperative care for, 137
preoperative preparation for, 133–134
radiation therapy for, 130, 133, 138
staging of, 130, 130t
surgical techniques for, *13, 14, 15, 16, 17,
18,* 128–138
for tumors above true pelvis, 134–137,
134, 135, 136, 137
for tumors of true pelvis, 137
symptoms of, 129, *130*
treatment of, 133
Retroperitoneum:
anatomy of, 1–5, *2, 3, 4, 84*
surgical approaches to,
eleventh-rib flank, 5

extraperitoneal transverse abdominal, 3–4
lumbodorsal, 5
midline abdominal transperitoneal, 2–3
subcostal flank, 3–4
thoracoabdominal extrapleural, 5
thoracoabdominal transpleural, 5
transverse abdominal transperitoneal, 2–3
twelfth-rib flank, 4–5
tumors of. *See* Retroperitoneal tumors
Rhabdomyosarcoma (RMS):
chemotherapy for, 444, 445, 446, 447–448
complications from treatment of, 448–449
histology of, 443–444
incidence of, 404, 443
neuroblastoma versus, 412
paratesticular,
metastases from, 448
treatment of, 448
as pediatric carcinoma, 402, 433
pelvic, treatment of, 445–448
radiation therapy for, 444–445, 446, 447–
448
staging of, 445
treatment of, 404
Rifampin, for bacillus Calmette-Guérin infection,
482
Right heart catheterization, vena caval extension
of renal cell carcinoma and, 72, *74*
RMS. *See* Rhabdomyosarcoma
Roentgenography, chest:
for bladder carcinoma, 235, 249, 254
for metastatic testicular carcinoma, 342
for neuroblastoma, 417
for radical nephrectomy, 37, 40, 43
for renal cell carcinoma, *586,* 590
for renal pelvic carcinoma, 89, 92
for ureteral carcinoma, 93

S-adenosylmethione (SAM), in measurement of
catecholamines, pheochromocytoma
and, 11
Sach's solution, in renal preservation, 55
Sacral promontory, nodes of, in lymphatic
drainage from prostate, 164, *164*
Sarcoma botryoides, non-surgical treatment for,
617
Schistosomiasis, bladder carcinoma and, 215
Schwannian spindle cells, histology of
neuroblastoma and, 412–413, *412*
Sciatica, inoperable carcinoma and, 617
Self-esteem, defined, 671
Self-image, defined, 671
Seminomatous testicular carcinoma, 306, 307–
308, 307t, *307,* 523
Senna, for constipation, 679
Sertoli cell tumor, pediatric testicular carcinoma
and, 432
Sexual function:
bladder carcinoma and, 672–673
evaluation of, 672
quality of life and, 671–672
self-image and self-esteem and, 671
sexuality and, 671, 672
penile carcinoma and, 673
prostatic carcinoma and, 149, 208, 673
renal cell carcinoma and, 673–674
testicular carcinoma and, 673
See also Ejaculation; Emission; Erection;
Fertility; Impotence
Shock, pheochromocytoma and, 11
Sigmoid colon, urinary diversion using, 302–
303, *303. See also*
Ureterosigmoidostomy

Sipple's syndrome, familial pheochromocytoma
and, 12
Small intestine, bladder substitution using, 295–
299, *295, 296, 297, 298, 299, 300*
Smegma, penile carcinoma and, 359
Sodium, renal dysfunction and, 665
Sonography:
for neuroblastoma, 418
for ovarian carcinoma, 600
for prostatic carcinoma, 596, 597
for renal cell carcinoma, 45
for retroperitoneal tumors, *598,* 601
for testicular carcinoma, 597, *598*
for uterine carcinoma, 599
for vaginal tumors, 599
See also Ultrasonography
Sphincter, artificial, continence of substituted
bladder and, 259
Spinal cord compression, radiation therapy for,
577, *578*
Spironolactone:
for aldosteronism, 9
for metastatic prostatic carcinoma, 502
Steatorrhea, urinary diversion and, 260
Stenosis:
infundibular, renal pelvic carcinoma and, 89
stomal,
as complication from pediatric cancer
therapy, 448
ileal conduit urinary diversion and, 263
ureteroileal, Kock pouch cutaneous urinary
diversion and, 282
ureteropelvic, renal pelvic carcinoma and, 89
Stentography, Indiana continent reservoir
urinary diversion and, 290
Steroid(s):
ketosteroids,
fractionated, virilizing tumors and, 10
secretion of, in adrenal carcinoma, 12
virilizing tumors and, 10
See also Corticosteroids; Dexamethasone
Stilphostrol. *See* Diethylstilbesterol diphosphate
Stoma, abdominal. *See* Urinary diversion, ileal
conduit
Streptozotocin, for metastatic prostatic
carcinoma, 511, 511t
Stress, surgical, presurgical medical evaluation
and, 654
Strictures:
intestinal, as complication from female pelvic
exenteration, 630
ureteral, as complication from radiation
therapy, 539
urethral carcinoma and, 363, 383
Studer reservoir urinary diversion, modified,
299, *299, 300*
Subserosal layer, of retroperitoneal connective
tissue, 1, 2, *4,* 142
Substance S, Cushing's disease and, 10
Succinylcholine, in transurethral resection, 225
Superoxide dismutase, in renal preservation, 55
Symptoms, in cancer patients, control of, 675–
680, 676t, 680t

Tachycardia, examination for, in presurgical
medical evaluation, 657
Tamoxifen:
for metastatic renal cell carcinoma, 26, 470t,
472t
for prostatic carcinoma, 461t
Tantalum-182, wires of, for bladder carcinoma,
535
^{99m}Tc MDP nuclear isotope bone scan, for
pediatric carcinoma, 403